CLINICAL ASSESSMENT FOR MASSAGE THERAPY

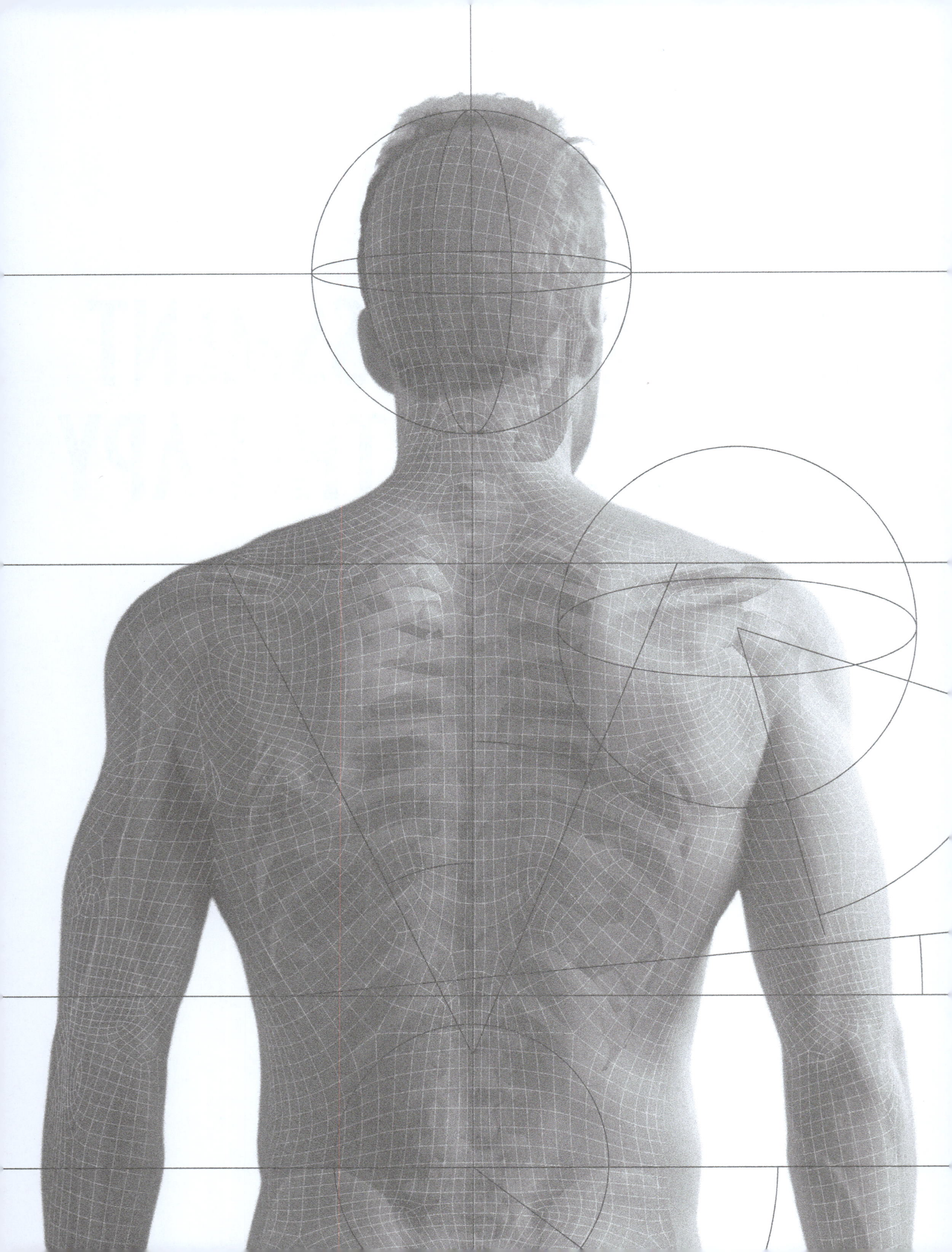

CLINICAL ASSESSMENT FOR MASSAGE THERAPY

A Practical Guide

David Zulak MA RMT

Foreword by Sandy Fritz BS MS LMT Board Certified NCBTMB

HANDSPRING PUBLISHING
Edinburgh

HANDSPRING PUBLISHING LIMITED
The Old Manse, Fountainhall,
Pencaitland, East Lothian
EH34 5EY, Scotland
Tel: +44 1875 341 859
Website: www.handspringpublishing.com

First published 2018 in the United Kingdom by Handspring Publishing

The authorised representative in the EEA is Hachette
Ireland, 8 Castlecourt Centre, Castleknock Road,
Castleknock, Dublin 15, D15 YF6A, Ireland

ISBN 978-1-909141-37-7

British Library Cataloguing in Publication Data
A catalogue record for this book is available from the British Library

Library of Congress Cataloguing in Publication Data
A catalog record for this book is available from the Library of Congress

Commissioning Editor Mary Law
Project Manager Morven Dean
Copy-editor Stephanie Pickering
Designer Bruce Hogarth
Indexer Aptara, India
Typesetter DSM, India
Printer CPI Group (UK) Ltd,Croydon,CR0 4YY

The Publisher's policy is to use paper manufactured from sustainable forests

This textbook is dedicated to my wife, Anne Wilson.
Without her support, love and inspiring example of determination,
this book would never have seen the light of day.
It is also dedicated to my extraordinary children,
Katie and James, for their sustaining love.

Contents

Contents *continued*

Contents *continued*

Foreword

To work with clients from an outcome goal process, it is necessary to be able to gather information about the client's health status. Physical assessment is an important part of the information gathering process. The client history and outcome goals will guide what physical assessments to perform. Physical assessment can also help provide screening for referral, especially if joint dysfunction is suspected. This book provides the information to learn a variety of assessment skills to better understand the condition of the various types of soft tissue and joints that may be related to the client symptoms.

Assessment seeks to understand not change. Assessment asks questions and interprets the responses to those questions. Asking a client to move a joint or hold against resistance are examples of the questions. The responses can be normal function, limited function, function with effort and so forth. We will not understand the client status without asking the questions first.

The assessment process is a skill. Too quickly we jump to interventions with intention to change function. We press on this and pull on that before we understand the bigger picture. I often identify massage therapists using too much intervention and not enough assessment. This text is focused on assessment. While guidance is provided toward choices for appropriate intervention, an intervention is only used once assessment identifies the conditions for a specific, unique individual and what outcomes for treatment are desired.

There are many types of physical assessment procedures. For the massage therapist, the ones used need to be effectively integrated into the massage session process. There is an expectation about the massage session by most clients. They want to lie on the table and be touched in a therapeutic way, experiencing a sense of satisfying pressure and movement. There is value in the general massage application. Performing too many physical assessment tests will not feel like a massage to the client. You need to intelligently pick and choose assessment methods. This text provides procedures to help you learn about your client. Remember all aspects of the massage session are assessment if you approach your client with mindful focus and pay attention to their response to the massage application.

Sandy Fritz BS, MS, LMT Board Certified, NCBTMB

Founder, Owner and Head Instructor

Health Enrichment Center

School of Therapeutic Massage Lapeer MI

March 2018

Acknowledgements

There are many people to thank for helping me make this book become a reality. I will begin by thanking all my students, who over the years taught me so much, who were so patient with me, and who encouraged me to pursue this project.

A large share of gratitude goes to Johan Overzet. Since meeting at the Sutherland-Chan School of Massage and Teaching Clinic in 1992, we have studied together, practiced our craft, debated, and advanced together. We both attended osteopathic courses together in Canada and helped each other survive the experience and be better manual therapists for it. The results of many of our debates over the years are scattered through this book. Johan has always been honest with me, whether in approval or criticism. That, above all, proves he is the truest of friends.

I would like to thank Anne Wilson MA for her invaluable editing skills over these many years. Also, I am indebted to Jackie Guanzon RMT and Ashley Marcos RMT for their efforts in serving as proofreaders for various parts of the book. Jackie also served as the principal model throughout the book, assisted by Antonella Licata, Darryl Hoogendam RMT, Justin Doherty RMT, Katrina Raney RMT, and Sara Hanson RMT.

I am grateful to my instructors at Sutherland-Chan School of Massage Therapy for their dedication to the profession and to their students. I wish to thank Debra Curties RMT and Trish Dryden MEd, RMT for their support and encouragement in my first attempts at teaching, which also occurred at Sutherland-Chan. My first co-teacher, the late Earl O'Neal PhD, RMT, who so generously shared his wealth of experience with me, is fondly remembered.

I am honored that Sandy Fritz MS, NCTMB has written the Foreword for this book. I have been inspired by her dedication to the profession of massage therapy, especially for her efforts over many years to improve the quality of education available for students and practitioners.

Of course, I need to thank those at Handspring Publishing who worked to bring this to print, including the publishers Andrew Stevenson and Mary Law. I especially wish to thank Mary for her kind support, advice and gentle reminders about deadlines over the last few years. Also, thanks go to Morven Dean (Project Manager), Bruce Hogarth (Designer), Stephanie Pickering (Copy Editor) and Hilary Brown (Marketing Manager); and to all those at Handspring Publishing who had a hand in producing this book.

Thank you all

David Zulak

Preface

My wide range of experience both as a student and as a teacher, in many different settings, from community colleges to universities and vocational colleges, has, I believe, given me an unusually thorough and deep perspective on, and understanding of, how to help others learn what they need to know within a post-secondary educational setting. As a massage therapy teacher, former program director and curriculum writer for schools of massage, and as a facilitator of workshops for massage therapists in assessment and techniques across Canada, I have listened to, watched, and learned from students of massage: their learning styles, their typical or atypical educational backgrounds, the life experiences they bring (or do not bring) to the classroom, and the many different reasons that brought them to the point of choosing this profession.

All of this experience and knowledge, gained over many years, has informed this guide. The design and style of this book, its voice if you like, is intended to help students learn the skills involved in assessment. It has been specifically written for students of massage and those practicing massage therapy. It is not meant to be academic, encyclopedic, or intimidating.

As a teacher faced with a student (or class) that performs badly my first thought has always been "how did I fail to communicate to them what they needed to know? How could I have taught this better? What else is it that they needed to know in order to understand and become proficient at assessment?" The answers to these questions built this book.

The book is deliberately written to be easily understood and therefore is not written with a typically academic or jargon heavy style. It does, however, include the proper terminology students need to know to continue their studies and to communicate with other health professionals. I have not written this book for academics or researchers, or for those who are already highly proficient in assessment. I have written it to assist students of massage therapy to quickly and efficiently learn the skills of assessment required of them by their schools, the regulators of the profession, and their future patients. Once they have learned what to do, how to do it, and why it is done a certain way, then they can read further, and continue to learn more about their profession or seek to specialize in treating specific types of patients, such as athletes, maternity clients, elder care, and so on.

The book's possible tendency to repetition, or "wordiness," is deliberate and intended to ensure that it includes all the information and clarifications that I have, over the years, learned many, if not most, massage therapy students need in order to learn the skills described. Further, I have seen over and over again in my career as an educator that if the student understands why they being asked to do something in a particular way rather than just memorizing the steps in some specific musculoskeletal test, they are both more likely to remember the procedure and (most importantly) will actually use these skills in their practice once they have graduated. Therefore, I have taken the time to fully outline the steps of each test and, when necessary, show them in a series of photographs. (I feel that a student's time is better spent on learning and practicing their assessment skills rather than expanding their reading comprehension skills!)

I have also provided, on occasion, some of the anatomical information needed when trying to understand the structures being tested and thus, how and why certain motions etc. are done in a certain way when doing a specific test. If one understands the anatomy of a joint or tissue that needs to be investigated, then the anatomy, the structure and function, of a joint or tissue will help one to remember how to do a test. Assessment is thinking anatomy. In other words, thinking through the implications of the structure and function of a tissue is how the various elements of assessment were invented or arrived at in the first place. If you actually forgot a test, or were never taught it, a firm grasp of anatomy and the physiology of movement would allow you to re-invent any musculoskeletal test, or maybe even create a new and perhaps better test!

As I said earlier, this is a teaching manual designed to introduce and provide the basics of the assessment skills required by our profession as massage therapists. My hope is that this manual can achieve this goal without traumatizing students so that when they have finished their training they will not only retain and use this information and these skills but will be both prepared and motivated to continue their learning of this essential element of massage therapy. Along with all instructors in massage therapy, I hope that our students come to realize it is only when they leave school that real learning begins.

David Zulak MA RMT

Massage therapy practitioner, instructor and author

Paris, Ontario, Canada

December 2017

Introduction

Clinical Assessment for Massage Therapy has been created to do what its title indicates, namely to help students of massage therapy learn the basics of clinical assessment. It is a manual for practicing massage therapists to recall, re-learn, or expand their assessment skills. It is designed specifically as a learning tool.

This assessment guide is written by a massage therapist specifically for massage therapists. Both students in massage therapy schools and those already in the profession need a book written with them in mind in order to help them be as effective and efficient as possible when treating injuries, impairments, and dysfunctions and ensure that the application of techniques and modalities remains both appropriate and safe for their patients.

The evidence base

A phrase often encountered when reading almost any written material in the health care professions is "evidence-based practice." In general, this evidence comes from three main sources: research, clinical practice, and client/patient values. Some authors consider that all sources of evidence should be valued equally while others prefer a hierarchy of values where research (especially double-blinded studies) rules supreme. I must disclose that I am of the former opinion, that evidence from a number of sources should be valued equally, especially within a manual therapy such as massage.

My principal reasons for not accepting research alone as the "gold standard" of evidence for manual therapies are, very briefly, as follows. When blinded research is being done on pharmaceutical medication, for example, the variables of the principal effective agent can be tightly controlled, as can the comparison agents (such as a placebo, or control group receiving no treatment). However, where manual therapies are concerned the variables around a technique or manipulation (for example) being investigated become very difficult to control. If a variety of agents/therapists are used ("inter-therapist") there is going to be variety in delivering the treatment modality (age, gender, physical conditioning, therapist-patient interaction, therapist's understanding of the modality, levels of training, etc.). Averaging out the data by mathematical probability models by necessity will ignore many of these variables and thereby make the results less relevant to actual clinical outcomes. On the other hand, restricting the variable (only one gender, age group, equal training and experience – if that is even considered a reasonable possibility) would mean that the results calculated would only apply to that restricted group of agents and, therefore, would be even less relevant to actual clinical outcomes.

If only one agent/therapist is used ("intra-therapist") in a study then, strictly speaking, the results of that study apply only to that individual (or their clones), resulting in even less relevance for the outcomes.

Mega-studies have their own issues. It must be remembered that the studies collected and found acceptable are rarely "replications" in the true sense. Without replication (as closely as is feasible) a research study cannot claim reliability. "Similar" or "related" is not replication. But more often than not mega-studies are just that: a collection of similar studies. Though each individual research study used may have calculated its own specific probability, without replication this probability for a specific result or conclusion remains in question. Combining a number of questionable conclusions does not somehow magically make that cumulative conclusion less questionable. While mathematical models used to calculate the results of such mega-studies may claim they impart reliability or validity to those results, such reliability can only be granted to the mathematics and not the content.

This is not an argument to discount evidence obtained from rigorous research. I only criticize the idea held by some that double-blind studies are the most acceptable evidence on which to base one's practice, and on the other hand, that evidence from clinical experience (both one's own and reports from others) is highly suspect. Both of these sources (research and experience) need to be treated equally and in turn need to take into account the client's/patient's social values and expectations (and consent) when applying such evidence-based treatment in order to strive for the best outcomes possible.

Outcome-based massage

My preference is for the term outcome-based massage. While evidence from many sources is used by a therapist in developing the most viable, effective and safe treatment plan for their patient, the outcome is made up from more than just this. The outcome, as noted above, is also based on the patient's expectations (personal and social), understanding (being informed), the therapeutic relationship (trust), and the consent granted. Treatment (which includes assessment) is therefore always more than evidence-based. Evidence-based practices are a necessary component for best practice in massage therapy, but they alone do not shape the outcomes achieved in clinical practice.

With respect to the research being done on manual assessment testing that is aimed at building an evidence base, much of that information requires a history of health care training or clinical experience in order to be of relevance to, let alone to be understood and appreciated by, any student of a health care profession. In light of the brevity of training that most massage therapists receive (and I include in this the lack of any preparatory education in the health sciences that the majority of massage therapy students possess upon enrolling), the information meant to be conveyed by evidence-based texts on manual testing may convey little to such a student body. In fact, it is only after they have completed their training, passed competency examinations, and acquired some clinical experience (beyond their public clinic experience during schooling) that most practicing massage therapists have the tools to explore and appreciate this information. Once a student has learned a specific test, and used it a number of times with a variety of patients (which often means after they have been practicing for some time), they can then use information on a test's reliability, for example, in a meaningful manner.

The reliability of a test is not just "this is a good test" or "this is a bad test." It is much more complicated than that. First of all, a test may be considered "reliable" in different ways. For example, research may show that test X may be fairly reliable when it finds a positive result (suggesting that a patient actually has the impairment being testing for). Yet it may be less reliable (or even unreliable) when the result is negative (concluding that the patient does not have the impairment tested for). In other words, a specific test may be able to get a large number of actual positive findings while getting almost no false negatives (a positive finding with no impairment actually present). So when the therapist gets a positive result when applying the test they can be fairly confident that the patient may well have the impairment being tested for. However, the test does not catch all instances of the impairment searched for, so that when the result of this test gives a negative response there are a significant number of false negatives (a negative finding with the testing, but the patient actually has the impairment).

The opposite may also be true: a specific test may not be very reliable when there is a positive finding (there are many occurrences of false positives, a positive found yet with the impairment tested for not actually present in the patient). But on the other hand, the test may be very reliable when a negative result occurs (very few false negatives that occur; the impairment is almost never present in those who test negative).

Of course, numerous variations or gradations of positive and negative reliability exist among the numerous tests available. Some tests may be fairly reliable when either a positive or negative result is found. Some tests could have very low or limited reliability when finding either a positive or negative result.

Having this information when one is already competent in assessment skills can be of immense help to the therapist in evaluating the reliability of the various tests they have in their repertoire. It can help them choose a specific test over another option (where both test the same structure or function), depending on the circumstances. In clinical practice it is not uncommon to run into the situation where the "best test" for X cannot be done because the patient (having some other impairment or pathology) cannot be in the recommended (optimal) positioning that a specific test requires in order to give a reliable result. Knowing how the variations to a test may affect its reliability, or knowing which other test may now be the only one available, is valuable. But such information requires the clinical situation combined with the experience of the therapist to be present in order to know how to apply and use such information. To a therapist in training, especially to massage therapy students, such information can be overwhelming and interfere with the process of learning the basic skills of manual testing. Indeed, for students of all manual therapies, this kind of information may prejudice their understanding of the various tests and methods of assessment they learn. Unfortunately the result of presenting some evaluations too soon, before the student has sufficient experience and skills to fully understand and evaluate the information, can be to make them more inflexible and less adaptive in their clinical application of those skills.

Further, the purpose of evidence-based assessment texts in large part is to present the evidence concerning the reliability of specific orthopedic tests for their diagnostic value. However, as there are issues around massage therapy and diagnosis, how this information is to be integrated and how to understand its utility to our profession needs further discussion within our profession. It is also an issue that needs to be discussed and negotiated with those health care professions that

protect their right and exclusivity to diagnose. Some of these issues are touched upon in Part I of this guide, which follows.

As already stated, this guide is designed to introduce and provide the basics of the assessment skills required by our profession as massage therapists. I hope readers will not only retain and use this information and these skills but will enrich their practice by their continued learning of this essential and fascinating element of massage therapy.

Common Abbreviations

AA, atlantoaxial
AC, acromioclavicular joint
ADL, activities of daily living
AF-ROM, active free range of motion
AIIS, anterior inferior iliac spine
AR-ROM, active resisted range of motion
ASIS, anterior superior iliac spine
CMC, carpometacarpal joint
CNS, central nervous system
CP, cerebral palsy
CT, computed tomography
CVA, cardiovascular accident
DDD, degenerative disc disease
DIP, distal interphalangeal joint
DJD, degenerative joint disease
DTR, deep tendon reflex
ERS, extended, rotated, side-bent
FRS, flexed, rotated, side-bent
GH, glenohumeral joint
ILA, inferior lateral angle
ITB, iliotibial band
IVD, intervertebral disc
LANL, lower motor neuron lesion
MCP, metacarpophalangeal joint
MI, myocardial infarction
MOI, mechanism of injury
MRI, magnetic resonance imaging
MS, multiple sclerosis
NSR, neutral, side-bent, and rotated
OA, occipitoatlantal
O-A, osteoarthritis
PF-ROM, passive forced ROM
PIIS, posterior inferior iliac spine
PIP, proximal interphalangeal joint
PNS, peripheral nervous system
PR-ROM, passive relaxed range of motion
PSIS, posterior superior iliac spine
QL, quadratus lumborum
RA, rheumatoid arthritis
ROM, range of motion
SC, sternoclavicular joint
SI, sacroiliac
SLR, straight leg raise
SOAP, subjective objective assessment plan
SP, spinous process
TFL, tensor fasciae latae
TIA, transient ischemic attack
TMJ, temporomandibular
TOS, thoracic outlet syndromes
TP, tender point
TrP, trigger point
TVP, transverse process
ULTT, upper limb tension test
UMNL, upper motor neuron lesion
VAT, vertebral artery test
VMO, vastus medialis oblique
WNL, within normal limits

Part I
Essentials of Assessment

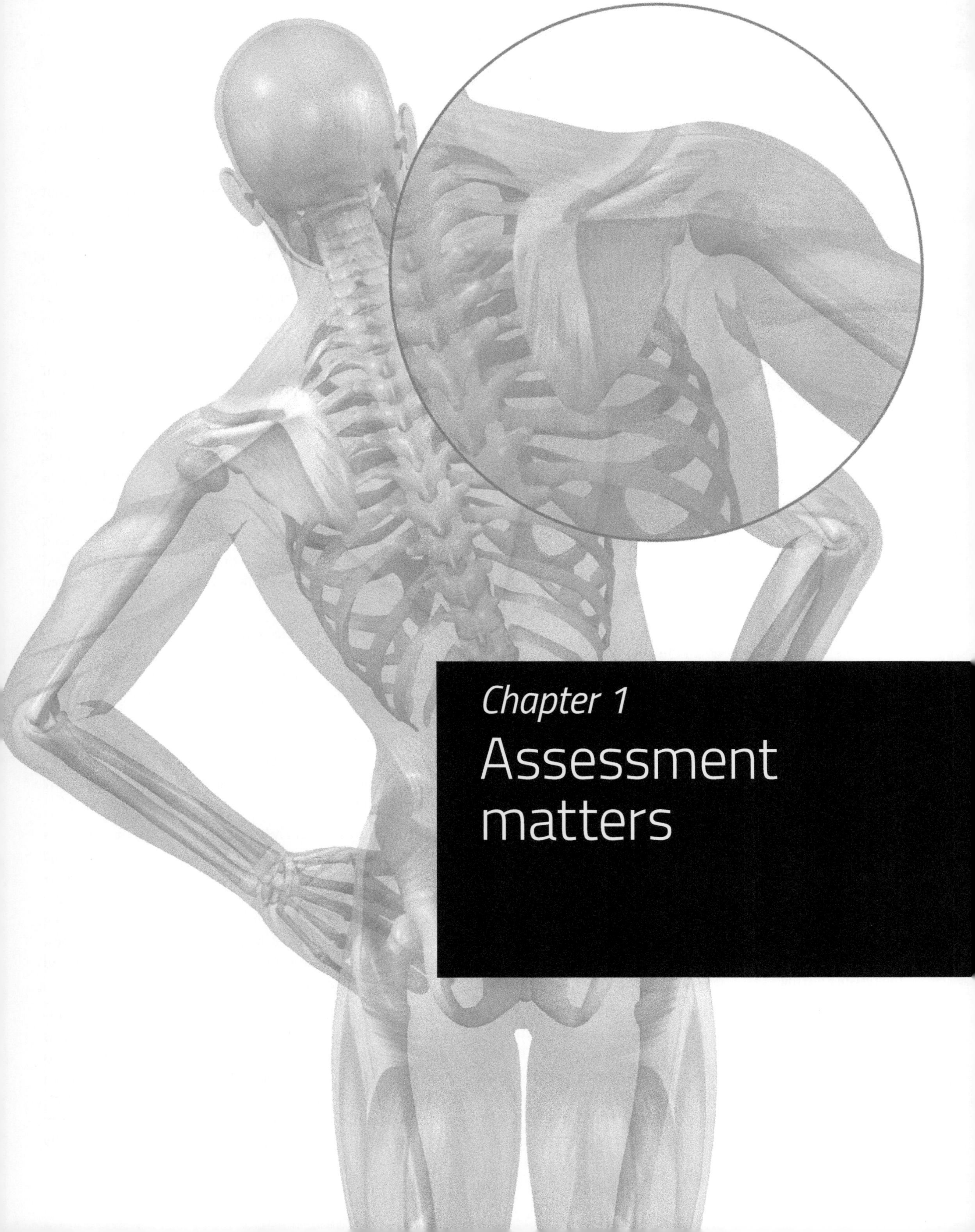

Chapter 1

Assessment matters

For many students, clinical assessment is an intimidating academic subject on a par with pathology or physiology. It is possible to approach assessment as a holistic, meaningful, and positive growth process as well as a solid medical procedural technique. I admit that I was not able to approach assessment this way as a student. I first recognized that assessment was part of the interconnected process of massage treatment through a conversion experience, if you will, just a few short weeks into my new profession as a massage therapist. It was mid-afternoon, and I was taking a case history from a new patient. My confidence as a therapist was being tested by my recent entry into the real world. I was missing the comfort of having a supervisor around from whom I could get assistance with assessing a patient. It was still very challenging. However, I am one of those people who likes to have a complete picture of what is going on before I proceed.

The patient and I got down to discussing her chief complaint. She told me that she had had a skiing accident the previous winter, injuring her shoulder. She had gone to the emergency room and seen an orthopedic specialist. At the hospital all the usual imaging studies had been done: X-ray, ultrasound, MRI. The diagnosis was a rotator cuff tear. The patient had been through two bouts of physiotherapy and had experienced no improvement. She told me she sometimes had her doubts about whether they got it right. When I asked the patient to point to where the pain had been coming from, she pointed to the back of her right shoulder around the area of her infraspinatus, teres major, and teres minor tendons. The patient had come to me to get help to relieve her pain and get strength and movement back in her arm.

Although I looked calm I had an inner moment of panic. "Right, these specialists could not help her, but somehow I am supposed to figure out what is going on?" Since I had no idea how to proceed, I did everything I could think of. I had her go through all active ranges of motion for the shoulders, bilaterally, as well as passive range of motion (assuming no joint involvement). The entire time I was thinking that I was not going to have anything to tell her. I then proceeded to isometric resisted testing. I was 10 minutes or so into this assessment (thinking she was probably becoming impatient and just wanted to get on the table) but I could not seem to stop myself from at least finishing the resisted testing.

Then, to my confusion and surprise, resisted external rotation that should have bothered an injured or dysfunctional infraspinatus and the teres muscles presented as normal. To my further surprise, resisted extension of the shoulder caused discomfort. When I asked the patient to point out where she felt the pain, she pointed to that same area of the tendons. This led to an even more panicky feeling on my part as I rapidly went through the possibilities in my head. Then an idea popped into my mind: I should test long head of triceps! So I did. I had the patient hold her upper arm in slight extension and resist my pushing her upper arm into flexion, and at the same time resist my attempt to abduct the upper arm. I was just beginning with gentle pressure and building slowly when the patient shouted: "That's it! That's where it hurts! That's what I injured." She had in fact been pointing to what I now know is the insertion of the long head of the triceps at the inferior tubercle of the glenoid fossa, which lies deep under the tendons of the infraspinatus and teres muscles as these pass over to insert on the humerus.

I was standing beside her thinking, "has her rotator cuff injury resolved, to be replaced by this other injury?" (I can be a bit thick.) All the while the patient was telling me that no one had ever done any of this testing with her. In fact, all anyone ever did was ask her a few questions and ask her to point to the site of the injury. After some further discussion with the patient (since I was reluctant to believe that I, as a newly graduate massage therapist, had accurately assessed her injury), I eventually had to bow to the probability that my patient originally suffered a severe strain of the long head of triceps, with the expected compensatory involvement of other tissues nearby and involved with the shoulder joint.

While I may have sounded matter of fact and confident when giving my assessment to the patient I was really quite stunned. I realized that by following the basic rules of orthopedic assessment the answer had just popped out at me. No feats of awesome intuition or analysis were required on my part. After the first treatment (she had 45 minutes left in her original hour), the patient felt a great deal of relief, and by the fourth visit she was pain-free. Following some simple strengthening exercises my patient was able to ski again that winter with no problem.

The patient was extremely happy that I took the time to assess her injury. She felt that I had listened to her. This bears repeating: *she felt listened to.* There are very few health care practitioners that spend an hour with the patient and have the time to really listen: to the patient, the story of their injury, and their healing process. The patient felt that by being thorough I had her best interests at heart. She was not in a rush to get on the table and get her massage; she wanted the best treatment *for her.*

Incidentally, it was also good for business: I have treated literally dozens of patients who have been referred to me by this patient. This experience was also good for building relationships with other health professionals. The patient's family physician was impressed and has, in turn, sent patients my way. My treatment was specific to her, specific to her injury, and the acuity or state of the tissue at the time I saw her. Though I specifically focused on her right triceps, and particularly the long head and its attachment onto the scapula, I also dealt with all the surrounding tissue and related structures, in light of what all of my testing told me. Her injury was unique simply because it was hers. Because the treatment was specific to her, it was the most effective treatment she had received for her injury.

Most of all I became a lifelong convert to the power of assessment. I discovered that assessment matters. Without it we are relying on what others tell us instead of trusting our own professional skill. With assessment our treatments are safe, targeted, effective, and massage therapy specific.

Assumptions can be misleading

It is essential to follow all of the steps of assessment from beginning to end before coming to a conclusion about the degree or type of injury or dysfunction. In the story illustrated earlier I could have assumed that the patient did indeed have a rotator cuff tear as diagnosed by other professionals and proceeded to treat the patient accordingly. Completing a full assessment according to a prescribed assessment protocol eliminates any tendency to jump to conclusions or treat based on assumptions, preconceived ideas, or diagnoses.

Assessment follows a basic protocol: case history taking and consent, range of motion testing (when appropriate), and any special or differential testing. Following this protocol or model of testing from beginning to end helps to eliminate errors. Put aside any guesses you may have along the way: they can be misleading; leave them until the testing is completed. Do not jump to conclusions! In turn, therapists should not only do the testing that would tend to support any prior guess or assumption, or a diagnosis made by another professional. Nor should you rely on another's assessment concerning soft tissue injury. Find everything out for yourself. Orthopedic assessment skills help give knowledge that is useful regardless of the techniques that are going to be employed in treating the patient.

I used to tell students that clinical assessment was 50 percent of our scope of practice, which is to assess and treat. I realize now that our profession cannot be divided up into percentages. To assess and treat is one seamless process. These subjects may be taught separately in school but that is part of the learning experience. In practice they cannot be divided.

What do we think we are doing?

Over the last several decades in North America massage therapy has been on a path toward becoming an integral part of the health care system. As a result, more and more emphasis has been placed on developing and refining treatments for soft tissue injury or dysfunction. Though relaxation massage and stress management will always be a part of our scope of practice, you just need to look at the curriculum of any school to see the growing list of conditions that we, as massage therapists, treat.

This direction in the profession has seen a variety of terms used to describe what we do: medical massage, therapeutic massage, orthopedic massage, and treatment massage, to name a few. In turn, massage therapists have toyed with different terms to describe themselves: bodyworkers, deep tissue specialists, or soft tissue specialists. This process of trying to define what we do, and the role we are to play within the health care environment, has resulted in a pithy statement regarding our scope of practice, the kernel of which is contained in the phrase: to assess and treat soft tissue injury and dysfunction.

Further, we assess and treat soft tissue injury and dysfunction with the goal of reducing pain or restoring function. In order to be therapists, truly to be treating people in order to help them recover from injury and to help them with their pain or provide palliative care, we need to know more than how to apply the diverse techniques such as Swedish massage, muscle energy, polarity, or craniosacral therapy. We also need to know why and when to apply these techniques. If we are to treat a wide variety of conditions we cannot rely on others to provide us with a ready-made assessment or diagnosis. Diagnoses provided by other health care professionals are often either too vague or too broad in their meaning, or do not help us as massage therapists to organize a clear plan of treatment for our patient. Further, if we do rely on another's diagnosis then we can fall into the trap of performing some memorized treatment routine that does not address a given patient's specific needs.

In order to use the techniques and the types of manipulations, along with other treatment modalities that we have learned, we need above all to be able to assess for ourselves the impairment or injury that the patient presents with. We need to determine for ourselves what tissues are impaired (and to what acuity) in the patient in front of us. A diagnosis, for example, of sciatica, does not necessarily help us to know specifically all the tissues that may be involved for our patient: the degree of impairment, the level of dysfunction, or any unsuccessful compensatory patterns. A diagnosis does not help us choose the appropriate techniques or modalities that are going to be the most effective for our patient. A diagnosis does not tell us what specific goals can be achieved in treatment.

Also, do not be led astray by some who might say that musculoskeletal assessment is antithetical to holistic or alternative approaches. A proper clinical assessment procedure in no way hinders or prevents a massage therapist from using whatever techniques they wish to explore; if anything, assessment provides the sure footing upon which specific techniques can be applied effectively, making you a better therapist. A strong grounding in clinical musculoskeletal assessment can help focus our intention and allow us to access the tissues of the body. If we cannot focus our intention, then we are often unable to be invited into the tissue and are left unable to assist the patient with their healing.

Many specialized techniques come with their own specific forms of assessment: craniosacral rhythms, energy evaluation, Traditional Chinese Medicine pulse diagnosis, and Hara palpation, to name a few. These assessment techniques often depend on either the technique employed or a specific model of human health, or both. However, no matter what techniques you use, clinical assessment can bring focus and direction to patient treatment. Understanding which soft tissues and structures are involved can help to bring all of our techniques together into a cohesive whole and maximize our effectiveness as therapists. Further, assessment techniques, from osteopathic to Traditional Chinese Medicine, need not be seen as being outside of classic orthopedic assessment. They can be employed as special tests or procedures. Indeed, they are tests designed to test specific structures, energies, or balances within the body.

Assessment is like drawing a map

For massage therapists, clinical assessment is the means by which we evaluate soft tissue and joint injury or dysfunction so that we understand how these physical structures are producing the pain and/or impairment the patient presents with. Its purpose is to provide the information upon which we can base our choice of the best way to treat the patient (or refer out). Clinical assessment is not diagnosis. We do not determine underlying pathologies or organ dysfunction. We are simply assessing or *describing* the condition of the musculoskeletal structure.

We map out range of motion, bilaterally compare the strength and length of muscles, and describe the feel of tissue. We note where there is pain, restriction, tension, or hypermobility. We are creating a picture of the individual that is before us so that we can find ways to lessen their pain, free their limbs, or help them cope with disabilities. Clinical orthopedic assessment for the massage therapist is the evaluation of soft tissue and its implications for the function of muscle and joints.

Massage therapists often see the body as an interdependent dynamic whole. We recognize that any change or dysfunction in any part of the body will, in a short time, affect other nearby structures. If not resolved quickly, the whole body can become involved.

Assessment is a methodology that allows us to draw a map of the pain, dysfunction, range of motion, tension, restriction, and limitations of our patient. It gives us an idea or picture of what is going on with the patient. This picture provides the groundwork for informed consent, treatment planning, goal setting, treatment, reassessment, medical/legal reports, and charting.

Assessment as the basis for being able to treat

To arrest, stop, or limit an impairment we must see what tissues or structures are involved and understand the condition of these tissues. We must understand what the normal condition is for the patient, so that we can resolve the pain or dysfunction. We must see our patients as unique individuals with unique treatment needs. This seeing is what we call assessment. In many ways, assessment is thinking anatomy. When we think through our anatomy we arrive at our manner of assessment. When learning a special test (such as a meniscus test for the knee), if you understand the anatomy and the biomechanics of the tissue and structures involved, then how to do the test becomes obvious.

How we think through or see anatomy accounts for the variations in testing across the variety of techniques and models that a massage therapist can employ. If you see the body as energy, you see how to assess it as energy. If you see the body as governed by its fascia, then that is how you see to assess. I do not think we need argue about which way of seeing is "right" or primary. I would rather provide a basis where they can stand together and work together for the benefit of our patients.

The whole purpose and intent of clinical assessment is to see and think our way into the body so that we may find the causes of pain or impairment in order to treat them, rather than just treating the symptoms. This is our ideal.

Being a detective

Let me be blunt. Many acute injuries are obvious in nature: primary injured tissue reveals itself as such by its swelling, redness, heat, bruising, bleeding, or loss of function. Assessment is much more difficult when a condition is chronic or has an insidious onset. At this point, assessment is like solving a mystery. When injuries are old or pain is chronic, we need to be shrewd and well-trained detectives. There are lots of red herrings, blind alleys, and disguises that may confuse us. In the chronic situation there are no easy answers and often no single assessment session is sufficient. It is in these cases that treatment and assessment are most clearly linked.

We can re-test various structures over several therapy sessions, or re-evaluate the results of our testing. We are palpating every moment that our hands are in contact with the patient. We observe endlessly and, by communicating with our patient throughout the treatment, our case history taking is a continuous process. By re-evaluating our previous treatments and the success of the remedial exercises and home-care suggestions we make assessment an ongoing activity.

Our attempts to understand the unique pain of our patient, and their unique reaction to that pain, are appreciated by our patients. In this way, through our dedication, we can always be successful. Through our assessment and reassessment we constantly see each patient anew through their own unique progress and so never find ourselves "doing the rotator cuff at three o'clock."

Assessment is not just the boring stuff that comes before the massage; it is the very heart and soul of treatment. If we say that we are health care treatment providers but cannot say precisely what it is that we are treating our patients for, in what sense are we therapists? We are among the last of the hands-on healers. Our profession and our training allow us the time and the techniques to treat each patient as a unique individual by seeing each patient's strengths, weaknesses, and possibilities.

Assessment really is a remarkable, holistic, meaningful, and positive process of growth that allows each patient to receive the treatment that they need and deserve. When assessment and treatment are two parts of one whole, massage therapists are really both holistic healers and medical professionals.

Isn't imaging technology better than manual assessment?

In the face of technology, health professionals have often acquiesced to employing or relying on machines, especially in the field of assessment. Are not X-rays, CT scans, or MRIs the truly objective base for making judgments about soft tissue pain and dysfunction? The short answer is, yes and no. For acute trauma-based injury, the answer is often yes. However, for chronic or recurring injury, the answer is often no. In a 1998 article in *Scientific American*, Dr Richard A. Deyo brought together some interesting studies about assessment when addressing the issue of low back pain.

Deyo concluded that: "at least for adults under age 50, X-rays added little diagnostic value to office examinations …" Further, referring to epidemiological research, it was "revealed that many conditions of the spine that often received blame for pain were actually unrelated to the symptoms … and multiple studies determined that many spine abnormalities were as common in asymptomatic people as in those with pain. X-rays can, therefore, be quite misleading." And lastly, "even highly experienced radiologists interpret the same X-rays differently, leading to uncertainty and even inappropriate treatment" (Deyo 1998).

Though hands-on assessments of the same patient by different health care professionals can also produce a variety of conclusions, the point is that X-rays are no more objective, and other than in trauma scenarios, often add little to case history taking and manual assessment skills. Nor are the new toys, CT scans, and MRIs, any better for soft tissue injuries. In one study that involved looking at pain-free individuals under 60 years of age (who had no history of back pain or sciatica), the "MRI found herniated discs in one fifth of pain-free subjects … Half of that group had a bulging disc, a less severe condition also often blamed … Of pain-free adults older than 60, more than a third have a herniated disc, visible with MRI, nearly 80 percent have a bulging disc and nearly everyone shows some age-related disc degeneration" (Weinstein et al. 2006).

Another study found two-thirds of pain-free individuals had disc abnormalities: "Detecting a herniated disc on an imaging test, therefore, proves only one thing conclusively: the patient has a herniated disc" (Deyo et al. 2009) Yet, to this day, if a person complains of low back pain and has an X-ray or imaging scan (often without any manual testing performed during an office visit) and a disc abnormality is found, that abnormality will often be said to be the cause of the patient's pain.

Another reason for the decline in the use of manual assessment skills concerns the changes happening in other manual professions. Many physiotherapists are becoming administrators of physiotherapy clinics. The same is true of occupational therapists. Paperwork generated by legislation and the health care system is moving them into supervisory roles, with assistants taking on the bulk of hands-on work. This distance from the patient means hands-on testing procedures can be overlooked and reliance may fall on the assessment the patient came to the clinic with from their physician or imaging centers.

As other professions give up manual testing skills and rely on imaging technology, we as massage therapists are in an enviable position. As manual therapists we have the palpation skills, the knowledge of soft tissue anatomy, and just as importantly, the time to spend with the patient. Who else is better suited or prepared to take up this craft of manual orthopedic assessment? As a profession we are positioned to take ownership of these skills and make ourselves invaluable members of the health care community. By affirming that assessment is integral to treatment, we have a valid claim to the title of therapist.

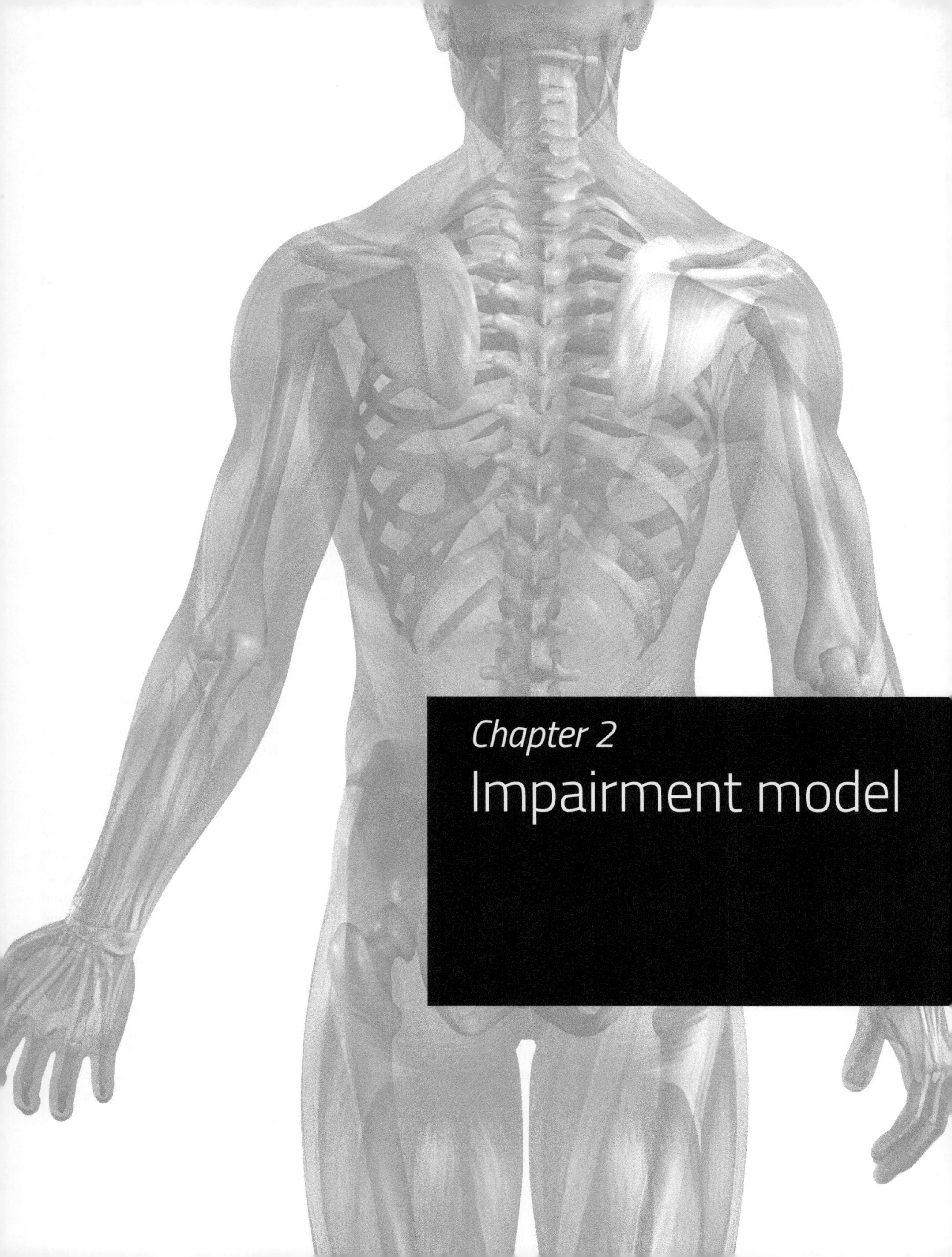

Chapter 2

Impairment model

This chapter provides a brief overview of the impairment model and how it can be used in massage therapy assessment.

Assessment versus diagnosis

Before discussing specific testing, or even an assessment protocol, or the steps of doing an assessment in general, I would like to give my perspective on the issue of just what it is we are doing when we are assessing, and how assessment differs from diagnosis. This should help clarify what we are doing when we assess and also help us see the necessity for being skilled in assessment as practicing massage *therapists*.

Unlike physicians, chiropractors, and physiotherapists, massage therapists are generally not considered to be diagnosing professionals. Legislation generally restricts diagnosing to those health care practitioners who have a much longer education, including a university degree. Sometimes students find the distinction between diagnosis and assessment difficult to understand. What does it mean when we say that a massage therapist needs to carry out the task of assessing soft tissue and joint injury?

Linguistically, diagnosis, which is from the Greek *gnosis*, meaning knowledge, implies understanding the cause of an illness or dysfunction. Through knowledge one ascribes a pathology. Assessing is from the Latin verb *assidere*, meaning to sit with or sit beside. In medieval times this term was used to denote establishing an amount, as in to evaluate. We use the word "assess" this way when we assess the value of a house or a tax on something. Assessing, in the health care field, implies measuring or establishing the level of something, usually function or dysfunction of the body or its parts.

Diagnosis is establishing the source of an underlying pathology, while assessment is creating a picture of the individual's function or dysfunction. If we are to be limited to assessing in the strictest sense, then the assessment describes impairments and outcome for massage therapy, replacing the diagnostic focus on conditions and syndromes. Therapists become focused on the goals and aims of treatment rather than on prognosis. These changes are not merely linguistic; they are practical changes that result in changes in practice.

A diagnosis given by a medical professional is useful to help that professional treat their patient. It will indicate whether the indicated pathology requires medication, surgery, splinting, or casting. It will establish a prognosis. The diagnosis will be useful to us to establish contraindications to treatment. But it does not stand in place of an assessment. We need to do our own testing in order to:

1. establish the impairments that are specific to the patient
2. decide on the outcomes that we can achieve through our techniques and modalities
3. present an assessment and treatment plan to the patient so that they can be informed about the reasonable goals and aims of treatment and come to a decision about how they want to proceed.

A well-structured assessment procedure can provide this. After all, without taking the measurements ourselves, how can we draw a useful map, or make a detailed plan of treatment? For that matter, without this detail how can we realistically say that we can adequately inform the patient and therefore receive from them an *informed* consent?

Further, we also must recognize that all too often the cause of someone's pain or dysfunction is never found: no specific diagnosis is ever made. This is most clearly seen in patients presenting with low back pain. The estimates of the cases where a cause of low back pain could be identified range from 10 to 20 percent (Hertling & Kessler 2006). Therefore, if we always need to definitively know the cause or be able to name the condition prior to treating the patient we would, more often than not, find ourselves with nothing to do, or at best perform some general routine with a few extra minutes on the area troubling the patient in the hope it would help. That is not therapy.

Assessing the patient's impairments and working on the outcomes related to them, with or without a diagnosis of the principal cause, means that we can always be of assistance to the patient. Optimally, it would be best to address the cause(s). But when the cause is not discernible we can still hope to address many of the troubling elements of their complaint. Even if the cause remains elusive, our assessment skills can provide us with a list of impairments that we may be able to address across a spectrum of outcomes: ranging from resolution of the dysfunction or pain to improving function slightly or at least maintaining it at the same level, or providing pain management. Therefore, even when we have only limited goals of treatment they are clear and we will be able to communicate them clearly to the patient.

In summary: we can say that an orderly assessment procedure allows us to establish the impairment(s) a patient suffers from, whether that is loss of movement, loss of strength, the experience of pain or discomfort with or without movement, etc. Some conditions we can interpret as impairments: after all, what is tendonitis but a descriptive term? Such descriptive terms only serve to imply a collection of signs and symptoms. Our own assessment lets us do the measurements, if you like, which allow us to draw up a detailed map of what ails our patient. We see for ourselves the amount of loss in range of motion (ROM); see exactly what motions result in pain; evaluate the difference of strength between paired limbs; generate suspicions about what tissues are or are not involved and about how acute they are. This information helps us draw a picture or map that allows us to chart, with our patient, the course of actions to take and so address the outcomes we hope to achieve through our course of treatments.

Impairments as impaired tissues or functions

Many massage therapists feel that they are only treating symptoms if they cannot find a cause for their patient's complaint. But, if we look at each symptom as having specific underlying impairments (specific impaired tissue structure and/or functions) to specific tissues (muscles, ligaments, joints, blood flow, or neurological issues) that present as pain, restrictions in motion, loss of strength, and the like, then we can almost always find ways to address them. Even when treating some of our most difficult cases we can always find some way to help, even if it is in a limited way. We have some potential benefit to offer. Further, as we deal with impairments such as pain and/or restriction of motion, the underlying causes may become more apparent as we progress through treatments.

Impairment model for clinical assessment

It is difficult to summarize the impairment model in a simple paragraph. Briefly, for massage therapy, an impairment is a change in the structure or function of the body from normal to a less functional state. As massage therapists our job is to treat the structures that have been changed for the worse and try to return them to their normal function again. A successful treatment is measured by achieving the goal (arrived at together with the patient) of the patient returning to their normal state of health. (This is an overly simple account, but there are other resources that are quite readable on this subject. For an excellent explanation of "impairments," establishing a patient's impairments, and how to arrive at appropriate outcomes for treatment, see *Outcome-Based Massage: Putting Evidence into Practice*, edited by Carla-Krystin Andrade, 2014.)

In general, there are four main levels within the Nagi model of disablement (Tovin & Greenfield 2001; see also the World Health Organization's International Classification of Functioning, Disability and Health):

1. *Active pathology:* a threat to the body's normal state and the internal responses to that threat. We can think of this as seeing things at a cellular level.
2. *Impairment:* any alteration or deviation from normal in anatomical, physiological, or psychological structures or functions. Seeing or thinking about anatomy and physiology.
3. *Dysfunction:* the inability to perform an action or activity in daily life in the manner performed by most people. Think activities of daily living.
4. *Disability:* a socially constructed term that is applied to those whose loss of (several) functions impact on them to the degree that they can no longer fully engage in critical social roles. The relationships between society and the individual.

Laboratory technicians and researchers, along with the bulk of medical professionals (doctors, nurses, etc.), are routinely involved in the treatment and cure of active pathologies. Physiotherapists, occupational therapists, etc. specialize in working with dysfunctions and rehabilitation. These health professionals certainly involve themselves in impairments. However, there seems to be an inherent tendency to compartmentalize or fragment the individual patient into systems and pieces. Level four also involves the realm of sociology, psychology, and the political sphere.

The place of massage therapists in this scheme of things is to deal with level two, or impairments. While other health professionals certainly deal with impairments in a variety of ways, massage therapists have carved out a niche as the manual therapists specializing in the musculoskeletal system with a whole-body, even holistic, approach. Yes, we work on the musculoskeletal system, but we can do so with an eye to the whole individual and their well-being.

Ideally, the whole purpose and intent of clinical assessment for a massage therapist is to find, whenever possible, the tissue or tissues involved in the impairment and gather information about the acuity of the impairment so it can be treated as directly and effectively as possible. Even without a diagnosis by treating the patient's impairment(s) we will be moving the patient toward healing. In fact, we never do treat a rotator cuff tear; rather, we treat the specific tissues involved in the patient who comes to us with shoulder problems. Therefore, *we are not treating conditions*, we are treating tissues.

While it is true that a diagnosis will imply a certain treatment approach, that approach can only be general in nature. To be specific in our treatment we need to see for ourselves the state of the tissues and how they and the patient have responded to (compensated for) having a particular impairment. To achieve specific outcomes, and in the order of priority that the patient wants, we need very specific knowledge. This is only achieved through a thorough assessment and is not possible if working only from a diagnosis that a patient received from another health care professional or that the therapist simply assumes is present.

Impairments and treatment plans

As we find the impairments that are affecting our patient we are also outlining our treatment plan. When composing a treatment plan, we need specific outcomes that we wish to achieve with the patient, and usually in a specific order or priority. Assessing the patient within an impairment model, rather than a syndrome or condition model, automatically gives the outcomes we seek to achieve. Finding a collection of impairments (not as a named syndrome) allows us to see our unique patient with a unique collection of concerns: range of motion limitations, levels of pain, weakness, apprehension. Together with the patient we can establish the priority of each impairment for them, thereby creating a unique treatment plan for that individual and their needs.

Massage therapists need to do their own testing in order to establish:

- the impairments that are specific to our patient, at a specific moment in time
- the outcomes available for massage therapy treatment and hence which techniques to use
- the creation of a treatment plan with options available for the patient to choose from.

This is exactly what a well-structured assessment procedure provides. Imagine a patient presents with a diagnosis from their physician stating that they have a rotator cuff injury. Having this diagnosis does not tell you how to treat that specific individual. Every muscle, ligament, and joint in the shoulder girdle needs to be compared to those on the patient's uninjured side. The impairment needs to be compared to what is normal for that patient. Naturally, "normal" for a frail elderly person, for example, is different than "normal" for a young triathlete, and goals for returning to health will differ for both of these individuals. As you find and grade deficits or impairments, the methods to improve health and function for your patient become your treatment plan.

Therefore, each treatment plan is unique and individual. Each plan is detailed and comprehensive. Each plan has clear outcomes and strategies for resolving the patient's impairment according to the patient's unique impairment, needs, and goals.

The impairment-based model (Box 2.1) includes the assessment, treatment plan, goal, treatment, and patient outcome. The model is focused on helping the patient return to a state of health. This health-based focus is very different from an illness- or pathology-based focus. As therapists it is our responsibility to assist our patients on their journey to wellness. Our assessment helps determine what that journey will look like.

Why we need to be competent at clinical assessment

To see ourselves as therapists, as professionals, we need to be competent at assessing soft tissue and joints, so that:

- we are able to develop treatment plans that are specific to our individual patients
- we have an objective basis for our record keeping of a patient's progress through treatment; that means that we assess prior to and reassess after each treatment
- we can design and monitor the effectiveness of the home care and remedial exercise programs that we give the patient
- we can help the patient understand their own condition
- we can provide the basic understanding and language that we need to be able to communicate with other health care providers with whom we are often involved
- we are able to present an image of competence to other professions and to insurance companies and the courts if called upon
- we can assess the treatment frequency and determine when to conclude treatment, as well as determine when to refer out.

Therefore, to lessen or alleviate an impairment or dysfunction, we must know what tissues or structures are involved, and understand the condition of these tissues within the context of what is normal for that patient, so that we can resolve the impairment.

Some general guidelines for assessment

The following rules need to be followed when performing an assessment; they are given here now so that the student can begin to get an overall view of what is to be done:

1. Begin with a thorough and thoughtful case history. This will help you rule out needless testing and save time.
2. Always observe and functionally test all muscles and joints bilaterally. Always begin with the non-impaired side if there is one. It is important to establish what normal is for your patient. This is your baseline.

SUMMARY

BOX 2.1 Impairments and associated techniques: simplified examples

Inflammation

- Pain – reflex techniques such as stroking, fine vibrations, low grade joint oscillations and cold applications.
- Edema – "superficial fluid techniques" – such as stroking, vibrations, effleurage, lymphatic techniques and appropriate hydrotherapy (e.g., cold, or contrast bathing).
- Tissue damage – appropriate techniques depending on the phase of tissue healing
  - acute: as above for pain and edema
  - subacute (light work), and
  - chronic (moderate to deep work): initially helping to align and prevent adhesions – effleurage, petrissage, PR-ROM, stretching, fascial techniques (e.g., frictions).

Restrictions/loss of ROM (as chronic)

- Adhesions: petrissage, myofascial techniques such as frictions, skin rolling, AR-ROM, stretches, etc.
- Joint dysfunctions: joint play, PR-ROM with over-pressure; muscle energy techniques, etc.

Neurological

- Spasticity: firm, slow pressure.
- Rigidity, atrophy: improve blood, lymph and nerve flow (both axonal transport and signaling) by assisting movement of fluids (effleurage, lymph drainage), or remove barriers or compressive sites with Swedish massage and/or myofascial techniques.

For these and others, cranial osteopathy (with appropriate instruction).

Central nervous system (alertness)

- Stimulating techniques: cranial osteopathy; improve blood flow by releasing compressive forces in the neck.
- Stress, anxiety: often inhibitory or relaxation techniques are used. This can include addressing immune suppression (from excessive cortisol levels).

Loss of muscle performance

Trigger point therapy, increasing tissue health, treating tendonitis/contractures with techniques such as those listed under adhesions (above).

Respiratory

Rib springing and mobilization techniques; intercostal work (raking); muscle energy.

Gastrointestinal tract

Abdominal massages, directional massage movement to assist peristalsis; visceral techniques.

Assisting immunity

Lymphatic techniques. Increase all fluids and nerve flow for general tissue health by removing barriers to flow (via petrissage or myofascial release), or by directly increasing flow via effleurage.

3. During the testing procedure, ask the patient the location of the pain, the nature of the pain, and any difference and/or changes in pain patterns.
4. Do not forget that the patient is your most valuable resource. If possible, have them point with one finger to the site of pain or injury. If need be, have them draw the boundary around the pain with their finger.
5. When asking if it hurts, ask where. After all, lots of testing can hurt, but not necessarily at the site of the chief complaint.
6. Try to arrange the order of testing so that the most painful test(s) are done last, otherwise the patient's apprehension after an experience of pain during a test will compromise or distort the results of those tests that come after.
7. Always support an injured limb in a secure neutral position.

8. Rule out the tissue and joint above and below (especially if observation or the case history suggest other joint involvement).
9. Be aware of nerve root ("radicular") or referred pain syndromes.
10. With chronic/insidious onset/diffuse and/or non-specific pain, an overall body scan may be necessary.

Review of what clinical assessment means for massage therapists

Clinical assessment is the means by which we evaluate soft tissue and joint injury or impairment so that we understand how these physical structures are producing the pain and/or impairment that the patient presents with. Assessment includes case history taking, and provides the basis or framework for treatment planning.

Clinical assessment is not diagnosis. We are creating a picture of the individual that is before us, not identifying pathology. As massage therapists we tend to see the body as a dynamic whole. We recognize that any change or dysfunction in any part of the body will affect other nearby structures, and ultimately, the whole body.

Chapter 3

Assessment protocol

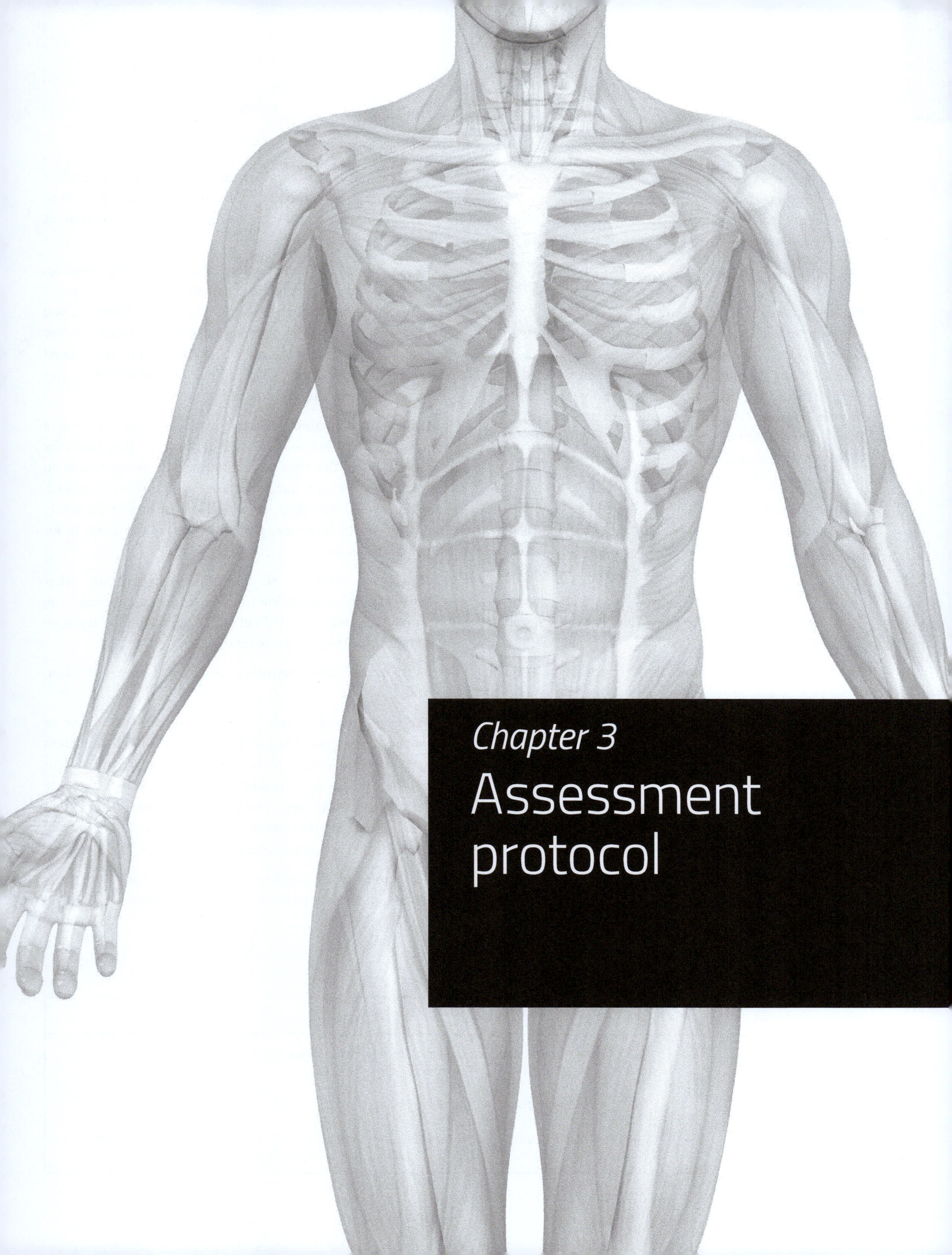

Chapter 3

This chapter begins with a very brief overview of a complete procedure (protocol) when doing an assessment. Each component of the protocol is then presented in more detail. These steps are further elaborated on throughout Part I and in Part II.

Brief overview of assessment protocol

1. **Patient intake** This is the all-important initial interview, or a re-interview of an established patient with a new injury or complaint. Active listening is our most important skill here. Give the patient the time to have their say, and repeat back to them what you have heard them say so that there is no misunderstanding. Most health care professionals agree that it is here that 90 percent of what we will need to know to help the patient happens. We therefore need patience to let the patient describe their symptoms.

The medical history information also gives us vital information about other potential causes, possibly pathological. With this we can know whether massage therapy is indicated or contraindicated. Further, it helps us to decide whether the patient needs to be referred out.

The interview consists of the categories of questioning shown in Table 3.1.

Pain/impairment questions Case history taking during the interview is asking relevant questions in a systematic and natural progression. It includes such things as the patient's own history of health, his or her family medical history, occupation, recreational activities, progressing to the patient's presenting condition.

NOTE: Keep your questions open-ended, or, to put it another way, try not to ask leading questions. Keep your questions simple. Listen attentively and clarify inconsistencies.

NOTE: THE IMPORTANCE OF CASE HISTORY TAKING CANNOT BE OVERSTATED!

2. **Consent** If any physical testing is appropriate, the patient needs first to be informed about what is to happen, to have any concerns or questions answered, and to give their consent before you can proceed.

3. **Observations** As mentioned, observations are ongoing, starting from the moment the patient walks into your clinic and continuing until the moment they leave. However, you may wish to carry out a formal postural assessment and/or gait analysis. Both of these are best done before any manual testing that may cause pain or discomfort and so distort your observations around posture and movement.

Inspection palpation You may wish to palpate the area of complaint, but should do so in a cursory manner. If we probe for the lesion site at this time we may cause pain or apprehension that will interfere with our manual testing to follow. Here such palpation would be called inspection and would entail gently feeling for tone, temperature (heat/coolness) of the tissue, or for edema in the tissue.

4. **Rule outs** While we are told in school about how other structures above and below the affected area may be referring pain to the area of the patient's chief complaint we are often *not* told how they can be ruled out.

Pain felt at the elbow may, in fact, be coming from the shoulder, or from the wrist.

The basic rule of thumb for ruling out the joint above or below the area you are going to investigate is to have the patient do active free movements of those joints and when a movement is pain-free, apply over-pressure (O-P). If no pain or recurrence of the impairment occurs, then you can assume (for now) that the joint tested with the rule out is not involved in the principal cause of the patient's chief complaint (see Hartley 2000a).

If that joint or surrounding tissue *is* involved in the patient's complaint, then these movements, with or without the O-P, will

TABLE 3.1
Categories of questioning

Personal information	Pain/impairment investigation
1. **Name and occupation** 2. **Medical history**	3. **Onset and duration:** causes, initial onset, how long have you had it, previous occurrences? Any medical attention at the time, etc. 4. **Site and spread:** location, radiation, referral 5. **Behavior and symptoms:** how has the pain changed or altered? Describe the pain as you first felt it, and now. What makes it better or worse: what time of day? Does it wake you at night, etc.?

often re-create the patient's symptoms. If either of these rule outs of the joints above and below re-create the patient's chief complaint, then that joint and surrounding tissue need to be investigated more fully, along with the original area the patient informed you of.

These rule outs take very little time, and are of immense help in preventing one from going down many blind alleys.

5. **Range of motion (ROM) testing** The usual order of testing in ROM testing is active free range of motion (AF-ROM), where the patient moves the affected area by themselves; then passive relaxed range of motion (PR-ROM), where the patient allows the therapist to move the joint or limb; followed by active resisted (isometric) range of motion (AR-ROM) testing, where the patient is instructed on how to move the limb but the therapist prevents any movement from happening (Table 3.2). However, if the patient lacks the ability to move the limb, then we may be involved with active assisted (AA-ROM) testing, where, in fact, we are helping the patient perform active free motions by removing the effect of gravity, for example.

If our case history taking or observations lead us to suspect a specific joint and its (non-contractile) tissues are principally involved in the patient's chief complaint, then we would change the order of testing to AF-ROM, AR-ROM and then PR-ROM, so as to follow the rule of doing the most painful test last whenever possible. If we suspect the injury is principally muscular, then the order of testing is the classic AF-ROM, PR-ROM and AR-ROM. Nonetheless, we always test AF-ROM, and always do so first.

NOTE: By this point in the protocol we should have mapped out the ranges of motion that are impaired, and noted and inquired about pain or discomfort, etc. Also at this point we should have some idea about what is going on. We may well be ready to provide our assessment to the patient at this point (see number 8 below). Alternatively, if we are suspicious of specific structures for which there is special or differential manual testing, we can proceed to do those as special tests.

6. **Special tests** Here is where we can – when it is appropriate or called for – do, for example, differential muscle testing. Where we can, if it is appropriate, do those special tests that test specific soft tissue (e.g., McMurray's meniscus test for the menisci of the knee). We should perform appropriate neurological tests or scans and test deep tendon reflexes (DTR). This is also the time to do any special testing for those different modalities we may employ, such as testing the craniosacral rhythms, Chinese medicine's pulse diagnosis, evaluation of energy flows via polarity therapy or Reiki.

7. **Direct palpation** Once all range of motion testing and special tests are completed, then we may choose to palpate the lesion site proper. We should again begin with a light palpation to re-test for any changes to temperature and/or edema that testing may have caused. Then we can proceed, with the patient's permission, to palpate deeper, to note the texture of the subcutaneous tissue, and to palpate the lesion site itself, if possible. Great care should be taken if you decide that this form of palpation is required.

CAUTION: Often deep palpation does not yield much information, and can re-injure or further injure fragile tissue.

8. **Assessment and treatment plan** Many of the orthopedic special tests and motion testing can result in our referring a patient out to get a confirming diagnosis for our suspicions of causes or pathologies that our testing implies. Nevertheless, we may also be able to proceed to work with the impairments found if no contraindications for treatment are apparent. If we remain within the impairment model, we can then proceed to establish outcomes that seem reasonable in light of our assessment and its findings. Having presented these outcomes or options to the patient, we can then arrive at a mutually agreed upon plan of treatment.

TABLE 3.2
Types of range of motion testing

AF-ROM	Investigates general function or ability (willingness) of the patient to perform specific actions. It does not tell us what types of tissues are involved
PR-ROM	Patient is passive and therapist moves joint(s) or limb. Designed to investigate joints and their (non-contractile) supportive tissues. At end-range, over-pressure (O-P) may be applied to fully test these tissues
AR-ROM	Isometric testing of muscle strength and integrity. As isometric, the non-contractile structures are not stressed (tested)

AF-ROM, active free range of motion; PR-ROM, passive relaxed range of motion; AR-ROM, active resisted (isometric) range of motion; O-P, over-pressure.

The benefit of an impairment-based model is that as impairments are found (such as restricted motion, pain, edema, etc.), these very impairments are what we will seek to resolve/treat. Therefore, they become the outcomes we seek to achieve. You use your clinical judgment to prioritize them and present that as a treatment plan to the patient.

Comments

The above represents an outline or protocol to follow when conducting an assessment (Figure 3.1). However, as I often tell students, we may not need to do it all at one time. When a patient presents with an injury or dysfunction, we certainly need to explore this by a case history taking specific to that patient's complaint, and do some brief observations. Further, the following can always be done:

Some inspection palpation prior to treatment, some rule outs, and then map out the patient's range of motion as best as possible, depending on the acuity of their injury or impairment. All of this can take as little as five minutes or so.

We then discuss the plan of action for this treatment (and possibly for the next several), providing a variety of optional plans, if reasonable. Post-treatment we can re-do some of the testing in order to see what we have accomplished (and have the patient see this as well) by re-testing affected ranges and asking "how does it feel now?" Tell the patient that we will possibly do some more testing next appointment and ask them to keep a mental note of how things go with their complaint until then.

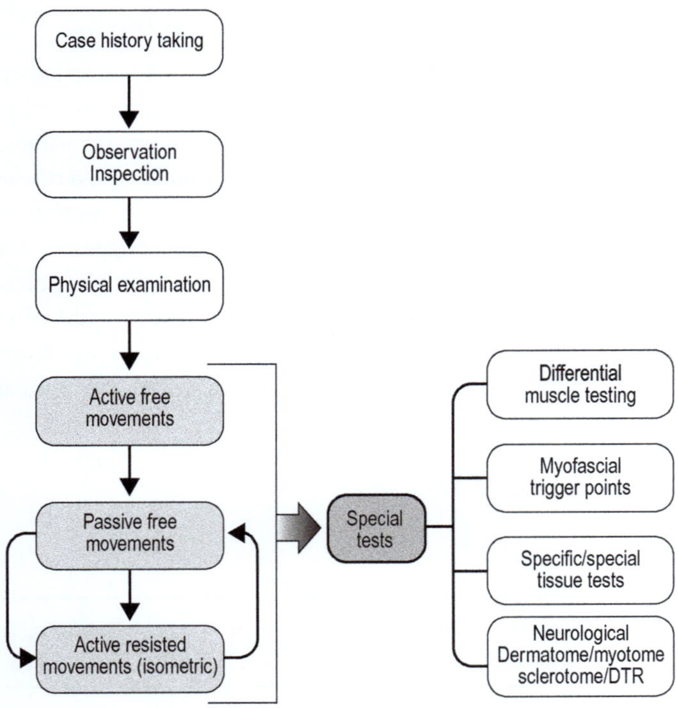

FIGURE 3.1

Clinical assessment protocol.

While writing up treatment notes, now that I have all of the information about what I have found during treatment and how the patient responded, I often take a few moments to re-evaluate the patient's condition, or to see if there is something I overlooked. I can often think of a few areas that I would like to explore through questioning or testing at the next appointment.

Therefore, when we itemize all of what we would do in an assessment it may seem like a lot and that would take too long; in reality, however, it is often quite manageable. Further, I have found that the patient appreciates this attention, and especially appreciates learning about what may be going on and why they are having the symptoms they are having. Even if no ultimate cause is found, addressing specific impairments and having an impact on them in turn gives the patient reassurance that they are moving forward.

Now that we have an overview of the principal elements of the procedure or protocol involved in obtaining an assessment, it is time to discuss each step in more detail.

Intake: forms, interviewing and case history taking

A misconception

One of the most common comments and concerns I get from massage therapists when teaching an impairment-based assessment protocol is that the patient would not accept their massage or treatment time being shortened so that the therapist could do more than one or two specific tests. There is an all too common assumption by massage therapists that the patient is in a hurry to "get on the table" and "get their massage." Nothing could be further from the truth for the patient with health concerns, whether those concerns are general or related to specific impairments.

I hear over and over again how much patients appreciate the fact that I take the time to help them understand what is causing their pain or dysfunction. In fact, based on patient feedback, it often seems that I am one of the very few health care practitioners who has taken the time to do the testing and explain my findings.

FIGURE 3.2 Sample intake form. With kind permission from ClinicSense.com©

INTAKE FORM

About You

Name

Sex

☐ Male ☐ Female

Address

City

State/Province

Country

Zip/Postal Code

Home Phone Number

Mobile Phone Number

Email Address

Marital Status

☐ Married

☐ Single

☐ Other ______

Birthday

Occupation

Employer or School

General Health Information

Family Doctor's Name

Family Doctor's Email Address

Family Doctor's Phone

Family Doctor's Address

Are you currently seeing other health care professionals?
(check all that apply)

- [ ] Chiropractor
- [ ] Physiotherapist
- [ ] Acupuncturist
- [ ] Massage Therapist
- [ ] Other ______________________
- [ ] Other ______________________

How would you rate your general health?

- [ ] Excellent
- [ ] Good
- [ ] Fair
- [ ] Poor

Please list any current medications and the conditions they are treating

Please list any major injuries, accidents or surgeries (including the approximate date)

Do you have any previous experience with Massage Therapy?

- [ ] Yes, my last massage therapy treatment was on Date ______________________
- [ ] No

Reason for visit

Primary complaint, cause and location of discomfort

When did the pain/discomfort start?

How often do you feel pain/discomfort

- [ ] Constantly
- [ ] Comes and goes suddenly
- [ ] Comes and goes gradually
- [ ] Other ______________________

How does the pain/discomfort feel

- [ ] Sharp
- [ ] Aching
- [ ] Throbbing
- [ ] Burning
- [ ] Tight
- [ ] Other ______________________

Pain/discomfort is brought on/made worse by

- [ ] Sitting
- [ ] Standing
- [ ] Lifting
- [ ] Bending
- [ ] Exercise/Physical Activity

Pain intensity

- [ ] Mild
- [ ] Moderate
- [ ] Severe

Pain/discomfort feels better with

- [ ] Ice
- [ ] Heat
- [ ] Anti-inflammatory medication
- [ ] Rest
- [ ] Activity

Health History

Head/Neck

- [ ] Whiplash
- [ ] Headaches/Migraines
- [ ] Concussion
- [ ] Ringing in Ears
- [ ] Hearing Loss
- [ ] Vision Problems
- [ ] Brain Injury
- [ ] Sinus Pain
- [ ] Other ______________________

Respiratory

- [ ] Asthma
- [ ] Shortness of Breath
- [ ] Chronic Cough
- [ ] Bronchitis
- [ ] Emphysema
- [ ] Sinusitis
- [ ] Frequent Colds
- [ ] Pneumonia
- [ ] Tuberculosis
- [ ] Smoker
- [ ] Other ______________________

Cardiovascular

- [ ] High Blood Pressure
- [ ] Low Blood Pressure
- [ ] Heart Attack
- [ ] Angina / Chest Pain
- [ ] Stroke
- [ ] Chronic Congestive Heart Failure
- [ ] Heart Disease
- [ ] Poor Circulation
- [ ] Phlebitis / Varicose Veins
- [ ] Pacemaker
- [ ] Hemophilia
- [ ] Family History of Cardiovascular Problems
- [ ] Other ______________________

Digestive

- [ ] Constipation
- [ ] Diarrhea
- [ ] Crohn's / Colitis
- [ ] Nausea
- [ ] Diverticulitis
- [ ] Ulcers
- [ ] Other ______________________

Nervous System

- [ ] Sensory Loss / Change
- [ ] Numbness / Tingling
- [ ] Spinal Cord Injury
- [ ] Thoracic Outlet Syndrome
- [ ] Carpal Tunnel Syndrome
- [ ] Sciatic
- [ ] Epilepsy
- [ ] Seizures
- [ ] Cerebral Palsy
- [ ] Parkinson's
- [ ] Multiple Sclerosis
- [ ] Neuralgias
- [ ] Other ______________

Musculoskeletal System

- [ ] Sprain / Strain
- [ ] Dislocation
- [ ] Arthritis
- [ ] Family History of Arthritis
- [ ] Tendonitis
- [ ] Bursitis
- [ ] Fractures
- [ ] Plantar Fasciitis
- [ ] Postural Deviation
- [ ] Degenerative Disc Disease
- [ ] Plates / Pins / Wires / Artificial Joint
- [ ] Other ______________

Other Conditions

- [ ] Cancer
- [ ] Diabetes
- [ ] Fibromyalgia
- [ ] Chronic Fatigue Syndrome
- [ ] Psychiatric Disorder
- [ ] Other ______________

Skin/Infections

- [ ] Infectious Skin Conditions
- [ ] Bruise Easily
- [ ] Hives
- [ ] Allergies / Hypersensitivity
- [ ] Dermatitis / Eczema
- [ ] Open Wound / Lesion
- [ ] Burns
- [ ] Acne
- [ ] Hepatitis
- [ ] HIV / AIDS
- [ ] Other ______________

Muscle/Joint Pain

☐ Jaw	☐ Left	☐ Right	☐ Both
☐ Neck	☐ Left	☐ Right	☐ Both
☐ Upper Back	☐ Left	☐ Right	☐ Both
☐ Middle Back	☐ Left	☐ Right	☐ Both
☐ Lower Back	☐ Left	☐ Right	☐ Both
☐ Shoulder	☐ Left	☐ Right	☐ Both
☐ Arm	☐ Left	☐ Right	☐ Both
☐ Elbow	☐ Left	☐ Right	☐ Both
☐ Wrist	☐ Left	☐ Right	☐ Both
☐ Hand	☐ Left	☐ Right	☐ Both
☐ Hip	☐ Left	☐ Right	☐ Both
☐ Leg	☐ Left	☐ Right	☐ Both
☐ Knee	☐ Left	☐ Right	☐ Both
☐ Ankle	☐ Left	☐ Right	☐ Both
☐ Feet	☐ Left	☐ Right	☐ Both
☐ Other ________	☐ Left	☐ Right	☐ Both

For Women

- [ ] Pregnant
- [ ] # of Children
- [ ] Gynecological Problems
- [ ] Other ______________

General

We like to recognize those people/organizations that refer patients to us. Please let us know how you found us:

- ☐ Doctor Name ______________________
- ☐ Friend Name ______________________
- ☐ Clinic website / Google
- ☐ Facebook / Twitter
- ☐ Advertisement
- ☐ Yellow Pages
- ☐ Other ______________________

☐ I hereby state that, to the best of my knowledge, my answers to the above questions are correct. I agree to and consent to assessment and treatment. I understand and consent that my medical information may be shared by the various care providers involved in my treatment.

☐ Treatments may be covered by extended health care plans. I understand that it is my responsibility to confirm the exact details of my coverage.

X ______________________ Signature

______________________ Date

Most massage therapists use a case history form, or an intake form, with new patients. These forms may vary greatly in length and in the amount of information and detail that the therapist wishes to gather initially, but they do have basic common elements.

Included here (Figure 3.2) is a sample of an extensive case history intake form. By looking through it carefully you can get a good idea about the breadth of information that you need to collect. This particular form is the basic template from an on-line office program (booking calendar, intake and treatment reporting, along with invoicing). The advantage of newer software and cloud storage is that the length of forms is not as much of an issue as when all forms were on paper and storage space could be an issue. There is more on record keeping at the end of this chapter. (The author would like to thank ClinicSense.com for permitting their intake form template to be copied here.)

Box 3.1 James Henry Cyriax (1904–1985)

See the website of the American Association of Orthopaedic Medicine for more information (http://www.aaomed.org/Cyriax-System-of-Orthopaedic-Medicine). Any online search of *James Henry Cyriax* will provide a wealth of information on Cyriax and his impact on modern orthopedic medicine. See also Cyriax's classic texts – *Textbook of Orthopaedic Medicine*, vols I and II – or the more recent summary: *Cyriax's Illustrated Manual of Orthopaedic Medicine*, Butterworth Heinemann, 1993. Cyriax coined the term orthopedic medicine and was a genius in developing the organized orthopedic model used widely today. For a succinct biography see https://www.ncbi.nlm.nih.gov/pmc/articles/PMC1478256/

Organization of a patient's intake

I want to mention just a few ways that this intake information may help us to develop some specific questions or areas of questioning that need to be organized before we begin to interview the patient.

I also want to make clear that the questions that arise out of the intake form may not be the first things we ask, but rather, are left until later when they may be more appropriate. There is a great temptation for all health care professionals to want to get straight to what they believe might be the heart of the matter. However, it is extremely rare to get all the information needed to understand the full context of the patient's issues from forms alone (or from medical test reports the patient may bring along with them). That understanding can only be achieved with an open mind, by not jumping to conclusions, and by beginning at the beginning.

Personal information

The first type of information that case history or intake forms gather is the patient's personal information. Those who follow in James Cyriax's footsteps (Box 3.1) have used the phrase "age and occupation" to name this category of information. Others affectionately refer to it as "the tombstone" – that short list of name, age, address, phone numbers, emergency contacts, and any other pertinent personal information required.

Even this type of information gives us some initial clues about what may be causing a patient's pain – for example, the patient's occupation can be a big clue. Some forms may even ask about recreational activities. Get us "in the ball-park," so to speak. All of this can at least supply us with some initial questions we may wish to ask concerning possible context and causes of pain (and other forms of impairments).

The patient may come in because their pain arose from a car accident or fall, but this personal information may still supply clues to: (1) how well they are healing, or not (i.e., how their activities of daily living – occupation, sports, recreation – could be affecting their healing); (2) any precipitating factors that may have led to them to being injured or made their injury worse (e.g., their job has them at a computer all day); (3) how they might prioritize their goals for therapy (i.e., they are more bothered by their headaches than by the wrist pain they have). These are just a few of the possible areas we might wish to explore during the interview with the patient, arising from their unique personal information.

Medical history

The next category or type of information gathered in an intake form is a general medical history – also affectionately known as "the organ recital" – any medical conditions concerning the heart, lungs, digestive system, kidneys, etc. We need to inquire into family history of any conditions. We certainly need this information to understand the indications and contraindications for massage and related modalities (e.g., hydrotherapy). In addition, specific to pain, we need to know if the patient's pain could be the result of an organ/visceral referral. Thus, for our understanding of the possible cause of pain, we need the medical history to rule out sources of pain that speak to a pathology that requires us to refer the patient out.

Categories of medical issues and specific issues to clarify If the patient indicates that they have a medical condition such

TABLE 3.3
Categories of medical issues and specific questions to ask

Category/system	Questions to ask regarding current history/recurrence
Heart/cardiovascular concerns	Hyper/hypotension; heart attack (myocardial infarction, MI); stroke (cardiovascular accident, CVA); transient ischemic attack, TIA (mini-strokes); thrombus, etc.
Lungs/respiratory problems	Asthma, bronchitis, pneumonia, emphysema
Digestive or gastro-intestinal system	Presence of swallowing difficulties, heartburn, appetite changes, nausea, vomiting, indigestion, constipation, diarrhea, abdominal pain, gas, hemorrhoids, liver and gall bladder disease. Assessment of palpable abdominal organs for pain, tenderness, discomfort and lack of motility
Urinary system	Presence of increased or decreased frequency of urination, infections, incontinence, kidney stones, kidney disease
Endocrine system	Presence of thyroid disease, diabetes, metabolic disturbances, changes in thirst, hunger, and perspiration
Senses	Problems with vision, hearing, taste, etc.
Nervous system	Numbness, tingling; epilepsy, nerve injury, or diseases of the central (CNS) or peripheral (PNS) nervous system, multiple sclerosis (MS), cerebral palsy (CP), anterolateral sclerosis (ALS)
Pathologies	There are several pathologies, conditions, or lifestyle issues often listed on intake forms or case history forms given to patients to fill out ahead of the interview: HIV, cancer, lupus, fibromyalgia, epilepsy Use of alcohol, recreational drugs; tobacco PMS; pregnancy Lifestyle choices Quality of sleep Depression or other mental health issues

as heart disease or asthma, then pursue that issue further. Table 3.3 lists the general medical categories and some of the most pertinent questions to ask within that category. The deeper your understanding of a pathology, the more detailed your questioning can become.

The importance of, and the need for, this information must be conveyed to the patient, with respect to any indications for massage therapy, or any precautions and contraindications (whether general or absolute) against.

Other areas to be discussed

- Other health care professionals involved in the patient's care.
- Current medications, whether prescription, over-the-counter, or supplements. These may alter examination findings (e.g., severity of pain).
- Past conditions (that the patient has recovered from): explain to the patient that past conditions may contribute to their current condition.
- Operations, hospitalizations, previous injuries and accidents.
- Family medical history: may provide clues to the patient's presenting complaint.
- Impairment and pain questions.

Many massage therapists end their case history form here, preferring to interview the patient for all the information about what brings them in for massage therapy. Others include some of the questions about pain or impairment on their intake forms. The form included in this section is an example. The therapist will review with the patient all the information given on a form during the interview. Further, the therapist will inform the patient that all medical information is held in the strictest confidence.

Charting and record keeping

Keeping good records is a must for massage therapists. Notes have to be taken of the interview with the patient, of their assessment and of each treatment. However, rather than interrupt the flow of discussing the protocol for assessment, charting and record keeping will be discussed at the end of this chapter.

A short history of pain and impairment

This is not about the nature of pain. It is about how to get a quick, efficient, but thorough case history of a patient's chief complaint that may include pain.

Interviewing the patient about their chief complaint

Some therapists "just go for it," and begin a long list of questions such as "what makes it better, what makes it feel worse," and so on. Certainly information will be gathered by this type of questioning, but usually in such a jumble as to limit the information's full utility. Also, the odds are that many pertinent questions may be skipped by accident. If this is the case, we may well miss important information and not only hamper how useful our treatments are, but possibly be led into implementing a completely wrong treatment plan, at best of no use, possibly even making things worse.

Organizing the questions of a case history regarding pain and impairments

A common tool taught to therapists to help them get the appropriate type and scope of questions asked is the acronym "OL' DR. FICARA," which stands for (as one variation has it): Onset, Location, Duration, Radiation, Frequency, Intensity, Character, Aggravation, Relieving, and Associated symptoms (Figure 3.3).

This is certainly better than "just going for it," but often the student does not understand (or is not taught) that there are different types of questions listed here – categories of information – hidden within this acronym.

Further, asking these questions in a specific order helps us organize and better understand the patient's pain and its possible sources, expressions, and gradations/acuity, etc.

Preferred method

The method I have found to be most useful goes back to James Cyriax and those who continued to develop his way of understanding orthopedic assessment. The first two categories of "age and occupation" and "medical history" are concerned with

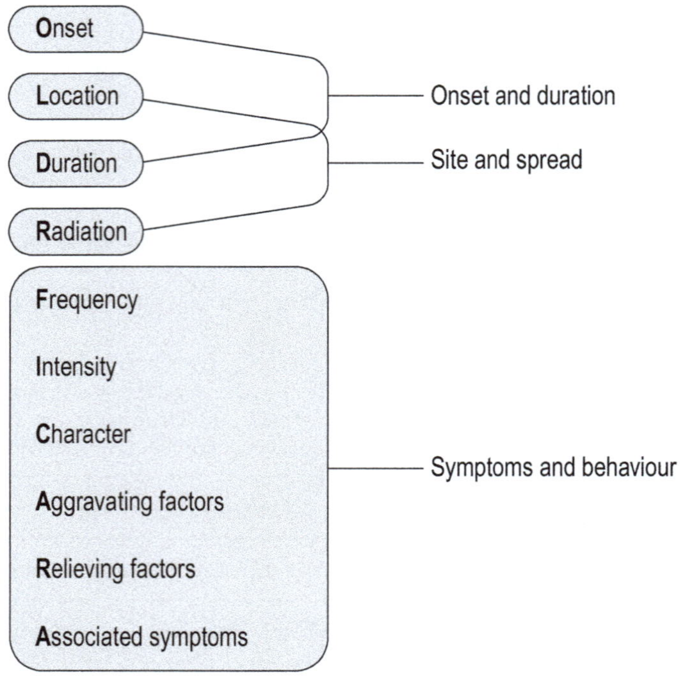

Note Some therapists use **OL' DR. FICARA** as an acronym to remember a number of questions, or types of questions relating to pain

FIGURE 3.3
Onset, Location, Duration, Radiation, Frequency, Intensity, Character, Aggravation, Relieving, and Associated symptoms.

exploring the intake form and gathering background information that will flesh out the basic context. The information needed for a thorough case history requires three more categories that explore the source and nature of the pain or any impairment:

- onset and duration
- site and spread
- symptoms and behavior.

NOTE: The last term is usually given as "behavior and symptoms," but I have turned it around so that it follows how I like to present the ordering of questions.

There are two reasons why this particular list of categories should be preferred. First, it nicely divides the whole range of possible questions into three basic categories or types that each speak to the source of pain in a different manner.

Onset and duration These questions deal with when and how the impairment happened – the possible origin or mechanism of injury (MOI); and any previous history of such. This talks to us about the mechanics of the injury and hence, gives us clues regarding the structures involved and the amount or acuity of the injury. One of its major purposes is to establish whether the impairment happened suddenly (i.e., trauma) or arose gradually over time. Also, we may get more information about predisposing factors; and we can inquire about initial treatments, medications or first aid received if that was necessary.

Site and spread These questions deal with where the impairment is – specific questions about the location of the pain, and if it travels or radiates/refers to anywhere else. This gives us clues such as whether we are dealing with superficial or deep structures as the source, as well as possible clues to types of tissues involved (muscle, connective tissue, nerve, etc.).

Symptoms and behavior These questions deal with what transformations to the impairment or pain have occurred over time, or how it has changed since onset. We can learn how the pain presented and expressed itself over time; clues to its present acuity; what is being done for it now, and by whom, and how it is responding; how activities of daily living are affecting recovery; and so on.

The second reason I like these categories concerns the order in which they are listed above. In this order, they provide a complete picture of the impairment, starting from the onset and up to how it is behaving today. Below is a summary of some of the questions that are asked in each category. The list does not include everything that can be asked. Its purpose here is to let you see the content and flow of each category of questioning and how comprehensive this approach is in getting a picture of the patient's chief complaint. With this information, the therapist can begin to formulate a plan of assessment.

With a comprehensive manual assessment, the therapist will be able to develop a comprehensive (and therefore appropriate and safe) treatment plan along with a home care regimen.

What follows are examples of questions from each category and the type of information that we are trying to elicit. Prior to questioning the patient about the onset, etc., provide them with a pain scale from zero to 10, with zero being no pain at all and 10 being the worst pain they can imagine. Do not have them grade it right now. Just tell them how to use this scale, and alert them that you will be asking them to give you a number, probably several times, during the course of the interview.

Onset and duration

With this category of questioning we want to know when the injury occurred. Was the onset sudden or gradual? How long has it been since the onset? Have you experienced the same or similar impairment previously? Do you know how you hurt yourself? When did you first notice the problem? Questions about the onset and duration of the impairment may be relatively limited in number.

A traumatic, sudden onset is often understood as an acute injury and so will have all of the hallmarks of one – most importantly, signs of inflammation, which are heat, redness, edema, and tenderness. The mechanism of injury (how the patient was injured) can speak to us about: (1) the degree of acuity and tissue damage, and (2) which tissues could be involved in the primary lesion. Are there secondary or other issues?

If there is a previous injury, you may want to investigate that occurrence as well, since it often happens that compensations to acute injuries can later become problems in themselves after the original injury has healed. Alternatively, with respect to a gradual onset, previous injuries may have set the patient up for the current impairment(s).

A gradual onset may imply a repetitive strain (cumulative trauma). In other words, the injury may have started at a cellular level, with healing not being able to keep up with wear and tear on the myofascial tissues, often resulting in a flare-up or acute-on-chronic situation. Whether acute-on-chronic (i.e., when a chronic condition "flares up") or chronic, we will be looking for some of the classic signs of chronic injuries: fibrotic, dense, and shortened tissues, or on the other hand disorganized, poorly maintained or repaired tissue, and either possibly with muscle weakness.

Whether the onset was sudden or gradual you will want to know about how the pain or impairment felt at the time (was it sharp, dull, etc., or weak, stiff, unstable, etc.?).

All of these sorts of questions help to provide the information that will enable us to ask questions that are more pertinent further along in the interview. Though there may be more questions that could be asked initially, we can get enough information about the mechanism of injury so that we can move on to site and spread.

Remember, you can always return to this category of questioning at the end, so do not over-question and get bogged down. More often than not, moving onto the next two categories of questions will help clarify the situation for you, or provide you with enough understanding of the patient's condition so that if you later return to "onset and duration" questions you will then be able to formulate clearer and more concise questions.

Site and spread

With site and spread questions, we want to clarify where they feel their pain or impairment. These questions can also initially be few in number; they focus on how specific the patient feels the site of the injury to be, and on any pain felt anywhere else in the body. This latter question should be asked in this straightforward way since the patient most likely does not know much about referral patterns, or possibly even that referral of pain can happen. Therefore, the patient is likely to not mention pains other than the chief complaint, as they often believe such pain is irrelevant to the issue.

Ask the patient:

- "Can you point a finger to where you feel the pain, or do you have to draw a boundary around it?" When the patient can point to a specific site for the pain or impairment, it is more likely to be a recent event (even acute or subacute) and in superficial tissue. If the patient has to draw a boundary round an area, then ask if the boundary is distinct or is it hard to gauge (vague). A distinct boundary implies that the impairment is often more on site, but deep, while a vague boundary could be referred pain.
- "If the pain travels or radiates anywhere else, could you please show me (draw for me with your finger) the path it takes to where it travels?" Ask yourself if the referral described to you follows the path of a dermatome or peripheral nerve, or is it following a specific type of tissue? Radiating pain with distinct borders suggests pressure on a nerve: if it is a nerve root, it spreads or follows a dermatomal pattern. If it is a peripheral nerve, then it travels along the path of that specific nerve.
- "Even if you think it is unrelated, have you, or are you, experiencing any pain anywhere else in your body ... (if so) ... Did you notice this before or since your current problem?" This speaks to possible referred pain/paresthesia, trigger points, etc. It may point to predisposing (pre-existing problems/pain), or on the other hand, to adaptive, compensatory problems arising since the onset of the current complaint.

Now that we have clarified the origin and the location of symptoms, we can go on to the almost unlimited category of questioning: the symptoms and behavior of the impairment. It is here that we really want to explore the nature of the pain and/or the impairment – what it is that they are *experiencing*.

Symptoms and behavior

Now we want to know what the patient is experiencing in terms of the characteristics of the pain or impairment, and how it has changed or evolved (i.e., its behavior) over time (days, weeks, months), and at various times of the day – how does it feel when they wake, throughout the day, at the end of the day and during sleep?

We may be tempted to explore the nature of the pain when dealing with the onset, or when dealing with the site and spread, but we should resist doing so. The main reason for resisting is precisely because the symptoms and behavior category of questions is so large. If we begin here, or enter into this realm before clarifying the onset and site issues, we may never get around to clarifying them at all. We could miss some very pertinent information contained in these two categories that is required if we are to give a safe and effective treatment.

Examples of symptoms and behavior questions include the ever popular (and first out of the mouths of students!) "What makes it better or worse? Is it worse or better at certain times of day? Worse or better after rest … or activity? Does it wake you up at night? Does it interfere with your daily tasks and activities? How?" And so on.

But even here we should order the questions somewhat. A good way to begin, after clarifying the site and spread, is to say something like: "Let us return to how the pain feels, especially how it may be different at different times or during different situations. So, first, in your own words please describe how the pain feels right now? How intense is the pain on a scale of one to 10?" This starts off with the symptoms. Once the patient has described the nature of the pain, then go into those behavioral or situational questions listed above – how the pain is altered by activities and the patient's specific living environment.

Terms patients use and what they may imply

Listed below are some common terms that a patient may use to describe their symptoms. The terms used can imply certain tissues as involved in their chief complaint. This, in turn, may help us prioritize which tissues need to be assessed. Note that similar descriptors can imply different types of tissues. These are "rules of thumb." They give clues to follow up on; they certainly are not "diagnostic."

Pain symptoms reported and their suspected origins

- Sharp, lancing, shooting pain: suggests a nerve lesion.
- Pins and needles, tingling: may imply ischemia of the peripheral nerves, often due to nerve compression or compression of blood flow.
- Dull, aching pain: deep somatic (not visceral) origin.
- Excruciating pain, unrelenting pain, intolerable pain, deep aching pain and boring pain: underlying localized pathology or systemic disorder. Refer out!
- Stiff, achy, muscle cramping or grabbing: typical of musculoskeletal disorders.

- Hot or feverish: implies inflammation.
- Sharp and burning, distributed along specific nerves: nerve root or peripheral nerve.
- Deep, boring, and poorly localized: may be due injury to bone.
- Localized (and with referred pain to other areas): joint.
- Diffuse, aching, and poorly localized, often referred to other areas: vascular issues.
- Dull, aching, poorly localized, and referred to other areas: muscle.

What the responses to symptoms and behavior questions can tell us

Changes in quality of the pain, or symptomatic picture, may offer many clues as to the nature and extent of the lesion:

- Continual reduction in pain and impairments implies healing.
- If the pain was improving prior to the treatment and stops improving or worsens immediately following the treatment the treatment needs to be re-evaluated.
- Lack of change over several treatments implies perpetuating factors (one of which could be the current treatment). An investigative reassessment is necessary. And a referral back to the primary physician would be in order, to rule out an as yet unknown pathology. Alternatively, sometimes the patient feels relief for a short period of time post-treatment, but this is brief and the impairments soon return as before. This can also imply other structural issues; for example, with a "whiplash" it might imply that though muscle pain in the neck is reduced along with a reduction in tone, an underlying injury to ligaments could be the issue. Muscle may re-tighten in a protective "holding and guarding" response to an underlying sense of instability in the cervical vertebra.

Worsening pain (prior to treatment and in spite of treatment) requires immediate referral out. Possible emergency measures may be needed. The treatment is not likely to be the cause if the pain was worsening prior to treatment.

Spasming that is not affected by treatment (either persisting or returning shortly after treatment) can be due to the holding and guarding that is stabilizing an unstable joint. You should suggest they get imaging done by a physician.

- However, calcium, magnesium or other nutritional deficiencies are often also a perpetuating factor in continued spasming (e.g., night cramping in the lower legs). Again, refer the patient to their primary health provider.
- Interference with blood supply or drainage of fluids can also be another possible cause. Refer out.

"When do you typically feel the pain?"

- Pain that does not decrease with rest but is not aggravated by movement (in other words, the pain is staying constant) is probably not muscular. The suspicion would be that the pain is arising from some pathologic process other than a common musculoskeletal disorder.
- Pain on rest which improves with movement is commonly due to mild inflammation. Movement helps the tissue to drain, reducing fluid pressure and removing irritating metabolites.
- Similarly, a disc lesion may often be aggravated by sitting (i.e., the back is in relative flexion), and walking will often give relief.
- Morning pain can be suggestive of arthritis, especially the inflammatory varieties, where edema has accumulated in the joints overnight.
- Morning stiffness that fades within a half-hour – "once I get moving …" – can suggest degenerative joint disease: osteoarthritis. This description is also common in developing (not yet acute-on-chronic) repetitive strain conditions.

Weakness in muscles When there is weakness with associated pain, the cause may well be due to a strain to the muscle. When there is weakness without pain, this is often due to a neurological issue. What the patient perceives as a muscle that "goes weak" or of a joint "giving way" is often due to instability in the joint. Due to an inherent instability within the joint, or its inert supportive tissues, the muscles that support that joint can suddenly go weak. This is due to a protective inhibitory reflex that turns these muscles off.

Awakening in pain Pain waking the patient at night can be from acute-on-chronic joint inflammation, or muscle tendonosis/tendonitis or compression syndromes (e.g., carpal tunnel). Rest (immobility) results in increased edema in the tissue involved, which leads to increased pressure, and increased compression of tissues within restrictive structures (tunnels, compartments and the like). Further, inflamed tissues will produce more chemical irritants and thereby stimulate pain receptors.

Pain from visceral or deep somatic sources is often accompanied by one or several autonomic symptoms: for example, tissue texture changes, sweating, goose bumps, etc., happening within a discrete area of the skin.

Dermatome and sclerotome pain Sclerotome pain (from bone or deep connective tissue) is typically felt as deep, aching, and poorly localized, whereas dermatome pain (felt as coming from a superficial source) is often sharp, sometimes shooting, and localized to defined dermatomal patterns on the skin.

When a tissue related to a particular sclerotome (or a sensory nerve root associated with an area of bone) is irritated, the patient may perceive the resulting pain as arising from any or all of the tissues innervated by the same segmental sensory nerve root. This is a result of the lack of precision in the central neural connections, and is not related to abnormal impulses "spreading down a nerve." Often there is nothing wrong with most of the area from which pain seems to arise.

A very important source of both dermatomic and sclerotomic pain is direct irritation of a nerve along its pathway as it carries afferent input from a particular area. This is properly referred to as projected (or radicular) pain, rather than referred pain. Such radicular pain can also come from irritation of a nerve root. Thus, an intervertebral disc protrusion or bony osteophyte may directly excite nerve fibers of a specific nerve root, sensory and/or motor fibers, producing symptoms or signs confined to the relevant dermatome, myotome, or sclerotome area. The symptoms or signs will vary, depending on the fibers affected. In most massage clinical settings, pain from the skin itself generally has a visible source: a "scrap," laceration, rash, or some skin condition (eczema).

Red flags

If the patient informs you of any of the following, you should treat these as situations where the patient should seek immediate medical help:

- The pain is unremitting; it never changes or abates regardless of activity or rest.
- Trouble breathing.
- Fainting spells or intense vertigo.
- Sudden weakness; slurred speech; sudden vision changes, loss of sense of balance.
- Chest pain that may radiate into the jaw and/or down the arm.
- Abdominal pain that is clearly not muscular – especially if just after eating.
- Sudden urinary incontinence, especially if it occurs after a fall; kidney pain is often felt in the low back area at the level of the 11th and 12th ribs.

Interviewing the patient

Some points to consider

- Note that it is important to practice asking questions. It is easy to get lost!
- Patients will bring up the subjects that are easiest to talk about. The patient may try to remain here and not go into areas you need to explore.
- It takes tactful questioning to explore potential related areas that may be difficult for the patient to talk about.
- When interviewing the patient, while all information gathered is important, emphasis should be placed on the portion with the greatest clinical importance.
- ***NOTE:*** Excellent listening skills are crucial. However, it is important to remember that you are in a gathering role in this new therapeutic relationship. Keeping the interview on track, as well as clearly understanding what the patient is telling you, is called "funnel sequencing."
- Symptoms are not absolute; things such as cultural, socioeconomic or language differences may cause different presentations or descriptors for similar conditions.
- Also remember that pain thresholds can vary greatly from individual to individual.

A good mnemonic for some of these points is "the rule of the five vowels" (A, E, I, O, U) for interviewing:

ATTENTIVE – reminds the interviewer to be attentive.

EVALUATION – refers to the weighing and sorting out of relevant information.

INQUIRY – the interviewer probes into significant areas requiring more clarification.

OBSERVATION – underlines the importance of non-verbal communication.

UNDERSTANDING – comes from listening to the patient's whole story, including their concerns and apprehensions; this will allow the therapist to be more empathetic.

Funnel sequencing

There are two types of questions used during case history taking: open-ended questions and closed-ended questions. Open-ended questions do not provide specific options for the patient to choose from. The patient is not guided to any answer, nor can they answer yes or no. Closed-ended questions, on the other hand, provide options for the patient to choose from. The patient may be directed to give certain kinds of answers or provide an answer that they feel the therapist wants to hear. Both of these two types of questions are employed when interviewing the patient. Open-ended questions cast a wide net, while close-ended questions are used, when necessary, to begin restricting the breadth of answers the patient is giving. The former prompt the patient to find their own words to answer a particular question, while the latter are used to bring a category of questioning to an end or stop the patient from "wandering" when answering. Using these types of questions can be thought of as funneling.

Open-ended questions do not restrict the patient's response. For example, ask about a patient's injury with: "Explain the circumstances of what brought you here" or "How did you hurt yourself?" This leaves it up to the patient to begin at the place they believe is most appropriate. The way in which the patient can answer is wide open with respect to their options.

Open-ended questions are helpful because they do not lead the patient to provide answers that they think the therapist might want to hear. They also prevent us, as therapists, from asking leading questions (based on a preconceived notion of cause) that will result in the patient responding as we want them to. We want the patient to give us *their* understanding of what has happened or is happening to them. We ask open-ended questions in order to get the maximum information, free of our pre-judgments and biases. As the patient does not have our training, they need the time to give us their version of what is going on, and why. In this way, we can be sure to have the appropriate information to be able to address the patient's concerns or issues, not just what we consider relevant.

By using open-ended questions, we are more likely to get a broader perspective of what is going on. We will also get information on how the lesion or injury is impacting the patient on many levels: not just physically, but also emotionally, and with respect to their daily activities, social life, employment issues and family. This information can make our treatment approach broader and more complex, in the sense of addressing the injury on many levels. We will definitely be more prepared to understand how to shape our responses to the patient's questions and needs, and so safeguard their emotional health, etc., to the best of our abilities and scope of practice.

A closed-ended question, on the other hand, asks the patient a question that can be answered with limited options or even just a yes or no response. The value of closed-ended questions is increased when they are employed correctly. Such direct questions can help calm the nervous patient, or help them focus on the issue under discussion. They can, in time, speed up the acquisition of pertinent information, or help clarify what may be seen as contradictory statements given in a patient's story. This type of questioning can be useful to pry more information out of a non-disclosing patient.

One of the best uses for closed-ended questioning is when the patient wanders off into information that is not relevant, or begins to repeat themselves. These types of questions help the therapist to take charge and bring the interview back on course. The following are ways that the therapist can help to control the flow of information and keep the interview on track.

Active listening

When you have completed a particular category of questioning then repeat, using the patient's own wording, what the patient has said so far. This is meant to ensure that we understand what the patient is saying, and that the patient feels that they have expressed themselves correctly. This is part of what is called active listening (see later in this section). We often begin this process by telling the patient something like: "Now, let me see if I have got this right …" Then you repeat their story back to them. Active listening can also be used at any point of the interview if you feel you are losing the thread of the story, feeling the patient is contradicting themselves, and so on.

Paraphrasing is repeating or echoing back, in your own words, sections of information to the patient when you feel that either a lot of information is already gathered and you wish to confirm your understanding, or you feel that you have missed something and need clarification (summarizing portions of a topic as you go along, if you like). This also lets the patient know that you are listening and following along; and it further helps by getting the patient to hear what they have actually said so far, and to confirm or alter the information.

Summarizing is sharing your understanding of the overall situation/condition of your patient. This is repeating back the whole storyline as you have digested it, but in a brief summary. Again, allow the patient to agree or alter this picture.

Therefore, in repeating back to the patient what we think they have said, we can ensure that we have got the story straight by having the patient confirm our understanding. For example, the patient may say either: "Yes, that's correct." Or, they can correct us by saying: "No, what I meant was …" Also, they can have the chance to alter/clarify their account: "No, no, that is not what I meant to say. It was more like …" or "Oh, I forgot to tell you …" At this point the patient may continue their account, now that they have been set back on course. You may then return to open-ended questioning if either you or the patient feels they have more to say on that specific issue or category of questioning. Alternatively, this is an opportunity to begin a new line of questioning, to move onto another category of questioning.

Open-ended questioning and funneling down to closed-ended questioning

The second thing we can do to "get back on track" (again, usually done after repeating back what the patient has said) is to "funnel down" to the closed-ended question. These are questions that may:

- be a change of topic, or have to do with a specific category of questioning
- have several options for an answer, or
- be as limited as a yes or a no answer.

This funneling is meant as a clarification tool, or to bring a patient back to the topic at hand.

We still first try not to overly direct the patient to a specific response, but we do give a narrower field so as to help the patient focus on specific aspects of their chief complaint: e.g., "How would you describe the pain that you feel today?"

If we still do not get a clear enough understanding, we may narrow the field by giving several optional answers, e.g., "Would you describe your pain as throbbing, numb, burning, achy, stabbing or deep?" Or, even narrower questioning, such as either/or types of questions: "You said it was throbbing, and also that it travelled down to your elbow. Does that referred pain in the elbow also throb or does it feel different? Do you experience these at the same time, or at different times?"

This narrowing down of the possible field of answers is what is meant by funneling. Funneling into narrower options and finally down to yes or no type questions results in asking leading questions. The patient is being directed to answer in a specific way. This can be used to clarify what the patient has been saying about a specific issue. Alternatively, it can be used to bring the discussion to a close on a specific category of questioning so that the interview can move onto other issues or categories of questions. This helps us bring to an end a discussion that is wandering off course or becoming repetitive.

Closed-ended questions are sometimes thought of as leading questions. They direct the patient to answer in a specific way. Examples of leading questions are: "Does your pain start here and travel to here?" "Does the arm feel like it is tingling?" This type of question will hopefully elicit a specific answer, which is meant to clarify or complete a line of questioning.

Leading questions To lead or not to lead, that is the question? It is not that we never ask leading questions, but rather that they are employed only after the more open-ended type have failed to gather all the information needed to develop a sound clinical impression – a hypothesis about what could be ailing the patient. And remember that every hypothesis needs to be tested. We need to be aware that we can question too closely or too long and lead the patient to give answers that may not be accurate, or even true, but only justify the answer we have already assumed to be true.

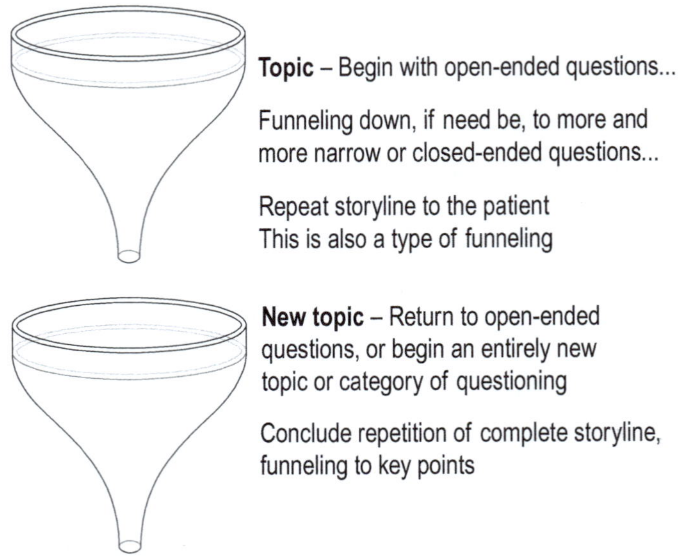

FIGURE 3.4
Funneling down and funneling out.

Funneling down and funneling out

Funneling in or down can be followed by funneling out (Figure 3.4). Let us say we need to clarify some points about the onset of an impairment and choose to funnel down to more specific questions. Once you have the information you need, repeat back your understanding to the patient. Either remain with the same topic, returning to open-ended questioning, or close off the last topic if you think it has been thoroughly covered and begin with a new line of inquiry with an open-ended question, as in moving from onset type of questions to site and spread questions.

If you follow this advice, you can get a correct, precise and complete history of the patient's pain or impairments.

At the conclusion of the interview you may want to briefly return to one or two of the categories of questions, if you feel you need to clarify something said earlier, or you may now have other questions about onset and duration, for example, that you now wish to ask.

Observations

Observations have been going on since you greeted the patient, they have continued through the intake process, through the treatment, and will continue until you see the patient out of the door. Nonetheless, at times we may wish to do a formal postural assessment and this would be best carried out before any manual testing that may cause discomfort or pain.

Inspection palpation is something we can begin at any time, including during the interview, when, for example, you may want to palpate for inflammation.

NOTE: Use the back of the hand to palpate for temperature. Do not do any deep or probing palpation at this time. Above all, it must be completely pain-free. If we probe for the lesion site at this time we may cause pain or apprehension that will interfere with our manual testing to follow.

Here such palpation is called inspection palpation and would entail feeling for tone, temperature (heat/coolness) of the tissue, or for edema in the tissue. We need to gather more than just visual information. In fact, we always learn more when we add palpatory experience to visual observations.

Observe the patient's body language when greeting the patient, escorting them to the treatment room and during the interview.

- Observe facial expressions: blank, happy, sad, tired, angry, in pain, drawn, or looking medicated (from painkillers, etc.), focused or distracted, to name a few. How is their coloring: pale, flushed, healthy, sickly, etc.?
- Observe body expressions, much the same as above. Do you notice, when they walk, stand or sit, that they are favoring or protecting a part of their body? Can they sit still or do they keep changing position (trying to get comfortable) or seem restless/agitated? Do they appear energetic or tired?

Finding your dominant eye

One important piece of information that is needed is finding out which is your dominant eye. The dominant eye is the one that we use to aim, or judge distance. The closer we are to what we are observing, the more important it is to know your dominant eye. Follow the instructions in the captions to Figures 3.5 and 3.6.

The therapist in Figures 3.5 and 3.6 is left eye dominant. (If you watch the person from in front as they do the test their arms and hands automatically align to their dominant eye.) On rare occasions, some say both eyes work (with the other closed), or neither (when either is closed). If so, they may have no dominant eye and they probably have difficulty judging depth and/or level in general.

The great importance of knowing which is your dominant eye becomes clear when you are checking levels, looking for

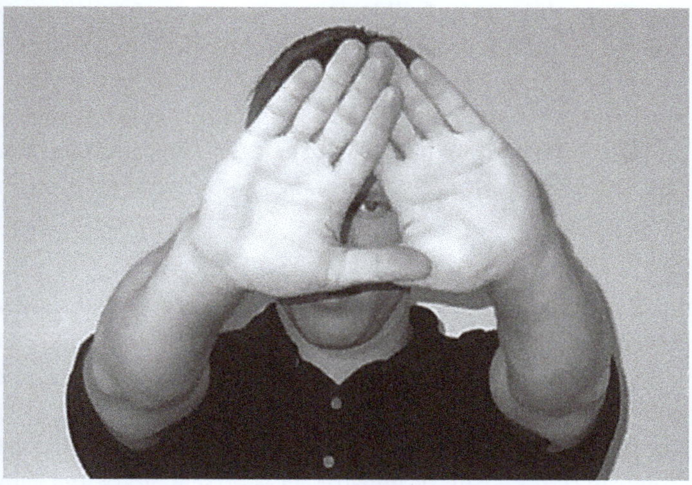

FIGURE 3.5 Finding your dominant eye 1

Open your hands and overlap them slightly, leaving a hole that you can look through. Raise your arms up to shoulder height, elbows extended. With both eyes open, look at some object on a wall that is about 12 feet away, such as a clock. Position your arms/hands so that you see the object with both eyes.

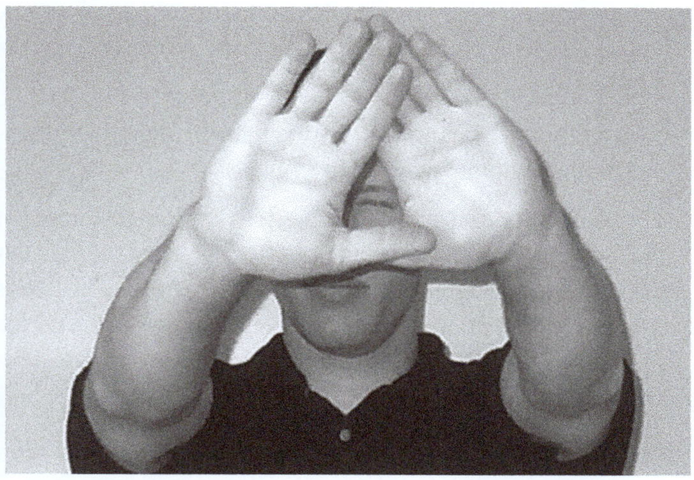

FIGURE 3.6 Finding your dominant eye 2

Now close one eye; let us start with the left eye closed. Do not move or shift your hands! Can you still see the object? Let us say that you can. Now close the right eye and open the left. Can you still see the object? In this example you should not be able to see it. Therefore, you are right eye dominant. However, it can be the left eye that is dominant for others, as it is for the therapist here.

asymmetries, etc. If you switch placing your eye in the patient's mid-line, you will get different findings at different times. However, if you always place your dominant eye in the patient's mid-line, then you will be much more accurate and consistent with your estimates. This is especially crucial when you are palpating landmarks, because the patient is so close to you. Again, if you watch someone else line themselves up to check iliac crest heights, for example, you will generally notice that the dominant eye is also slightly forward compared to the other eye, i.e., the therapist slightly rotates their head so that their dominant eye is forward.

The most organized forms of observation are performing a postural assessment, and/or a gait analysis. For the time being, we will make just a few brief comments about their value. Later, we will deal with both of them in greater detail.

Postural assessments, gait analysis, and any motion palpation or range of motion testing of specific regions of the body are essential for finding muscle imbalances, along with structural or functional asymmetries. In terms of locating and evaluating impairments, these structured observations have been said to rely on finding the following:

- **A**symmetry
- **R**estriction (to motion, whether of joints, tissues or of any elements of the circulatory and lymphatic systems or nervous system)
- **T**issue texture changes (trophic changes, signs of inflammation, or autonomic nervous system signs).

These observations are known collectively under the acronym ART. Sometimes an "s" is added (ARTs) to represent the patient's subjective reporting of pain, etc. However, the capital letters represent what are considered objective findings (ART) and the "s" is left in lower case specifically because it is subjective information (Chila 2010; DeStefano 2011).

Visual inspection: examples

A – Landmarks: using bony landmarks, the general alignment and positions of structures is assessed.

R – Differences in motion from the norm, or when compared bilaterally.

T – Soft tissues: observe contours, comparing bilaterally. Look for edema, hyper-/hypotrophy

- skin: look for rubor, cyanosis, shininess, loss of hair, or patches of hair, etc.
- scars: from injury or surgery.

Rule outs

Once you have decided which joint or region of the body you are going to investigate as the source of the patient's chief complaint, you must rule out the joint above and the joint below. It is imperative to determine whether those joints/areas could be referring into the area of the chief complaint. If this rule out testing does not reproduce the patient's chief complaint, then that joint is said to be "ruled out" and not in need of immediate further testing.

As an example, if the elbow is the area of the chief complaint, then both the shoulder and the wrist must be ruled out as possibly being involved before the elbow itself is tested. This is done to make sure that the structures or tissues of the shoulder or wrist are not referring symptoms into the elbow. Keep in mind that the patient may experience pain or other symptoms or impairments with the rule out testing itself. If the rule outs do not provoke or reproduce the chief complaint, they are set aside for the time being and may be tested at another time.

However, these secondary issues may be involved indirectly or partially in the primary complaint. Though we may immediately continue to focus on the primary reason for the patient being there, we will sooner or later need to address these issues too. Often they can be "milder" than the primary issue but may well be predisposing factors for it, and/or perpetuating factors if not dealt with. Again, we need, in the end, to address the whole. Therefore, the information gathered from rule outs when negative (i.e., they do not reproduce the chief complaint) are not discarded and tossed aside, but rather are very important with respect to getting at all the causes (direct or indirect) of an impairment.

These rule outs, or quick tests, stress the principal tissues involved in each of those joints to be ruled out. Therefore, you begin by having the patient do specific AF-ROM tests of that joint. When the end-range of each movement is reached, ask if the patient is experiencing any pain (even if other than their chief complaint). If no pain or impairment is present, grasp and support the limbs or structures and tell the patient to relax and let you move it. You will apply O-P (over-pressure) as if/when performing passive relaxed range of motion (PR-ROM) testing. This stresses the inert or non-contractile tissues of that joint.

Once O-P has been applied, again ask the patient if they feel any pain or impairment. If there is no pain, move to the next anatomical motion and rule it out. If the patient does experience pain, ask if it is the same pain as they came to see you about, or something different. If you get a positive reproduction of their chief complaint when doing a rule out, that joint now needs to be included in your protocol of testing and considered ruled in. After all, a chief complaint may include more than one joint.

More on range of motion testing

The most important rule for range of motion (ROM) testing is that the unaffected limb or side (when this is the case) is tested first. This establishes what is normal for this particular patient. The impaired side is compared to this and not to some conceptual ideal (which is often called "normal range of motion"). This is done in AF-ROM, PR-ROM, and AR-ROM. Not doing this comparison and comparing the impaired motion to some ideal standard may well skew expectations of the patient and also cause the therapist to try and reach a goal that may not be appropriate for that patient.

Active free range of motion (AF-ROM) testing

AF-ROM testing tells us mostly about ability, mobility, and function of a specific joint and the tissues involved in its motion. The patient moves the joint voluntarily and by doing so, AF-ROM determines: the joint's range of motion; the patient's willingness to move it; which motion produces pain; the quality of control over movements; it may also give some idea about the stability of surrounding tissues.

We may observe restriction to range of motion as well as structural asymmetry side-to-side for the limbs (bilateral comparison). During AF-ROM the patient may tell us of pain happening with certain motions. AF-ROM reveals which actions or functions are impaired; however, it does not help us to differentiate between the types of tissues involved in the impairments. This is because both contractile and inert tissues are involved, such as muscle (contractile tissue) or ligaments, joint capsule or articular surfaces (non-contractile or inert tissues). With AF-ROM, as with all testing, we are trying to reproduce the pain/dysfunction that is troubling the patient. We are looking at pain and function (activities, occupational or recreational stressors, etc.).

Remember, we compare, when applicable, the impaired side to the unimpaired side or limb. Therefore, we ask the patient to perform these actions on their "good side" first to find out what is normal for them; only then do we ask them to move the impaired side.

Passive relaxed range of motion (PR-ROM) testing

PR-ROM is meant to inform us about the condition of the non-contractile tissue involved in the joint. As the name implies, the patient should be relaxed and allow the therapist to move the limb or joints and tissues. Theoretically, if the patient does not engage the musculature, then PR-ROM only stresses, and so tests, the non-contractile tissues. Therefore, we now begin to be able to differentially test between contractile and non-contractile tissues involved in the patient's chief complaint.

Passive forced (passive O-P)

Classically, what follows is the application of over-pressure (O-P) if the joint is taken to end-range and there is no pain or impairment found. O-P is meant to be the gentle application of a light forcing of the joint to see if it will move a little bit further past the end-range. This adds a slight additional stress on those non-contractile tissues, to further test them. For example, O-P applied to a joint in a specific direction will apply stress to specific ligaments or a specific part of the joint capsule. If the O-P produces pain or impairment to function, then we can conclude that some non-contractile tissues are involved in the patient's chief complaint. Further, knowing our anatomy, we can know which non-contractile tissues were stressed.

End-feel

When we apply O-P, we are attempting to clarify the end-feel. This is what is felt by the therapist when they passively move the patient's joint slightly past the available range of motion.

There are several types of end-feel:

- *Bony end-feel*: bone on bone, an abrupt hard stop to movement when two hard surfaces meet.
- *Capsular end-feel*: a leathery resistance, with only the slightest give at the end of range. Normal range of motion is available.
- *Soft-capsular end-feel*: sometimes called a boggy end-feel. The end-feel is soft because the joint capsule is swollen. It often feels as though you are pushing into a balloon filled with water. There is a loss to the amount of normal range for that joint.
- *Springy block end-feel*: often has a muscular rebound away from the end of range due to a loose body or an intra-articular displacement.
- *Soft tissue approximation end-feel*: tissue meeting tissue ends movement.
- *Muscle spasm end-feel*: a hard leathery feel, with no give and with some push back.
- *Empty end-feel*: the patient stops the O-P from happening because pain or apprehension prevents them from moving further. Therefore, the therapist cannot get to an end-feel.

A number of these can be normal end-feels. The extension of the elbow is usually a bony end-feel. The biceps brachii pushing into the forearm is soft tissue approximation. The type of normal end-feel for each joint is given in the appropriate chapter of the text. However, any of these can be abnormal when encountered when they are not expected.

Joint mobilization testing

A physiological motion in a synovial joint is some combination of a roll, spin, slide, and traction or compression, which the patient can do voluntarily. On the other hand, an accessory motion is the occurrence of just one of those motions individually, which the patient cannot perform as a voluntary action. These accessory motions can be performed on a joint by a therapist during PR-ROM, while stabilizing one side of the joint and moving the other. Slide is the most commonly employed accessory motion in joint mobilization testing, and is also used as a treatment technique.

In joint mobilization the therapist holds one bone still while gliding the other one back and forth several times to check for its ability to slide. The application of movement is roughly 90° to the fixed, unmoving bone's joint surface. The technique is applied when the joint is in an open packed position (when the ligaments and capsule are loose). Further, a slight traction is applied to the joint. This traction is just enough to hold the joint's surface apart, as if one bone is floating just off the surface of the other. This avoids grinding the surfaces together. The amount of slide the therapist wants to feel in a normal joint is about 1/8th of an inch (2–3 mm).

As an assessment technique, the therapist checks first the uninvolved joints (on the unaffected side of the body) and then the involved synovial joints for this small amount of sliding movement. If, when testing a restricted joint, this amount of motion is not palpated, then at least some of the joint's restriction is due to tightness/shortness in the joint capsule and ligaments. If a joint is hypermobile and the slide seems excessive, then the joint capsule and ligaments may have been over-stretched. If the joint play is excessive, yet it is a restricted joint in AF-ROM, that would imply that the surrounding supportive muscles are hypertonic in order to protect the joint. In a similar way, if the joint play appears normal, but restriction to AF-ROM is observed, then any restriction is coming from outside of the joint (extra-articular).

For more detail on this topic, and for the system of grading the amount of movement, see below, "Assessing joint play with joint mobilization."

Active resisted range of motion (AR-ROM) testing

AR-ROM speaks to us about the integrity of contractile tissue. In order to do this, the therapist prevents the patient from moving the joint while the joint is held in its mid-range (i.e., neutral or resting position) as the patient contracts the muscles intended to provide movement for a specific range of motion. However, we do not let any motion take place, hence the test is isometric. By not allowing movement, the joint capsule and other inert tissues receive little or no stress. In fact, because the testing is performed in mid-range, the capsule and ligaments should be lax. Since a concentric contraction often brings the joint surfaces together, the capsule and ligaments become even more lax during isometric testing.

In summary:

- The joint with the muscles we wish to test is placed in its mid-range.
- The therapist instructs the patient that they are to *slowly build up to* their full strength over a period of five seconds. If pain occurs, they are to inform us, and they can stop if they want.
- The patient holds the maximum contraction for about five seconds, and then is told to slowly relax the muscle over five seconds.
- This method of testing should reveal the amount of strength the patient has, as well as the quality of their strength. Is it constant? Is there a jumpiness, or lack of fine motor control?

In many cases, the therapist tends to ask the patient to resist their effort to move their limb. This is the best way to ensure that the increase in resistance is slow, as is the release. Further, this is often helpful for the therapist who is concerned that the patient will overpower them, allowing movement that will ruin the test, or hurting themselves, or even the therapist.

AR-ROM: look for strength or weakness, ask about pain

- Strong and painful – mild strain.
- Weak and painful – severe strain.
- Weak and painless – rupture, or nerve damage (a red flag).
- Strong and painless – normal.

Active resisted tests are first looking to see if the pain or dysfunction is in the contractile tissue. But, remember that muscle weakness (while it may be due to atrophy, fatigue, strain or pain apprehension), may also be due to nerve involvement, vascular insufficiency, or some other impairment or pathology.

By now we have mapped out the ranges of movement that are impaired, and noted and inquired about pain or discomfort, etc. Therefore, at this point we should have some idea about what is going on. We may well be ready to provide our assessment to the patient. On the other hand, if we are suspicious of specific structures for which there are special or differential manual tests, we can proceed to do those. These are referred to as special tests.

Special tests

Special tests are tests that have been designed to assess specific tissues: specific ligaments or tendons; meniscal pads in joints; bursae; nerve roots, etc. They can also be seen as techniques that may help us palpate or observe tissues too deep or unavailable for normal observation or range of motion testing.

Special tests include:

- Differential muscle testing.
- Specific soft tissue tests that are not done during range of motion testing. They are considered special because they usually require movement through several anatomical planes. They are designed to test a specific tissue or structure. Further, they often have special names like Patrick's test, McMurray's meniscus test, tennis elbow test, etc.
- Neurological tests or scans; tests of deep tendon reflexes.
- Any modality's specific tests such as testing the craniosacral rhythms, assessing by pulse diagnosis, or evaluation of energy flows. These specific modality tests should be done at this time.
- Palpation of myofascial trigger points (TrP).

Once all range of motion testing and special tests are completed, we may choose to palpate the lesion site proper. This specific palpation of a site known to be painful is always done last. We should again begin with a light palpation to re-test for any changes to temperature that testing may have caused and for changes in edema. We can then proceed, with the patient's permission, to palpate deeper to note the texture of the subcutaneous tissue, and to palpate the lesion site itself, if this is possible. This is a good time to perform any palpation for TrPs.

Comments on ROM testing

The above represents an outline, or protocol, to follow when conducting an assessment. We do not need to do it all in one visit, though, and often we cannot because of the patient's level of acuity. When a patient presents with an injury or dysfunction, we always need to explore this by taking a case history specific to their complaint and do at least some brief observations, a little inspection palpation if called for prior to treatment, some rule outs, and then map out their range of motion as best as is possible, depending on how acute their injury or impairment is. However, we can always do AF-ROM, because, even if the patient cannot do the movement, that is the available AF-ROM. With practice, all of this can take as little as five minutes or so.

A further point needs to be made. As with all testing, which tissues are sought to be the primary focus of testing while isolating others from being tested can be an ideal hoped for. For example, passive relaxed range of motion testing ideally seeks to isolate and just test non-contractile tissues, specifically joint ligaments, capsules, and articular surfaces. But when applying over-pressure at end-range we can at times place stretch on an impaired muscle and produce pain. This is why it is important to have the patient point to where they feel the pain or other symptoms. Pointing to or describing where they feel the pain can help the therapist (who knows their anatomy well) realize that a tissue other than the one expected was stressed during the testing. This can help reduce the number of false positives.

The same can be true for active resisted range of motion testing. While preventing motion (isometric) in the joint we test the contractile tissues (muscle) and seek to keep stress off of the non-contractile elements around the joint. Nonetheless, while tension may be reduced on ligaments and capsules by the contractile force bringing the joint surfaces together, if the joint surfaces (or a meniscal pad between them) are brought together, compressed, with AR-ROM, and if these are impaired/injured they may well produce an experience of pain or discomfort during the test. But again, having the patient point to exactly where they feel the pain (and say where they feel it) can help with this as well.

Assessment and treatment plan

Again, some of the orthopedic special tests will result in referring a patient out to get a confirming diagnosis for the causes or pathologies our testing suggests. However, we may proceed to work with the impairments found if no contraindications for treatment are apparent.

If we remain within the impairment model, we can then proceed to establish outcomes that seem reasonable to achieve in light of our assessment and its findings. Having presented these outcomes or options to the patient, we can then arrive at a mutually agreed upon plan of treatment.

Impairments and treatment plans

As we find impairments, and if we understand the techniques that treat certain kinds of impairments, then we are finding the treatment plan that is automatically best for the patient. The evaluation of how effective our treatments are is done by specific re-testing that looks at the impairments we are addressing with those techniques (Figures 3.7, 3.8).

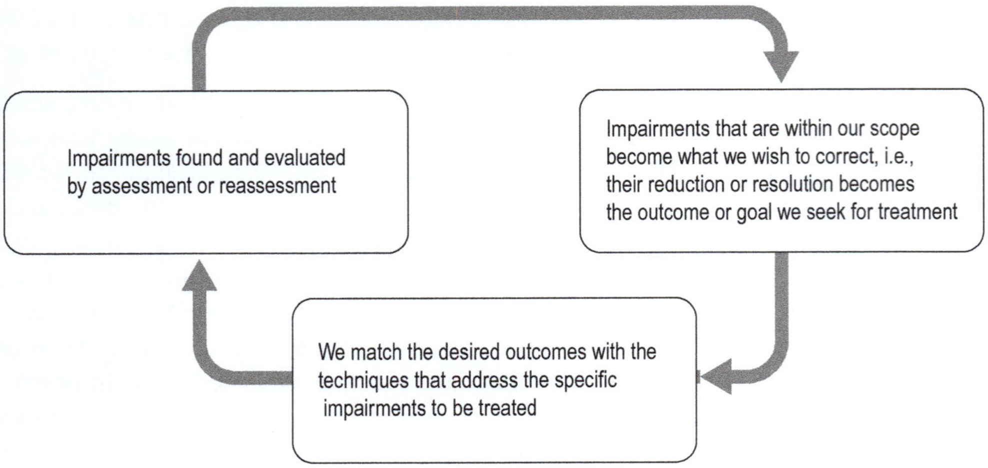

FIGURE 3.7
Impairments and goals.

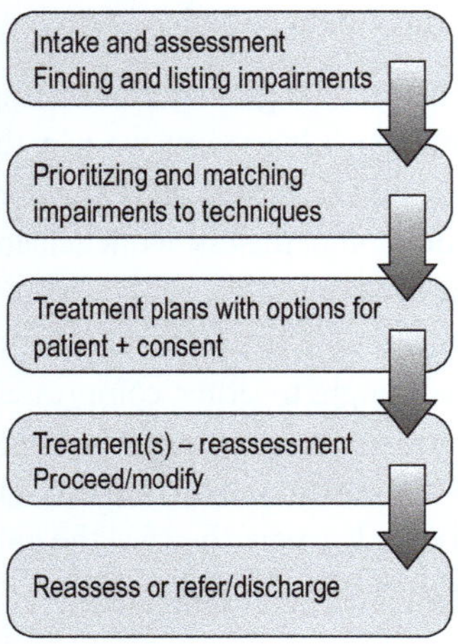

FIGURE 3.8
Finding impairments and devising treatment plans.

Charting and reporting

Writing up notes or charting your patient's appointment and treatment is required by law in most jurisdictions. For every appointment with a patient you need at a very minimum to record the reason for that visit (their goals or chief complaint), your observations and findings/assessment, and the treatment carried out.

These notes are not meant to be long and involved as that would be too time consuming for the therapist, especially in a busy practice. Nonetheless, they need to be sufficiently thorough that an accurate history is available for each treatment. Further, that record has to be understandable by a third party. Almost all health care practitioners use some sort of shorthand or abbreviations when writing up their notes. Even though many of these are shared or would be understood by members of the same profession, often a therapist will fall into the habit of using many abbreviations or symbols that work for them. For this reason, the therapist should have an ongoing list of their shorthand with explanations.

Accurate records are needed when a therapist is asked, for example, by a patient's lawyer or insurer for a letter outlining (summarizing) the patient's history of treatment (i.e., a medical-legal report). Usually the request is for a specific issue, for example when treating a patient for a motor vehicle accident, or for a specific period of time. On the other hand, you could be asked to provide copies of, or all, your original notes regarding each and every appointment: assessment notes, treatment notes, etc. (Hence the need for a list explaining abbreviations and symbols used.)

Consent for release of information

Remember, the patient needs to give their consent before you either speak to another person about their appointments or provide any written material about them. While verbal consent can be acceptable for some things (depending on the legislation governing any specific jurisdiction), it would be wise to always get written consent from the patient prior to providing any records or any information about the patient to a third party. Further, never ask for some sort of general consent that would allow you to communicate with anyone; consent of this kind should always specify exactly who is allowed to receive such information. This could be more than one person (e.g., a lawyer and his staff).

Without specific consent to do so, even mentioning by name a patient that you are treating to anyone else can be a breach of confidentiality. This includes the patient's immediate family or close friends.

Legal issues aside, having a written history that charts a patient's course of treatments over a number of appointments is really the only way to be consistent in carrying out a plan of treatment.

SOAP notes

Recording assessment results and treatment notes requires some use of shorthand or symbols. The most common way of organizing all of this information is referred to as SOAP notes: that is, **S**ubjective, **O**bjective, **A**ssessment and **P**lan of treatment.

Subjective information is what the patient says to you about their reason for being there, what you learn from them during the interview, etc. Even if they tell you the results of medical tests or another health care practitioner, these are subjective. (You need to see copies of medical tests or communication with their other providers to treat these as more objective information.)

Objective information comes from your own testing or findings; it includes positive or negative findings of testing (including palpation done during treatment).

Assessment is recording the impairments found; the overall picture you have put together from their case history form, interview, and testing.

Plan of treatment. This includes both short term and long term goals/outcomes that you and the patient have agreed to pursue during a course of treatments. As treatments occur this part of the notes records the specific treatment that day and reference to how the course of treatment is proceeding (i.e., report any adjustments that may be made to the plan depending on how the patient is responding to treatment, etc.).

Recording your assessment findings

When doing an initial assessment, a therapist should have a separate page or tab from the health history form on which to record their assessment findings. These assessment forms can be relatively simple, or jammed with information. Many students and newly graduated therapists prefer forms that list all the tests, specifically the so-called special tests. This helps them to ensure they have not left out any testing. However, such lists are often only useful for those who do not understand how the tests work, what the tests are actually examining, and what information the tests are really telling us. If this is the case, then such lists are not really useful at all, except to help students find their way through an oral-practical exam. They can look informative, but their functionality is questionable. Therefore, while such a list by region or joint may be useful for students as study notes, practicing therapists should avoid them.

With respect to reporting continuing assessments as a treatment plan proceeds, this is usually done within the treatment portion of a note. Alternatively, one of the many advantages of software programming is that for each appointment there is a set of tabs or boxes for each of the four parts of a SOAP note. Notes are easily comparable from treatment to treatment.

Charting on paper or online?

Templates for SOAP note taking are readily available with a quick search of the Internet. There are numerous examples available online that a therapist can download and print at little or no cost. Many therapists will look at several examples and then take the best ideas from each and put together a template that suits their needs. They print out them out and fill one in for each appointment and place it in the patient's file.

However, more and more massage therapists are turning to medical software designed for manual therapists to do their SOAP note charting. Some programs may already have built into the software program ways of speeding up note taking (such as boxes to tick, or tags that can be placed on anatomical images, etc.); some may just have a space in which you can type your notes, or have some combination of both. Though software-based charting is the inevitable future for massage therapists (as it is for all health care providers) it is not yet clear what this will look like and exactly how it will function. A simple Internet search of the phrase "SOAP charting for massage therapy" will bring up a wide spectrum of possible platforms and software available to the therapist. A therapist needs to take into consideration not just the qualities and benefits of any particular method but also whether it complies with regulatory requirements of their specific governing bodies, legislation and jurisdiction.

Short-hand

Many of the most common abbreviations or symbols used in notes have been around for several decades and were employed to save time when everything was written in longhand and to reduce the amount of paper that needed to be physically stored. However, the use of these shortened forms may not always be convenient – or even possible – when they are being typed into a laptop or tablet. Therefore, what is included here is a list of some short forms or symbols that are meant only as suggestions, and a number of which may be impractical, depending on which medium a therapist employs in their record keeping. They may be useful as a guide for reading old paper charts.

Various governmental bodies or massage therapy associations regulating the practice of massage may have their own specific standards and forms of charting and recording of assessments and treatment notes that they wish followed.

Box 3.2 lists some examples of abbreviations that could be used when writing up your notes. All of these may be used when writing longhand; however, many (i.e., those using symbols) are not practical for typing on a tablet or laptop.

Box 3.2 Suggested abbreviations for SOAP notes

The follow are suggestions only. Many different types of medical practitioners, from different schools and different countries, have developed their own versions, as have individuals. The important issue is that a practitioner's notes have to be readable by others in the medical profession. Some may be self-evident, but it is a good idea to make a "key" – a list of the short-forms/symbols and their meanings – that could be copied and given when your notes are to be read by others. These could be fellow practitioners in a group practice, or when for legal reasons you are required to submit copies of your original clinical notes.

General terms

IVC	informed verbal consent
CHx	case history
CC	chief complaint
Assess	assessment
Tx	treatment
TxPl	treatment plan
Impt	impairment
ROM	range of motion
AF-ROM	active free ROM
PR-ROM	passive relaxed ROM
PF-ROM	passive forced ROM
AR-ROM	active resisted ROM/isometric muscle testing
WNL	within normal limits
ADL	activities of daily living

Palpatory findings/clinical impression

HT	muscle hypertonicity (as classifying dysfunction)
Spsm	spasm
H↓T	muscle hypotonicity
TrP	(myofascial) trigger point
TP	tender point
Atphy	atrophy
↓Jt	hypomobility/decreased joint ROM
X Jt	joint locked
↑Jt	joint hypermobility
X↓	sensation referred from
↓X	referred to
+++	tension: mild + mod ++ severe +++
\\\	texture/fibrosis: min \\ mod \\\ very fibrous \\\\
XXX	painful/tender: mild X mod pain XX severe XXX
↓Temp	decreased temperature or colder
↑Temp	increased temperature or warmer
Inflmm	inflamed/inflammation
Edema	edema

Posture and body planes

↶↺↻↺	torsion/rotation (context dependent)
↗	elevation/superior/higher/more/lengthened
↙	depression/inferior/lower/less/shortened
Prtrct	protraction
Rtrct	retraction
↙mm	shortened muscle
mm↗	lengthened muscle
Cntrc	contractured muscle (mm) or ligament (lig)
→I	medial
←I	lateral
O	anterior
●	posterior/dorsal
prox	proximal
dist	distal

Body areas

Cr	cranium
face	face
jaw	mandible
C/Sp	cervical spine
T/Sp	thoracic spine
L/Sp	lumbar spine

Scrm	sacrum	
Rbcg	ribcage	
Abdm	abdomen	
O/A	occipitoatlantal junction	
A/A	atlantoaxial joint	
C/T-Sp	cervicothoracic junction	
T/L-Sp	thoracolumbar junction	
L5/Scr	lumbosacral junction	
plvc	pelvic	
plvcgrd	pelvic girdle	
shldr	shoulder	
	shdrgrdl	shoulder girdle
	GH	glenohumeral
	AC	acromioclavicular
	SC	sternoclavicular
	Scap	scapula
UpEx	upper extremity	
	arm	humerus
	4/arm	forearm
	hand	hand
	digit (#)	fingers
	MC	metacarpals
	DIP	distal interphalangeal joint
	PIP	proximal interphalangeal joint
LwEx	lower extremity	
	thigh	thigh
	leg	leg
	ft	foot
	MT	metatarsal
	toe (#)	toes
	DIP	distal interphalangeal joint
	PIP	proximal interphalangeal joint

Active movement and treatment positioning

flxn	flexion
extn	extension
SB	side-bent/lateral flexion: L= left; R= right
Rot.	rotation: L= left; R= right; O= anteriorly; ●= posteriorly
abd→	abduction
→add	adduction
sup'n	supination
pron'n	pronation
evrs'n	eversion
invrs'n	inversion
sup	supine
prn	prone
Sdly	side-lying
h	seated
O__^_	crook-lying (supine), with knees bent

Subjective responses

mild	mild
mod	moderate
svr	severe
Px	pain
Px⇒	referring/traveling
!!!	throbbing
cnstnt	constant; freq frequent; sldm seldom or never
intrmt	intermittent
AFX	affects, influences
↑	increase
↓	decrease
Δ	change
Δ̶	no change
↑S/S	aggravates symptoms/signs
↓S/S	decreases symptoms/signs

Conditions

Imprt	Impairment
CC:	chief complaint
CHx	case history
HA	headache
MGRN	migraine
WAD	whiplash associated disorder (I, II, III, IV)
TMJ	temporomandibular joint syndrome
Tndop	tendonitis/tendinopathy
DDD	degenerative disc disease
DJD	degenerative joint disease
TOS	thoracic outlet syndrome
CTS	carpal tunnel syndrome
RA	rheumatoid arthritis
O-A	osteoarthritis: mild; mod (moderate); svr (severe)
OsteoPh	osteophytes

Modalities and miscellaneous

Mx	massage
SwMx	Swedish massage
Rlx	relaxing
Tx	treatment
Strk	stroking
Vibf	fine vibrations; Vibc coarse vibrations
Eff	effleurage
Petr	petrissage
Kn	kneading
M-Strip	muscle stripping
JtMobs	joint mobilizations (Grades: I, II, III, IV)
Oscil	joint oscillations (Grades: I, II, III)
RkShk	rocking and shaking
Rhythmobs	rhythmic mobilizations
Tapt	tapotement: I = light/tapping; II = moderate (open hands); III = open fists; IV = pounding (closed fist)
MFR	myofascial release
ME	muscle energy technique (MET)
NMT	neuromuscular therapy
CrSr	cranial-sacral therapy
PRT	positional release/strain-counterstrain (S-CStr)
MLD	manual lymph drainage
TrP tx	trigger point therapy/treatment
Acpr	acupressure/Shiatsu
ART	Active Release Technique
REM-EX	remedial exercise
Hydro	hydrotherapy
ACUP	acupuncture
HotSt	hot stone massage
MEDs	medications
PRN	when needed (from the Latin *pro re nata*); can apply to medicines, hydrotherapy, stretching/exercises (*remex*) or treatments

Practitioners:

MD	medical doctor
D.O.	osteopathic physician
MT	massage therapist
Chiro	chiropractor
OT	occupational therapist
PT	physiotherapist
RN	nurse
RNP	nurse practitioner
DOMP	Diploma of Osteopathic Manual Practice (or variations thereof), not a physician

Chapter appendix

Assessing joint play with joint mobilization

This last section is a brief and generalized summary concerning the purposes and application of joint mobilization. (For more detail see Edmond 2006; Hertling & Kessler 2006; Kisner & Colby 2012.) What is presented here is in no way intended as instructional; always learn any joint manipulation from a qualified instructor.

Assessing joint play with mobilization is a passive relaxed technique that can not only increase or restore range of motion of a restricted joint, but can also be used for pain reduction and for increasing joint tissue health. The heart of the technique is the application of glide in specific directions and grades of pressure, the intent of which is to increase the slide between two joint surfaces. Remember that slide is what is happening in a moving joint, while glide is what the therapist performs in order to perform an assessment of the quality and quantity of that slide. There are five basic movements within a synovial joint: roll, slide, spin, distraction, and compression.

Roll

This is the action of one joint surface rolling on another. If this were the only movement available in a joint, then it would move like a rolling ball, or a rocking chair on the floor. The ball, for example, has to move across the surface in order to keep rolling. Therefore, happening on its own, rolling would require a great deal of laxity to both the joint capsule and the ligaments, as the moving bone would be required to move across the adjoining joint surface. Note that the direction of movement of the bone is in the same direction as is the rolling of its surface.

Slide

This is the action of one joint surface sliding on another. When a joint has slide available, if a moving bone is rolling the action of rolling can only happen while the moving bone slides in the opposite direction. For example, think of abduction of the glenohumeral joint with the head of the humerus rolling on the glenoid surface superiorly while the humeral head slides inferiorly. You can see, then, that slide permits a bone to move "in place."

Spin

This is one joint surface rotating on another which, again, requires glide so that the moving bone "stays in place" and does not travel (skate) across the non-moving bone's surface. In the example of the shoulder, while the humerus moves through 90° of abduction, it rotates (spins) externally.

Distraction

This is movement of the joint surfaces away from each other, as occurs, for example, when there is no load on the arm and the shoulder is swinging freely as a person walks.

Compression

This is when two articular joint surfaces are pushed together: think of a person doing a push-up. Another example of compression is when the capsule of the shoulder is twisted, pulling the two joint surfaces together. This is also common when there is musculature contraction across the joint, or when the muscles of a joint spasm.

Glide and slide

A physiological motion in a joint is some combination of the five motions on the previous page and an action that the patient does voluntarily. An accessory motion, on the other hand, is the occurrence of just one of roll, glide, spin, traction, or compression. A patient cannot perform any one of these motions on its own as a voluntary action. These accessory motions can only be performed passively on a patient while stabilizing one side of the joint and moving the other. Glide is the most commonly used motion in joint mobilization techniques, though the others can be used in specific situations. For purposes of being brief, we will outline the methods and grades of mobilization with respect to glide.

Joint mobilization technique has the therapist hold one bone fixed (unmoving) while the other bone is glided back and forth several times. The application of movement is roughly 90° to the fixed, unmoving bone's joint surface. The technique is applied when the joint is in an open packed position (when the ligaments and capsule are at their loosest). A slight traction is applied to the joint; however, not so much that the joint capsule is pulled tight, but just enough to hold the surfaces apart. Glide should not occur with the surfaces pressing or resting on each other. It should only occur when the two surfaces are incrementally apart, as if the moving bone is floating just off the surface of the other. This avoids grinding the surfaces together. If too much traction is applied, all of the slack in the joint capsule is taken up and there is no longer enough slack to permit mobilization by glide.

While gliding the joint, the amount of slide that should be felt in a normal joint is about 1/8th of an inch. This availability of motion is known as "play," more specifically, joint play. Therefore, you may encounter the terminology "joint play assessment," which is an alternate name for joint mobilization testing, the term used in this and other textbooks.

Whether being used to assess or treat, the key to successful joint mobilization is that the patient must be relaxed. The patient must not hinder the process by holding and guarding the joint. To understand whether assessment or treatment by joint mobilization is appropriate for your patient, see the list of contraindications at the end of this section.

When using joint mobilization as an assessment technique, the therapist checks the involved synovial joints for the amount of movement (play) available.

- If the appropriate amount of play is not felt when testing a restricted joint, some of restriction can be attributed to tightness/shortness in the capsule and ligaments (intra-articular impairment).
- On the other hand, if a joint is hypermobile and the slide seems excessive, then the joint capsule and ligaments may have been over-stretched, leaving the joint unstable. Therefore, if the joint play is excessive, yet restriction to the joint is observed in AF-ROM, that would imply that the surrounding supportive muscles are hypertonic in order to "splint" (protect) the joint.
- In a similar manner, if the joint play appears normal, but restriction to AF-ROM is observed, then any restriction is coming from outside the joint, i.e., extra-articular.

Next, we will take a look at the grades of glide employed in assessing joint play. Note that the glides appropriate for assessment are those listed as grades I, II, and III. All of these descriptions are expressed in terms of joint mobilization as a treatment modality. To assess the joint play available in a joint, you would begin with grade I, in order to prepare the joint for testing. Then, you would increase the amplitude to grade II – and only then, if appropriate, move on to grade III. The higher grades are strictly for treatment purposes, not for assessment!

Grades of joint mobilization

Listed here are the five grades of joint mobilization, employed in standard practice worldwide, as devised by the Australian physiotherapist Geoffrey Maitland. Remember that you always start with grade I and move your way through the grades without skipping any of them. Once you have reached the highest grade available, you must re-do the grades in reverse order from that point.

Grade I Gentle oscillations at the start of joint motion; i.e., at the neutral point in mid-range/resting position. The oscillatory (back and forth) motion is more like vibration, as you are gliding the moving bone only 1/32nd of an inch, or so (25 percent of the total 1/8th inch of slide available, on average).

- This grade is very useful during acute stages of joint injury. It can be used in almost any situation. (See contraindications at the end of this section.)
- Both grade I and grade II oscillations are referred to as low-amplitude and low velocity.

Grade II Gentle oscillations from neutral that move no more than 50 percent of the normal total slide available with any given synovial joint.

- Both grade I and grade II are used to reduce the patient's experience of pain. The primary mechanism for this is the activation of the mechanoreceptors, the joint's proprioceptors. (See Pain gate theory, p. 48.)
- Further, the activation of these proprioceptors relax the muscles that cross that joint: (1) by the reduction of the sensation of pain; and (2) the rhythmic "on/off" (contract/relax) signals generated by activation and deactivation of stretch reflexes in the muscles. This may be produced by the inhibition of the antagonist, due to the activation of the agonist, and then a quick reversal of roles, over and over again, during the oscillations.
- Both grade I and grade II increase joint tissue health via increased synovial fluid movement between the synovium and the articular surfaces.

Grade III These oscillations occur near the limit of a joint capsule's mobility during glide. The degree of motion is considered moderate amplitude and low velocity. The purpose of grade III is to encourage restricted joint capsules and ligaments to loosen.

- Stretch is a term often used in textbooks when describing the purpose of grade III mobilization. However, for many students this may imply a greater degree of amplitude and force than is actually meant. Terms such as "encourage," "coax," or "convince" tissues to lengthen (give way) may be more helpful for students in understanding the quality and quantity of the force needed for this grade.
- As with grades I and II, the encouragement to release restriction relies on the oscillations to be free of any discomfort. This will assist in reducing pain and relaxing the musculature of the joint. If done with too much force (trying to push through the motion barrier), the therapist will activate the muscles' stretch receptors and actually reduce the motion available due to increased muscle tension.

- The end result of grade III oscillations is intended to be an increase in range of motion of the joint by a lengthening or loosening of the capsule and other connective tissue structures. This would lead you to believe that the capsule had been stretched (as if the barrier had been pushed through) when, in fact, the motion had stopped just before engaging the barrier.
- This grade should never be used in acute stages of injury/inflammation. However, it is excellent for chronic stages.

Grade IV These small amplitude and low velocity oscillations are done up to the limit of movement of the joint capsule and its supportive connective tissue. These rhythmic oscillations are pushing, very slightly, through the barrier of restriction. This grade is to be used:

- only if no inflammation is present
- only if the oscillations are not painful (mild pain is okay) for the patient
- only when preceded by grade III oscillations to ensure the joint is ready for stretching
- only when grade III causes no discomfort and when muscles are deemed to be of appropriate tone, relaxed and healthy.

Grade IV must not be used to stretch the capsule beyond its normal physiological limit, otherwise injury may result. The therapist must be experienced with using grades I to III in order to have a good feel for generating various amplitudes, and must also have developed a keen sense of the physiological limit of capsules of various synovial joints.

Remember, once again, that to help prevent post-treatment inflammation, achiness or reflex muscle spasming, you must follow grade IV with grades III, II and I in this reverse order. You should ice the joint after treatment, since there is always a possibility it was injured or inflamed by treatment.

Grade V This grade of mobilization is not within a massage therapist's scope of practice. It is a small amplitude, high velocity thrust at the end of range. It is not performed as an oscillation. It is meant to break adhesions in the connective tissues of a joint. This type of mobilization is used by chiropractors, osteopaths, or specially trained physiotherapists and physicians.

Grades of traction

There are three grades/degrees of traction, as devised by Professor M. Kaltenborn:

1. Used for the reduction of pressure from the joint's surfaces, without actually separating them. This causes a reduction in pain.
2. Takes up the slack of the fibrous capsule. In other words, this pulls the joint surfaces apart (distraction/decompression) until the end-range of the joint is felt in the fibrous capsule.
3. Involves stretching of the capsule and the soft tissue around the joint, in order to restore full motion to a restricted joint.

Traction (distraction/decompression)

Tractioning of the joint capsule, ligaments, and musculature should be done with the joint open packed (roughly mid-range or in a position of rest/comfort). The distraction is perpendicular to the treatment plane, which is at the center of the concave joint surface, when present. You need to be knowledgeable about the specific joint's articular surface orientation in order to apply traction in the appropriate direction. An example is the shoulder joint, where the articular surface of the glenoid fossa faces roughly 30° inferiorly, laterally (abduction), and anteriorly (flexion), a position referred to as "scaption." Therefore, for the arm (humerus) to be at 90° to the glenoid fossa, it must be abducted and flexed at approximately 30°.

- Use body-weight instead of muscular strength to do the tractioning.
- Apply traction only in chronic situations, for improving tissue health, etc.
- Traction can be sustained, or applied momentarily, releasing and re-engaging over several cycles.
- Sustained tractioning can provide a gentle stretch to joint structures.
- Cycled tractioning will create a pump-like action in and around the tissues involved in a joint.
- Traction can relax muscle tissue, and help remove connective tissue trigger points.

Compression

- The starting position for compression is also in the open pack position, with the moving joint at 90° to the stabilized joint surface.
- A sustained compression (from 1 to 90 seconds) can be applied if pain-free. This can assist in postural release techniques to further shorten tissues, or to facilitate a quicker relaxation response.
- Short oscillations (from 1 to 10 seconds of compression and release), when pain free, can assist in improving or maintaining the health of joint articular cartilage. This is achieved by gently pushing some synovial fluid out of the cartilage on compression and then, on release of compression, the articular cartilage will re-absorb synovial fluid: this creates a pump-like movement in and out of the cartilage, flushing out older fluid and replacing it with nutrient rich synovial fluid.

Rules for application of joint mobilization

- The patient must always be relaxed.
- Explain the procedure and receive consent.
- Assess before and after use, when using modality for treatment.
- Stop mobilization/assessment if it is painful.
- Always finish with grade I and II.
- Contact with both sides of the joint should be as close to the joint as is possible.
- Ensure the grip on the tissues is as comfortable as possible for the patient.
- When using glide, motions are parallel to joint surfaces.
- When distracting or compressing a joint the motion is perpendicular to the joint plane.

Indications for using joint mobilizations

- To reduce pain (via mechanoreceptors).
- To reduce muscle hypertonicity or spasming.
- To restore mobility to restricted joints.
- Can improve proprioception through stimulation of receptors that transmit position and motion.
- Assist in improving health of intra-joint tissues (through stretching) and nutrient exchange in articular cartilage.
- Restores or preserves extensibility and tensile strength in articular tissues.
- Post assessment, and especially treatment, responses can include ache or pain. Advise use of ice, along with AF-ROM, to reduce any pain or stiffness.

Rhythm and duration of oscillations: treatment

- Three to six sets when treating. One or two sets when assessing. Pause for several seconds in between sets. The higher the grade, the longer should be the pause.
- Oscillations should be smooth and rhythmic.
- For grades I and II oscillations are two to three per second, though grade I can be higher. Grade III, as a higher amplitude, can be reduced to one to two oscillations per second to help sustain control and so not move through the restriction barrier. Grade IV and distraction can be sustained for six to eight seconds for the purposes of stretching. Compressions can be held for three to six seconds to maximize the amount and depth of fluid exchange in articular surface.
- Each set for grades I and II is generally one to two minutes in order to achieve pain reduction and a relaxation/inhibitory response.
- Each set for grades III and IV is generally 20 seconds, up to a minute.

Contraindications

Universally contraindicated

- Any undiagnosed/unassessed lesion.
- Active inflammatory or infective arthritis.
- Malignancy/tumors.
- For mobilization of vertebrae when there are herniated discs with nerve compression, and prolapsed or sequestered stages of degenerative disc disease (DDD).
- Metabolic bone diseases.
- Joint ankylosis.
- Bone fracture.
- Internal derangement.
- Cauda equina lesions.
- Cervical spine with patient who has vertebrobasilar insufficiency.

Contraindicated for grade III and higher

- Patient's inability to relax.
- Inflammatory arthritis (currently not in a flare-up).
- Osteoporosis (during grade I/slight and early grade II/moderate osteoporosis).
- Congenital, or induced bone deformities.
- Vascular disorders on-site.
- Ligamentous rupture or laxity.
- Joint effusion.
- Total joint replacement.

NOTE: Use of grade I (or even II) may be permitted in order to reduce pain and assist with tissue healing and health.

Used with caution

- During pregnancy.
- During illnesses, such as the flu (that may have tissues dehydrated and/or with muscle hypertonicity and/or pain).
- When there is bony/fused rotoscoliosis.
- With patients who are "fragile," or in poor general health.

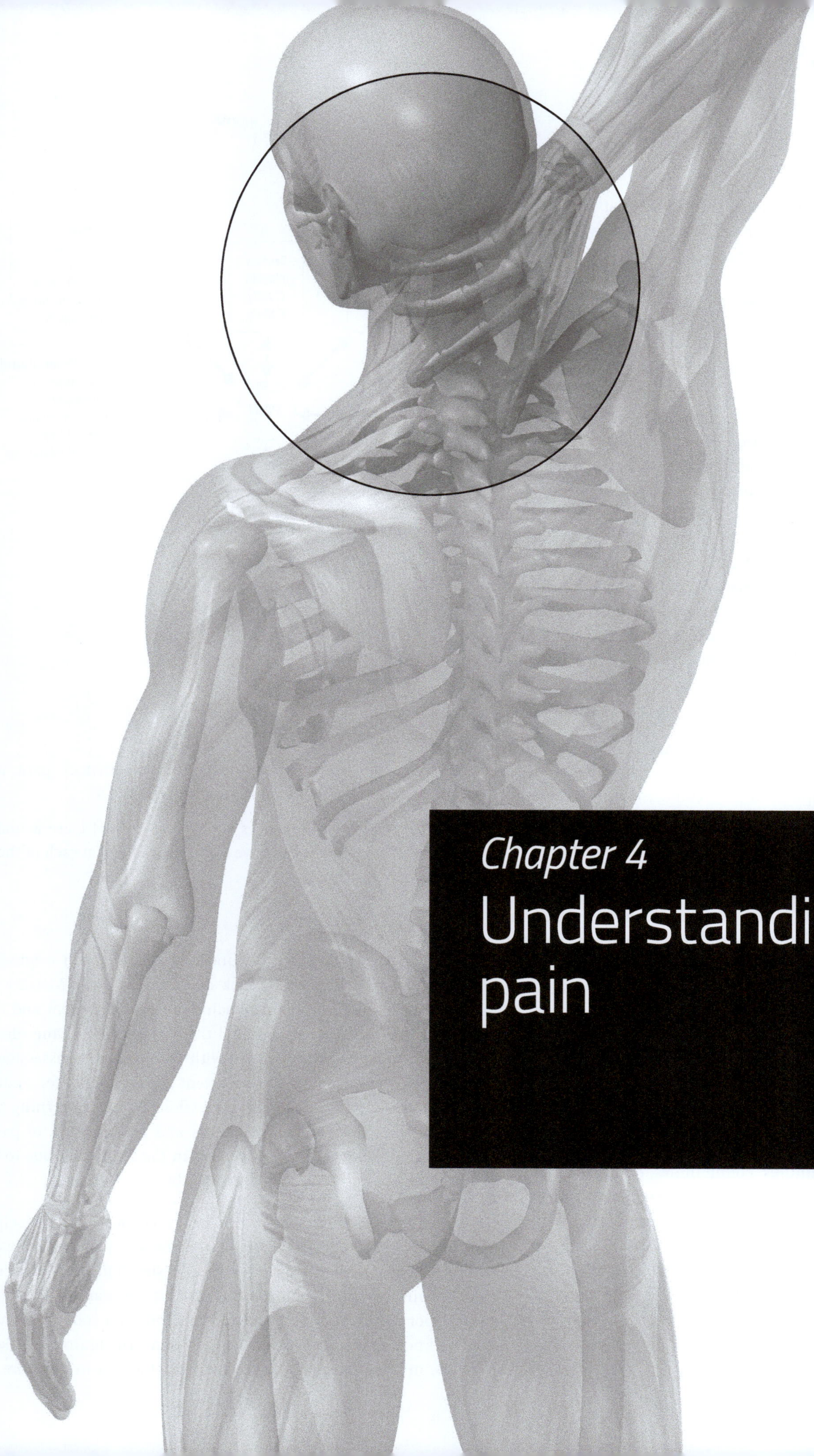

Chapter 4

Understanding pain

Patients come to therapists with the hope that we can reduce or eliminate their pain. Pain is not a straightforward response to injury, but a complex process mediated by individual experience, social values, and context. It is also necessary, since it is the body's alarm system for alerting us to when something may be wrong. As Ronald Melzack put it:

> Pain is a personal, subjective experience influenced by cultural learning, the meaning of the situation, attention, and other psychological variables. Pain processes do not begin with the stimulation of receptors. Rather, injury or disease produces neural signals that enter an active nervous system that (in the adult organism) is the substrate of past experience, culture, and a host of other environmental and personal factors. These brain processes actively participate in the selection, abstraction, and synthesis of information from the total sensory input. Pain is not simply the end product of a linear sensory transmission system; it is a dynamic process that involves continuous interactions among complex ascending and descending systems. (Melzack & Katz 2013)

Above all, as noted, pain is a subjective experience. More than just an awareness, pain is a perception, an interpretation concerning its origins, quality, intensity, and meaning. Therefore, although the perception of pain can arise with tissue injury, it does not have to. For example, think of a time when you might have cut yourself but did not notice until later, or when you noticed you had a bruise but could not remember having bumped into something. Or consider phantom pain, where a person will continue to feel pain in an amputated limb. A person can sometimes experience pain when something traumatic happens to someone else. From these examples and others we know that pain is a complex issue, involving the whole person: physically, mentally, socially, and spiritually. This is often referred to as the biopsychosocial pain model. (See the website of the International Association for the Study of Pain (IASP) for a good discussion of these issues, www.iasp-pain.org/.)

The experience of pain is ultimately unique to every person. However, certain cultures, communities, or social groups may share an understanding of pain and, therefore, within these groups an individual can have an experience of pain that others in that group can sympathize with or relate to. Cross-cultural understanding is sometimes more difficult. The meaning of pain is community mediated. For body builders and marathon runners muscle pain has a different meaning than it has for people with multiple sclerosis. Context and community can change the meaning and language of pain.

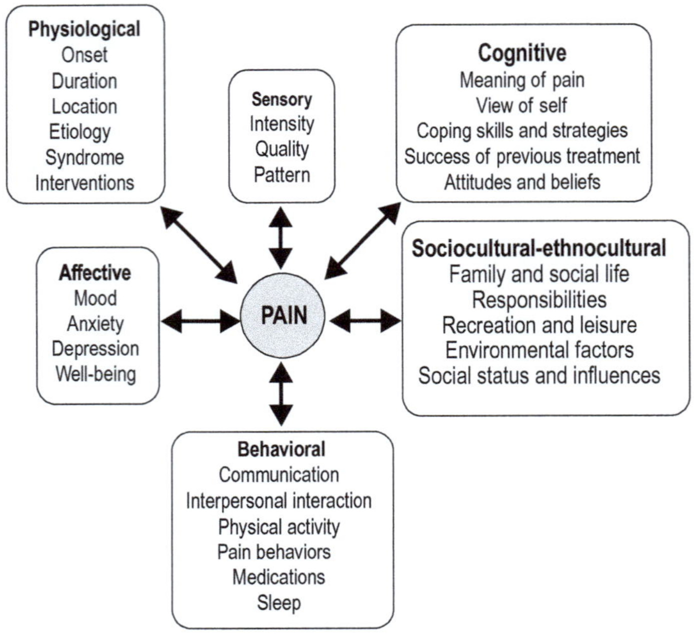

FIGURE 4.1

Influences on the experience of pain.

The influences on how a person experiences pain are numerous. Figure 4.1 explores some of these.

NOTE: All of the influences shown in Figure 4.1 are actually two-way paths. Pain can have a disabling effect on each of these spheres of influences.

The pain gate theory

The pain gate theory is an understanding of pain originally developed by Ronald Melzack and Patrick Wall (Melzack & Wall 1965). As a *model* it remains the most prevalent and the most useful theory for manual therapists to use in the therapeutic situation when dealing with pain, for either assessment or treatment. It remains a persistent general theory for understanding the nature of pain, even while details concerning the instigation of pain, the mediators and transmission of pain, and the roles of the higher centers in the brain continue to be researched and are updated frequently.

Put very simply, the pain gate theory operates on the principle that the brain has to prioritize information. It would be overwhelmed if it had to process everything simultaneously. In terms of pain, if you are sitting too close to a fire, for example, it is more important for you to get that information from your brain than to know that your neck muscles are sore. The brain prioritizes the information that you receive, allowing you to be aware of the most relevant information. In more neurological terms, pain gate theory starts with the idea that pain fibers in general are unmyelinated, or slow-transmitting fibers, while many other sensory fibers (such as skin receptors for pressure, cold, or heat) are myelinated, or fast-transmission fibers. It is thought that the central nervous system (CNS) can only process so much information at a time. Therefore, for self-protection, the body will prioritize the information that is allowed into the brain when there is a multitude of sensations coming in. Under normal circumstances, signals from the fast fibers are always sent unhindered to the brain, while signals from the slower fibers will usually be conveyed as a lower priority. The system is very similar to priority shipping; the most important messages are sent faster.

However, when there is a barrage of information coming into the CNS from one or more nerve roots, flooding a particular spinal level, the slow nociceptor's (pain) signals will often be inhibited or blocked from continuing up into the higher centers. A gate into the pathway to the brain has been closed for these slow fibers. Signals from the fast fibers continue to be conveyed so that the body can respond to external emergencies.

The experience of pain cannot always be inhibited or blocked, especially when the injury or lesion is intense, or when it represents a danger that is threatening the individual. Nonetheless, in the clinical setting (or any safe setting for that matter), actions like increasing skin sensation (such as hot, cold, and touch), along with stimulating the fast fibers of joint receptors (such as in passive movements, or joint mobilization), can be used to inhibit the sensory transmission of pain. Colloquially we refer to this as providing a *distraction*. How well these inhibit or distract us from the experience of pain can provide important information about the nature of the lesion. For example, often, with chronic low-grade pain, the person can be distracted from experiencing the pain. However, acute pain may override any attempt to inhibit it.

Further, how the individual experiences the pain can alter how well it can be blocked. A sharp biting pain may be harder to ignore than a deep ache. The sharp pain is often from a recent severe injury, while the ache could be from something healing but still in need of attention. Therefore, how the person describes the quality of their pain can give us clues as to its chronicity or its stage of healing. The intensity or quantity of the pain can help to assess the degree of injury (severe, moderate, or mild). Yet always remember that how the person is dealing with their pain is modified by the influences of culture, family, mental state, and the meaning they ascribe to pain.

The more recent models of pain also add the idea that signals from the brain (for example, from the limbic system, the prefrontal cortex, and the cerebellum, the higher centers of the nervous system) can contribute to modulating the experience of pain; they can inhibit the feeling of pain or intensify the experience of pain (Melzack & Katz 2013). Therefore, the perception of pain can be highly dependent on the context, on a person's history, experiences, social roles, physical and emotional health.

The therapist needs to be aware of all of this when conducting an inquiry into a patient's current experience of pain. Most importantly, the therapist needs to be able to translate how the patient speaks about pain in order to gain valuable clues or suspicions about possible physical causes of the pain (the degree of the injury or lesion, its location, etc.) and which factors may be modulating the experience of pain. All of this information will guide how the therapist will assess and treat that specific patient's concerns.

Terminology and definitions

Let us look at some of the most common medical terms used to describe pain, pain sensitivity, and decreased pain sensitivity, and their meanings.

Pain is an unpleasant sensory and emotional experience associated with actual or potential tissue damage, or described in terms of such damage.

Pain types

Acute pain Sharp, bright, site-specific pain considered to be limited to 24 hours to several days following injury. When orthopedic in nature, the problem is often observable by eye, or by imaging. X-rays, ultrasound, CT and MRI scans can all be useful for showing the internal details of acute orthopedic issues. Acute pain is more amenable to revealing its source since, generally, we need only look for the inflamed and lesioned tissue. Usually this pain is chemically based due to released or produced metabolites specifically created by the inflammatory process.

Subacute pain This type can still be sharp and bright, but usually only when the tissues are challenged. Otherwise, the experience of pain can undergo many changes from intense to dull and achy, and anything in between. This is the stage when tissues are setting the stage for healing, and carrying out most of the healing work. Tissues remain fragile, and re-injury is the greatest threat at this point. Signs of inflammation diminish throughout this stage. The length of time for the subacute stage depends on the type and amount of tissue damage.

Chronic pain Chronic pain is defined as pain lasting more than three (or six) months beyond the expected healing time, and it may continue indefinitely. Chronic pain is harder to observe with the human eye. Studies have shown that imaging technology is often not any better than manual testing at discovering its source, and that it may, in fact, be more misleading (Deyo 1998). Inflammation can be minor, or absent. Therefore, chronic pain requires a bit of detective work to discover: clues may be uncovered slowly, sometimes over the course of several visits. Chronic pain may also present as referred pain; in other words, where the pain is felt may not be where the problem is. This referred pain is often experienced as a deep achiness, with vague and undetermined borders.

Chronic pain is often thought to come from previously injured tissue (such as in sudden trauma) being unable to complete the healing process. On the other hand, it may also arise from repetitive strain or cumulative trauma that culminates in an expression of pain and impaired function. In this latter situation, it is surmised, tissues never get a chance to fully heal during rest. It can be thought of as *a debt*, where the everyday stresses and strains on tissue are not completely repaired during the day's rest cycle (sleep and rest). Yet the patient may not yet be experiencing pain. If the tissue keeps experiencing this type of stress and strain day after day, then slowly but surely a debt gets built up until it goes too far. The tissue finally generates a significant inflammatory response (e.g., tendonitis) in which the amount or concentration of chemical mediators produced are sufficient to generate, for example, pain, edema, and activation of a local immune response (mast cells and the like). Other expressions of this cumulative trauma have been thought to create trigger point (TrP) development in muscles and connective tissue. Another is seen in tendonosis, where healing is so delayed that the connective tissue elements become disorganized (through continual breakdown) and seem to forget how to re-organize themselves into healthy tissue.

An important quality of nociceptive (pain) receptors is that they do not accommodate – that is, they do not become accustomed to, and stop sending, the sensory information. A common example of sensory nerves that do accommodate are many skin receptors (for example, when we put on clothing we become accustomed to the feel of the cloth touching our skin and are no longer aware of it after a short time). One way pain fibers avoid accommodating is by emitting special neurotransmitters and other similar substances that keep the receptor site sensitive. The most well-known of these is substance P.

In long term chronic pain cases, the sensory endings of the nociceptive nerve will begin to multiply (Mense & Simons 2001). We do not get more nerves growing, but we can get more nerve endings to grow. In this way, the patient can literally become more pain sensitive over time, to the point where even light touch can be felt as painful. This ability of the nerve endings to multiply is a curse for chronic pain sufferers. They have grown more pain receptors that can emit more self-irritating chemicals. This may be one way that chronic pain may perpetuate itself, even if the original cause disappears.

Acute-on-chronic Acute-on-chronic pain refers to illnesses or injuries where episodes of pain alternate with episodes of relative wellness. There are two categories of acute-on-chronic pain of interest to manual therapists. One is a pathological or disease-based pain, and the other is injury-based pain. The diseased-based pain is associated with relapsing/remitting illnesses that have a cyclical disease course of alternating periods of relative wellness and inflammation or pain. The other cause of acute-on-chronic pain is injury-based pain with a cycle of healing that can be interrupted by re-injury or re-inflammation.

The most obvious example of pathological acute on chronic pain would be rheumatoid arthritis, where the pathology is always present, but runs in cycles (dull, achy pain most of the time, but prone to acute flare-ups). A more common example for massage therapists of injury-based acute-on-chronic pain would be when a patient is suffering a bout of tendonitis that fades for a while, but then returns with intensity.

Terms implying increased sensitivity

The following terms are concerned with changes in pain interpretation that occur in the central nervous system (CNS).

Hyperalgesia An increased pain response to a stimulus that is normally painful (i.e., a reduced threshold with an increased or exaggerated response).

Allodynia Pain caused by a stimulus that does not normally provoke pain (reduced pain threshold: and the stimulus and response are of different sensory modalities). For example, normal tactile stimuli evoking pain, such as a light stroking manipulation of the skin, is felt by the patient as severe burning pain. The sensation disappears if the stimulus is removed.

Hyperpathia An exaggerated pain response to normal stimuli in damaged neural tissue, which remains even after the stimulus is removed.

Causalgia A syndrome that occurs after a traumatic nerve lesion, where any sensation in the area is felt as burning nerve pain. This is often combined with vasomotor and pseudomotor dysfunction and later trophic changes in the tissue affected. This is often thought of as a dysfunction involving the autonomic nervous system (ANS).

Dysesthesia An unpleasant abnormal sensation from an otherwise innocuous/normal stimulus. This is not normally perceived as pain as such. It could be, for example, the sensation of a breeze on the skin producing a sensation of ants crawling under the skin or a prickly sensation. This interpretation of normal sensations that would usually be accommodated to (that we can forget about) may not necessarily be accommodated to in this situation, but persists and becomes annoying.

Hyperesthesia A painful syndrome characterized by an abnormally painful reaction, especially to repetitive stimuli.

Terms implying decreased sensitivity

The following terms are concerned with changes in interpreting pain that are occurring in the CNS.

Analgesia Absence of pain in response to stimulation that would normally be painful.

Hypoalgesia Diminished pain in response to a normally painful stimulus (increased threshold and decreased response).

Terms designating other types of pain

The following terms apply to pain that is neither exaggerated nor suppressed.

Anesthesia Usually used to refer to an induced state in which the person is unaware of pain; often from a pharmacological source.

Paresthesia A response to a normally painful stimulus that generates an alternative sensation, for example, light touch creating the sensation of water running over the skin. Threshold and response can be the same, but the response is a different kind of sensation than normally expected.

Central pain Pain initiated or caused by a primary lesion or dysfunction in the CNS. For example, a lesion in the spinal cord.

Referred pain Pain perceived at a site different from its point of origin (but usually innervated by the same spinal segment or nerve root). It is difficult for the brain to correctly identify the original source of pain. It can be alone or concurrent with pain located at the origin of the noxious stimuli. It can also mask the true origin of the nociceptive stimuli. It can be applied to pain that arises from somatic structures (joints, bone, ligament, etc.) as well as viscera. In muscles it can often occur with a deep muscle. As a rule of thumb, the more superficial the lesion the more likely the site of pain and the lesion will be the same. We almost always know where a paper cut is on the skin; it is where we feel the pain. On the other hand, the deeper the tissue or structure the more likely we are to have some variance between where we feel the pain and where the lesion or impairment is. A well-known example of referred pain is heart muscle pain during a heart attack being felt in the jaw or shoulder.

Radicular pain Pain originating from a nerve root lesion. It is not uncommon for such pain to often be felt at the end of a dermatomal area (the most distal point that the sensory nerves associated with that nerve root extends to).

Radiating pain Pain that intermittently travels away from a site of injury or impairment ("starts at my shoulder and shoots down my arm and into my hand"). It may travel in a specific direction or it may spread out from a central point. It can be from a radicular or a referred pain source.

Neuritis Pain sourced in a peripheral nerve, and felt in the peripheral nerve's area of innervation.

Sclerotomic pain A sclerotome is an area of bone or connective tissue innervated by a single nerve root. Pain in any tissue shared by the same nerve root can either refer pain into the bone, or (the more common use) refer bone pain into more superficial tissues.

Dermatomal pain Dermatomes are the areas of skin innervated by a specific nerve root. Deeper structures sharing the same nerve root may express their pain through their corresponding dermatome. Radicular pain felt superficially will only be perceived as being within the area of skin it specifically innervates, its dermatome.

Terminology for pain from other sources

Myofascial pain Any pain sourced in the musculoskeletal system can be called myofascial: any pain from muscle and its component parts.

Muscle spasm or guarding The sudden involuntary full contraction of a muscle. The causes of spasm and guarding vary from a metabolic imbalance (for example, low electrolytes, which can occur after excessive fluid loss from perspiration, or overuse that depletes the muscles' nutrient stores), to a protective spasm (sometimes call *muscle guarding* or *splinting*) that is a reflexive quick shortening of muscles around an area of trauma that is intended to stabilize the structures involved by preventing further movement (that may worsen the injury, etc.). This may be viewed as a protective reflex rigidity. When persistent, such guarding may cause blood vessel compression and give rise to pain now sourced in the muscles involved due to ischemia causing local and referred pain. A spasm maybe so strong that the muscle will injure itself by causing micro-tearing within the cell's contractile mechanism. Colloquially, a painful spasm is called a cramp.

Trigger points A trigger point is a small, local point of irritation in a muscle that is thought to be responsible for (set off) a significant response, either locally or at a distance.

A short review of trigger point theory

After several decades of acceptance by physicians and manual therapists, the evidence for trigger point theory has recently been re-evaluated and found lacking (see Quintner et al. 2015; see also Paul Ingram's *Trigger Point Doubts* at https://www.painscience.com/articles/trigger-point-doubts.php).

The validity of the science around the trigger point theory is a debate that will go on for years. Nonetheless, as long as the outcome of trigger point therapy is pain relief, trigger point therapy as a useful clinical model of myofascial pain and as an approach to treating such pain remains a valuable clinical tool. Therefore, we will review the standard understanding of what trigger points are, and how they are, and how they are assessed.

According to Travell and Simons, a trigger point (TrP) is a focus of hyperirritability in a muscle or its fascia that is thought to be involved in many cases of myofascial pain. There are three types of trigger points (Travell et al. 1999):

- *Active TrP*: symptomatic with respect to pain; it refers a pattern of pain at rest and/or on motion that is specific for the muscle.
- *Latent TrP*: non-symptomatic with respect to spontaneous pain; it is only painful when palpated.
- *Satellite or secondary TrP*: develops in response to overload, shortened range, or referred phenomena caused by trigger point activity in another muscle.

In clinical practice trigger points are best known for their referral of pain. This referral is what distinguishes them from tender points (T-P), where the pain or tenderness is usually at the site of the lesion, due to damage of tissue. The trigger point is not seen as necessarily injured tissue. This distinction needs to be clearly understood by the therapist. Treating trigger points and tender points in the same manner can cause the treatment to be at best ineffective (as when treating a trigger point as if it was a tender point), or injurious (as can happen in aggressively treating a tender point as if it was a trigger point). This is why it is essential to assess trigger points and tender points accurately.

Treating a trigger point as a T-P will either create no change, or it will turn an active trigger point into a latent trigger point. In other words, with respect to the latter, it may well inhibit a trigger point's symptoms from being felt, but it will most likely re-activate at some point.

As a T-P implies, there is injury and usually some level of inflammation present; therefore, treating it like a trigger point, especially via compression and/or stretch, can further injure the lesioned tissue. In turn, this may install a trigger point in the tissue that will remain present once the injury heals.

Criteria needed to assess the presence of a TrP

- A palpable taut band within the muscle (if the muscle is accessible).
- Finding a specific, discrete nodule within the taut band that the patient reports as painful to the touch.
- Palpation of this nodule with pressure recreates the patient's chief complaint. This occurs with an active TrP. Continued pressure on a pain-free latent point may irritate it and turn into an active TrP.
- A painful limit to full stretch during range of motion testing: during AF-ROM, PR-ROM, and often during AR-ROM when full generation of strength is attempted. (Some weakness in the muscle with a TrP is common. This response occurs with both active and latent TrPs.) Note: These actions (i.e., the assessment itself) may make a latent TrP active.

Confirming criteria

- Presence of a local twitch response within the taut band of muscle fibers. This can sometimes be observed by eye, and always with palpation.
- Pain or altered sensation (paresthesia) within the area of the body that is considered the referral area for that TrP. This is generated by compression of the nodule within the taut band.
- Some restriction to ranges of motion (ROM), especially during ROM-testing, are observable.

Listening to the tissue: how pain speaks to us and what it might be saying

Region-specific information will be found in other chapters. For example, in the lumbar spine chapter you will find more on how pain comes from intervertebral discs (discogenic pain). What follows are a few generalizations that will help the student begin to develop an appreciation of what can be learned from the patient's description of pain through case history taking. (There is also a chapter on case history taking, where the meanings of common words or phrases that patients use are discussed fully.) The following information is a brief overview of the terminology used by health care practitioners when talking about pain. Students should look to their pathology textbooks for more in-depth information on the neurology of pain.

Somatic pain

Somatic pain is a very general term that means pain coming from any tissue in the body (*soma*). Pain can result from pathology of muscle, joint, ligament, bone, nerve, or viscera. Pain that is experienced as sharp and well-localized usually arises from superficial structures such as skin. Pain of deep somatic origin, from organs (viscera), bone, or deep muscles, for example, has a deep aching quality and it is often hard to locate or pinpoint exactly where it is coming from. In addition, deep somatic pain is often associated with autonomic phenomena such as increased sweating, pallor, or reduced blood pressure, and is commonly accompanied by a subjective feeling of nausea and faintness.

Some characteristics or common descriptors are given later.

Muscle pain's clinical features

Muscle pain is experienced in a variety of ways. Muscle pain is often described as achy. Patients may also report feeling stiff or tight. Patients with deep muscle pain may describe the pain as similar to that of a bruise. Muscle pain is experienced in a variety of ways. Muscle pain might also be described as sharp and sudden, sometimes due to trigger points.

Four common responses found during active resisted muscle testing and their implications are listed below:

- Strong and painless: all is well.
- Strong with pain: minor strain/damage, micro-tearing.
- Weak with pain: moderate to major strain/damage, tearing of muscle fibers.
- Weak and painless: usually implies either a neurological lesion or the rupture of muscle. Refer out.

Crepitus in muscle Crepitus is the term used for that "crunchy" or "snapping" noise that comes from tissue when the patient moves a joint or limb, or when the therapist moves that tissue. Though often used with respect to joint impairments it can occur in fibrotic tendons and is, therefore, not distinctive for impairments within the joint. Crepitus in a muscle, without pain, is a minor impairment. It occurs as the muscle rolls or slides over bone, for example. For example, the levator scapula is a muscle that often produces crepitus around the upper medial angle of the scapula. However, the fibrotic nature of the connective tissue in the muscle may be symptomatic of muscles that are overused or often under strain. Therefore, they may be occasionally a source of pain or a sense of tightness or tension.

Crepitus with pain (occurring in a muscle tissue) when the patient moves implies degenerative changes in the tissue. Pathology is possible, so refer out as well as treat.

Characteristics or common descriptors of muscle pain

Spasm types:

- Tonic spasm describes a painful, persistent muscle contraction that will suddenly or gradually release.
- Clonic spasm describes a painful series of muscle contractions and relaxations, each following the other, sometimes very briskly (like shivering), or somewhat less quickly (like shaking).

Cramp A lay term often used to describe a muscle spasm (tonic or clonic) that happens in the limbs, as in "leg cramps;" also used in such phrases as menstrual cramps, stomach cramps (colic), and the like. Therefore, when the patient uses this term it requires further investigation.

Strains An over-stressed muscle system causes physiological breakdown to the structure and function of the muscle.

- First degree strains, or mild strains, designate trauma to muscle that is at a cellular level ("micro-tearing"). Stiffness and discomfort may last up to five days. This often occurs in muscles during eccentric contraction, or when on stretch. It may take several hours for the patient to be aware of pain. Pain coming on during activity or exercise may imply greater micro-tearing, or that the muscle has exhausted its fuel supply as well. No more than 25 percent of fibers are thought to be involved in a first degree strain.
- Second degree strain (moderate) is felt often as the injury occurs. It is felt as a sharp, tearing sensation, possibly followed by a sensation of burning. This then resolves into a diffuse ache, which may generate referred pain (such as a TrP). It can be brought on either by sudden movement, usually with exertion or over-stretch, or by overuse (gradual onset). The more severe the strain, the greater the number of contractile units that are likely injured, with more tearing of the muscle's connective tissue components occurring as well (gross tearing), with 25 to 75 percent of fibers affected.
- Third degree strain (severe) is often described as a rupture or complete tear. In lay terms this is a torn muscle. The term is used if some fibers do in fact remain intact, but more than 75 percent are torn. Pain is often intense at the time of the

rupture and will usually make the person unable to continue any activity. Pain can fade rather quickly if the muscle is completely ruptured but the muscle's function is gone.

Repetitive strain A gradual onset strain caused by repetitive motion. It has also been called *cumulative trauma*. It may take days or months of overuse for symptoms to first appear. There is an increase in pain over time: it usually begins being painful post-activity, progressing to pain during activity (and usually after as well). In severe or acute cases it will begin to wake the patient from sleep. Weakness in the muscles involved becomes manifest after the appearance of pain.

Pain may decrease in intensity if the activity is stopped or decreased for several days; however, it will flare up again once the same (or similar) activity is resumed or increased. Examples are the various forms of tendonitis and tendonosis that can develop in numerous muscles in the body. If edema is produced then the patient can develop syndromes such as carpal tunnel or tennis elbow, for example.

Tendonitis versus tendonosis or tendinopathy

It is important to make a distinction between the terms tendonitis and tendonosis. Painful and dysfunctional tendons that have previously been diagnosed as tendonitis are now having the term tendonosis being applied instead. This is due to the findings of histological studies done in the late 1990s on painful tendons (such as in tennis elbow) which show a lack of neutrophils and other classical inflammatory substances in these painful tendons. Hence the move to omitting the "-itis" from the designation.

The term tendonitis is now generally reserved for an acute injury that resolves quickly over a week or two, while the chronic situation (3–6 months) is called tendonosis.

Tendonosis is characterized by degeneration of the once organized collagen fibers in the tendon into a disorganized condition, leading to weakening of the tendon and making it prone to tearing or rupture if never resolved. A complexity to this understanding is that without inflammation being present in all or most stages of tendonosis, trying to explain the experience of pain by the patient becomes problematic. The designation tendonosis may be more accurate, but it has actually made the impairment more puzzling. However, new research suggests that although not all inflammatory chemicals are present (as would be present in a joint suffering from rheumatoid arthritis, for example), it may be an error to think that the tendon is not inflamed in any way throughout all stages of the pathology. Nonetheless, tendonosis will most likely remain the preferred term, though what that implies may change as research continues (see Rees et al. 2014).

TABLE 4.1
Sprains: tissue tearing classification

Grade of tearing	Degree of sprain	Amount of tearing/injury
Minimal	First degree	Less than one third of fibers torn or in need of repair (i.e., tissue failure)
Partial	Second degree	One third to two-thirds of fibers torn or fail
Complete	Third degree – Partial rupture	A tear or failure of more than two-thirds of tissue, but there is continuity in the remainder of the tissue
	– Complete rupture	There is no longer any continuity. The latter can be painless after it occurs since no tension is placed on that specific tissue (though others around it may have suffered injury)

Manual testing will generate a positive result in cases of either tendonitis or tendonosis. Both can present as painful, usually decrease the range of motion in the joint involved, and may cause weakness in the involved muscles. Therefore, for the time being, both terms (-itis or -osis) may be used in this text, but are usually meant to imply tendonosis.

Sprains and ligament pain

A sprain is an injury to a ligament(s) typically of traumatic onset, with pain increasing post-trauma over several hours due to joint effusion. Movements that stress the ligament are painful locally (conversely, a total rupture may become painless post trauma) (Table 4.1).

Any accompanying muscle spasm that occurs post ligament trauma (splinting to protect injured tissues) that continually recurs (even after treatment) may speak to instability of the joint due to ligament laxity.

Bone pain

Bone pain is generally described as deep, dull, and intense; it may be so intense as to disturb sleep. Bone pain may be trauma related but need not be. Typically, pain here is not related to movement, unless a fracture is present; then the pain will be described as sharp. Continuous, deep, boring-like pain needs immediate referral out as this may imply a serious pathology is present. Do not treat until the patient has been cleared by a physician.

Joint pain and impairments

Joint pain is felt in and around the joint; it is often described as achiness or stiffness. It can also be felt as sharp, which is often accompanied by weakness. This can mean there is an injury to the articular surface, the presence of a loose body in the joint, and/or a tear to the capsule or ligaments. It can be described as either increasing (moderate to severe impairment), or decreasing (mild impairment) with activity.

Decreased range of motion in the joints may be due to:

- muscular hypertonicity/contracture
- muscle injury or fibrosing
- trigger points
- scarring of the joint capsule
- bony deformities
- inflammation or joint effusion.

Joint effusion This means fluid retention within the joint capsule, or swelling. Swelling within a joint presents with a capsular pattern of restriction. Certain ranges of a joint will decrease for a specific joint in a specific order. This is due to the fact that many joints in the body have fibrous capsules that have a twist in them (when in neutral) or other characteristics that produce distinct patterns of loss of range when the capsule swells. Capsular patterns are mentioned for the major joints of the body in the appropriate chapter.

Joint clicking May be heard upon joint movement. Examples of causes of persistent joint clicking would be the degenerative joint disease (DJD) of osteoarthritis, and the derangements of a knee or temporomandibular joint (TMJ) meniscus. Occasional clicking can be due to tendon snapping over bony surfaces (especially of hypertonic muscles), or it may be due to cavitation (i.e., release of gas that has built up in the joint). Clicking implies a short quick sound (like snapping your fingers), often occurring in a specific spot in a range of motion. Other words used by patients are popping or snapping. *If pain occurs with clicking that is a red flag and a referral to seek medical attention should be advised.*

Joint crepitus Often described by the patient as a creaking or cracking sound upon movement. Usually occurs on active movement, sometimes on passive movement. Most often it is due to joint surface wear or tendon/sheath adhesions or roughness. With respect specifically to joints, coarse crepitus (sounding like a creaking stair) implies severe osteoarthritic changes, while fine crepitus (walking on crisp snow or dry leaves) implies minor osteoarthritis.

NOTE: Joint noises associated with movement are more clinically important when they are accompanied by pain or instability. *This is a red flag and requires the patient to be referred to a physician.*

Nerve pain: nerve roots and peripheral nerves

Nerve pain, also known as nociceptive pain, is pain sourced by the noxious stimulation of pain receptors or compression or injury along the course of the nerve. Nerve pain is most often described as sharp, intense, or like an electric shock.

Nerve root entrapment Entrapment of the sensory portion of a nerve root produces pain that is often described as mild or tingling. When more intense it may be described as a sharp, shooting pain or as a distinct numbness. Nerve entrapments tend to be felt as constant or as radiating along a well-delineated path traveling distally or away from the site. The constant sensation implies a persistent entrapment (or pathology of the nerve). The sudden and/or shooting type implies intermittent entrapment, where the nerve root is impinged upon during certain movements and released on other movements. The path or area of the sensation occurs within the specific dermatome of that nerve root. If long term and chronic, the pain may be described as a deep dull ache.

Entrapment of peripheral nerves The words used to describe peripheral nerve entrapment are much the same as for nerve roots. It arises from the pressure on the peripheral nerve somewhere along its path through the body (e.g., carpal tunnel syndrome: pain/numbness/weakness in thumb and first finger as the median nerve is compressed in the wrist). If persistent, these sensations can also evolve into a deep achy pain or numbness.

Differentiating sensory and peripheral nerve entrapment is generally a matter of noting the area of the body affected. Nerve root entrapment produces its effects in the specific dermatomal area for that nerve, while peripheral nerve entrapment sensations will occur within the area enervated by it. To compare the areas of dermatomes to the areas of peripheral nerve enervation see the chapter on the cervical spine (for the upper body maps) and the chapter on the lumbar spine (for the lower body maps).

NOTE: The sensation that is described as "pins and needles" or tingling often arises from a non-neural source. The patient may describe a limb "going to sleep" if they have been sitting, lying down or holding a position for a long time. They get a tingling or pins and needles sensation in a limb that may also be accompanied by weakness that fades over several minutes when they move again. The most common cause of this is that (1) there has been a compression of the blood supply to the area, reducing blood flow to it; (2) once the person moves or shifts position the sudden increase or return of blood flow to the area produces the sensation of pins and needles; the degree of weakness is due to the length of time the blood was reduced enough to leave the muscle tissue starved and depleted of the nutrients it needs to produce the energy required for motion.

Decreased nerve conduction The following is the usual progression of two types of loss that occur when nerve conduction is decreased. The range of sensory and motor loss correlates to the severity of the compression or injury of the peripheral nerve involved. The progression given begins with minor compression symptoms and progresses to severe compression symptoms.

- *Sensory loss:* decreased nerve conduction in sensory nerves present in the following symptom progression. Loss of: vibration sense, light touch, perception of hot and cold, deep touch.
- *Motor loss*: decreased nerve conduction in motor nerves present with the following symptom progression: Loss of: deep tendon reflexes (stretch reflex), muscle strength.

Visceral pain Pain arising from organs is visceral pain. As a deep somatic structure, an organ will produce diffuse pain that is referred to the body wall. Organ pain is experienced in the more superficial areas of the body (superficial muscle and skin) that the organ shares a nerve supply with (see Figure 4.2). Therefore, diffuse intersegmental (spinal) pain and/or dysfunction may have a visceral origin.

RED FLAGS Because organs can refer into the body wall therapists need to keep in mind which superficial structures of the body represent referral areas for visceral pain when treating patients. For example, when treating someone for low back pain that seems to be located over the lower ribcage, remember that the kidney can refer into this area. Ask the patient about any changes to urinary issues (especially blood in the urine). Further, if treatment and home care are not making any real change to the symptoms in the area then referring them to seek medical attention is necessary. Of course, any abdominal

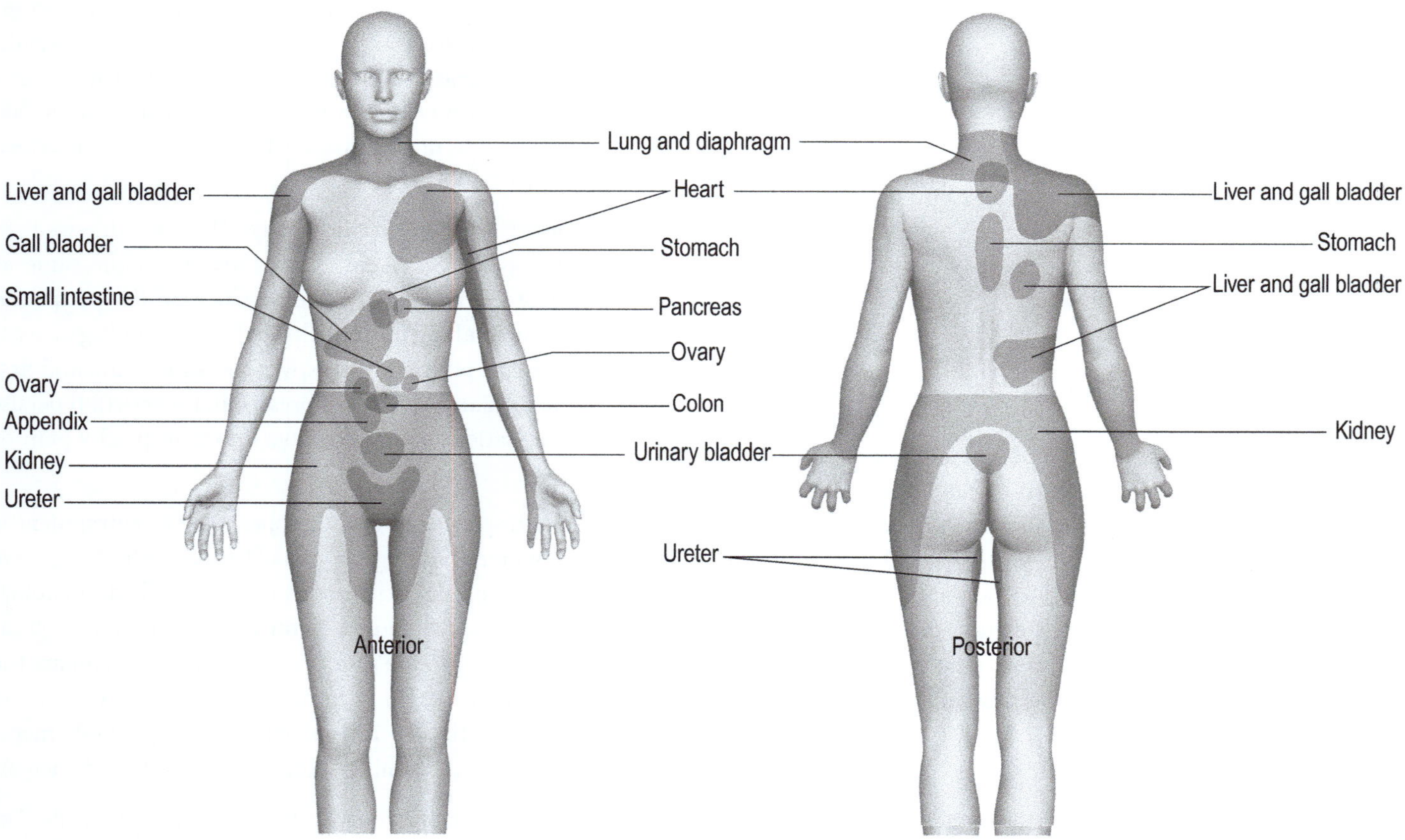

FIGURE 4.2

Visceral pain map.

pain described as excruciating, unrelenting, deep, or boring suggests a serious lesion and could be a medical emergency.

Conclusion

Pain is a complex human experience mediated by personal experience, genetics, and culture. It can be acute, subacute or chronic. It can occur in nerves, bones, muscles, or ligaments. Pain can be sharp or dull, excruciating or mild, persistent or intermittent. Pain can represent serious pathology or a welcome stage in the healing process. The professional language that we use to talk about pain might be very different than the language our patients use to talk about pain. Our patients know that pain places limits on their lives; they seek massage therapy treatment as a means to manage and relieve pain.

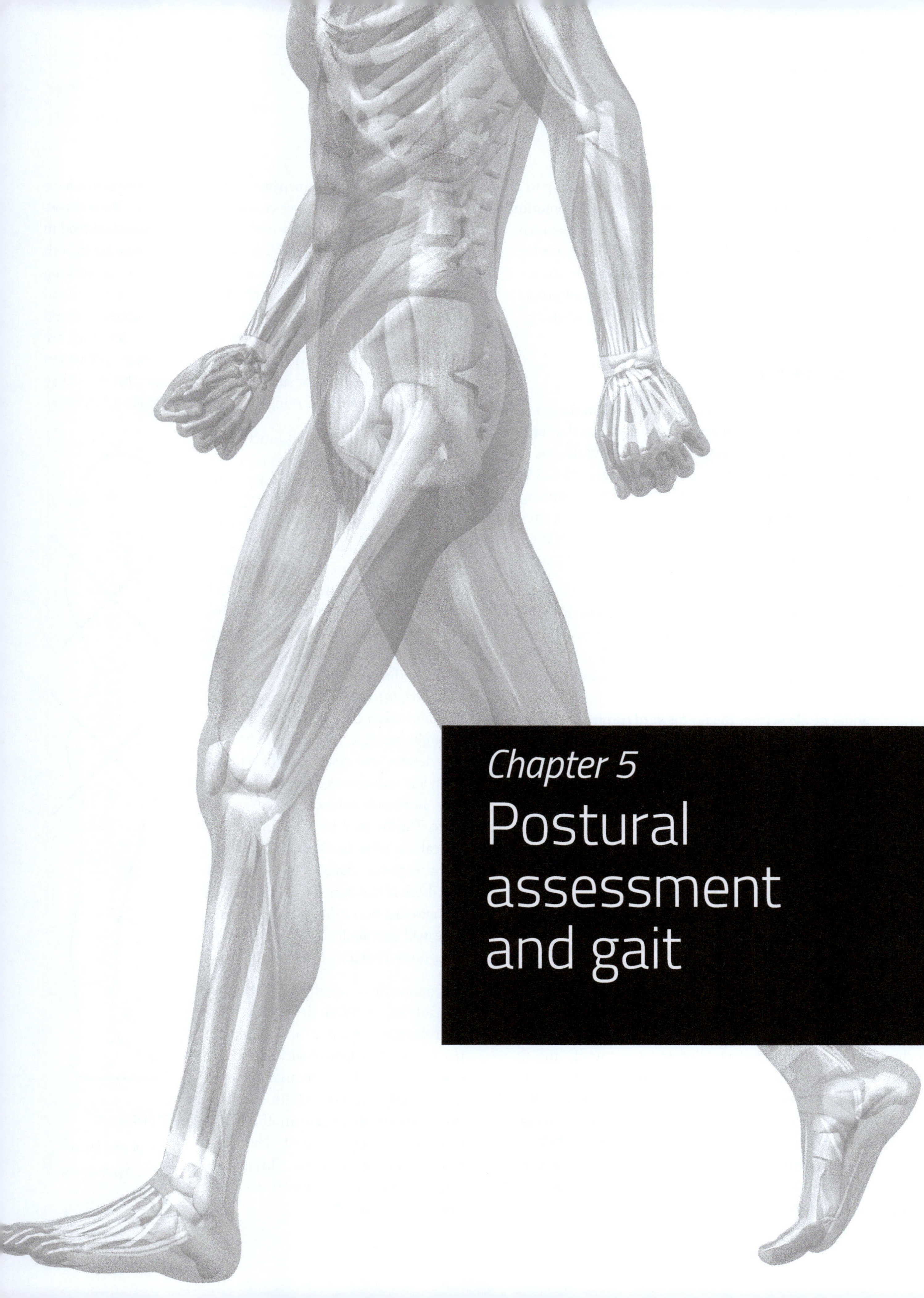

Chapter 5

Postural assessment and gait

Posture refers to the position of the body in relationship to gravity. Gait refers to the motion of limbs during locomotion (walking and running). Posture and gait are both dependent on the interaction and coordination of muscles as they adapt the body to the forces (such as gravity) that compose the environment in which it lives. Assessing posture and gait provides information about the way a patient's muscles are working together.

Muscle balance and posture

The overcoming of gravity is the primary determination of the balancing act that the musculature performs to hold us upright. Other influences include bony structures, pathologies, emotional stressors, and pain. Occupational or recreational activities also influence posture (Ward 2003). The balancing act between all the elements of the body occurs within the environment, the context, in which it lives. The way in which the body is whole and healthy is determined in many ways by how it is within the greater whole we call our world.

Our posture and movements are dependent on muscles working in coordination. For the shoulders to be in a place from which they get the maximum movement with the least stress on all the tissues involved all muscles, front and back, side to side, above and below, have to be in balance in order to hold the shoulder girdle neither too far forward (protracted or shoulders rolled forward) nor pulled too far back (retracted), neither too elevated nor too depressed. This balance not only has to be there in static posture, but also during all the motions that the shoulder can perform. Of course, for the shoulders to be in balance the thoracic and cervical spine and the skull have to be in their balanced positions, and so on through the whole body. The skull, cervical and thoracic spine also depend on the shoulders being in balance. Posture and motion depend on an exquisite, complex dance between structure and function.

Changes to posture affect our musculature by altering the balance between muscles, making some muscles short and others long. When the relationship between muscles that are balanced against each other (agonist and antagonist, flexor and extensor, etc.) becomes imbalanced, posture and function of the body must change, usually for the worse. Shortness in muscle and tissue pulls body parts out of a balanced position, but this requires weak and long muscles to permit this to happen (Kendall et al. 2005). Imbalance occurs when one muscle becomes too high in tone and shortens as it tightens. The result is that its balancing/opposing musculature often lengthens and becomes weaker. The opposite is also true: if a muscle weakens and lengthens, then the opposing muscle becomes short and tight.

Janda and Jull have shown how this occurs in patterns that have become known as the upper cross syndrome and the lower cross syndrome (Figure 5.1). Janda noticed that the muscles that tend to tighten are the ones responsible for sustaining our posture in both static and dynamic states. These muscles are always *on*, or working (except when the person is asleep). Many of the muscles that tend to tighten (but not all) are two joint muscles. The muscles that tend to go weak and long are referred to as *phasic* muscles. They are muscles that work only to perform specific tasks when called upon but are not responsible for sustaining our posture. Therefore, they can often be *off*, or not working, a lot of the day (Janda & Jull 1987).

Changes to posture and function are often the predisposing factors leading to injury or overuse syndromes. Examples are: headaches, low back pain, rotator cuff strains, thoracic outlet syndromes, and patellar femoral pain syndromes. On the other hand, muscle imbalance can be the result of traumas as the body tries to protect itself through splinting, or as we compensate for temporary losses of function. If the injury persists for more than one or two days, the body often adapts to its new posture and function and takes this as the new normal. Though antalgic movement patterns may lessen and disappear the body is often left with changes due to the alterations in muscle balance that have taken place. The longer it takes an impairment to heal, the more likely it is that the body will accept the changes to its function and think of this as normal. The postural changes that occur due to muscle imbalance will eventually affect other structures (even changing the shape of bone).

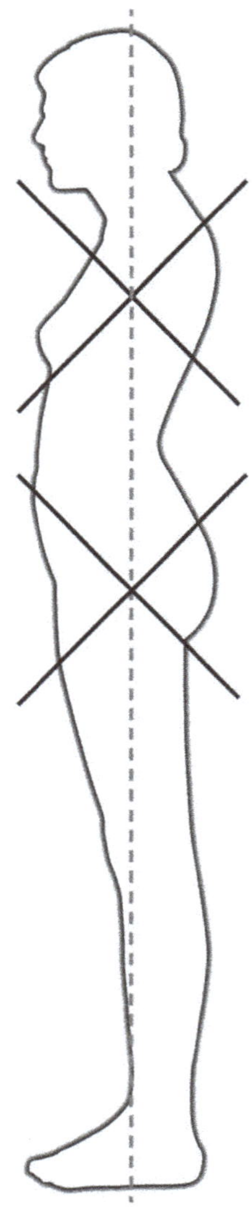

FIGURE 5.1
Upper and lower cross syndromes.

Compression syndromes that are a result of postural deviations affect neurological, vascular, and lymphatic tissues creating neurological signs and symptoms, and/or vascular changes that directly affect the health and function of tissues. Joints are another structure affected by postural deviations, resulting in misalignment. This leads to degenerative joint change, or to a predisposition to injury.

Visceral organs also undergo stress when there are deviations to posture which affect the shape and orientation of the abdominal cavity (e.g., from an anterior pelvic tilt). Visceral changes include the tractioning of bile ducts, rotations of organs leading to possible physiologic alterations in function, and tractioning or compression of sympathetic nerves or ganglia.

Thoracic outlet problems, and other acquired nerve compression syndromes, are often the product of muscle imbalances. The neurovascular bundles can become compressed in the tissue's connective tissue elements, or between structures (bone, etc.) that are pulled out of position by muscle imbalances (Box 5.1).

Lung capacity and function can be affected by postural deviations in the cervical spine and the ribcage: scalenes shorten and lift the first two ribs, making them insufficient to come into play when axillary capacity for the lungs is required due to increased demand. Changes of the ribcage mechanics can do the same, sometimes fixing some of the ribs in an inhaled or an exhaled position.

Muscle imbalance and the resultant postural deviations are often the primary reason for degenerative joint disease (such as osteoarthritis), especially in the spine, pelvis and lower limbs, and for degenerative disc disease in the spine. There is the obvious situation of changes to the curves of the spine, rotations of limbs, etc.

INSIGHTS

Box 5.1 Axoplasmic flow

Though it is somewhat of a digression, there is one important point that I would like to make here. Compression of neural tissue does not just affect nerve conduction per se, as in conduction down myelin sheaths. What is also affected by compression is axonal flow (or axoplasmic flow), the movement of substances through the nerve cell's cytoplasm and down the axoplasm. This includes mitochondria, lipids, proteins, some organelles, and the like. Due to the length of the axon, there is a fast and a slow transport system, both of which need to be functioning correctly if nutrients are to be supplied to all areas of the cell in a timely manner. The axon terminals appear to possess ribosomes (which were probably transported there from the cell body), which can produce proteins. In this way, the terminal endings can make at least some neurotransmitters on site, from raw materials supplied by the transport system. Further, materials are sent back up the axon (retrograde transport) for breakdown, some parts are recycled, and others may be discarded by the cell body.

Tensegrity

Trying to understand how all of this balancing takes place within a classic mechanical model of blocks, pulleys, and arches quickly becomes either too complex or too simplistic. A subtler way to understand the interplay between structure and function is to be found in what is called the *tensegrity* (tensile/tension integrity) model, a term coined by the inventor and architect Buckminster Fuller. When looking at human architecture, it proposes that the spine should not be looked at as merely a column, or a set of blocks that are stacked one on top of the other with increasing compressive forces accumulating as we go down the spine. Rather, tensegrity is meant to explain how, when we add the ribs and muscles to the picture, the forces are distributed by the tension in the muscles and fascia, through their attachments on the ribs and vertebrae, in a way that reduces the compressive forces going through the spinal column. In other words, weight can be transferred out to the body wall. (See Myers 2014 for a good introduction to the term tensegrity.)

Creating an imbalance in the tension throughout the body's trunk will change the dynamics of tensegrity within the thorax, causing exponential stress on some muscles or connective tissue (cables) while others go lax and no longer do their job. Those taking the strain suffer from tensile overload – tendonitis, shortness, and hypertonicity. Those that are lax suffer atrophy. The bones (struts) suffer from the changes in tension, with weight shifting on or off them. This can affect their shape, their growth, and the level of the bone's density.

Further, due to the development of muscle imbalances, the ribcage no longer functions (as struts) to carry the trunk weight outward. Therefore, we have an exponential change in the compressive forces traveling down the spine. Further, these forces are no longer evenly distributed in the spine but shift about, passing unevenly through anterior surfaces of thoracic vertebrae facet joints in areas of lordosis, uneven stresses on the cartilaginous disc layers, etc. In fact, if this tensegrity, or integration through balanced tension, were not natural to the body we would all suffer at an early age from degenerative joint and disc diseases, tissue contracture, resulting changes to lung capacity, changes to the environment of the visceral organs, blood flow, and on and on.

Tightness versus tautness

There is an important palpatory observation we need to keep in mind when investigating the musculature for shortness and excessive length. Muscles are palpated as lax, as relaxed, as having normal tone, or as taut. We often make the common mistake of calling all taut muscles *tight*, but what we are really feeling is tautness. We need to check the length of a muscle before we can say it is tight, because tightness implies a short, even contractured muscle. However, muscles can be long and taut. If a muscle is stretched, it becomes taut. If we have confused tautness with tightness, we can make the mistake of thinking a lengthened taut muscle is tight and therefore *short*, and proceed to lengthen an already overly long muscle. This could result in making the patient's postural deviations worse.

For example, patients with a forward head and shoulders posture often have an excessive kyphosis: tight pectoralis and posterior cervical muscles, with weakened and lengthened rhomboids, middle and lower trapezius muscles. The patient often enjoys the mid-thoracic area being worked during massage and the therapist often mistakes the tautness of these muscles as tightness and proceeds to relax and lengthen these muscles further. This may make the patient feel temporarily better but, in fact, it only makes their shoulders roll forward more and exaggerate their kyphosis.

One further consequence of the contracturing of a taut muscle, like the hamstrings of a patient with an anterior pelvic tilt, is that the muscle loses its elasticity. So, though the hamstrings may have become frozen in a slightly lengthened position, they usually will appear as short on a length test (which requires the muscle to stretch). Again, patients with these taut hamstrings love them being worked on, but if the therapist treats them in a manner that lengthens them, then the anterior pelvic tilt will increase, making things worse. Therefore, the need is for a careful and comprehensive postural analysis with landmarking.

Consequences of muscle imbalance

We can go beyond the muscles mentioned by Janda and Jull and see further implications. As an example, in the upper cross syndrome, long rhomboid major muscles allow the serratus anterior muscles to go short. The connective tissue component shortens as well over time and so the serratus ends up contractured (as with the patient whose scapulae you cannot lift off the ribcage or mobilize well).

Further, if you lengthen the pectoralis, the sternocleidomastoid and posterior cervical muscles and then strengthen or "wake up" the inhibited rhomboids and lower traps and add tone to the deep neck flexors, those shoulders will still not go back if those serratus anterior muscles (along with the latissimus dorsi and teres major) are not lengthened as well. In order to get a complete response, you need as complete a picture as you can get.

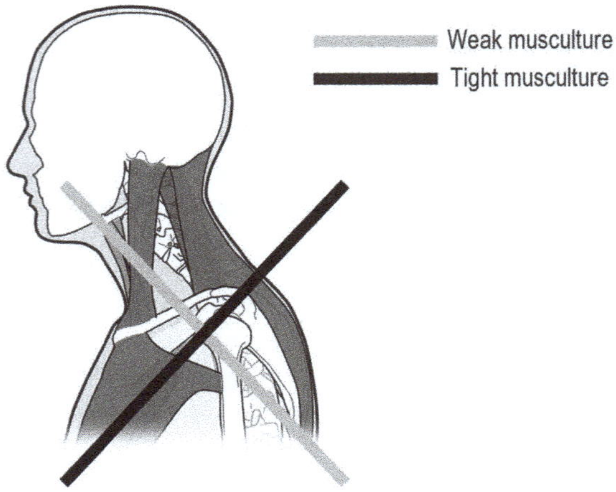

FIGURE 5.2 Upper cross syndrome

Tight muscles (dark line): suboccipitals; upper trapezium and levator scapulae; sternocleidomastoid and scalenes; teres major, latissimus dorsi, and teres minor; pectoralis major and serratus anterior. Weak muscles (lighter gray line): deep flexors of the neck; rhomboids, infraspinatus, and teres minor; middle and lower trapezium. (Janda & Jull 1987).

Observations and inspection: upper cross syndrome

The upper cross syndrome (Figures 5.2 and 5.3) produces the shifts in structures shown in Figure 5.3 by changing the length and strength of muscles.

Observations made of a forward head posture and hyperkyphosis: hyperkyphosis in the thoracic spine means that the upper and mid-thoracic spine is more flexed than normal while the lower thoracic segments are more extended. The increased flexion in the upper and mid-thoracic spine stretches the musculature on the back at these levels, making them long and therefore weaker/inhibited. In turn, the upper and middle ribs are depressed, leaving the ribcage fixed and held as if the person is always exhaling, thereby decreasing lung capacity. This shortens the pectoralis major and minor, pulling the shoulders forward with scapula protracted.

Lower cross syndrome (one cause of hyperlordosis)

For the lower cross syndrome, the classic short (and tight) and long and weak muscles are organized as described in Figure 5.4. This is a bilateral anterior pelvic tilt, which is one of the most common muscle imbalances found in the clinical setting (Janda & Jull 1987).

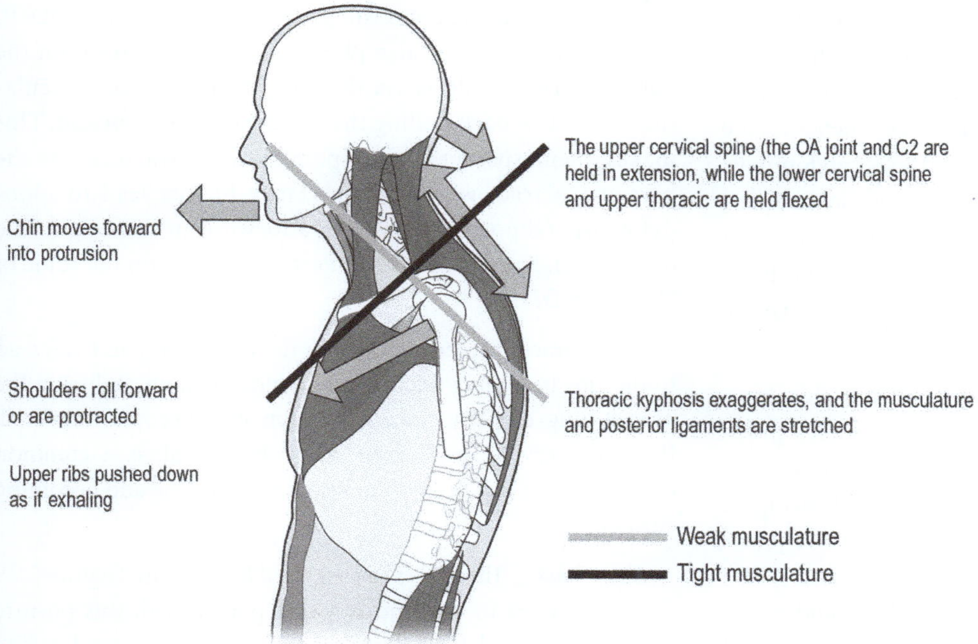

FIGURE 5.3

Shifts in structure in the upper cross syndrome.

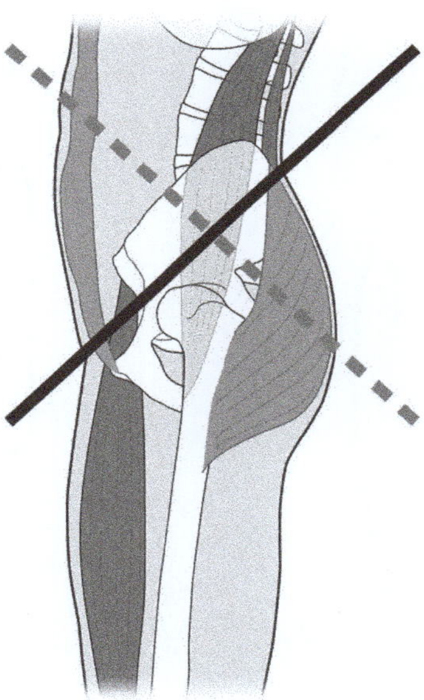

FIGURE 5.4 Lower cross syndrome

Short, tight and facilitated muscles (dark line): lumbar erectors, quadratus lumborum; iliopsoas, rectus femoris, and tensor fasciae latae; thigh adductors; piriformis. Lengthened, weak, and inhibited musculature (broken line): rectus and transversus abdominis; gluteal muscles; vastus medialis, lateralis, and intermedius (of quadriceps). (Note that hamstrings are not included in either listing because they are properly referred to as "taut," not tight and short. Taut means lengthened, but hypertonic. The hamstrings are stretched because they are the only muscle preventing the pelvis from rotating further anteriorly. Over time, they contract and will appear "short" when tested for length).

Other common postures and their faults

Other common postural faults are described below and in shown in Figures 5.5 to 5.8. Again, these are usually the product of muscle imbalances. Each chapter in this text has some further discussion on these and other postural impairments that occur from muscle imbalance or structural lesions (see Kendall et al. 2005; Magee 2014; Mitchell 2001, 2004, 2005).

Normal posture Here, the ear sits roughly over the shoulder, the shoulder sits over the trochanter, and the gravity line runs just behind the patella and just in front of the malleoli (Figure 5.5). The spine has its proper elongated S-shape that provides a spring to cushion the joints and structures of the spine.

Military posture This is named for the classic "head up, stomach in and chest out" position of a soldier at attention

(Figure 5.6). It requires the person to extend their low back (increasing the lumbar lordosis) while lengthening or flattening the thoracic kyphosis as they protract their shoulders. Often, the chin is lifted, extending the upper cervical spine. Therefore, the low back and mid-back erectors are short and tense, abdominals are tense, rhomboids and lower traps short and tense. The sub-occipitals are short and tense, along with the scalenes (holding the first two ribs up). The pectoral muscles are short and tense as well (lifting the ribs and sternum while lowering the clavicle onto the ribs beneath it).

The military posture, and any posture that generates hyperlordosis of the lumbar spine, produces many problems. For the joints of the low back, this hyperlordosis closes the facet joints and they become weight- or load-bearing. If chronic, then the occurrence of osteoarthritis in these joints becomes more likely. The posterior intervertebral disc (IVD) becomes loaded as well, leading to poor nutrition and hence compromises the health of the disc. This makes the IVD more likely to degenerate (degenerative disc disease, DDD). The excessive lordosis also places an increased strain on the narrow pars articularis via the attachments of the musculature of the low back pulling the vertebrae into extension. This makes them susceptible to spondylolysis (fractures of the pars articularis), which, in turn, may further lead to spondylothesis (slippage of a vertebra forward in relation to the one below). See Chapter 12 in Part II for more on the topic of IVDs and DDD.

The thoracic flatness along with the expanded chest can lead to the ribs becoming fixed in an inhaled position, reducing the overall lung capacity since exhalation may become restricted. Posterior cervical pain, especially suboccipital, is a common occurrence for this posture, developing over time and becoming chronic.

Sway back This refers to a forward hip posture (Figure 5.7). The sway refers to the tendency of a person with this posture to sway back and forth (i.e., anteriorly and posteriorly). The

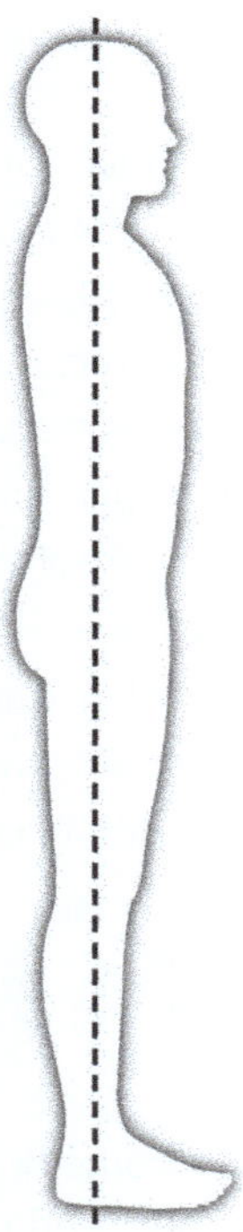

FIGURE 5.5

Normal posture.

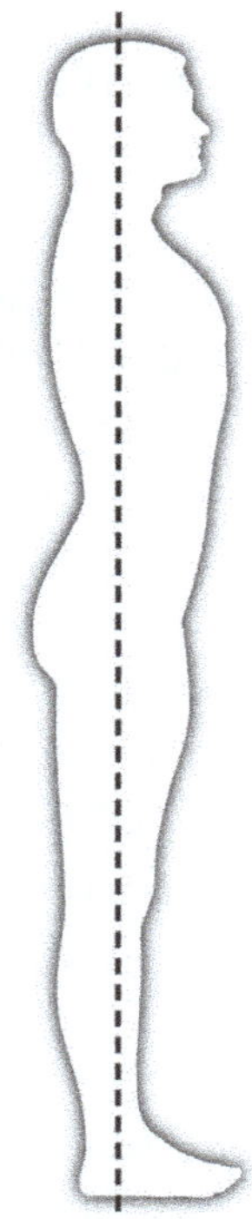

FIGURE 5.6

Military posture.

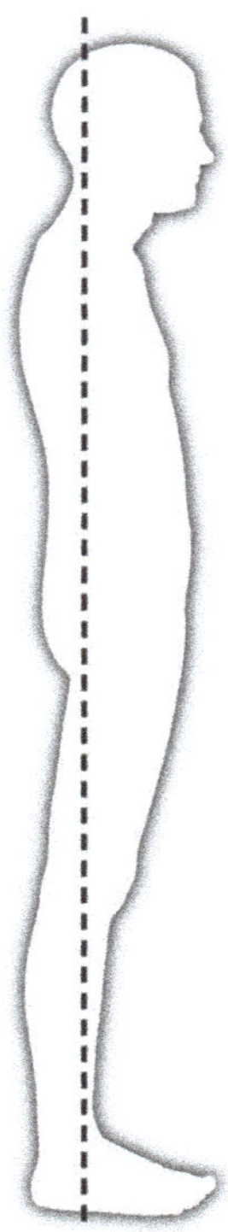

FIGURE 5.7

Sway back posture.

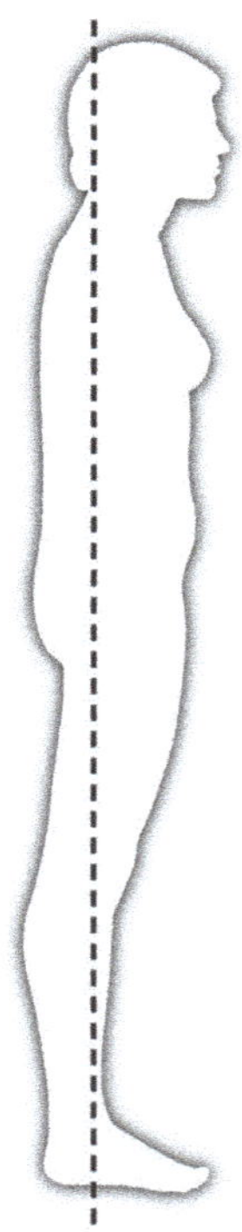

FIGURE 5.8

Flat back posture.

reason for this is that with the hips thrust forward their weight will shift onto the toes. This creates a feeling of imbalance so the musculature of the legs and hips will alternate in tension, causing the person to sway back to front as they remain perched on their toes (Kendall et al. 2005). The lumbar spine is extended (hyperlordotic) at the lowest lumbar vertebrae, which are sitting on posteriorly rotated hips. The hip joint is in extension, as are the knees. (The thoracic kyphosis and cervical lordosis are also exaggerated.) The first one or two lumbar vertebrae and lower thoracic vertebrae are often flattened and resist motion. This adds to the compressive force on the lowest hyperextended lumbars.

Muscles creating sway back posture:

- Tight and hypertonic muscles: lumbar erectors, quadratus lumborum; hamstrings and gluteus maximus (for the knees: vastus medialis, vastus lateralis, vastus intermedius).
- Weak and inhibited: abdominals, except for internal oblique which may be hypertonic (Kendall et al. 2005), iliopsoas, rectus femoris.

Common hyperlordotic issues:

- Posterior thoracic fatigue is a common complaint from patients.
- Neck pain with impairments to cervical motion occurs frequently.
- Protracted shoulders set up the shoulders for rotator cuff injuries.
- Knee tissues and joint structures are under constant strain.

Flat back This posture occurs when there is a greatly reduced or absent lordosis in the lumbar spine (Figure 5.8). There is also an increased upper thoracic kyphosis and forward head posture. Because the lumbar spine curve is decreased – flattened – the body will compensate for this by throwing the head forward (upper thoracic hyperkyphosis and upper cervical hyperlordosis). Often, the whole body tilts forward, resulting in the toes grabbing the ground and the toe flexors, therefore, contributing to a pes cavus (high arch) in the foot.

Therefore, the pelvis-lumbar complex has:

- the lumbar spine flexed, resulting in stretched low back erectors
- a posterior pelvic tilt with extension of hip joint; tight and short hamstrings, abdominals, with a lengthened rectus femoris and iliopsoas.

The flat back, or lack of lumbar lordosis, on top of the posteriorly rotated hips results in degenerative disc disease due to the lack of a natural springiness that comes from a proper lordotic curve. The forward head posture produces cervical pain from strained muscles, overloaded facet joints and spasming suboccipital muscles. This is a recipe for chronic headaches or migraines.

General postural examination

Introduction

The classic postural examination is done standing. We will explore seated, supine, and prone examinations as well. These could all be done as an initial or detailed postural examination, or done separately, depending on the information needed.

The author would like to point out that in his own practice he prefers to include some motion in a postural examination. The motion included can be found in the section of this book detailing examination of the spine (Chapter 10).

The topic of gait analysis is a separate section later in this chapter but many therapists (including this author) would incorporate this in a postural examination as well. However, it is often only included when the patient's condition and goals warrant it. Therefore, the therapist has a lot of flexibility in how they do their postural assessments, and can have several options available depending on the patient's condition and needs, and the therapist's clinical judgment.

If possible, use a plumb line, especially if you are just learning these skills. With experience, many therapists develop quite a trained eye and no longer need a plumb line. The plumb line should begin, or be centered, in the anterior and posterior views, exactly in the middle between the two feet. In the lateral views, the plumb lies just behind the malleoli of the ankle.

What are we taking note of?

We are noting orientation and asymmetries of structures in vertical (sagittal), frontal (coronal), and horizontal (transverse) planes (Figure 5.9). Take note of rotation and/or side-bending of one or both limbs, hips, shoulders, and in the truck and head. Bilaterally compare levels of paired structures, bulk of tissues, length, and proportions.

Points to remember as you begin your postural assessment

1. When you find structures or levels that appear to be asymmetrical or not level, then always check above and below that area/structure for its cause or compensations. Rarely does an impairment stand alone.

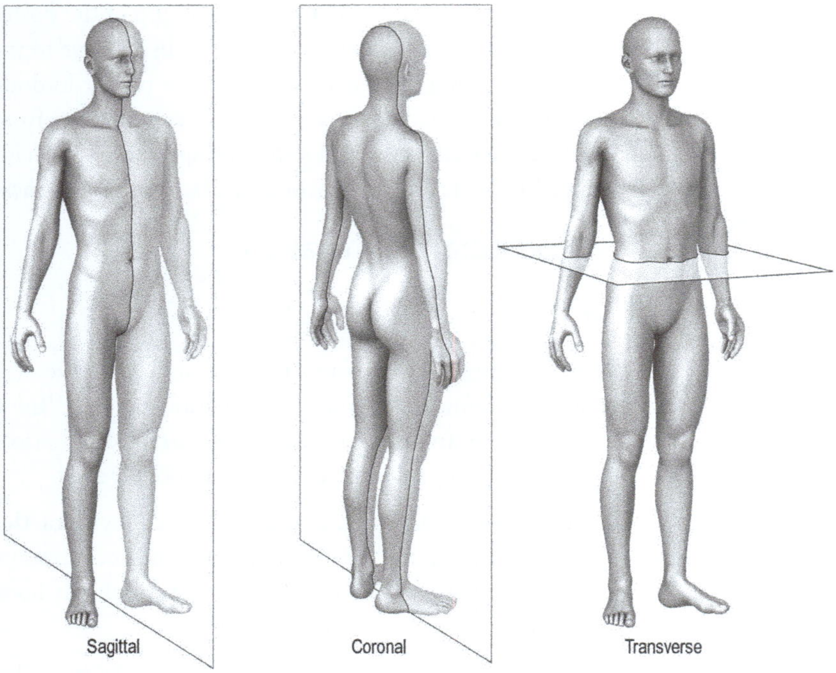

FIGURE 5.9
Anatomical planes.

2. Be sure you are not being misled. Is something that appears higher or lower, more anterior or posterior, rotated and/or side-bent actually the issue or cause of the asymmetry? Alternatively, is the other side possibly out of position? For example, one elbow, the left, is farther from the body than the other. This can imply that the trunk is side-bent left, moving the left shoulder farther from the mid-line. This can certainly be true sometimes. However, on the contralateral right side, a protracted shoulder may make the right arm lie closer to the body, making the normal space (on the left) appear as if it was abnormal. Experience helps sort these out. Therefore, along with looking at the surrounding structures and tissues to see which areas show impairment or compensation, also look to the body as a whole to give you the appropriate answer.

Standing postural exam

NOTE: Much of the information from a standing postural examination is needed to compare with supine and prone examination so that we are not misled by what we see when the patient is on the table in those positions. The major difference for these instructions about a standing postural assessment is that the author considers it important that the patient should be standing in a natural pose when doing a postural assessment. Only after seeing the patient in this more natural position, should the patient be asked to have their feet together, etc., as has been traditionally done.

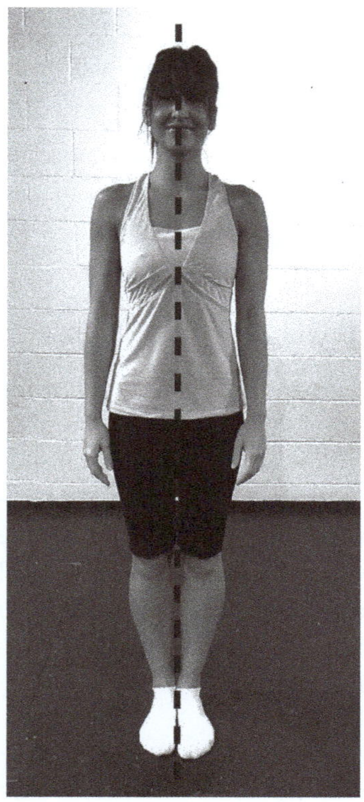

FIGURE 5.10
Artificial pose.

An artificial pose, such the one shown in Figure 5.10, can be instructive, but not until after you have observed the patient in what is a more natural posture for them. You see more clearly

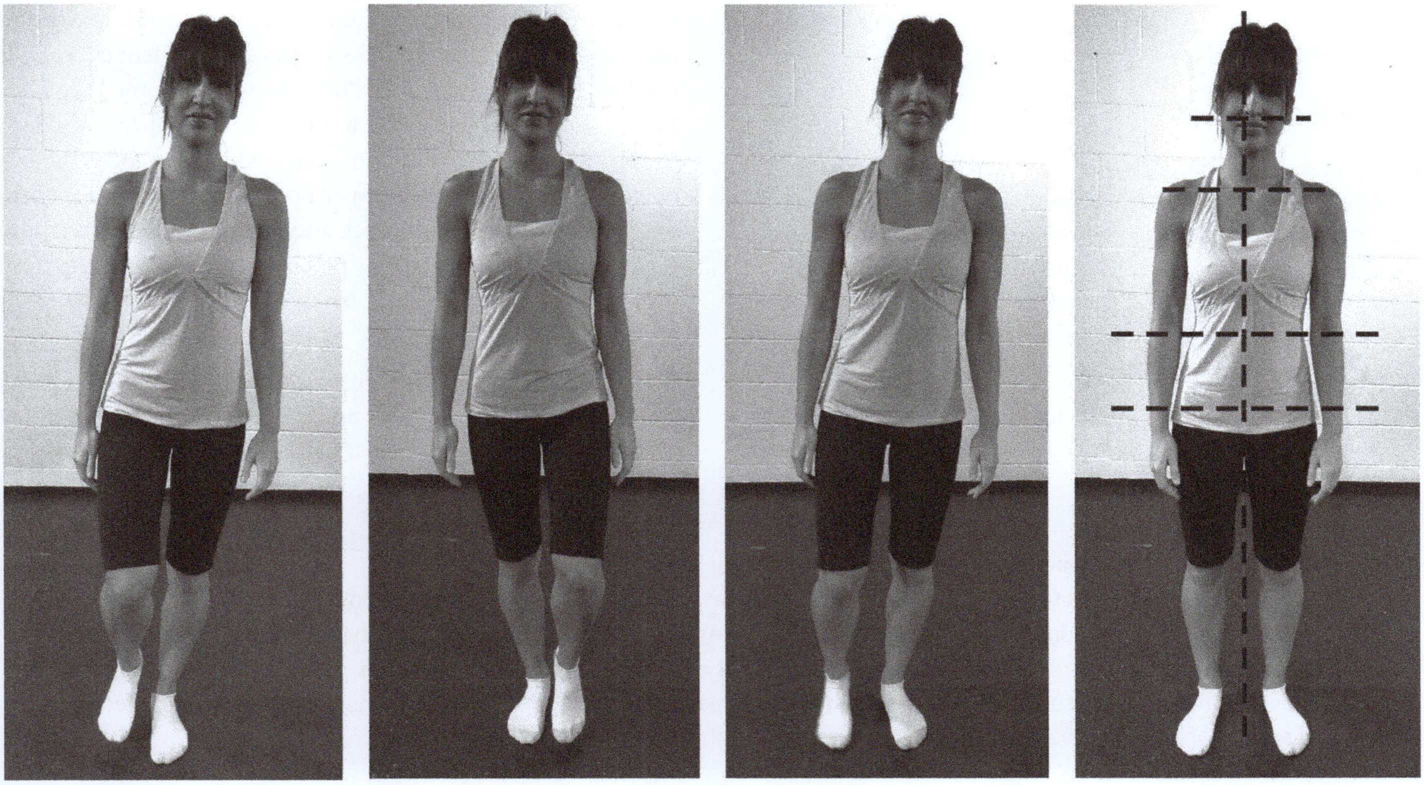

FIGURE 5.11 Establishing a natural posture

To assist in establishing a natural posture instruct the patient to look up slightly (you do not want them watching their feet) and take a couple of steps, while staying in place. Then, tell them to stop and do not alter their position.

their holding patterns, their asymmetries, etc., in the natural pose. The artificial pose is just that, artificial.

Therefore, once you establish a more natural pose (Figure 5.11), do not correct the patient's feet positions, head position, etc. You are trying to have them stand as they naturally do, or as near to it as they can, even though they are in a clinical setting.

Note the differences in where the plumb line runs up the body in the artificial pose versus the more natural pose.

Plumb line

The plumb line, with the ideal posture, should run up equidistant between the knees, through the pubis symphysis, navel, mid-sternum, center of the neck, through the chin, nose, and between the eyes. Check for levelness of knee creases, PSISs, greater trochanter heights, iliac crest heights. Check the levels of the patella, side shift in hips (pelvic obliquity), and level of greater trochanters, ASISs, and iliac crest heights, waist, levels of clavicles, acromions, jaw orientation, ear and eye levels.

NOTE: In the four parts of Figure 5.11, the patient leans to the left. The shoulders seem level, but the contours of the upper shoulders are not the same. However, the left hand is more inferior than the right. The right iliac crest is slightly higher (this would all be clearer in real life). She does seem to compensate for this somewhere along the way, as the shoulders seem level from this view. Yet, at the cervical spine she again bends to the left, and does not compensate at the suboccipital region (head).

IMPORTANT: If you compare the artificial pose (Figure 5.10) with the more natural posture (Figure 5.11), in the former, you do not see the tilt of the whole body to the left, but only a slight tilt in the cervical spine or head. The tilt of the body and head is even clearer when the patient is walking in place; the head will lean left, but not right (it only comes back to being straight). *It is* *important to watch the patient as they walk in place and not just look at them once they stop moving.*

Initial observations

First, observe the natural orientation of the whole person. Take note of obvious asymmetries. Many students take too long to do their assessments because they waste time trying to observe or find minute differences. At this point in the assessment, it is suggested that any small differences (under 1/8th of an inch) should be ignored for now. We may concern ourselves with these minor differences once we palpate landmarks.

It is then useful to look at the lower body, hips and down to the feet, and focus there for several seconds, noting the orientation of structures (rotation of limbs or trunk and head) and any asymmetries side to side (level, bulk, length, etc.). If need be, then check and focus from knee to feet, and then knee to hip, for a few seconds each. Observe the upper body, hips to top of the head. Again, you can divide your focus, after a cursory view of the whole upper body, into looking from hips to shoulders, shoulders to neck and head, then arms. It is suggested that your observations begin at the feet since it is from here that the body can first begin to become unbalanced or asymmetrical.

CAUTION: Though you may observe an asymmetry in one place, you cannot prejudge the issue and assume that the cause for that is in (or completely in) that very structure or tissue. It could be

TABLE 5.1
Common asymmetries and some consequences
Presented here is a partial list of (common) asymmetries and an example or two of what they might mean. Keep the caution in this section in mind. (See the appropriate chapter for more on these possible connections/consequences.) The more assessment you do, and the more you understand your anatomy and joint motions, the more you will understand how varied and numerous are the possible implications of asymmetry. This does not really make things more difficult, rather the more specific and effective (not to mention safer) you will be able to make your treatments.

Asymmetry	Consequences
One foot rotated in or out (normally foot is turned out 7–15°)	If foot is turned out, it may be pronated. This, in turn, may show up at knee as a valgus knee on that side. If turned in, foot may have a high (and possibly more rigid) arch, which could create a varus orientation at knee. (See Chapters 7 and 8 for more information)
Knee observations as above; observe patella orientation	Valgus knee will put strain on medial collateral ligament and meniscus of knee; varus would put strain on lateral ligament and meniscus of knee. Increased strain means increased risk of injury
Hips unlevel	Could be from a real bony leg length difference or, more likely, from a muscle imbalance side to side and anterior to posterior. When one-sided, or more on one side than the other, pelvis is unlevel. In turn, sacral base is tilted. This causes spine to side-bend and rotate to correct for this, i.e., it produces a scoliosis. Further, unlevel hips may imply a sacroiliac joint impairment. Rotations in trunk can lead or be due to spinal lesions or impairments
Rotations in trunk can lead to or be due to spinal lesions or impairments	This can increase strain on sacroiliac joints, change orientation of shoulders (which always leads to some sort of problem there or in arms), or neck issues
One shoulder more protracted (and usually lower)	This leads to imbalanced strain of rotator cuff muscles. Some muscles become longer (stretched), some shorter, with inevitable consequences to: (1) muscle tissue health and (2) poor mechanics for shoulder motion and, hence, an increased risk of osteoarthritic changes in joint
Side-bent cervical spine	This will stretch (facet) joint and muscle tissues on one side, and shorten muscle and compress joints on the other side, leading to neck pain. Further, a side-bent cervical spine can compress one side of joints and muscles involved in conjunction of skull and spine (occipital-atlanto joint) leading to suboccipital headaches
Rotation or side-bending of head	Will impact immediately on occipital-atlanto joints, and atlanto-axial joint below that, not to mention what can happen in the cervical spine as a whole

compensation from a structure/tissue that is above or below. In other words, it could be the result or consequence (a secondary or tertiary impairment) of some other (original) impairment.

Compensations are often an appropriate response by the body; they are the body's attempt to compensate for impairments, or for asymmetries (length or size differences) that are structural or functional. It will be rare to find anyone who is symmetrical. After all, humans are right or left handed, have a right or left lead foot. These inevitably create minor (and usually acceptable) compensations, and for this reason are often called a "successful compensatory pattern" (Chila 2010; Zink & Lawson 1979). Wellness and health are not negatively affected. The effect of a slight dip in the right shoulder can be seen in a slight tilt of the head to the left, a slight side-bending of the upper thoracic spine, a slight anterior tilt of the right pelvis, etc. There is a gentle compensation going through the body, side to side, back to front. An "unsuccessful compensatory pattern," on the other hand, is not side to side, etc., and often the postural balance is quite skewed, with marked differences side to side. More on this later.

Much of this information will be needed to compare with the supine and prone examinations or, even more importantly, when treating the patient, so that you are not misled by what you see when the patient is on the table in those positions. In other words, when the patient is prone or supine, gravity will change the orientation of rotations, side-bending, etc., from those seen during the standing postural exam. Therefore, you may need to consult your point-form written notes.

Some common asymmetries are described in Table 5.1

Standing lateral view

Most therapists will look at the patient from each side, to get a lateral view (Figure 5.12). If possible, depending on the room available to you, try to move yourself to look at the patient from each side. If you need the patient to turn sideways, then have them take one or two steps in place to re-establish their natural posture.

The plumb line should be positioned just behind the lateral malleoli and then the therapist is to note where the following landmarks are (i.e., whether they are behind or in front of the plumb line): the patella, the greater trochanter, the glenohumeral joint and the ear canal. In the *ideal* posture we would find that the plumb line continues to be just behind the patella, through the greater trochanter, through the middle of the glenohumeral joint and the external meatus (ear canal) of the ear.

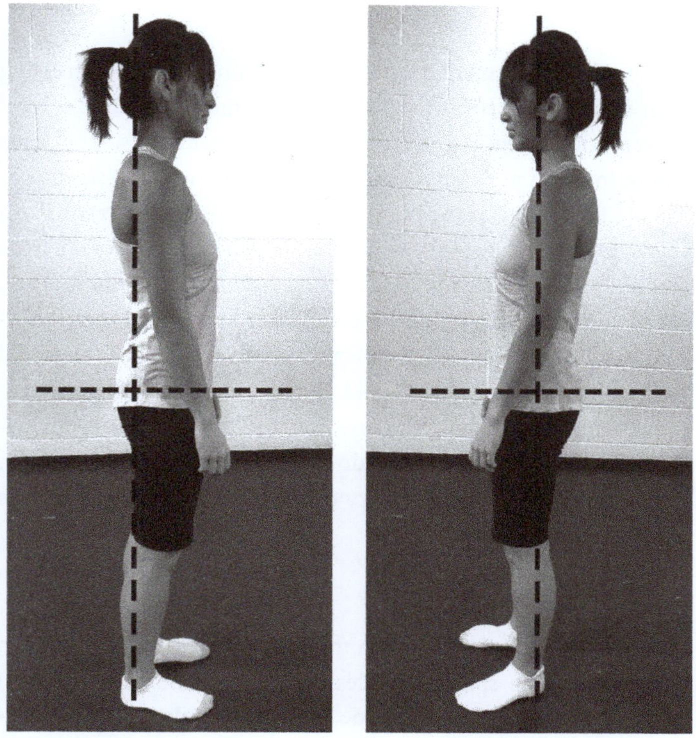

FIGURE 5.12 Standing lateral view

Observe the patient from each side. Note how the plumb runs through expected landmarks. If the patient must turn, have them turn to one side and re-establish natural pose, then make your observations. Then have the patient turn to the other side and repeat re-establishing the natural pose, and then make your observations.

One of most important levels to observe is from the PSIS to the ASIS. Normally, the ASIS is 5–15° lower to a horizontal line running through the PSIS (posterior to anterior). Women, in general, tend to have a greater pelvic tilt anteriorly than men. A tilt of more than 20° implies that the innominate is anteriorly rotated, while one of zero or less (i.e., the ASIS is higher than the PSIS) implies that the innominate is posteriorly rotated (a much rarer finding).

NOTE: In Figure 5.12 you can see how the patient's body as a whole rotates to the left (the right side's landmarks from the knee up are significantly forward of the plumb line compared to the left view). Her right innominate (hip bone) is anteriorly rotated. This will make a leg functionally longer (see Chapter 9 for more on this) as the acetabulum moves slightly anteriorly and inferiorly, making that hip joint lower.

Detective work

As you make a mental note of suspicions while progressing through the postural assessment, you may find that several observations begin to suggest certain possibilities. You keep these in mind as you proceed through your whole testing protocol. To put the same point another way, positive results can become linked together, or coalesce, which can help you develop more specific concerns as you move along with your testing. These, in turn, can guide which specific areas need more thorough investigating with specific testing. Further, postural testing may indicate which detailed testing may not be appropriate or necessary at this time, helping you avoid uninformative testing and meaning you do more efficient testing in a much more rational order. You carry out your detective work by this process.

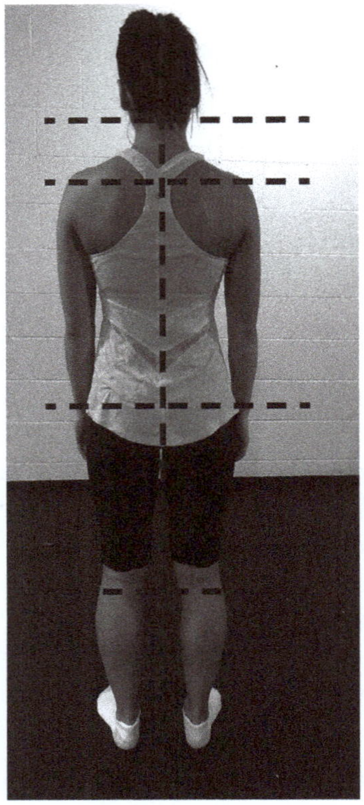

FIGURE 5.13
Posterior view

Have the patient turn with their back to you and have them establish a natural posture. Start between feet, followed by the gluteal cleft, lumbar spine, thoracic spine and ribs, neck and head. Observe the arches of the feet, the orientation of the Achilles tendons, knee creases, etc.

Posterior view

The plumb line starts between the feet, through the gluteal cleft, up through the spinous processes (lumbar, thoracic, cervical) and anion on the occipital bone, and the scapulae should be relatively equidistant from the mid-line (Figure 5.13). Check first if Achilles tendons are straight or on an angle (valgus or, much rarer, varus), then check the levelness of knee creases, PSISs, waist creases, lower angles of scapulae, acromions, occiput and ears.

Palpating and checking landmarks

Once you have made your cursory observations, move closer to the patient and begin palpating bilateral landmarks. Again, start at the feet. Check levels side to side. Though some possible interpretations are presented below, they are only meant as examples. Each chapter later in this text provides more detailed and thorough explanations for such findings.

REMEMBER: Use your dominant eye when checking landmarks, especially as you must be close to the patient. (See instructions on finding your dominant eye in Chapter 3, Figures 3.5 and 3.6.)

Sitting behind the patient Landmark and palpate the levels of the arches of the feet (Figure 5.14), the orientation of the Achilles tendons (Figure 5.15), creases of the knee fossa (Figure 5.16), ischial tuberosities (Figure 5.17), trochanters (Figure 5.18), PSISs (Figure 5.19), iliac crest heights (Figure 5.20), (creases of) waist, inferior and superior angles of scapulae (Figures 5.21, 5.22), acromions (Figure 5.23), mastoid processes (Figure 5.24).

The transverse arch runs across the foot at the heads of the metatarsals. This arch helps the foot to toe-off using the big toe when walking or running. The bone of the big toe is quite large and made to take that stress. When the transverse arch falls, the patient is more likely to toe-off on the second toe, which, being smaller, is prone to stress fracture. Also, not coming off the big toes interferes with the efficiency of walking or running.

In other positions for observation and palpation, supine or prone, for example, you may note that there is a callus under the head of the second metatarsal. This is a sign that the foot is toeing off that toe. This also occurs to those who have Morton's foot (in whom the head of the second metatarsal is further forward than the first or big toe). Further, the fall of the transverse arch can lead to a compression syndrome between the metatarsal heads that pinches a sensory nerve that will grow into a neuroma (see Chapter 7).

There are several possibilities for unlevel ischial tuberosities: (1) there is a bony difference in leg lengths, or a difference in functional leg length; (2) a lower ischial tuberosity on one side may mean that that side's innominate is posteriorly rotated, or that the higher side's innominate is anteriorly rotated; (3) the sign of a *hemi-pelvis*, i.e., that one side of the pelvis (one of the innominates) is literally smaller than the other side. In this last situation, though the ischial tuberosity is higher on a side, the iliac crest on that side would appear level or even lower than the other side's iliac crest height. (See Chapter 9 for more on all of these, and other findings.)

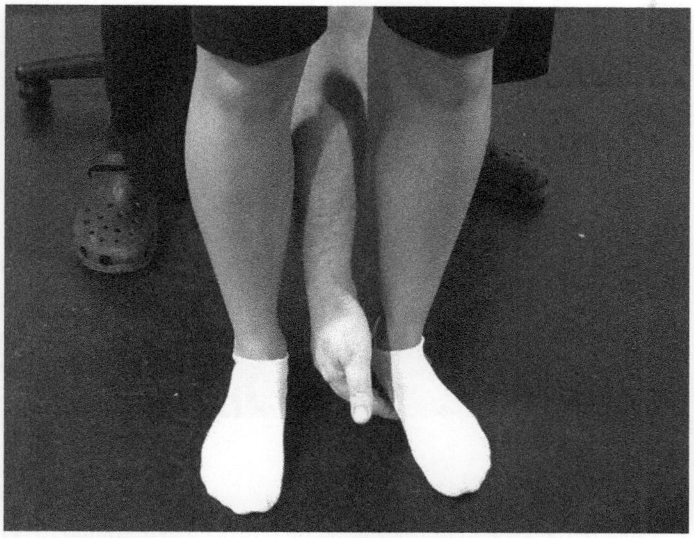

FIGURE 5.14 Arches and feet

Slip the tips of the index and middle fingers as far as you can under one (longitudinal) arch, then the other; compare heights. Note if forefoot (one or both) looks wider than the other (or than normal). If so, then anterior transverse arch may have fallen. (Will check further in prone or supine.) It is best for therapist to be seated behind the patient, or down on one knee.

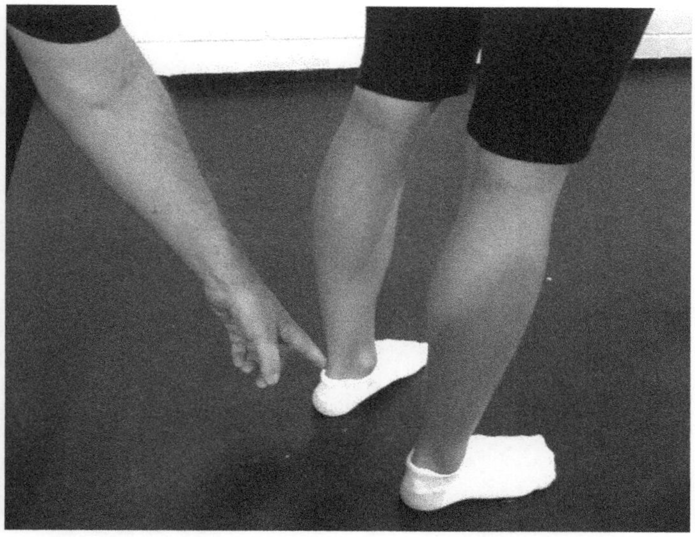

FIGURE 5.15 Achilles tendon

Note the orientation. Normal is vertical. A valgus orientation means that the insertion on the heel is more lateral than it is superiorly at its origin. This implies pronation of the hindfoot. (You can imagine a valgus orientation of the Achilles tendon if you roll your body-weight onto the inside/medial edge of your feet, i.e., pronate your feet).

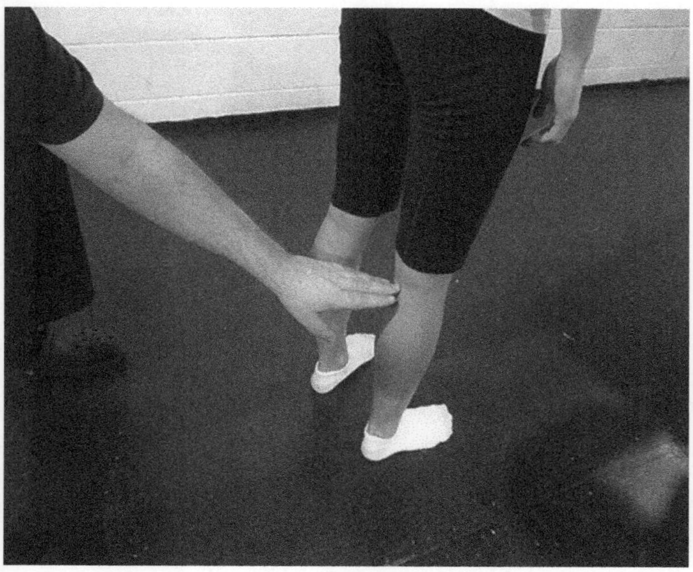

FIGURE 5.16 Knee creases

Note the orientation of the crease at the back (fossa) of the knee. Horizontal? Slightly angled? Compare both sides. May speak to a valgus or varus orientation, or leg-length issue, etc.

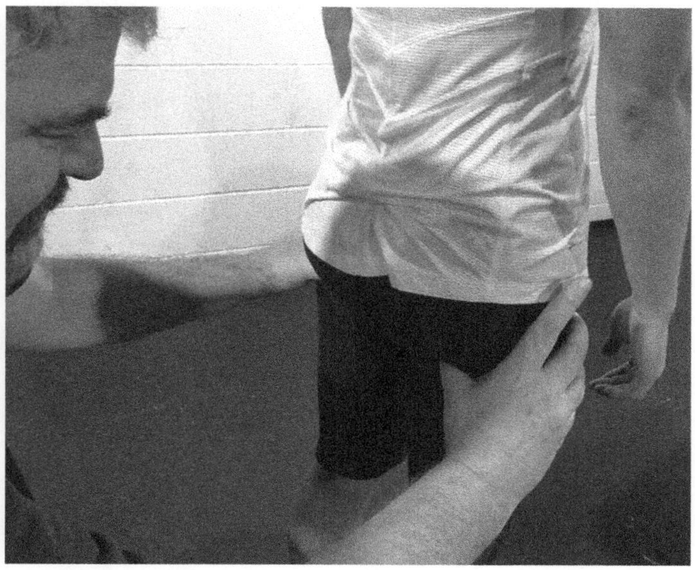

FIGURE 5.17 Ischial tuberosities

Palpate for superior insertion point for hamstrings, where posterior thigh meets gluteus maximus. Need to go deep with pressure directed slightly superiorly.

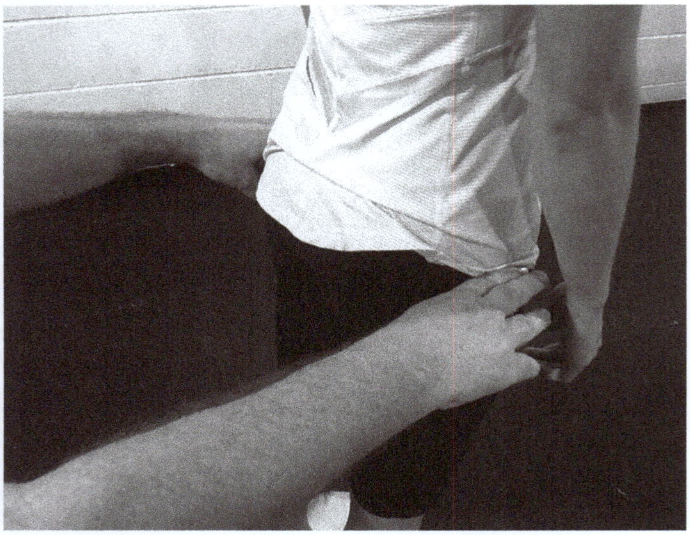

FIGURE 5.18 Greater trochanters

Place edge of index fingers on top of greater trochanters.

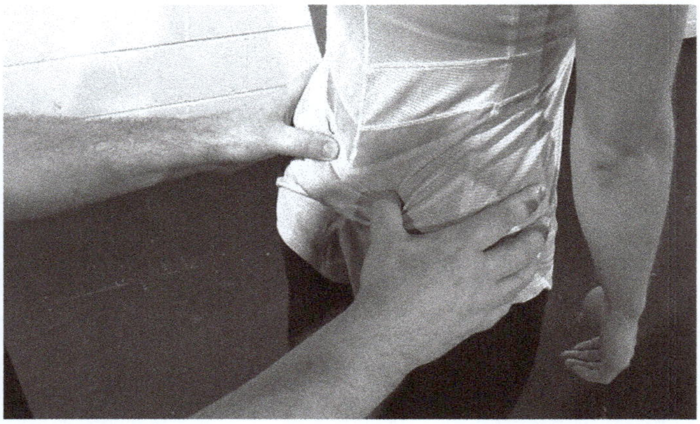

FIGURE 5.19 PSISs

Palpate PSISs bilaterally with thumbs. Tuck edge of thumbs under PSISs in order to compare accurately.

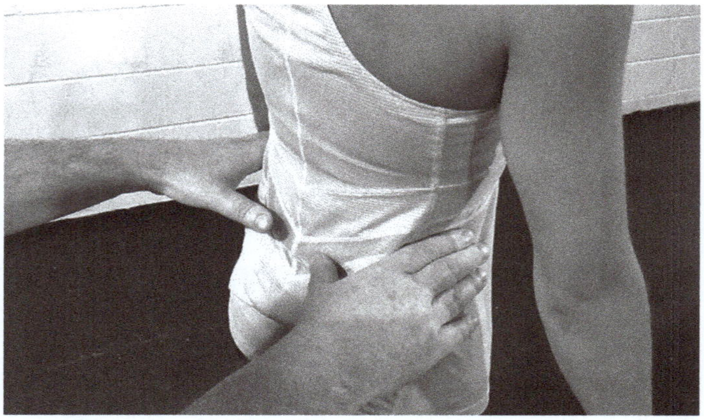

FIGURE 5.20 Iliac crests

Place index fingers on top of iliac crests at most lateral point.

INSIGHTS

Box 5.2 Compensatory structural patterns versus the asymmetry of tensile forces within the body

Sometimes, therapists will go right to the hips, and if the iliac crests appear level they will assume all is well with the lower limbs. Assuming that if there are inequalities they must be successfully compensating for each other, since the hips are level, is a very misleading assumption that could leave you wandering for several treatments trying to understand what is going on and finding no answer. It is not appropriate to assume that compensations that are alternating are benign. They may be benign, but it is possible they are not. What is important is the flow of tensile forces as they move up and down the body. It is these variations of tension (and laxity) that precipitate many impairments or injuries. In fact, someone could look relatively balanced visually, but the imbalance and asymmetry of tension/laxity could still be happening and wreaking havoc on several tissues and joints in the body.

The ischial tuberosities, the PSISs and the iliac crests can call have several possible explanations for their unequal heights. Chapters on the hip and innominate (Chapter 9) and the sacro-iliac joint and pelvis (Chapter 11) have more much on this. As there are numerous, interconnected reasons, we will leave them for discussion in those specific chapters.

However, there is a good possibility (even when inequalities were found in the lower limbs) that the trochanters nevertheless palpate as level. Hidden in those lower limb inequalities may lurk some compensations that leave the hips level (Box 5.2). Or the asymmetries seen may be the body's way of compensating for unequal bone length in the lower limbs. To repeat: like any good detective, you need to be thorough in your investigation.

The PSISs can be very large. Therefore, to try and gauge their level may be misleading if you place your thumbs on their large posterior surface. It is best to tuck your thumbs under the PSISs in order to assess their levelness one to the other. Practice finding this site quickly as it is an area that very commonly needs to be palpated

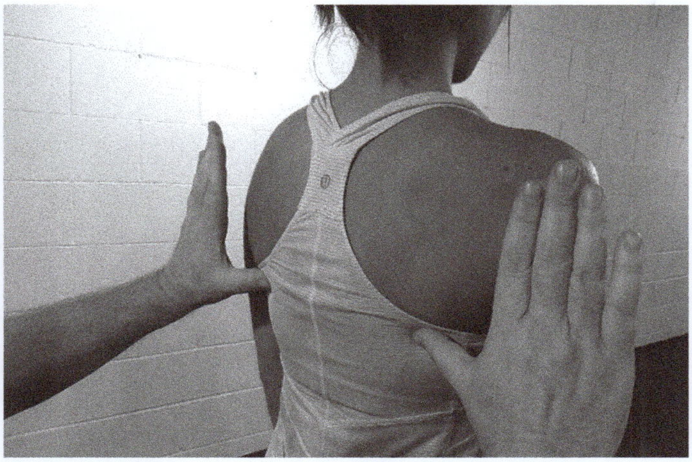

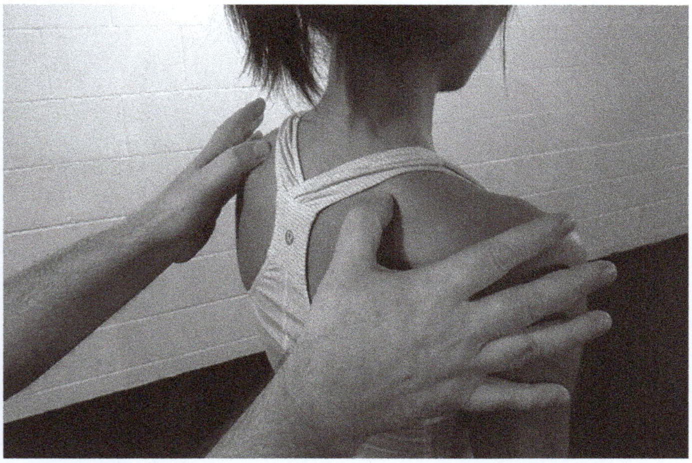

FIGURES 5.21, 5.22 Scapulae

Place the pad of the thumbs under the inferior lateral angles; also compare angles from the mid-line (spine). Further, check the superior lateral angles: they should be only slightly closer to the mid-line than the inferior ones. Palpating these angles and observing the distance of each scapula's medial border from the spine can give clues about curvatures in the spine, or just commonly hint at a protracted (forward) or retracted (drawn back) shoulder.

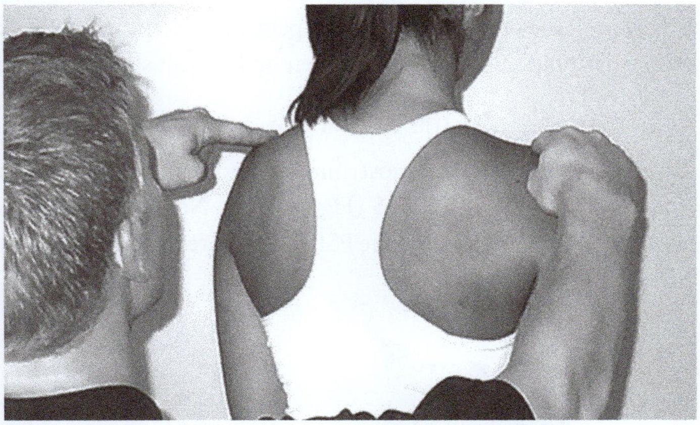

FIGURE 5.23 Acromions

Place the pad of thumbs under inferior lateral angles; also compare angles from mid-line (spine). Further, check superior lateral angles: they should be only slightly closer to the mid-line than inferior ones.

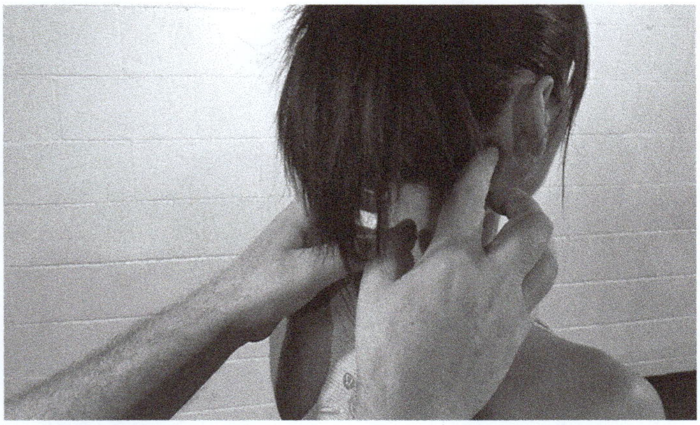

FIGURE 5.24 Mastoid processes

Palpate with tip of index fingers (or pads of thumbs). This helps to establish how level the base of the skull is.

in numerous tests. Some therapists will first find the iliac crests (laterally) and follow their edges down to the PSISs. See below.

NOTE: The levelness of the iliac crest heights may point to there being no serious lower limb inequalities, or that there are successful compensations for inequalities/impairments. They are successful in that things become level, but these compensations may be failing and producing impairments locally and at a distance. It is through the direction and intensity of the tensile forces that compensations above and below are produced. This is what allows a seemingly minor impairment or asymmetry to have such large effects at great distances from that source.

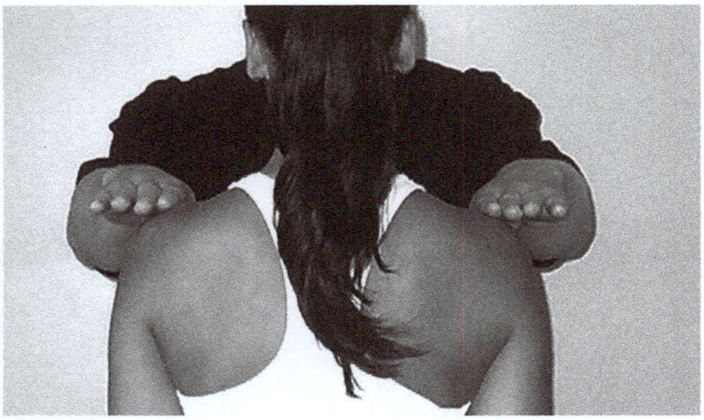

FIGURE 5.25 Head and acromions anterior view

Check orientation of head and levels of acromions.

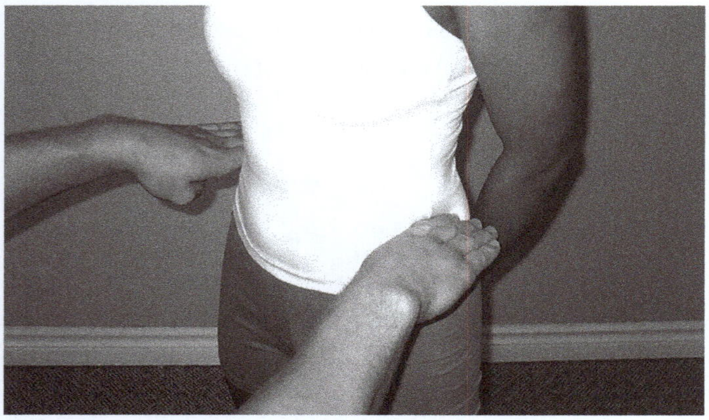

FIGURE 5.26 Iliac crests

Palpate superior lateral edges of iliac crests.

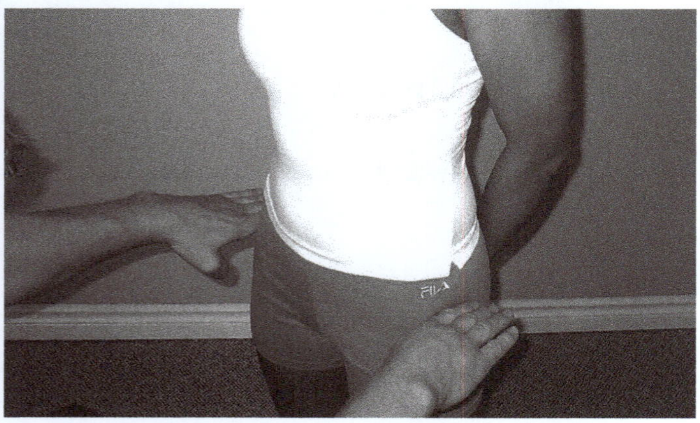

FIGURE 5.28 Greater trochanters

Palpate and landmark the superior edge of the trochanters.

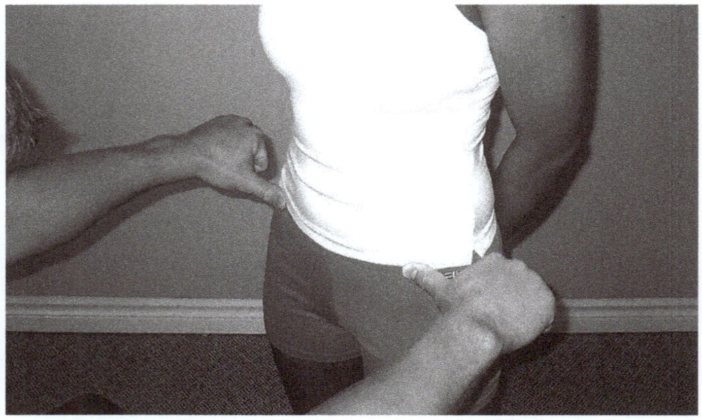

FIGURE 5.27 ASISs

Palpate under side of ASISs.

Anterior landmarking

The primary landmarks to check from the front are the head and acromions (Figure 5.25), iliac crest heights (Figure 5.26), ASISs (Figure 5.27) and the greater trochanter heights (Figure 5.28). Also check the inferior angle of the patella, and repeat the check of the orientation of the feet and their arches (not shown).

Landmarking from the side

From this position, the most import landmarking is done to the ipsilateral ASIS and PSIS (Figure 5.29). Normally, the ASIS should be 5–15° lower than the PSIS. Any more than that amount

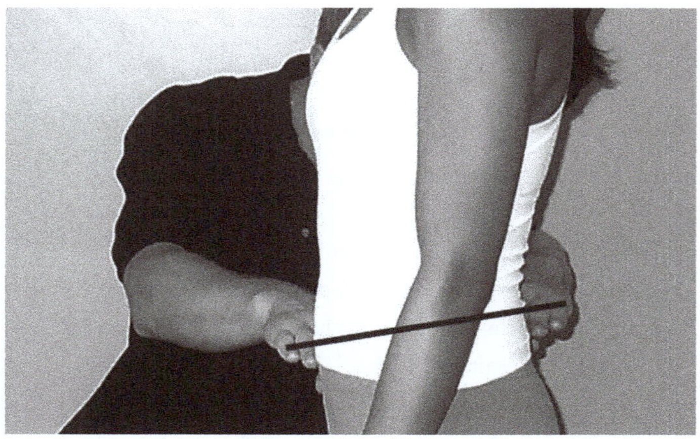

FIGURE 5.29 ASIS and PSIS levels

Tuck edge of one index finger under inferior edge of ASIS and other hand's index finger under inferior edge of PSIS. Estimate levelness or slope. Check both sides and compare.

INSIGHTS

Box 5.3 Postural challenges for stability

Just prior to having the patient sit, you may wish to do a specific postural challenge (Figures 5.30 and 5.31). This is done to evaluate the stability of the patient's overall natural posture.

A patient who has their weight on the heel of the foot will feel that they will topple backward more easily. Often these patients will have a flat back and posteriorly rotated innominates/pelvis. If a patient seems to be more willing to topple forward they have their weight on their toes. In this case, the patient's overall posture, when seen with a plumb line from the side, will show the hips and shoulders to be forward of the plumb line.

Some patients will easily sway back and forth several times with seemingly no preference, either for forward or backward. This implies a sway back, where the lumbar spine is extended (hyperlordotic) at the lowest lumbar vertebrae, which are sitting on posteriorly rotated hips. In addition, the hip joint is in extension, as are the knees. The thoracic kyphosis and cervical lordosis are also exaggerated. (See Chapter 12 for more on this.)

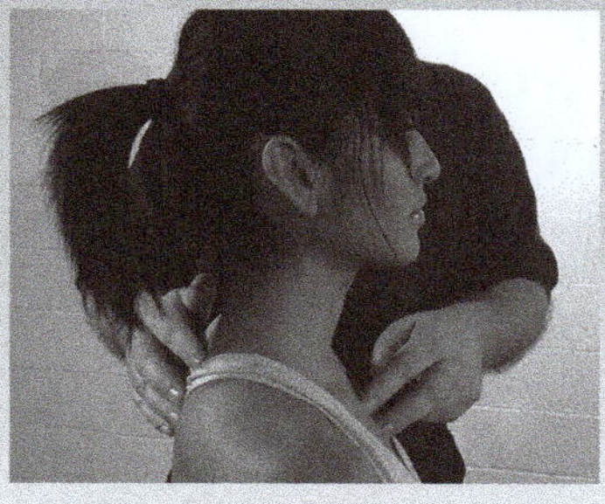

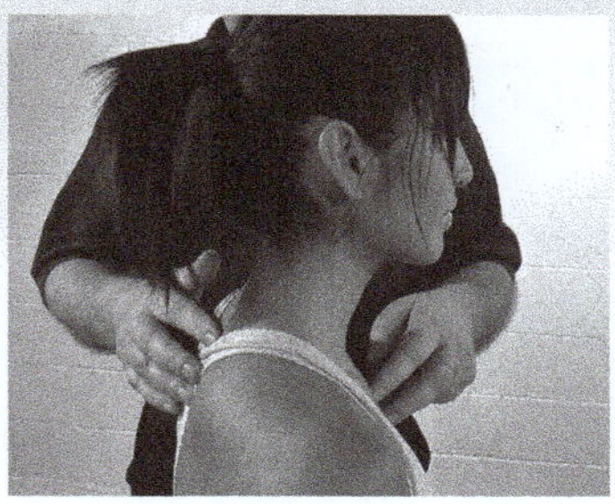

FIGURES 5.30 and 5.31 Anterior–posterior challenge

Place a finger or two on the manubrium and a couple of fingers on and below the C7 vertebrae. Very gently push the patient about 1/2 inch backward and then forward. Observe how well patient can keep their balance and whether they were willing to more easily go forward or backward (or topple).

of anterior rotation and the innominate is said to be anteriorly rotated. If the angle back-to-front is zero or higher (than level), the innominate is said to be posteriorly rotated. You must check both sides, as there usually is a difference. This is invaluable information to have to understand what otherwise might appear as contradictory findings of other landmarks and postural positioning (see Chapter 9 on the Hip and innominate).

See Box 5.3 for postural challenges for stability before commencing your seated examination. See also Box 5.4, below.

Seated postural examination

Important: Note, when the patient sits down, if any of the previous landmarks change orientation, one to another. If some, or most, alter, then this implies that many sources of postural asymmetries found with this patient have come from the lower limbs (hips down). However, if the asymmetries remain, then their sources will be found in the upper body (from the pelvis up).

Asymmetry

If the asymmetries in the trunk do remain, and the iliac crest heights are unlevel, then you may wish to slide a lift (shim) under the ischial tuberosity on that low side. If the patient's left iliac crest is lower by 1/4 of an inch, place a lift of similar height under the left ischial tuberosity and see if the asymmetries stay the same, lessen or disappear. (When using a lift or shim, have the patient sitting on a firm surface.)

If things become (more) level, then our problem is within the pelvis. Either a hemi-pelvis (one side smaller than the other) or, a severe rotation of one innominate to the other. There are two possibilities for this unilateral rotation:

1. A severe anterior rotation of one innominate can shift the ischial tuberosity posteriorly, making that side's innominate seem lower when sitting.
2. Alternatively, a severe posterior innominate will shift the ischial tuberosity anteriorly, making that innominate seem higher when the patient is sitting.

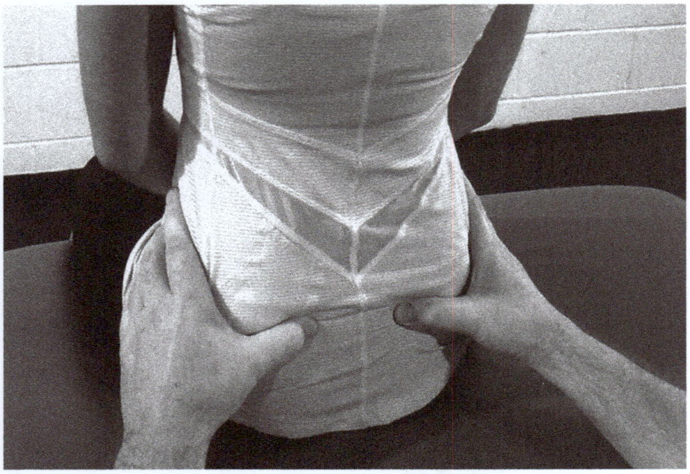

FIGURE 5.32 Check PSISs

Landmark PSISs by placing a thumbs under them.

One hint for unequally rotated hips is a difference in heights of the PSISs (Figure 5.32).

Proceed to re-check the iliac crest heights, angles of scapulae levels and their distance from the spine, as well as the acromion and occiput levels. All of this should take less than 30 seconds.

Rationale for continuing postural assessment in supine and prone

Usually most postural examinations end at this point. The therapist would now try to put together the numerous observations made so far and inter-relate as many as possible into some suspicions.

For example, the patient presents with the pelvis rotated left and the right iliac crest and trochanter appear high, yet the right ASIS is low. This would imply that the right innominate is rotated anteriorly, which also makes it slightly internally rotate (inflare). In turn, the right leg could be functionally longer. However, the right leg is slightly shortened by the right valgus knee, the weight shifted over the left leg and with the right hip also shifted anteriorly (leaving the right leg on an angle which shortens its overall height.)

To help compile these possibilities into suspicions, we may need a little more information. A lot of this can come from supine and prone comparisons of landmarks. Further, even if everything appears different, since we most often treat patients laying on a table, we need to note these changes so that when we treat we can tell if our treatment is producing the results we want as we work, and not have to wait until the end of the treatment to reassess and find if we were successful. Otherwise, we run the risk of continually missing the mark for our outcomes.

INSIGHTS

Box 5.4 Posturally challenging the chief complaint: exploring how the chief complaint fits into the whole

Just prior to having the patient sit, you may wish to do a specific postural challenge (Figures 5.30 and 5.31). This is done to evaluate the stability of the patient's overall natural posture.

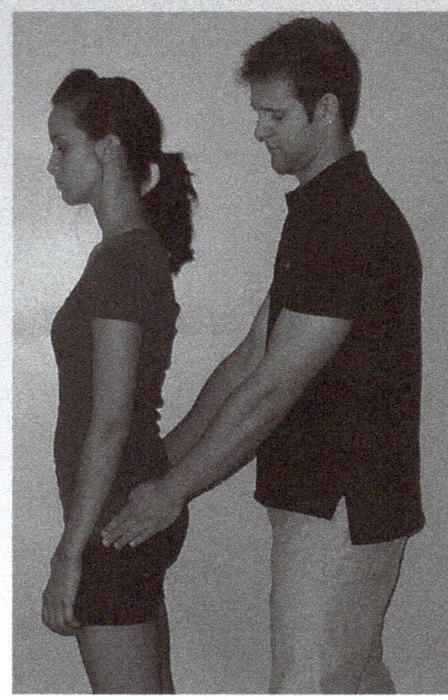

FIGURES 5.33

Observe and gently correct the patient's posture.

As a final step of observation and inspection, look at how the patient naturally stands and correct their posture with gentle movements, if possible (Figure 5.33). For example, push the patient's hips back, unlock hyperextended knees, reposition a forward head over the shoulders and note what changes occur above and below. If the patient can briefly sustain this corrected position, the tension or pain that they may now experience will point to areas that need to be included in your assessment and treatment (i.e., injured, contractured, or weakened/stressed tissues or structures, muscle imbalances, etc.). This will help reveal problems that have a global effect as well as being intimately connected to specific impairments.

Supine landmarking

NOTE: Supine and prone landmarking, while giving more information, may be too much information for a new student. Most of the implications of what is found here will be much better understood once the hip and innominate, and the sacroiliac joint and pelvis chapters have been mastered (Chapters 9 and 11). You will often find these instructions re-occurring there with much more detailed explanations available because the anatomy and physiology (functioning) of the tissues and joints are explained in greater detail.

However, for more experienced students, or for practicing massage therapists, this information may be of use as presented here (Figures 5.34, 5.35). As with the standing patient, we can assist the patient to lie in their natural orientation: the patient is crook-lying. Ask them to lift their hips off the table, and then let them drop back down to the table. The musculature around the pelvis will pull according to their current tautness (short or long) so leave the patient lying supine according to their muscle balance. This overcomes most deviations that are simply caused by the patient lying down or after turning over from a prone position. Have the patient let you passively pull each bent leg into extension. Begin your observations in supine from this point.

Check ASISs (Figures 5.36–5.38)

Findings

- Check if ASISs are level in superior–inferior direction (horizontal plane). This helps us uncover innominate rotations (anterior or posterior). If one ASIS is lower than the other, then that innominate is anteriorly rotated, or the other is posteriorly rotated. Your results above, from the standing side view assessment of PSIS-ASIS levels, will help decide which is which. (See further testing in Chapter 9.)

NOTE: Compare these results with the malleoli levels seen above. This could provide a clue for a functionally long or short leg being present, or the possibility of a bony leg length difference. If the difference seen right to left in the malleoli is matched by the difference right to left in the ASISs, then we may have a functional leg length difference. This is going to have repercussions from the arches of the feet to the levelness of the eyes! Again, there is much more detail on this in Chapters 9 and 11.

- Check if heights of the ASISs from the table are symmetrical (anterior–posterior direction). This may help confirm rotation in the pelvis. ***NOTE:*** It is wise to rely more on the standing assessment's findings of the direction of rotation than on the supine or prone findings. When patients are lying down, the upper or lower body-weight may cause the body part to roll opposite to its standing orientation.
- Distance from the mid-line using the umbilicus gives us clues to inflares or outflares. When the ASIS is closer to the mid-line than its pair, it is called an inflare (or internal rotation of the innominate). When the ASIS is farther from the mid-line that the other, it is in an outflared position (or external rotation of the innominate). Determining which is which will depend on further testing

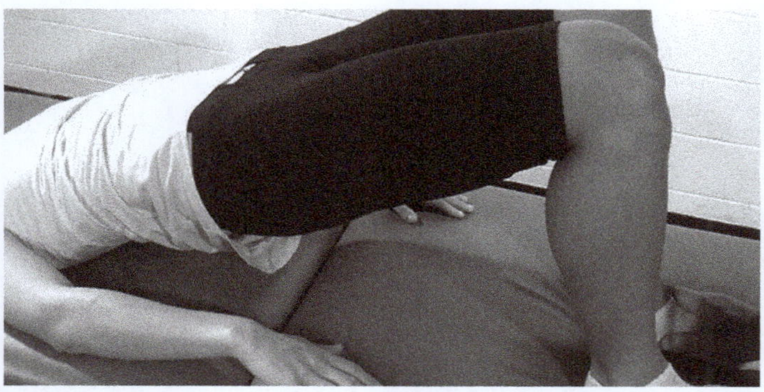

FIGURE 5.34 To achieve a natural position in supine

Crook-lying with hips raised, the patient drops the hips back onto the table and lets the therapist passively straighten one leg at a time. The therapist applies less than one pound of traction momentarily. This traction is not meant to travel past the knees, and is used only in an attempt to negate some inequalities brought about by lowering the legs from crook-lying.

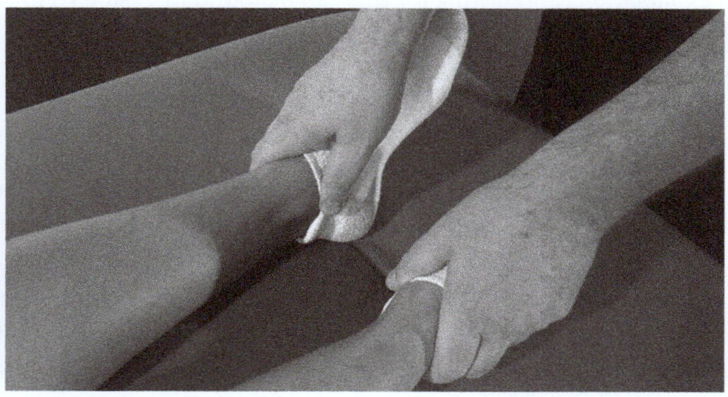

FIGURE 5.35 Natural position supine – ankles

The thumbs need to be under the bottom edge of the malleoli. Observe medial malleoli levels. Note if one leg appears longer/shorter, or equal. You will want to compare your findings here with those found regarding levels of ASISs.

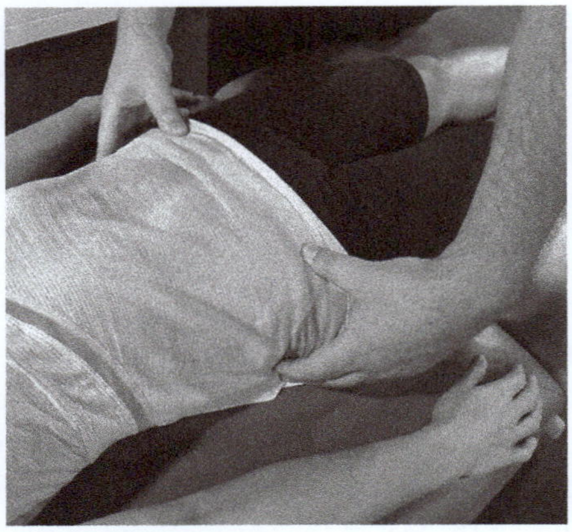

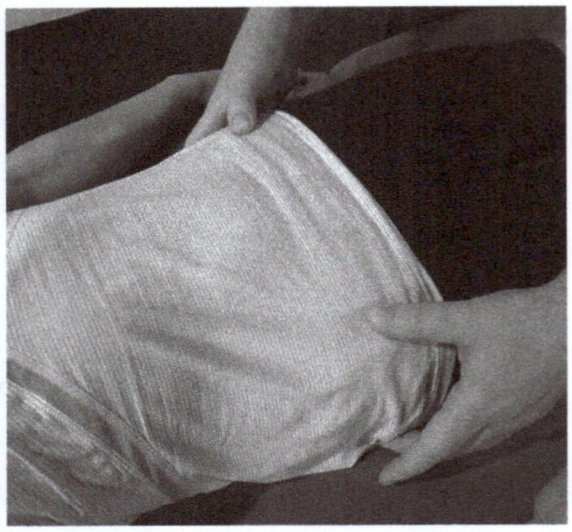

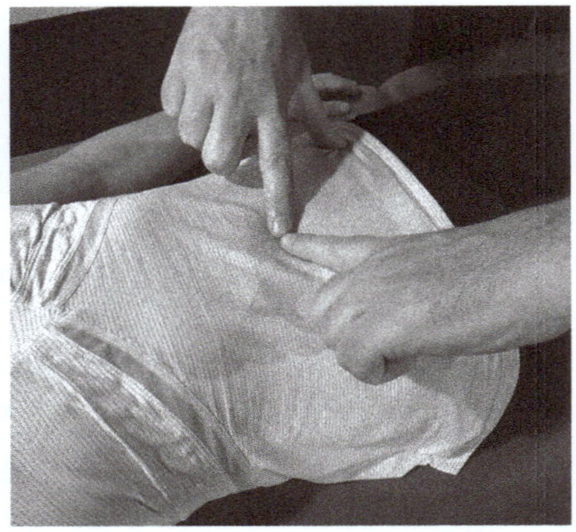

FIGURE 5.36, 5.37 and 5.38

1. **Level of ASISs horizontally.** Have the thumbs under the ASISs.

2. **ASISs heights from table.** Place the thumbs on the anterior surfaces of the ASISs.

3. **Check for inflare/outflare.** Place the thumbs under the ASISs and reach with the index fingers to the umbilicus (navel). Compare distances one side to the other.

and evaluation (covered in detail in Chapter 9). You may have checked for inflares and outflares in the same manner when the patient was standing, but still check when the patient is supine to understand how the body is responding to being supine.

These flares can appear on their own (due to muscle imbalance, etc.) but usually accompany hip rotations: anterior rotation with an inflare and posterior rotation with an outflare. (Further explanations and testing for this can be found in Chapter 11.)

Checking for rotations: a general fascial examination of the trunk and upper body

Introduction to advanced observations

Students should leave the following until they are proficient in postural assessment (in particular) and general orthopedic assessment skills (in general). A more advanced set of observations would be as in Figures 5.39, 5.40. ***NOTE:*** The picture for uncompensated patterns does not actually match the pattern shown. On the other hand, the compensated pattern shown is more like the patient's real pattern.

If asymmetries are found, how does the body compensate? When one area of the body is out of balance, note if the compensations above and below the impairment site are alternating one side to another, or front to back; these are considered moderately successful compensations. On the other hand, do several compensations in a row run the same direction, which is a sign of an uncompensating response, usually indicating a more serious lesion or set of lesions?

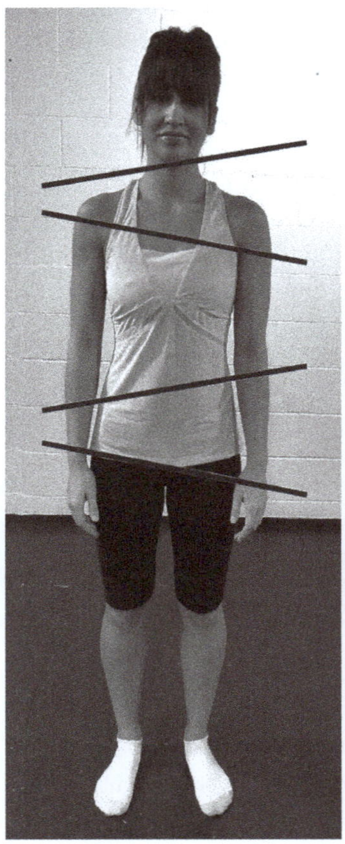

FIGURE 5.39
Compensated pattern

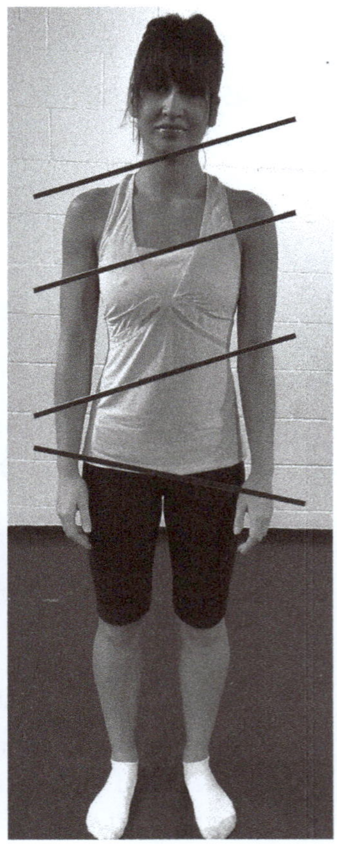

FIGURE 5.40
Uncompensated pattern

For example, if the right hip is higher than the left, a compensating body would have the lumbar spine side-bend right over the higher side. The thoracic spine may compensate, slightly curving left. This leaves the shoulders in a more normal position than the hips.

Using the same example of a higher right hip, an uncompensated body may side-bend also to the right, exaggerating the shoulder asymmetry, forcing the neck and head to try to compensate.

NOTE: Compensatory patterns are discussed in most chapters, looking at how impairment at specific areas may impact on the body as a whole.

Fascial examination Part I

Static assessment of general myofascial patterns (Figures 5.41–5.45, Box 5.5)

We can bilaterally compare the heights (off the table) of the hips (ASISs), lower ribcage, upper ribs, anterior shoulders, and left and right occiput. In other words, check the heights of all of these from the table, comparing one to the other.

NOTE: An alternating pattern is common, and shows the body is compensating efficiently. In this case, a patient may be symptom free, or at worst present with minor pain or impair-

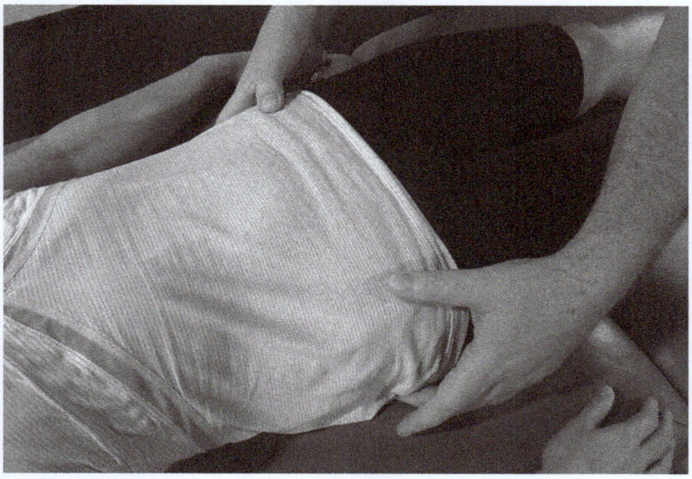

FIGURE 5.41 1. ASIS heights

Note which ASIS palpates as higher off table.

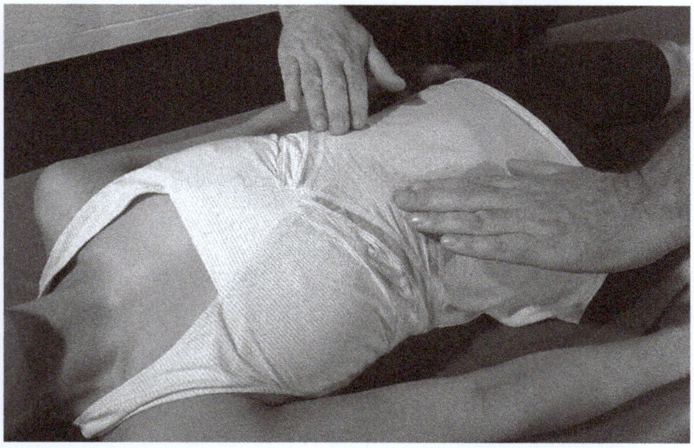

FIGURE 5.42 2. Lower rib heights

Use the lower ribs to compare bilaterally their heights from the table.

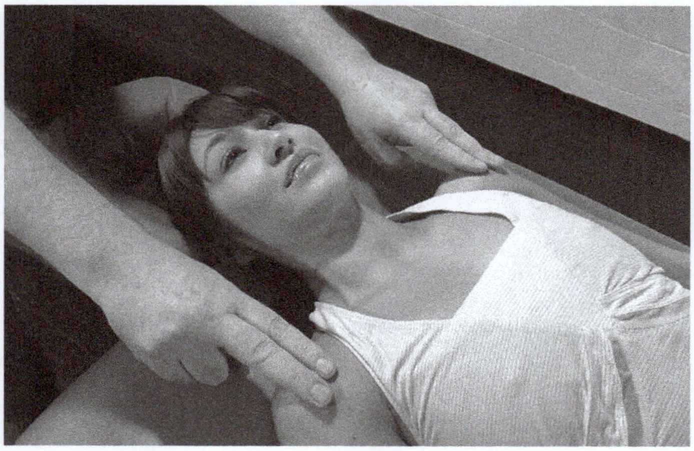

FIGURE 5.43 3. Anterior shoulder heights

Place finger pads lightly on the anterior surface at the head of the humerus.

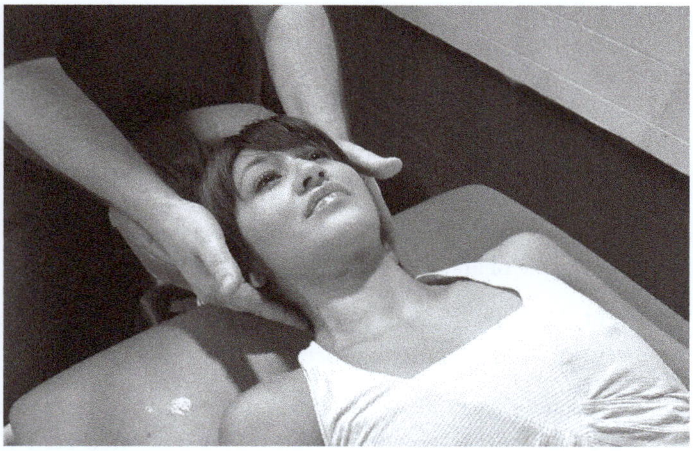

FIGURE 5.44 4. Occiput heights

Check with a single finger pad under each side of the occiput. For greater accuracy, use the mastoid processes.

INSIGHTS

Box 5.5 Upper ribs heights

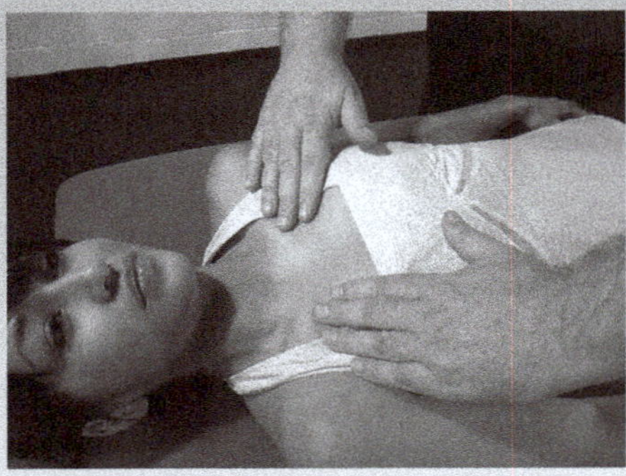

FIGURE 5.45 Upper ribs heights

Finger pads over ribs two and three just below clavicles. See important note below.

NOTE: The reason why you may want to include this area in the landmarking and checking for heights and rotation is because this is a very common area for rib impairment. Further, it reveals the state of the upper thoracic vertebrae, which act as a base for the cervical spine. In fact, many manual therapists, especially osteopaths, consider the first few thoracic vertebrae as functionally part of the cervical spine.

This idea of linking the upper thoracics as part of the cervical spine complex makes it even clearer why the shoulder girdle is used to check the cervical-thoracic junction between C7 and T1. The shoulder girdle is then seen as hanging from a muscular and connective tissue sling, which runs from the occiput down to T3 or T4. The shoulder girdle can then be imagined as a horizontal bar (or coat hanger) extending outward that exaggerates any rotation in this transition zone (just like the ribs can reveal the more subtle rotations or side-bending of the thoracic vertebrae).

The upper cross syndrome, with its protracted shoulders and forward head posture (hyperlordosis of the cervical spine), compresses the upper chest, increasing the torsional forces generated on the anterior portion of the ribs, while increasing the kyphosis in the thoracic region. See the beginning of this section on posture for the upper cross syndrome, and note how well it matches the sympathetic response posture described above.

Further, the upper ribs can be torsioned by the tensile forces generated between the lower ribs being rotated one way and excessive rotation of the shoulder girdle in the opposite direction during use of the upper limb. Excessive rotation of the shoulder girdle in the same direction as the rib predisposes the shoulder girdle, ribs, and/or lower cervical spine to eccentric strain. This makes the upper ribs a very common area for rib motion impairments.

Therefore, it is easy to imagine these upper ribs, the shoulder girdle, and the lower cervical spine as a highly interconnected area and transition zone between the upper cervicals (and head) and the trunk. Further, this interconnectedness has consequences in the origin of thoracic outlet syndromes (TOS), for example.

You can think of the arms as long levers that can put enormous strain and torsional forces through the ribs and upper thoracics if the person performs unbalanced or awkward activities with them, such as pulling, lifting, reaching, etc.

ment. However, if all of one side is high, the pattern cannot be alternating. In this case, a patient usually presents with high degree of pain or impairment.

An example of an alternating pattern is:

Right ASIS higher; **Left** lower ribs higher; **Right** shoulder higher; **Left** occiput/mastoid process higher.

A so-called uncompensated pattern is when two or more of these landmarks are not alternating. This is often seen in patients who present with moderate to severe pain.

Now, compare directions of rotation from one set of landmarks to the next. By noting rotations and their sequence (opposite or same direction), we can see the overall fascial patterning in the pelvis, trunk, shoulder girdle, and head and neck. Be sure to use light touch when landmarking. After all, you do not want to push unequal sides down into the table.

Fascial examination Part 2

Motion palpation of rotational bias at spinal junction zones

No one is without some rotations in the spine or trunk, and this is simply due to handedness. What is telling is whether the rotations generally alternate one level to the next. There are four transition points in the spine that need to be checked. This is done by engendering gentle rotations to the left and right at specific spots. ***NOTE:*** We mentioned in Part I the reasons why and how we could at times be misled about rotations when checking heights of landmarks of a supine patient. The following testing is more reliable as we are checking the quality of motion of structures and tissues.

To check the mobility of these transition zones, simply place two or three fingers under each of the areas listed below. Rock gently and relatively slowly each portion of the body by lifting one side and then the other a 1/2 inch to 1 inch). Look for ease and quality of motion on one side or the other. The side toward which an area of the body is more willing to roll, i.e., it moves toward it with ease, is the direction the myofascial tissues are pulling that side toward (which in supine shows as moved anteriorly). In turn, resistance to movement on one side implies that this side is not being pulled anteriorly, and is probably being pulled posteriorly.

Place your hands/fingers under the:

1. pelvis while observing the quality of pelvic rotation. Check by gently rocking the pelvis up and down, i.e., the lumbosacral junction
2. lower thoracic ribs while observing motion around the waist, i.e., the thoracolumbar junction
3. shoulder girdle while observing the preferred motion direction at the cervicothoracic junction
4. occiput while testing the mobility and preference for rotation at the atlanto-occipital junction.

In the order listed above, check the heights off the table of the specific landmarks. The body is rotating to the side that compares lower at each of the landmarks. If the rotations alternate between the sets of landmarks, the patient is considered to be "compensated." This implies successful accommodation (for now). Therefore, the patient may be asymptomatic or they may suffer from minor to moderate lesioning or impairment.

If the rotations are not always alternating, then the thought is that the patient is *uncompensated*. This is usually found in patients with severe lesions or impairments, often, but not always, trauma-based. Gordon Zink D.O. is the originator of these observations. In his clinical practice (mostly in hospitals), he noted that the uncompensated patient often suffered from some systemic pathology, or an organ, gland disease process, while the compensated did not. An outline of Zink's proposal can be found online in a dissertation on compensating and uncompensating patterns (Pope 2003).

Compensating, uncompensating and rotations: seeing fascial tension directions

The most important information that this can give is to see if the patient is compensating successfully, i.e., are the rotations alternating as we proceed up from the pelvis.

These rotations are accompanied by side-bending (see Fryette's rules of spinal motion in Chapters 10, 12). Side-bending, in turn, lifts one side and its tissues superiorly (creating a convexity on that side) while the other side's structures and tissues are moved inferiorly (concavity on that side). Convexity in the ribs opens up the spaces between the ribs, while concavity compresses several ribs.

Remember in general we can say that the motor for the postural asymmetries we will discuss is muscle. What we are going to describe below is the fascial tensions that can be generated by muscle imbalances. If chronic, these postures will change the length and tension within the overall fascial complex that the body is wrapped in. Therefore, for the purpose of treatment, we not only would have as an outcome the re-balancing of muscle length and strength, but also the overall fascial web as well. If we focus only on muscle we cannot get the results we seek in treatment.

Therefore this analysis speaks about the rotations at special areas of the spine, namely what has been called the transitional joints or areas of the spinal column. Further, it speaks to the tension found in the fascia as a response to these rotations that have become postural due to sustained muscle imbalance.

A very common example of an alternating pattern and an attempt to balance tensile forces is the one below. These observations could commonly be seen in a right-handed person with a right lead foot.

Anterior landmarking

At the pelvis The right hip is often more anterior (off the table) than the left, implying the pelvis (at the lumbosacral junction) is rotated left. This creates an increase in tension of the tissues and fascia between the ASISs.

NOTE: The anterior rotation of the right hip (innominate) is principally ascribed to tight hip flexors: a short and tight rectus femoris tensor fasciae latae (TFL) and the iliopsoas. More is involved than this, but we will leave that aside for now. In turn, the ilium, being attached to the inside of the right innominate and inserting on the lesser tubercle of the femur (medial) along with the psoas, will internally rotate (inflare) the innominate. This inflare is also helped by the TFL.

The right ASIS is closer to the mid-line than the left. In turn, the PSIS on the left is also found to be closer to the mid-line (see Chapter 9). This creates tension and torsional forces running round the pelvis. There is an always an attempt at a balance of forces within any structural asymmetry. The following have similar consequences.

At the ribcage The left lower ribs are higher than the right, implying that the lower ribcage is rotated to the right at the thoracolumbar junction. A myofascial twist, i.e., torsion, is established (from lower ribs to shoulder girdle) in the ribcage, opening some ribs and closing others in a criss-cross pattern: opening the lower left ribs (as if inhalation was happening there) and closing the right lower ribs (as if exhaling). However, the upper left ribs are closed/compressed (exhaled) and the right upper ribs are opened (inhaled). How so? This is because of the next observation: the shoulder girdle is rotated left.

At the shoulder The right shoulder is higher than the left, implying that the cervicothoracic junction (and hence, the cervical spine) is rotated left. (Protracting the right shoulder, tipping the shoulder slightly down, retracting the left and lifting it. The cervical spine above the shoulder girdle often bends and rotates to the left.)

At the head The left mastoid process (or left side of the occiput) is higher off the table, implying that the occiput/head is rotated to the right – at the atlantoaxial joint. Further, the occiput is tipped to the right at the occipital-atlanto joint (by the left condyle of the occiput going into flexion and the right into extension. The consequence of this later adjustment or compensation is for the left space between C1, the atlas, and the occiput to be opened, while the right side's space is closed, possibly compressing neurovascular tissues, etc.).

Uncompensating patterns and ill health However, you may find that one or more of these levels do not compensate in an alternating pattern to the one above or below and we then have what is called an "uncompensated pattern." Two or three junctions may be rotating in the same direction. These tensile forces amalgamate into serious torsions passing through joints above and below as well as on site.

Serious compensatory impairments may multiply, and these forces further traction and/or compress the neurovascular-lymphatic tissues, interfering with their flow. This interference with fluid movements added to all these torsional forces distorting the musculoskeletal posture must inevitably affect the organs of the body. This may explain why Gordon Zink D.O. found his patients with serious health problems and diseases often had uncompensating patterns (Chila 2010).

Prone landmarking

To perform prone landmarking, you can purposely have the patient lie prone; or you may choose to wait for a time when specific testing has the patient lying prone. When you do, check the following: levels of plantar surface of heels (Figure 5.46), ischial tuberosities (Figure 5.47), PSISs (Figure 5.48) (and height

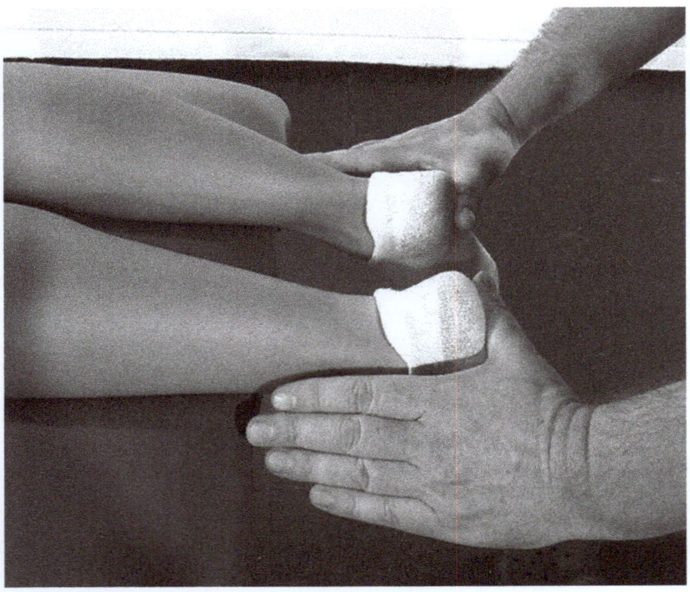

FIGURE 5.46 Heel levels

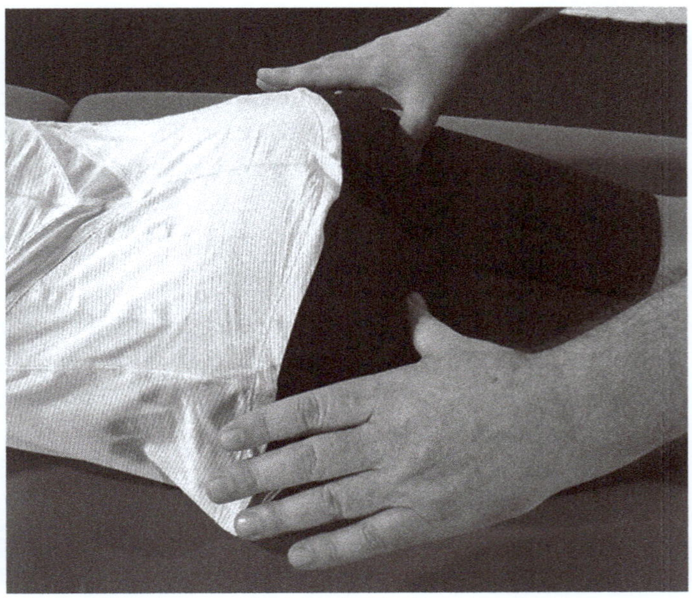

FIGURE 5.47 Ischial tuberosities

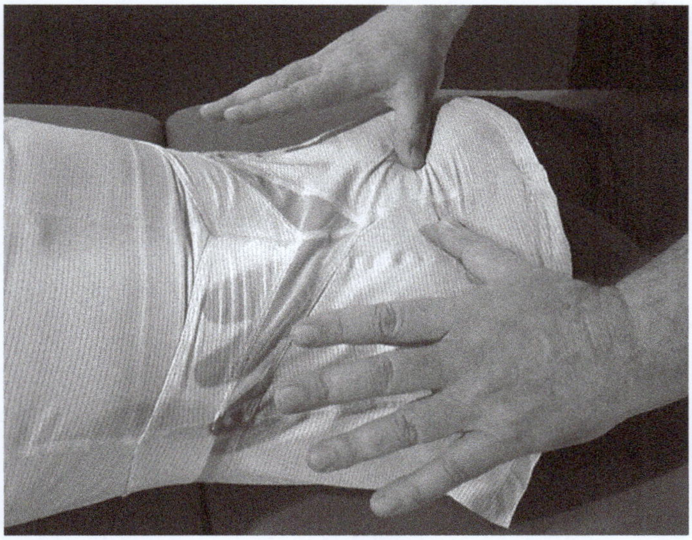

FIGURE 5.48 PSISs

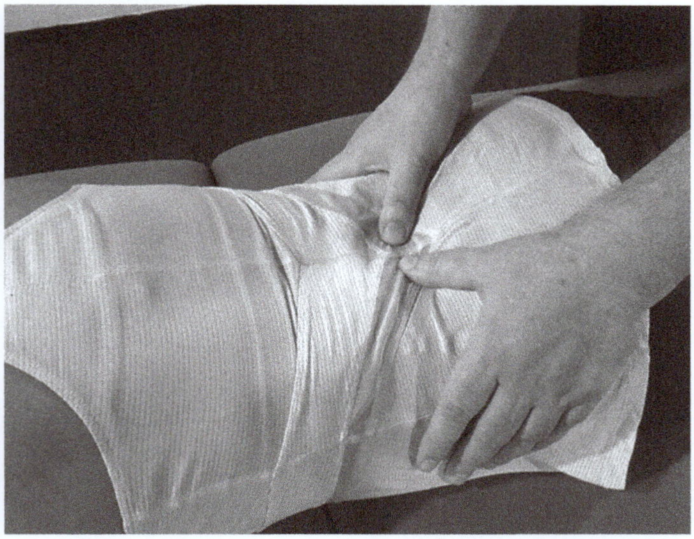

FIGURE 5.49 Lateral curves

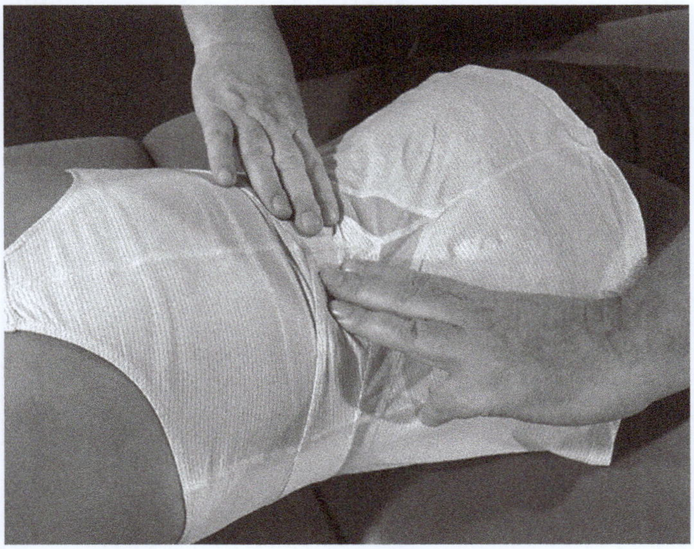

FIGURE 5.50 Tissue bulk of erectors

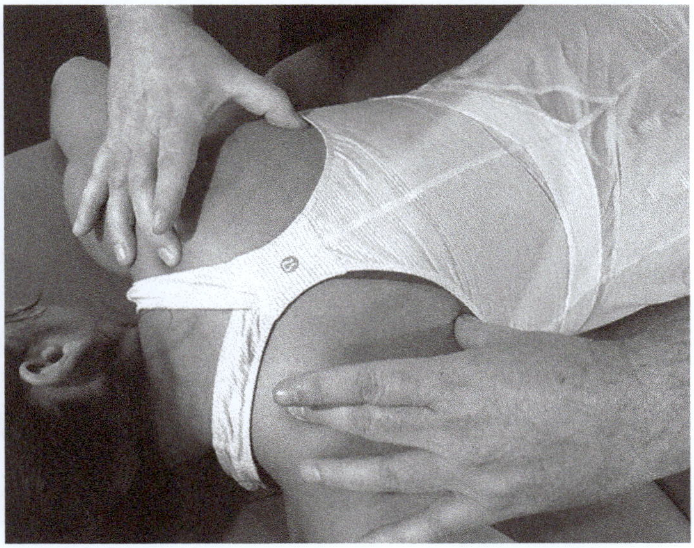

FIGURE 5.51 Scapular orientation

from table), and the lateral curves in the spine (Figure 5.49), tissue bulk of the erector spinae (Figure 5.50), and scapula orientation (Figure 5.51).

Compare your results of prone landmarking with supine, as well as with the results of your standing postural assessment.

Gait analysis

NOTE: This section of the introduction, which is concerned with the assessment of gait, is divided into two parts. Part I is the classic way of analyzing gait, with a few additions. Part II is a different approach to gait analysis, which attempts to see gait within the context of the whole body.

Part I: Classic gait analysis

Introduction

Every standard text on general orthopedic testing will have the basic information on the terms used when analyzing how the patient is walking. These are the classic divisions:

Stance phase

- Heel strike (Figure 5.52).
- Foot flat (Figure 5.53).
- Mid-stance or single leg stance (Figures 5.54 and 5.55).
- Heel-off (Figure 5.56).
- Toe-off (Figure 5.57).

Swing phase (Figure 5.58)

- Initial swing (acceleration).
- Mid-swing.
- Terminal swing (deceleration) (Figure 5.59).

REMEMBER: Just like a standing postural assessment, try to get as many views from various directions as possible. Also, do not try to see everything at once. First, look at the feet as they

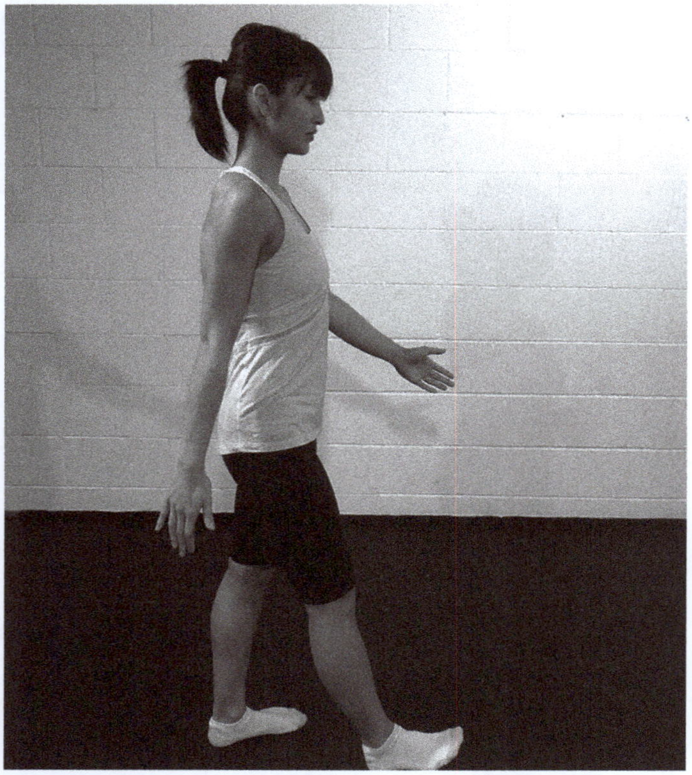

FIGURE 5.52 Heel strike

Also known as loading response. The hamstrings have eccentrically contracted to slow the leg down, and the heel comes to a stop barely above the ground. The landing of the heel should be soft. The tibialis anterior eccentrically controls the lowering of the foot. The externally rotated tibia begins internally rotating and causes the hind-foot (the subtalar joint) to pronate while the tibialis anterior still holds the forefoot (the tarsals, metatarsals and phalanges) in supination. This causes the ligaments of the foot and the plantar aponeurosis to go slack (untwist the foot) so that it can accommodate to the ground, thus allowing the foot to absorb some of the shock of hitting the surface it is walking on. At this point, the center of gravity is at is lowest point during gait.

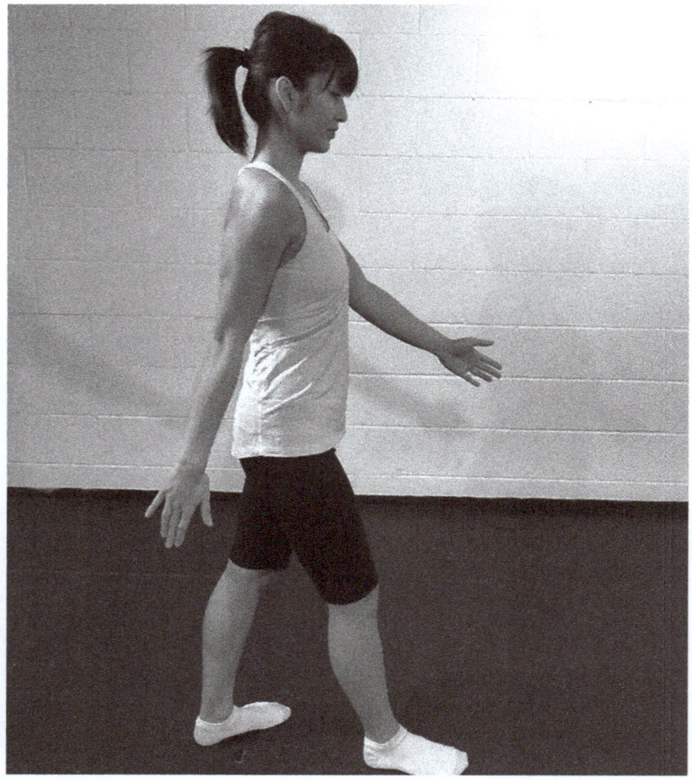

FIGURE 5.53 Foot flat

Foot accommodates to contours of surface. The tibia continues its internal rotation as the foot moulds to the ground. The forefoot will now begin to pronate (full adaptation of the medial longitudinal arch begins). The plantar flexed ankle (plantar flexed as it is ahead of the rest of the leg) now starts to dorsiflex as the tibia begins to come over the foot. Moving now toward mid-stance, the hip also begins to extend, from its flexed position, to bring the trunk forward, and the once externally rotated (at heel strike) hip starts to internally rotate as well, i.e., the internal rotation that started at the hind foot and moved through the tibia, has now reached all the way up to the hip.

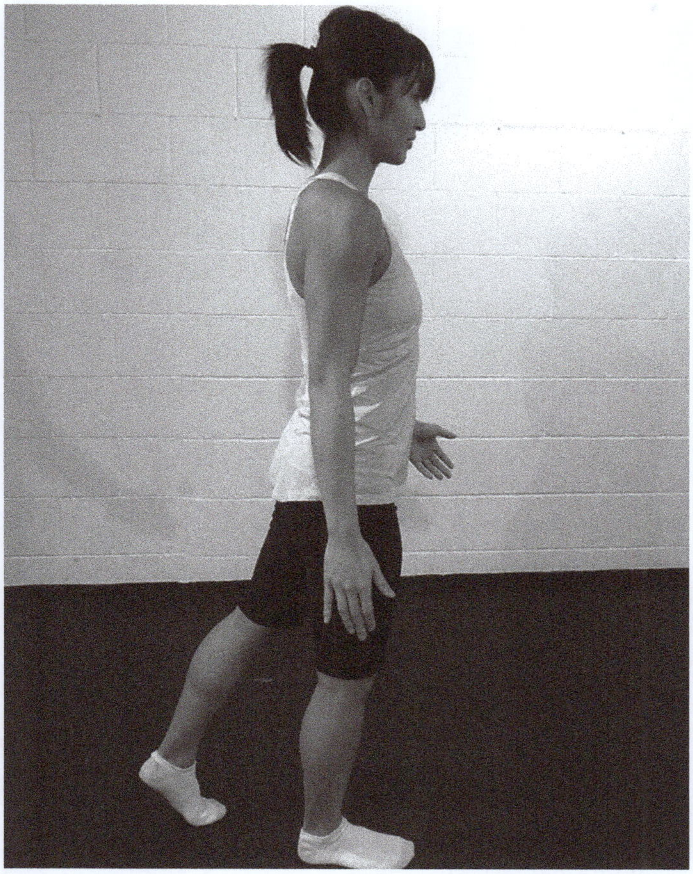

FIGURE 5.54 Start of stance phase
Weight is shifted onto stance leg.

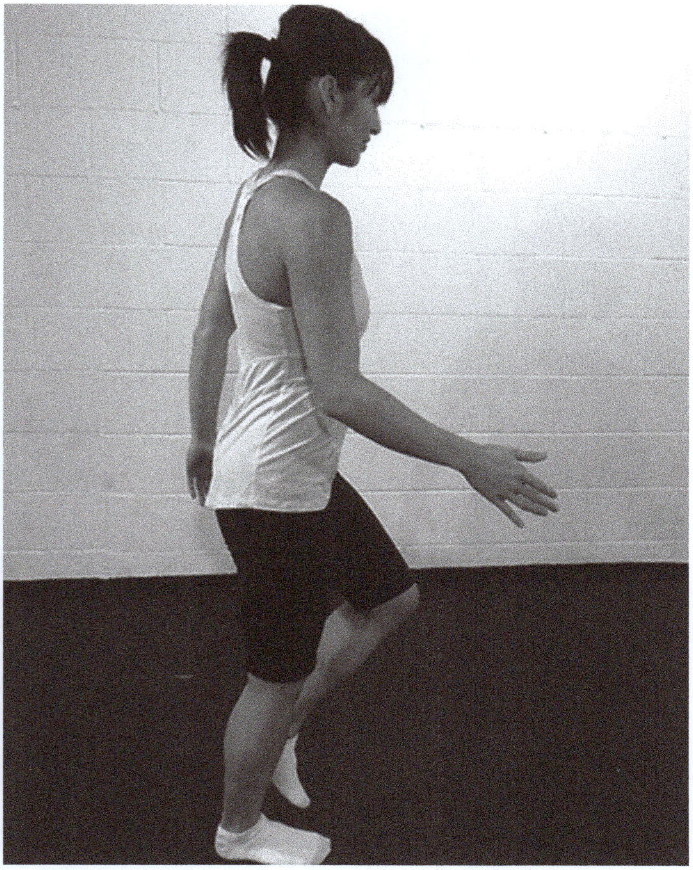

FIGURE 5.55 Mid-stance or single leg stance
Weight all on stance leg.

walk back and forth, then note the knees as they walk back and forth. Then watch the hips, and so on up the body. Lastly, watch all areas working together.

Impairments (Figures 5.52 and 5.53) Foot slap occurs if the tibialis anterior is weak or inhibited. Peroneal nerve lesions are the most common cause of this. Heel spurs will cause a person to avoid heel strike and come down on the flat of their foot or on their toes. Extension lag or the inability of the quadriceps to extend the knee will cause the patient to come down on a flat foot – the tibia will not internally rotate and so the foot will not untwist in order to accommodate itself to the ground.

A fixed (rigid) ankle from joint swelling, or anything causing decreased range of motion of the ankle's mortise joint, will mean the foot cannot plantar flex and therefore it also cannot weight-bear until mid-stance. As a result, the patient will usually hop onto a foot that has a rigid ankle.

The body moves over the stance leg as the trunk is drawn forward by the extensors of the hip. Though the leg is straight, the knee is not locked. Moving into mid-stance: when the hip is extended to 10°, the once straight but unlocked knee begins to flex. The tibia now begins to externally rotate, which means the hindfoot begins to supinate while the forefoot is still pronated and the foot begins twisting, i.e., the opposite of when the foot "untwisted." This is the start of what is known as the windlass effect (Box 5.6), the start of the tightening of the plantar aponeurosis.

Impairments (Figures 5.54–5.56) A locked knee in mid-stance causes a loss of cushioning for the knee, hip and trunk. The gait looks very stiff or exaggerated. Pain may be present with a structural flat foot (pes planus). Over-pronation of the foot will cause a lax or functional pes planus. Either type will jeopardize the stability of the stance, which, in turn, generates muscle guarding due to the body's apprehension of instability. This results in hypertonicity of muscles in all compartments of the leg. The loss in the transverse arch may lead to corns, calluses, or neuromas that cause pain during weight-bearing.

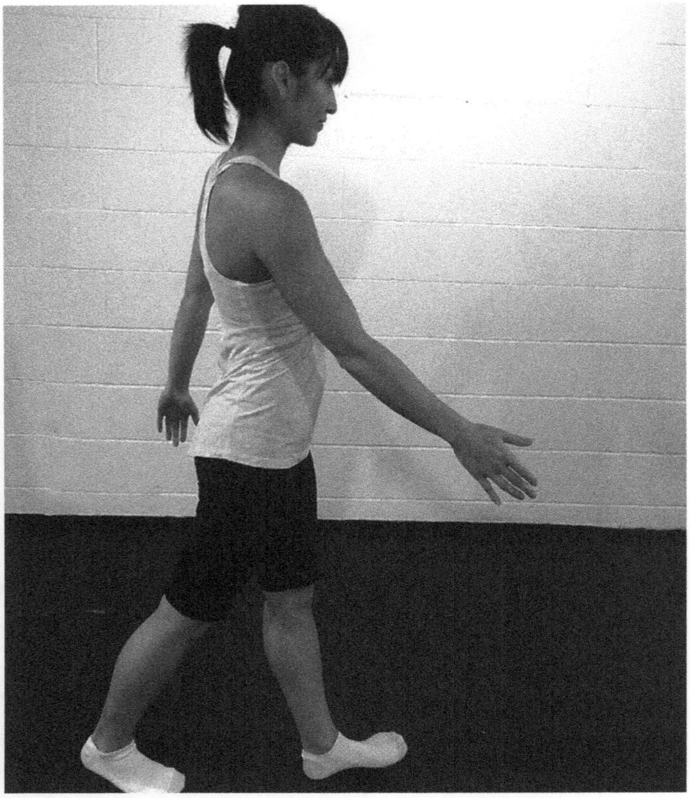

FIGURE 5.56 Heel-off

Heel comes off the ground.

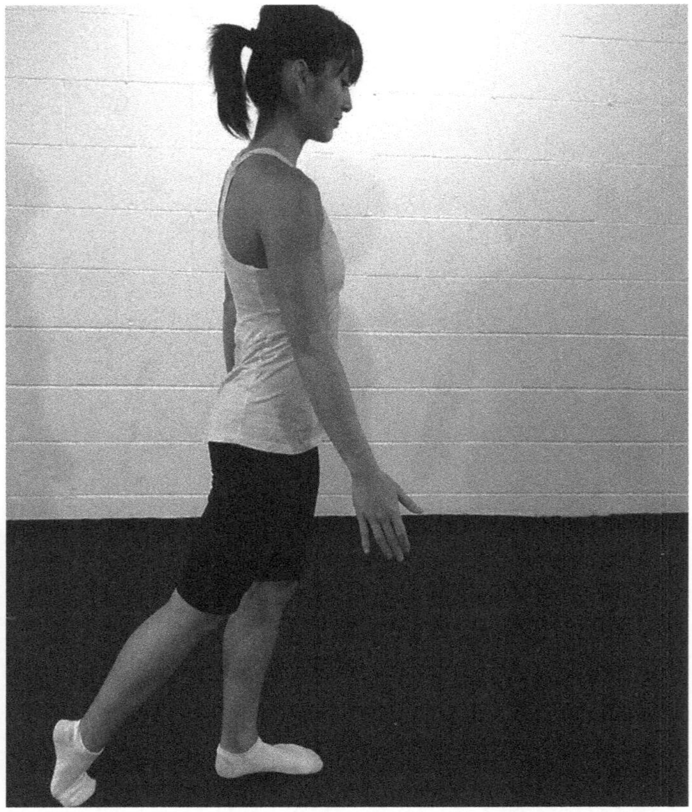

FIGURE 5.57 Toe-off

Toe-off, aka "push-off," occurs.

Trendelenburg gait Weak hip abductors will cause the swing leg's hip to drop, or have the person side-bend over the stance leg to hold up the swing leg.

As the ankle plantar flexes, the weight of the body shifts from the outside of the foot, across the metatarsal heads, and to the first toe. The hip reaches its maximum internal rotation. The center of gravity in the body rises about 1 inch. As the metatarsophalangeal joints extend, the aponeurosis is pulled tight and the windlass effect comes into full force. The foot has now become a rigid lever. This leads to maximum efficiency of the plantar flexors to thrust the body forward. The hip shifts from extension and begins to flex.

Impairments (Figure 5.57) Gastrocnemius-soleus weakness will prevent efficient toe-off. Hence, the patient will not so much push off on a flat foot as lift the foot prematurely using hip and knee flexors as well as elevators of the ipsilateral hip.

A ***rigid metatarsophalangeal joint*** of the first toe will also prevent the patient from toeing off correctly, and the person will instead go off the lateral side of the foot, or even off the whole foot. The same effect happens with a bunion on that joint.

INSIGHTS

Box 5.6 Windlass effect

This is a key function of the foot during gait. It refers to the changes in tension on the foot's plantar ligaments as it enters, holds, and leaves the stance (weight-bearing) phase of walking. The arch of the foot is not meant to be rigid and inflexible. It is designed to mold to the surface it is on. When the heel strikes the ground, the foot is lowered under the control of the tibialis anterior muscle, working eccentrically. The ligaments of the foot will soften, allowing the arch and the bones to mold to the surface they are moving onto. As the foot moves to "toe-off," these ligaments tighten as the arch leaves the ground to stabilize and hold the arch so that the maximum amount of the mechanical energy of the plantar muscles flexing goes into moving the body forward. To see that this works to our mechanical advantage, we need only talk with those who have an arch or two that has fallen. They lose mechanical efficacy and not only does the foot have aches that are painful from the joints and ligaments, but the plantar muscles need to work extra hard to walk and thus tire easily.

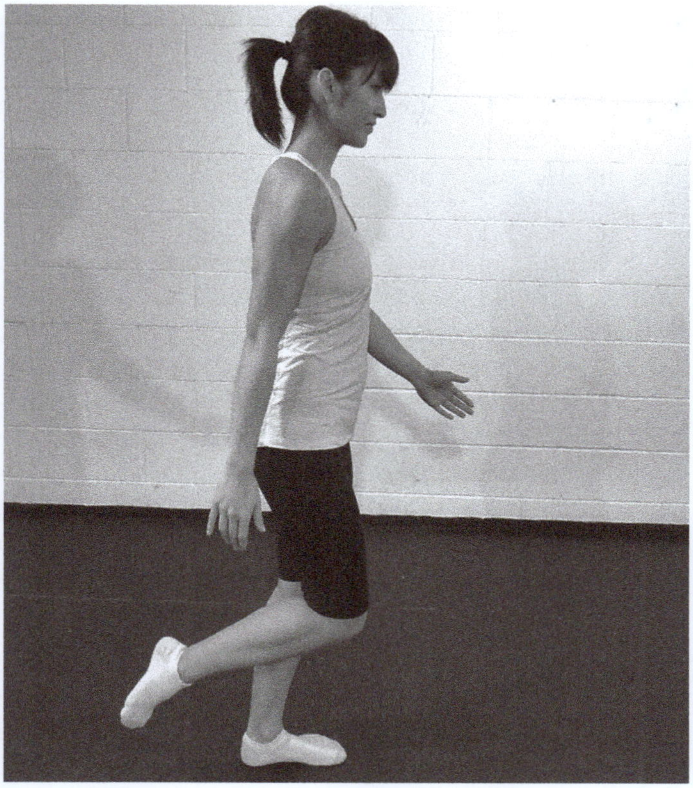

FIGURE 5.58 Swing phase

Swing leg accelerates forward.

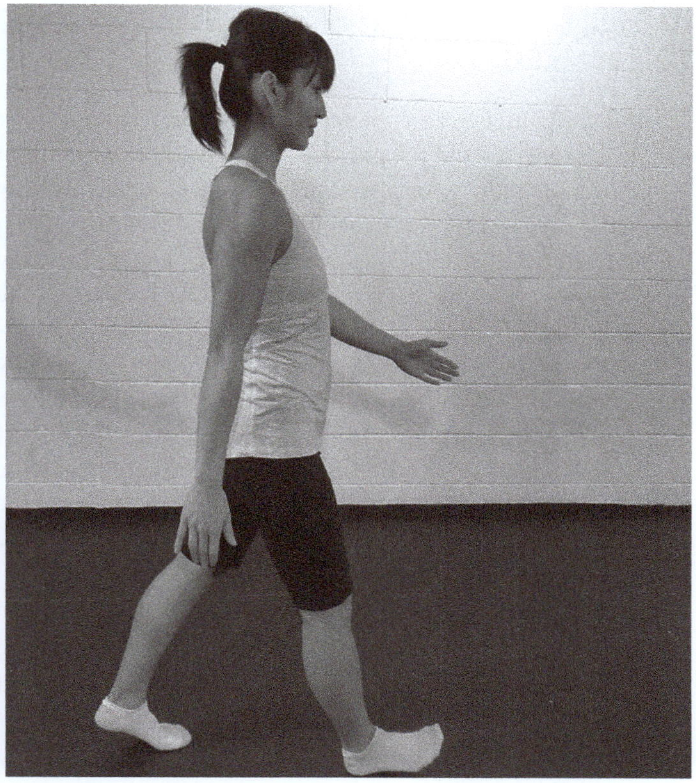

FIGURE 5.59 Terminal swing

Deceleration of swing leg.

A ***fallen arch***, or a ***pes planus***, does not permit the twisting of the intrinsic ligaments of the foot and arch (the windlass effect) and so some of the force of push off is lost. The gastrocnemius-soleus tire easily. Long walks become very tiring for the lower legs, as does standing for a long time.

The initial and mid-swing phase is sometimes called the open kinetic chain stage of gait, because motion happens without any weight on the limb. The ankle dorsiflexes to help the foot clear the ground as it swings forward. The knee is flexed to 65° to also help the foot clear. The hip flexors are engaged to throw the leg forward. The hip becomes flexed and remains medially rotated and now becomes slightly raised as well: all of this assists the foot to clear the ground. While the knee remains flexed, the ankle and phalangeal joints return to neutral, leading to an unlocking or untwisting of the metatarsal joints (forefoot). The aponeurosis is slackening, unlocking the arch.

Impairments (Figure 5.58) Hip flexor weakness (L2) will cause the patient to lurch the trunk backward to use tissue stretch to help throw the leg forward (gluteus maximus lurch – posteriorly rotating pelvis).

Steppage gait Tibialis anterior (L4) is unable to hold the foot dorsiflexed so the patient excessively flexes the knee to help the foot to clear the ground.

Impairments (Figure 5.59) Thumping heel occurs when a person's heel(s) hits the ground hard with a thump. The hamstrings may be short, stopping forward momentum of the foot too soon. The heel is higher off the ground than it should be and so drops, causing the heavy step. If the hamstrings are long and weak, the leg will overshoot and the heel will drive itself into the ground, creating a jarring effect as the person walks. Either way, the person often makes an audible thump when walking on some surfaces.

The hip begins to externally rotate as it moves from mid-swing. It reaches its maximum flexion at 30–40°. The hamstrings are now eccentrically engaged to slow down the forward momentum of the leg. This provides a soft landing for the heel. As the knee moves to become fully extended (but unlocked), the tibia externally rotates. The foot is supinated and the arch is softened to allow the foot to be able to mould to the ground. Heel strike is next.

Now, repeat the assessment of gait on the other side of the body.

Part II: Gait – an alternative view and analysis (Figure 5.60, 5.61)

Walking is a full body action, from the temporalis to the flexor digiti minimi. Most of the musculature in the body is working (contracting) either concentrically or eccentrically, directly propelling the body or stabilizing structures so that gait can occur. A healthy human is capable of walking all day. The body is designed to employ contracting muscle, and also access the recoil inherent in myofascial connective tissue. Below is a simplified model of the tensile relationship occurring in the body during gait. For example, on right heel strike, I imagine walking to be like two cylinders, one on top of the other, turning toward each other for 30–45°. By the time of heel strike on the right, the tension in the lower body to turn left and the upper body to the turn right has reached its maximum.

In the front of the body

On right heel strike, the solid diagonal line is contacting in the front. It represents the flexors (of the ankle, hip, the internal and external obliques, pectoralis major and minor, and the flexors of the arms).

- The right leg is forward, while the opposite shoulder is also coming forward. The shoulder and arm are flexed as well.
- The right lower body is turning to the left, while the upper body is turning to the right.

While the other side's diagonal broken line (representing the opposite flexors) lengthens, the muscles are contracting eccentrically.

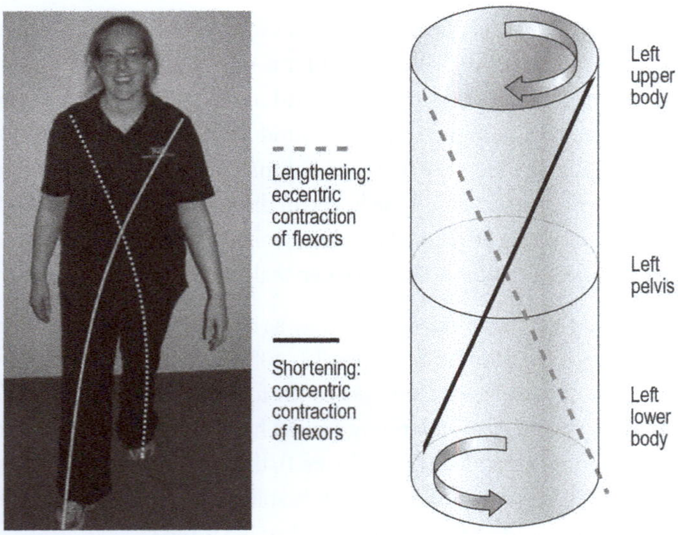

FIGURE 5.60 Anterior view, right heel strike

- The left leg is posterior, while the opposite shoulder has also gone posterior.
- The lengthening or stretch of the left upper body over to the right shoulder reaches its maximum. This generates tension in the myofascial connective tissue, some joint capsules, ribs and ligaments.

This connective tissue can store energy which, as recoil, can assist in propelling the body forward when it is needed. Therefore, as the person progresses from heel strike on one side (e.g., on the right) and is moving toward heel strike on the other side (the left), this stored energy will be combined with the concentric muscle contraction of left hip flexors, etc. It is as if the opposing rotations within the body load a spring (elastic material), which it then uses to assist muscles in alternately moving each side of the body forward. Therefore, the muscular force to take each step is not all used up with the step, but much is recycled via this connective tissue recoil.

Just to digress a bit, the eccentric contraction is happening in the lengthening muscles in order for the body to achieve smooth rhythmic motion while walking. Therefore, all of the muscles are always working, concentrically or eccentrically. They are not turning on and off but switch smoothly from shortening to lengthening under exquisite control, like a dance. This is happening from the temporalis assisting the jaw to remain properly positioned as motion moves through the body, while the head remains forward looking; to the digiti minimi controlling the baby toe's motion from weight-bearing to repositioning to become once again adaptive to the surface the body is walking on.

From behind

The right latissimus dorsi and other extensors of the shoulder pull the right shoulder back, and rotate the trunk (anterior view) to the right, while the arm extensors pull the arm into extension.

- While the other side's diagonal broken line (representing the opposite set of extensors) lengthens, the muscles are contracting eccentrically.
- The right extensors of the leg, the right piriformis, and the left latissimus, along with the left arm are lengthened, or on stretch. The right quadratus lumborum has finished working concentrically and is beginning to work eccentrically.

Imagine the two contracting lines working together

- These two lines of concentric contraction cross the body from opposite sides: one anteriorly (right foot to left shoulder) and one posteriorly (from the left foot to right shoulder).

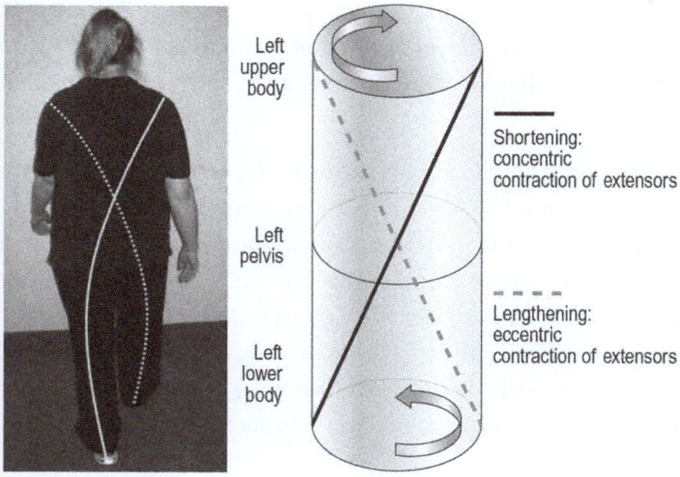

FIGURE 5.61 Posterior view, right heel strike

- An anterior diagonal line of contraction from the right hip flexors (and across the abdomen, up into the left shoulder) is matched with a contraction of the posterior diagonal left hip (etc.) extensors. These two propel the right leg forward. This has the lower body rotating left (in the anterior view).
- Further, this is matched by the trunk musculature rotating the trunk to the right (anterior view) and the left shoulder musculature swinging the arm forward: the two contracting lines thus turn the upper body to the right.

Imagine the two lengthening lines working together

- These two are diagonal across the body: the anterior lengthening line runs from the left foot to the right shoulder, and the posterior lengthening line runs from the back of the right heel to the back of the left shoulder.
- At the same time as the contracting diagonal lines are working, the two lengthened diagonal lines have stored some of that energy used and will now use it to assist the left leg and the right shoulder to come forward as the body moves toward left heel strike.

Each step we take uses direct muscle contraction assisted by connective tissue recoil to move forward. This relationship makes walking a smooth alternating action, which can be sustained easily for long periods of time.

The diagonal lines shown in Figures 5.60 and 5.61 are not, of course, flat, but are three-dimensional curved lines. The anterior and posterior concentric/shortening contracting lines are actually concave; while the anterior and posterior lengthening (eccentrically contracting) lines are curved convexly.

Visualization experiment

It is hard to show the two concave and two convex lines on a two-dimensional page. Therefore, it is best if the reader stands still in a right heel strike pose and imagines the following:

The front of the body As you look down at the front of your body you can visualize the concave (shortening) line running from the right foot, up the leg, up across the abdomen (from the right hip to the left lower ribs), to the left shoulder, and the swing of the left arm forward. In turn, you can imagine the (lengthening) convex line running from the left foot, up the left leg, moving from left to right (through the obliques) across the abdomen, and into to the right shoulder, while permitting the right arm to swing posteriorly into extension.

The back of the body You then should imagine the posterior concave (shortening) line from the left heel, up to the hip, across the gluteus maximus and aponeurosis into the right low back, and up into the right shoulder, extending the right shoulder. Now imagine the posterior (lengthening) convex line from the right heel, up the leg, across the aponeurosis (right to left), up into the back toward the left shoulder, letting the left arm swing forward in flexion.

- If you now walk in slow motion, you can visualize how these lines alternate side to side and front to back as you walk. Also, it is relatively easy to visualize the recoil happening from the shoulders, in concert with the swinging of the pendulum-like arm movements, and see how both can play a large role in moving the body forward during walking.
- Therefore, the trunk is not just pulled along by the hip flexion of the right, and pushed from behind by the extension and toe-off. As the left arm swings forward along with the shoulder pulling itself forward (on right heel strike), the trunk is moved forward by the momentum of this mass of tissue. In a sense, we could say that the trunk is moving itself forward through its portion of the shortening/contracting lines and the lengthening diagonal lines.

Pelvis and abdomen: transition area for the contracting diagonal lines

Let us discuss the structures and tissues that contract and shorten across the front of the body, and then across the back of the body.

In the front of the body In this example of right heel strike, with the flexors of the hip contracting, the right internal oblique, working in concert with the left external oblique, directs the tension across the abdomen over to the left upper trunk.

- The right internal oblique's attachment on the right iliac crest and inguinal ligament pulls that right hip (innominate) up in front while posteriorly the tension from the stretching tissues (especially the connective tissues) draws the posterior iliac crest down. This results in the posterior rotation of the right innominate.

In the back With the extensors of left the hip contracting, the transition to the right trunk begins with the left gluteus maximus. The contracting force passes into the left quadratus lumborum and across the low back aponeurosis, continuing up through the aponeurosis into the right latissimus dorsi and into the right shoulder.

- The stretch of anterior connective tissues within the hip flexors (iliopsoas and rectus femoris) and the iliotibial band pulls down on the left anterior portion of the innominate. This results in the anterior rotation of the left innominate.
- The left forward shoulder and trunk, rotating right, stretch the left quadratus lumborum, etc., and lift the posterior iliac crest upward, assisting in the anterior rotation of the left hip.

Reminder: Much more detail and explanation concerning the movement of the hips and pelvis and muscle involvement is to be found in Chapter 11. See also Box 5.7.

Stumbling

What we have described so far concerning gait has assumed that all body parts are working together in a coordinated manner. However, injury, muscle imbalance, or physical asymmetry can throw a wrench into this wonderful clockwork movement. I hope that having read this far, it is clear that any impairment in any part of the body must influence, to some degree, one's gait. A shoulder injury that limits the swing of the arm will affect directly the motion of the contralateral hip and leg (and indirectly, everywhere). Even something as seemingly harmless (to gait) as forward (protracted) shoulders will affect the storage and use of potential energy from the lengthening diagonal lines. A tight hamstring on one side will decrease the length of stride on one side and further, impact on the efficient use of energy expended by the antagonist flexors.

Alternative whole body or comprehensive analysis of gait

In many ways, therefore, it is helpful to see gait as a whole body process, especially when looking for the source, or sources, of impairments to gait. In turn, it is suggested that one of the most helpful ways to perform a gait analysis is to imagine the diagonal lines, convex and concave, as the patient walks.

In brief, the following is the order for testing gait with this alternative model. When you notice an impairment with gait, note whether it is most apparent when the structure or area is a shortening or lengthening line and whether it is most obvious from a posterior view or an anterior view. If equally obvious from front or back, then choose one to begin your assessment with. Whichever line it is, whether anterior or posterior, start with your observations focusing on that line first.

Observations in brief

NOTE: When observing a patient walking (toward or away from you) either from an anterior or posterior view, do so in the following manner:

1. Look at the line as a whole.
2. Focus down to region, then specific site.
3. Look now at structure when line changes (from shortening to lengthening, or vice versa). However, now observe structure or tissue specifically on site, then regionally, and finally as a whole line.
4. Lastly, take a lateral view.

Observations in more detail

Look for asymmetry of movement in general, and only then focus more closely on portions (regions) of both the shortening and the lengthening diagonal lines to identify the (specific) location of the problem. To evaluate an impairment's nature and its impact, scan down the diagonal line associated with that structure/tissue.

1. First as a contracting/shortening line, watch the whole line, anteriorly, then posteriorly (or vice versa).
2. Only after seeing the line as a whole in action, begin to focus on parts (regions) of the line. Narrow down to observing the distinct impairments visible during gait. If possible, identify any effects that this impairment seems to be having on other regions of the body involved in that diagonal line. Again, anteriorly and posteriorly.

The advantage of finding two or more asymmetries of motion, impaired motion, or what have you, is that one is less likely to be led astray. All too often, the compensatory (or secondary) impairment is more obvious than the original cause or issue. Seeing the whole line as a continuum enables a more comprehensive or whole-body analysis. This also provides available optional sites to investigate and treat if the treatment of what seemed the principal impairment does not rectify the patient's complaint. You know where to begin looking as you reassess.

I have often found in my clinical practice that the fish I most often catch are red herrings! Nevertheless, once you have those out of the way (or have minimized them), the real culprit will stand out.

3. Throughout the gait analysis, also look at the tissues involved in impaired movements seen in the shortening line and how they, in turn, function or behave during a lengthening/energy storing line. This, too, may reveal other culprits or reveal more about a specific impairment noted previously.
4. You also need to look at the posterior matched contracting line: when problems are seen in one region and, for example, very clearly in an anterior line, there will have to be repercussions in the posterior lines. Again, what may seem subtle or minor from an anterior view could, with a posterior view, reveal itself to be a major impairment.

INSIGHTS

Box 5.7 More than you may want to know about the motion within the pelvis and the sacrum ... at least for now

All of this (both information and theorizing) is explained more fully in Chapter 11.

Continuing with our example of right heel strike: the symphysis pubis (with its articular disc) permits the right abdominal internal oblique (via its attachments) to pull the right ramus of the innominate to rotate superiorly (right innominate as a whole rotating posteriorly). The left ramus rotates inferiorly (as the left innominate rotates anteriorly). However, things are not so simple at the back of the pelvis.

Torsional forces must pass through the sacroiliac joints. The motion of these joints is minimal, but crucial. Due to the orientation of the sacroiliac joints, and the fact that there are two joints here, somehow the sacrum has to accommodate the two opposing motions of the right and left innominates. In a sense, the sacrum is forced to squirm between these moving innominates. With a right heel strike, the right side of the sacral base (the right superior portion of the sacrum) will move anteriorly relative to the posteriorly moving right innominate. It is not so much that the sacrum moves as it resists moving with the innominate. On the left side, the left sacral base resists moving anteriorly with the left innominate; it moves slightly posteriorly relative to the left innominate rotating anteriorly.

As the right innominate rotates posteriorly, it is also moving inferiorly. The innominate, by necessity, will drag the sacrum along somewhat, tilting the sacral base to the right. This is assisted by the left innominate's posterior portion moving superiorly (as the innominate as a whole rotates anteriorly), slightly lifting the left sacral base. (The shape of the sacroiliac joints also makes the sacrum move in this manner, but see Chapter 11 on the sacroiliac and pelvis for more on this.)

This combined action through the sacroiliac joints results in the sacral base on the right being anterior and inferior in relation to the right innominate. To tip anteriorly and inferiorly like this, the left inferior lateral angle of the sacrum will move posteriorly and slightly superiorly. From this response of the sacrum to right heel strike, the sacrum is said to rotate over a diagonal axis that runs from the upper corner of the left sacroiliac joint to the inferior portion of the right sacroiliac joint. By the time we reach left heel strike, the innominates will have reversed their rotation and so too will the sacrum: the sacral base will be tilted to the left, over a diagonal axis running from the superior edge of the right innominate's sacroiliac joint down to the inferior portion of the left sacroiliac joint.

Imagining

Alternatively, we can envision the motion of the pelvis as primarily the movement of the innominates, while the sacrum tries to hold its position in space in the coronal plane, resisting moving its sacral base anteriorly or posteriorly. Yet, the sacrum does rotate slightly by tilting a little right (during right heel strike) then left (on left heel strike) as we walk. Could we not then imagine and think of the sacrum as only rotating slightly right and left, back and forth, rocking side to side, around a sagittal (anterior–posterior) axis? It works like the axis of a hairspring in an old spring-driven watch, or the axis of a pendulum in a clock, making this axis the still point around which the whole body moves as it walks. Muscles need to work extra hard to walk and thus tire easily.

Take the time

Though it may seem tedious to have the patient walk back and forth seven, eight, or more times, the amount of information you will gather and the completeness of your picture regarding the patient's chief complaint will be comprehensive and will save you a lot of time in the end. Your assessment will be more complete, and so your treatments will be more effective and impressive in their results. Further, the patient will be safe from unsuitable or erroneous treatment.

Taking it to the next level

Once you have found asymmetry of movements, impairments, or imbalances that seem to emanate from a specific region of the body by scanning a diagonal line and have located the focus of the disturbance to gait, you can begin to analyze that region through classic range of motion testing (ROM). Based on that information, you can move onto the specific special tests that are applicable.

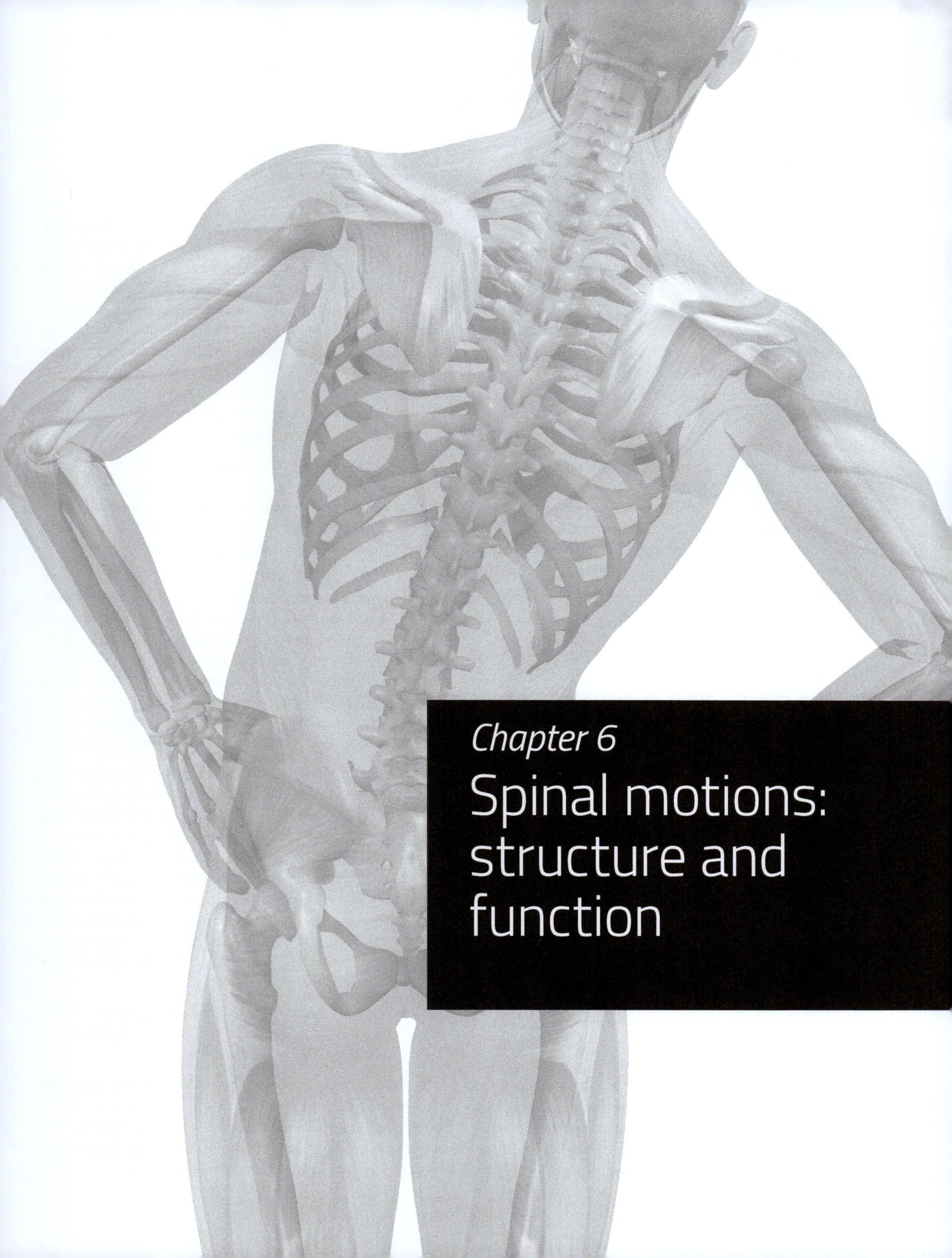

Chapter 6

Spinal motions: structure and function

Chapter 6

NOTE: *This short chapter on spinal motion does require the reader to have some basic knowledge of the anatomy of the spine.*

The living spine

Though the subject of the spine can be an enormous topic, my purpose in this chapter is to provide a general overall picture of the living spine, that is, the spine in motion. I want to describe some of the ways in which the spine functions according to the nature of its structure, and also show how its structure and function can become impaired or dysfunctional. What follows must by necessity be general in nature. Further, I will skip details of pathological changes that may occur over time or those due to disease processes.

The usefulness of looking at the spine in this way is that it helps the therapist imagine or visualize those structures intrinsic to the spine and how they function. I call this type of exercise *thinking anatomy*, that is, thinking through the implications of the structure and function of the musculoskeletal system. Structure (anatomy) permits and informs function, and function (physiology) shapes structure. With this perspective we can envision how the body seeks balance, successfully or unsuccessfully.

Spinal curves, discs, and facets

The spine acts as a spring or shock absorber for the trunk and head. Looking at the spine in profile, we see the familiar curves. These curves allow the spine to act as an S-spring. Pressure from above or below compresses the structure, but not like the loading of a solid column. Rather, the curves become exaggerated; absorbing the stress from the load, while the springiness inherent in it (via intervertebral discs, ligaments, muscles, living bone, etc.) pushes back. When the load is removed, the spine can lift itself back into it original shape, even without muscular action. This assumes that the load was not so great as to deform inert tissue or injure and impair muscle function.

Some of this absorption of forces comes from the intervertebral discs (IVDs). The intervertebral disc is a polyaxial joint. It can accommodate any direction of motion, including shear forces, as well as compression and decompression. The ball-shaped nucleus pulposus at the interior of the IVD is a gel contained within numerous layers or bands of cartilaginous tissue. This makes it uncompressible, and it cannot lose volume as long as those surrounding layers remain intact. When under pressure it pushes back, acting as a self-righting mechanism for the spine, and this ability also allows the annular fibers around it (which can deform) to re-inflate. Further, the nucleus, as uncompressible, acts as the axis of motion between vertebrae, as a swivel-type joint. It remains gel-like until middle age, when it then becomes fibrosed. As a result, it loses its capacity to recoil to pressure, and so the cartilaginous layers can more easily lose their height.

The annular fibers, being cartilaginous, can lose water when under pressure and can therefore be compressed with a resulting change in shape. This compressibility provides some of the *give* within the spine, so that it can work as a shock absorber that helps accommodate the compressive forces exerted on the disc. Therefore, the fibrous portion of the IVD, as compressible, can have its shape altered when under stress. When the load or stress is removed these annular fibers reabsorb water, re-inflating. The principle motor driving this re-inflation is the nucleus pulposus. However, if the layers are put continually or forcibly under stress their integrity can begin to break down.

Constant or frequently recurring compression or stress will prevent the annular fibers from taking back their water, leaving them dry and brittle. Then the gel-state nucleus itself will flatten as it begins to push its way outward through the cracks and breaks in the annular fibers and force the layers in front of it to bulge, or *herniate*.

In the lumbar spine, the nucleus is not in the center of the disc, but is positioned slightly posterior in order to better accommodate the compressive force when the spine is in neutral. In other words, because the lumbar's anterior (lordotic) curve puts more mechanical stress on the posterior portion of the disc, the nucleus, being slightly posterior to center, is better able to provide support. Therefore, as the lumbar curve exaggerates under load, the posterior-positioned nucleus provides protective support.

However, with flexion of the lumbar spine the compression of the anterior portion of the disc pushes the nucleus even more posteriorly. If the posterior cartilaginous layers are weakening (losing their integrity) then the nucleus will begin to shift even more posteriorly, causing the weakened layers to bulge, or herniate. The posterior longitudinal ligament (which is quite narrow at the lumbar spine) often helps sustain the integrity of the most posterior fibers of the disc, and so the bulging nucleus often rolls out around this ligament and moves to the side, moving in a posterior lateral direction. This puts it on a collision course with the neural foramen and the spinal nerve at that level.

In the cervical spine, C2 to C7, the nucleus pulposus is also slightly posterior within the IVD, and therefore functions, or dysfunctions, much like the lumbar spine.

The thoracic vertebrae have their nucleus pulposus generally more centered within the IVD. The lowest thoracic vertebrae, being slightly extended (beginning the lordotic curve in the low back), can have the nucleus slightly posterior; the flexed vertebrae of the thoracic kyphosis have it more centered.

We have talked mostly about flexing and extending portions of the spine. Side-bending functions in much the same way, with the nucleus acting as an axis over which side-flexion occurs. These three motions, of course, do not only move in a seesaw fashion; there is, in addition, some shearing occurring as the vertebra above slides in the direction of flexing, extending, or side-bending. This shearing action can cause more stress to the annular fibers than compression alone.

However, rotation is even more stressful on the IVD's annular fibers. As the layers of annular fibers run (in general) in alternating diagonal directions, the stress/tension running through the fibers during rotation will be resisted by some, while others are actually made lax. With fewer fibers resisting the forces, they are more likely to break down. Further, rotation also pulls the vertebral bodies closer together. This also reduces their ability to be shock-absorbers.

Facet (zygapophyseal) joints are meant to be slightly gapped or minimally weight-bearing when the spine is in neutral (or, as some say, the facet joints *idle*, as the engine of a motor vehicle idles, neither engaged nor in use but ready to be used). This slight gapping occurs the closer the curves of the spine are to being ideal. The structures involved in facet joints (bone, articular cartilage, synovial fluid, joint capsules, ligaments, muscle) all contribute to the weight-bearing ability through the area; yet the articular surfaces can remain gapped in the thoracic and lumbar spine. The weight is distributed throughout the structure, where even the fluid in the joint can hold the joint surfaces apart, with the fluid playing a supporting role as forces move through the joint structures.

However, as the curves exaggerate, the lordotic curves (normal in the cervical and lumbar portions of the spine) go into extension and the facet joint surfaces approximate and become weight-bearing. These stresses going into the articular cartilage, similar to the cartilaginous annular fibers, lose fluid – it is literally squished out of them. This fluid mixes with the free synovial fluid within the capsule, making the capsule balloon, which still helps the joint, as a whole, resist the forces that are pressing through the bony facet process. However, the internal pressure of the fluid in this weight-bearing situation will stress the synovial and fibrous capsules and prevent nutrients from entering the synovial cavity. Therefore, the longer this hyperlordosis persists, or the more extreme and forceful the extension: (1) the more quickly the articular surfaces will begin to break down and suffer other osteoarthritic changes; (2) the more likely it is that an injury can occur to the capsules; (3) the greater the chance for injury to occur to the intrinsic spinal ligaments and (fourth layer) musculature, with some overstretched and some left shortened; and (4) the poorer the nutrition within the joint.

Now, when the spine moves from neutral into extension, side-bending/flexing, and rotating the facet surfaces not only compress but are also going to glide one over the other. This glide, or skating, also stretches the capsules, and will lengthen some supportive joint tissues while making others lax. Flexing the spine gaps the joints but generally stretches most of the facet joint tissues. Therefore, adding rotation or side-bending to a flexed spine can take ligaments and joint capsules past their tolerance and they will begin to sprain or tear these tissues, while deep intervertebral muscles will undergo strain.

Fryette's rules of spinal motion

I would now like to discuss what are commonly referred to as Fryette's rules of spinal motion. The first two were formulated by Harrison Fryette D.O. while a third was added by C. R. Nelson D.O. They have also been call Fryette's laws or principles (Chila 2010). I like to use the term "rules," as they really should be taken as rules of thumb. They are informative about how the spine can move, but as is common with many living things, the spine does have a tendency to appear not to know the rules, or to choose at times to ignore them.

Remember too that every individual person's spine is itself individual and unique. No two facet joints are absolutely identical from one person to another, nor are any individual's two facet joints in their spine exactly identical. Each has at least some small, possibly trivial, differences, while others can be shaped quite differently and so function differently, all to varying degrees. Even the adjoining facet joint surfaces can have different shapes (e.g., one may have a slightly convex surface while its partner may be basically flat), be of differing sizes, or even differ in orientation one to another.

Definitions and observations

We first need a couple of definitions and observations.

A motion segment of the spine is defined as two adjacent vertebrae and all the joints between them. Between the typical spinal segment there is the IVD joint and two facet joints. When the motion under observation is between two vertebrae we are talking about segmental motion. When we are discussing several vertebrae moving we speak of group motions: these are clarified in Fryette's rules of spinal movements. Those rules were meant to specifically apply to both the thoracic and lumbar spine, but not the cervical.

A couple of observations:

1. Spinal movements are coupled. This means that any motion of the spine impacts on any other motion and, further, that some

motions generally accompany each other. With respect to the last point, it has been proposed that side-bending and rotation are always coupled in the spine.

2. The motions are named from the perspective of the vertebra above, with reference to the one below. Therefore, to say that a vertebra is side-bent and rotated is to say that relative to the vertebrae below, the vertebrae above is side-bent and rotated.

Fryette's rules

These rules have been shown to be especially valid for the lumbar spine (Bogduk 2012; Chila 2010; Mitchell 2004).

*1. **Fryette's first rule of spinal movements:*** when moving from neutral, the spine side-bends first and then rotates in the opposite direction.

Comments

Neutral here means the spine is neither flexed nor extended. Side-bending occurs in the frontal or coronal plane. Rotation happens in the transverse plane. When speaking of motions in neutral, side-bending occurs before rotation.

Kapandji (2008) says the following, to explain how this coupled movement in opposite directions occurs:

> This automatic rotation of the vertebrae … [When side-bending/lateral flexion occurs] … depends on two mechanisms – compression of intervertebral discs and the stretching of ligaments. The effect of disc compression is easily displayed on a simple mechanical model … If the model is flexed to one side, contralateral rotation of the vertebrae is shown by the displacement of the various segments off the central line. Lateral flexion increases the internal pressure of the disc on the side of movement; as the disc is wedge-shaped its compressed substance tends to escape toward the zone of lower pressure, to rotation, i.e., contralaterally … Conversely, lateral flexion stretches the contralateral ligaments, which tend to move toward the mid-line so as to minimize their lengths … It is remarkable that these two processes are synergistic and in their own way contribute to rotation of the vertebrae. (Kapandji 2008)

*2. **Fryette's second rule of spinal movements:*** when the spine is non-neutral – when in flexion or extension – rotation happens first, and then side-bending, both in the same direction.

Comments

When the spine is working normally in flexion or extension, rotation precedes side-bending. As these occur in the same direction we do not get the synergistic (compensating) motions we get when the spine is in neutral, thus the stresses of lengthening of some supportive tissue and the amount of compression on others are greater. If we then add in rotation/side-bending it is not surprising that the tissue may exceed their tolerances and become injured.

However, even when having started in neutral lumbar spine, impairments, when they do occur, are likely if the order of vertebral motion is not synchronized. For example, if the spine is first in neutral and the patient side-bends and rotates and then flexes or extends the chances of an impairment or dysfunction increase substantially as each additional plane of motion occurs. Knowing the order of movements that produced the patient's injury helps the therapist understand how the patient became lesioned. This information comes from a thorough case history taking, if the patient can remember the motion or even the final position they got into when their impairments were caused.

*3. **Fryette's third rule of spinal movements:*** introducing motion to a vertebral joint in one plane automatically reduces its mobility in the other two planes.

Comments

This rule is fairly self-evident. It is important, however, for understanding how injuries occur. Again, if the patient's spine is moved following the second rule as the vertebrae are flexed, some degree of motion is no longer available for side-bending and rotation. If, however, the person moves the spine into extremes in any of the three planes, as we noted above, this greatly increases the chances of injury. If the IVD and facet joints are driven too far, then injuries to the joint structures themselves and/or to the intrinsic muscles of the spine are likely to occur.

The first rule is often referred to as *type I motion*. Type I dysfunctions usually occur as a group (as in a scoliosis, for example). Therefore, they are referred to as a group or neutral dysfunction, where a number of vertebrae side-bend one way and rotate in the opposite direction. A functional scoliosis means that the scoliosis may disappear when the patient flexes or extends the spine (i.e., the scoliosis will decrease or disappear in moving in one direction, while it may exaggerate when moving in the other – which one happens in flexion or extension depends on several issues). However, in a bony (or pathological) scoliosis the vertebrae can be rotated and side-bent either to opposite sides or to the same side; they will not be following Fryette's rules, and this scoliosis usually does not change significantly.

The second rule is *type II motion*. Type II dysfunctions occur most often when the spine is already flexed or extended and then side-bending and rotation are added. These dysfunctions usually occur in isolation, in a single segment strain, with lifting and twisting, as an example. In other words, they are often segmental dysfunctions, generally not in several segments in a row (as a group). However, it is quite possible to have several segmental dysfunctions, one on top of the other, but each should be treated as individual motion segments. Again, this will help us understand how to test for these types of lesions, and to understand the results of such testing.

Note that when the spine seems in neutral, if the person has hyperlordosis or hyperkyphosis (excessive curves), or flattened curves (hypo-), then that portion of the spine is not in neutral and will function as type II motion, leading to type II impairments. So, for example, if a patient with a lumbar lordosis due to an anterior pelvic tilt now rotates or side-bends, the joints involved will follow the second rule (type II motion) rather than the first rule (type I motion).

Considerations

Of special note: The spine is a continuum.

Though we refer to portions of it as the lumbar, thoracic, and cervical spine, many structures undergo graduated changes as we progress up the spine from the sacrum to the occiput. It is true that there are transition points, predominately where the ribs come into play: the cervicothoracic (C7–T1) and thoracolumbar (T12–L1) junctions. (We are ignoring the lumbosacral and occipital-atlantal junctions, as we are removing the spine from its context of the body as a whole. These are covered in other chapters.) The ribs have real impact, but we will also get to that later.

The point here is that the rules apply fairly consistently to the lumbar spine, and up into the lower thoracic spine. However, as the facet joints slowly but progressively change their orientation as they move up the spine, these rules are going to become less consistent as we move into the upper half of the thoracic spine, until the point where they no longer apply to the cervical spine at all. Gradation in spinal structure (shape) results in a gradation of function, and a graduation of how predictive these rules of Fryette's are.

The cervical spine, from C2 to C3, tends to move usually with side-bending and rotation occurring to the same side, either in neutral or when the cervical spine is flexed or extended. This is due to the orientation of the facet joint surfaces. However, these vertebrae can be made to move opposite to each other under special circumstances. Hence, Fryette's rules just do not apply to them. Further, the unique shapes of C1 and C2 means they move in their own unique way. There, structure informs their function, and vice versa.

Do all spinal lesions occur in these ways?

No. *Lesions, by nature, may show patterns, but unusual traumas, severe blows or an unusual structuring or shape to the vertebrae can result in atypical patterns.* The rules of spinal movement are meant to help explain common clinical findings. However, because everyone is unique, joint shapes differ from person to person. *Any lesion may present as unique.* You may, on a rare occasion, find a group dysfunction where the lumbar or lower thoracic vertebrae seem rotated and side-bent to the same side, for example. Alternatively, a segmental dysfunction could have the motion segment rotating and side-bending in opposite directions. After all, lesions are lesions because things have gone wrong! Lesions know no rules. The joints in the spine can be forced into moving (functioning) in ways that do not conform to their shape (structure). Thus, we need to know how to accurately palpate and test the joints of the spine and, more importantly, not make assumptions about how things should be and, thus, forgo the testing. We need to be open-minded enough in order to be prepared to find the unexpected.

How the spine contributes to holding the body upright

Let us look at how the spine contributes to holding the body upright, how it bears the weight of the trunk, head, and upper limbs. Often the spine is still thought of, or described, as a column (hence the classic name spinal column) that works mechanically, like a pillar, supporting all this weight. However, this is no longer considered an appropriate model. This is where one of the many important jobs the ribs perform comes into play. Rather than only transferring weight and other stresses onto the spine, the ribs can distribute a lot of the weight of the upper body outward, to the body wall.

This transfer of weight and forces outward is referred to in the concept of *tensegrity*. The term tensegrity was coined by architect, engineer, and scientist R. Buckminster Fuller, who was the original designer of the geodesic dome. He said his inspiration for that design came from the structures within the living cell, its cytoskeleton. The word "tensegrity" is a contraction of the phrase "tensional integrity." Tensegrity describes the forces at work in a structure that is formed by a network of compressive, rigid elements interconnected through tensile or elastic elements, which give the structure its overall integrity. Due to the elastic property of the interconnections, when one element of the tensegrity structure is shifted (moved and/or loaded), this shift is spread throughout the whole structure. All the other elements shift as well, adapting and compensating by morphing into a new configuration. By yielding in this way to these shifts such a structure is more accepting of the forces or loads applied, without breaking.

Acting in this way, the ribs, and all the other tissues and structures of the spine working together, disperse stresses and strains that would cause them to snap if they were a rigid structure. Therefore, the ribs also help the body absorb the forces of walking, running, weight-bearing, reaching, pulling, etc. This is in addition to their duties of being the bellows for breathing and fluid movement (as part of circulatory system, especially for venous and lymph flow through the trunk). The qualities of tensegrity also help the ribs, and their related tissues, be even more effective in nurturing and protecting the organs within the trunk.

By looking at the spine in this way, by seeing its function as guided by its structure, and how its function can shape structure, the therapist is better equipped to understand how the spine works and how it gets into trouble. We can only see this way if we are looking at the spine as a living, changing, and adaptive system.

Part II
Regional Assessment

ANKLE AND FOOT: CHAPTER OVERVIEW

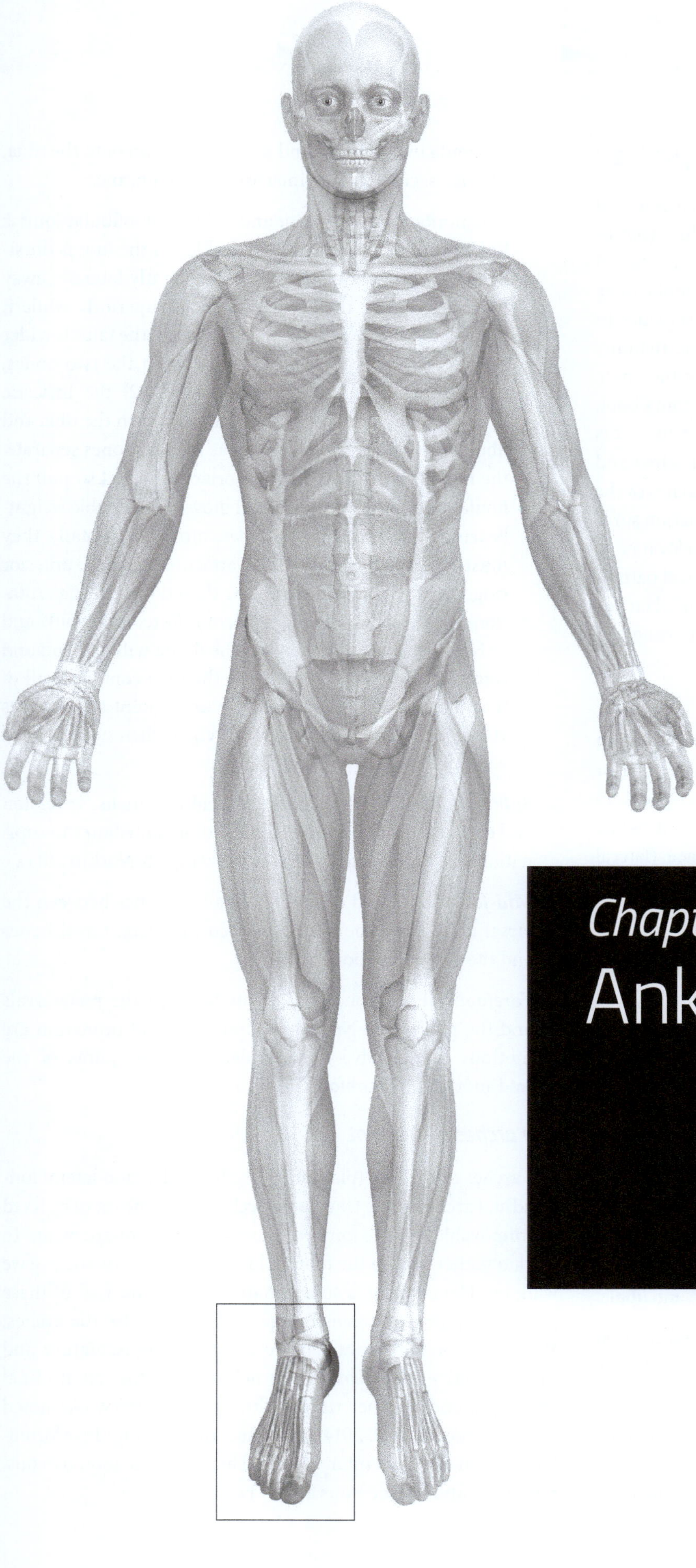

Chapter 7

Ankle and foot

Clinical implications of anatomy and physiology

The following are some anatomical observations that have clinical implications. Understanding the functional relationships (physiology) between the structures and tissues of the ankle (anatomy) will help explain how structures of the lower leg and foot can be injured, and help us understand how orthopedic tests work to provide the information that they do. Please review the anatomy of the joints and muscles involved in the function of the ankle and foot. It is suggested that the reader have an anatomy book at hand to more easily understand the information given in this section. For example, Schuenke et al. (2014) have a succinct and highly informative section on the plantar vault and arches of the foot, osseous, muscular, and ligamentous. The information summarized here has been chosen because of its direct relevance to orthopedic testing and understanding of the mechanical pathologies of the ankle. (See also Agur et al. 2014; Dutton 2012; Hartley 2000b; Hertling & Kessler 2006; Hoppenfeld 1976; Levangie & Norkin 2011; Magee 2014; Schuenke et al. 2014.)

Four main areas of the ankle and foot

1. ***Talocrural joint:*** the ankle joint proper. A synovial joint between the superior surface of the talus and the inferior surface of the distal tibia. The distal tibia also provides the medial surface (the medial malleoli) of the joint, while the distal fibula provides the lateral joint surface (lateral malleoli). Only dorsiflexion and plantar flexion are considered to happen at this joint. This joint is reinforced on the medial side by deltoid ligaments (anterior and posterior tibiotalar, the tibionavicular, and tibiocalcaneal), and on the lateral side by the anterior talofibular, calcaneofibular, and posterior talofibular ligaments.

Tibia and fibula interaction

- The junction between the distal/inferior tibia and fibula is composed of a superior sydnesmosis joint portion whose rough surfaces are held together by strong ligaments: an anterior and posterior tibiofibular ligament; an interosseous ligament internal to this joint, and further by an anterior transverse ligament. They are also held together by an interosseous membrane that runs between the length of the shafts of the tibia and fibula.
- Just inferior to this syndesmosis joint is a synovial portion between the tibia and fibula, which is continuous with the talocrual joint.
- The junction between the superior (proximal) tibia and fibula is a plane/gliding joint and is synovial. It too is reinforced with anterior and superior ligaments that run from the head of the fibula in a superior and medial direction onto the tibia, and is also secured by the interosseous membrane.

  The motion of the superior and inferior tibiofibular joint is linked to the movement of the ankle. As the foot is dorsiflexed, the distal fibula moves ever so slightly, laterally, away from the tibia at the ankle and slides superiorly while it rotates internally. This occurs because: (1) the talus is wider at the front, and as it moves up between the two bones, those bones are pushed slightly apart; (2) the inelastic fibers of the interosseous membrane between the tibia and fibula are on oblique angles and as the two bones separate, the fibers have to move more horizontally and so pull the fibula superiorly. The fibula will move on the stable weight-bearing tibia; and (3) as the fibers move horizontally, they must simultaneously pull their attachment on the anterior ridge of the fibula in a medial direction (internal rotation). Therefore, as the foot is plantar flexed, the fibula and tibia come closer together and the fibula will descend and rotate back out externally. Since the tibia comprises all of the superior bony portion of the ankle joint and it takes 90 percent or more of the body's weight when standing and walking, it is only the fibula that moves.

2. ***Subtalar joint:*** between the talus and calcaneus. Inversion and eversion occur here; hence this joint contributes to supination and pronation of the foot (Levangie & Norkin 2011).
3. ***Mid-foot:*** composed of many joints and bones between the tarsal bones; and the joints between the distal tarsal bones and the metatarsal bones.
4. ***Forefoot:*** all the bones and joints between the metatarsals and the phalanges. Note that supination and pronation are motions that involve the subtalar joint, the joints of the mid-foot and the forefoot.

The arches of the foot

The arches of the foot (plantar vault, the medial and lateral longitudinal arch and the transverse arch) are not meant to be fixed or immovable. All the joints of the ankle and foot are meant to work together to help the foot mold to the ground or surface we walk on. Hence there is some small laxity between all of these joints, including between the bones that comprise the arches. We need to remain aware of how both the musculature and the connective tissue sometimes help to hold the longitudinal arch rigid and at other times, allow it some laxity. (As noted above, Schuenke et al. 2014, have a succinct and highly informative section on the plantar vault and arches of the foot, osseous, muscular, and ligamentous anatomy.)

The anterior tibialis is extremely important in providing muscular assistance for the integrity of the medial longitudinal arch. For example, when the foot moves from heel-strike to weight-bearing (mid-stance), the tibialis not only works eccentrically to control the lowering of the foot to the ground, it also controls how much give the arch will allow so that the foot will mold to uneven ground. It will also assist in pulling the arch up to make it rigid when we toe off. The anterior tibialis not only assists in the control of pronation and supination of the whole foot it also balances with the tibialis posterior by exerting a pull down on some the bones within the arch. The peroneus longus is another crucial muscle; along with the brevis, it helps control supination and pronation, and as a result, how the foot molds to the ground. The other muscular support of this arch comes from the flexor hallucis longus and the flexor digitorum longus, as well as the intrinsic muscles of the foot. Further, without all of this muscular support the arch would fall and the navicular (keystone) would tumble down towards the ground.

When reviewing the muscles of the foot, examine how they assist in helping the foot adapt to the surface upon which it presses. Note also the role that both the shape of the bones and the connective tissue play in the function of the foot.

With respect to the connective tissue support of the medial arch, the most well-known tissue that is supportive of the arches of the foot is the plantar fascia. It can be compared to the string of a bow, with the bow being the bony arch. It is important to remember that its distal attachments on the foot are onto the proximal phalanges. As such, when the foot is moving from heel-strike toward mid-stance, the fascia/aponeurosis can have a little laxity (with the phalanges in neutral or even slightly flexed). However, when the foot moves from mid-stance to toe-off, and the phalanges go into extension, the arch is pulled tight by both the plantar fascia and the flexors of the toes, resulting in the longitudinal arch becoming rigid. Therefore, the arch can have enough laxity to be adaptable to the ground and yet can be made rigid enough to enable the full force of the plantar flexors to drive toeing off effectively and efficiently (without losing some of the force that occurs if the arch is lax). This is sometimes referred to as the windlass mechanism, or windlass effect. This efficiency of muscular force through the rigid arch (when toeing off) is what allows humans to walk all day, if need be. Windlass is a term used in sailing or boating; referring to what otherwise would be called a pulley, or using something as a pulley (like the mast of a sail boat) by wrapping a rope around it to make it easier to pull.

The transverse or metatarsal arch is helped to sustain itself by the keystone shape of the metatarsal rays, and it is principally held by the adductor hallucis and the lumbricals. This arch readily flattens as body-weight passes through it during the gait cycle (when going into toe-off). Therefore, this also helps the foot mold to the ground.

NOTE: When a person has a flat foot, or fallen arch (a pronated foot or pes planus), weakened toe flexors (and often tibialis anterior) no longer help the arch go rigid and as a result the plantar fascia structure fails. The flexors alone cannot sustain the integrity of the transverse arch. This results in a loss of efficiency of muscular effort, and as a result the person's lower legs will tire more quickly when walking and standing.

Inversion and eversion, pronation and supination

Strictly speaking, when talking about the foot, the terms inversion and eversion apply to the motion happening at the subtalar joint. Supination and pronation happen through several joints: subtalar, tarsal, and metatarsal joints (hindfoot, mid-foot, and forefoot).

The terms supination and pronation can be used when speaking of AF-ROM in the foot. They are actions that the person can actively do. They include inversion and eversion of the hindfoot but also require many more movements of joints throughout the foot. These other movements include adduction and abduction, which describe some of the motions of the mid-foot and forefoot. Hence, supination and pronation imply multiple movements at multiple joints. Therefore, the terms inversion and eversion (when used in reference to the foot) refer to: the motion strictly between the calcaneus and the talus, and motions that can only be done in isolation from other motions of the foot by PR-ROM.

Therefore:

- hindfoot (subtalar) *inversion* with mid-foot and forefoot *adduction* = supination
- hindfoot (subtalar) *eversion* with mid-foot and forefoot *abduction* = pronation.

Range of motion for the ankle and foot

Ankle/talocrual joint

Dorsiflexion 20–30°

Plantarflexion 40–50°

Forefoot

Pronation 20°

Supination 40°

See the Appendices at the end of the book for charts and tables on muscles (muscle origin, insertion, innervation, action, and synergists), joints (actions ranges, muscles used, tissues stretched and compressed), a table on capsular patterns (of restriction, open packed/resting positions, and close packed positions) and several charts on neurological testing where any such testing would involve this chapter's region.

The protocol (Box 7.1) begins with the case history.

> **Box 7.1 Protocol**
>
> Case history (specific questions)
>
> Observations
>
> Rule outs
>
> Active free range of motion (AF-ROM)
>
> Passive relaxed range of motion (PR-ROM)
>
> Active resisted range of motion (AR-ROM)
>
> Special tests

Case history (specific questions)

The following are some examples of specific questions concerning the knee that build on the basic case history questions as presented in Part I, Chapter 3.

- Have you noticed any changes in performing daily activities due to your ankle(s) or feet? Sports? Are there any actions or positions that you are in during the day that you think may be contributing to the problem?
- Describe the nature of the pain. Note:
  - aching pain, though often mechanical, may indicate degenerative changes as well
  - sharp, "catching" pain implies some mechanical problem
  - pain at rest is often overuse and inflammatory in nature
  - pain during activity is often structural or mechanical.
- If swelling in the joint has occurred you need to ask about the speed with which the joint swelled. Did it come on gradually or suddenly? Is there any bruising?
- In the patient's own words, have them describe what is wrong with their ankle or foot. Note if your patient uses terms such as:
  - snapping: taut ligaments or tight tendons crossing the joints; may imply those that pass behind and around under either malleolus
  - grinding (crepitus): implies initial stages of osteoarthritic changes within the joint
  - creaking (gross crepitus): implies severe osteoarthritic degeneration
  - catching or locking: implies mechanical dysfunction of the joints ligaments and/or musculature
  - giving way or becoming weak on weight-bearing: may imply neurological or vascular issues as well as mechanical.

Be sure to ask the following:

- Do you have diabetes or any circulatory conditions?
- Have you ever injured this ankle before?
- Does the temperature or sensation change in one or both of your feet?
- Do you have deep pain in your calf?

Observations

Regional assessment within the context of the whole

As with every area of the body being investigated by orthopedic testing (specific view), remember to always look at the joint or tissue being examined within the context of the surrounding joints and structures (regional view). What is the interplay of impaired tissues or structures with the rest of the tissues in that region? In turn, take into consideration the global view: how are that joint and that region affecting the whole body? How is the whole affecting or influencing the region and the specific site(s) of impairment(s)? Just as with treatment, the approach to assessment also moves from general to specific and back to general.

Not all the preconditions for an impairment exist on site and/or in the surrounding region; they can come from the totality of the body of the person and their environment.

Standing postural examination

Remember: Observation begins the moment a patient enters the clinic. Perform a postural scan from each side and from the front and back. Deformities are visible signs of impairment that result from either severe genetic or long-term conditions. These deformities will have caused clear compensatory changes to the structures in support of those areas.

Note obvious deformities and consider their implications. Is the deformity a contributing factor to the patient's chief complaint?

Have the patient stand in a natural pose. To assist in this, instruct the patient to look up slightly (i.e., you do not want them watching their feet) and take a few marching steps on the spot. Do not correct the position of feet, head, and so on: you are trying to have the patient stand naturally.

Note the general orientation of the upper body, especially rotations and side-bending of the shoulders or spine. Note the general orientation of the hips. Look to see if the hips are shifted right or left over a leg or for a unilateral or bilateral pelvic tilt. Note the proportions of tissue bulk and orientation of the thigh and lower leg (rotations throughout the course of the limb down to the feet, for example, varus or valgus of knees). To review the components of a full postural assessment see Part I, Chapter 5.

Postural examination of the foot

- From behind, note whether the Achilles tendon is straight up and down or whether it is off at an angle – which could imply a pronated hindfoot.
- Take the index and middle fingers of one hand and try to slide them under the arch of a foot. Use the same two fingers (of the other hand if not different in size) and repeat, trying to slide them under the other arch. Note any differences between the two feet.
- Compare the width and shape of the forefoot of each foot, especially at the metatarsal arch across the metatarsal heads. Does the arch seem present or does one or other (or both) forefoot appear wide and flattened when weight-bearing?
- With the patient high-sitting, note any changes to the arches of the feet. Do the longitudinal arches still seem fallen (structural pes planus)? Do they now look normal or at least have more of an appearance of an arch, which would indicate a functional pes planus? Does the transverse metatarsal arch return when not weight-bearing?

See also Box 7.2.

Box 7.2 Posturally challenging the chief complaint: exploring how the chief complaint fits into the whole

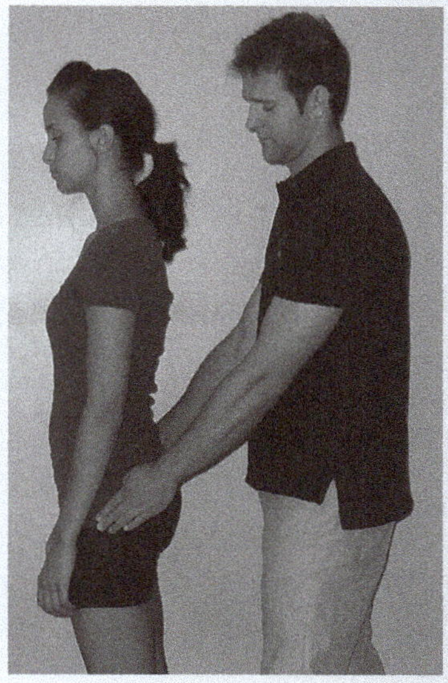

FIGURE 7.1

Observe and gently correct the patient's posture.

As a final step of observation and inspection, look at how the patient naturally stands and correct their posture with gentle movements, if possible (Figure 7.1). For example, push the patient's hips back, unlock hyperextended knees, reposition a forward head over the shoulders and note what changes occur above and below. If the patient can briefly sustain this corrected position, the tension or pain that they may now experience will point to areas that need to be included in your assessment and treatment (i.e., injured, contractured, or weakened/stressed tissues or structures, muscle imbalances, etc.). This will help reveal problems that have a global effect as well as being intimately connected to specific impairments.

Rule outs

Guidelines for rule outs of joints above and below chief complaint

Once you have decided which joint or region of the body you are going to investigate for the source of the patient's chief complaint, you must first rule out the joint above and the joint below. It is imperative to determine whether the joints/areas above and below the primary joint or region could be referring to the impaired joint or tissue. If this testing does not reproduce the patient's chief complaint, then that joint is said to be ruled out and not in need of immediate further testing (Hartley 2000b).

The patient may experience pain or other symptoms or impairments with the rule out testing but if they do not provoke or reproduce the chief complaint then they are set to one side for the time being and may be returned to at another time. These quick tests stress the principal tissues involved in each of the joints to be ruled out. They primarily focus on the non-contractile elements.

Begin by having the patient do specific AF-ROM tests of the joint in question. When the end-range of each AF motion is reached, ask if the patient is experiencing any pain (even if other than their chief complaint). If none is present, grasp and support the limbs or structures and tell the patient to relax and let you move them. You now apply over-pressure (O-P) as if/when performing passive relaxed range of motion (PR-ROM) testing. It is O-P that stresses the inert or non-contractile tissues of that joint.

Having applied the O-P, again ask the patient if they feel any pain or impairment with the O-P. If there is no pain, proceed to the next AF motion and continue as above. If the patient does feel pain, etc., further clarify by asking if the pain (or whatever the impairment is) is the same as what they came to see you about, or something different. If you get a positive reproduction of their chief complaint when doing a rule out, then that joint now needs to be included in your protocol of testing for the chief complaint – it is considered ruled in. A chief complaint may include more than one joint. If you get pain with or without other impairments but these are not part of the patient's chief complaint, then record them but return to your testing of the area indicated by the patient's complaint. These extra findings can be investigated further at a later date. If neither joint reproduces the patient's chief complaint during either the AF or the PR with O-P portion of these rule outs, then move on to the regular AF-ROM testing of the joint or structures that are the focus of the day's testing.

- *The following joints must be ruled out before testing the ankle to ensure that their structures are not referring symptoms to the ankle and/or foot. The following tests are all done supine with knees bent (crook-lying).*

Knee

Have the patient actively flex and then extend the knee. If active movements are pain-free apply O-P in each range to challenge the joint and its supportive tissue (Figures 7.2, 7.3).

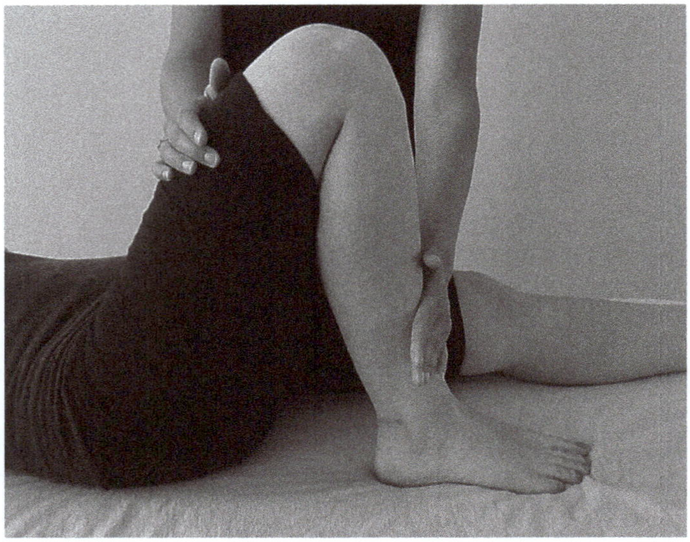

FIGURE 7.2 Knee flexion O-P

If there is no pain on actively flexing knee tell patient to relax and allow you to take it to end-range. If there is still no pain apply gentle O-P.

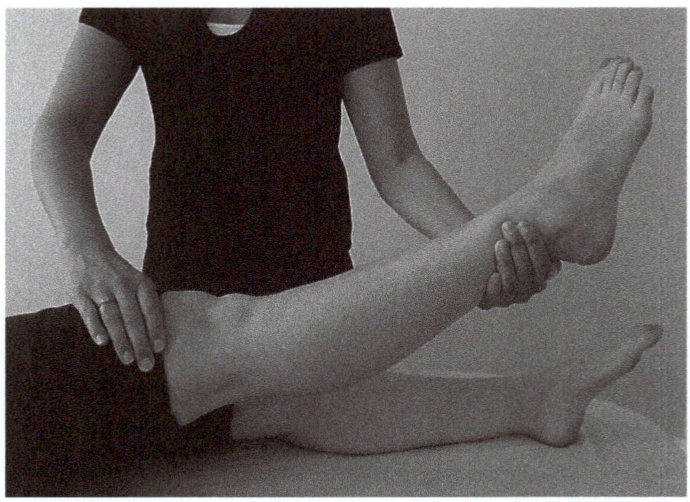

FIGURE 7.3 Knee flexion O-P

Have patient extend knee. If pain-free, lift leg (above ankle) several inches off table so it goes into full extension. If patient is still pain-free apply gentle O-P into further extension.

Superior tibiofibular joint

Rule out by passive anterior/posterior glides (i.e., joint mobilization). These movements are best done with the knee flexed at 90° with the patient supine on the table. Only a small movement (3–3.5 mm or 1/8 inch) is available. Simply note if it moves or not (Figure 7.4).

If the patient's ankle is not in an acute or subacute phase you may wish to also palpate the head of the fibula: with the patient still in the position in Figure 7.4, palpate the head of the fibula with your thumb and index finger and have the patient actively dorsiflex and plantar flex the foot. Note: as the patient dorsiflexes, the fibula should lift up (move superiorly) and roll forward slightly. Restriction of motion of the fibula is a common cause of restricted dorsiflexion of the ankle.

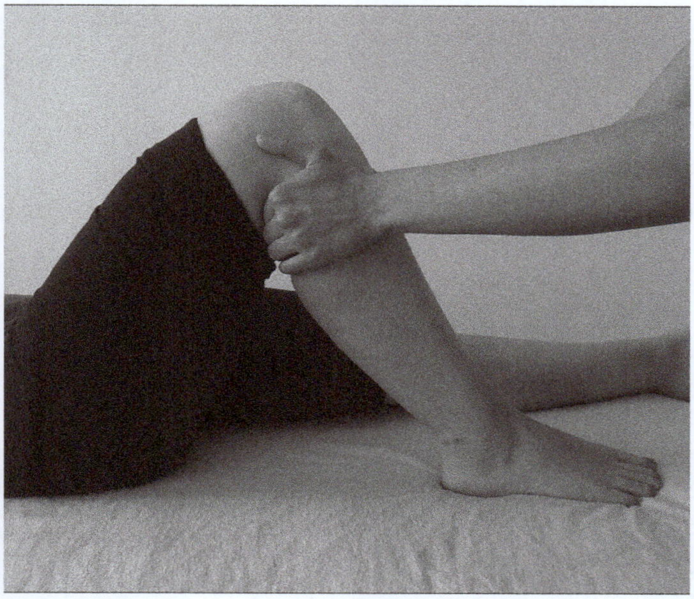

FIGURE 7.4 Testing superior tibiofibular joint

The patient is supine with knees bent, crook-lying. Note that the foot is plantar flexed to loosen the ankle joint. Place the heel of one hand on the anterior portion of the fibula near the superior end of the bone so that your thumb can rest against the head of the fibula. Stabilize the tibia with the other hand. Now, lean into the fibula and see if you can note if slight movement is available. The fibula should glide slightly posteriorly. Now, with your fingers that are behind the fibula, draw it forward. Do you note it moving forward? You may need to repeat two or three times to get an adequate sense of motion.

Rule out structures below the ankle (distal to) (the metatarsophalangeal and interphalangeal joints) by active free flexion and extension of the toes. Be sure to stabilize across the metatarsals so that the ankle does not move. You would only do this rule out if you were sure only ankle joint structures were injured and do not suspect muscular involvement. This might be too much of an assumption to make at an early stage of assessment and therefore this rule out is not suggested for use in every case.

If neurological signs and symptoms have been noted when taking your case history, rule out the lumbar spine. To rule out the lumbar spine have the patient actively forward flex then laterally flex. Then have them rotate their trunk left and right. If the movement has been pain-free at the end of their active free range of motion apply slight O-P. Next have the patient extend their low back. *Remember to never apply O-P in extension of the spine.* If extending the back does not cause a recurrence of neurological signs and symptoms, do the quadrant test (see Chapter 12 for details). The quadrant test is designed to maximally close the facet joints and, therefore, also the neural foramen of the lumbar spine on the side to which the patient bends. The test may tell you one of the actions that is involved in producing the symptoms, but as so many tissues are involved in the maneuver, it is not highly specific.

The positive sign we are testing for here is the re-creation of the patient's neurological symptoms in the lower limb. Have the patient rotate slightly to one side, place their hand on the back of that thigh and slide their hand down toward the back of their knee.

Range of motion testing (ROM)

Perform the following range of motion testing (compilation derived from: Dutton 2012; Hartley 2000b; Hertling & Kessler 2006; Hoppenfeld 1976; Magee 2014; Petty 2011; Starkey & Brown 2015).

Active free range of motion (AF-ROM)

The talocrural joint, the subtalar joint, and the joints of the forefoot are all being employed in AF-ROM. There are a couple of options when doing active free range of motion of the foot and ankle. If the patient is able to weight-bear, then you can do some quick testing with the patient standing. This method is shown first. These are referred to as quick tests (Hoppenfeld 1976) (Figures 7.5–7.8).

Assessing AF-ROM on the table (Figures 7.9, 7.10)

If the patient is limping and/or experiencing ankle pain take the more conservative approach and perform the tests in a non-weight-bearing position. Have the patient supine with the ankles off the table.

Supination and pronation

Supination and pronation happen through several joints: subtalar, tarsal and metatarsal joints (hindfoot, mid-foot, and forefoot). These terms, supination and pronation, are specifically reserved for AF-ROM in the foot. For this reason we have not used the terms inversion and eversion here, which belong to the subtalar joint proper. (Other terms used are: adduction/abduction. These terms are usually reserved terms for forefoot motion.) These will be tested separately with PR-ROM (Figures 7.11, 7.12).

Quick tests for the ankle

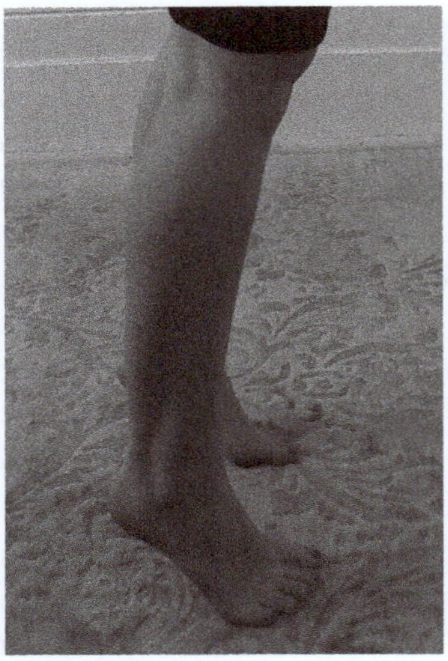

FIGURE 7.5 Plantar flexion
Standing on toes

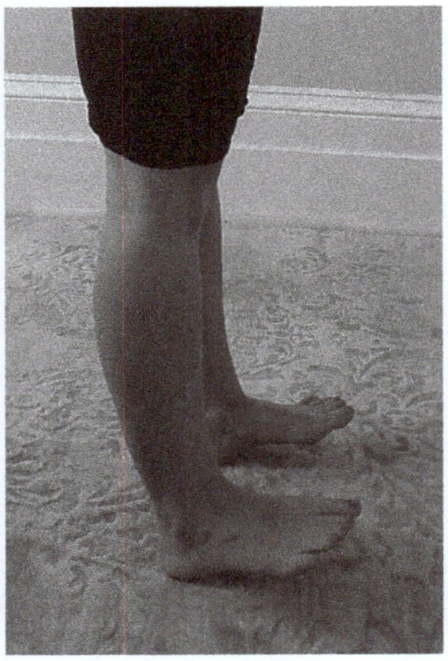

FIGURE 7.6 Dorsiflexion
Standing on heels only

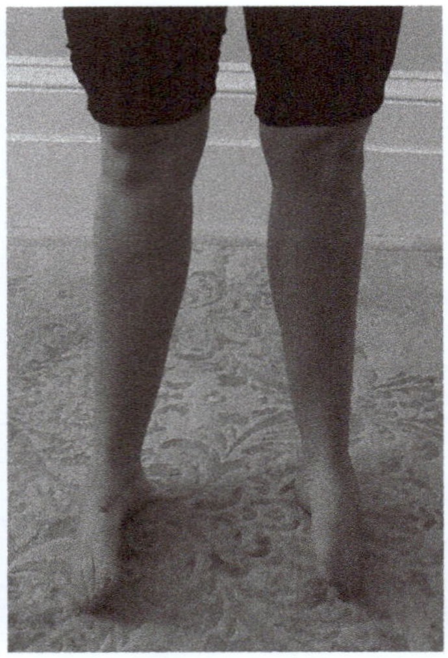

FIGURE 7.7 Supination
Rolling onto lateral edge of feet; knees coming further apart; varus

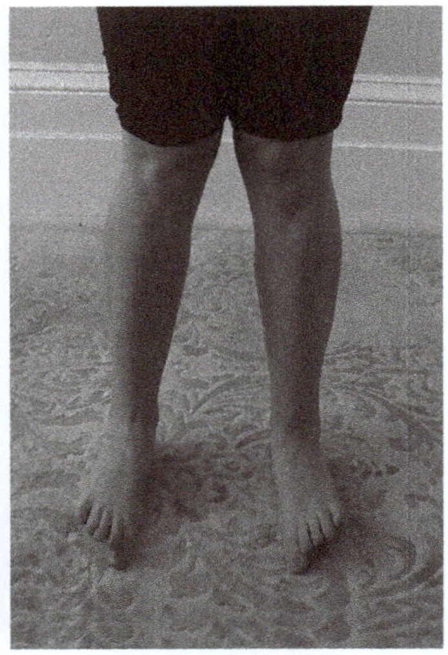

FIGURE 7.8 Pronation
Rolling onto inside edges of feet; knees coming together; valgus.

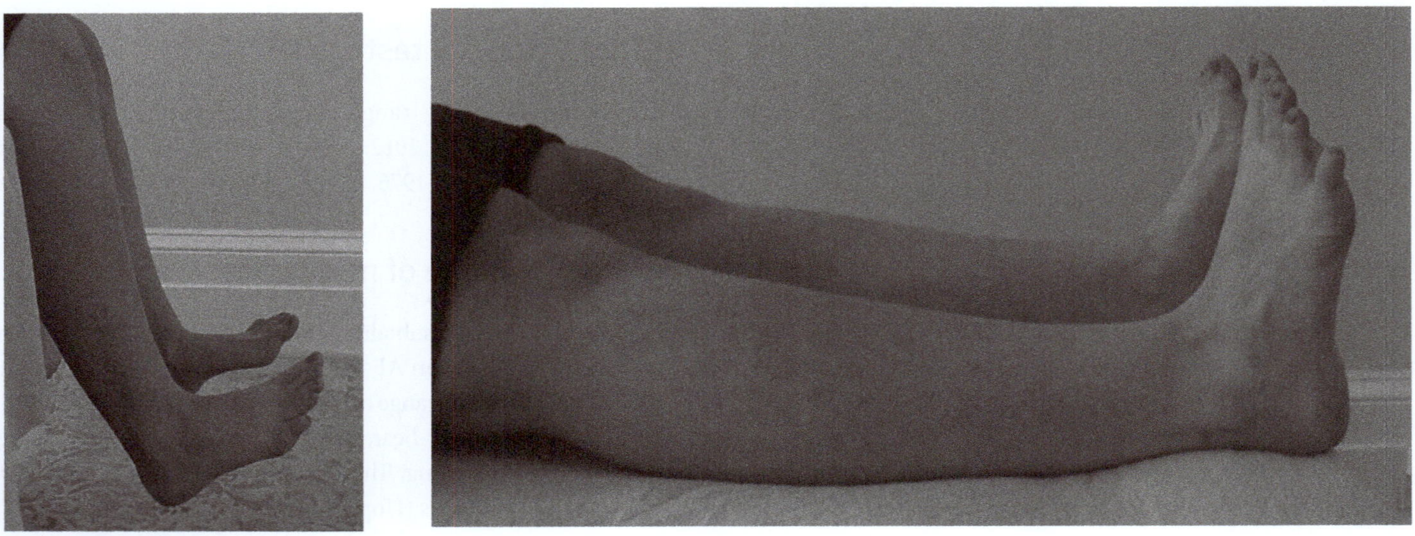

FIGURE 7.9A and B Dorsiflexion 20–30°
Patient lifts feet and points them toward head. Note: 10° of dorsiflexion is minimum needed for normal gait patterns

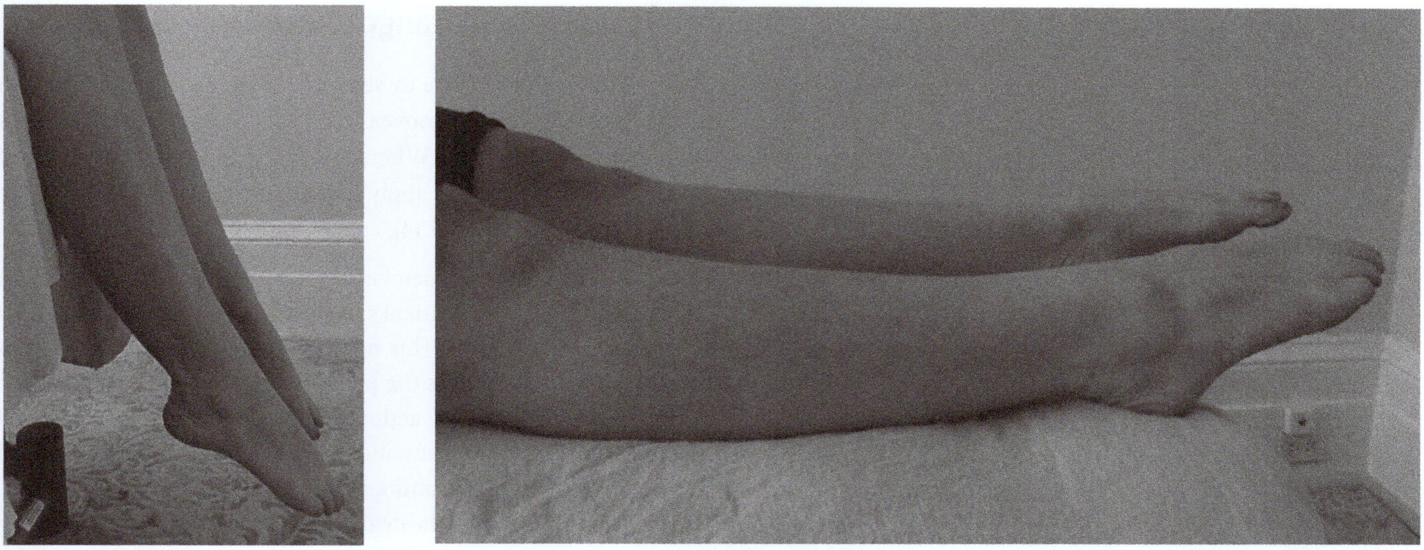

FIGURE 7.10A and B Plantar flexion 40–50°

Have patient point their toes.

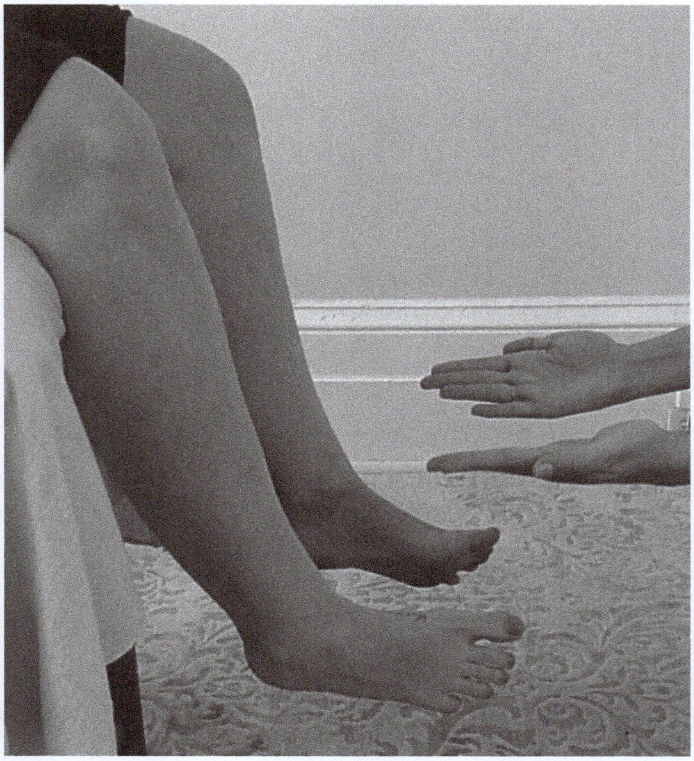

FIGURE 7.11 Supination

Ask patient to turn soles of feet inward (toward each other) while you demonstrate with hands.

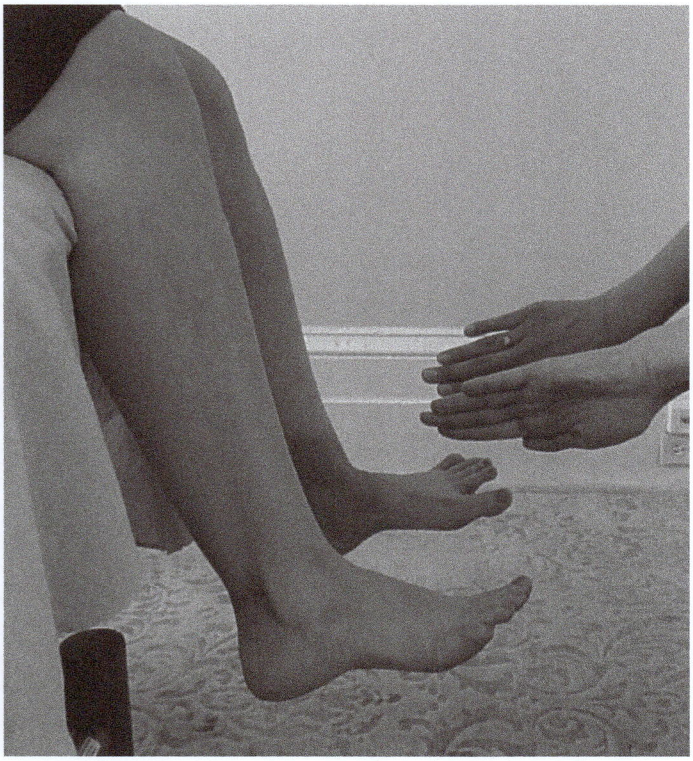

FIGURE 7.12 Pronation

Ask patient to turn soles of feet outward while you demonstrate with hands.

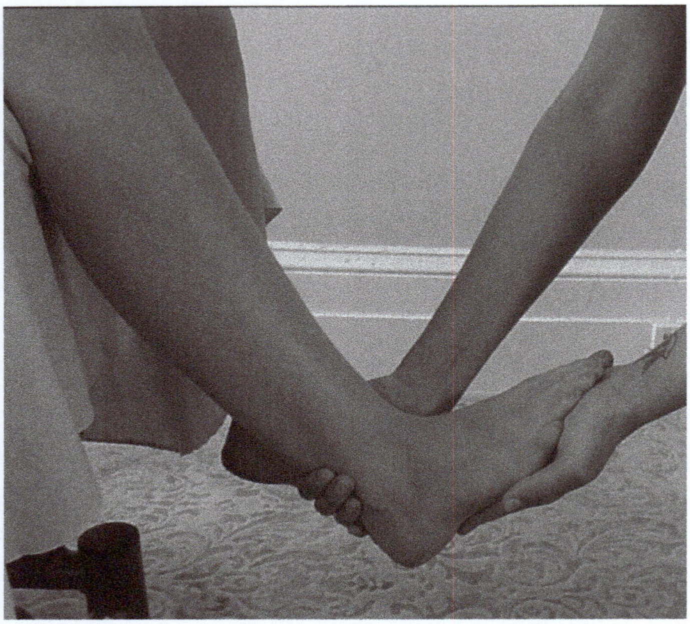

FIGURE 7.13 Dorsiflexion

End-feel is generally tissue stretch due to Achilles tendon.

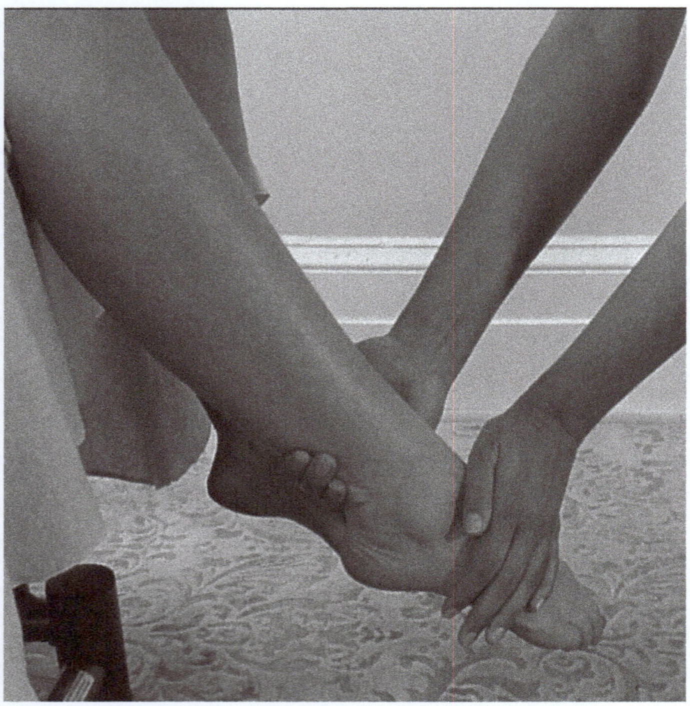

FIGURE 7.14 Plantar flexion

End-feel is generally bony as talus contacts tibia-fibula mortise (may also be tissue stretch if dorsiflexors of foot are shortened or tight).

Passive relaxed range of motion (PR-ROM)

Have the patient supine or seated high enough so that you can easily and confidently move their feet. Take note of any crepitus as you move the joint. When end-range has been reached, and only if there is no pain, apply slight O-P to determine the joint's end-feel (Figures 7.13, 7.14).

It is important to remember to have a towel roll ready so it can be placed under the patient's thighs just proximal to the knees when doing PR-ROM. This negates tightening of the gastrocnemius muscle and allows the knees to be slightly flexed. Have the patient do the following actions and see if they reach the normal degrees of movement (the patient may also prefer to be high-seated to perform these tests, although it is more difficult for the therapist to accurately note the degree of movement in this position):

- dorsiflexion: end-feel is normally tissue stretch
- plantar flexion: end-feel is normally hard/bony
- forefoot adduction: end-feel is normally tissue stretch
- forefoot abduction: end-feel is normally tissue stretch
- subtalar inversion: end-feel is normally hard/bony
- subtalar eversion: end-feel is normally hard/bony.

Subtalar joint and forefoot

There are four other movements of the foot we need to explore. These cannot be done actively by the patient in isolation but require the therapist to passively move them (Figures 7.15–7.18).

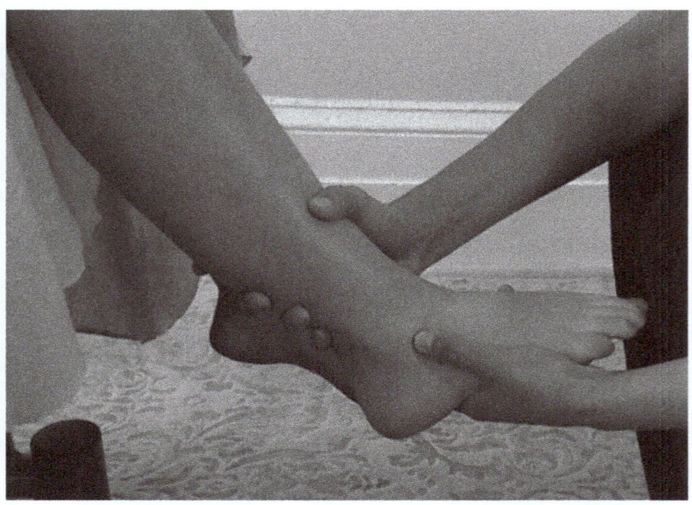

FIGURE 7.15 Forefoot abduction 10°

Stabilize heel, grasp metatarsals as group while abducting forefoot. End-feel is tissue stretch (supportive connective tissue).

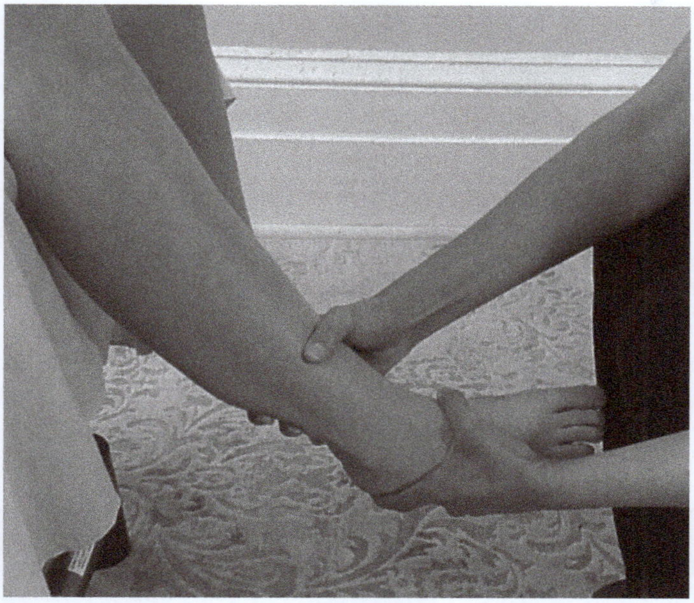

FIGURE 7.16 Forefoot adduction 20°

Stabilize heel, grasp metatarsals as a group and adduct forefoot. End-feel is tissue stretch.

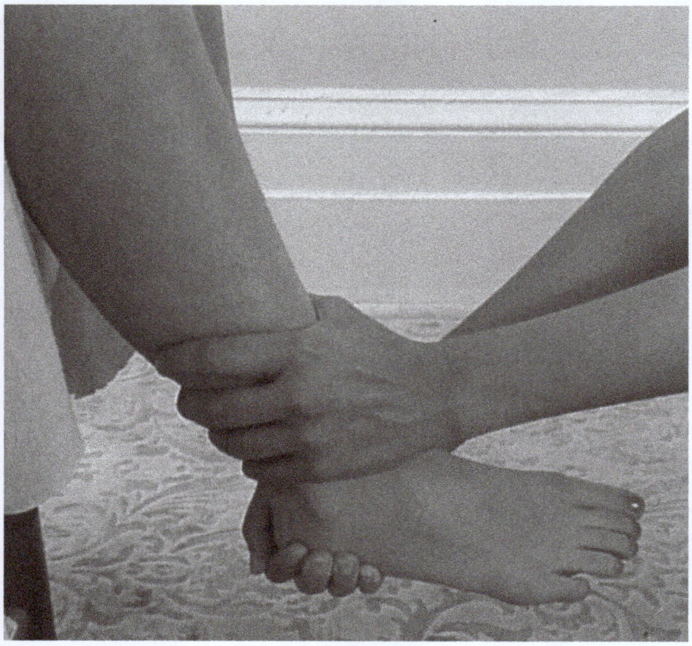

FIGURE 7.17 Subtalar inversion 5°

Patient high-sitting or supine. Stabilize above ankle with one hand, and grasping firmly onto heel, apply pressure in a medial direction trying to invert heel. Support foot in neutral with forearm. End-feel should be hard/bony.

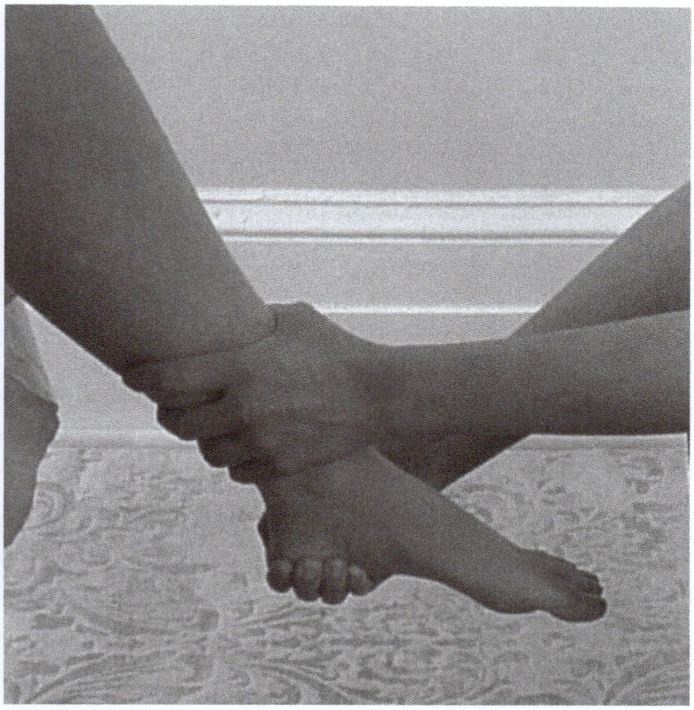

FIGURE 7.18 Subtalar eversion 5°

With patient in same position, apply pressure in a lateral direction attempting to evert heel. End-feel should be hard/bony.

Forefoot abduction and adduction The movements here take place through the tarsal and metatarsal joints.

The movements of subtalar inversion and subtalar eversion occur between the talus and calcaneus joint. This joint may be injured any time the heel is fixed while there is medial or lateral movement of the leg (with the weight of the body on it), placing excessive shear force through the joint.

Assessing joint play movements of the ankle

Note excess motion or a complete lack of motion (or "bind"); have the patient tell you immediately about any discomfort, pain, or altered sensation during and after each application of mobilization. These tests in general are going to be stressing ligaments. The therapist may want to wait until after ligament testing is complete (see special tests below) before assessing joint play available in the ankle and foot (Figures 7.19–7.23).

The therapist needs to keep in mind that restrictions found in joint mobilizations (or assessing joint play) need not necessarily come from intrinsic structures of the joint (joint capsule ligaments) but may also be restricted by hypertonus in muscle(s) that prevent movement in either general or accessory joint motions under assessment. In the ankle, this can most often be seen in the talocrural joint where excessive tone in the gastrocnemius and soleus coming through the Achilles tendon interfere with the ankle's dorsiflexion and anterior draw of the talus.

The ideal position for mobilization movements of the foot is with the foot off the end of the table.

CAUTION: You may wish to put a hand towel folded several times under the lower leg right at the end of the table (not illustrated below). Though padded, many treatment tables can still have a hard edge just under the padding and since a number of these mobilizations can apply pressure towards the ground the patient's leg could be pressed through the padding and into a hard edge on the table. Also note that all of the mobilization tests except the talar rock can be done with the patient supine. Though more force could be applied in some movements by having the patient prone, etc., having them move about can be uncomfortable and time-consuming without getting significantly clearer responses from the testing. Testing may be compromised or ruled out by the presence of edema or bruising in the ankle or foot or by the patient feeling pain as leg, ankle, or foot is grasped.

For more on general application and instructions, see the joint mobilization section in Chapter 3. (For additional information and for optional positioning of patient or limb and variations or additional tests see also: Edmond 2006;

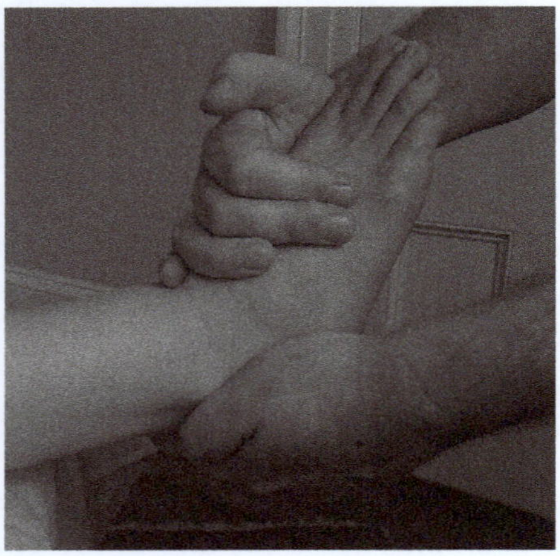

FIGURE 7.19 Distraction/decompression of the talocrural joint

Grasp the heel and dorsum high up on the foot and apply long axis traction to the ankle. Use your body-weight by leaning back rather than trying to pull through the shoulders and arms.

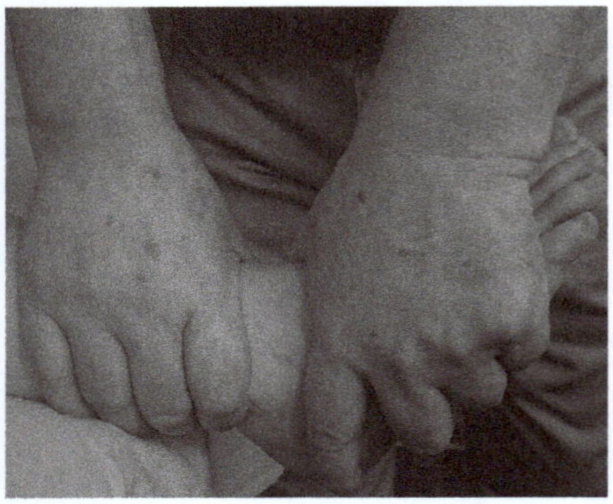

FIGURE 7.20 Anterior-posterior glide through the talocrural joint

Stabilize the lower leg by gently but firmly pressing the lower leg above the ankle into the table; grasp and encircle the dorsum of the mid-foot so that your index finger and thumb are just below the malleoli. Distract talocrural joint slightly and apply a downward (posterior) force shearing through the talocrural joint; hold momentarily (asking about pain, etc.). Release the shear force and then draw the foot upward (anteriorly), hold momentarily, etc., release. If painless then repeat several times. (If you feel not enough force can be applied drawing the foot anteriorly then cup the heel and draw it anteriorly.)

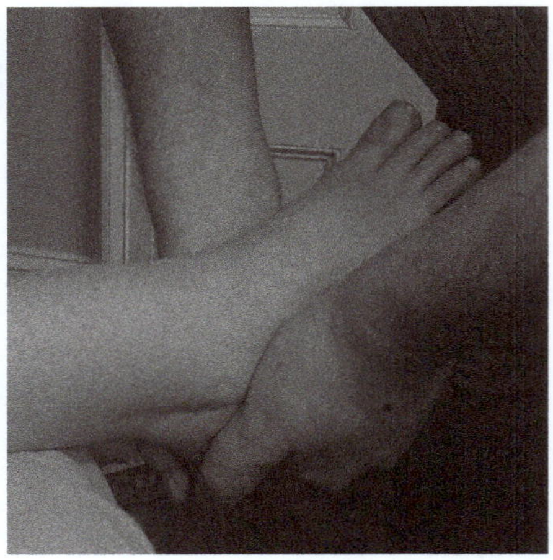

FIGURE 7.21 Shear and side tilt of subtalar joint

Grasp the calcaneus medially and laterally and hold firmly. Distract and then: (1) apply a side-to-side motion (shear) through the subtalar joint (but do not let the leg slide side to side on the table); (2) tilt the calcaneus (on the talus) medially and laterally (inverting and everting the hind-foot).

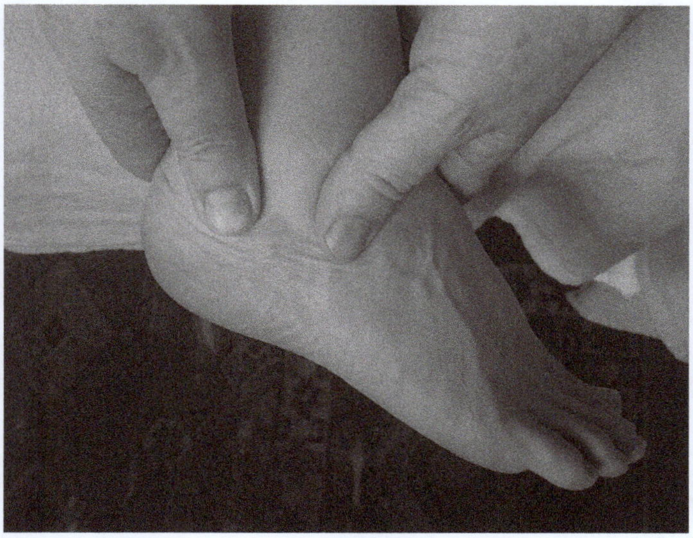

FIGURE 7.22 Plantar or talar rock test

The patient is side-lying with the knee and hip slightly flexed. The therapist has his or her back to the patient. Grasp the foot, placing both thumbs just below the lateral malleoli. Slightly distract the joint (both the talocrual and subtalar joints will distract). Slowly flex and extend the ankle (keep the joint distracted). At the very end of flexion and extension it is *normal* to feel a "clunk;" this may be from subtalar joint motion between the talus and calcaneus that is thought to be required for a full range of motion in flexion and extension of the talocrual (ankle) joint (Hertling & Kessler 2006; Magee 2014).

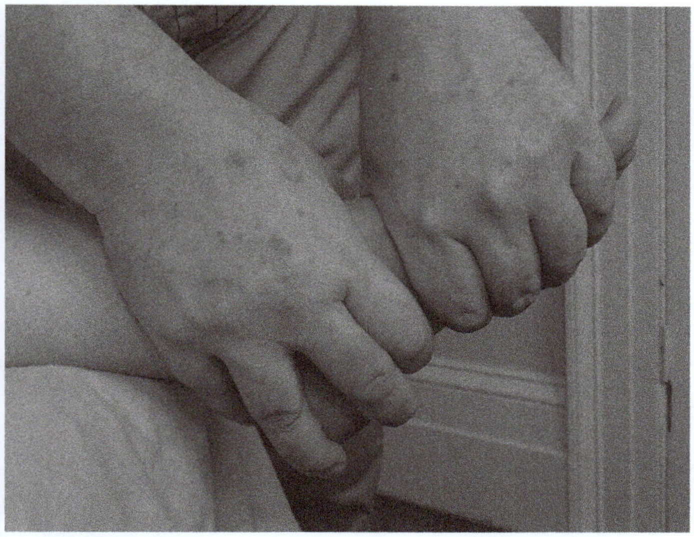

FIGURE 7.23 Superior-inferior glides and rotation to mid-tarsal and tarsal-metatarsal joints

(1) Carefully landmark and place the web-space of one hand over the talus and navicular (just distal to the malleoli) and the other hand over the cuneiforms. Have the thumbs and fingers reach under the medial and lateral arches of the foot. With distal hand apply an inferior and then superior shear through the mid-tarsals. Repeat three or four times. If pain-free then with the distal hand apply a rotatory force medially and laterally) through the mid-tarsals. (2) Shift the hands so the proximal hand is stabilizing over the cuneiforms and the distal hand is over the base of the metatarsals. Apply inferior and superior shears. Then apply the rotatory motions through the tarsal-metatarsal joints. (Shears/glides and rotation contribute to pronation and supination.)

Hertling & Kessler 2006; Kaltenborn 2006; Kisner & Colby 2012; Magee 2014; Starkey & Brown 2015.)

Metatarsophalangeal and interphalageal joint play assessment (Figures 7.24, 7.25)

Interphalangeal joint assessment (Figure 7.26)

The photos show some of the testing of the great toe. The therapist can then proceed to test the other four toes in the same manner. Of course, there will be one more step required as the other toes have proximal and distal interphalangeal joints (PIPs and DIPs). The testing of these simply proceeds as above.

Active resisted range of motion (AR-ROM)

CLINICAL NOTE: Have the patient begin the following isometric testing using only a portion of their strength and then, during a count of 5, build up until maximum exertion is reached. If the therapist is concerned that a patient may overpower them they should tell the patient to resist their pressure with only equal counter-pressure, and have the patient match the increasing pressure being applied by the therapist during a count of 5. The patient is supposed to immediately tell the therapist if pain is felt. If pain is felt stop the isometric testing to prevent further injury to involved tissues. The patient needs to reach full exertion,

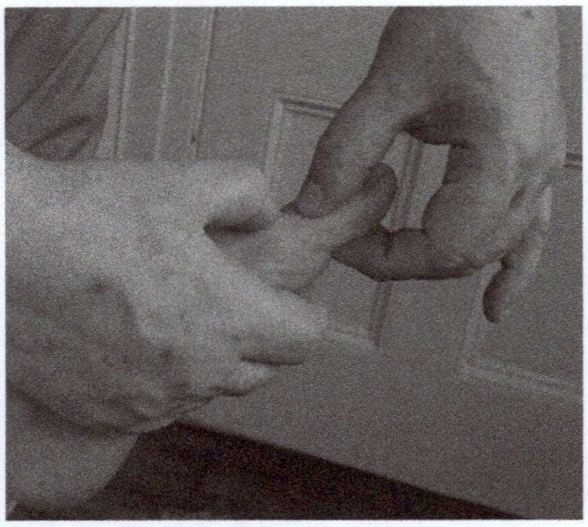

FIGURE 7.24 Metatarsophalangeal and interphalageal joint play assessment

(A) *Metatarsophalangeal distraction.* With one hand grasp with thumb and index finger the metatarsal head and with the other hand grasp the proximal phalange. Apply long-axis traction. Begin gently increasing traction, release slowly. Then gently compress the joint surfaces and again distract. Repeat several times. Compressing assists palpation of the amount of maximum play between the joint surfaces.

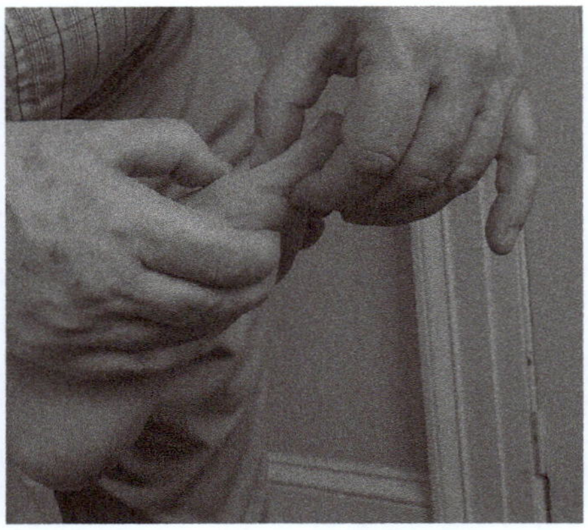

FIGURE 7.25

(B) *Metatarsophalangeal superior-inferior glides.* Position hold as above with slightest traction ("dis-engagement" of joint surfaces) then apply an inferior glide and then superior.
(C) *Metatarsophalangeal medial-lateral glides.* Hold as in (B) and apply gentle glides side to side. Alternatively, the therapist may shift the distal hand's finger position so that thumb and index finger are on the medial and lateral sides of the phalange.
(D) *Metatarsophalangeal rotation.* Hold as in (B) or (C). Alternative hold: using the distal hand rotate the joint medially and laterally.

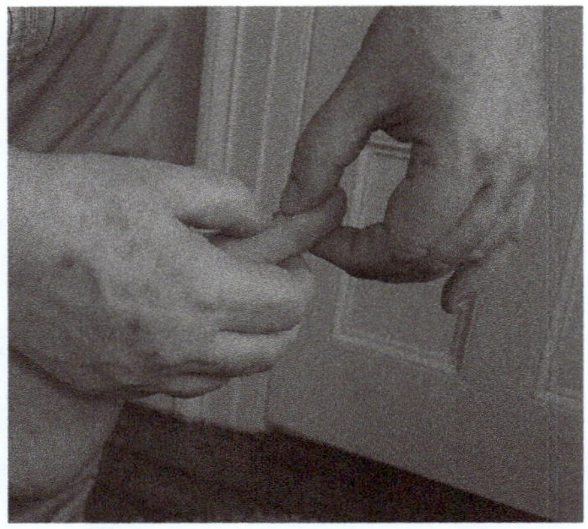

FIGURE 7.26 Interphalangeal joint assessment

Joint play assessment continues now by repeating these movements to assess the great toe's interphalangeal joint. All of these movements are repeated to test the interphalangeal joint as were used on the metatarsophalangeal joint. The proximal hand stabilizes the proximal phalange while the distal hand holds and moves the distal phalange of a joint.

if possible, to see if (1) there is full strength followed by pain, which indicates a mild strain to the tissues; or (2) weakness is encountered without any pain, which is a neurological red flag. Any sign of neurological involvement requires a referral back to their primary physician. If the patient is told to use only part of their strength then both (1) and (2) could be missed.

If the patient can perform strength testing while weight-bearing, do as follows (see quick testing).

Have the patient perform each of the actions in Figures 7.27–7.30 while they walk back and forth (see also Figure 7.31). If it is necessary to help the patient keep their balance, place your hand on their shoulder and follow along with them as they walk. Even if you let the patient walk back and forth on their own, stay close and be ready to assist them to stay upright. Note: these are not isometric tests but since the musculature of the legs is very strong isometric testing may be impractical as the patient often overpowers the therapist.

Perform the tests as follows:

First, have the patient go up onto the toes while standing on both feet to test plantar flexion. Hold for 5 seconds, repeat 10 times. If there is no discomfort or fatigue, then repeat the test with the patient using only one foot at a time. Remember to test

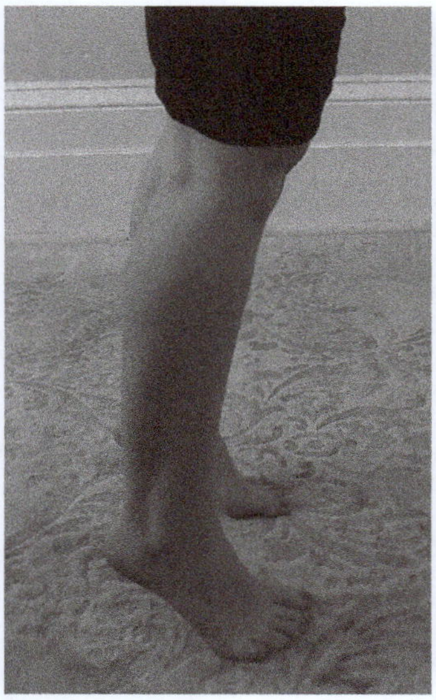

FIGURE 7.27 Plantar flexion
Stand on toes, then walk.

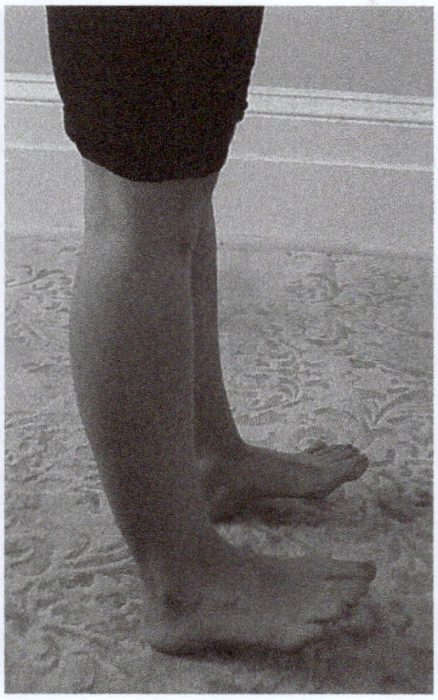

FIGURE 7.28 Dorsiflexion
Stand on heels, then walk.

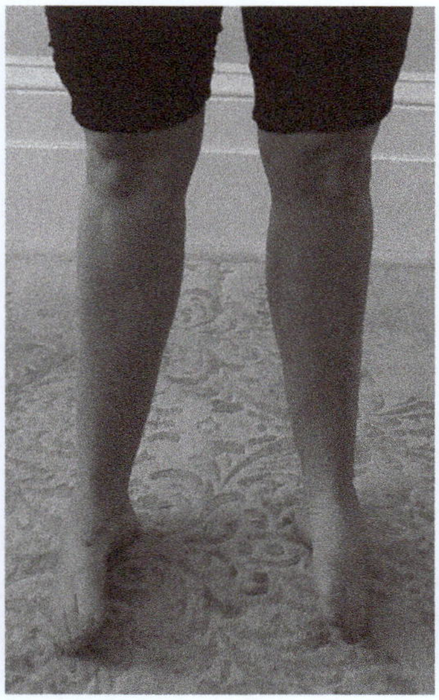

FIGURE 7.29 Supination
Roll onto lateral edge of feet, knees coming further apart (varus), then walk.

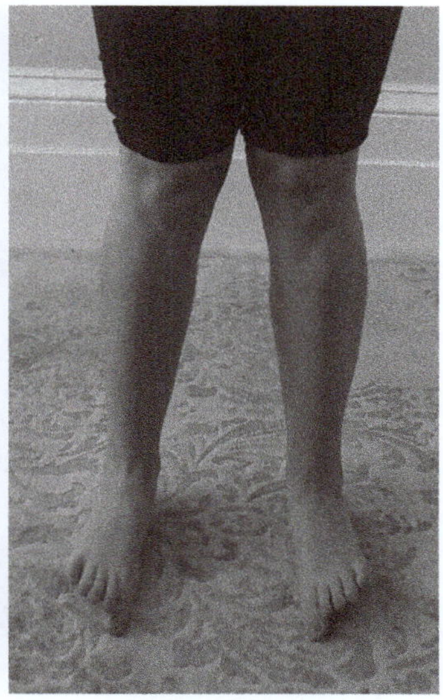

FIGURE 7.30 Pronation
Roll onto inside edges of feet, knees coming together (valgus), then walk.

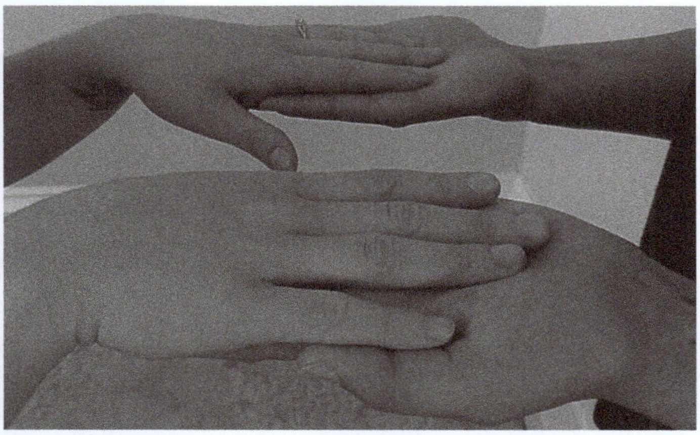

FIGURE 7.31 Assisting with weight-bearing
If the patient cannot walk back and forth, perform the test by supporting as follows: hold out your hands palms up and tell the patient to place their hands on top of yours. While the patient performs these actions (as shown previously) standing in one spot, you can notice weakness or fatigue by the patient putting pressure into your hand. It will be felt in one hand on the weak side, or onto both hands if bilaterally fatigued or weak. Difficulty with balance will cause the patient's pressure to alternate in amount. They may move side to side and/or forward and back. Have the patient report any pain or sense of weakness.

the unaffected side first. Plantar flexion is tested differently than other three motions because strength of plantar flexors usually requires time to fatigue before unilateral weakness will even begin to show.

To test the other three motions, have the patient perform and hold each motion (dorsiflexion, supination, and pronation) for 20–30 seconds. To prevent any further injury, always do these three AR-ROM tests bilaterally.

Non-weight-bearing AR-ROM testing

If the patient appears acutely injured, or is unable to do the AR testing weight-bearing, then do the following: with the patient supine (or high-sitting), tell the patient to hold a position while they resist you moving their foot. Remember to increase the amount of pressure slowly. Move toward maximum yet pain-free exertion. Test dorsiflexion, plantar flexion, pronation, and supination in this progressive manner (Figures 7.32–7.35).

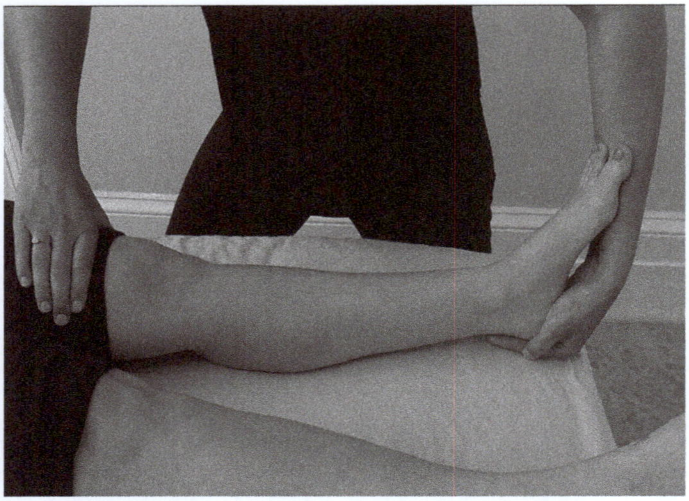

FIGURE 7.32 **Resisted plantar flexion**

Have the patient's ankle in neutral position. To test all plantar flexor muscles as a group, have the patient's legs extended. Stabilize the thigh with one hand, and with other, cup the heel and have your forearm under the patient's foot. Tell the patient to hold this position as you try to dorsiflex the foot.

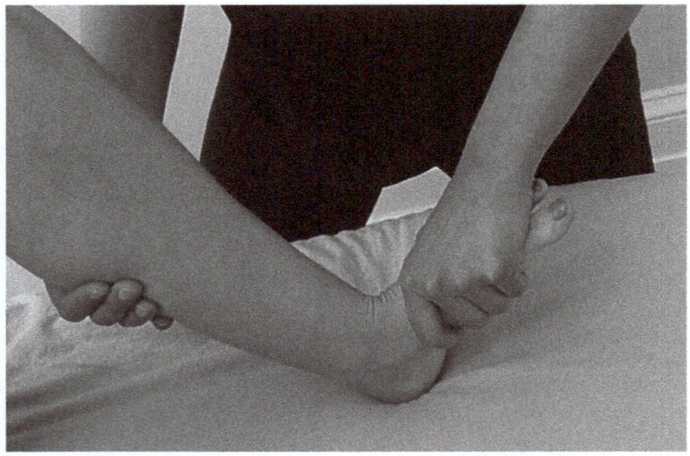

FIGURE 7.33 **Resisted dorsiflexion**

Stabilize above the ankle with one hand, and apply pressure or resistance with the other hand across the metatarsals. Have the ankle in neutral position. It is best to have the knee bent and use the heel on the table as the axis of movement. This prevents excessive movement or exertion by the patient of tissues above the knee.

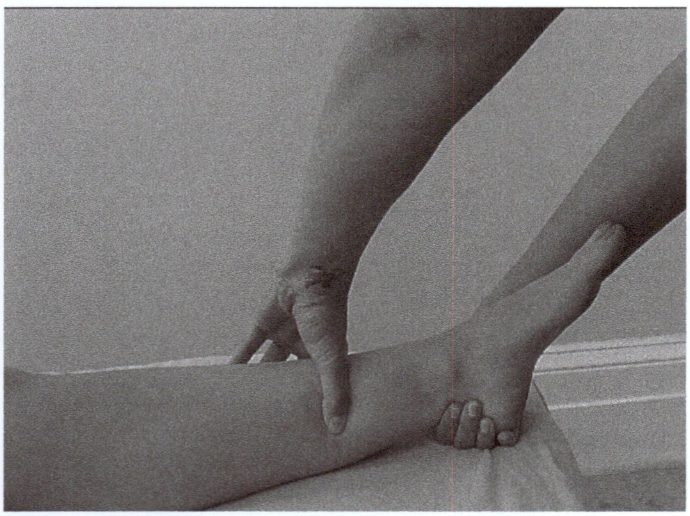

FIGURE 7.34 **Resisted supination**

With the ankle in neutral position, stabilize the lower leg above the ankle, then have your other hand cupped around the calcaneus and lateral border of the patient's foot against the inside of your forearm. Have them try to hold this position while you try to invert the hindfoot and adduct the forefoot (i.e., bring the foot into supination).

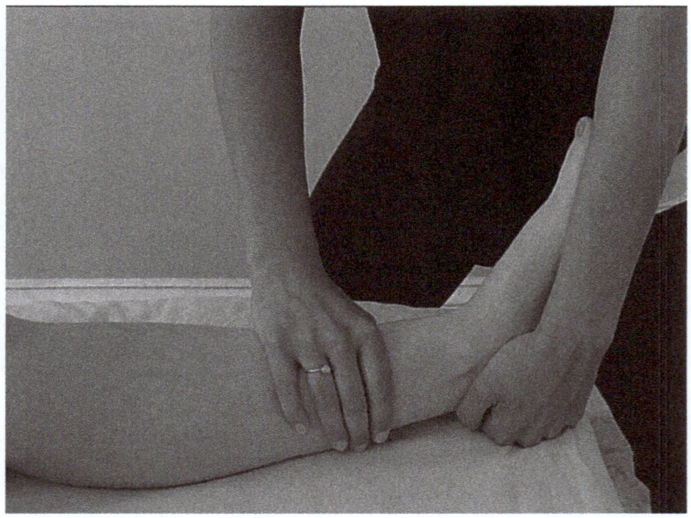

FIGURE 7.35 **Resisted pronation**

With the ankle in neutral position, stabilize the lower leg above the ankle, then have your other hand cupped around the calcaneus and medial border of the patient's foot against the inside of your forearm. Have them try to hold this position while you try to evert the hindfoot and abduct the forefoot (i.e., bring the foot into pronation).

Special tests

Differential muscle testing

The therapist uses differential muscle testing on those muscles that have been possibly implicated as impaired during AF- or AR-ROM testing, or by the patient's description of pain and/or dysfunction (see Part I, Chapter 3; see also Kendall et al. 2005 for a comprehensive exploration of and instruction in muscle testing; see and compare: Dutton 2012; Hartley 2000b; Hertling & Kessler 2006; Magee 2014).

Differentiating between soleus and gastrocnemius (Figures 7.36–7.38)

Though these two muscles share the same tendon, the gastrocnemius crosses the knee while the soleus does not. Because of this, one is often more hypertonic and/or more painful than the other. Which muscle is affected depends on many factors, such as daily activities, knee and ankle issues, etc.

We can also stress the tibialis posterior specifically (Figure 7.39). It can be highly involved in plantar flexion when patients exert

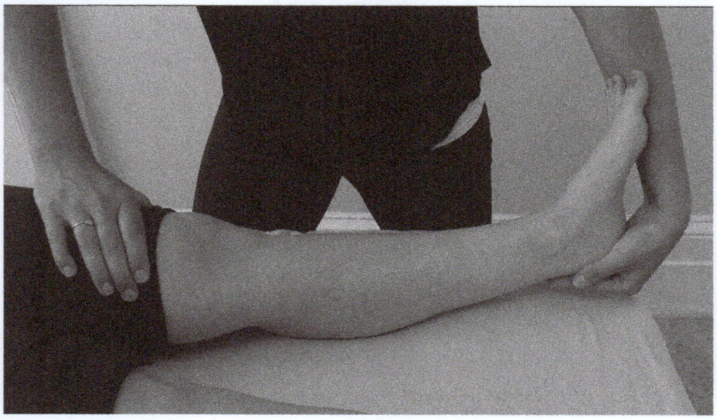

FIGURE 7.36 1. Testing both muscles

Stand at the side of the table and reach back to cup the patient's calcaneus with the hand while the forearm is under the patient's foot. Have the patient's foot close to neutral and either resist the patient's attempt to plantar flex or have them hold this position and try to dorsiflex the foot.

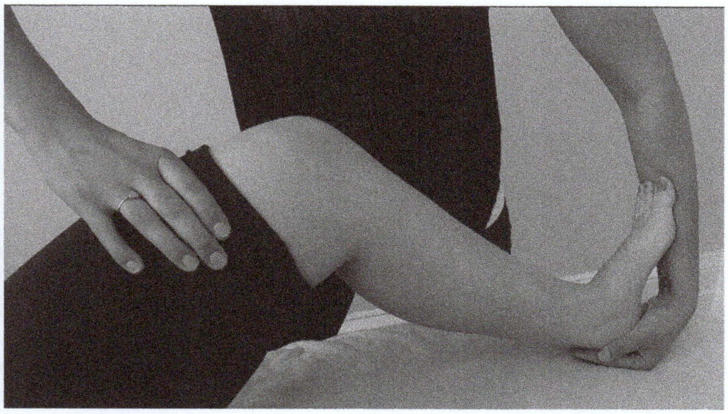

FIGURE 7.37 2. Stressing soleus

Keep the position of the resisting hand as in the first picture, but now the knee is bent slightly, making the gastrocnemius less efficient so the soleus muscle becomes the prime mover. Compare the results of the two tests.

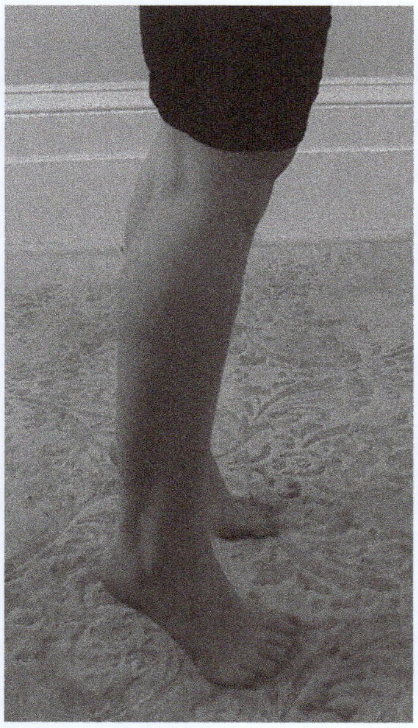

FIGURE 7.38 Differentiating in standing

First, have thepatient stand on the toes for a minute or more (or they can go up on toes repeatedly if more fatiguing is required). Second, to make gastrocnemius insufficient and stress soleus more, have the patient flex the knees slightly. Compare results of these two testing positions.

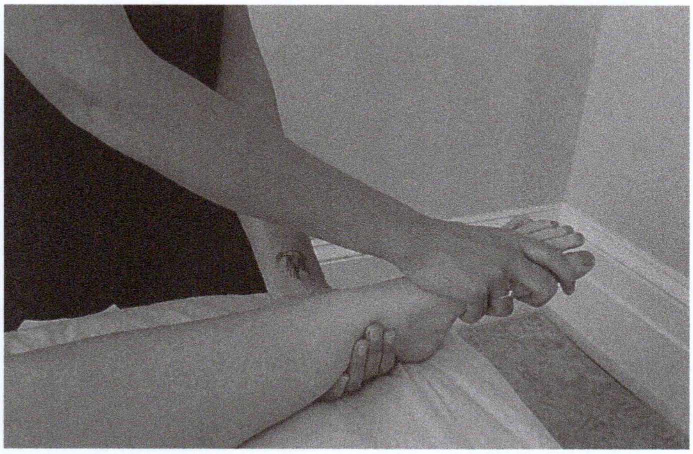

FIGURE 7.39 Testing tibialis posterior

Plantar flex and invert the foot for the patient and then try to dorsiflex and evert the foot as the patient resists.

themselves while walking long distances or running, and especially climbing stairs. The tibialis anterior can also be stressed specifically (Figure 7.40).

Testing fibularis (peroneus) longus and brevis

These muscles both evert and plantar flex the foot (Figure 7.41). The fibularis muscles are commonly injured (eccentric muscle strain) when the patient sprains the lateral ligaments of the ankle. They are often tender on palpation when patients suffer chronic ankle and foot ailments.

The fibularis (peroneus) tertius helps to evert and dorsiflex the foot (Figure 7.42). Therefore, we can resist the patient performing these motions simultaneously; or we can place the foot in inversion and dorsiflexion and have the patient resist our attempt to move it out of that position. The latter is preferred.

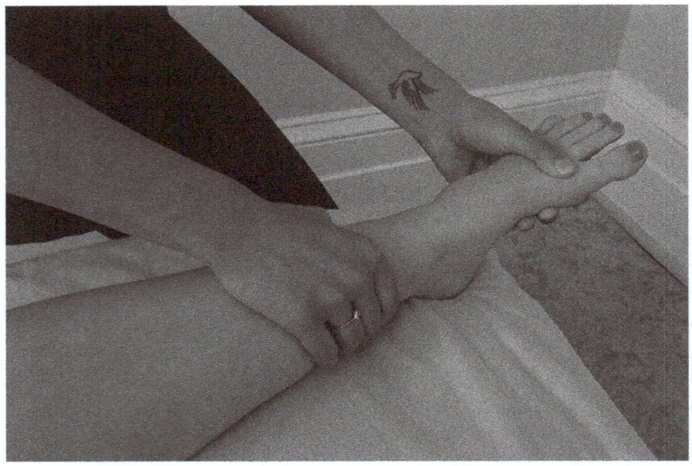

FIGURE 7.41 Testing fibularis longus and brevis

Passively evert and plantar flex the foot. Next, have the patient resist dorsiflexion and inversion. Note: you cannot differentiate between longus and brevis as they are too close together and the fibers run in the same direction.

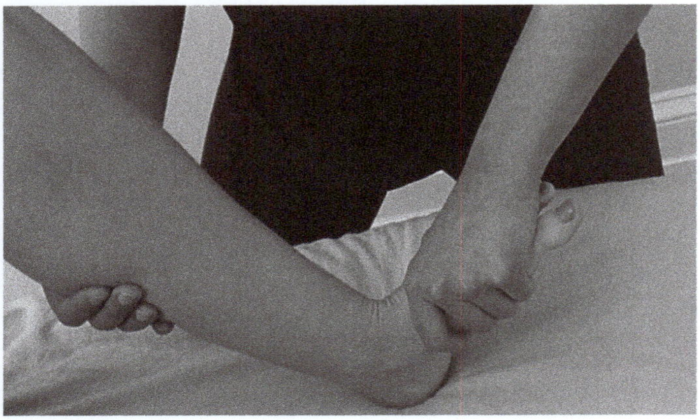

FIGURE 7.40 Testing tibialis anterior

Dorsiflex and invert the foot. Ask the patient to hold this position. As they resist, try to plantar flex and evert the foot.

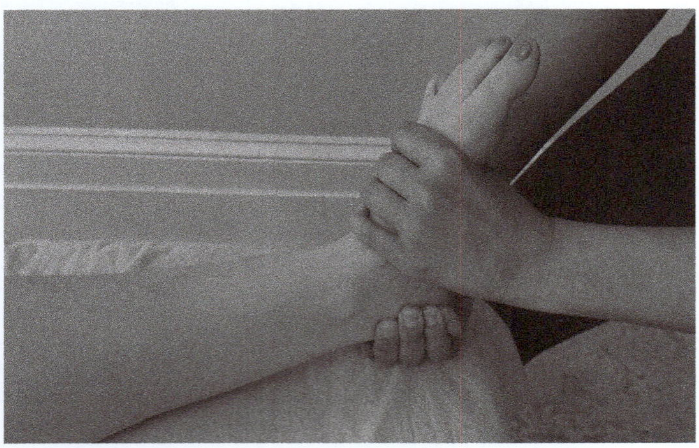

FIGURE 7.42 Testing fibularis tertius

Evert and dorsiflex the foot for the patient. Then have the patient resist you trying to invert the foot.

Testing the long flexors of the toes

The long flexors and extensors of the toes also need investigation here, as they can contribute to talocrural joint motions, as well as their principal task of moving the phalanges (Figures 7.43–7.46).

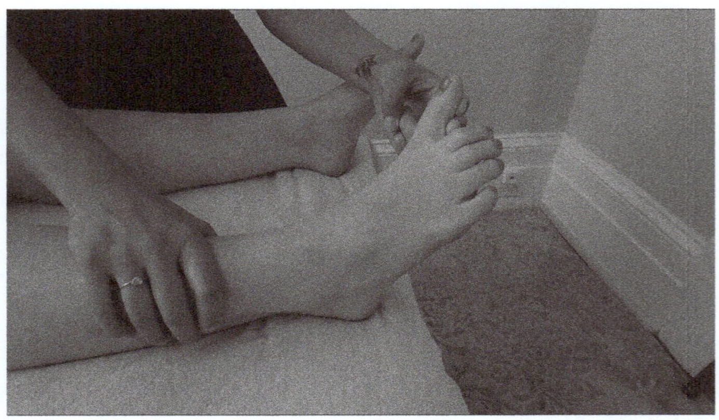

FIGURE 7.43 Testing flexor hallux longus

Flex the patient's big toe for them, then try to extend the toe by pressing up on the distal phalange. It should be strong enough to resist.

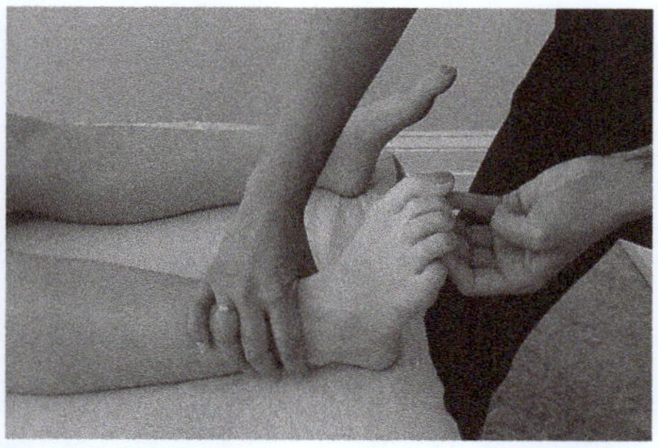

FIGURE 7.44 Testing flexor digitorum longus

Flex the toes for the patient and then have them resist you trying to extend them. Your pressure should be exerted at the distal phalanges.

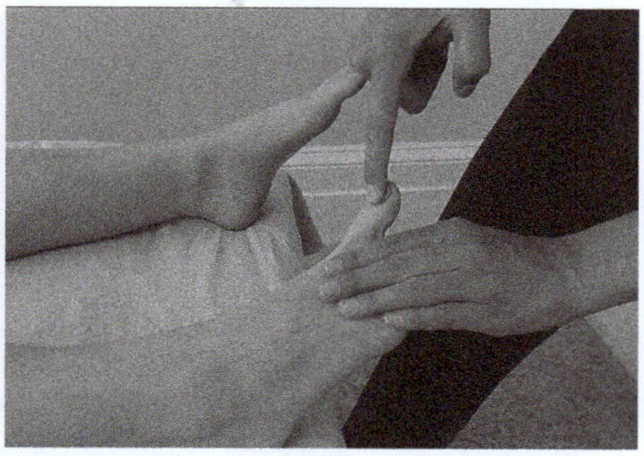

FIGURE 7.45 Testing extensor hallux longus

Lift the big toe into extension. Have the patient hold extension while you try to flex the toe. The patient should be able to resist. Weakness without pain suggests a problem with the L5 motor nerve.

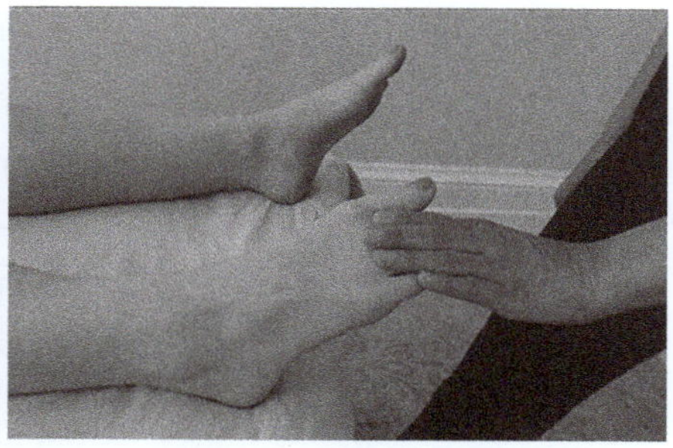

FIGURE 7.46 Testing extensor digitorum longus and brevis

Extend the patient's toes for them. Ask the patient to try to extend the toes further as you resist. To stress brevis more, dorsiflex the foot to make longus insufficient and then have the patient extend.

Ligament tests

Talar tilts

These passive tests are designed to stress the primary ligaments of the talocrural joint in an orderly and systematic manner (Hartley 2000b).

Medial (deltoid) talar tilts (Figures 7.47–7.49)

This medial ligament is fan-shaped and made up of three portions. It does not tear easily. In fact when the test is positive, it is more likely a periosteal tear or an avulsion fracture than an actual tearing of the ligament itself. With an avulsion fracture, the joint is then hypermobile on the medial side.

Lateral talar tilts (Figures 7.50–7.52)

The three tests shown in Figures 7.50, 7.51, and 7.52 test ligaments on the lateral side of the foot.

Anterior draw test (Figures 7.53, 7.54)

This is another way to test the anterior talofibular ligament. The name comes from the movement performed during testing. Besides testing for injury to the ligament, the advantage of this test is that it will show instability from a ruptured anterior talofibular ligament. A ruptured ligament may not elicit pain that is specific to that ligament's location.

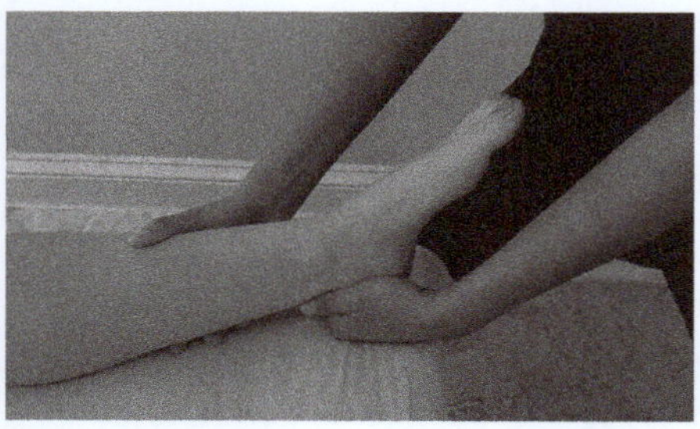

FIGURE 7.47 1. Middle fibers

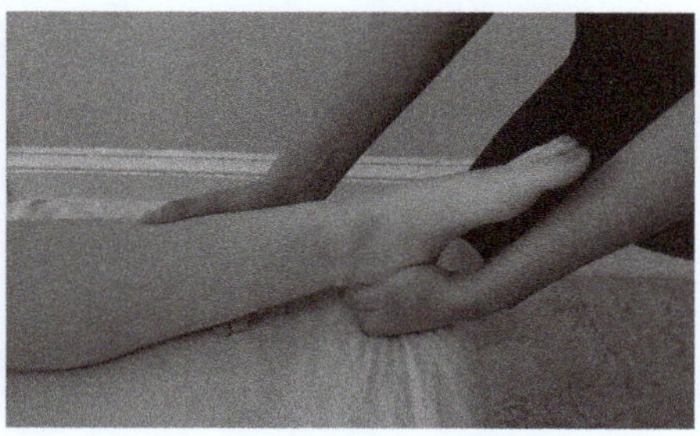

FIGURE 7.48 2. Anterior fibers

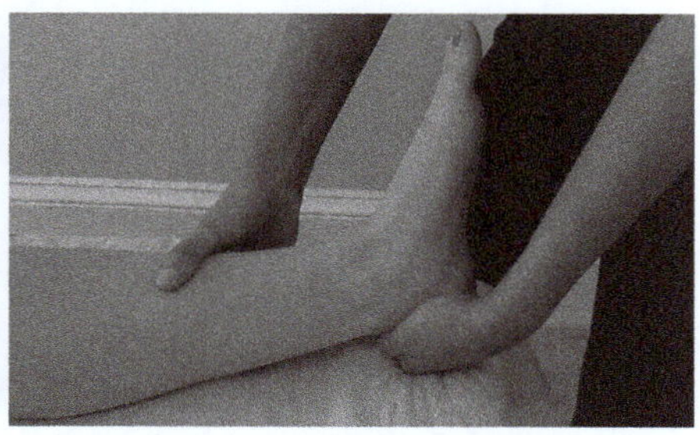

FIGURE 7.49 3. Posterior fibers

Have the patient's foot in neutral. Support the leg above the ankle and grasp the calcaneus. (1) With the foot in neutral, slowly evert the foot, testing predominately middle fibers. (2) Slowly plantar flex and then evert the foot to test anterior fibers. (3) Dorsiflex and evert the foot to test posterior fibers. A positive sign is pain or excessive movement.

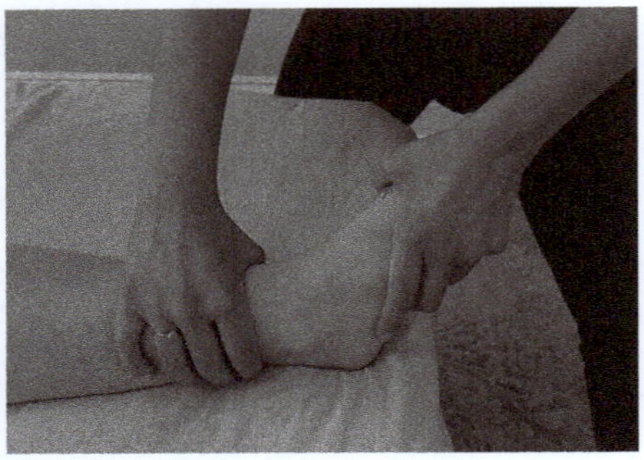

FIGURE 7.50 Anterior talofibular ligament test

Passively move the patient's foot into plantar flexion and inversion. A positive sign is pain is felt along the ligament or at its attachments.

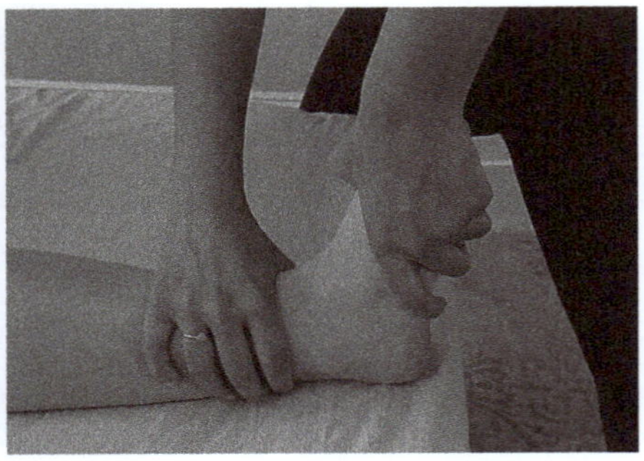

FIGURE 7.51 Testing calcaneofibular ligament

The patient's foot is in slight dorsiflexion. Bring the foot into inversion. Pain felt along the site of the ligament is a positive sign. This strong ligament is often injured only after the anterior talofibular has already lost its integrity.

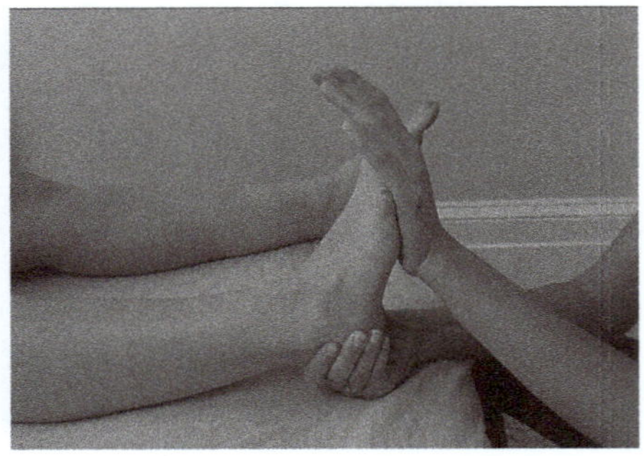

FIGURE 7.52 Posterior talofibular ligament test

Passively dorsiflex the foot. With the other hand, grasp the calcaneus, and invert the foot while drawing the heel posteriorly.

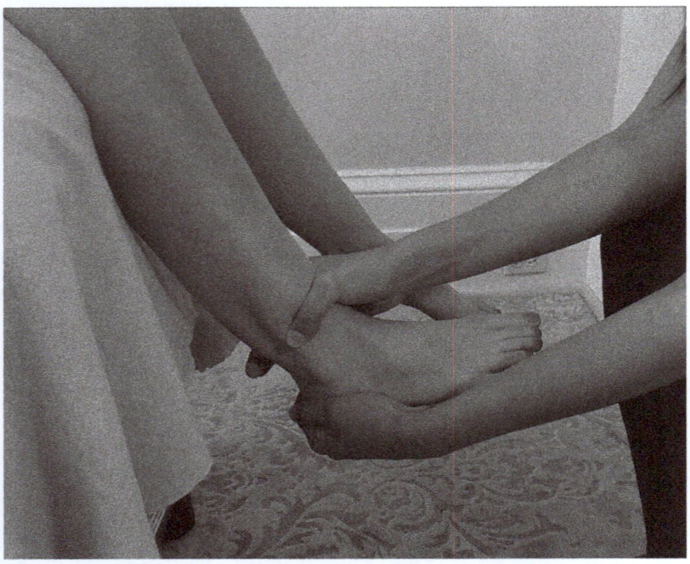

FIGURE 7.53 Anterior draw test of ankle

With patient high-sitting, stabilize the lower leg with one hand just above ankle and cupping the calcaneus with the other hand; now, draw the heel toward you, thereby placing a stretch on the ligament. A positive sign is pain (where the ligament is located) and/or hypermobility of the joint seen and felt by the heel moving forward.

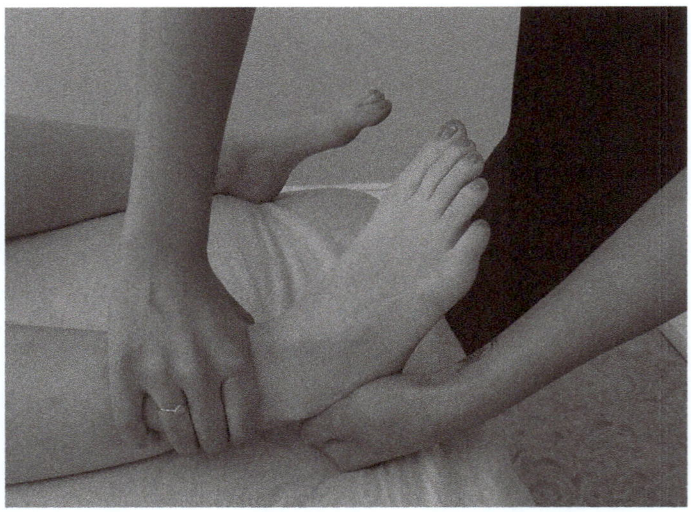

FIGURE 7.54 Alternative positioning for anterior draw test

You can perform the test with the patient in a supine position. Place a towel roll or pillow under the knee to release any tension in gastrocnemius and soleus (not shown here). While stabilizing the lower leg, cup the calcaneus in other hand and draw it forward. A positive sign is pain felt along the course of the ligament, and/or hypermobility noted as the head of the talus moves forward, sometimes with a "clunk." Note: without the towel roll under the knee, gastrocnemius-soleus can be in spasm and prevent the calcaneus from moving forward.

Wedge test (Figure 7.55)

This tests the integrity of the anterior inferior tibiofibular ligament (which helps hold the tibia and fibula together). It can be injured by jumping down from too great a height, or having the foot excessively dorsiflexed. The test is meant to push the head of the talus up between the tibia and fibula, putting tension on the ligament between them, reproducing the action that caused the sprain. It is good to perform the wedge test as it eliminates the anterior talofibular ligament as the source of the pain.

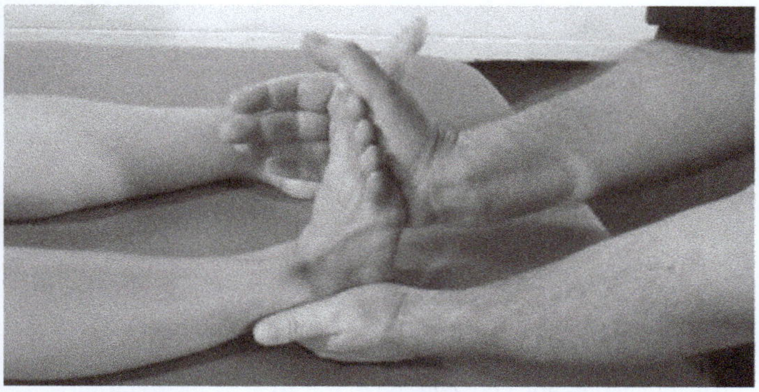

FIGURE 7.55 Wedge test by dorsiflexion

If the patient agrees, you can passively dorsiflex the foot and apply O-P. This will cause a larger anterior portion of the talus to press the malleoli apart, putting tension through the anterior inferior talofibular ligament. The patient is then instructed to point to the exact place where pain is felt if the test is positive.

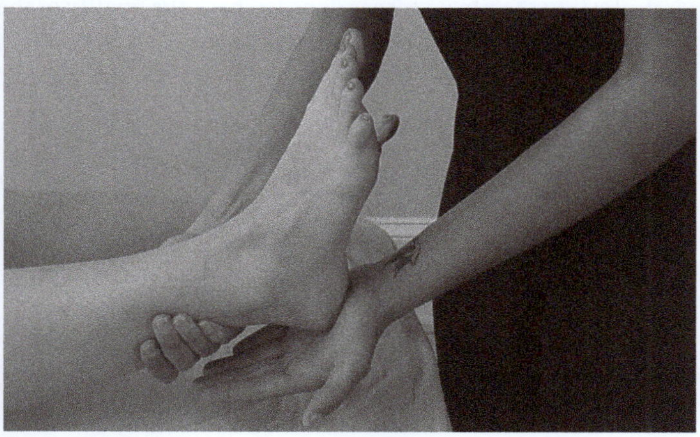

FIGURE 7.56 1. Mild provocation

With one hand, apply pressure to the bottom of the calcaneus superiorly.

Alternative wedge test (Figures 7.56, 7.57)

This is a progressively provocative testing of the anterior inferior tibiofibular ligament. If the patient is apprehensive about the dorsiflexion test, you can do the following. Have the patient's foot in neutral while they are supine with the ankle off the table.

Achilles tendon rupture test (aka Thompson's test) (Figure 7.58)

This is a simple classic test that has been used to see if the Achilles tendon has ruptured. However, if it has totally ruptured, the gastrocnemius (and soleus) often "slides up" into a ball shape, giving the back of the leg a distinctive look. The test is required only if there is a partial rupture.

With a complete rupture of any tendon, remember that there may be no pain present, as the nerves themselves can be severed. The patient may complain of having had the sensation of a ball rolling up the back of the leg, or that it felt like someone kicked them, or felt a slithering sensation up the calf. These sensations are caused by the muscle shortening when its attachment is ruptured.

Squeeze test for Morton's neuroma (Figure 7.59)

This is to test for the presence of a neuroma between the metatarsal heads, usually between the third and fourth metatarsals. This is called a Morton's neuroma.

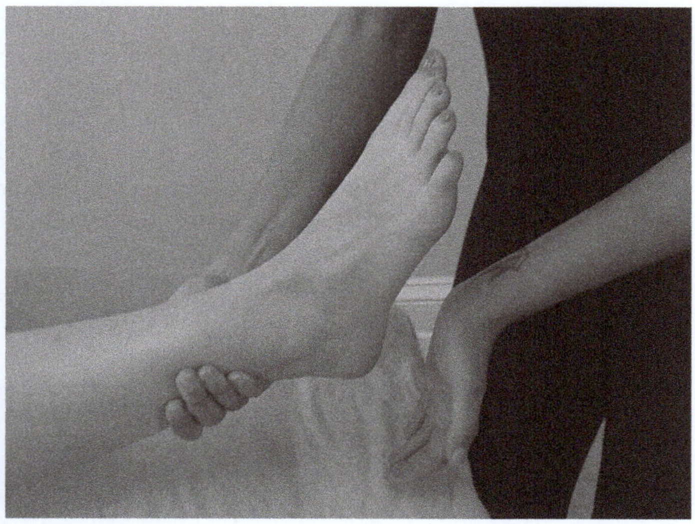

FIGURE 7.57 2. Moderate provocation

If the procedure in 1. produces no pain at the site of the ligament, then you may increase provocation by hitting the bottom of the heel with a quick, mild blow or tap.

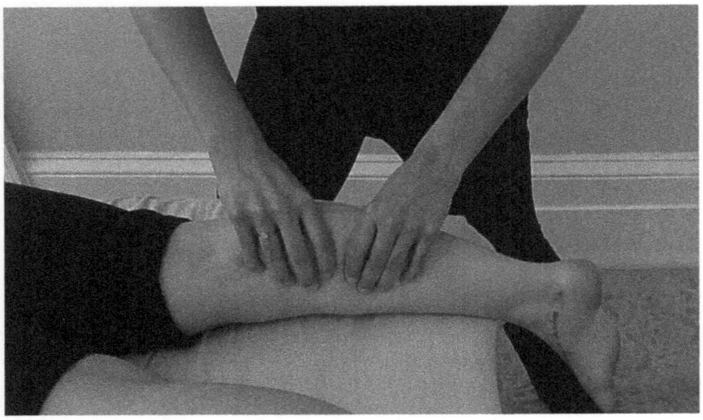

FIGURE 7.58

Have the patient prone with feet off the table. With both hands, squeeze the calf and look to see if the foot plantar flexes. If it does not plantar flex, the test is positive and that means that there is a severe tear or complete rupture of the Achilles tendon. (Refer the patient to their doctor or emergency department.)

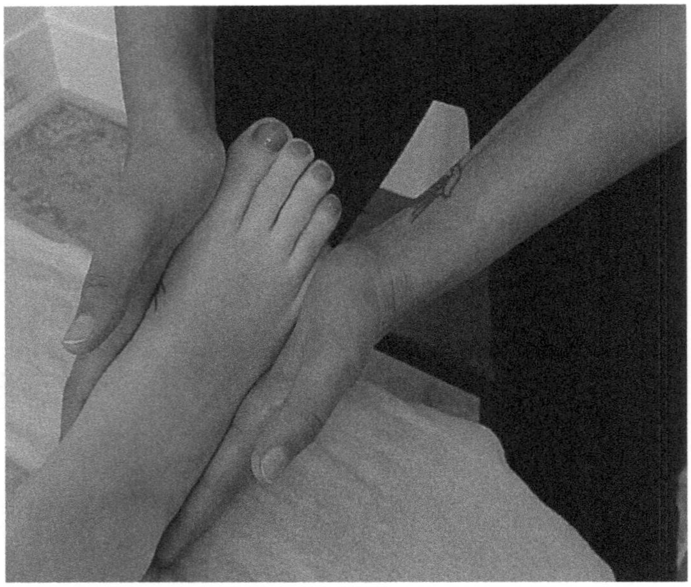

FIGURE 7.59 Squeeze test for neuroma

Encircle the forefoot with both hands while keeping it relatively flat, and squeeze the metatarsal heads together. Do not let the forefoot arch with the pressure applied. If this creates a sharp pain between second and third, or third and fourth metatarsals, then the test is positive.

Testing for tarsal tunnel syndrome (Tinel's sign) (Figures 7.60, 7.61)

Tarsal tunnel syndrome is when there is swelling in the tendon sheaths, compressing the tibial nerve behind the medial malleoli. This causes pain, usually felt into the bottom of the foot. The patient may experience weakness of intrinsic muscles of the plantar surface of the foot. The compression occurs in a "tunnel," the "walls" of which are made up of the tough connective tissue of the retinaculum of the ankle as it wraps around the lower portion of the malleoli, and by both the bony malleoli and the bony calcaneus. This is much like the carpal tunnel in the wrist. The syndrome usually occurs in those who go "en pointe," such as dancers, and gymnasts. The tibialis anterior, flexor digitorum, and hallucis muscles are overused, to the point where the sheaths behind the malleoli swell and compress the tibial nerve.

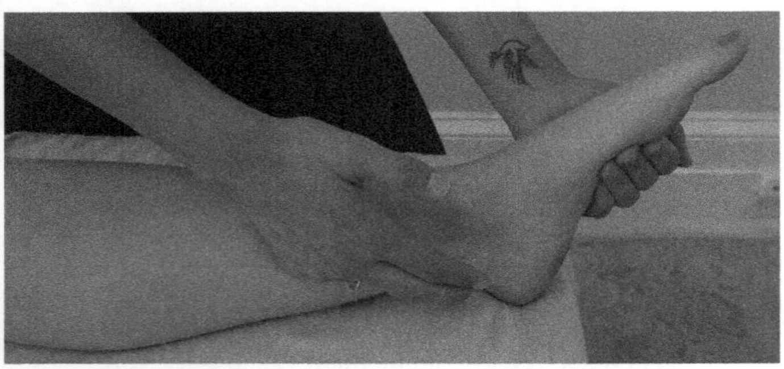

FIGURE 7.60 1. Positioning for tarsal tunnel test

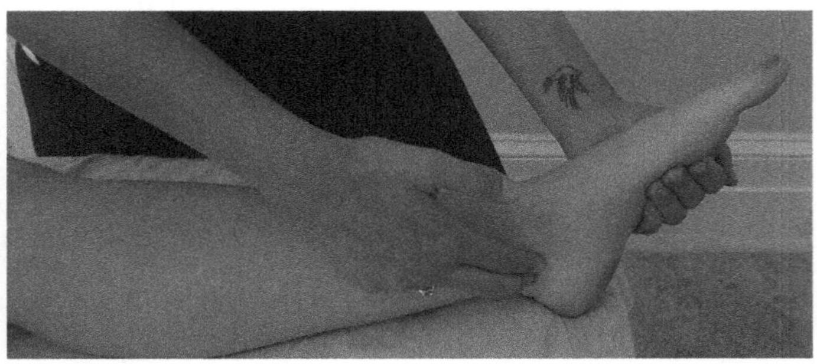

FIGURE 7.61 2. Tapping over tarsal tunnel

Using either the tips of the index and third fingers held together, or a reflex hammer, percuss (tap) several times behind the medial malleoli. A positive sign is pain and or paresthesia felt distal to the area tapped.

Testing for pulses in the foot (Figures 7.62, 7.63)

If the patient's foot feels cold, or is blue, edematous, or numb/tingling, then test for appropriate blood flow into the foot.

1. Testing the tibial pulse is done to check the quality of the blood flow into the bottom (plantar area) of the foot. This pulse is fairly strong and highly palpable in most people.

2. Testing the dorsal pedal pulse assesses the quality of blood flow into the dorsum of the foot. The pulse is palpated just laterally to the external hallux longus tendon as the arterial vessel passes over the talus and navicular bones. To locate the hallux longus tendon, resist the patient's attempt to extend their big toe. The tendon becomes very prominent.

Homans' sign (Figures 7.64–7.66)

Testing for Homans' sign has traditionally been done for thrombosis. Pain felt deep in the calf or popliteal fossa of the knee is an indication to do the test. The onset often begins after a period of immobilization of the leg(s), for example, after hospitalization, prolonged illness, immobilization of a lower limb because of a fracture, etc. It may also be present as an ache in the calf that becomes more intense with movement of the limb, for example, walking or climbing stairs. It may reveal itself as "intermittent claudication" (a cramp-like pain).

The patient may report being able to walk a certain distance and then pain in the calf appears and grows until they must rest. The pain will go away, but if the activity is resumed the pain will reappear at

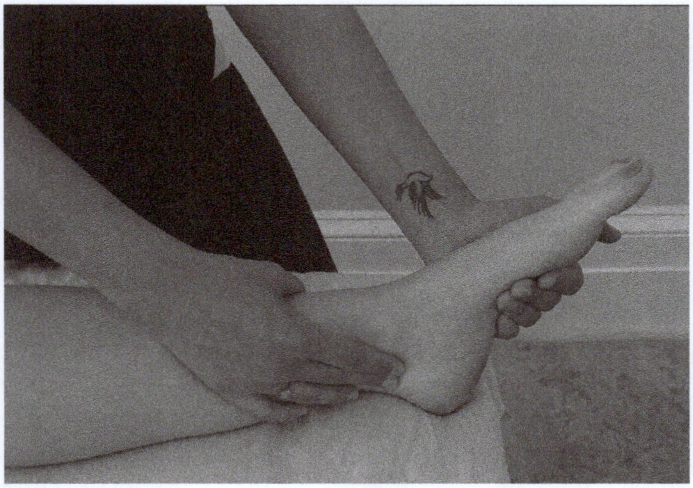

FIGURE 7.62 1. Testing tibial pulse

Palpate lightly about 1 inch above the medial malleoli.

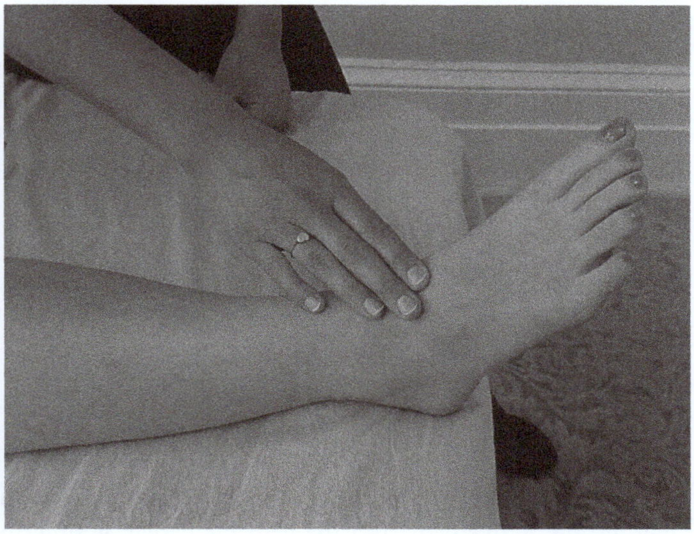

FIGURE 7.63 2. Testing dorsal pedal pulse

Palpate over the dorsal pedal artery.

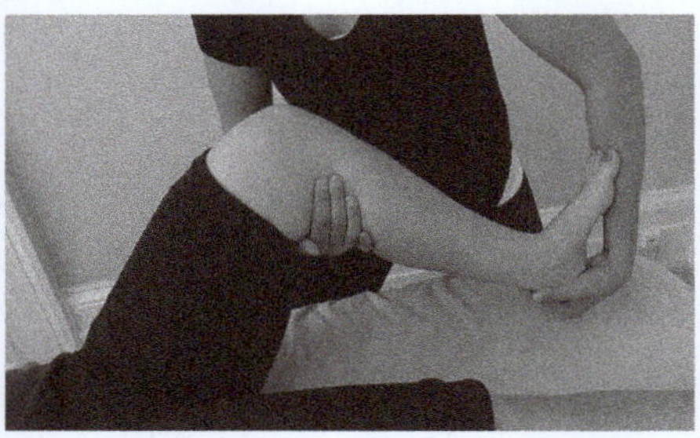

FIGURE 7.64 1. Positioning

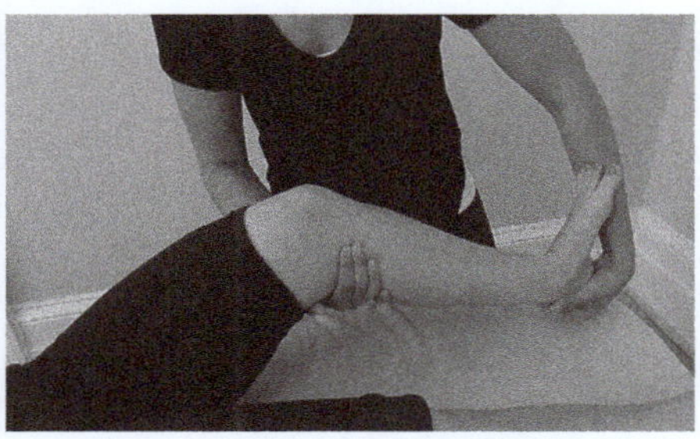

FIGURE 7.65 2. Dorsiflexion and extending knee

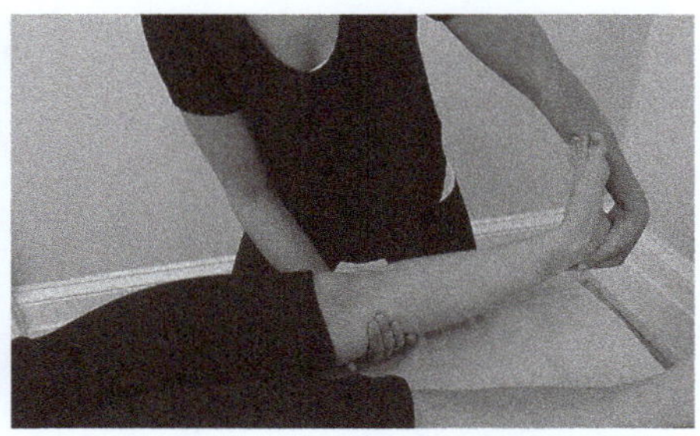

FIGURE 7.66 3. Final position

With the patient supine (though can also be prone), have the knee bent 45°, dorsiflex the foot, then slowly extend the knee. This will increase pressure inside the posterior compartment of the lower leg where thrombi are often situated. If pain is felt upon extension of the knee, then test is considered positive. This is considered a medical emergency and a contraindication to any treatment by a massage therapist. When performing this test, or whenever you are suspicious of a thrombus, do not palpate for a lesion.

consistent intervals, always getting some relief with rest. Blood flow is being impeded, and with increased requirements demanded by activity, the muscles undergo hypoxia and become painful.

The test itself is not conclusive, but may only reinforce a suspicion of the existence of a deep vein thrombosis (DVT). If the therapist is suspicious, it is not wise to do the test as it has been traditionally done, with palpation of the thrombus, as this may cause an embolism. Below is a description of a modified version of this test.

NOTE: The jury is still out about the efficacy of this test.

Physicians who specialize in blood clotting disorders and have orthopedic experience tend to not have much faith in Homans' sign, but prefer to rely on case history taking, followed by blood work. If you are suspicious of thrombosis, do not treat the area, and refer the patient to their physician for a diagnosis.

Specific ROM testing of the toes

Active range of motion of the toes:

Flexion: 45°

Extension: 70°

Metatarsal-phalangeal and phalangeal joints (toes)

The following tests can be used if the therapist believes the toes are the source or part of the pain the patient is suffering from. For completeness, have the patient flex and extend all the toes and note any restrictions of movement. Have them tell you if these motions cause any pain. If they do cause pain or discomfort, remember to ask them to clarify whether the pain being experienced is or is not the same as their chief complaint. To help clarify if the impairment is sourced in the joint perform PR-ROM testing; and to see if the impairment is from muscle perform AR-ROM testing of the toes.

AF-ROM flexion and extension of all toes (Figures 7.67, 7.68)

NOTE: If the ankle and foot move properly (i.e., normal toe-off for correct gait), the big toe must have at least 35–40° of extension, even if only passively. Have the patient focus on actively flexing and extending their big toe. The other toes will also flex and extend, but having the patient focus on the big toe helps them to show the maximum AF-ROM available.

Have the patient slowly repeat flexion and extension of all the toes (as above) several times while you observe the quality and quantity of motion in the 2nd to 5th metatarsal-phalangeal joints.

Passive relaxed range of motion (PR-ROM) of forefoot

If AF-ROM was negative, then flex and extend all of the toes as a group in PR-ROM. However, be sure to specifically test the first phalanges (big toe). It is here in PR-ROM that you should see the real joint range of the big toe. Flexion equals 45°; extension equals 70–90°. Make sure that in extension the toe has the required minimum of 35–40° of movement required for normal gait.

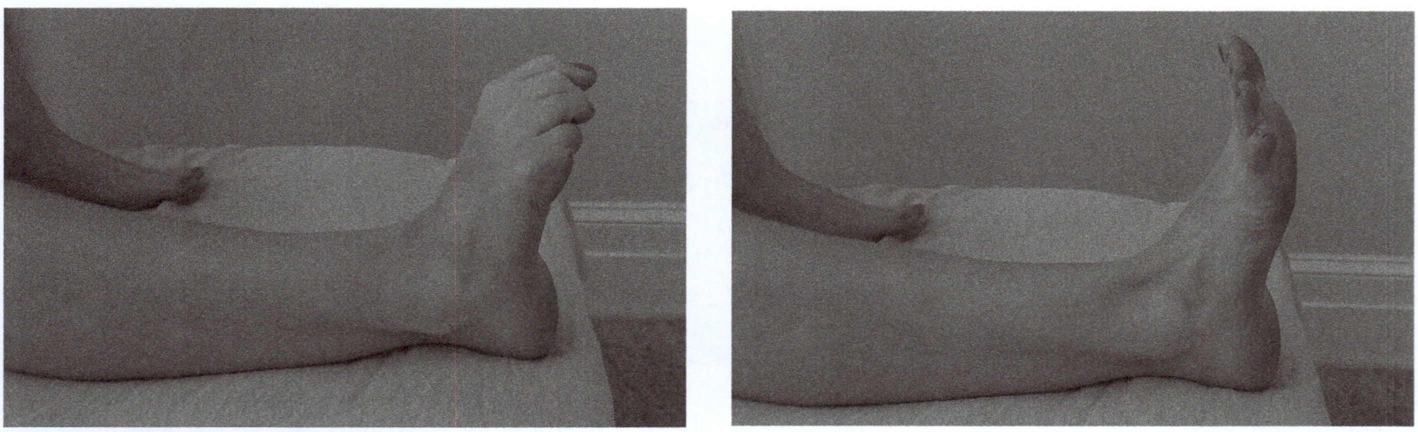

FIGURE 7.67 **Note 1st metatarsal-phalangeal joint**
(A) Flexion 45°; (B) extension up to 70–90°.

If the patient does not have the minimum motion in the big toe, they will be shifting their weight and begin to toe-off laterally onto the second or third toe. The heads of those metatarsals cannot sustain such stress (weight). A callus will build up under the head of the second and even third metatarsal which, if seen, is suggestive of this problem. Also, the threat of stress fractures developing in these much thinner metatarsals is high.

Group flexion and extension of phalanges (Figures 7.69, 7.70)

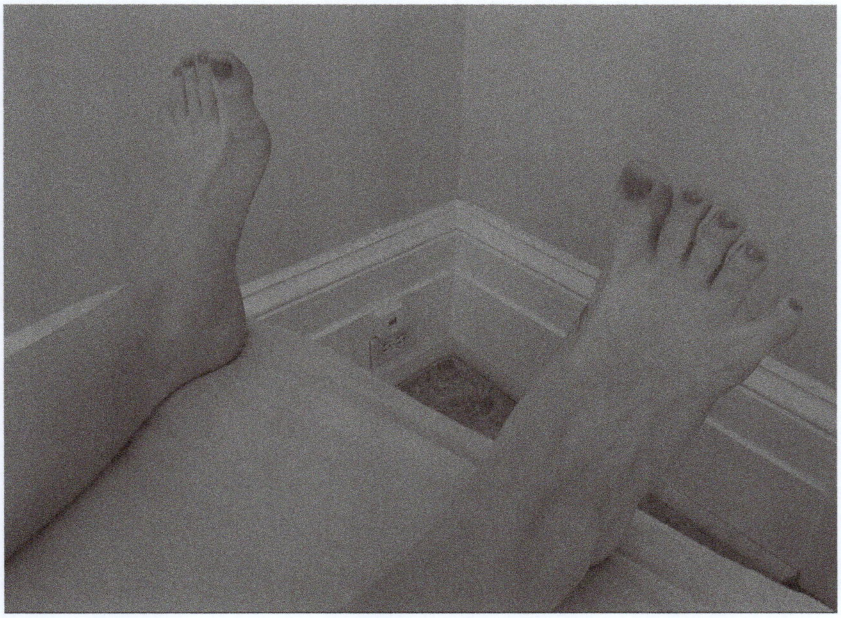

FIGURE 7.68 AF abduction of phalanges

Have the patient spread their toes, noting the quality and quantity of motion.

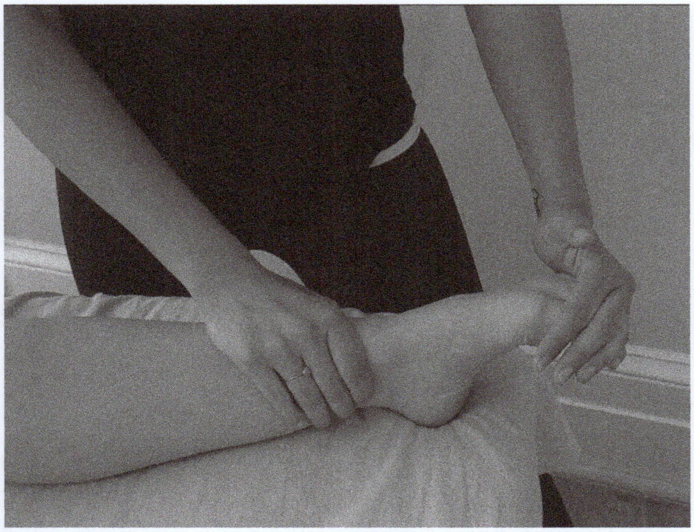

FIGURE 7.69 Metatarsal flexion 45°

Push toes via distal phalanges into flexion.

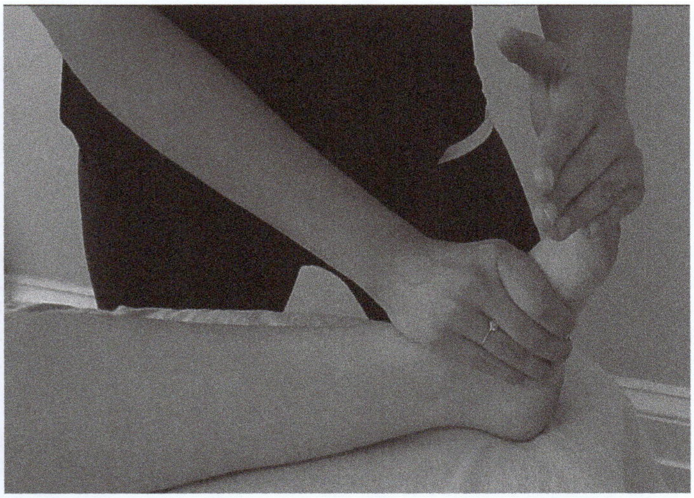

FIGURE 7.70 Metatarsal extension 70–90°

Push toes via distal phalanges into extension.

Big toe flexion 45° (Figures 7.71, 7.72)

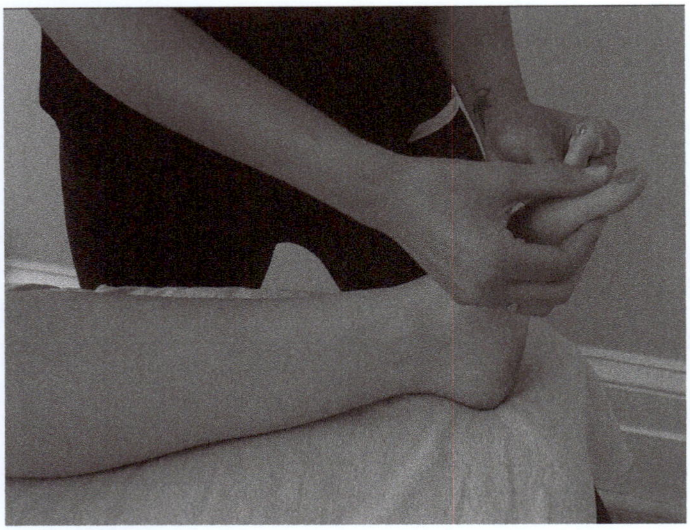

FIGURE 7.71 Proximal metatarsal-phalange

Stabilize metatarsals. Grasping the proximal phalange, push the metatarsal-phalange joint into flexion.

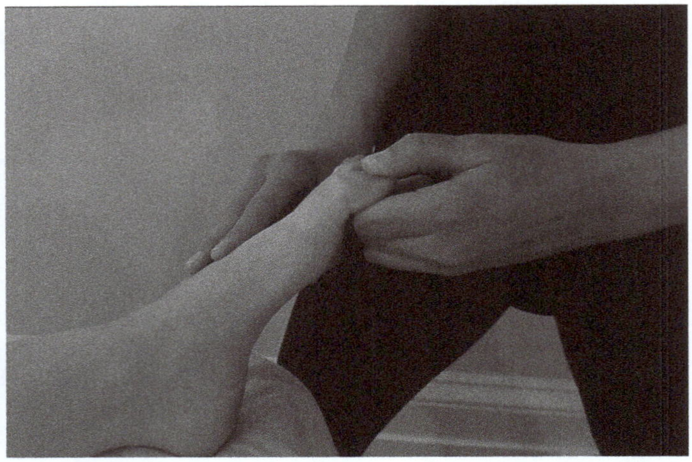

FIGURE 7.72 Distal interphalangeal joint

Stabilize the proximal phalange and grasping the distal phalange, flex the distal joint with your thumb as your first two fingers resist motion in the proximal phalange. (The therapist has had to move away the hand holding first phalange to show distal joint movement.)

Big toe extension 70–90° (Figures 7.73, 7.74)

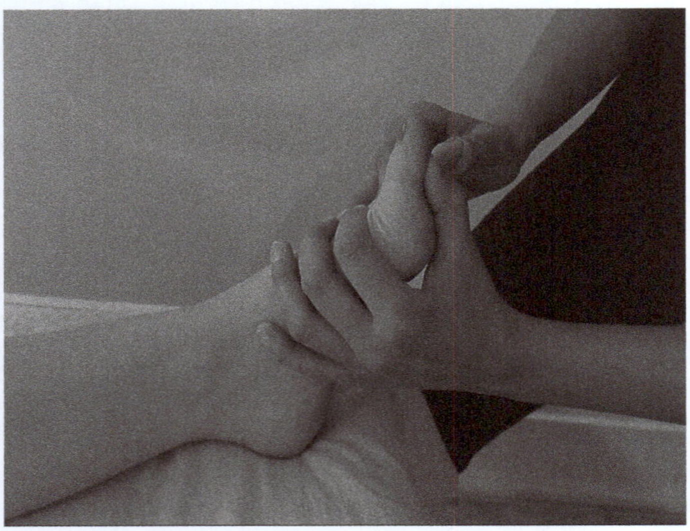

FIGURE 7.73 1st metatarsal-phalangeal joint 30–50°

Stabilize the metatarsals and lift the proximal phalange into extension.

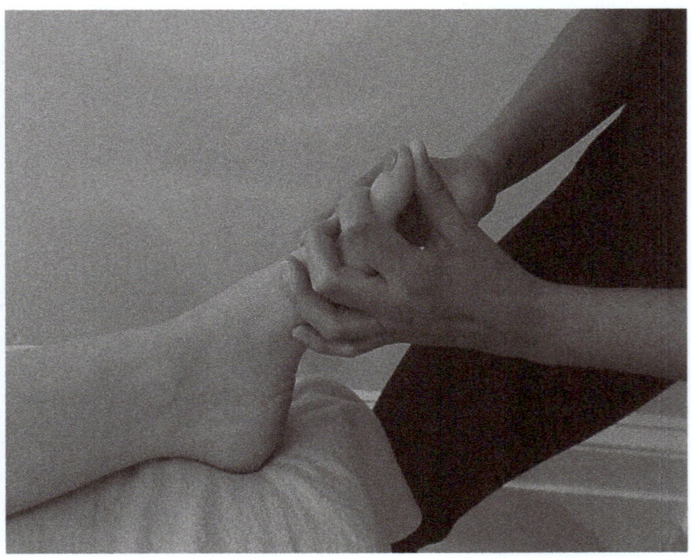

FIGURE 7.74 Interphalangeal joint 20–40°

Stabilize the proximal phalange, grasp the second phalange and lift the joint into extension.

PR-ROM Of 2nd to 5th phalanges (Figures 7.75, 7.76)

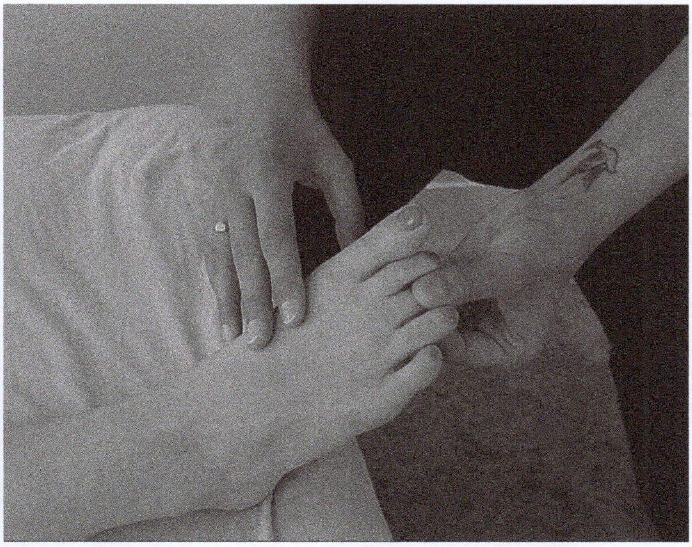

FIGURE 7.75 Example of PR-ROM digit flexion

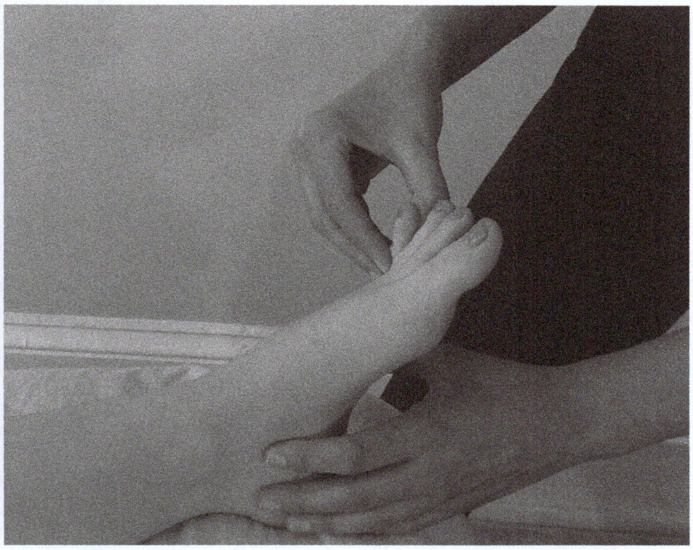

FIGURE 7.76 Example of PR-ROM digit extension

End-feel for all the toes is generally tissue stretch on extension, and often tissue approximation in flexion. Extension happens primarily at the metatarsal phalangeal joint, while the end-feel of the proximal and distal phalangeal joints is firm, or leathery, due to the extensor expansion.

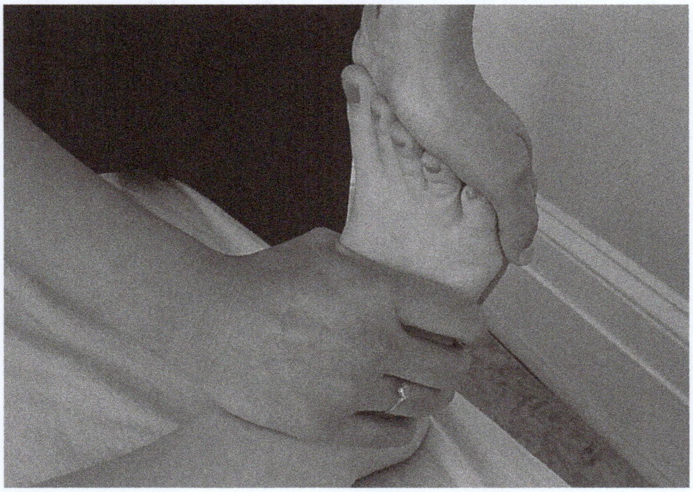

FIGURE 7.77 AR-ROM digit flexion

To test flexors of toes, you can use the palm of your hand against the underside of the patient's toes, with the toes in slight extension, and have them try to curl their toes against your resistance. Or, you can have them flex their toes (scrunch up your toes) and you can apply pressure in order to try to extend (or "uncurl") them.

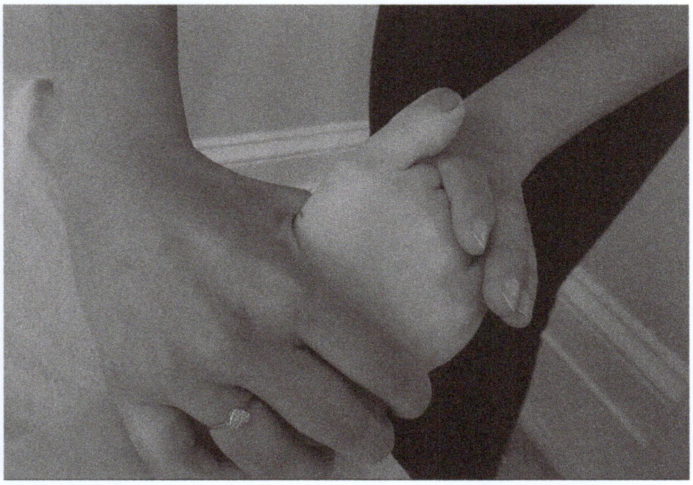

FIGURE 7.78 AR-ROM digit extension

Stabilize across the metatarsals and place your other hand across the superior surface of all of toes and then passively move the toes into slight flexion and have the patient try to extend the toes. Or, you can have them extend their toes (point your toes toward your head) and then have them try to resist your pressure to bring them into flexion. This tests the extensors of the toes.

If AF-ROM or PF-ROM of all the toes has produced pain or impairment of movement, test each toe individually by passively flexing, extending, and side-bending medially and laterally.

Test each joint in the following order: (1) metatarsal phalangeal joint; (2) proximal phalangeal joint; (3) distal phalangeal joint. Always stabilize the bone just proximal to the one you have grasped.

Active resisted range of motion (AR-ROM) of forefoot (Figures 7.77-7.80)

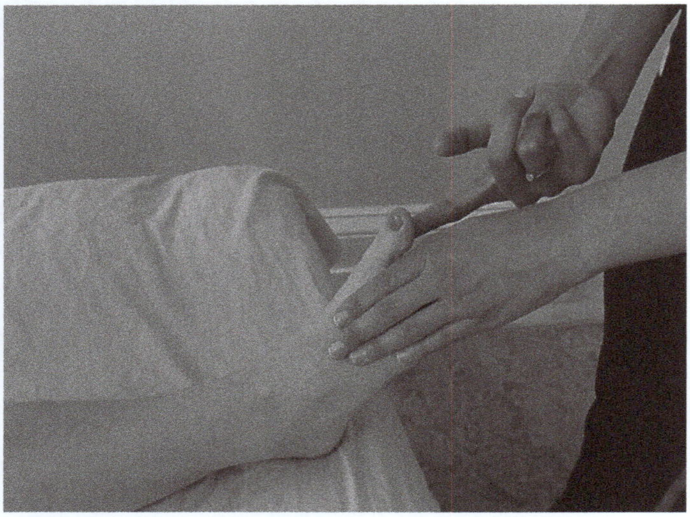

FIGURE 7.79 AR-ROM big toe flexion

This test is especially important if the patient has shown signs of not toeing off correctly when walking. Place the toe in neutral and ask the patient to resist you extending it.

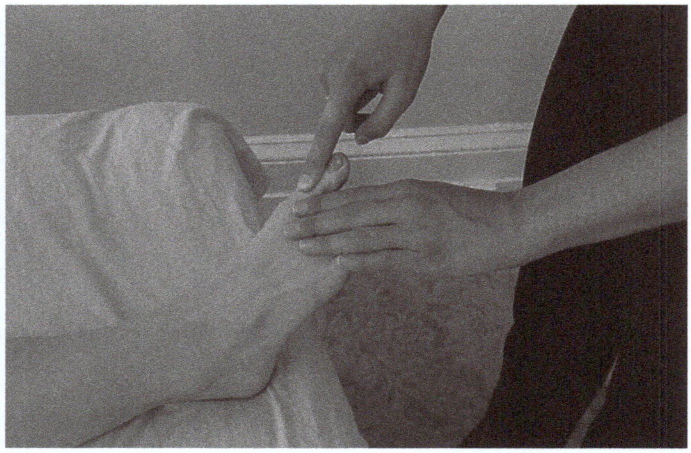

FIGURE 7.80 AR-ROM big toe extension

Stabilize across the metatarsals. Place your index finger over the nail on the patient's extended big toe. Ask them to hold it there as you begin to apply pressure. This tests the integrity of the extensor hallucis longus and is also a test for nerve root L5 (a myotome test).

KNEE: CHAPTER OVERVIEW

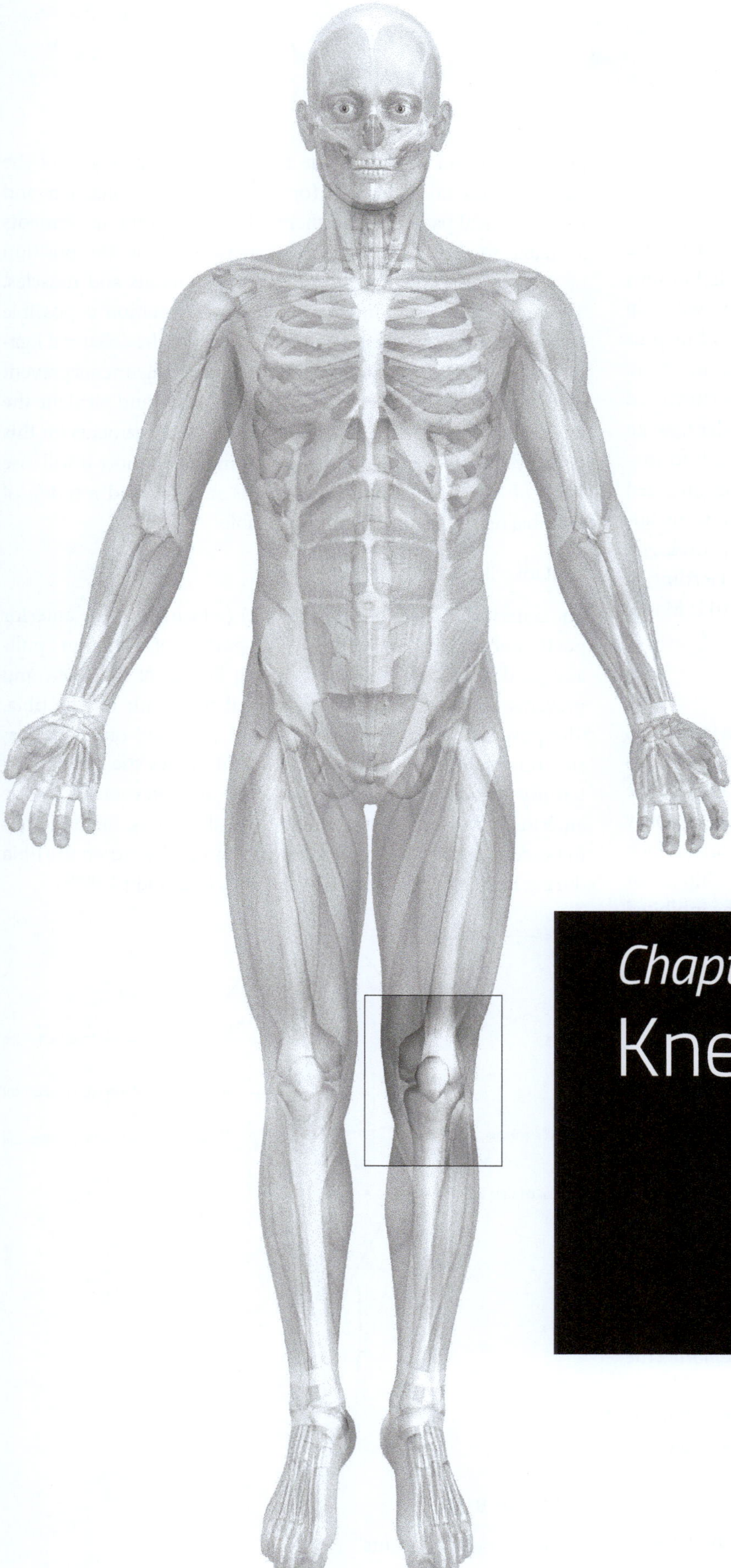

Chapter 8

Knee

Clinical implications of anatomy and physiology

The following are some anatomical observations that have clinical implications. Understanding the functional relationships (physiology) between structures and tissues (anatomy) will help explain how structures of the knee can be injured and help us understand how orthopedic tests work to provide information. Please review the anatomy of the joints and muscles involved in the function of the knee. It is suggested that the reader have an anatomy book on hand to more easily understand the information in this chapter. The information that has been summarized here has been chosen because of its direct relevance to orthopedic testing and understanding of the mechanical pathologies of the knee (see also Dutton 2012; Hartley 2000b; Hertling & Kessler 2006; Hoppenfeld 1976; Levangie & Norkin 2011; Magee 2014; Schuenke et al. 2014).

Review of the musculature

Extensors Quadriceps (in extension the tensor fasciae latae helps to lock the knee). For clinical reasons the quadriceps muscle is best thought of as made up of two different groups of muscle: the three vasti muscles, all of which are single joint muscles solely involved in flexion of the knee, and the rectus femoris, which crosses both the knee and hip. The rectus femoris as a hip flexor can often be short and tight while the three vasti can be inhibited and weak.

Flexors Biceps femoris, semimembranosus, semitendinosus; assisted by the gastrocnemius, sartorius, gracilis; weakly flexed by popliteus.

Rotators with knee flexed Medial rotators of the tibia: semimembranosus, semitendinosus, gracilis, sartorius, popliteus.

Lateral rotators of the tibia: biceps femoris, tensor fasciae latae.

Popliteus unlocks the knee by laterally rotating the femur on the weight-bearing tibia. This slackens the muscles that cross the knee and its ligaments, removing compressive forces in the knee.

A complex joint

Three joints make up the knee complex; the *tibiofemoral*, the superior *tibiofibular*, and the *patellofemoral*. Our principal concern is with the tibiofemoral and patellofemoral joints, but the superior tibiofibular joint will be addressed during PR-ROM.

Tibiofemoral joint

The tibiofemoral joint is the largest joint in the body. Its synovium is extensive, communicating with many bursae and pouches around the knee. The two bones, the condyles of the femur and the tibial condyles (or plateau), are not congruent and have meniscal pads between them. There are several movements available to the tibiofemoral joint, depending on the position of the two bones, which are guided by ligaments and muscles. The more the knee is in extension, the less rotation is possible between the tibia and femur. In full extension, the collateral ligaments prevent lateral rotation and the cruciate ligaments prevent medial rotation. Hence, when weight-bearing and straight the knee is quite stable, relying on both muscle and ligaments for this stability. However, as the knee is flexed more and more it will lose some of its muscular and ligamentous support, and rotation of the tibia on the femur becomes available.

Cruciate ligaments (Figure 8.1)

The anterior cruciate ligament (ACL) (attached on the anterior portion of the tibia and the posterior portion of the femur) pulls and guides the femur forward during flexion of the knee, and prevents excessive posterior motion of the femur on the tibia. The posterior cruciate ligament (PCL) (attached on the posterior tibia and anterior femur) pulls and guides the femur posteriorly during extension of the knee and prevents excessive anterior movement of the femur on the tibia. Thus, the two work in tandem to move the femur forward and backward on the tibia during flexion and extension of the knee (Kapandji 1986b).

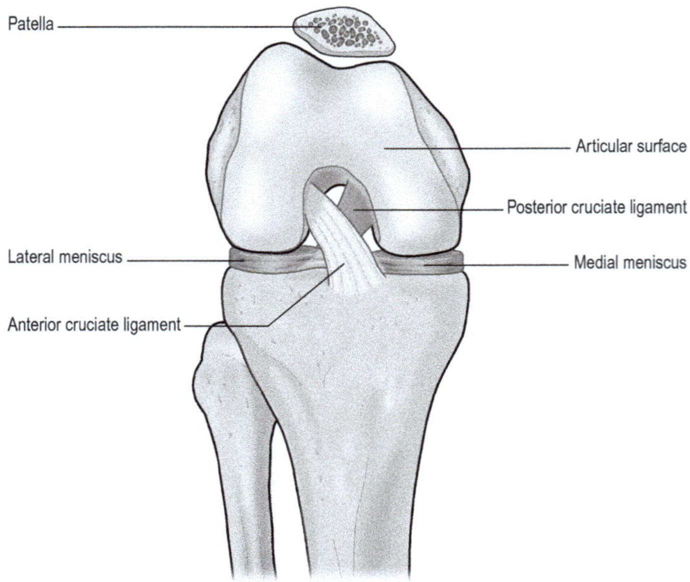

FIGURE 8.1

The cruciate ligaments.

It is not so much that this guiding actually pulls the femur anteriorly or posteriorly, but rather that the ligaments hold the femur from moving anteriorly or posteriorly off the tibial plateau. This keeps the articulation of the knee joint occurring within only a small range of excursion on the tibia (i.e., keeping the meniscal pads from shifting too far anteriorly or posteriorly), while at the same time allowing the large and lengthy articulating surface of the femur to glide and move within the meniscal pad and on the surface of the tibial plateau. The femur can therefore roll while, to all intents and purposes, its contact on the tibia remains almost stationary.

Further, because the anterior attachments of both cruciates are slightly more medial than their posterior attachments, they will also tend to direct the femur to rotate medially very slightly on hyperextension of the knee (i.e., when the knee is locked when standing). Hyperextending the knee increases the tension on these ligaments as they begin to hook around each other where they cross. This pulls the joint surfaces tightly together. The knee is unlocked by the popliteus muscle moving the femur in lateral rotation, back to neutral, so that flexion can occur. However, during lateral rotation of the tibia during flexion the cruciates will move apart from each other and provide the laxity within the knee required for such rotation.

Collateral ligaments (Figure 8.2)

The medial collateral ligament of the knee is also known as the tibiofemoral ligament as it runs from the medial side of the medial epicondyle of the femur onto the medial side of the tibia. It is continuous with the fibrous joint capsule and through that linked to the medial meniscus. Running up and down, the superior attachment is slightly posterior relative to the inferior attachment on the tibia. It becomes taut on knee extension and slack on knee flexion.

The lateral collateral ligament of the knee runs from the lateral epicondyle to the head of the fibula. Its superior attachment is slightly posterior to the inferior attachment on the head of the fibula.

As with the medial collateral, it, too, is taut on extension of the knee and lax during flexion. Therefore, as flexion of the knee increases the lateral-medial stability provided by these ligaments decreases.

NOTE: Lateral (external) rotation of the tibia is checked by both the lateral (fibular) and medial (tibial) ligaments. The cruciate ligaments resist medial/internal rotation of the tibia. A helpful phrase to remember which ligament checks which tibial rotation is "*lateral* rotation stopped by *collateral* ligaments;" medial rotation is, therefore, checked by the cruciate ligaments.

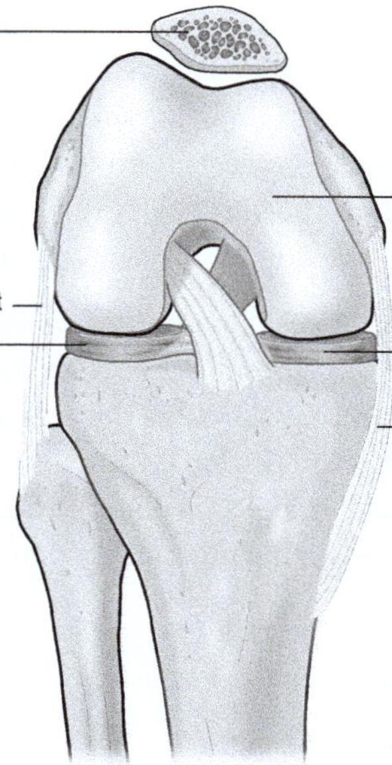

FIGURE 8.2
The collateral ligaments.

Injuries to the collateral ligaments are more likely to happen when they are under strain, such as when the tibia is laterally/externally rotated (e.g., during valgus orientation of knee, which especially stresses the medial collateral). As valgus orientation of the knee occurs more often (even if it is only a momentary positioning) than a varus orientation, this is one reason that the medial collateral ligament is more often injured.

Medial/internal motion of the tibia stresses the cruciates where they cross. Lateral/external rotation takes some tension off the ligaments. The ACL is usually injured when the leg is hit from the lateral side and the foot is planted on the ground – the classic occurrence is the football tackle. In such an injury, though the ensuing valgus orientation does produce lateral rotation of the tibia, nonetheless, the tibia is driven forward but the foot cannot move, injuring the ACL while also stressing the medial collateral ligament. Because the medial collateral ligament is attached to the joint capsule, it will often tear the capsule (and its capillaries, etc.), which is how blood is able to enter the joint.

Further, the medial meniscus (see below) has attachments to the medial ligament and capsule, which hold it fixed, while the valgus movement of the knee has it pinched between the medial condyle of the femur and the tibia. Add the tibia moving anteriorly and the meniscus will almost certainly be torn. Thus, three tissues, the medial collateral ligament (and joint capsule), the medial meniscus, and the ACL, can all be injured in the same trauma. This has been referred to as "the terrible triad" since recovery from all three tissues being injured at once can have a poor prognosis for anyone, especially professional athletes (Magee 2014). Many a career has been ended by this triad, but surgery for any one of the three individually is often very successful.

The posterior cruciate is often injured in soccer. If a running player's foot strikes the ground rather than the ball, the tibia is driven posteriorly, tearing the posterior cruciate. Or again, in football, a tackle from the front through the tibia will do the same. However, many people continue to function quite well without an intact PCL, as the muscular support often takes over its function.

Functions of the menisci

The menisci serve several functions:

- They act as shock absorbers, spreading the stresses over a larger area and protecting the condyles of the femur and tibia from wear.
- They aid in nutrition and lubrication of the joint by assisting in moving the synovial fluid within the joint capsule.
- They make the joint surfaces more congruent.
- They reduce friction during movement.
- They prevent pinching of the joint capsule (by not allowing the capsule to move between the tibia and the femur).
- They participate in the "screw home" mechanism by participating in guiding rotational motions in the knee.

The medial meniscus is crescent- or C-shaped; the lateral meniscus is similar, but its ends almost meet. The ends of the C-shapes are sometimes called the anterior and posterior horns of the meniscus. At each of these ends or horns the meniscal pad is thin. The pads are wedge-shaped (with a slightly concave surface that cups the condyle of the femur, which it sits under), with the thickest portions of the menisci at the medial and lateral sides of the knee. The pads possess no nerves; pain felt is from the tearing of their supportive coronary ligaments. The two menisci are attached to each other by the transverse ligament of the knee.

The rounded shape of the articular surface of the femur fitting into the cup-shaped meniscal pad helps hold the menisci in place under the femoral condyles as the femur glides on the plateau of the tibia.

During extension of the knee, the menisci are further assisted to move anteriorly, pulled partly by the fibers of the meniscopatellar ligament, and the lateral meniscus is further assisted by the meniscofemoral ligament fibers. As the femur rolls into extension, it pushes the patella anteriorly and superiorly, tightening the meniscopatellar ligament, which in turn pulls on the transverse ligament of the knee, pulling both menisci forward. Also, the posterior cruciate ligament tightens as the knee extends, pulling on the meniscofemoral ligament, which tugs the posterior horn of the lateral meniscus forward.

During flexion of the knee, the medial meniscus has fibers from the semimembranosus tendon running to its posterior aspect, which help move the meniscus posteriorly, keeping it under the condyle. The popliteus has fibers to the posterior area of the lateral meniscus, and performs a similar function. The more firmly attached medial meniscus slides anteriorly and posteriorly during flexion only half as much (1/8 inch) as the more loosely attached lateral meniscus (1/4 inch).

The medial meniscus is more often injured than the lateral. Some of the reasons for this are as follows:

- The knee is more likely to undergo a valgus stress during injury (blows to the thigh and leg usually come from a lateral direction, severely compressing the meniscus).
- The medial meniscus is more securely fixed in place and is therefore more easily torn as it is unable to shift about under extreme pressure and at end-range motions of the knee.
- Combined with the fact that the medial meniscus has fibrous attachments both to the medial collateral ligament and to the medial joint capsule, the following can occur: when tension is placed on those structures, the medial meniscus can be pulled into positions that may cause the meniscus to be further pinched between the bones.

Patellofemoral joint

The two principal purposes of the patella are: (1) to prevent friction between the quadriceps tendon and the femoral condyles; (2) to act as an anatomic pulley that increases the efficiency of the quadriceps muscles. Both of these functions require the patella to move, and move along a track provided by the trough-like shape of the distal femur's condyles.

During flexion of the knee, the patella slides down (relative to the femur) into the intercondylar notch (onto the inferior surface of the condyles); while in extension, the patella will position itself between the (anterior surface) of the condyles.

During rotation of the tibia on the femur, the patella will rotate on medial rotation of the tibia (when the knee is flexed). The inferior apex of the patella rotates medially. On lateral rotation of the tibia, the apex rotates laterally.

Though the shape of a patella can differ between individuals, overall it is usually a basic oval shape, broader at the superior portion and more pointed at the inferior end (the apex). The anterior surface is convex overall. The posterior surface is slightly V-shaped, which helps to keep the patella tracking between the condyles during the various movements between the femur and the tibia. There are several articular surfaces (facets) on the underside of the patella which, during proper tracking, articulate with the corresponding surfaces of the condyles.

If the orientation of the patella is altered by either too much tension (shortening) or too little tension (lengthening) of the quadriceps, then these patellar facets will not be aligned correctly and osteoarthritic changes will occur. This is commonly referred to as a chondromalacia of the patella, a "softening of the underside of the kneecap." This results in a reflexive inhibition of the quadriceps muscles and the patient will speak of the knee giving out occasionally.

It is estimated that during normal gait the patella is forced back upon the condyles by about two-thirds of one's body-weight. Going uphill or up stairs, this increases to two times one's body-weight, while going downhill or down stairs this pressure increases to three-and-a-half times. If the patient, when asked when they feel their knee will not hold them up, replies "it usually occurs coming down stairs" we can assume that mild osteoarthritic changes (chondromalacia) are occurring. If they say that going up or down the stairs brings on their symptoms, then moderate damage has occurred. Severe degenerative changes are occurring when walking on a flat surface brings on these symptoms.

The principal muscle whose inhibition is most crucial for the development of chondromalacia by improper tracking of the patella is the vastus medialis, more specifically a segment of that muscle referred to as the vastus medialis oblique (VMO). As the heads of the femur are wider apart than the knees during standing and walking, the bulk of the quadriceps muscles run down to the knee on an oblique angle. Therefore, there will be a pull to the lateral side of the knee. However, the patella must run or track straight up and down (just as the femoral condyles are oriented). The vastus medialis (and VMO) is the only one of the four quadriceps muscles that is oriented in such a way as to pull the patella medially. Therefore, the patella is lifted by the muscles of the quadriceps pulling from both medial and lateral directions, which results in the patella lifting straight up.

It is thought that the VMO needs to contract before the other three muscles in order for the patella to be able to track vertically. After all, the other three muscles are larger and outnumber the vastus medialis. If any injury or inhibition occurs that affects the VMO, then tracking problems begin and osteopathic changes result. To restore proper tracking, both the strength and the timing of the VMO need to be corrected.

The patella will dislocate, usually laterally, when it rises up and over one of the sides of the trough or valley created by the shape of the condyles. Possible reasons for this type of dislocation are a weakness in the VMO and/or a sudden contraction of the quadriceps while the tibia is externally/laterally rotated. The patella is driven right up and over the lateral condyle, and this is extremely painful.

The lateral condyle of the femur has a longer and steeper orientation that usually helps prevent this.

Superior tibiofibular joint

The junction between the superior tibia and fibula is a plane/gliding joint and is synovial. It has sometimes been found to be continuous with the popliteus bursa (and hence, potentially with the synovium of the knee). It is reinforced with anterior and superior ligaments that run from the head of the fibula in a superior and medial direction onto the tibia. It is further secured in place by the interosseus membrane running between the length of the shafts of the fibula and tibia.

The motion of the superior tibiofibular joint is linked to the movement of the ankle. As the foot is dorsiflexed, the fibula moves laterally away from the tibia at the ankle and slides superiorly while it rotates internally. This occurs because:

- the talus is wider at the front and as it moves up between the tibia and fibula the tibia and fibula bones are pushed slightly apart
- the inelastic fibers of the interosseous membrane between the tibia and fibula are on oblique angles, and as the two bones separate the fibers must move more horizontally, and as a result, pull the fibula superiorly (the fibula will move on the stable weight-bearing tibia)
- as the fibers move horizontally, they must simultaneously pull their attachment on the anterior ridge of the fibula in a medial direction (internal rotation). Conversely, as the foot is plantar flexed, the fibula and tibia come closer at the ankle, the fibula will descend and rotate back out externally.

Active range of motion of the knee

Flexion 135°

Extension (−5°)–0–15°

Medial rotation 5°

Lateral rotation 5°

Chapter 8

See the Appendices at the end of the book for charts and tables on muscles (muscle origins, insertions, innervation, actions and synergists), joints (actions, ranges, muscles used, tissues stretched and compressed; another table on capsular patterns of restriction, open packed/resting positions and close packed positions) and several charts on neurological testing where any such testing would involve this chapter's region.

The protocol (Box 8.1) begins with the case history.

> **Box 8.1 Protocol**
>
> Case history (specific questions)
>
> Observations
>
> Rule outs
>
> Active free range of motion (AF-ROM)
>
> Passive relaxed range of motion (PR-ROM)
>
> Active resisted range of motion (AR-ROM)
>
> Special tests

Case history (specific questions)

The following are some examples of specific questions concerning the knee that build on the basic case history questions as presented in Part I, Chapter 3.

Have you noticed any changes in performing daily activities due to your knee(s)? Sports? Are there any actions or positions that you are in during the day that you think may be contributing to the problem?

Describe the nature of the pain. Note:

- aching pain, though often mechanical, may indicate degenerative changes
- sharp, "catching" pain implies some mechanical problem
- pain at rest is often overuse (inflammatory in nature)
- pain during activity is often structural or mechanical.

If swelling in the joint has occurred, you need to ask about the speed with which the joint swelled. If the joint began to swell immediately it can mean that blood is a large component of the fluid present. If it took some time (several hours, for example) for the swelling to gradually increase, then it is more likely due to an increase in synovium. Nonetheless, ask the patient if they have seen a physician. If you believe that blood is a possible component of the fluid, you need to refer the patient out and have them seek immediate medical attention as they may need the knee aspirated (drained). Blood is corrosive to articular cartilage. (For the palpatory signs of blood in joint effusion, see Rule outs: joint effusion, p. 141).

Have the patient describe in their own words what is wrong with their knee. Note if your patient uses terms such as:

- snapping: implies taut ligaments or tight tendons crossing the joint
- grinding (crepitus): implies initial stages of osteoarthritic changes within the joint
- creaking (gross crepitus): implies severe osteoarthritic degeneration
- catching or locking: implies mechanical dysfunction of the ligaments and or meniscus
- giving way or becoming momentarily weak: implies patellar dysfunction.

If the patient reports a giving way of the joint ask if it feels like the knee will give way when going up stairs/uphill or down stairs/downhill. If it is felt going up/down hills or stairs it may mean retropatellar lesions. As noted above, when walking up a set of stairs or uphill, the pressure exerted by the patella against the condyles of the femur is roughly two-and-a-half times body-weight, compared to seven-tenths of body-weight when walking on a level surface. Walking down stairs, the force is three-and-a-half times body-weight. Normally when osteoarthritis or chondromalacia begins in the retropatellar area it will usually first be noticed when going down stairs, etc. Then, it will progress and be noticed going up as well as down. In acute and late-stage osteoarthritis, the pain will be present in level walking.

Asking questions about activities that provoke pain can provide important clues to possible pathologies.

- "It popped and then it hurt." This implies an anterior cruciate ligament tear, or possibly an osteochondral fracture (usually edema/swelling occurs soon after). Refer to the patient's physician.
- "My knee feels weak all the time." Often implies a complex ligamentous and joint impairment causing instability. *The patient should seek physician's referral for imaging.*

Observation and inspection

Landmarks

Review your anatomy so that you can landmark the tibial tuberosity, the joint margins, and the tibial plateau or tibial condyles, as well as the head of the fibula.

Further, use landmarks to gauge the orientation of the pelvis to the feet. Check anterior superior and posterior superior iliac spine (ASIS and PSIS) levels, and check the symmetry of the iliac crest, trochanters, ischial tuberosity heights, medial and lateral malleoli, and arches of the feet.

Regional assessment within the context of the whole

As with every area of the body being investigated by orthopedic testing (the specific view), remember to always look at that joint or tissue within the context of the surrounding joints and structures (the regional view). What is the interplay of impaired tissues or structures with the rest of the tissues within that region? In turn, take into consideration the global view: how is that joint, and the surrounding region, affecting the whole body; and how is the whole affecting or influencing the region and the specific site(s) of impairment(s)? Just as with treatment, the approach to assessment also moves from general to specific and back to general. Not all the preconditions for an impairment exist on-site or in the surrounding region. They can come from the totality of the body, the person, and their environment (the global view).

REMEMBER: Observation begins the moment your patient enters your clinic. Perform a postural scan of the patient from each side and from the front and back. Observe how they naturally stand and include a quick gait analysis. Deformities are visible signs of impairment that result from genetic, severe, or long-standing conditions. These deformities will have caused clear compensatory changes to the structures in support of those areas. Note obvious deformities and consider their implications. Is the deformity a contributing factor to the patient's chief complaint?

Orientation of the patella

The following are common descriptive terms used for describing the orientation of the patella as seen during a postural examination:

- *fish eye patella* face (are turned) laterally
- *squinting patella* appear turned medially
- *patella baja* is used to describe patella that are lower than normal; usually due to inhibited or weak (lengthened) quadriceps
- *patella alta* are patella that sit higher than normal; usually due to short quadriceps. Observed from the side, the patella may ride high enough to expose the fat pad that usually hides behind the lower aspect of the patella. This will appear as a double "hump" or "camel sign."

Orientation of knee

The following deviations in orientation can be unilateral or bilateral. They speak to the relationship of the femur to the tibia:

- *Genu valgus* orientation of the knees (Figure 8.3A) is often the result of medially rotated femur and laterally rotated tibia. This can occur, for example, because of an increase in the Q angle, an antetorsion or retroversion of the hip, or pronation of the foot. This is colloquially referred to as knock-knee. This stresses/strains the structures/tissues on the medial side of the knee, while compressing the lateral structures such as the lateral meniscus.
- *Genu varus* orientation of the knees (Figure 8.3B)is normal for infants but usually disappears with growth. The most common reason for this is rickets or other such bone pathologies where the bones literally bow (hence, the term bow-legged). Mild to moderate occurrences can be due to genetics which result in retrotorsion, anteversion of the hip, and pes cavus. A varus orientation of the knee will compress the medial portion of the knee while stressing the lateral structures.
- *Genu recurvatum*, or hyperextended knee, can be the result of excessive laxity in the ligaments of the knee. It can be found bilaterally when there is a severe anterior pelvic tilt.
- *Fixed-flexed knee* has the patient standing with one or both knees slightly flexed. This can be due to a muscle imbalance, deformation of the knee joint, or a swollen knee joint.

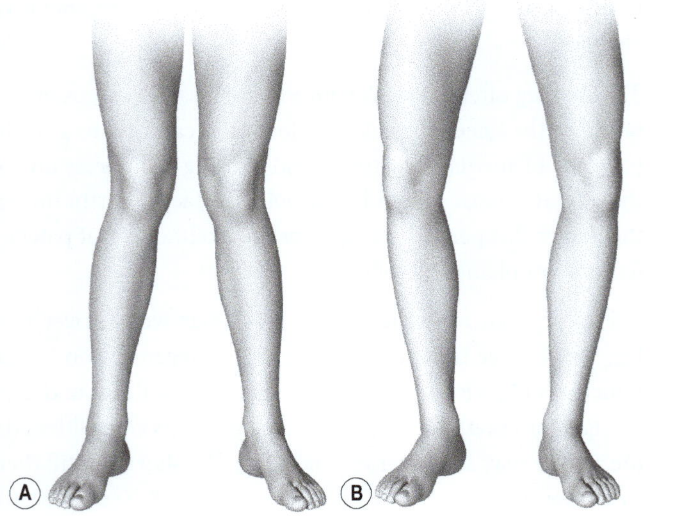

FIGURE 8.3

Genu valgus and genu varus.

- *Medial tibial torsion.* This is often due to a muscle imbalance (short semimembranosus and semitendinosus which may be accompanied by a short medial head of the gastrocnemius) and will usually result in squinting patellae. Feet will toe in (if the femur is positioned in neutral).
- *Lateral tibial torsion* is often due to a muscle imbalance (short biceps femoris which may be accompanied by a short lateral head of the gastrocnemius, and a short/tight iliotibial band (ITB)) and will tend to produce fish-eye patellae. The feet will toe out (if the femur is positioned in neutral).

Leg length and anterior/posterior rotation of hip or innominate: consequences for the knee

A leg-length difference (structural or functional) is likely to create muscle imbalances in the hips and lower limb whether between muscle groups (flexors and extensors) or between the two lower limbs (such as in adductor lengths and tone). Unlevel hips, and so an unlevel sacral base, continue the imbalances up into the spine. Further, the pelvis may drop on one side due to either: (1) a (contralateral) weak gluteus medius; or (2) the contralateral leg being longer, either structurally or functionally, resulting in a pelvic shift that moves the weight over one or other leg (Chila 2010; Hertling & Kessler 2006; Pope 2003).

Other possible consequences are:

- The short leg often will hyperextend the knee in order to make it functionally longer (while the long leg's knee will often be slightly flexed when standing). The hyperextended knee is more susceptible to injury from trauma or degenerative changes.
- The long leg often presents with a compensating valgus orientation of the knee. The valgus orientation can lead to a strain (stretch) of medial structures, and loading (compression) of the lateral meniscus and lateral joint surfaces. Furthermore, the longer this persists, the greater the likelihood that patellofemoral problems will follow.
- A long leg can have the person shift their weight over that leg, which over time may cause quicker degeneration to the structures of its knee. However, if the long leg flexes and uses a valgus orientation of the knee to shorten its overall length, the weight may shift over the short leg. The short leg will then suffer the consequences (Chila 2010; Hertling & Kessler 2006). For further details on this topic, see Chapter 9.

Femoral torsion

Femoral torsion/medial rotation of the femur can be the result of bony deformities of the hip. It may also be due to muscular imbalance, with tight medial rotators of the hip. This medial rotation of the femur results in squinting patellae. The feet may also be medially (or internally) rotated (pigeon-toed). Again, all of this may lead to patellofemoral dysfunction, chondromalacia, and medial collateral ligament sprains.

Femoral retroversion

Femoral retroversion or any chronic lateral rotation of the femur leads to fish-eye patellae. This results in a higher degree of susceptibility to patellar subluxations and dislocations, leading to a genu varum and making the patient more susceptible to lateral collateral ligament problems and medial knee compression issues. Further information on torsions and retroversions can be found in Chapter 9.

Pronated feet

Pronation of the feet will cause internal tibial rotation, leading to added stress on the patellofemoral joint, the patellar tendon, lateral joint structures, and medial meniscus.

Bursa

Note swelling in any of the bursae of the knee. The bursae most noted by observation are frontal, as listed below:

- Suprapatellar bursa (continuous to the synovial joint capsule): swelling in the suprapatellar pouch may be contained only in that area, or given that it is an extension of the joint capsule, the swelling may also be intra-articular in nature.
- Prepatellar bursa: sits right on top of the patella and just under the skin covering the knee. It becomes inflamed from crawling on the knees or a blow on the patella. This was once known as housemaid's knee because kneeling on a hard floor is one cause.
- The superficial infrapatellar bursa lies between the skin and the patellar tendon.

The bursae that are deeper and less observable are as follows:

- The deep infrapatellar bursa lies under the infrapatellar tendon and the tibia.
- The anserine bursa lies between the tibia and the inserting tendons of the gracilis, sartorius, and semitendinosus (which all unite to form the pes anserine).

There are numerous posterior bursae that are continuations of the synovial capsule. These are behind the tendons of both the medial and lateral gastrocnemius tendons, and the popliteus, for example. These bursae separate muscular tissues from the capsule and/or bone. Any of these may swell and the muscle/tendon may pinch it so that the swelling remains only at the site as the bursa no longer communicates with the capsule. They are referred to as a popliteal or Baker's cyst. These are palpated in the popliteal fossa with the knee flexed. When present, a Baker's cyst will restrict flexion of the knee.

As mentioned at the start of this chapter, the suprapatellar bursa and the gastrocnemius bursa are extensions of the synovium of the knee joint capsule. On knee extension, pressure from the stretched gastrocnemius pushes the fluid out of the posterior portion of the synovial capsule and inflates the suprapatellar bursa, and when the knee flexes, the quadriceps tendon pushes the fluid back into the gastrocnemius bursa (both medially and laterally). There are other bursae in the knee, but these are the ones most commonly inflamed.

Intracapsular edema

If the swelling becomes intracapsular, and the more edema there is, the more the knee will want to assume a resting position of 15–25° of flexion. This allows for the greatest size of the synovial cavity to hold the maximum capacity of fluid. This position is also called a position of comfort for an injured knee.

Atrophy

It is important to have the patient contract the quadriceps muscles bilaterally when observing for atrophy of the muscle. Particularly observe the vastus medialis, which can appear as a hollow or divot in the middle of the muscle. The vastus medialis is crucial for proper patellar tracking. (For further information on observation and inspection of the knee see: DeStefano 2011; Dutton 2012; Hartley 2000b; Hertling & Kessler 2006; Hoppenfeld 1976; Magee 2014; Starkey & Brown 2015.) See also Box 8.2.

Rule outs

NOTE: Inflammatory arthritis, e.g., rheumatoid arthritis (RA), should be ruled out through case history taking. The tell-tale signs for RA are bilateral joint pain, especially if found in other pairs of joints in the body, such as the hips or hands. If the RA has been destructive to the joint, there are palpable changes to the involved joints and eventual observable deformation (Grossman & Porth 2014). Refer the patient out if they have not seen a doctor about this presentation and received a diagnosis. Caution must be exercised with any joint suffering from RA. Joint tissue becomes fragile over time in cases of RA. Over-pressure (O-P) or any stress to the joint and its supportive structures needs to be avoided. Active free range of motion (AF-ROM) and gentle passive testing, along with pain-free palpation is often the extent of testing.

Box 8.2 Posturally challenging the chief complaint: exploring how the chief complaint fits into the whole

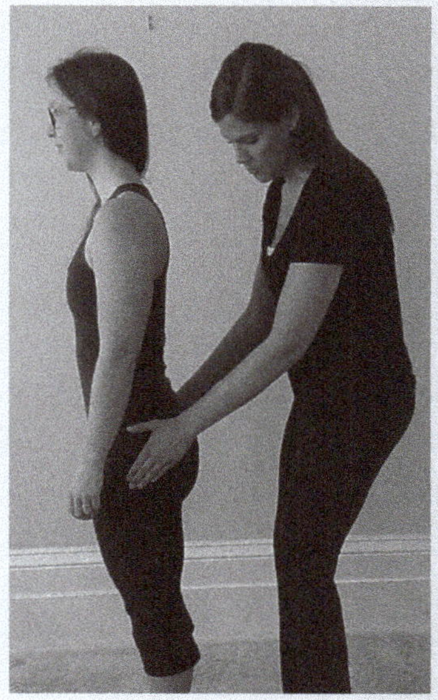

FIGURE 8.4

Observe and gently correct the patient's posture.

As a final step of observation and inspection, look at how the patient naturally stands and correct their posture with gentle movements, if possible (Figure 8.4). For example, push the patient's hips back, unlock hyperextended knees, re-position a forward head over the shoulders and note what changes occur above and below. If the patient can briefly sustain this corrected position, the tension or pain that they now experience may point to areas that need to be included in your assessment and treatment (injured, contractured, or weakened/stressed tissues or structures). This will help reveal problems, that have a global effect as well as being intimately connected to specific impairments.

If the patient has RA then the joint effusion tests presented in the text are compromised: if you find joint effusion/swelling you cannot distinguish that from the swelling due to an arthritic flare or from an injury.

The following joints need to be ruled out before testing the knee to ensure that their structures are not referring symptoms into the knee. Note, however, these rule outs cannot be performed if the knee injury is acute. Rule outs are required mostly in chronic situations or when the source of impairment to the area of the chief complaint is not obvious.

Ruling out the joints above and below (Box 8.3)

Hip Active hip flexion with O-P and medial rotation with O-P (Figure 8.5). These two actions place enough stress through the joint surfaces, capsule, and supportive tissue to elicit the patient's chief complaint in the knee if the hip is the source of that complaint.

Foot and ankle With the knee flexed and comfortable (use a towel roll under the thigh), have the patient perform active plantar flexion, dorsiflexion, inversion, and eversion, from neutral. Follow each pain-free movement with O-P, and return the joint to neutral and have the patient proceed to the next movement. However, since the gastrocnemius and plantaris cross the knee, some of these ankle movements may well engender a response in knee structures (as is shown in the AF-ROM section of Chapter 7, on the ankle).

If neurological signs and symptoms have been noted when taking your case history, rule out the lumbar spine. To rule out the lumbar spine, have the patient actively forward flex, then laterally flex, and then have them rotate their trunk left and right. With every movement that has been pain-free, apply O-P at the end of their active free range of motion. Then have the patient extend their low back. ***NOTE:*** Remember: *never apply O-P in extension of the spine.*

If extending the back does not cause a recurrence of neurological signs and symptoms, then do the quadrant test instead of O-P. The quadrant test is designed to maximally close the facet joints and the neural foramen of the lumbar spine on the side to which the patient bends.

The positive sign we are testing for here is the re-creation of the patient's neurological symptoms in the lower limb. Have the patient rotate slightly to one side, place their hand on the back of that thigh, and slide the hand down toward the back of their knee.

Fractures

To rule out fractures of the long bones (the tibia, fibula, and femur). If there is no obvious deformity use a reflex hammer to tap the bone at a distance from where the patient complains of pain, thus avoiding the potential fracture site. Alternatively, have the patient supine, raise the injured leg into a straight leg

INSIGHTS

Box 8.3 Guidelines for rule outs

Once you have decided which joint or region of the body you are going to investigate for the source of the patient's chief complaint, you must first rule out the joint above and the joint below. It is imperative to determine whether the joints/areas above and below the primary joint or region could be referring to the impaired joint or tissue. If this rule out testing does not reproduce the patient's chief complaint, then that joint is said to be ruled out and not in need of immediate further testing.

Remember, the patient may experience pain or other symptoms or impairments with the rule out testing, but if the chief complaint is not provoked, then they are set aside for now and may be returned to later. These quick tests stress the principal tissues involved in each of those joints to be ruled out. They primarily focus on the non-contractile elements. Therefore, you begin by having the patient do specific AF-ROM tests of that joint. When the end-range of each AF motion is reached, ask if the patient is experiencing any pain (even if other than their chief complaint). If no pain or impairment is present, grasp and support the limbs or structures and tell the patient to relax and let you now move it. You will now apply O-P as if performing passive relaxed range of motion (PR-ROM) testing. It is O-P that stresses the inert or non-contractile tissues of that joint.

Having applied the O-P, again ask the patient if they feel any pain or impairment with the O-P. If no pain/impairment is experienced, proceed to the next AF motion and continue as you did above. However, if they do experience pain, etc., then further clarify by asking if this is the same as the pain/impairment they came to see you about or something different. If you get a positive reproduction of their chief complaint when doing a rule out, then that joint now needs to be included in your protocol of testing for the chief complaint; it is now considered to be ruled in. Remember that a chief complaint may include more than one joint.

If you get pain with or without other impairments, but these are not part of the patient's chief complaint, then record these, but return to your testing of the area indicated by the patient's complaint. These extra findings can be investigated further at a later date. If neither joint reproduces the patient's chief complaint during either the AF or the PR with O-P portion of these rule outs, then proceed onward to do the regular AF-ROM testing of the joint or structures that are the focus of the day's testing. (See Hartley 2000b for more details on rule outs.)

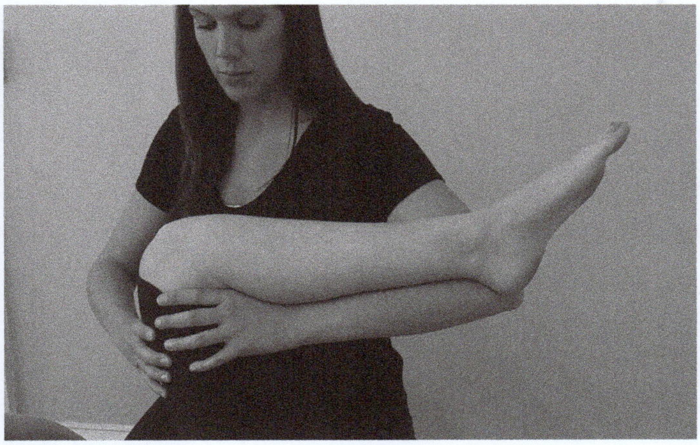

FIGURE 8.5 Ruling out hip

Have patient flex hip and knee, asking them to try to bring their knee to your shoulder. If pain-free, then apply O-P from distal thigh (but not with a hand on knee). If necessary, support lower leg to protect knee.

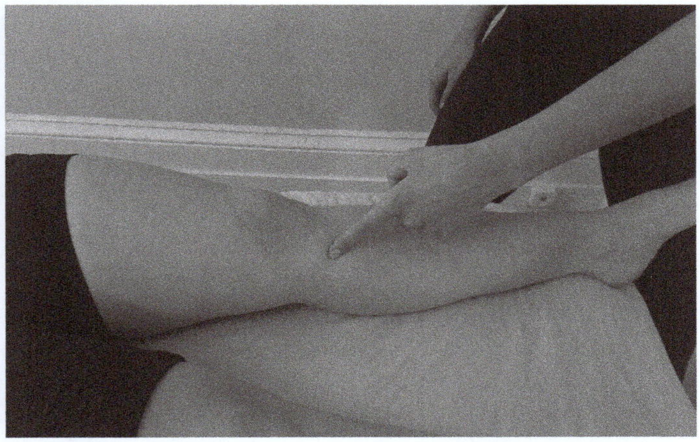

FIGURE 8.6 1. Inspection site for minor edema

This is the site where minor edema pools, and from where wiping begins.

raise at 30° and firmly tap the inferior surface of the calcaneus, directing the force upward into the leg. Having the foot dorsiflexed and the leg extended puts the ankle and knee joints in a close packed position which will transmit the force of the blow all the way up the leg causing pain at the fracture site. For example, the edges of a stress fracture will vibrate and generate a painful response (Hartley 2000b).

Joint effusion

The tests for joint effusion described below are done prior to ROM examination. We need to know prior to testing the knee itself whether there is edema present, the approximate quantity, and whether there is the possibility that this edema contains blood. If blood in the edema is suspected this is a red flag and the patient should be referred out immediately to have the knee drained. See previous case history questions concerning swelling in the knee and the clues that the patient may provide that blood is or is not present. Why do the testing if the swelling is obvious? The testing can help to determine if blood is a major component of the fluid present in the knee.

Perform these effusion tests with the patient supine and the knee in extension, or with as little flexion as possible. Moderate to major effusion will prevent full extension of the knee. Further, as ROM testing and the special tests can irritate many structures, it is wise to also do the wipe test (for minor effusion) before and after a testing protocol, to note if such testing has caused joint effusion where none had been noted earlier, or if it has increased an effusion already present. Note that even minor joint effusion may reflexively reduce the strength of the quadriceps by 30 percent.

Wipe (or sweep) test (Figures 8.6–8.11)

Minor edema in the knee can easily be overlooked. It is observed as puffiness on the medial side of the knee just below the patella (Figure 8.6). It is thought that even a teaspoon of extra fluid in the knee can cause inhibition of the VMO fibers of the vastus medialis muscle, whose function is crucial for proper patellofemoral tracking. Impairment to this muscle's function creates an imbalance within the quadriceps group, which is thought to be a principal cause of patellofemoral pain syndrome.

Watch the medial side of the knee, just below the patella, to see if there is any fluid or increase in swelling. The area will slightly swell and may even pulse two or three times, with a wave-like motion, as edematous fluid flows back into this lowest point of the synovial capsule. This is best for testing slight to moderate effusions.

Fluctuation test (Figures 8.12–8.14)

This is the preferred test for moderate effusion in the knee, but will also work on gross effusion. It is performed by alternating pressure below and above the patella, *moving fluid back and forth from the inferior area of the joint capsule to the superior area.* If fluid motion is palpable, the test is positive for swelling in the joint. The fluid must be felt to move up and down across the joint

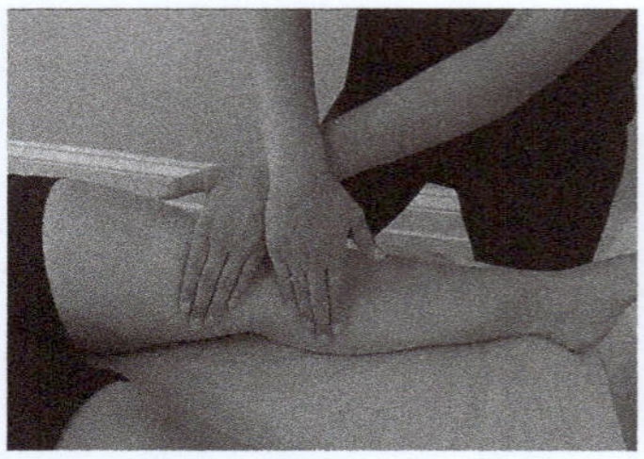

FIGURE 8.7 2. Beginning wipe test

Using fingers of one hand, begin stroke or wipe, inferior to superior, medial to patella, below pocket of edema. Use constant, firm pressure.

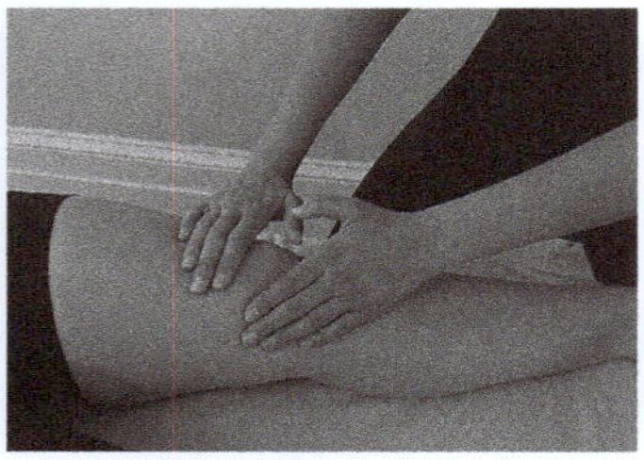

FIGURE 8.8 3. Continuous wiping up medial side

Stroke upward three or four times, with alternating hands, on medial side of knee. Purpose is to move fluid superiorly up through joint capsule toward suprapatellar area.

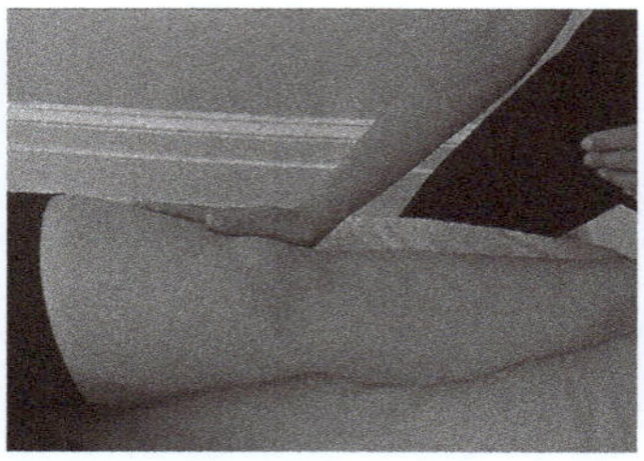

FIGURE 8.9 4. Wiping up and over patella

With a continuation of the last stroke on medial side, wipe firmly over suprapatellar "pouch" (bursa) toward lateral side of knee.

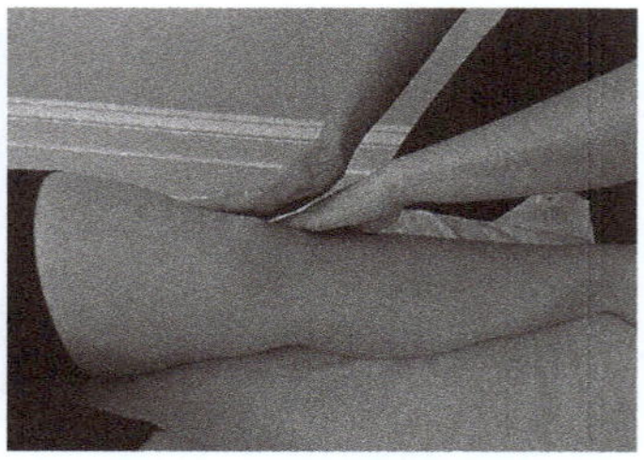

FIGURE 8.10 5. Wipe down lateral side of knee

Continuing stroke (without interruption), wipe downward on lateral side of knee.

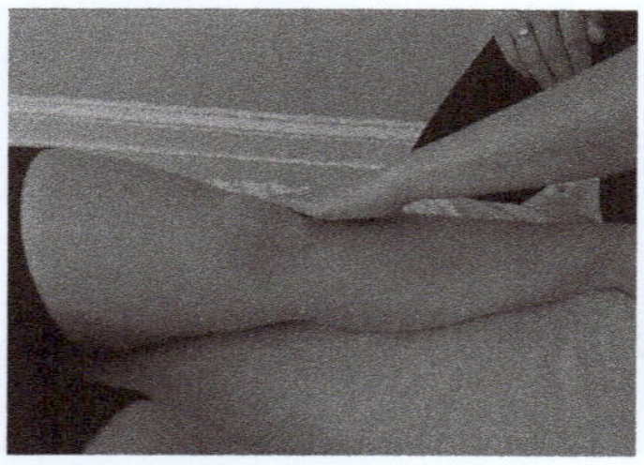

FIGURE 8.11 6. Finish stroke just below patella

Bring fluid down to infrapatellar area. Hold pressure of fingers there while observing medial infrapatellar area.

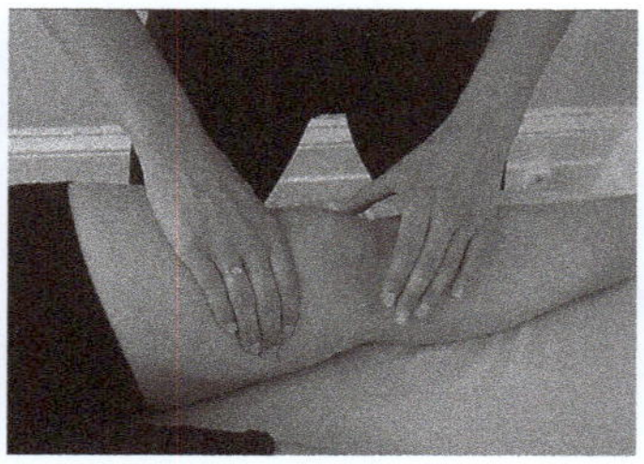

FIGURE 8.12 1. Hand positioning for fluctuation test

Place one hand over suprapatellar pouch, and other hand just below patella over infrapatellar tendon area.

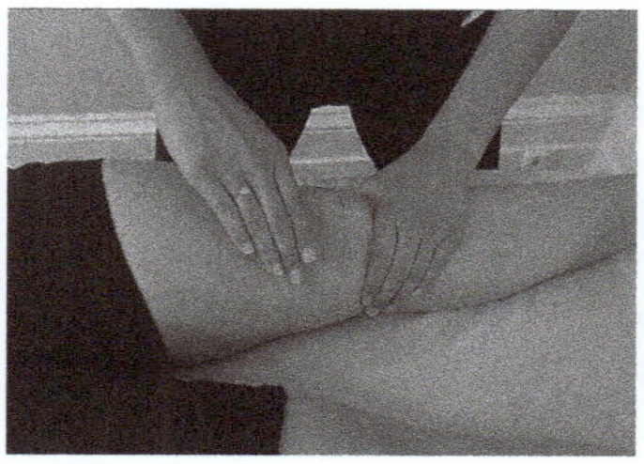

FIGURE 8.13 2. Milking fluid back and forth

Gently milk, or press one hand, then other, rhythmically while noticing movement of any fluid.

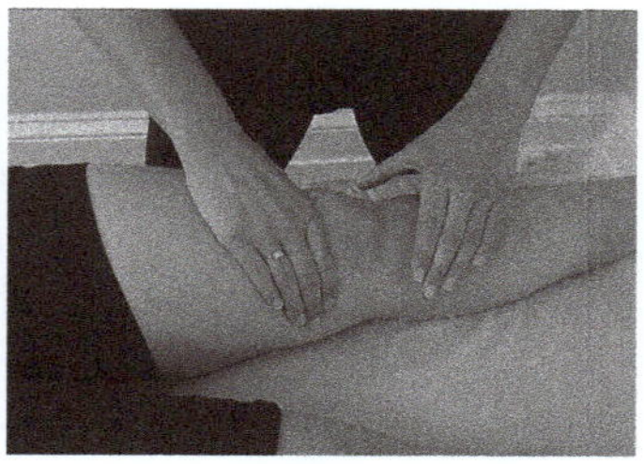

FIGURE 8.14 3. Repetitive milking or fluctuation

Repeat fluctuation test, moving fluid back and forth across joint line.

line of the knee. Otherwise it may only be an infrapatellar bursa, for example, that is swollen, and you cannot move the fluid to a position above the patella. Note that clear effusion (just synovial fluid) moves like water, whereas a thick or jelly-like movement means that there is blood in the joint. In the latter case, refer out to have the joint aspirated as soon as possible.

Patellar tap test (ballottement test) (Figure 8.15)

This test is best for gross effusion in the knee joint. When the knee is severely swollen, the therapist may not be able to move the fluid if the capsule is taut due to the amount of fluid it contains, or the patient will not tolerate the increase in pressure. This test has been called the tap test, not because the patella is tapped, but rather that when the floating patella is pushed down onto the condyles of the femur, the condyles are tapped by the patella. The patella is floating off the condyles because it is attached to the joint capsule which is swollen sufficiently to have expanded and lifted the patella away from the condyles. Again, even more so than in the case of the fluctuation test on the previous page, the swelling of the knee is usually obvious, but the test is done to ascertain whether or not the fluid contains, or is, blood. If you suspect blood, refer out for immediate medical attention.

In a positive test, you will feel a descending and then floating sensation. A "tap" may be felt as the patella sinks through the swelling while making contact with the condyles prior to floating back up once pressure is removed from the patella. The therapist in Figure 8.15 shows the use of the thumbs to press down, but that is done here only to show the action. The broader pressure of the palm is better as a smaller area of contact can "rock" or "tip" the patella rather than push the whole patella down. The floating action is palpable. If unsure, then repeat the test using the thumbs in the center of the patella to push down, and see if you can observe the action.

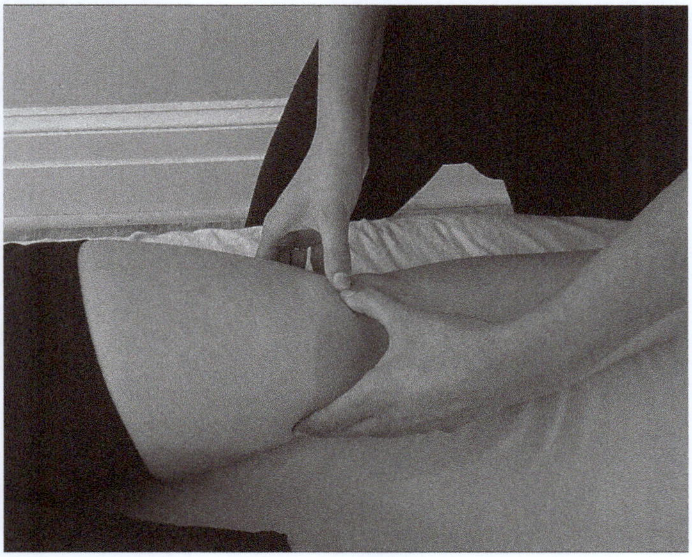

FIGURE 8.15 Patellar tap test

Place the palm of one hand over the patella, then gently press the patella down into tibiofemoral joint. Release pressure while sustaining light contact on patella. Palpate to see if the patella floats up on release.

If there seems to be a delay or hesitancy in the patella floating back up, then there may well be blood present. If the patella immediately returns to where it started after the pressure is released, then it is more likely to be synovium.

Pushing gently into gross edema with one finger can also be a test for blood. If a recent swelling acts like "pitted edema" there can be blood present. In pitted edema, when you remove the pressure a "pit" or "divot" remains in the tissue. When it is blood, the divot will disappear after a second or two. Again, this requires the patient to be referred out to see if immediate aspiration of the joint is required.

Range of motion testing (ROM)

Perform the following range of motion testing (compilation derived from: Dutton 2012; Hartley 2000b; Hertling & Kessler 2006; Hoppenfeld 1976; Magee 2014; Petty 2011; Starkey & Brown 2015).

Active free range of motion (AF-ROM)

Active knee flexion 135° (Figure 8.16A–C)

The therapist can place their hand over the patella (not shown) while the patient flexes the knee, to feel for crepitus. Patellar crepitus that begins around 30° of flexion may indicate problems with the retropatellar surface. However, crepitus without pain may well be benign.

NOTE: Tight hamstrings may be involved in many of the following tests, contributing to their positive signs. Therefore, the

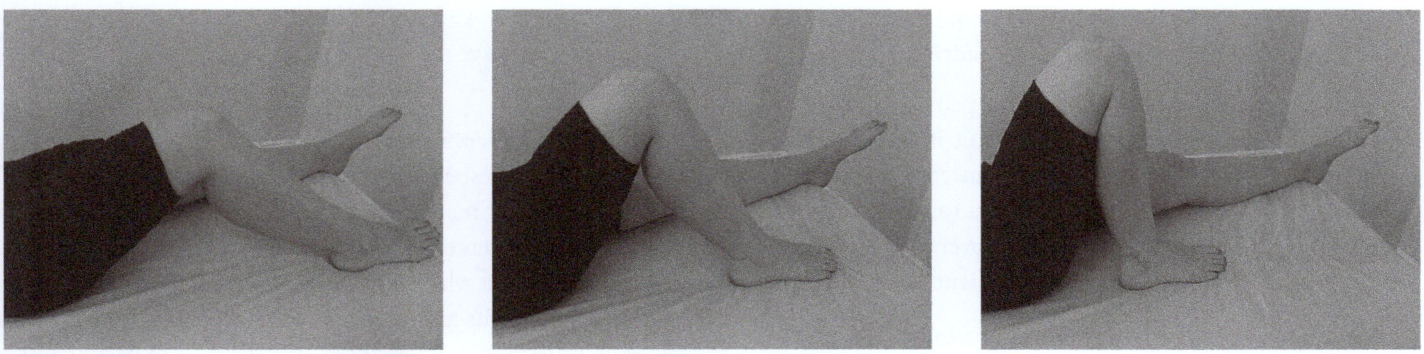

FIGURE 8.16A–C AF-ROM supine knee flexion

With the patient supine, ask them to lift foot slightly off surface of table and take their heel toward their buttock.

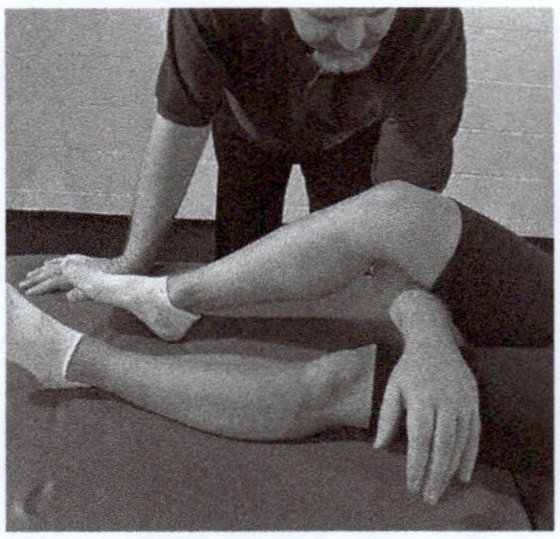

FIGURE 8.17 1. Starting position

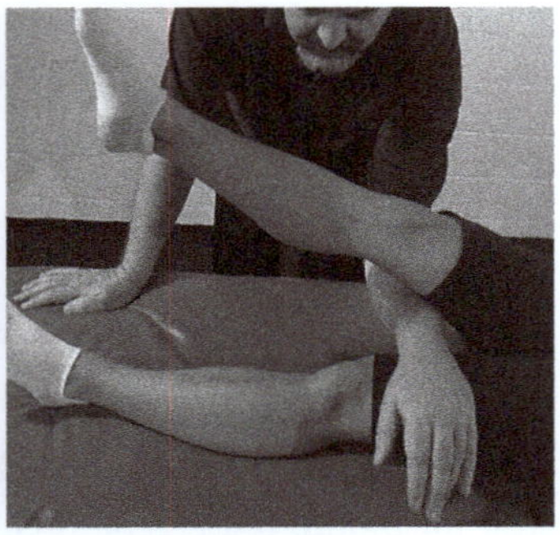

FIGURE 8.18 2. AF-ROM extension of knee

Patient starts with knee in slight flexion. Next, observe degree of extension as patient holds extension for 5 seconds.

length and tightness of hamstrings should be tested now, but only if there is no contraindication to full knee extension due to joint swelling or pain.

Perform a straight leg raise (SLR) on each leg to test hamstring length. Hip flexion of 75–85° with the knee in extension would be considered within normal length for the hamstrings.

Active knee extension 0–15° (Figures 8.17, 8.18)

This can be done with a patient high-sitting or supine. If the patient is supine, place your forearm or a towel roll on the table under the patient's now flexed knee and have them extend the knee from that position, if possible. Place the forearm under the thigh, proximal to the knee with the palm of your hand on the opposite thigh. Have the patient hold the extension for at least 5 seconds. Prime movers are the quadriceps.

Note the quality of movement of the patella and its tracking. Jerky movements of the patella or crepitus in the patella during the last 20–30° of extension can be caused by a weak vastus medialis or by a tendency for the patella to sublux. This is best observed by lightly placing a free hand over the patella and palpating its quality of movement as the patient extends the knee.

Quadriceps inhibition test (quadriceps lag sign) (Figure 8.19)

A special test you can do now is the quadriceps inhibition test. The test consists of an observation made as the patient tries to extend the knee and hold it for 5 seconds (Hertling & Kessler 2006).

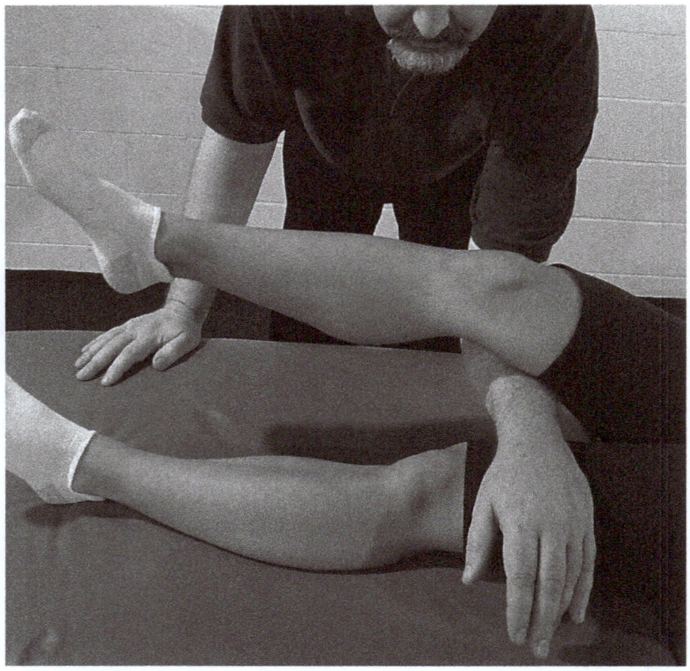

FIGURE 8.19 Quadriceps inhibition test

With the patient seated or supine, observe what happens as they fully extend knee. Observe whether the patient can get knee into full extension and if they can hold it there for more than a few seconds. Positive signs are: (1) the inability to get the knee into full extension, while reporting there is no pain, etc., and the patient telling you they either feel weak or just cannot hold the position; (2) the patient can achieve full extension but cannot hold leg and it quickly drops down to 5–20° of flexion. Quadriceps is then either suffering from atrophy (which should be visible/palpable), or it is inhibited by tight hamstrings (reciprocal inhibition), or neurologically (as with a L3 nerve root impingement).

A further observation: if there is atrophy to the vastus medialis muscle, especially of VMO, a sulcus or "hollow spot" just superior and medial to the patella will appear and/or be palpable, in the center of where the vastus medialis muscle is. It is most apparent when the muscle is working, as in AF extension of the knee. Its appearance usually accompanies a positive lag sign, especially if the weakness has been there in the muscle long enough for atrophy to occur. Weakness in this muscle is also often accompanied by a presentation of patellofemoral pain syndromes because of the crucial role it plays in proper patella tracking.

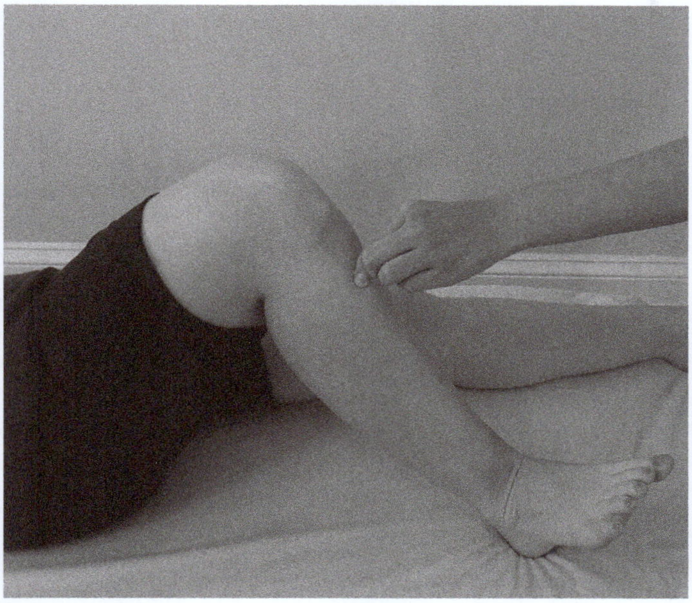

FIGURE 8.20 1. AF-ROM external (lateral) rotation of tibia (30–40°)

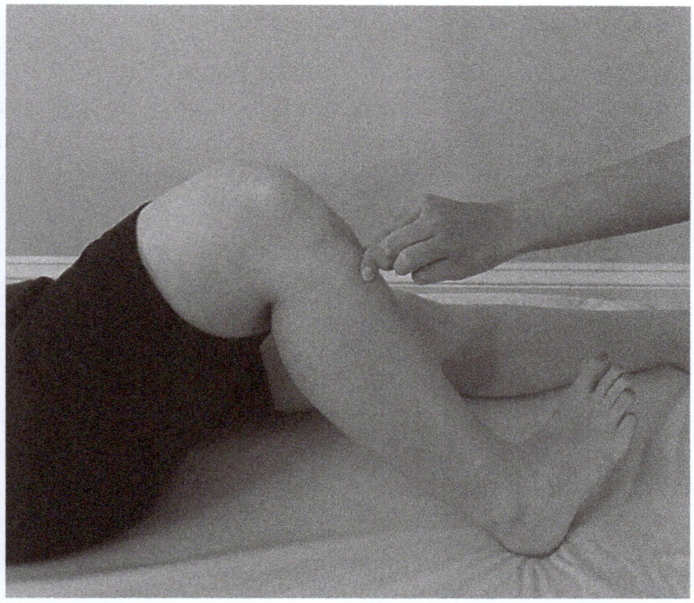

FIGURE 8.21 2. AF-ROM internal (medial) rotation of tibia (20°)

Palpate tibial tuberosity to gauge motion.

Active medial and lateral rotation of the tibia (Figures 8.20, 8.21)

With the patient crook-lying or high-sitting, and the knees flexed at 90°, have the patient rotate their feet inward (tibia rotates medially) and outward (tibia rotates laterally). The knee needs to be flexed, as rotation cannot occur in extension due to muscle and ligament stabilization of the knee. You may wish to stabilize the femur to prevent it from abducting or adducting during tibial rotation. Watch the lower leg, not the feet. It is best to palpate the tibial tuberosity and observe the motion of the tibia by this landmark while the patient internally and externally rotates the tibia.

Note especially if the patient seems to lack rotation one way while the other direction seems very full or even excessive. This may imply that the patient's tibia is already rotated in the range most lacking. For example, if the patient seems to have excessive medial rotation, but has little or no lateral rotation, the tibia may already be laterally rotated. Since the knee is to be flexed 90° for this testing, the tibial tuberosity should be aligned straight under the "apex" of the patella (i.e., the pointed or V-shaped lowest portion of the patella). Note if it is not properly positioned and in which direction is it being held rotated. (See the Helfet test in the section on special tests. It can be done at this time, or when doing passive testing of tibial rotation.)

The patient may have rotated the tibia medially or laterally to compensate for changes occurring below (e.g., pes planus/cavus) or above the knee (e.g., short femur ipsilaterally or unilateral anterior pelvic tilt). Other causes of tibial torsion include shortening, spasm, or contracture of either the biceps femoris (lateral rotation) or of the semimembranosus/tendinosus and popliteus (medial rotation).

Since the cruciate ligaments will have to twist around each other when the tibia of the flexed knee rotates medially this is when most injuries to cruciates occur, especially the anterior cruciate ligament (Magee 2014; Schuenke et al. 2014).

Passive relaxed range of motion (PR-ROM)

Have the patient supine or seated high enough that you can easily and confidently move their knee. Ask the patient to relax during PR-ROM, and especially when applying O-P. Note any crepitus, as you move the joint. When end-range has been reached, and only if there is no pain, apply slight O-P to determine the joint's end-feel. Be sure to stabilize above the joint and remember that, when O-P is applied: (1) do not change the basic orientation of the joint; and (2) try not to engage or move other surrounding tissues or structures more than necessary.

Passive knee flexion (Figures 8.22, 8.23)

An alternative method for O-P is to lay the extended leg on the table, hold the thigh down on the table while you lift the lower leg (at the ankle) into hyperextension. Many therapists feel that with this latter positioning they can better gauge if the patient has a knee that can hyperextend. It is said that men usually have 0–5° of hyperextension available, while women often have 5–10° of hyperextension available (Magee 2014). Hyperextension of 15° or more should be considered as hyperextended, genu recurvatum.

Passive lateral and medial rotation of the tibia (Figure 8.24)

Have patient crook-lying; knees at 90°. Place both hands around the superior portion of the lower leg, so that your thumbs are on either side of the tibial tuberosity. Rather than grip too tightly with the fingers, lean onto the tibia (and fibula); thereby the thenar eminences will have a firm hold that will not twist the skin rotating the tibia. The therapist should rotate their whole torso, and not use their wrists. It is the collateral ligaments that restrict lateral (external) rotation; it is the cruciates that restrict medial (internal) rotation. Excessive motion or pain while rotating could imply injury to the appropriate ligaments. (See Special tests.)

Joint mobilization

Joint mobilization is an extremely valuable tool in assessing the intrinsic mobility of a joint under investigation. We are looking for a small amount of joint-play within the joint that permits the necessary motions of glide, roll, and/or spin that are required for proper motion of the joint surfaces and appropriate ability for the joint surfaces to distract (separate from each other). Further, other mobilizations test for pain (such as compression test) and/or reflexive apprehension (specifically in shear tests). (For further details and instruction see Part I, Chapter 3. Also, see the following for more information, optional positioning of patient or limb, variations, and additional tests: Edmond 2006; Hertling & Kessler 2006; Kaltenborn 2006; Kisner & Colby 2012; Starkey & Brown 2015.)

Passive patellar movement (patellar glides) (Figures 8.25–8.28)

The following passive movements of the patella should be available when the supine patient is relaxed. Have the knee flexed to 20° or so with a pillow or towel roll under the distal thigh

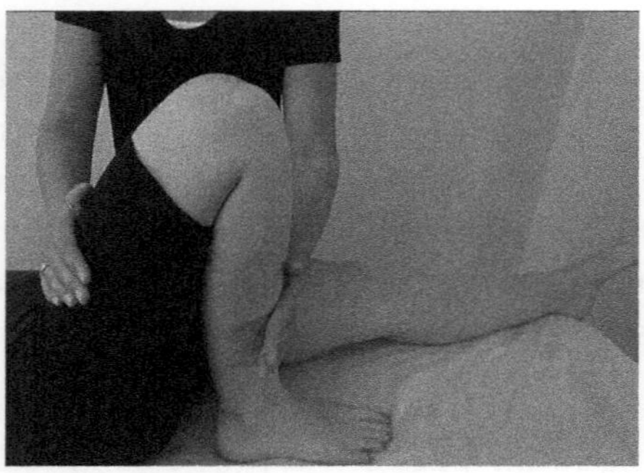

FIGURE 8.22 1. PR-ROM knee flexion 135–150°

With the patient supine, place one hand on the patient's thigh and with other hand hold the tibia above the ankle. Bring the knee into flexion while lifting the foot slightly off table. If there is no pain, apply O-P with your hands placed just above and below knee. End-feel is tissue approximation or tissue stretch (usually from tight quadriceps).

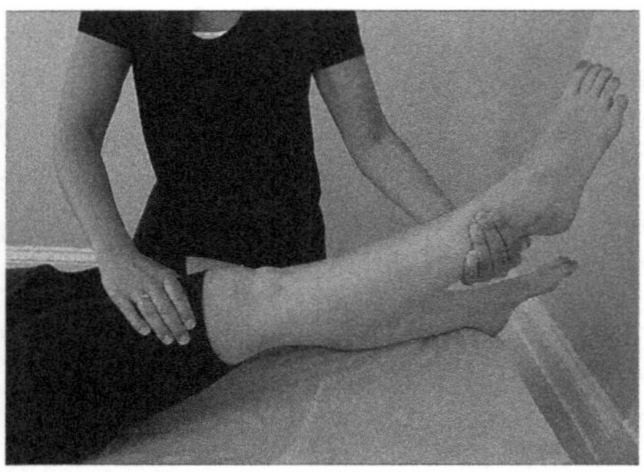

FIGURE 8.23 2. PR-ROM extension of knee 0–15°

Bring the leg into full extension. Stabilize the thigh and apply O-P. You should experience a firm muscular end-feel.

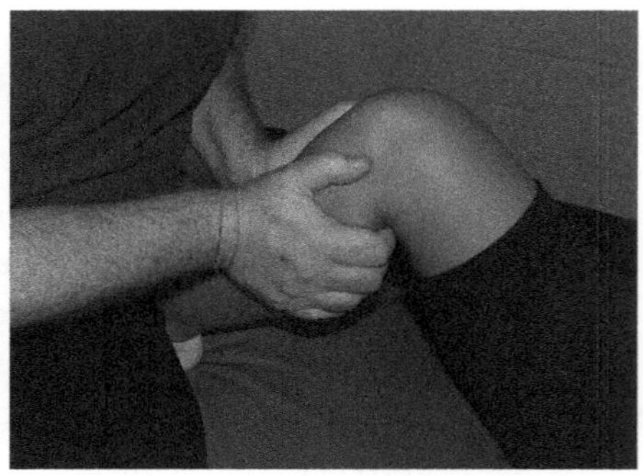

FIGURE 8.24 PR-ROM lateral (30–40°) and medial (20°) rotation of tibia

Turn the tibia medially/internally into end-range; if pain-free apply O-P. Then do the same turning the tibia laterally/externally. There should be a ligamentous or leathery end-feel. It is best to repeat the rotations several times in each direction. This version of passive O-P avoids putting stress through the ankle.

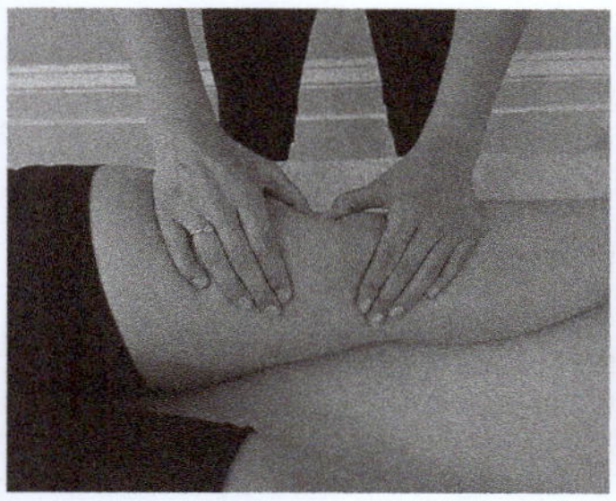

FIGURE 8.25 **1. Medial patellar glide**

With the tips of the thumbs/fingers press on the lateral side of the patella in a medial direction.

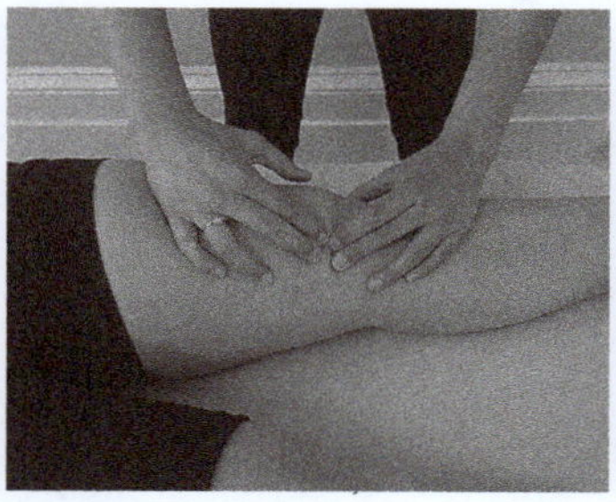

FIGURE 8.26 **2. Lateral patellar glide**

Push the patella laterally. This is sometimes called the patellar apprehension test, since the patient will not want the patella moved in this direction if they previously experienced a lateral dislocation. There is a protective reflex contraction of the quadriceps muscle.

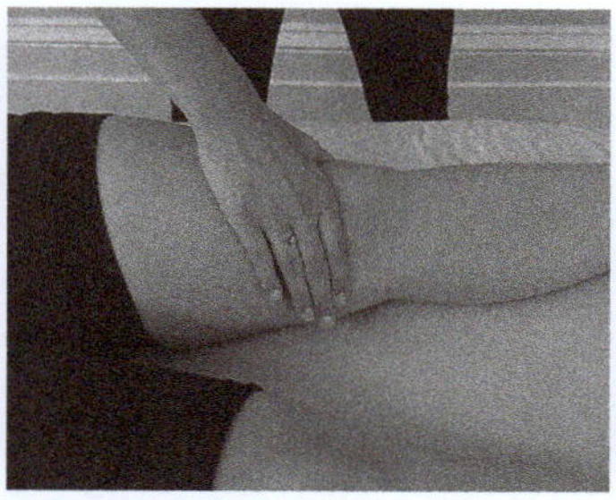

FIGURE 8.27 **3. Inferior patellar glide**

The therapist attempts to push the patella inferiorly. Only a slight motion is available. ***CAUTION:*** *Try to avoid pushing the patella down into the femur while pushing inferiorly. Otherwise you may "grind" the patella into the bone, causing pain.*

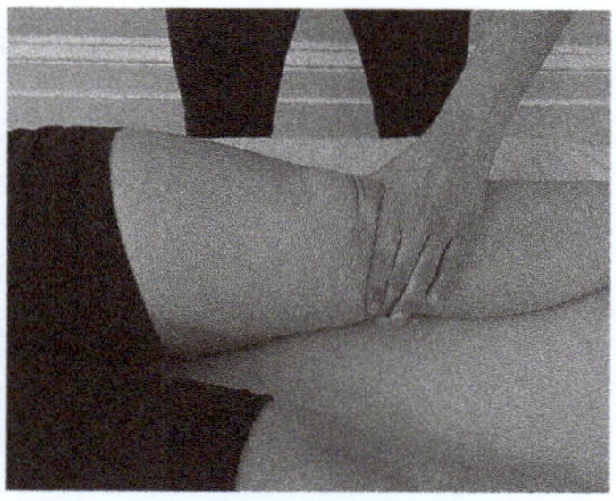

FIGURE 8.28 **4. Superior patellar glide**

The therapist attempts to push the patella superiorly. Only a slight motion is available.

so as to relax the musculature around the knee. Note crepitus and/or apprehension in the patient observed as they contract their quadriceps to prevent movement of the patella. At the end-range, apply a slow and very small amplitude O-P. Perform these glides of the patella gently in the following directions.

Lifting the patella (Figure 8.29)

The patella can also be lifted off the condyles of the femur and moved side to side. You should be able to get some decompression, which is a lifting or floating of the patella off the condyles. If the patella seems welded to the femur the quadriceps may be hypertonic. If there seems to be too much laxity then the quadriceps may be weak, inhibited, or suffering from atrophy. Lifting the patella on a number of patients in different stages of health and strength will give you the experience needed to be able to judge laxity or hypertonicity of the quadriceps.

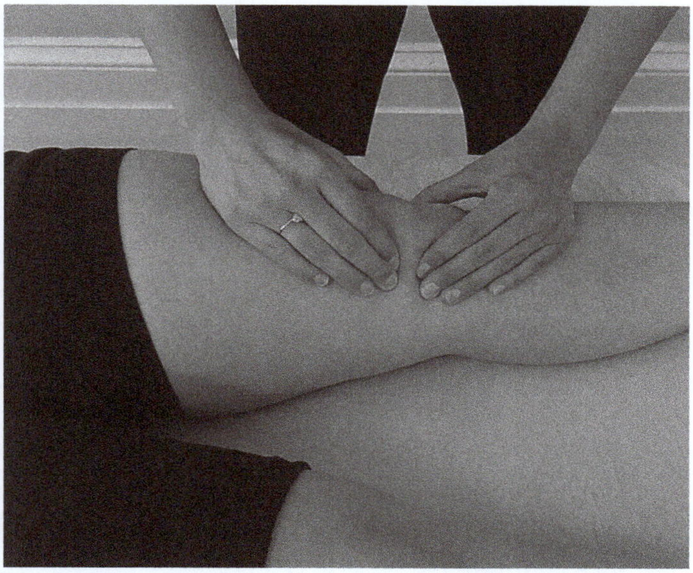

FIGURE 8.29 **5. Lifting patella**

Grasp patella at four corners, using thumbs and index fingers. Lift.

Superior tibiofibular joint glide (Figures 8.30, 8.31)

Test the superior tibiofibular joint when exploring the causes of lateral knee pain. When the ankle dorsiflexes, the front of the talus, which is wider anteriorly than posteriorly, pushes the distal fibula laterally. This also causes the fibula to move superiorly and internally rotate (see Part II, Chapter 7, Ankle and foot).

Anterior/posterior tibiofemoral glide (Figures 8.32, 8.33)

These glides are versions of the draw tests for the anterior and posterior cruciate ligaments (ACL and PCL), respectively. End-feel is ligamentous. (See next section on special tests.)

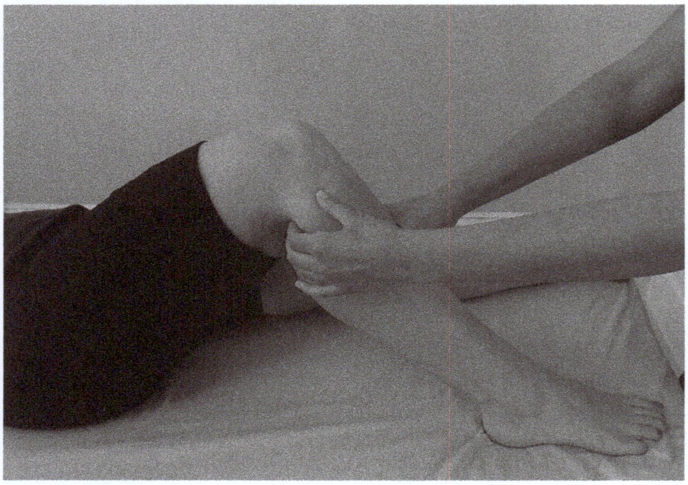

FIGURE 8.30 1. Superior tibiofibular glide positioning

Place two fingers behind the head of the fibula (you can also hold the fibular head between the thumb and index finger). Hold the foot/ankle in neutral. Plantar flex the patient's foot and note if the head of the fibula moves slightly inferiorly and rolls slightly externally. (You may not feel this very slight motion.)

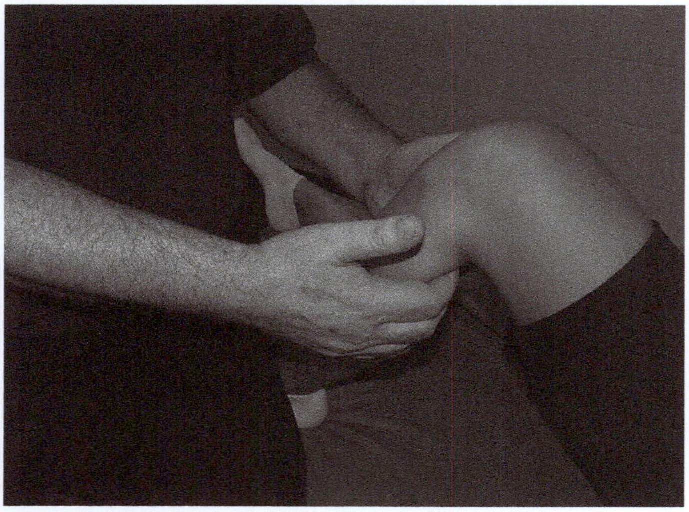

FIGURE 8.32 1. Anterior tibiofemoral glide

Sit on the patient's foot and cup your hands around the tibia. Lean backward, gliding the tibia anteriorly.

Tibiofemoral joint shear test (Figure 8.34A, B)

This test seeks to place a lateral and medial shear force through the joint margin. To achieve this shearing force, the therapist's hands need to be close to the joint line. End-feel is ligamentous.

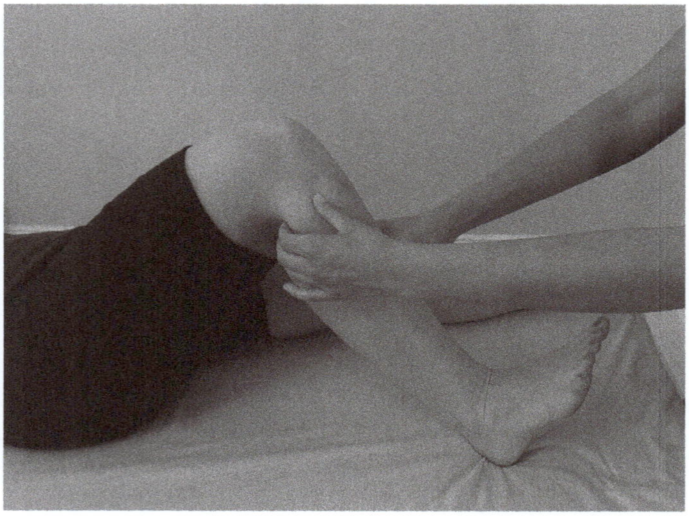

FIGURE 8.31 2. Dorsiflex ankle while palpating

Dorsiflex the foot and note if the fibular head moves slightly superiorly and rolls slightly forward (rotates internally).

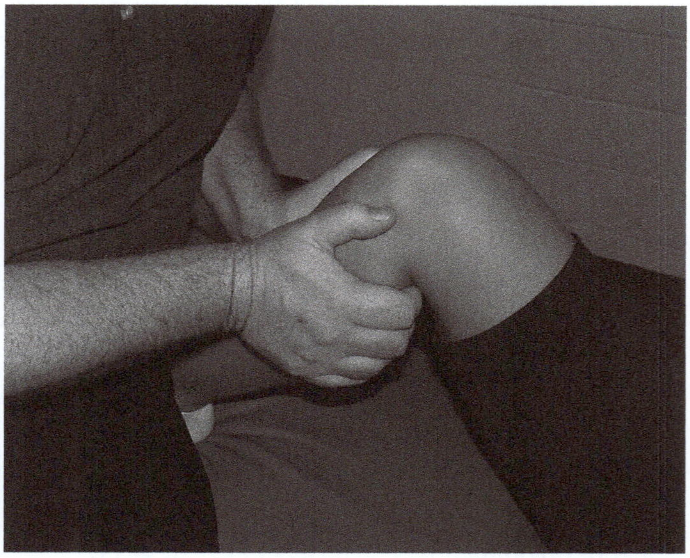

FIGURE 8.33 2. Posterior tibiofemoral glide

Stabilize the femur with one hand and with the other grasp the anterior surface of the tibia just below the knee. Press the tibia posteriorly.

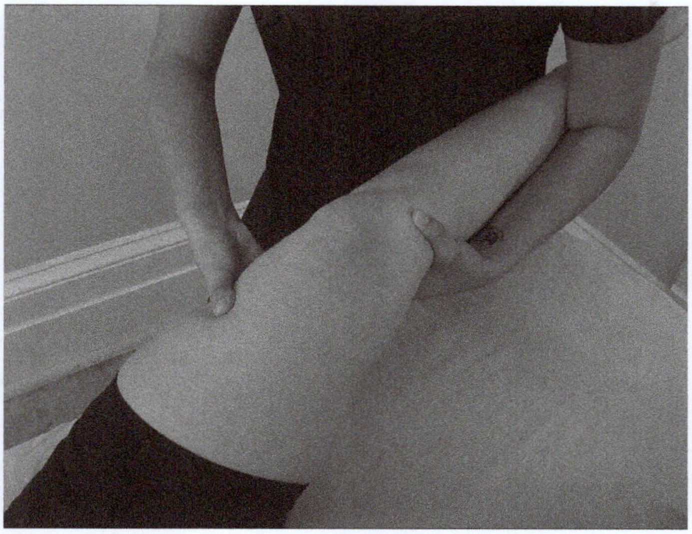

FIGURE 8.34A Lateral shear of tibiofemoral joint

With the patient crook-lying, lift the leg above the ankle until the knee is at 20–30° of flexion. Hold the ankle between your arm and trunk and use that hand to cup the medial side of the proximal tibia as near as possible to the joint line. Stabilize the lateral side of the femur at the epicondyle area. Push the tibia laterally as you push the femur medially.

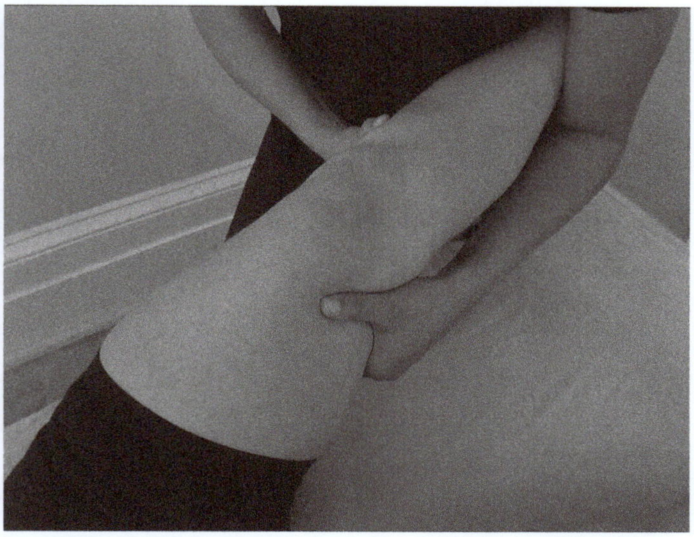

FIGURE 8.34B Medial shear of tibiofemoral joint

The patient is crook-lying, with the knee at 20–30° of flexion. Hold the ankle under your arm and use a hand to stabilize the medial side of the epicondyle of the femur (i.e., above the knee). Cup the other hand over the lateral side of the proximal end of the tibia, as close to the joint line as possible. Have the head of the fibula sitting in the palm to minimize pressure on it. Push the femur laterally as you push the tibia medially.

NOTE: These are not the same (or as specific) as the varus and valgus stress testing for the collateral ligaments.

Distraction (decompression) of tibiofemoral joint (Figure 8.35)

This action gaps the tibiofemoral joint. Repetitive distraction and compression will improve joint nutrition, and can reflexively relax the muscles crossing the joint (as long as the motion is pain-free). Use your body-weight and rock back away from the joint when tractioning or decompressing it.

Try not to pull using your shoulders. To compress the joint, simply rock forward, pushing the tibia toward the femur.

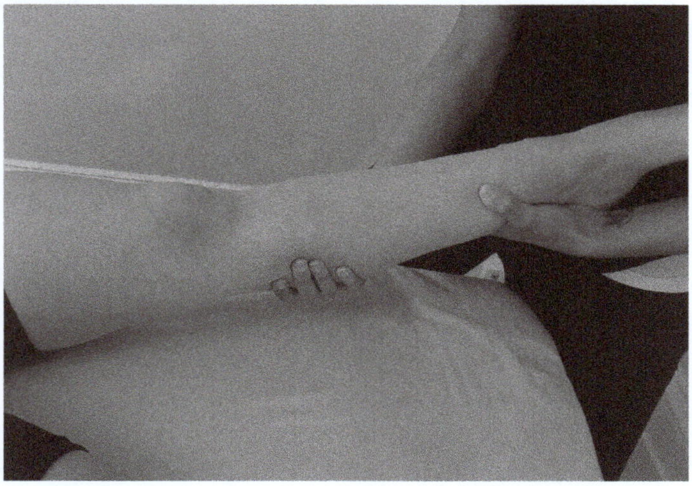

FIGURE 8.35 Tibiofemoral joint distraction

Place a pillow or towel roll under the patient's knee so that it is slightly flexed. Traction the tibia away from the femur. This can be followed with compression.

Active resisted range of motion (AR-ROM) (Figures 8.36–8.38A, B)

See Part I, Chapter 3 for a discussion of active resisted testing and what we learn from such testing, including a grading scale 0 to 5 (see Kendall et al. 2005 for a truly comprehensive exploration and instruction in muscle testing; see and compare: Dutton 2012; Hartley 2000b; Hertling & Kessler 2006; Magee 2014; Petty 2011).

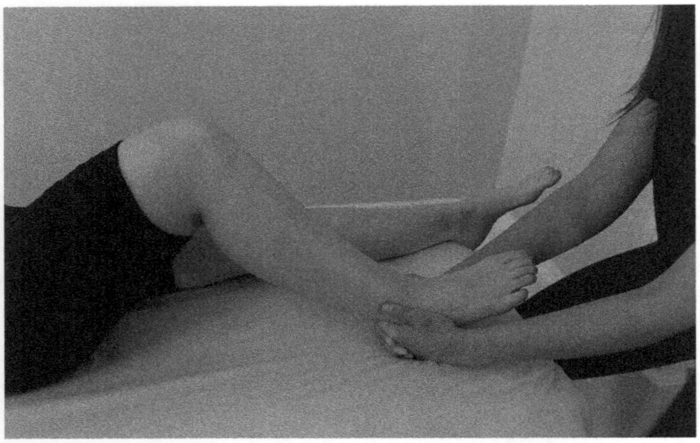

FIGURE 8.36 AR-ROM knee flexion

With the patient crook-lying, grasp the heel of the leg to be tested and lift slightly off the table. Ask the patient not to let you move them. Slowly increase pull until you feel muscle working maximally. Hold this for about 5 seconds and slowly release.

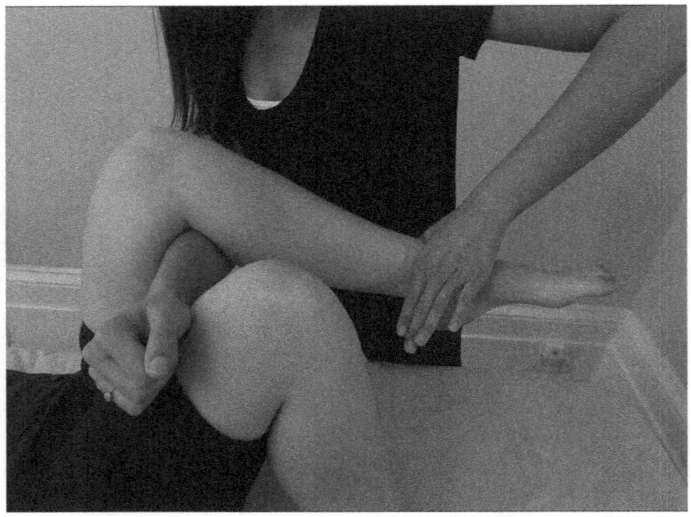

FIGURE 8.37 AR-ROM knee extension

Lift one leg into extension and place your forearm under the patient's thigh with the distal end of your forearm resting on the other thigh just above the patient's knee (if there is no injury to the quadriceps or swelling in that knee). Passively lower the extended leg over your forearm, slightly flexing the knee. In this position, ask the patient not to let you move them into more flexion.

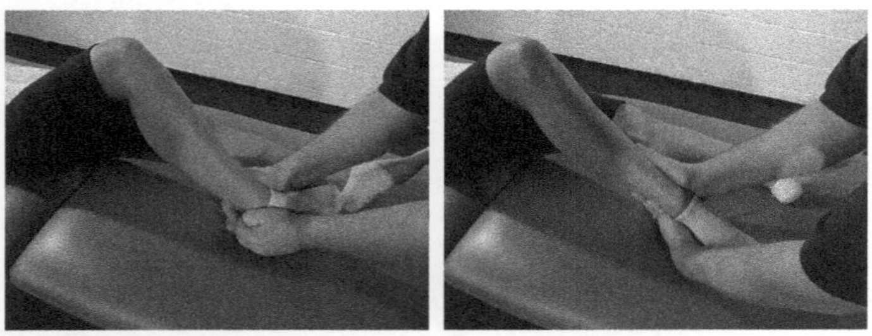

FIGURE 8.38A, B AR-ROM tibial rotations

With the knee flexed, dorsiflex the patient's foot, leaving the heel on the table. Rotate the tibia medially slightly and ask the patient to try and rotate back while you stabilize the tibia by holding it mid-shaft and through the ankle. This tests the strength of lateral rotation. Then, rotate laterally and repeat to test medial rotation.

Testing is done with the patient in the crook-lying position, as it is safer for the patient's low back and stops them from using upper body-weight to compensate for weakness in the muscles being tested.

Special tests

Differential muscle testing

The therapist uses differential muscle testing on muscles that have been implicated as impaired during AF-ROM or AR-ROM testing, or when the patient's description of pain and/or dysfunction implicates the muscle (see Part I, Chapter 3). Positive signs for impairment are as for AR-ROM testing: pain and/or weakness (Kendall et al. 2005).

Hamstrings (Figures 8.39, 8.40)

By turning the tibia medially or laterally while resisting knee flexion, you can test the medial or lateral hamstrings. This is very important as the ability to laterally and/or medially rotate the tibia will be affected by the relative length and strength of each set of hamstrings, and such a muscle imbalance will affect gait from heel strike to toe-off.

Soleus versus gastrocnemius (Figures 8.41A, B, 8.42A, B)

If these muscles do not seem acutely impaired, do the following testing standing. If you suspect acute impairment, then do the testing supine.

- If pain is present with extended knee and with bent knee, and the pain is the same in each, it is probably the soleus that is at fault.

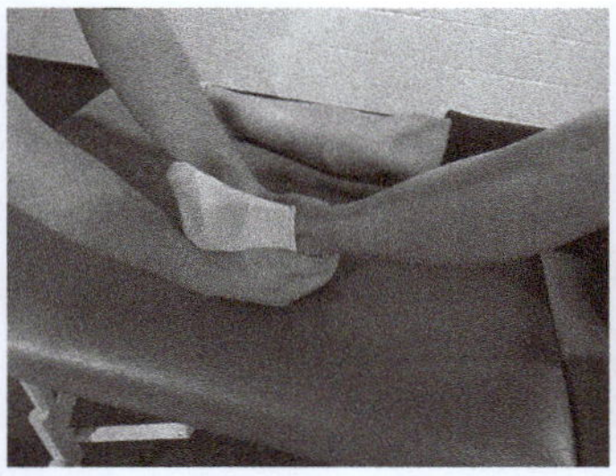

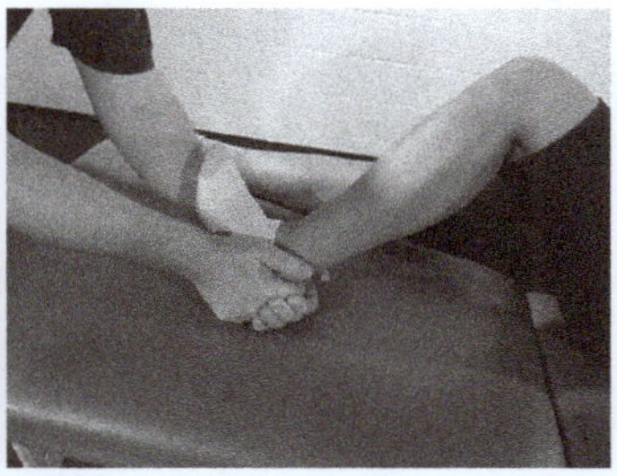

FIGURE 8.39 Specific test biceps femoris

Have the patient crook-lying. Turn the lower leg laterally to shorten the biceps femoris long and short head. The patient brings the heel to the buttock as the movement is resisted. This specifically tests biceps femoris.

FIGURE 8.40 Specific test semimembranosus/ tendinosus

If lower leg is rotated medially, semimembranosus and semitendinosus are tested specifically.

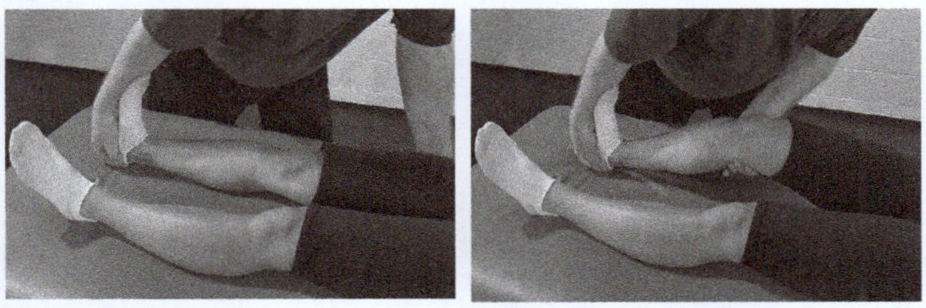

FIGURE 8.42A, B Supine testing of gastrocnemius and soleus

(A) With the knee extended and the ankle slightly plantar flexed, cup the calcaneus and have forearm under the patient's foot. Instruct the patient to hold this position as you attempt to dorsiflex the foot. (B) Flex the patient's knee 40–60° and repeat thetest.

- If pain is present with extended knee and with bent knee, and the pain is different with each, then both muscles are involved.
- If there is pain present with the extended knee, and there is none (or very little) with the knee flexed, then the gastrocnemius is the injured muscle.

Remember that a two-joint muscle is more likely injured (or more severely injured) than a one-joint muscle. Also, it is not uncommon to find that these muscles differ in strength.

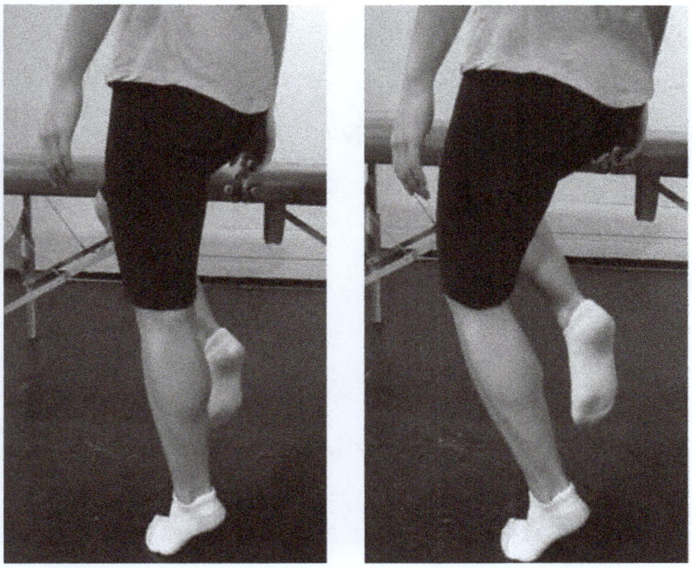

FIGURE 8.41A, B Standing testing of gastrocnemius and soleus

With the patient standing on one leg, knee extended, instruct the patient to go up on the toes. Have them repeat this several times. Now have the patient flex the knee slightly and repeat toe-raises. Compare the results. (The patient may need assistance with stabilization or balance).

Quadriceps (Figures 8.43, 8.44)

Though not a resisted differential muscle test per se, it is still a good idea to differentiate the rectus femoris from the three vasti muscles by length testing. It is not uncommon for a patient to have a tight rectus femoris while the rest of the quadriceps are hypotonic or weak. The main reason the rectus femoris can be more hypertonic is that it also works as a hip flexor. Have the patient side-lying (testing the leg that is superior) with the hips and knees bent. In this position, the rectus femoris is made lax.

Usually, the first sign of a tight rectus femoris is pain, a burning sensation, or a stretch felt just below the attachment of the muscle onto the anterior inferior iliac spine (AIIS). ***NOTE:*** The patient often increases the lumbar curve and anteriorly rotates the hip when trying to stretch the rectus femoris, thus hiding its shortness by bringing the origin closer to the insertion and avoiding putting a stretch through the muscle. Observe how most people do the "runner's stretch" and note how they usually hyperextend the low back as they grasp their ankle and pull it to the buttocks. Most people keep the low back hyperextended (hyperlordotic) as they stretch rather than flatten the lumbar spine (a posterior pelvic tilt) as they should.

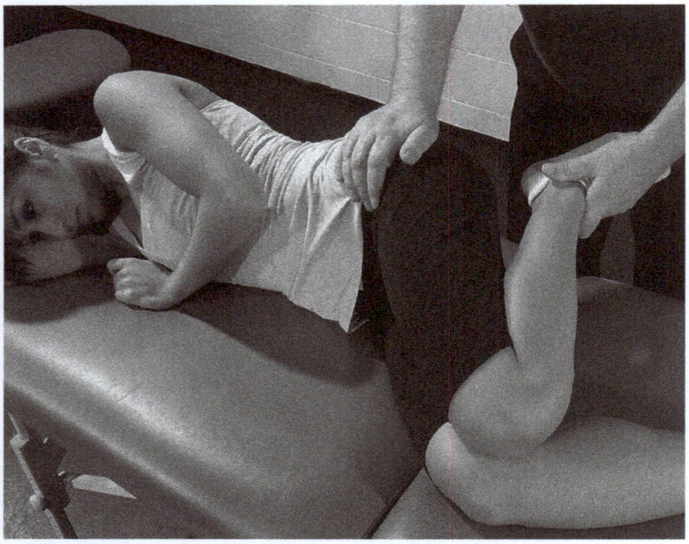

FIGURE 8.43 Testing the length of the three vasti muscles
Bring the heel as close as possible to the buttocks. Ask about pain or stretch.

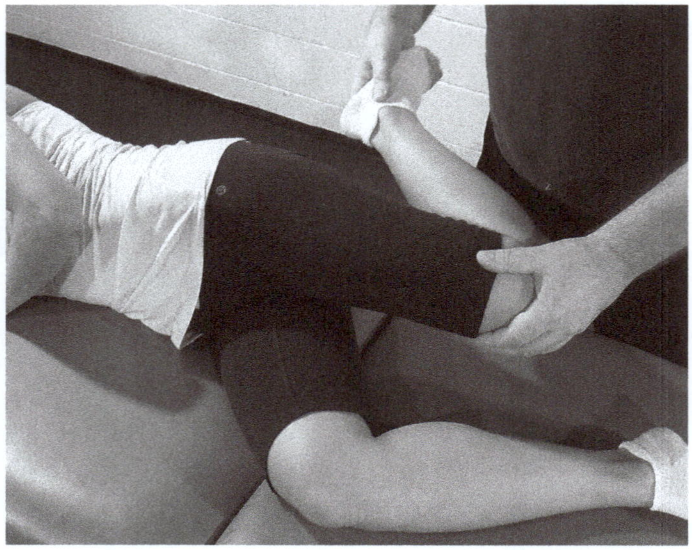

FIGURE 8.44 Testing the length of rectus femoris
Bring the hip back into neutral as in standing, or even slightly into hip extension. Ask the patient to keep the lower back flat and again flex the knee. Compare results with the previous test.

The rectus femoris should be thought of as separate from the three vasti muscles for the purposes of assessment specific to the knee, the hip, or for analyzing posture around the pelvis and lower extremities. The rectus femoris crosses the hip and the knee, and as mentioned, it can be tight and short while the rest of the quadriceps can be long and weak. Thus, the rectus femoris and the vasti muscles can be in entirely different states of impairment or conditioning.

Other special tests

Modified Helfet test (Figures 8.45, 8.46)

This tests the "screw home mechanism" that allows the knee to lock. With the patient high-sitting or crook-lying, palpate the tibial tuberosity and note if it is centered under the midline of the patella. When the knee is extended by the patient the tibial tuberosity should be closer to, if not in line with, the lateral border of the patella. This shows that the tibia has externally rotated, as it should. If the quadriceps is not strong enough to bring the knee into full extension (see quadriceps inhibition test), the therapist may assist the patient in achieving full knee extension to see if the tibial tuberosity has moved laterally.

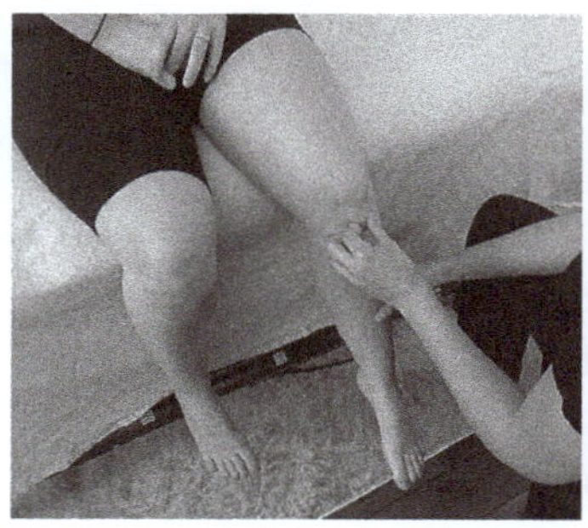

FIGURE 8.45 1. Modified Helfet test
Landmark the tibial tuberosity and apex of the patella.

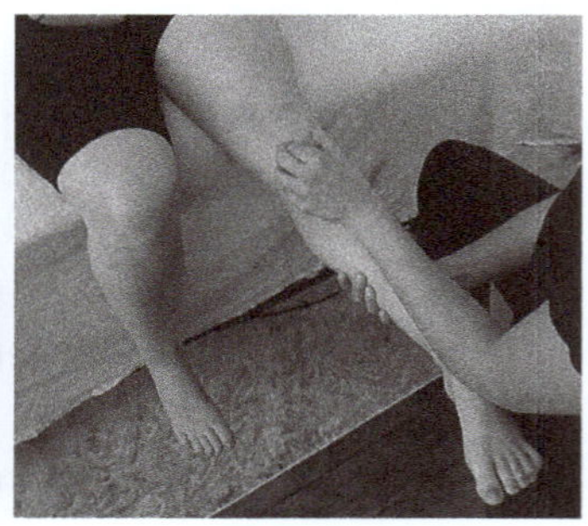

FIGURE 8.46 2. Modified Helfet test
Have the patient extend the knee and landmark both again.

If the tibia does not rotate, the hamstrings, especially the semimembranosus and semitendinosus, may be too tight (hypertonic) and short. There is also the possibility that there may be a loose body preventing movement, but in this case pain would usually be present with full extension of the knee (Hertling & Kessler 2006; Magee 2014). The positive sign is an impaired or non-functioning screw home mechanism.

Ligament integrity tests

The valgus and varus stress tests for the knee are *not* the same as a shear test (see the description of joint glides in the PR-ROM section of this chapter). These two tests (Figure 8.47A, B) are meant to gap one side of the joint while the other side is compressed.

Note that lateral rotation of the tibia is checked by both the lateral (fibular) and medial (tibial) ligaments. As noted earlier, the phrase that helps you to remember which ligament checks which rotation is "lateral rotation stopped by collateral ligaments." Therefore, medial rotation is checked by the cruciate ligaments. Injuries to the collateral ligaments are more likely to happen when they are under stress, when the tibia is laterally/externally rotated (e.g., valgus orientation of knee, especially stressing the medial collateral).

Valgus stress test (Figure 8.47A)

When done at 0° of extension/flexion this test is intended to assess the medial collateral ligament and posterior medial capsule sprains. However, the joint is stabilized in extension by the muscles crossing it and if they are hypertonic or in spasm stress to the collateral ligaments may not be sufficient to adequately test them. As a result, testing with the knee in full extension is likely to produce confusing, non-specific results. For example, a protective spasming/splinting by muscles can be due to a protective reflex generated by the instability of the joint caused by ligamentous laxity. This muscular support is capable of holding the joint fixed, even though the ligament is injured or stretched.

Therefore, the test is more specific for stressing non-contractile medial tissues at 15–30° flexion since this positioning slackens the muscles that help stabilize the medial knee (sartorius, gracilis, semitendinosus, semimembranosus, medial gastrocnemius) and places more stress on the medial collateral ligament along with the anterior superficial fibers of the joint capsule. The positive sign is pain and/or gapping of the medial joint margin, implicating the medial collateral ligament (and possibly the fibrous capsule). The test is also good for checking joint instability when performed while palpating the medial joint margin. A positive sign for instability is excessive movement.

Varus stress test

This test has also traditionally been done at 0° of flexion/extension when testing for strain of the lateral collateral ligament and a posterior lateral capsule sprain. Zero degrees of flexion/extension will stress the iliotibial band and the tendon of the

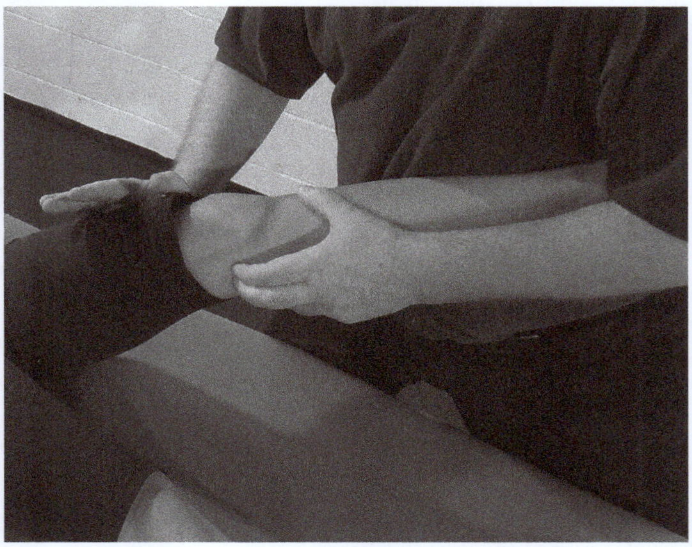

FIGURE 8.47A Valgus stress test of knee

The patient is seated or supine. The knee is flexed 15–30°. The ankle is tucked against the therapist's trunk while the medial joint margin is palpated by fingertips (not shown here). The other hand is just above the knee on the lateral thigh. The therapist turns their trunk toward the knee, pulling the proximal tibia laterally while pushing the thigh medially.

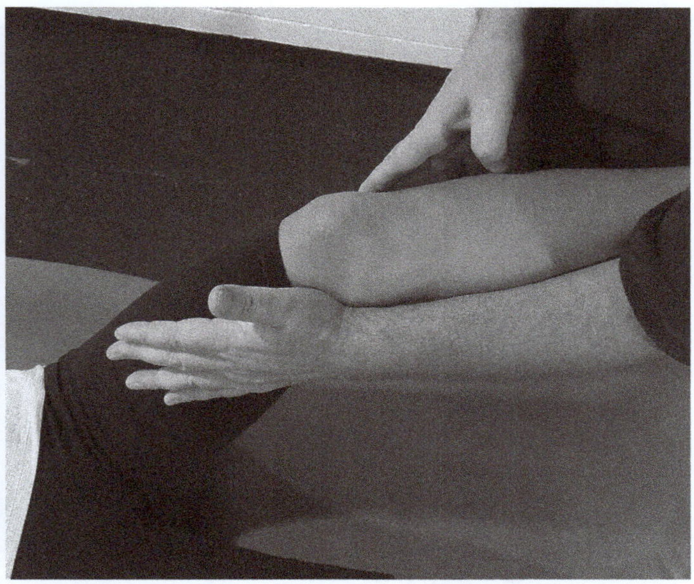

FIGURE 8.47B Varus stress test of knee

The patient is seated or supine. The knee is flexed 15–30°. The ankle is tucked against the therapist's trunk while the lateral joint margin is palpated by the fingertips. The other hand is just above knee, on the medial thigh. The therapist turns their trunk away from the knee, pulling the proximal tibia medially while pushing the thigh laterally.

biceps femoris. By testing at 15–30° of flexion with the muscular component and the ITB removed, the varus stress test specifically stresses the lateral collateral ligament and the lateral capsule. Palpate the lateral joint margin while doing the test if you wish to get a more clear and palpable result for joint instability, and not just for a sprain to the ligament. The positive signs are excessive gapping of the lateral joint margin and/or pain.

REMEMBER: If the joint margin opens significantly, it implies that more than just the collateral ligaments are involved and that other intrinsic (and possibly extrinsic) joint structures will have been impacted.

Apley distraction test (Figure 8.48)

While this test has been used to check both collateral ligaments, it tends to produce unclear results. Its best use is in concert with the Apley compression test (see under meniscus testing below). Nonetheless, we will present it here.

With the patient prone, the therapist places a knee on the patient's posterior thigh to stabilize the femur, and then distracts (tractions) the joint. This has traditionally been followed by rotating the tibia, first in a lateral direction and then medially. The positive sign is pain that is site-specific to the ligament, implying that it is strained but not ruptured. Since many other structures could also be the cause of pain this test tends to be unspecific.

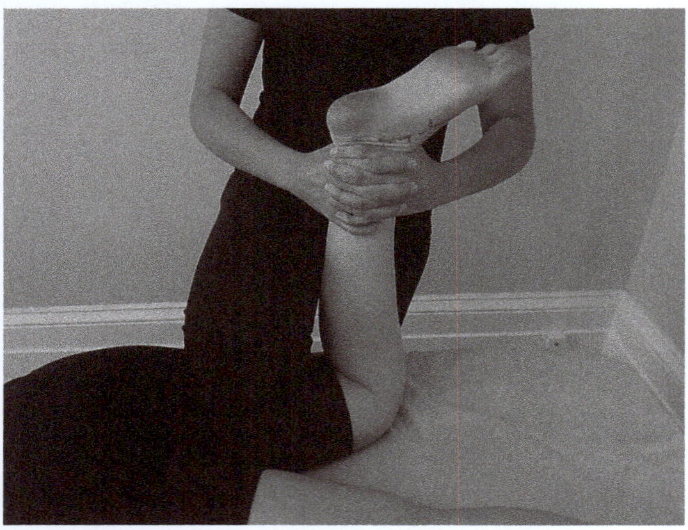

FIGURE 8.48 Apley distraction test

The patient is prone. Flex the knee 90°. Place your knee on the patient's posterior thigh for stabilization. Grasp the leg just proximal to the ankle and rotate the tibia first in one direction, then the other. Take to end-range and apply slight O-P.

NOTE: What makes this test poor is that is only useful with acute ligament strains, which you should not be provoking in this manner. Further, the test may render a false/negative result with respect to minor or moderate strains.

Draw tests (cruciate ligament testing)

These are tests for the anterior and posterior cruciate ligaments. Other tests, such as the Lachman's test, are becoming more common, but they require a developed skill of timing to perform correctly; this level of skill only comes with constant use of such a test. Unless a massage therapist deals mainly with athletes they do not have the opportunity to test knees enough to warrant learning a test like Lachman's. Therefore, we are presenting the draw test as the preferred test for the purposes of this manual.

Avoiding false positive results Proper landmarking is vital so we do not get false positives for cruciate ligament strains and ruptures. Injury to the anterior cruciate ligament (ACL) is much more common than to the posterior cruciate ligament (PCL). However, if we have not landmarked properly and are not palpating correctly we can be fooled into thinking we have an ACL tear when, in fact, it is a PCL tear.

How does this occur? It can happen when the patient has a PCL tear and is then positioned for testing in the crook-lying position (supine) with the knees bent. The tibia can fall posteriorly (or more likely is pulled posteriorly by the hamstring muscles). Before we even begin testing we may not have the tibia and femur in a neutral position. Therefore, when we push posteriorly we do not notice laxity due to a ruptured ligament. But when we draw the tibia forward we feel movement that appears excessive, but we are only moving the tibia back through neutral into the end-range for an intact and uninjured ACL. This movement may make us incorrectly decide the patient has a torn ACL when, in fact, they have a torn PCL (Hartley 2000b; Magee 2014). In order to prevent such a false positive, we will describe the landmarking and palpating necessary for cruciate testing to be accurate (see anterior draw test below).

What we need to do first is to look for what has been called the *sag sign*, an observation made during the set-up for the draw tests, which is intended to prevent misreading the movement noted during testing. Further, the sag sign is itself part of confirming that the posterior cruciate ligament is torn.

Anterior draw test (anterior cruciate ligament) (Figures 8.49, 8.50)

Have the patient crook-lying on the table. After telling the patient about what you are going to do, sit on their foot to stabilize it.

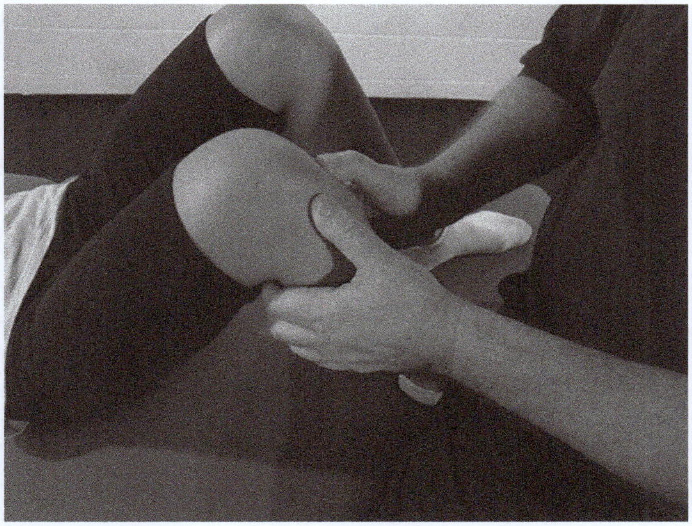

FIGURE 8.49 Palpate hamstring tendons

Use index fingers to press up into hamstring tendons. Note tension.

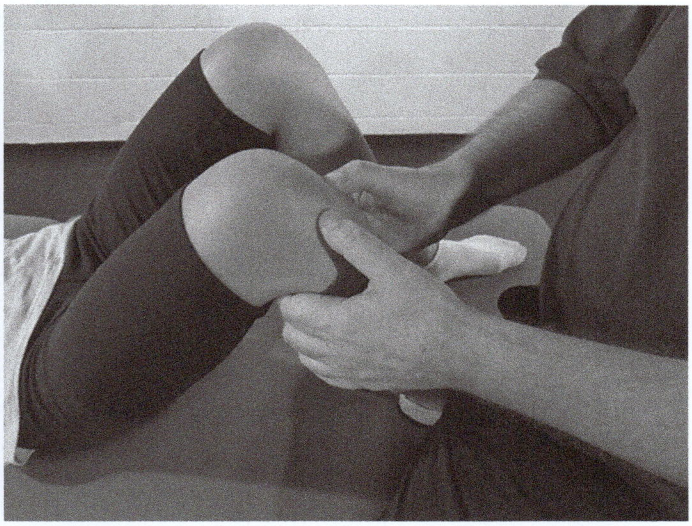

FIGURE 8.50 Anterior draw test

Lean back and draw the tibia toward you. The positive sign is excessive forward movement.

Place the fingers of both hands behind the tibia and the thumbs of each hand on either side of the infrapatellar tendon. Palpate first by pushing gently with the thumbs onto the edge or lip of the tibial condyle (tibial plateau). You should be able to clearly feel the edge of the tibial condyle and a slight hollow space above that will be felt on either side of the tendon. This space is created by the curved condyles of the femur.

The sag sign is present when you cannot clearly feel the anterior border of the tibial condyle because the tibia has "sagged" or "fallen" posteriorly due to a torn or absent PCL.

Next, with the index fingers of each hand (which should be positioned on the posterior-lateral aspect of the tibia), palpate the tension on both the medial and lateral hamstring tendons (Figure 8.49). This is done by simply lifting each hand and pressing into the tendons with the index fingers.

If the tension seems high (a hard cord-like feel) in these tendons, then the hamstring may be in spasm. You would then get a false negative when you attempt to draw the tibia forward against the spasming hamstrings that will hold the tibia in place, even though the ACL may be torn. However, one advantage of the draw test is that the knee is quite flexed (providing greater chance for laxity to the hamstrings) while Lachman's and other tests often have the knee in only slight flexion. You can ask the patient to try and relax the muscles of the leg in case they are apprehensive about the test, or are holding the leg in position for you (even though they need not do so).

It is also a good idea to practice palpating the hamstring tendons in the crook-lying position on a number of patients who have no ligament impairments of the knee in order to familiarize yourself with a sense of the usual levels of tension in hamstring tendons. Only once this landmarking and palpation has been done, and neither sag sign nor spasming hamstrings are present, do you continue with drawing the tibia forward.

To test the anterior cruciate ligament, draw the tibia forward by leaning back and using your body-weight (Figure 8.50). Do not pull forward using muscular exertion. Lean back slowly to add more weight and gently increase the pull on the structures without jerking the joint. This provides a smooth anterior glide of the tibia on the femur. Keep palpating the tibial plateau throughout the test (as well as noting if tension increases in hamstrings).

There is usually a small amount of joint play available. If the cruciate is intact, there should be a firm stop as you lean back and the pull goes through the whole lower limb. The positive sign is excessive movement, which is confirmed by palpating the edge of the tibia and feeling it more distinctly than before the anterior glide was introduced. It will feel like you can place the tips of the pads of the thumbs on top of the tibial condyle/plateau.

Palpation of the change in the relationship between the tibia and the femur is essential to establishing a positive sign for joint laxity. The positive sign of pain may be present during the anterior drawing of the tibia if the ligament is strained and partially torn, but not ruptured. Sufficient tearing will reveal some laxity within the joint. On the other hand, excessive movement and no pain implies a complete rupture.

Posterior draw test (posterior cruciate ligament) (Figure 8.51)

After having done the anterior draw test, keep your grasp and palpation on the tibial condyles as above. To produce a posterior glide and test the integrity of the posterior cruciate ligament simply lean forward. The push here comes through the thenar eminence portion of your hands. Slowly lean forward to gently add weight to safely increase the pressure on the ligaments. PCL tears are not nearly as common as ACL tears. The positive sign is excessive movement. Also, as you palpate the joint during testing, the condyles of the femur will become more distinct as you lean into the leg and the edge of the tibia will become less distinct. Pain may accompany the test if the ligament is strained but not ruptured.

Lachman's test for anterior cruciate ligament (Figure 8.52)

This is an alternate test for the anterior cruciate ligament. This test's advantage is that it can be done, and movement palpated, even if there is significant edema in the joint. Nonetheless, if there is edema, it is best to test with caution. The test is done with the leg in only 10° or 15° of knee flexion to help reduce the stabilization caused by the muscles, especially the hamstrings. This test is considered slightly more sensitive and specific than the draw test (Cleland & Koppenhaver 2011).

Stabilize the thigh with one hand and draw the tibia forward with a quick but smooth anterior draw. Follow with a posterior shift, then alternate back and forth several times. The motion can be thought of as wobbling or creating a wave-like motion through the joint by moving the tibia forward and back two or three times in succession. The accent is on the anterior draw, letting gravity assist in the posterior direction. The positive sign is excessive forward movement. Pain may accompany the test if the ligament is strained but not ruptured.

Lachman's test works very well and is fairly reliable, especially when performed just after the injury occurs. Hence, athletic therapists and sports trainers prefer this manner of testing the anterior cruciate, especially when they are on site when the injury has occurred. With practice, the skilled practitioner can also test the posterior cruciate.

There are some variations to how Lachman's test can be done. The version shown here (Figure 8.53) is sometimes called the ***quadriceps active test*** (Starkey & Brown 2015) or the dynamic extension test. You can place one of your forearms (or a towel roll) under the thigh to flex the patient's knee for testing. The patient can simply lift their heel off the table (i.e., extend their leg) as you watch and palpate for the positive sign of the tibial plateau moving anteriorly. The tibia is drawn forward by the pull of the quadriceps.

You can add further assistance to overcome tight hamstrings by applying resistance just above the ankle instead of palpating the knee. Then have the patient try to extend their knee. The quadriceps will have to work harder and so will exert more force on the inferior common tendon, resulting in a pull on the tibial tuberosity. This may shift the tibia anteriorly if the anterior cruciate ligament is torn. This increased exertion of the quadriceps may also generate a higher level of reciprocal inhibition to counter the hypertonic or spasming hamstring muscles. However, this active

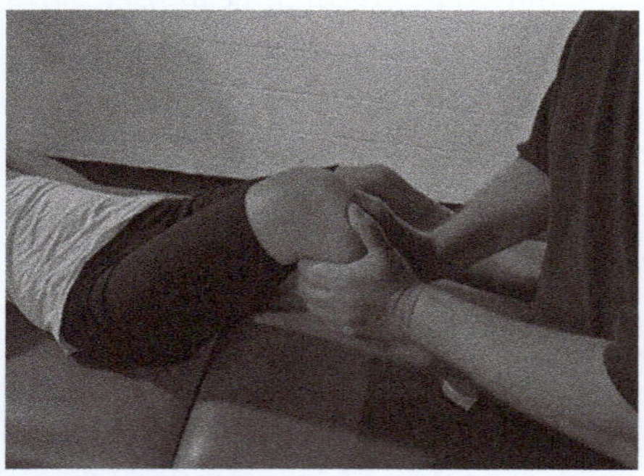

FIGURE 8.51 Posterior draw test

Lean forward, pushing the tibia posteriorly. The positive sign is excessive movement, the condyles of femur moving forward, and possibly pain.

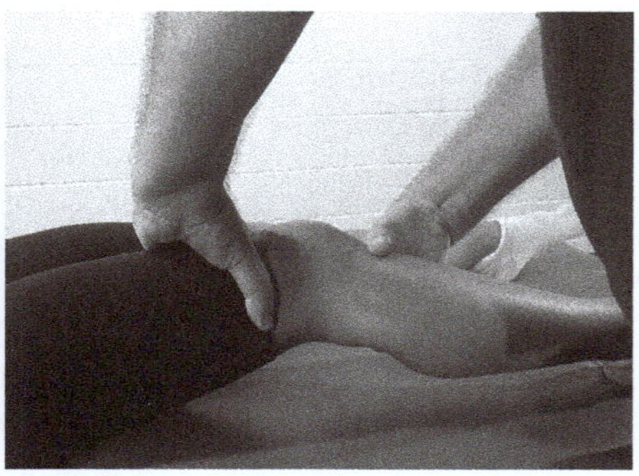

FIGURE 8.52 Lachman's test for anterior cruciate

With the knee in slight flexion, stabilize the femur. Draw the tibia back and forth.

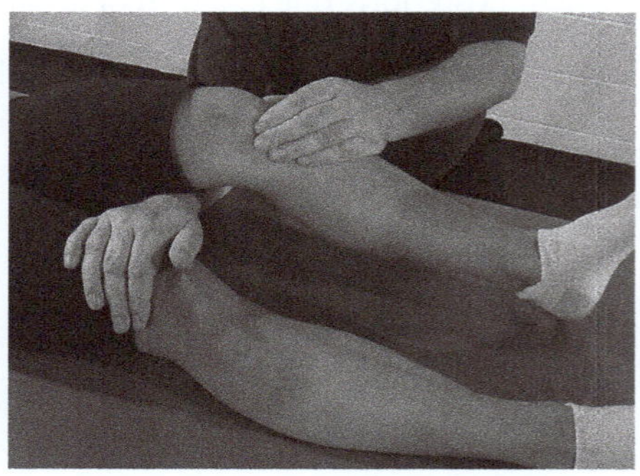

FIGURE 8.53 Quadriceps active test

Have the patient extend the flexed knee as you palpate. Observe whether the tibial condyle/edge comes forward.

resisted version requires observation alone to see the positive sign of anterior movement of the tibia on the femur.

Meniscus integrity tests

Apley compression test (Figure 8.54)

This test is useful in testing for meniscal injury if the patient's knee is not able to flex past 90° without pain. Though it can be a specific test (i.e., it is fairly accurate for finding those who do not have a lesion, finding a true negative) it does have a low sensitivity (i.e., it can produce a lot of false positives) (Starkey & Brown 2015; compare with Malanga et al. 2003 who rate the test as quite poor in both sensitivity and specificity).

After doing this compression test it is useful to now do the Apley distraction (decompression) test (see above). This can help prevent some false positives. For example, if one gets a positive result to the compression test and the suspicion is for a meniscal tear, tractioning the joint and then rotating it medially and laterally while the knee is at 90° should relieve or remove the positive signs found. If it does not, then it may be less likely that there is a meniscal tear; in other words, the positive finding of the compression test may be a false positive.

McMurray's meniscus test (Figures 8.55–8.65; Box 8.4)

This test is often done very poorly, or even incorrectly. Please read the text carefully! If done correctly, it is the preferred test. It will

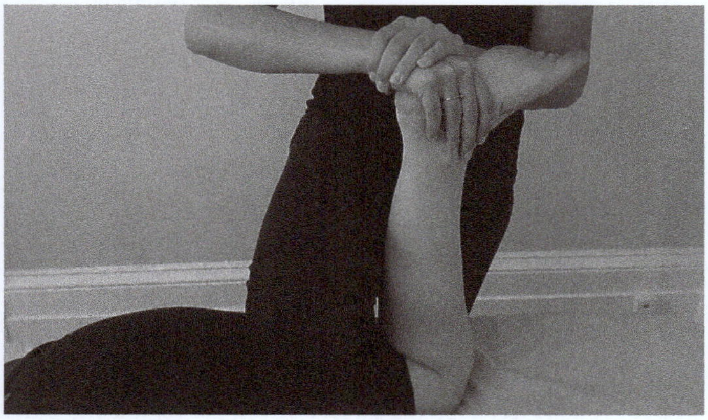

FIGURE 8.54 Apley compression test

With the patient prone and the knee flexed to 90°, grasp the patient's foot in one hand and with other hold the tibia proximal to the ankle. Be sure to place pressure straight down into tibia and lean on the heel with one hand while you rotate the tibia internally and externally. The positive sign is pain, clicking, or catching.

INSIGHTS

Box 8.4 How much stress should you apply during the McMurray's meniscus test?

Something that seems to baffle students attempting the McMurray's meniscus test is how to apply a valgus or varus stress through the knee and how much pressure to use. The test seems complicated in that you are to palpate at the knee, hold the lower leg or foot and also apply a valgus/varus stress through the knee. Figures 8.55 and 8.56 show that when the lower leg (tibia) is externally rotated (heel facing in or medially, toes away from the mid-line) and there is no stabilization above the flexed knee, the leg as a whole, and the knee specifically, falls outward or laterally. However, if you simply hold the knee in line with the hip and ankle, you are automatically applying a valgus stress through the knee, and with the appropriate pressure.

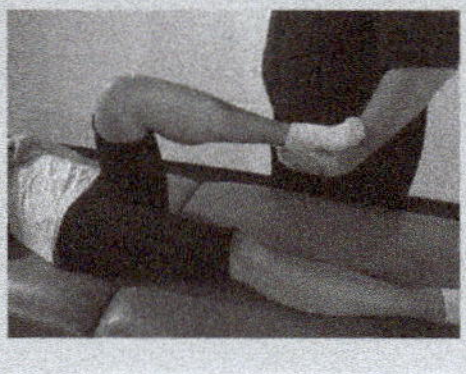

FIGURE 8.55

Unsupported knee with internal rotation.

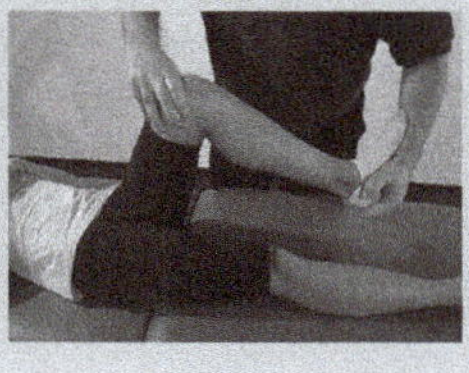

FIGURE 8.56

Supported knee provides valgus stress.

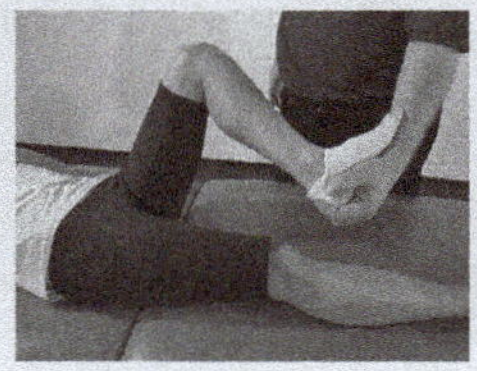

FIGURE 8.57

Unsupported knee with external rotation.

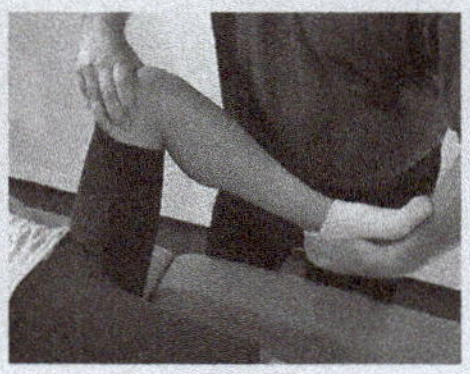

FIGURE 8.58

Supported knee with varus stress.

Figures 8.57 and 8.58 show that when the lower leg (tibia) is internally rotated (heel out laterally, toes toward mid-line) and there is no stabilization above the flexed knee, the leg as a whole, and the knee specifically, fall inward or medially. However, if you simply hold the knee in line with the hip and ankle, you are automatically applying a varus stress through the knee, and with the appropriate pressure.

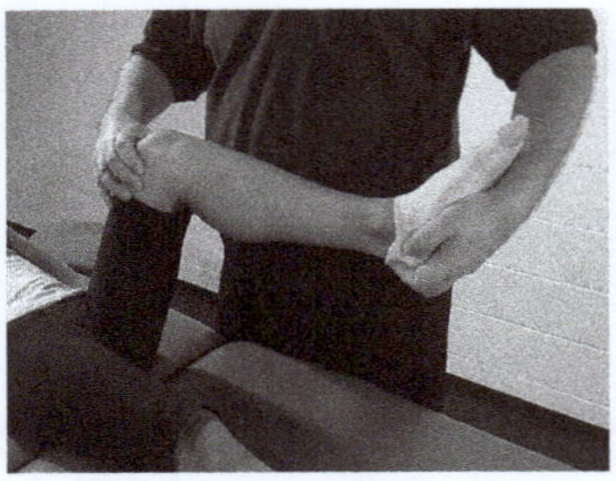

FIGURE 8.59 1. Palpating joint margin

Grasp the patient's thigh just above the knee with one hand and if possible, palpate medial and lateral joint margins with the fingers. Use the thumb and index finger. Throughout testing, make sure the pads of these fingers rest on the epicondylar edges of the femur, while the tips are at the joint margin. Being close to the joint margins improves palpation of crepitus.

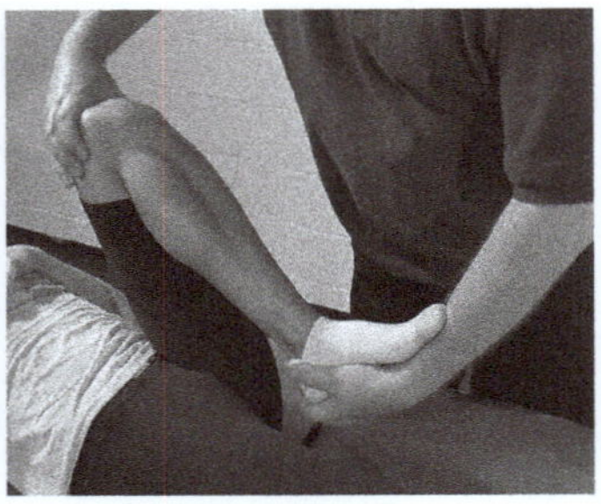

FIGURE 8.60 2. Positioning for first stage of test

With the other hand, grasp the heel of the foot and bring the patient's knee into full flexion, or as close to full as the knee permits. If the patient cannot flex the knee close to full flexion, the test could be compromised. Maximal flexion is needed to be able to place sufficient pressure through the posterior lip or section of both meniscal pads (posterior horns of the meniscus). Otherwise, posterior tears or injury to the meniscus that have changed its integrity or shape will be missed.

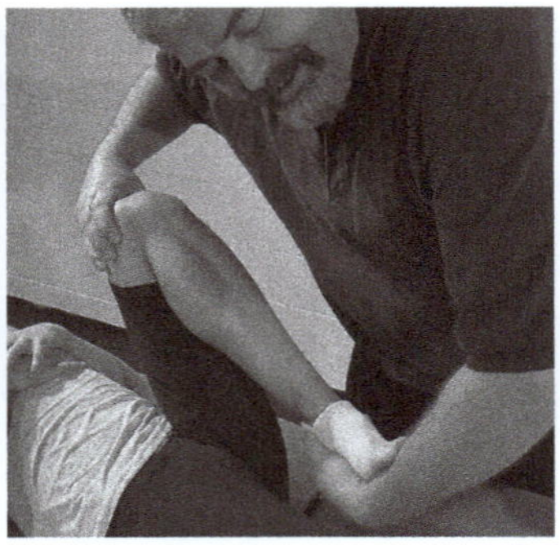

FIGURE 8.61 3. Testing posterior horns of meniscus

While continuing to palpate the joint margins for crepitus or tenderness, place an ear close to the knee to listen for clicking or snapping. Rotate the tibia internally and externally while the knee is fully flexed. This tests the posterior horns or ends of C-shaped menisci. This action squeezes the posterior portion of the menisci between the condyles of the femur and tibia, while the condyles of the femur sweep or slide over the posterior section of each pad.

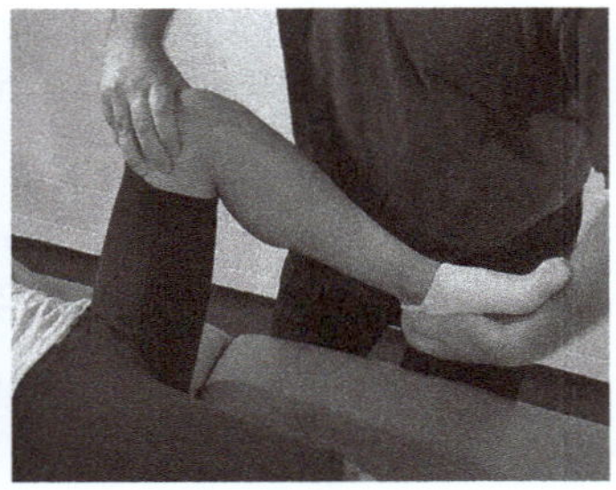

FIGURE 8.62 4. Stage two of test

Internally rotate the tibia with the knee still flexed (the heel of the foot faces away from the mid-line of the body). Holding this internal rotation of the tibia, extend the patient's knee. Keep the knee in line with the hip and ankle by firmly pulling the knee laterally, hence creating the required slight varus stress. Extend the knee slowly and palpate for bumps or skips during knee extension.

CAUTION: *Although you are straightening the knee, stop short of taking it into full extension as this could injure tissue.*

challenge more of the meniscal pad and can replicate the injury process. Though it is not necessarily more accurate than the Apley compression test (Starkey & Brown 2015), it can give a lot of palpatory information about the non-contractile tissues of the knee. It should be done after testing the collateral ligaments and the cruciates, hence its placement in this protocol for the knee.

This test requires a fairly full range of knee motion to perform it correctly. For the test to be effective, the therapist needs to be diligent in doing the actions described. It is important to pay attention to the text and not just the pictures. Position the patient in supine (the patient may need to be crook-lying to take the pressure off the knee). This test is an excellent example of how the specific quality of the motions during testing allows you to indirectly palpate deep into tissues not available for direct palpation. You will be palpating the meniscal pads of the knee through the condyles of the femur.

NOTE: You are not applying a varus stress, per se. It is more that you are simply holding the knee from wanting to fall in a medial direction. This forces the lateral condyle of the femur to exert pressure down into the lateral meniscus as it sweeps the whole inside edge of the pad. The testing procedure reproduces similar conditions or stresses under which the injury to the lateral meniscal pad may well have occurred, as in doing a deep knee bend.

When learning this test, and for purposes of understanding how much of a varus stress is needed, practice this part of the test several times, but let the knee move in or out as it wants

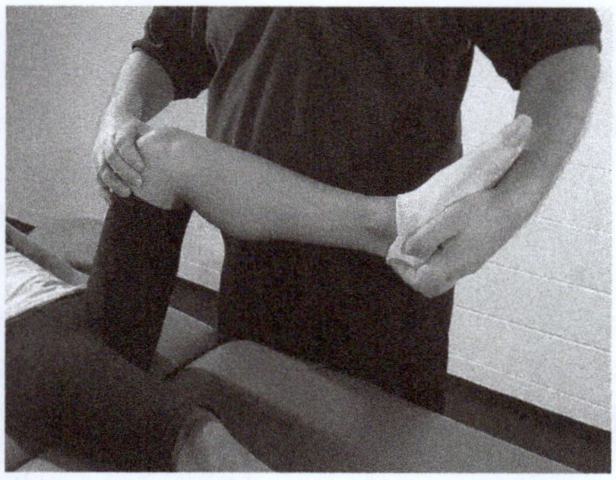

FIGURE 8.63 5. Resetting the knee

Bring the knee into 90° flexion and internally and externally rotate the tibia two or three times again. This will gently reset knee, ensuring that structures are repositioned properly.

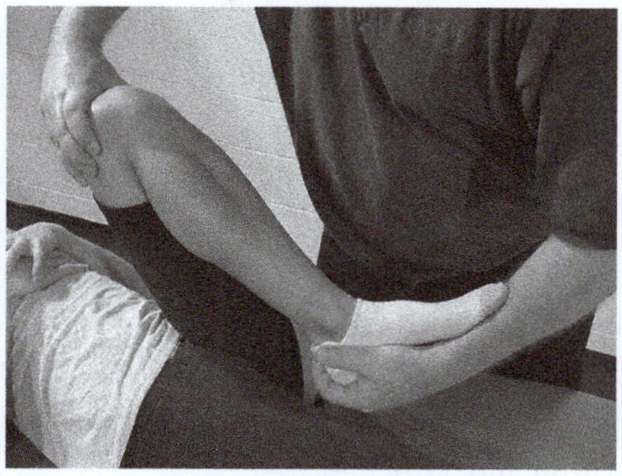

FIGURE 8.64 6. Preparing for testing medial meniscus

Bring the knee into full flexion and internally and externally rotate two or three times so the femoral condyles are exerting pressure through the posterior portions of the meniscus (see number 3).

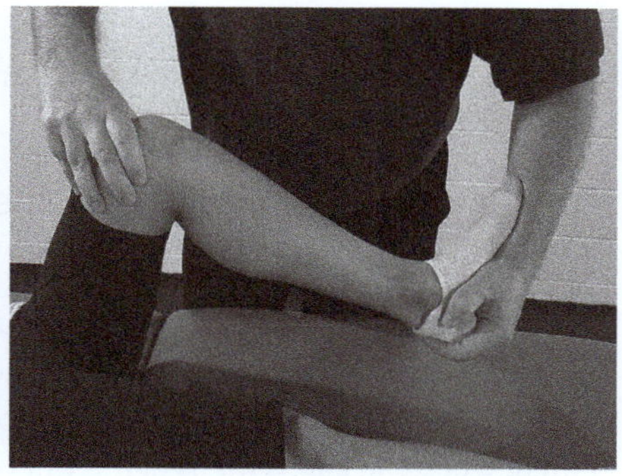

FIGURE 8.65 7. Testing medial meniscus

Test the medial meniscus by externally rotating the tibia (the heel of the foot is turned in toward the mid-line of the body). Apply a valgus stress to the knee, preventing it from falling out away from mid-line, as you again bring the knee into extension (but avoid going into full extension, as above). Positive signs include clicking, crepitus, skipping, etc.

(see Box 8.4). Get a feel of the varus pressure. Further, extending the knee increases the pressure between the tibia and the femur. With these actions, the lateral femoral condyle sweeps over and presses into the wedge-shaped surface of the meniscus from its most posterior portion to the most anterior. As full extension of the knee itself creates a great deal of compression of the joint surfaces, avoid going into full extension while the tibia is held rotated and the knee is in a varus position. This precaution is required in order to avoid injuring the meniscus or other joint structures.

When performing the test as it should be done, the motion should feel smooth. A sense of roughness and bumps or skips while extending the knee from a fully flexed position are positive signs for this test and imply injury to the meniscus. There are compressive forces through the lateral tibial and femoral condyles which makes these bumps or stutters palpable in the hand holding the heel. It is also possible to feel or hear crepitus, popping or clicking. However, ensure you are not feeling patellar crepitus! This underlies the importance of having proper positioning of the palpating hand holding the knee.

RED FLAGS: Pain is not a sign of injury to the meniscus itself, as the pads are aneural. Rather, it can imply a tear to the coronal ligaments of the meniscus, a loose body floating between the femur and meniscal pad, or a tear in the meniscus that leaves a *flap* of tissue still attached to the meniscus but when folded over acts like a loose body; the latter two put pressure into the hard bone of the condyle of the femur, which is neural. Late-stage osteoarthritic changes to the articular surface or a stress fracture of the femoral condyle would also produce pain. For these reasons, refer out to physician to have appropriate testing (e.g., X-rays, ultrasound, etc.). You should repeat steps 2 through 4 a couple of times, palpating for positive signs.

As discussed concerning the varus pull, it is more about holding the knee in line as you bring the leg into extension, rather than specifically forcing the knee into a valgus orientation. Keeping the knee centered as you extend it applies enough of a valgus stress for the test to work. The medial meniscus will now have the pressure of the medial condyle of the femur sweeping through the length of the inside surface of the pad. You should repeat steps 6 and 7 a couple of times. Positive signs are the same as mentioned above. Injury to the medial meniscus can also involve the medial collateral (tibial) ligament and so it too may be tender on palpation.

Lastly, having completed the testing, remove the rotation of the tibia, remove any varus or valgus stress, and place the limb into a position of comfort for the patient.

Palpation of the coronary ligaments (Figures 8.66, 8.67)

This may give a clue to an injury of a meniscal pad. The coronary ligaments are thickenings of the fibrous joint capsule where it attaches to the anterior portion of the tibial plateau. Often, when the pad is injured, it is out of position and a thicker portion of the meniscus becomes trapped or pinched momentarily between the femur and the tibia. It may move in a way that stresses and injures the coronary ligament's attachment to the pad.

Box 8.5 Mnemonic to remember what is being tested

Heel Out ... Pull Out ... Tests the Outside meniscus

Heel In ... Push In ... Tests the Inside meniscus

In other words:

- When the heel is out (internal rotation of the tibia), pull out, or hold, the knee in mid-line (varus pressure). This tests the outside (lateral) meniscus.
- When the heel is in (externally rotated tibia), push in, or hold, the knee in mid-line (valgus pressure). This tests the inside (medial) meniscus.

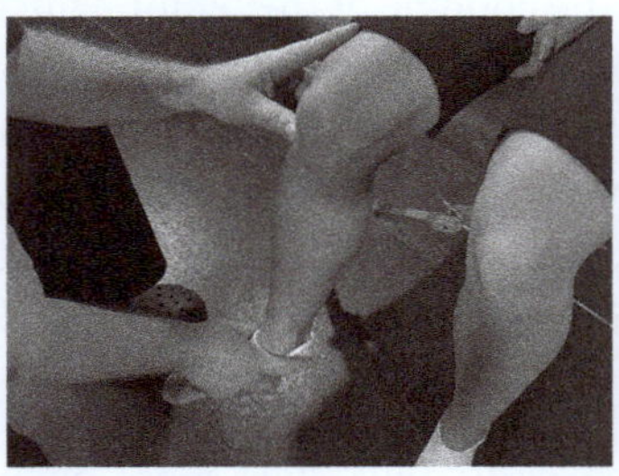

FIGURE 8.66 Lateral coronary ligament palpated

Rotate the patient's tibia laterally while palpating the lateral coronary ligament at the anterior joint margin, lateral to the quadriceps tendon.

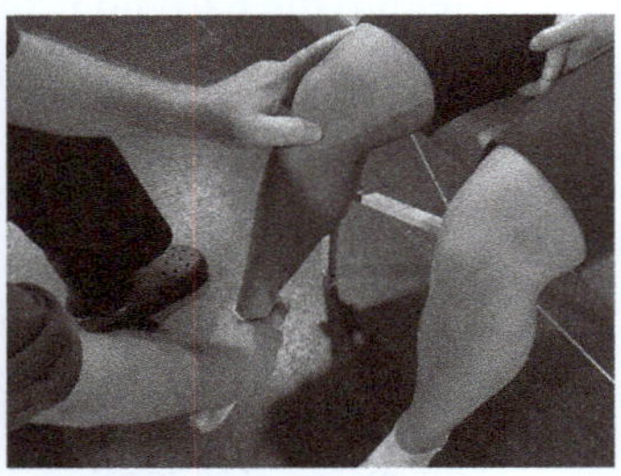

FIGURE 8.67 Medial coronary ligament palpated

Rotate the patient's tibia medially while palpating the medial coronary ligament at the anterior joint margin, medial to the quadriceps tendon.

Have the patient high-sitting or crook-lying. When the tibia is internally rotating on a flexed knee, the medial meniscus is held anteriorly by the medial femoral condyle. This in turn pushes the coronary ligament forward as well, making it easily palpable. The medial meniscus is slightly more mobile than the lateral meniscus, which makes it easier to palpate through the coronary ligament. It also makes it more prone to injury. If the coronary ligament has been injured it will be tender. This usually implies that there is also an injury to the meniscus.

Turning the tibia externally pushes the lateral meniscus and its coronary ligament forward. Pressing into it with a finger pad may elicit tenderness if the coronary ligament has been stressed or injured. This, in turn, may imply that the meniscal pad to which it is attached is also injured.

The value of this test is that it may add weight to a positive finding of either the Apley compression-decompression test or McMurry's meniscus test. Therefore, it may be best to see this as a companion test to either of those two meniscal testings, rather than a stand-alone test.

Patellofemoral tests

Patellar apprehension test (Figure 8.68)

Dislocation of the patella is very painful and the patella often returns to its proper position on its own. Therefore, if the dislocation reduced itself, then the patient may not always be sure about what has happened, but will have experienced severe pain. This test is meant to confirm that a dislocation has occurred. A history of dislocations will cause the quadriceps to reflexively

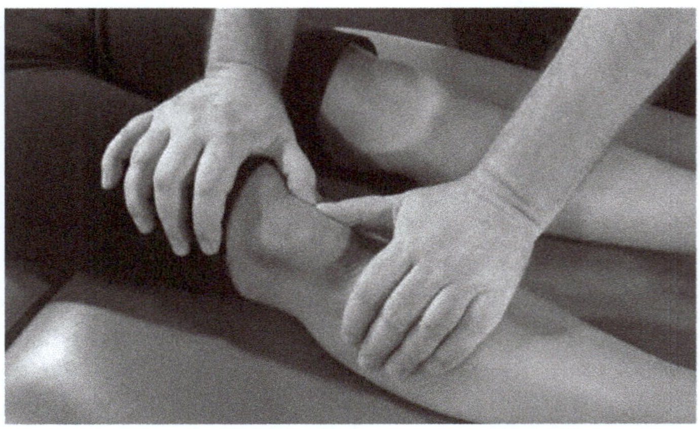

FIGURE 8.68 Patellar apprehension test

The knee is flexed 20°. Glide the patella laterally. Positive sign is patient apprehension, tightening of the quadriceps.

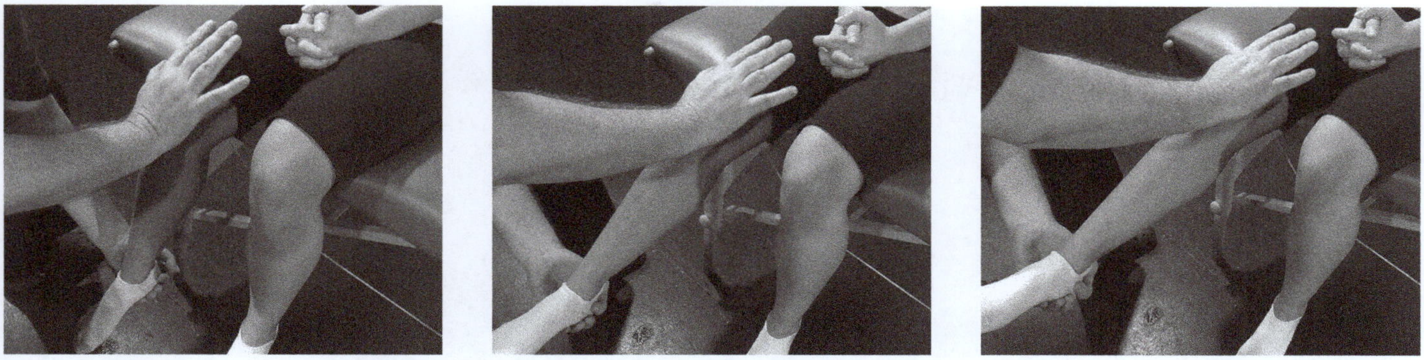

FIGURE 8.69A–C Patellofemoral compression testing

Gently compress the patella into flexed knee at 90° (A), 45° (B), and 15° (C) of knee flexion. If pain-free, repeat with the patient isometrically contracting the quadriceps at each step (Hertling & Kessler 2006).

contract and prevent movement. The positive sign is the apprehension seen on the patient's face and the spasming of the quadriceps to prevent the lateral movement.

Patellofemoral compression tests (Figures 8.69–8.71)

The following tests are used to detect so-called patellofemoral pain syndromes. The usual cause of the pain syndrome is osteoarthritic change happening to the underside of the patella (the retropatellar surface) due to improper tracking. This test can be done at 90°, 45°, and 15° of knee flexion. This test can be done passively by the therapist, who applies increasing pressure very gently over the patella; or, for further provocation, the therapist can ask the patient to contract their quadriceps isometrically (using only part of their strength) at each of the degrees of knee flexion while the therapist applies some pressure over the patella. Resist movement at the patient's ankle.

Though the test is for patellofemoral pain syndromes, it will also be positive for a chondral fracture, for pre- or suprapatellar bursitis, and quadriceps tendonitis (if the quadriceps is contracted by the patient). However, the positive sign for patellofemoral pain syndromes is pain that is felt to be on the retropatellar surface, often described by the patient as "a deep ache in the bone" or "under the knee cap."

A way of applying even more provocation if the above testing does not reproduce the patient's symptoms is to apply compression to the patella while the patient actively extends the knee and the therapist applies some resistance (an isotonic contraction) (Figures 8.70, 8.71). The extension of the knee begins from a position of 90° of knee flexion. The patient is high-sitting and the therapist puts the palm of their hand over the patella. The other hand holds the leg near the ankle and applies a slight resistance as the patient extends their knee under this light load

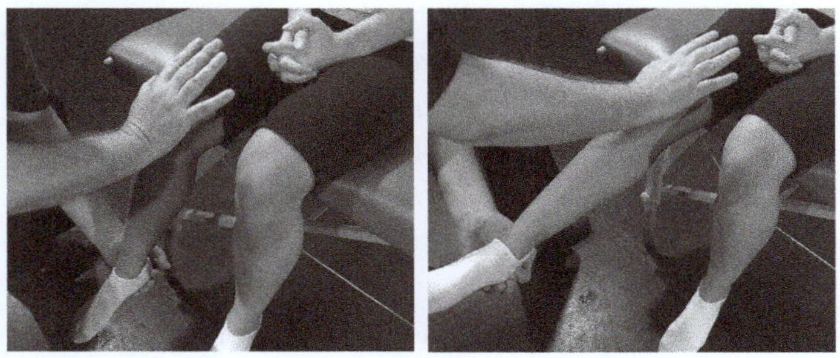

FIGURE 8.70, 8.71 Isotonic patellofemoral test

The patient's knee is at 90°. Place one palm on the patella, and the other hand resisting movement just above the ankle. Instruct the patient to extend the knee while providing moderate resistance.

First do this test by having the patient straighten their knee while simply palpating over the patella for crepitus, a "stuttering" of the patella, and have the patient report any pain or discomfort.

Second, if no pain was felt by the patient, only then does the therapist lean gently onto the patella with the palm of their hand (using *partial* body-weight, not muscular effort). This provides sufficient provocation to elicit a positive sign of pain, crepitus, or a palpation of roughness. It can be repeated with increasing pressure on the patella until the symptoms are reproduced.

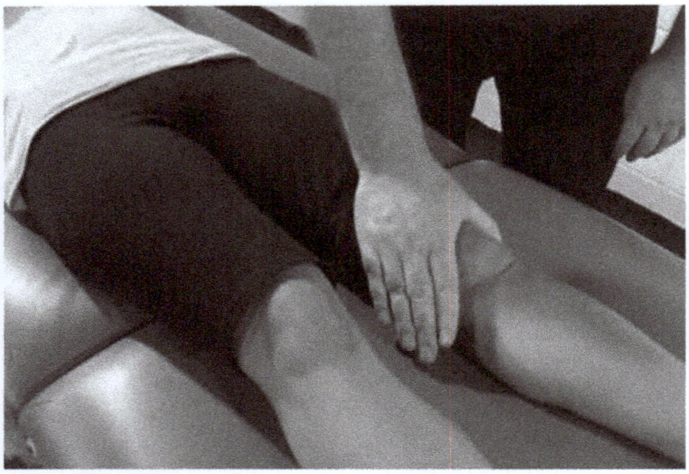

FIGURE 8.72 Clark's test

With the patient supine, trap the upper patella with the web-space of the hand and apply pressure toward the lower leg. Have the patient contract quadriceps. The patient may feel pain or may not be able to contract quadriceps due to reflex inhibition. Pain may be lessened somewhat when the test is done in 20° of knee flexion by placing a towel roll under the thigh.

Clark's test (patellofemoral grind test) (Figure 8.72)

CAUTION: This is a classic orthopedic test for chondromalacia. Though we describe Clark's test here, we are suggesting that this test *not* be performed. The reason for this is that it can cause excessive pain and/or false positive results. The test, by its nature, does not allow for normal tracking of the patella and consequently almost always causes some pain. It is better to do the testing as shown above for patellofemoral pain syndromes. The reason we have included the test is that it is still in use by some manual therapists and physicians and still commonly taught in massage therapy programs. Also, when you talk about testing of the patella with your patient, they may well show signs of apprehension due to a previous experience with this test. Reassure them that you have alternate means of testing. (See also Magee's 2014 discussion on this test and similar testing.)

Some other special tests

Iliotibial band friction syndrome test (Noble's compression test) (Figure 8.73)

This test is also known as the runner's knee test. The patient's knee is slightly flexed while the patient is supine. The therapist puts pressure on the ITB with their thumb about an inch above the lateral epicondyle of the femur. While maintaining this pressure, the leg is passively extended. The test is positive if the patient complains of pain when the knee is around 30° to 10° of flexion. When the knee goes into full extension and the tibia laterally rotates (the screw home mechanism), the tension is released slightly from the iliotibial band. Therefore, in full extension the pain may (in mild cases) lessen or disappear.

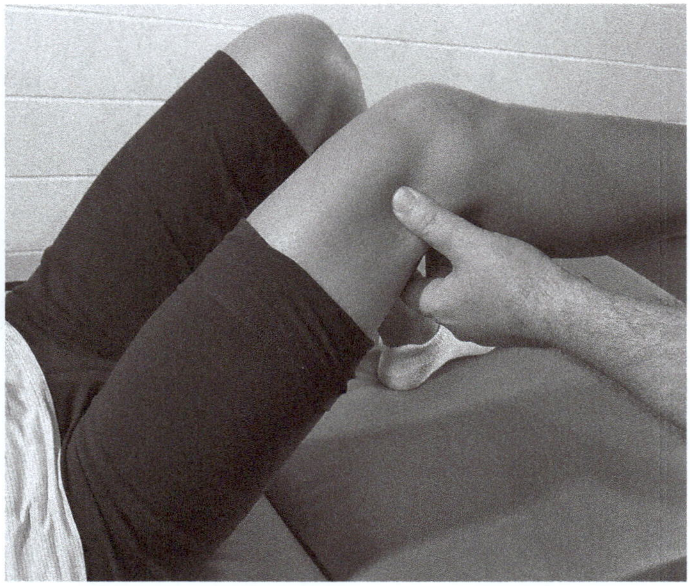

FIGURE 8.73 Iliotibial band (ITB) compression test

With the patient's knee slightly flexed, apply pressure against the ITB just proximal to the lateral epicondyle of the knee. Passively extend the patient's knee. The positive sign is pain.

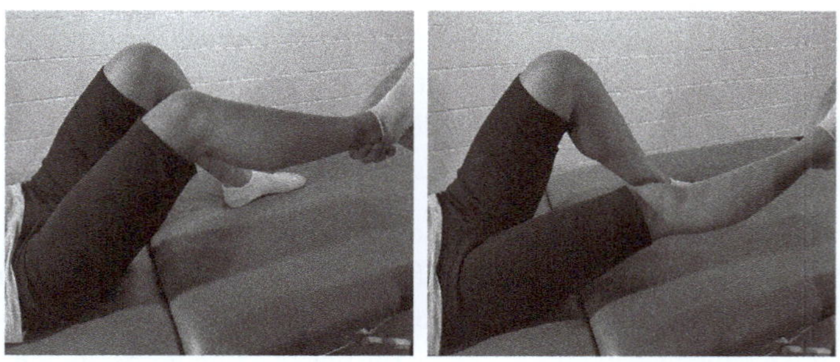

FIGURE 8.74A, B Bounce home test

The patient is supine. Flex the hip slightly. Now flex the knee to 45°. While supporting patient's heel, let the knee drop into extension. The positive sign is the knee bouncing out of extension and/or remaining in slight flexion.

Bounce home test (Figure 8.74A, B)

Often done to test for a torn meniscus or loose body within the knee joint. In this test, the patient is lying supine and the therapist flexes the knee to 40° or 50°. With one hand under the heel of the foot, the therapist lets go of the thigh and allows the knee to drop into extension. A positive sign is that the leg will not go into or stay in full extension, but bounces out of extension.

The bouncing back into flexion occurs because the compression of a loose body between the femur, meniscal pads, and tibia causes the hamstring to reflexively contract (usually accompanied by pain) and pull the knee out of extension. This end-feel is sometimes referred to as a "springy block." This could be considered a muscle spasm end-feel. The knee may also bounce out of extension due to swelling in the joint. Thus, the test is not conclusive for a loose body; its value may be questionable. (Note, however, that Magee 2014 finds the test useful even though there is no significant research evidence to support its diagnostic value.)

HIP AND INNOMINATE: CHAPTER OVERVIEW

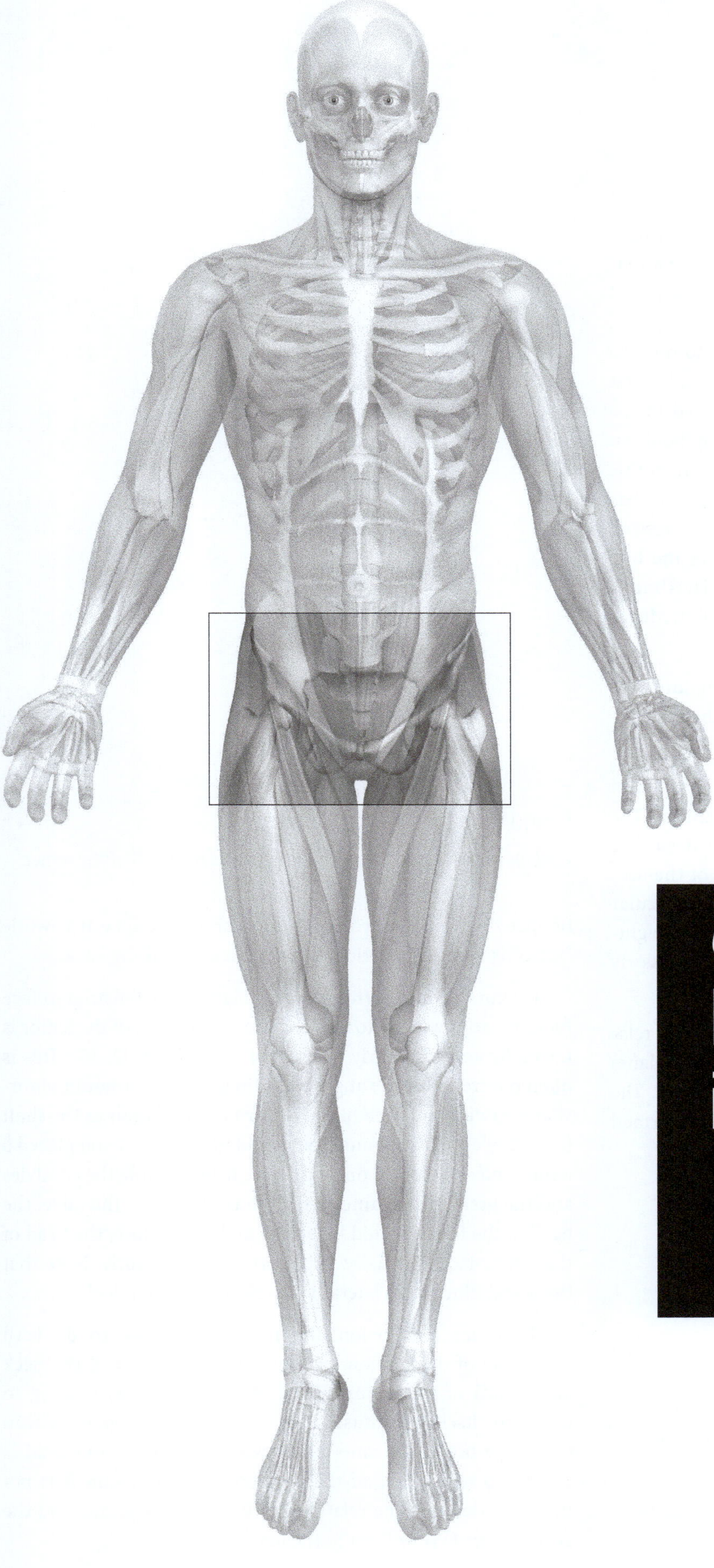

Chapter 9

Hip and innominate

Clinical implications of anatomy and physiology

This section provides some anatomical observations that have clinical implications. Understanding the functional relationships (physiology) between structures and tissues (anatomy) will help explain how structures of the hip and pelvis can be injured, and help us understand how orthopedic tests work to provide the information that they do. It is suggested that the reader first review the anatomy of the joints and muscles involved in the function of the hip and pelvis and keep an anatomy book on hand to more easily understand the information given in this section. The information that has been summarized here has been chosen because of its direct relevance to orthopedic testing and understanding of the mechanical pathologies of the hip. (See Agur et al. 2014; Dutton 2012; Hartley 2000b; Hertling & Kessler 2006; Hoppenfeld 1976; Levangie & Norkin 2011; Magee 2014; Mitchell 2001, 2005; Schuenke et al. 2014.)

The hip joint is the head of the femur in the acetabulum. The hip joint is also known as the coxofemoral joint or the acetabulofemoral joint.

Three bones, which make up the innominate (os coxa), meet and form the acetabulum: the ileum, pubis, and ischium. The joint surface (lunate surface) is a horseshoe-shaped surface that covers the anterior-superior-posterior surface of the acetabulum and its labrum. The superior surface of the articular cartilage takes most of the stress when the joint is weight-bearing. The acetabulum faces laterally and slightly inferiorly and anteriorly.

The neck of the femur is normally angled about 125° in relation to the shaft of the femur (in the frontal/coronal plane) (Figure 9.1). This is referred to as the angle of inclination. The following abnormal angles of inclination would be confirmed by X-ray or other imaging:

Coxa valgum: if greater than 125° of inclination.

Coxa varum: if less than 125° of inclination.

Antetorsion/retroversion, retrotorsion/anteversion: twisting and turning

Antetorsion and *retrotorsion* are structural deviations (twists) within the anatomy of the femur, while *anteversion* and *retroversion* can be thought of as relational terms between the components (bones) of the joint. Thus, "*-versions*" are the consequences of the "*-torsions*."

Etymologically, torsion (from the Latin, *torsio*) means twist or twisting, while version (*versio*) means turning or to turn or face. Further, "ante" is anterior or facing forward, while "retro" is what is posterior or going back or looking back.

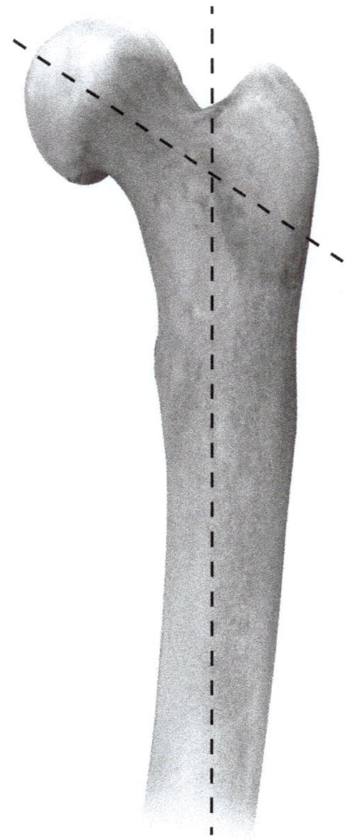

FIGURE 9.1

Angle of inclination between the neck and the shaft of the femur.

Antetorsion and retrotorsion (Figure 9.2) Twisting to face forward, and twisting to face backward. The neck of the femur is normally angled slightly forward of the shaft by 12–15°. This is often referred to as the angle of declination – the amount of torsion (or twist) the neck of the femur has in relation to the shaft (or condyles) of the femur. You would notice this if you placed a femur anterior side up on a table (see below): while the condyles and the greater trochanter are all in contact with the table, the head of the femur would be off the table. Therefore, the head of the femur faces medially, superiorly, and anteriorly. Note that the acetabulum faces laterally, inferiorly, and anteriorly.

The terms antetorsion and retrotorsion have to do with this angle of declination, or twist from the norm of the neck (and head) of the femur. Think of these terms as relating to the femur itself, and thus, to the orientation of its parts within the single bone. The amount of twist in the neck and head is compared to the face of the long bone of the femur. It is not meant to describe the relationship between the femur and the acetabulum. (We will get to the latter shortly.)

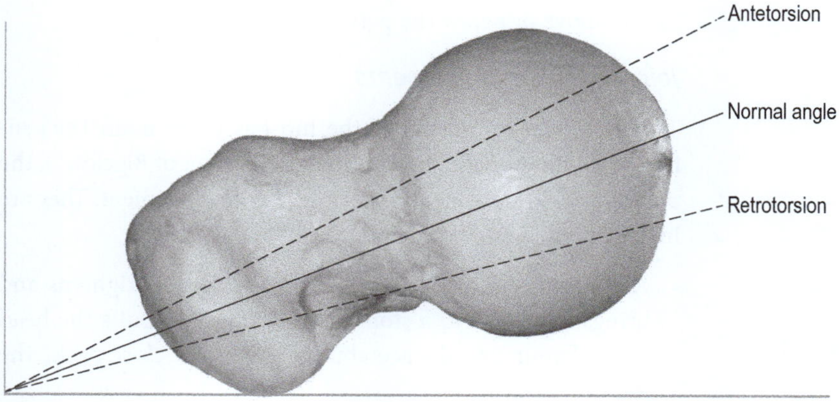

FIGURE 9.2
The angle of declination/torsion.

Femoral antetorsion is when the angle of torsion or twist is greater than normal, for example, 25° or more. The neck of the femur is twisted more than normal causing the head of the femur to be more anterior than normal with respect to the shaft of the femur.

Femoral retrotorsion is when the angle of declination/torsion is less than normal, for example, 8°. The neck of the femur is twisted more than normal causing the head of the femur to be less anterior than normal (twisted backward) with respect to the shaft of the femur.

Anteversion and retroversion: turning out, turning in

Anteversion and retroversion refer to the orientation of the joint surfaces relative to one another.

The head of the femur does not usually sit in the acetabulum at 90° (it does not sit square, or at a right angle to the acetabulum). It normally rests in the acetabulum with the head of the femur turned slightly so that it faces more anteriorly than posteriorly. The consequence of this is that some of the head's articular surface is more exposed anteriorly than posteriorly. This is referred to as normal anteversion, and the rotation from a right angle is 15° of anteversion.

Note, however, the term anteversion, in orthopedics, is generally used clinically to mean hyper-anteverted, or anteverted more than normal. Therefore:

- anteversion of the hip means that the articular surface of the head of the femur is turned excessively anteriorly within the acetabulum, exposing more of itself anteriorly
- retroversion of the hip is when the head of the femur is turned posteriorly within the acetabulum and exposes less articular surface anteriorly than normal.

Antetorsion and anteversion If *the femur* is antetorsioned then its head will expose more of its forward surface as it is turned anteriorly, i.e., *the hip joint* is anteverted.

Retrotorsion and retroversion If the femur is retrotorsioned then its head will expose less of its surface and be turned posteriorly, i.e., the hip is retroverted.

Consequences of versions and torsions

Antetorsioned hip If a femur is antetorsioned, but the head is oriented normally within the acetabulum, then its thigh (shaft) will be *internally* rotated. When standing, the patient's knees will be in a valgus orientation, with pronated feet. Therefore, the patient would present during ROM testing as having restricted external rotation of the hip and excessive internal rotation. This is because the therapist will roll the thigh *externally* until the femur/thigh is facing forward, and begin from there to measure rotation. This starting position for ROM measurement has the femoral shaft (and thigh) facing straight forward, but the joint has been externally rotated to achieve this look. The joint is now anteverted.

Retrotorsioned hip If the femur is retrotorsioned, but the head is oriented normally within the acetabulum, then its thigh (shaft) will be *externally* rotated. While standing, the patient will present as having varus knees and supinated feet (pes cavus arch). During ROM testing the patient appears to have less internal rotation and greater than normal external rotation. This is because the thigh/femur is *internally* rotated (in the hip joint) to make it appear neutral leaving the hip joint retroverted.

In summary

Antetorsion and retrotorsion are structural, bony orientations, while anteversions and retroversions speak to the resulting changes in orientation within a joint *because* of the torsion present.

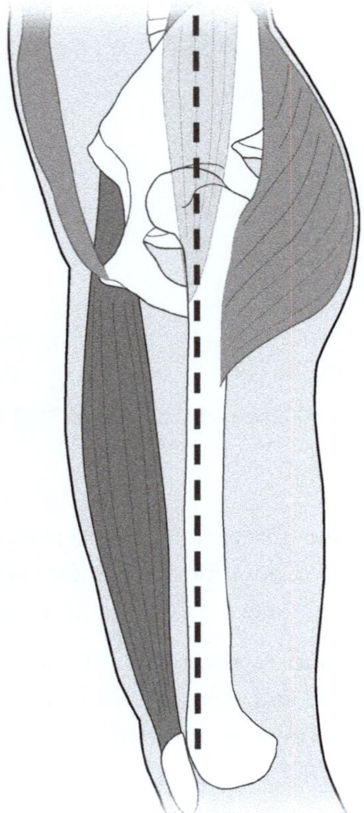

FIGURE 9.3
The line of gravity running through the trochanter.

We will be able to tell from some manual tests that the overall relationship between the two bony structures of the joint may not be normal. Therefore, checking for the overall orientation of the hip joint in relation to the frontal plane is said to be "checking for anteversion or retroversion of the hip," even though this issue includes antetorsion or retrotorsion. Some textbooks, articles, and therapists will, in fact, speak of checking for antetorsion or retrotorsion of the hip. The testing for this is found later in this chapter, under Observations.

NOTE: The trochanter has the line of gravity running through it when you are laterally viewing the ideal posture (Figure 9.3). However, the center of the acetabular-femoral (hip) joint is positioned slightly in front of that line. Therefore, torsions and versions will influence the orientation of this joint to the gravity line, and in turn, the position of the pelvis as a whole with respect to the gravity line. Often, this forces the pelvis to tip either anteriorly or posteriorly in order to compensate. The consequences of these changes of orientation of the joint and the structure of the femur will influence all that is above or below the pelvis.

Joint capsule and ligaments

The fibrous joint capsule of the hip has three main thickenings: the iliofemoral ligament (the "Y ligament of Bigelow"), the pubofemoral ligament, and the ischiofemoral ligament. They are in a spiral or twisted orientation.

- As the thigh extends, the twist in the capsule tightens and brings extension to a stop. The twisting also pulls the head of the femur into the acetabulum: this will "close pack" the joint.
- When the hip is flexed, the capsule untwists, providing a greater range of motion that is stopped either by muscular tissue stretch (such as the hamstrings and gluteus maximus) or by soft tissue compression (the thigh up against the trunk). This laxity in the capsule allows the femur to move very slightly out of the acetabulum: this is "open packed." Not surprisingly, therefore, hips are most often dislocated when the hip is flexed.

Musculature

Review the origin, insertion and actions of the following muscles of the hip, listed here as the primary muscles of each action:

- ***flexors:*** iliopsoas, rectus femoris, tensor fasciae latae
- ***extensors:*** gluteus maximus, hamstrings – semimembranosus and semitendinosus, and the biceps femoris (longus and brevis)
- ***abductors:*** gluteus medius and gluteus minimus
- ***adductors:*** pectineus, adductor brevis and longus, adductor magnus, and gracilis
- ***external/lateral rotators:*** obturator internus and externus, gemellus superior and inferior, quadratus femoris, and the piriformis
- ***internal/medial rotators:*** shared by several muscles of the hip.

Considerations of bony structures: torsions and versions

What follows is an exploration of a few possibilities of what can go wrong with not only the hip but all the structures both above and below it. It is not meant to make the therapist feel helpless in the face of unknowns or as if they have been presented with too many possibilities. Rather, the purpose is to provide a few examples of what can go wrong so as to better understand and appreciate the structure and function of the joint, and expanded treatment possibilities. Further, it may help the therapist realize they must keep an open mind and not jump to conclusions.

If the hip remains retrotorsioned without compensation, the femur will be externally rotated. If all remains equal, the foot would also be externally rotated. A few possibilities for compensation follow:

- If the foot is "turned out" externally the result would be that the foot is more likely to be pronated and have a lowered longitudinal arch. This will functionally shorten the leg causing numerous pelvic and spinal compensations above the pronated foot.
- However, the tibia may compensate by rotating internally, and result in a pes planus foot and a varus orientation to the knee.
- The patient may compensate for retrotorsion by medially/internally rotating the leg (femur), by retroversion, so that the shaft of the femur and the rest of the leg is facing forward as if normal. Therefore, the hip would be retroverted in order to correct for a retrotorsioned femoral head. This can have a degenerative effect on the hip joint itself, as in early osteoarthritis. Certainly, the mechanics for a gait pattern that such a possibility presents do not bode well for not only the hip joint itself, but for all the joints and tissues of the lower extremity, and further, for tissues up into the spine.

If the torsion of the hip is relatively normal but the hip is (hyper-) anteverted the femur and structures below are initially externally/laterally rotated. This will tend to have the foot externally rotated (if the structures of the knee do not compensate or deviate). As mentioned above, the longitudinal arch of the foot is placed under great stress in this position and is likely to fail and fall.

- However, the tibia may internally rotate giving a varus orientation to the knee and produce a pes cavus orientation to the foot.
- Both of these possibilities will create an unlevel pelvis, affecting the spine (C- or S-curvatures) and will have an impact on gait.

Pelvic floor

Some of the tissues contributing to making up the pelvic floor include:

1. the hip bone (os coxa or innominate), pubic bone, sacrum, and coccyx
2. the obturator internus and the gemelli going from the posterior-superior portion of the greater trochanter, obliquely downward posteriorly to wrap around or attach to the ischial tuberosity; making up the lateral wall of the pelvis
3. the piriformis, running from the posterior-superior portion of the greater trochanter over to the medial border of the sacrum, composes much of the posterior wall
4. the funnel or bowl of the pelvis is composed of the levator ani muscles and the various coccygeus muscles
5. the connective tissue surrounding these muscles (such as the tendinous arch – the fascial covering of the obturator internus muscle); and various ligaments (such as the sacrotuberous ligament, sacrospinous ligament, etc.).

Bursa

An important source of pain or snapping that arises in the inguinal area is the bursa underlying the iliopsoas tendon as it passes over the pubic bone. The painful movement can be on flexion or external rotation of the hip when acute bursitis is present. After a bout or two of bursitis the bursa will enlarge as it fills with fibrous material from exudate, and the tendon will create a snapping sound or sensation as it slides laterally on external rotation of the hip.

Trochanteric bursitis is usually caused either by a direct trauma to the bursa overlying the greater trochanter (such as a fall onto the outside of the hip, or a blow to the area) or by a taut iliotibial band (ITB) frictioning the bursa as it slides over it during such activities as walking or running.

Another bursa that can be a problem is under the tendons of the hamstrings just before they insert onto the ischial tuberosity. Just as with the trochanteric bursa the ischial bursa can become inflamed by trauma (such as a fall onto the sitting bone), or by excessive tension or tautness in the tendons causing extreme compressive forces that pinch the bursa between the tendon and bone. The latter can occur, for example, in a standing person who is continually bent forward (or repetitively bending forward, as in reaching at a work table) in a manner that requires the hamstrings to hold the pelvis/hips from tipping anteriorly.

True hip joint pain is actually most often felt in the groin area, which is just anterior to the joint. When most people refer to "hip pain" they are usually referring to the area of the greater trochanter.

Muscle balance issues to note

Tensor fasciae latae (TFL) and iliotibial band (ITB)

Remember that the tensor fasciae latae and the iliotibial band not only aid in hip flexion and abduction, but also assist external rotation of the tibia. When shortened, the iliotibial band can play an important role in holding a pelvis or innominate anteriorly rotated, and also hold the tibia in external rotation (creating a valgus orientation of the knee). A tight ITB can hold the hip (innominate) slightly abducted or externally rotated (i.e., an outflare) where the ASIS of that innominate is further from the mid-line than normal. (See Box 9.1. Further definitions and explanations are located in Chapter 11.)

Tight versus taut hamstrings

The hamstrings can be tight (short and hypertonic) or they can be taut (long and potentially fibrosed). The latter situation often arises when the hamstrings are chronically working to prevent further rotation of an anteriorly rotated pelvis. In both situations the hamstrings will appear short when tested for length. Both situations are often assumed to be tight muscles upon palpation, and the therapist will try to release and lengthen both situations. But loosening taut hamstrings before the antagonist muscles holding an innominate or pelvis in anterior rotation are lengthened will only exacerbate that anterior rotation. Therefore, it is advised to release all other tight postural muscles and activate all inhibited muscles involved prior to treating taut hamstrings.

Gluteals

The gluteus maximus muscle (and the posterior portion of the gluteus medius) extends the leg but when the legs are fixed it also extends or posteriorly rotates the pelvis. (This happens to help to lift the trunk from a flexed position, working along with the erector spinae group of muscles, etc.) Inhibition or weakness in the gluteus maximus leaves the hamstrings as the only group of muscles to hold the pelvis level anterior-posteriorly, a battle which the hamstrings will lose.

Impairment to the gluteus minimus and medius results in the patient being unable to hold the pelvis level side to side in a horizontal plane during gait, therefore, the non-weight-bearing side of the pelvis falls or moves inferiorly.

Impairments to innominates and effect on posture and function

We need to understand impairments to the innominates in order to fully comprehend what is happening in the hip as a whole and the implications that such impairments may have for the body above and below the hip. (**Note:** Innominate dysfunctions or impairments are discussed further in Chapter 11.)

Box 9.1 Comprehensive assessment of the hip

All too often the examination of the hip does not take into account the various positions of, or impairments to, the innominate. As a result, the therapist cannot assess the hip comprehensively. How are we to understand how a hip is impaired if we only look at what is happening to the femur? We need to take note of how the musculature pulls and twists and torsions the innominate out of neutral, and alters the orientation of the acetabulum. Otherwise how can we possibly understand or correct hip impairments?

An innominate can be rotated anteriorly or posteriorly; or it may have an outflare (where the ASIS is further from the mid-line than normal) or an inflare (the opposite of an outflare). An innominate can be unilaterally shifted superiorly (an upslip) or inferiorly (a downslip). Further, these changes in orientation of the innominate can often be coupled together.

Note also that one innominate could be anteriorly rotated with an inflare, while its opposite may be posteriorly rotated with an outflare. Also, the whole pelvis can be rotated left or right, or sit unlevel in the horizontal plane. Remember that these deviations from neutral can have their source in the pelvis or as compensations for impairments and dysfunctions to joints and tissues above and below the pelvis.

All of these (see Chapter 11 for fuller definitions, etc.) must affect the orientation of the acetabulum, which in turn must have an impact on how the hip joint functions.

We need to draw the line somewhere when initially looking for causes and consequences of hip impairments, otherwise we will have to take every bone in the body into consideration when assessing any joint, and that would be too cumbersome. But in this instance we are only asking the therapist to consider the other bone (innominate) that is half of the hip joint.

Nevertheless, it is worth repeating that historically, most texts have ignored the innominate and its impairments when discussing the assessment of the hip joint. This text will attempt to begin to address this omission. We will introduce some of the innominate dysfunctions here, and will discuss them in even greater detail in the sacroiliac section of the text (Chapter 11), where they more commonly receive attention (from osteopaths, chiropractors and physiotherapists).

Consequences of innominate rotations

The pelvis can rotate anteriorly, which will increase the lordosis of the lumbar spine (hyperlordosis). It can also rotate posteriorly, which decreases the lordosis (hypolordosis or a reversed lumbar curve). Hyperlordosis will strain the structures of the lumbar spine by loading the facet joints, compressing intervertebral discs, and/or stressing the bony ring of the arch around the spinal column. Hypolordosis (flat back) prevents the lumbar spine from functioning efficiently as it transfers weight down the body and impairs its ability to cushion the spine (like a spring) when forces come up from the legs and pelvis (as happens with walking, running, or jumping).

What has been said so far has to do with bilateral anterior or posterior rotations (or tilts) to the innominates. However, the innominates of the pelvis move opposite to each other during gait. During heel-strike, the innominate on the ipsilateral (same) side is rotating posteriorly, the leg is externally rotated and the innominate will also slightly externally rotate. This action causes the ASIS to move superiorly and laterally, and the PSIS to move inferiorly and medially. (See gait analysis in Chapter 5, and also Chapter 11.)

Meanwhile, the other innominate rotates anteriorly as the foot is toeing off. Also, the innominate internally rotates slightly medially (i.e., the ASIS will move inferiorly and medially and the PSIS moves superiorly and laterally). The medial rotation of the innominate matches the medial rotation of its extending leg which is toeing off. Therefore, persistent changes to the orientation of the innominate have an impact on gait.

Unilateral rotation of innominate and consequences for the lower limb

One side of the pelvis can become fixed in an anterior or posterior rotation. This is then referred to as a unilaterally anteriorly/posteriorly rotated pelvis. Note that being in a fixed position does not mean that the innominate no longer moves during gait, for example, but rather its "neutral" has shifted anteriorly or posteriorly; the hip rotates from this new "norm." The ability for rotation may change (for example, have less motion in one direction or the other, depending on a number of factors). An imbalance in the musculature of the hip (usually in this case in the hip flexors) is often the primary cause of this. (Note also that the whole pelvis, for example, could be anteriorly rotated, but the right side may rotate anteriorly even more than the left side. This may happen to the right side if it has even shorter hip flexors. Therefore, a "unilateral rotation" can refer to the relative positioning of one innominate to the other.)

The impact of one innominate becoming fixed in a rotation more than the other side (or even both rotated in opposite directions to each other) means, for example, that the pelvis as a whole is rotated in one direction as the person stands. This in turn adds rotation to the lumbar spine, as the person compensates for the rotated pelvis by rotating the lumbar spine in the opposite direction so that they face forward. In concert with all of this the sacral base for the spine is held "torsioned" (tilted and rotated). And when a group of lumbar segments are rotated in one direction they will often side-bend in the opposite direction, resulting in a functional (i.e., non-structural), rotoscoliosis. (See Chapters 11 and 12.)

Further, when one innominate rotates anteriorly the acetabulum on that side is moved forward and down relative to neutral or the opposite hip. This causes that leg to become functionally longer, and that hip joint and thigh to move anteriorly. This will further un-level the sacral base.

Examples of compensation by shortening structures in the long leg

- The tibia may help the leg compensate by laterally rotating and create a valgus orientation of the knee in an attempt to shorten the long leg. The development of knee problems, especially on the medial side, is sure to follow.
- The body may further try to compensate by having the foot pronate. In fact, the lateral rotation of the tibia itself often results in the foot pronating.
- This effectively shortens the distance from the ground to the top of the tibia. Such pronation, of course, leads to foot and ankle problems.
- Such changes in the compensating leg are usually accompanied by the person now shifting their weight over the other leg. With the weight now shifted over the short leg, its knee joint can undergo extra stress and strain, as does the arch of that foot. Thus, the knees and feet on both sides may undergo deleterious changes, but for different reasons, and in different ways. In this scenario, it is not uncommon to see that the short leg will have a slightly extended knee (while the long leg often has the knee slightly flexed).

Example of a long leg not compensating On the other hand, the functionally longer leg may not compensate, causing the hip with the anterior rotation to become higher than the other. This, too, unlevels the sacral base and leads to a scoliosis in the low back. Further, if the right hip is anteriorly rotated (which is very common in right-handed people), the upper body via the lumbar spine will often side-bend over that long leg. After all, the person is not going to walk around with their trunk tilted off to the left! Now the body has shifted the weight over to the right.

In either case, when the weight shifts over to one side, it can cause the hip on that side to become predisposed to posterior rotation. This is because the acetabulum is slightly in front of the normal center of balance (or lateral plumb line) and the trunk's weight above that innominate slowly exerts pressure on it to rotate posteriorly. This effect will help to reverse (or lessen) an anteriorly rotated leg that has had the upper body's weight swing over it. However, if the weight has shifted over the "short leg," that will only drive the short leg's innominate more posteriorly and result in exaggerating the disparity of functional length between the two legs.

If the innominate unilaterally rotates posteriorly, then the acetabulum goes up and backward, functionally shortening that leg. Like anterior rotation, this also unlevels the sacral base and contributes to the spinal compensations of side-bending and rotations (i.e., rotoscoliosis). In this situation, the knee may take on a varus orientation in an attempt to lengthen the leg. This varus knee is accompanied by internal rotation of the tibia, which usually leads to a supinated foot (pes cavus). The pes cavus, in heightening the arch of the foot, further assists in increasing the functional length of that leg. However, structures and tissues at the lateral knee will begin to undergo chronic strain and degeneration. Meanwhile, structures intrinsic to the foot can become rigid into a pes cavus (and prone to injury such as stress fractures to the metatarsals); or the rigid arch may over time begin fail due to the stresses placed on it and eventually collapse (into a pes planus).

Thus, unilateral rotations of the innominate can have a huge impact above the pelvis on the low back and the ascending spine, and in turn, on the joints below the pelvis. Therefore, careful landmarking and postural observations are crucial to unravelling the extent and kind of potential compensations that can occur due a rotated pelvis (either bilaterally or unilaterally).

Of course, the rotation of the pelvis itself can be a compensation or consequence of impairments from above (especially the lumbar spine) or from impairment in the lower extremity. Thus, our skills as "assessment detectives" need to be highly developed precisely because we see so many patients whose list of impairments and compensations have been developing and interacting over several months or even years.

With an anteriorly rotated pelvis the hip flexor muscles will be shortened and hypertonic as the hip is always in a slightly flexed position, even when standing. Conversely, a posteriorly rotated pelvis and hip can leave some hip flexors long and weakened. Similar (but contrary) changes occur to the hamstrings. (With a little thought the consequences for the muscles in and around the hip, pelvis and low back can be worked out.)

Further, the innominate being held malpositioned for long periods of time can lead to osteoarthritic or other degenerative changes to the hip joint.

All of this gives more meaning to a line from an old song: "...The thigh bone is connected to the hip bone; the hip bone is connected to the back-bone..."!

For more on adaptation to leg length differences see Chila (2010), DeStefano (2011) and Mitchell (2001, 2005).

One last point Most joints in the body work synergistically. Which means that in order for almost any joint in the body to function normally the surrounding joints may need to move in some manner, to some degree, in order for the principal joint to have its full range. Therefore, when investigating a joint we must take note of the surrounding joints. It is the living body we are assessing when doing AF-ROM, and not some discrete anatomical piece of it in isolation. In normal movement of the hip (acetabulofemoral joint) there needs to be small movements in the sacroiliac joints, in the pubic joint, and in the lower lumbar vertebrae (via the iliolumbar ligaments). Also, consider that we need the knee to flex if full hip flexion is to be seen. Only through experience with range of motion testing can we come to learn what is acceptable motion in the surrounding tissue and joints.

Active ranges of motion of the hip

Flexion: 110–130°

Extension: 10–20°

Abduction: 30–50°

Adduction: 20–30°

Internal (medial) rotation: 30–40° (with hip and knee flexed to 90° each)

External (lateral) rotation: 40–60° (with hip and knee flexed to 90° each)

See the Appendices section at the end of the book for charts and tables on muscles (muscle origin, insertion, innervation, action and synergists), joints (actions, ranges, muscles used, tissues stretched and compressed); another table on capsular patterns (of restriction, open packed/resting positions and close packed positions) and several charts on neurological testing where any such testing would involve this chapter's region.

Box 9.2 Protocol

Case history (specific questions)

Observations

Rule outs

Active free range of motion (AF-ROM)

Passive relaxed range of motion (PR-ROM)

Active resisted range of motion (AR-ROM)

Special tests

The testing protocol (Box 9.2) begins with the case history.

Case history (specific questions)

Where do you feel pain?

- Lateral hip: often implies muscular or related tissues that attach to the greater or lesser trochanter.
- Inguinal region: could indicate the involvement of the iliopsoas, or could indicate involvement of the hip joint.
- Gluteal pain can be from lateral rotators, gluteal muscles, and/or the sacroiliac joint.

Do you notice any snapping or clicking noises? Where do you "feel" that?

- Snapping in the area of the greater trochanter can imply trochanteric bursitis and/or iliotibial band tautness.
- In the inguinal region could imply pectineal/iliopsoas bursitis.

Have you ever experienced a sudden sense of weakness in the hip that then passes?

- This can imply a protective reflex inhibition of the musculature in response to joint stress.

Have you ever had an inguinal hernia or experienced any previous groin strains?

Observations

Regional assessment within the context of the whole

As with every area of the body being investigated by orthopedic testing (specific view), remember to always look at that joint or tissue within the context of the surrounding joints and structures (regional view). What is the interplay of impaired tissues or structures with the rest of the tissues in that region? In turn, take into consideration the global view: how is that joint and region affecting the whole body? How is the whole affecting or influencing the region and the specific site(s) of impairment(s)? Just as with treatment, the approach to assessment also moves from general to specific and back to general.

Not all the preconditions for an impairment exist on-site or in the surrounding region; they can come from the totality of the body, the person and their environment.

Remember: observation begins the moment a patient enters the clinic. Perform a postural scan from each side, and from the front and back. Deformities are visible signs of impairment that result from severe genetic or long-standing conditions. These deformities will have caused clear compensatory changes to the structures in support of those areas. Note obvious deformities and consider their implications. Is the deformity a contributing factor to the patient's chief complaint?

NOTE: Though most of what follows is in the introductory chapters as well, particularly Chapter 5, we repeat a lot of it here because of the crucial importance of the information gained during a postural exam with respect to properly interpreting and understanding any of the testing presented here concerning the hip. For some of these, see the section on the clinical implications of anatomy and physiology at the beginning of this chapter.

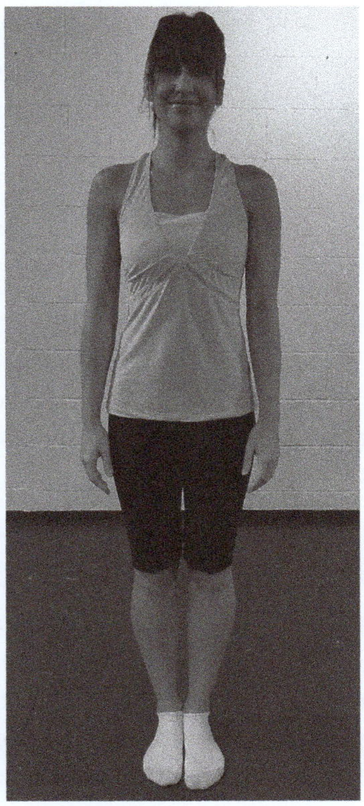

FIGURE 9.4 Standing postural exam

Have the patient take some steps in place without looking at their feet. This will give you their natural stance, the way they support themselves normally.

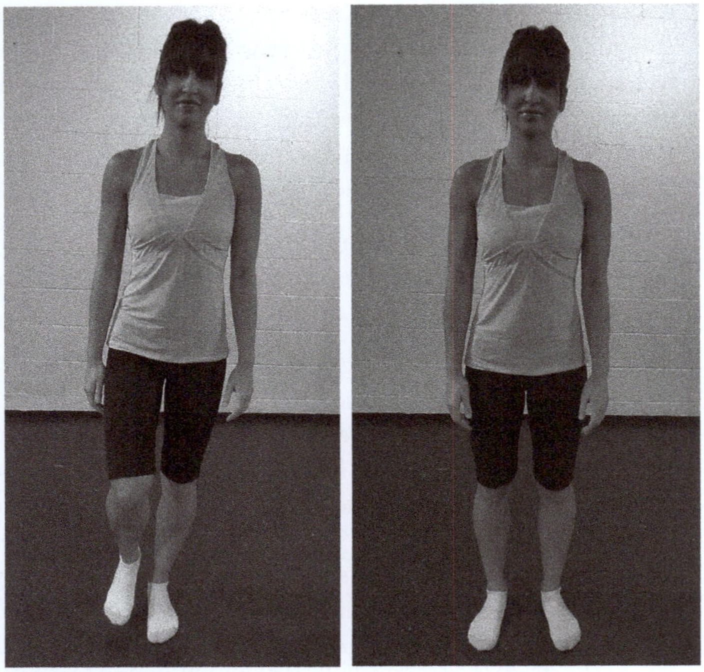

FIGURE 9.5A, B **Walking in place: natural posture**

Have the patient take some steps in place without looking at their feet. This will give you their natural stance, the way they support themselves normally.

1. Note the general orientation of the upper body, noting rotations and side-bending of the shoulders or spine.
2. Note the general orientation of the hips, thighs, knees, tibias, ankles, and feet. Look to see if the hips are shifted right or left over a leg.
3. Note the proportions, tissue bulk, and orientation of the thigh and lower leg. Look for rotations of the limb down to the feet, varus or valgus angulations of knees or ankles and arches of the feet.
4. Note any pelvic obliquity. Is one ASIS higher than other or one PSIS higher than other?

- Anterior rotation of innominate is a forward torsion of the innominate on the sacrum, where the ASIS is lower and the PSIS higher on the same innominate.
- Posterior rotation is where the PSIS is lower and the ASIS higher on same side.
- If both ASIS and PSIS on same innominate are higher than the contralateral innominate then we have what is called an "upslip" of the innominate on the sacrum. The hip joint and its innominate have been pushed superiorly while the opposite hip has not. There is a shear through the pubic symphysis and sacroiliac joint. This is confirmed by finding that ischial tuberosity is also higher on that side, which is often caused by jumping down from a height onto one leg, for example. This will make legs appear to be of unequal length since one iliac crest will be higher (on upslip side) than the other.

CAUTION: Much of this information about standing examination should be compared with supine and prone examination so that we are not misled by what we see when the patient is on the table in those positions. Most impairments occur and have their effects when the patient is weight-bearing. Further, if the patient is standing artificially straight during this examination then we may see neither what is causing their chief complaint nor the compensations they have undergone (see Chapter 5) (Figures 9.4, 9.5A, B).

Standing postural exam

Anterior view (Figures 9.6–9.9A, B)

Posterior view (Figure 9.10)

Besides observing the pelvis and legs, note if the lumbar spine is curved left or right. Also re-check the iliac crest heights and trochanter heights, etc., to confirm anterior view findings. Observe lordosis of the low back and lateral plumb line or gravity line to see how the pelvis sits with respect to that (see postural assessment in Chapter 5).

Lateral view (Figures 9.11, 9.12)

Observe whether there is an anterior pelvic tilt (usually accompanied by a hyperlordosis) or posterior pelvic tilt (usually with a flat back/hypolordosis). Normal tilt is 5–15° (women tend to have more tilt than men). Check from *both* sides in order to evaluate if one innominate is more anterior/posterior than the other.

Postures due to muscle imbalances

Two examples of muscle imbalance patterns that result in impaired postures are shown in Figures 9.13 and 9.14.

NOTE: Sway back refers to the tendency of a person with the posture shown in Figure 9.14 to sway back and forth (i.e., anteriorly and posteriorly). The lumbar spine is extended, sitting on posteriorly rotated hips, and the hip joint is in extension, as are the knees. For other postures that can affect the hip, see Chapter 5.

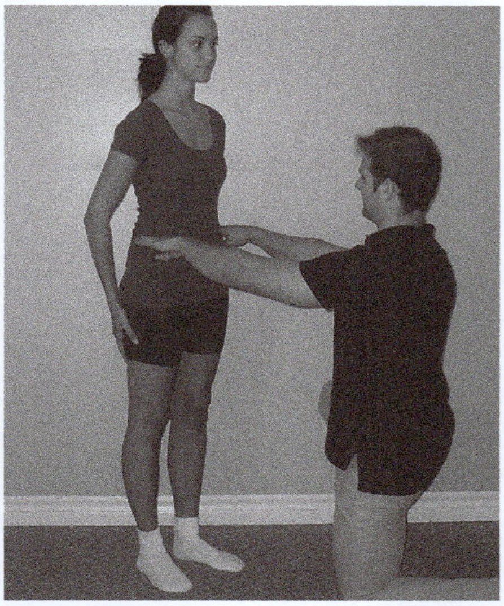

FIGURE 9.6 Check iliac crest heights

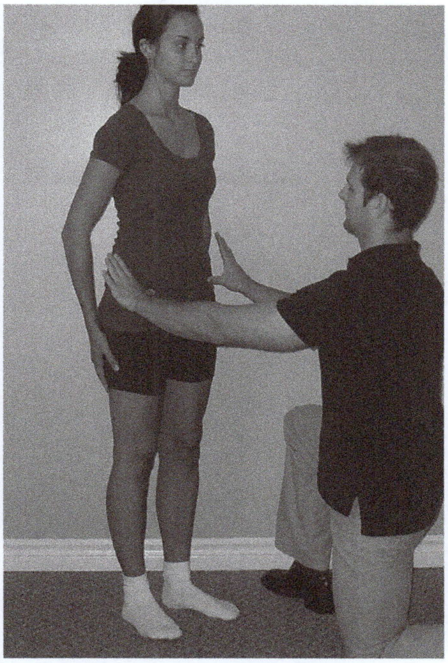

FIGURE 9.7 Check ASISs

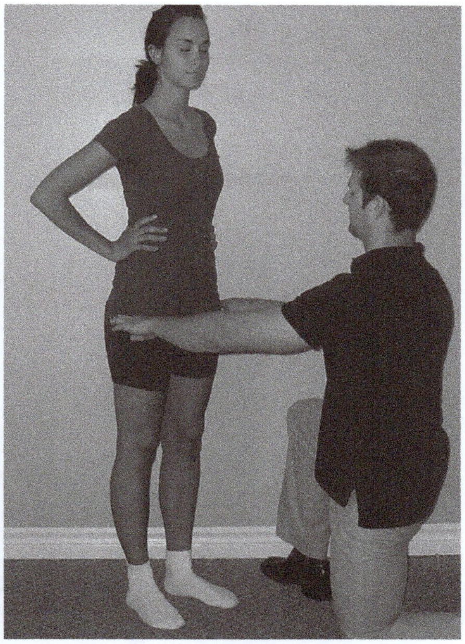

FIGURE 9.8 Check greater trochanter

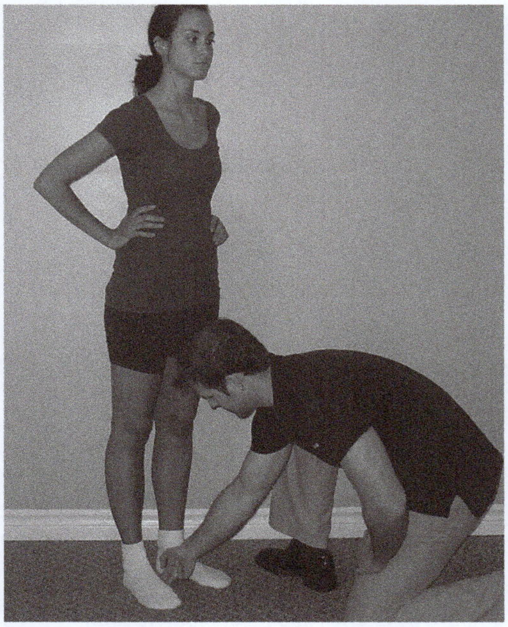

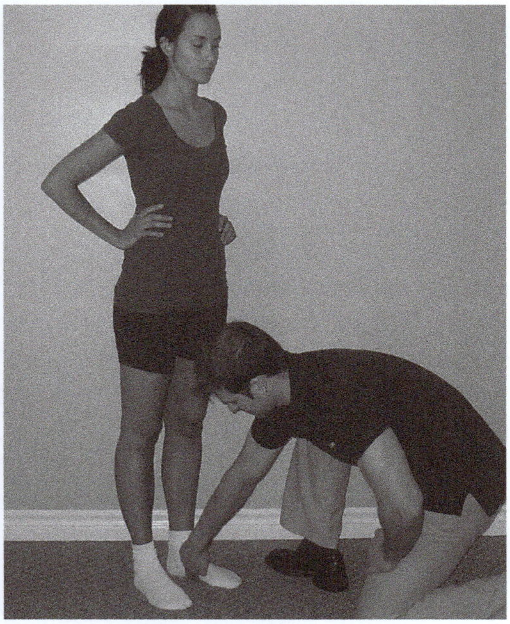

FIGURE 9.9A, B Check arches of feet

Postural examination and landmarking in supine, prone, and side-lying

NOTE: The following postural examination positions are given here though they are not necessarily done at this time. They can be used when the therapist has the patient in any of these positions (supine, prone, or side-lying) when doing specific testing. In other words, when you first have the patient assume any of these positions to do other tests, take the time to do the observations mentioned here prior to carrying out the specific testing intended. The landmarking and observations should only take a minute or less to do.

REMEMBER: When the patient is recumbent on the table (as opposed to upright), gravity affects the body differently. With

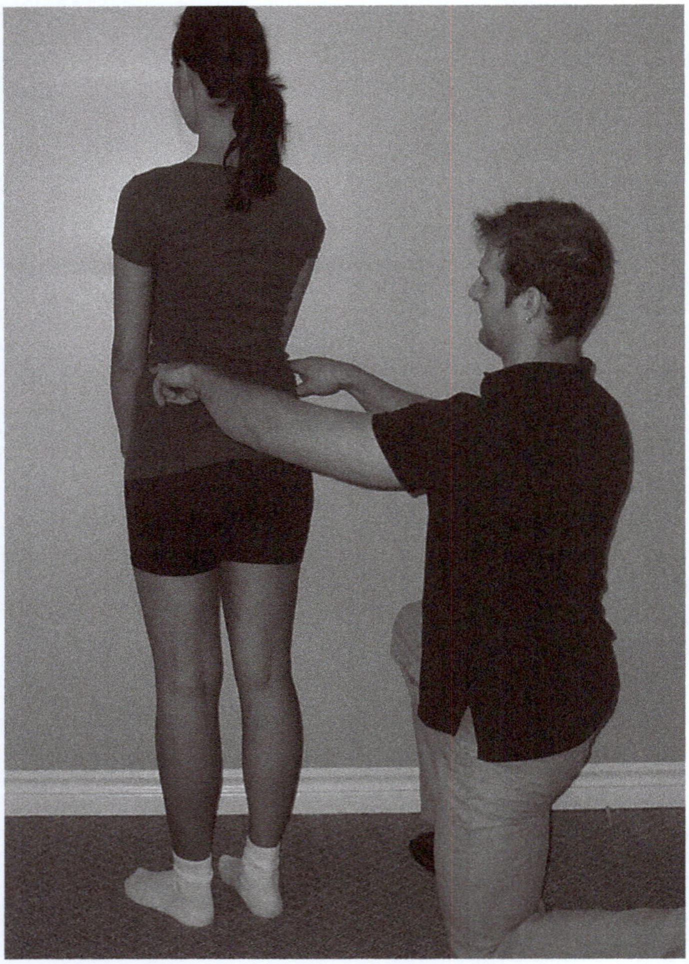

FIGURE 9.10 Check PSIS levels

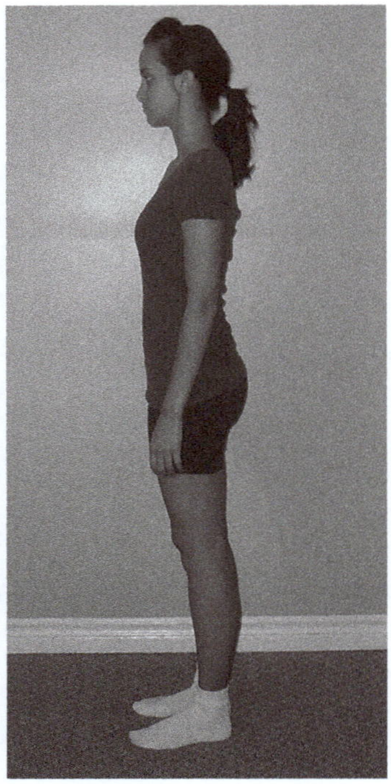

FIGURE 9.11 Lateral view

Observe the lateral curves of the spine, the position of the body over the feet (is the upper body leaning forward?), etc. (Again, see Chapter 5, postural assessment, for details.)

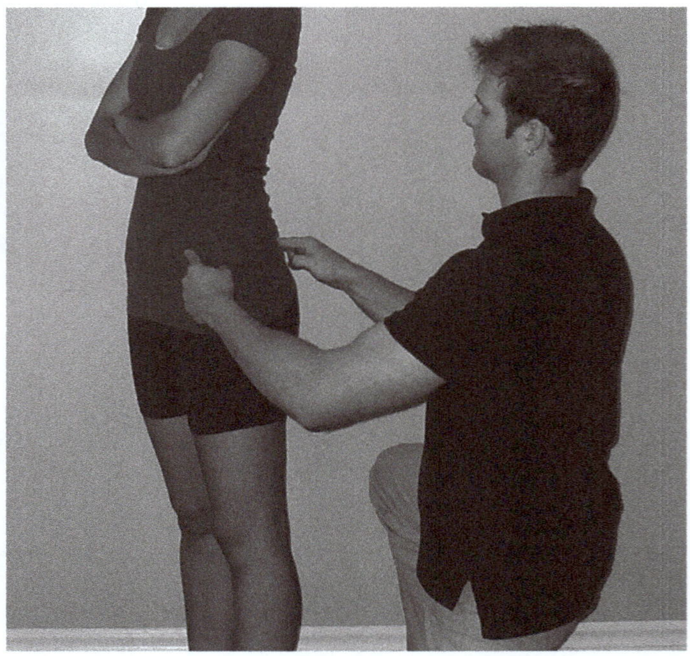

FIGURE 9.12 Compare PSIS and ASIS levels (pelvic tilts)

Observe whether there is an anterior pelvic tilt (usually accompanied by a hyperlordosis) or posterior pelvic tilt (usually with a flat back/hypolordosis). Normal tilt is 5–15° (women tend to have more tilt than men). Check from *both* sides in order to evaluate if one innominate is more anterior/posterior than the other.

gravity not exerting its effects from the head down, a new pattern of positioning is created that will be reflected in changes to the landmarks. Therefore, you can expect to find different results than the ones seen in the standing exam. The important point to remember is that you need to evaluate each finding considering the position that the patient is in, and think through what is too short (and pulling) and what is too loose (what allows the part to be pulled out of alignment).

Supine postural exam

It is best to normalize the hips prior to landmarking and palpating structures around the pelvis and the hip as the patient may not be lying straight on the table. Do the following if the patient is able: have the patient crook-lying (supine with hips and knees bent). This is usually a position of comfort for the patient. Have them lift their pelvis off the table a few inches for

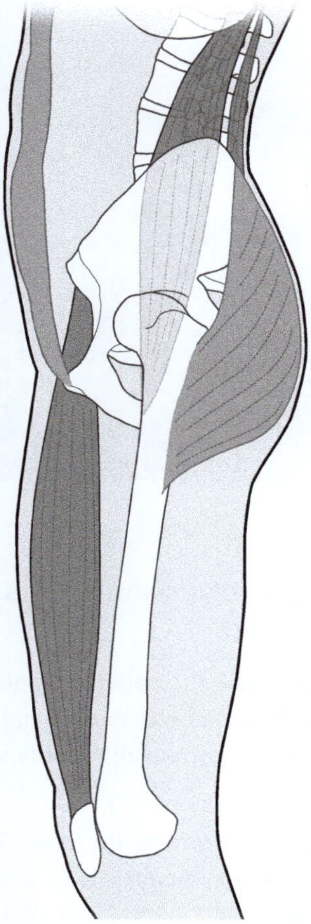

FIGURE 9.13 Anterior pelvic tilt with hyperlordosis

Tight and facilitated/hypertonic muscles: lumbar erectors, quadratus lumborum, iliopsoas, piriformis, rectus femoris, tensor fasciae latae, adductors, hamstrings, especially biceps femoris.
Weak and inhibited muscles: rectus abdominis, transversus abdominis, gluteals, vastus medialis/lateralis.

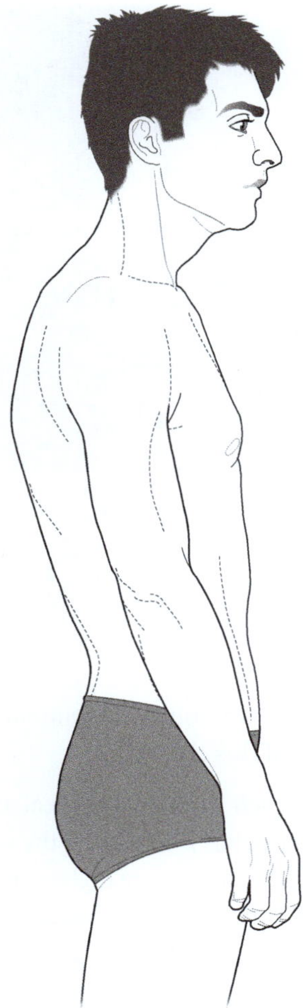

FIGURE 9.14 Sway back

Tight and facilitated/hypertonic muscles: lumbar erectors, quadratus lumborum, hamstrings, gluteus maximus.
Weak and inhibited muscles: rectus abdominis, transversus abdominis, iliopsoas, rectus femoris.

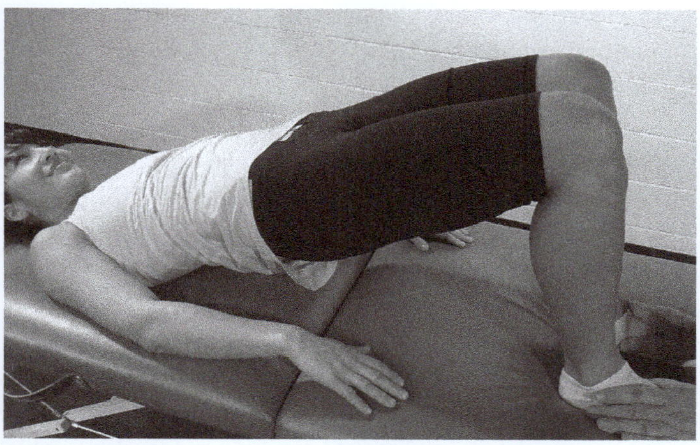

FIGURE 9.15

Normalizing the hips prior to landmarking by engaging the musculature.

just a few seconds (a count of "1, 2, 3") and then instruct them to let their hips drop lightly back down to the table (Figure 9.15).

Have the patient relax and let you move their legs (Figures 9.16 and 9.17). Proceed to extend each leg one at a time. The active lifting of the pelvis off the table engages the musculature in and around the pelvis which will pull the hips, etc., into what is the normal position for that patient.

Once the patient lets the hips drop back to the table the musculature can relax and the patient should then allow the therapist to passively straighten the legs. This has the effect of aligning the patient into what is their neutral position. In this way, you can more accurately palpate for asymmetries that are actually present in the body and not be misled by those that are just incidental to how the patient happens to be lying at that moment.

Now, observe the following:

1. Note the relative heights of the iliac crests and ASISs bilaterally. Compare these with the relative position of the medial malleoli. For example, if the right ASIS is lower than the left, do you find a corresponding asymmetry between the right and

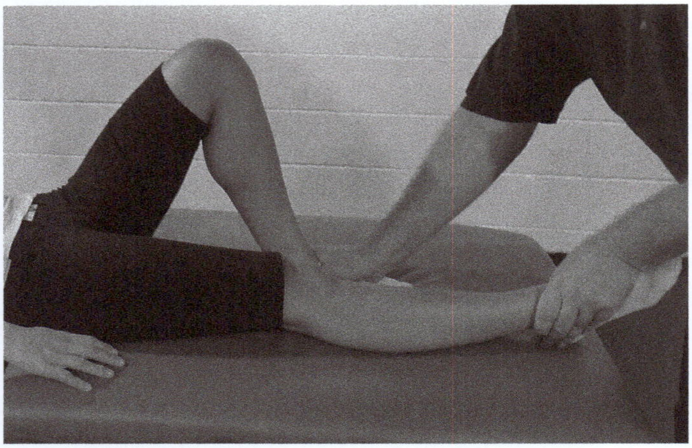

FIGURE 9.16
Extend the patient's legs one at a time.

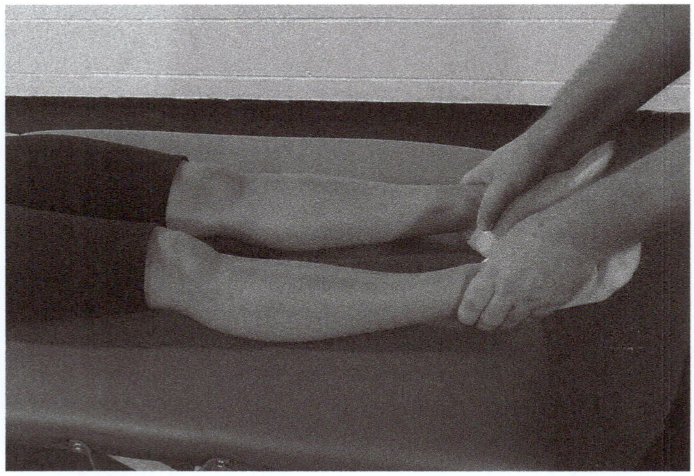

FIGURE 9.17
The patient allows the therapist to passively straighten the legs.

left medial malleoli? (See *Unilateral rotation of innominate* in clinical implications at the start of this chapter.)

2. Check for rotation (to the right or left through a vertical axis) of the pelvis, where one side of the pelvis is higher off the table than the other (i.e., one ASIS and trochanter are higher off the table on one side than the other). However, observing this only in the supine (or prone) position may be misleading, a false positive. If the appearance of rotation to the right or left occurs only when the patient is supine (and was not present when they were standing), then this may imply that it is the patient's trunk that is rotated. It may be that when the patient lies down the weight of the trunk causes it to level itself and the rotation now appears in the pelvis. On the other hand, the weight of the trunk or legs could pull the pelvis out of a rotated position that would show when standing but disappear when the patient lies supine.

Therefore, the need for careful observation during a standing postural exam, even if brief, cannot be over-emphasized. The information learned with a standing postural observation is needed for comparison with what we observe when the patient is lying supine. Otherwise, during treatment, for example, when we notice rotations while the patient is on the table, we may make erroneous assumptions about postural asymmetries and muscle balance.

Note any outflare of the innominate, where one ASIS is further from the mid-line than the other, which often accompanies external rotation of the femur. Also, note any inflare, where one of the ASISs is closer to the mid-line than the other; this is usually found with an internally rotated femur on that side.

3. See if you can slide your hand under the patient's lumbar spine. If you can, it often implies that the patient has a hyperlordosis that is being held by chronically shortened tissues.

4. Palpate the distance between the table and the posterior aspect of the greater trochanters. Asymmetry here could imply an anteversion or retroversion of the head of the femur(s), especially if the pelvis itself is level with the table. If you suspect anteversion or retroversion refer to the prone postural examination below.

Side-lying postural exam

Check the tension of the gluteus medius and minimus, the tensor fasciae latae (TFL), and the iliotibial band (ITB). You can also palpate the tension in the quadratus lumborum, erector spinae, and transverse abdominis on the side that is up.

Prone postural exam

1. Check the tone of the gluteus maximus, the lateral rotators (especially the piriformis), and the hamstrings. Compare the tension on the sacrotuberous ligaments and levels of ischial tuberosities. Note that when one sacrotuberous ligament palpates taut compared to the other it could imply a sacroiliac joint or innominate impairment/malalignment. One ischial tuberosity palpating higher can imply that that side of the hip is anteriorly rotated and/or held flexed. Further, you often notice that the buttock on that side looks higher than the other.

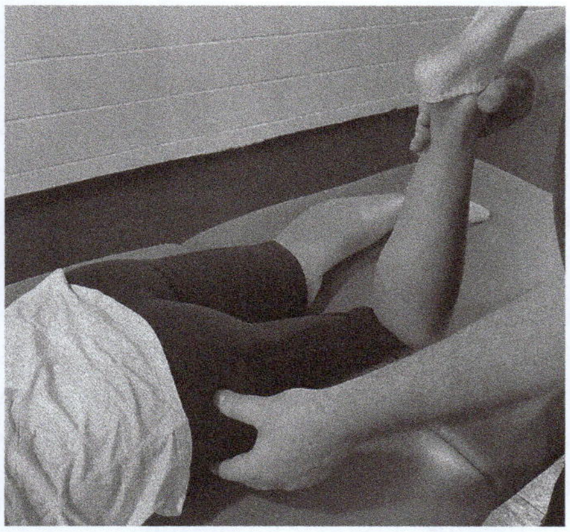

FIGURE 9.18 1. Landmark and position patient

Locate and place fingers under greater trochanter.

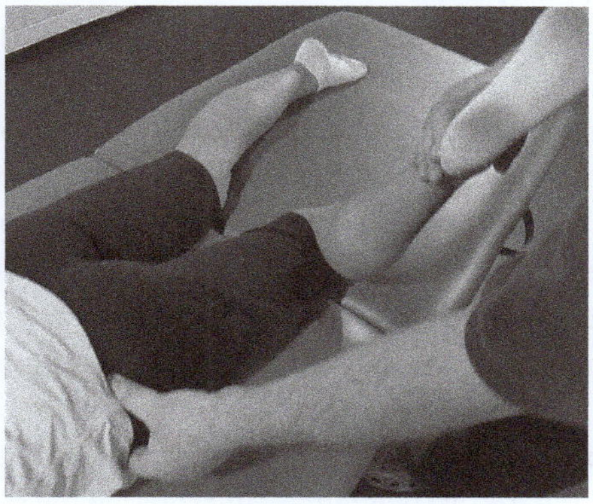

FIGURE 9.19 2. Internally/externally rotate hip

Palpate greater trochanter and by internally and externally rotating hip locate when trochanter feels parallel to table.

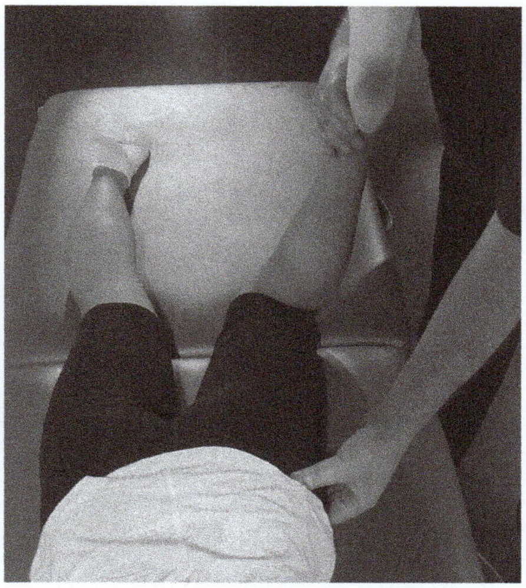

FIGURE 9.20 3. Observe angle of hip

Observe angle that lower leg is in. If it is angled out about 8–15° then hip is within normal range. If it is clearly less than 8° then it is probably retroverted. If you go obviously more than 15° then the hip is probably anteverted.

2. Carefully observe and note if the buttock on one side is, or appears to be, higher than the other. This could imply a shortness/contracture in the ipsilateral rectus femoris or a unilateral anterior rotation of the innominate (due to rectus femoris and iliopsoas shortness, SI joint impairments, or rotation of the lumbar spine). However, note the earlier comment about trunk rotation shifting to the pelvis in the supine postural examination.

Palpating for anteverted/retroverted hip (Figures 9.18–9.20)

To test for an anteverted hip in the prone position, flex the patient's knee (if no knee impairments prevent you from doing this) and palpate the anterior and posterior surface of the trochanter with the thumb and fingers. As you continue to palpate internally rotate the thigh/femur by moving the lower leg out toward you – *do it slowly!* When you have rotated the thigh 8–15° the trochanter should feel level. If you need to rotate much more than 15° the hip may be anteverted. If you go much less than 8° then it may be retroverted. Compare both sides.

Box 9.3 describes a final step of observation you may wish to perform and some general observational notes are set out below.

Box 9.3 Posturally challenging the chief complaint: exploring how the chief complaint fits into the whole

NOTE: *The following postural challenge testing should only be done once the therapist has finished all the testing that they are going to do on that day, as it may provoke pain or other symptoms that may interfere with the tests planned for later.*

As a final step of observation and inspection, look at how the patient naturally stands and then, if possible, correct their posture with gentle movements. For example, push the patient's hips back, unlock hyperextended knees, re-position a forward head over the shoulders, and note what changes occur above and below. If the patient can briefly sustain this corrected position, the tension or pain that they now experience may point to areas that need to be included in your assessment and treatment (injured, contractured, or weakened/stressed tissues or structures). This will help reveal problems that both have a global effect and are also intimately connected to specific impairments.

Note the following observations at any time during testing or treating:

Note pilomotor (goose bumps) or sudomotor (perspiration) responses by tissues or the appearance of subcutaneous trophedema (thickened subcutaneous tissue, i.e., an orange-peel look and texture to the skin). Any of these may indicate an autonomic (sympathetic) response. These responses in the skin travel through the ventral ramus of a nerve root and innervate the dermatomal area of that nerve root and generate a motor and visceral (e.g., sweat glands) response. If not occurring from appropriate stimulation (such as heat or cold), then it often implies a response to pain or injury: (1) on-site, which includes underlying tissues in that area (such as muscle or fascia); (2) from anything innervated by the associated nerve root, its rami, (such as that spinal level's joint capsule), associated autonomic ganglion (e.g., visceral referral), or the associated spinal cord segment; and/or (3) a myofascial trigger point.

Also note that pain coming from the hip joint itself often shows up in the groin, the superior frontal-medial thigh or inguinal area. If the patient points to the greater trochanter while complaining of pain from the hip, it is usually a sign of musculature origin.

Rule outs

The joints above and below where the patient feels pain (or any impairment) can be the actual source of the chief complaint. Therefore, we need to rule out both the joints above and those below that area. This is the role of rule outs, which are active free range of motion (AF-ROM) tests of the joints above and below with some over-pressure (at end-range if the AF is pain-free). If this rule out testing does not reproduce the patient's chief complaint then that joint is said to be ruled out and not in need of immediate further investigation. We can then begin testing the joint or area in which the patient experiences pain and impairment with some confidence that the source may well be found there (Hartley 2000b).

The patient may experience pain or other symptoms or impairments with the rule out testing but if they do not provoke or reproduce the chief complaint then they are set aside for the time being and may be returned to at another time. These quick tests stress the principal tissues involved in each of those joints to be ruled out. They primarily focus on the non-contractile elements.

Of course, the acuteness or the nature of the patient's impairment can sometimes prevent them from moving those joints without involving or affecting the suspected area.

Complications when ruling out the joints above and below the hip

The hip, pelvis, and lumbar spine areas of the body work in a closely interconnected manner. In fact, there is a term for this: lumbopelvic motion. The musculature shared by, and involved in, these areas is sometimes referred to as the core musculature. Working the core usually involves stressing the hip-pelvis-lumbar complex. Ruling out the joints above and below any of these joints becomes difficult, if not impossible, with respect to certain ranges of motion. Observation and palpation, along with a thorough case history, combined with a general understanding of how these all function together anatomically, are all crucial to either deciding whether or not to perform the rule outs (individually or collectively), and for interpreting the results of the rule outs done for the hip.

Ruling out the lumbar spine and the sacroiliac (SI) joints often involves moving the innominate (ileum, etc.). Thus, they can compromise hip testing proper. Use your clinical judgment to decide if you wish to use any of these rule out tests. Or alternately, use one or more of these tests at a later date when you feel they will minimally compromise the hip but will be helpful in checking for involvement of the sacroiliac or lumbar joints with the patient's chief complaint.

Though our view is that rule outs are done prior to regular manual testing, we can make an exception in this case precisely because of the interconnectedness of the hip-pelvis-lumbar complex, and also because the three rule outs have the patient in three different positions. Moving between the rule out positions described on the following pages will often affect the hip, possibly irritating or aggravating the impairments.

If you wish to perform rule outs then wait to do so until the patient assumes each position during the regular progression of your testing, as in the following examples:

1. Rule out the lumbar spine when the patient is standing.
2. Rule out the sacroiliac joints when the patient is supine.
3. Rule out the knee when it is safe and convenient to have the patient side-lying.

Remember that with each action you have the patient perform, or that you carry out, always ask about pain or any other symptoms that they may have experienced, and ask if this is part of the persisting problem – i.e., does it match the chief complaint?

Ruling out the lumbar spine

It is often impractical to rule out the lumbar spine as many active free movements of the lumbar spine cannot be done without stressing the hip joint by potentially moving the innominate.

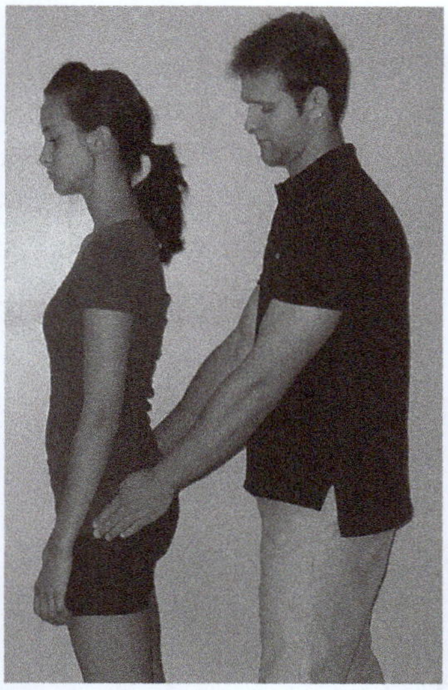

FIGURE 9.21 **1. Landmark over ilia and greater trochanter**

Have the thumbs on the iliac crests and the fingers over the greater trochanter.

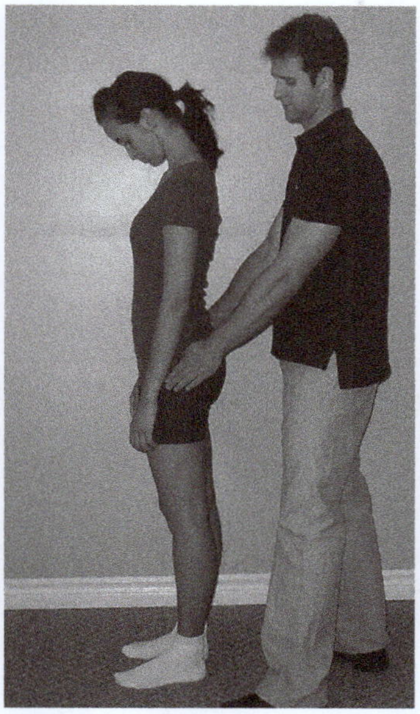

FIGURE 9.22 **2. Have patient begin flexion**

Have the patient slowly flex the neck, then curl the thoracic spine. Then have the patient begin to flex the lumbar spine. Once you notice the hips about to move have the patient stop.

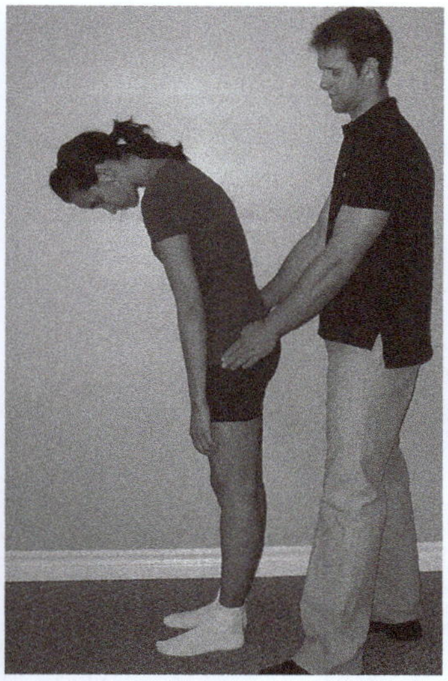

FIGURE 9.23 **3. Note if lumbar lordosis has changed**

When the patient has reached relative end-range of lumbar motion (just before moving the hips), note if the lumbar spine was able to actually flex or is still in lordotic curve.

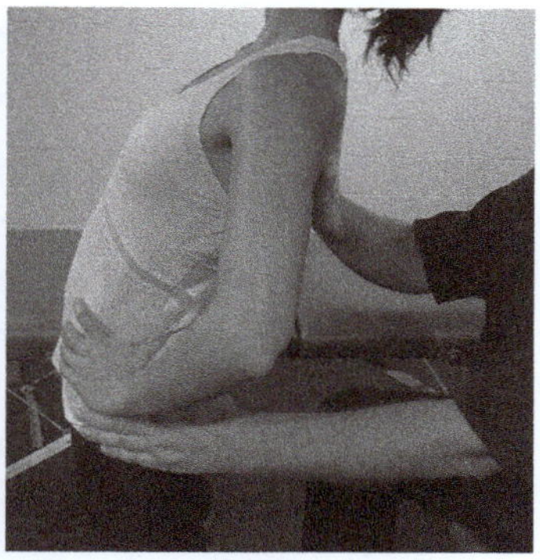

FIGURE 9.24 **4. Test extension of low back**

Have the patient return to neutral from flexion, then extend the low back.

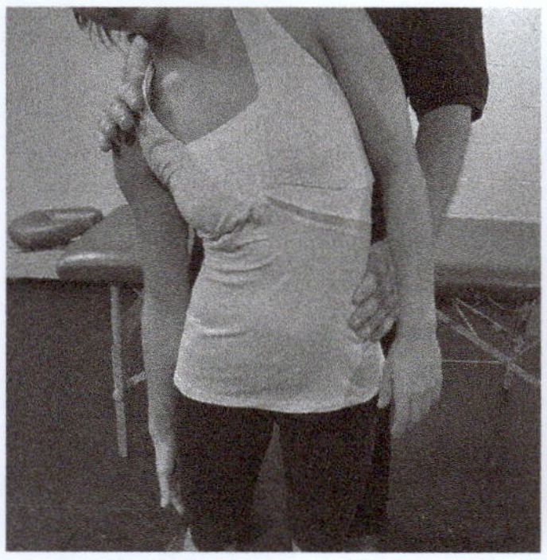

FIGURE 9.25 **5. Check side-bending of lumbar spine**

Have the patient side-bend. Keep your monitoring hand for hip motion on the opposite hip. Check side-bending to the other side.

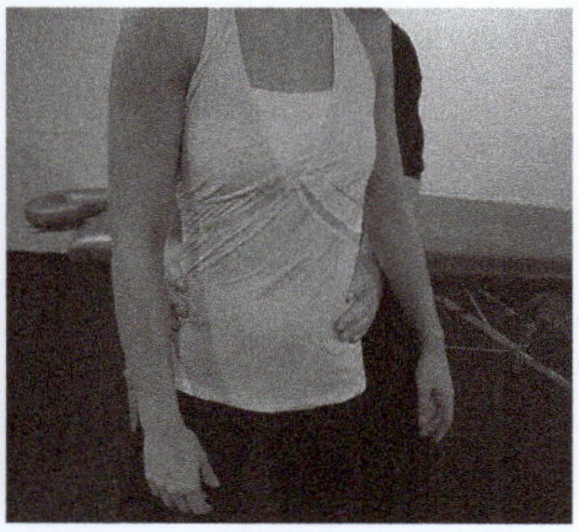

FIGURE 9.26 **6. Check rotation of low back**

Complete this set of motions with rotation. Have both hands on the patient's hips to monitor motion.

The therapist needs to pay close attention to when the movement of the lumbar spine begins to move down into the pelvis. Stop the patient before this occurs. Therefore, end-ranges of the lumbar spine will usually not be reached. Over-pressure will only force the movement through the pelvis into the sacroiliac joints and hips, and so it is not performed.

Have the patient do the AF-ROM flexion of the lumbar spine shown in Figures 9.21–9.26 while you are standing behind with your hands on their hips. This will enable you to note when the hip begins to move.

Rule out of the sacroiliac joints

The sacroiliac joints should be ruled out in non-acute stages of hip impairments using anterior and posterior gap tests and shear (rock) tests. See Chapter 11 for details of the anatomy of the SI joint. Be aware that these tests rely on putting pressure through the innominate, which may alter this hip joint structure and cause pain. The patient is in a supine position for all of these tests.

Gap tests (Figures 9.27–9.29)

Shear tests (rock tests) (Figure 9.30)

You are trying to move the innominate in a manner that will have it shear through the joint line. To rock the pelvis keep the hands over the ASISs, with heel of the hand on the ASIS to PSIS and the fingers over the lateral portion of the hip. With the elbows still held flexed so that the forearms are 30–45° to the table (roughly the angle of the joint surfaces of the sacrum and innominate), push one hand at a time in an alternating manner toward the table on an oblique angle. You are directing the force toward the mid-line but as if the target is two or three inches below the patient's sacrum. It is often called the rock test as the therapist usually alternates back and forth two or three times.

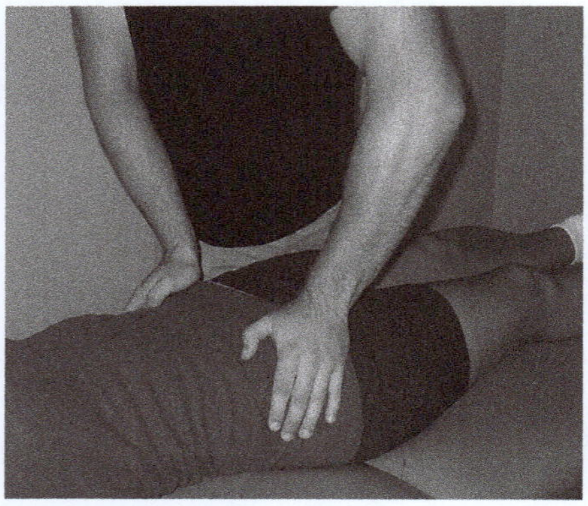

FIGURE 9.27 1. Landmarking prior to gap test

Using the palms of your hands, locate both ASISs.

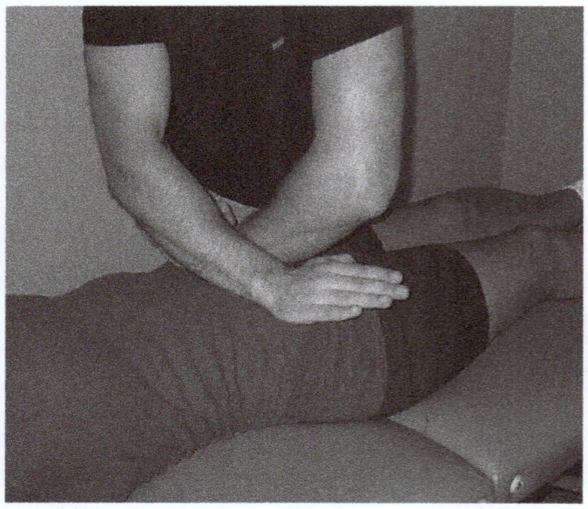

FIGURE 9.28 2. Hand position for anterior gapping test

Cross the forearms and place the heels of the hands on the inside edge (medial side) of the ASISs. Gently using body-weight, push them apart. This gaps the anterior portion of the SI joints and stresses the anterior sacro-iliac ligaments.

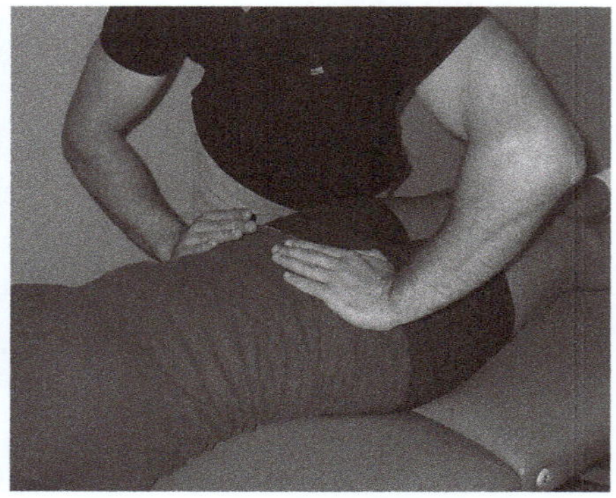

FIGURE 9.29 3. Hand position for posterior gap test

Uncross the forearms and with elbows bent place the heel of each hand on the outside edge of the ASISs. Push the ASISs toward each other, stressing the posterior sacroiliac ligaments, gapping the posterior portion of the SI joints.

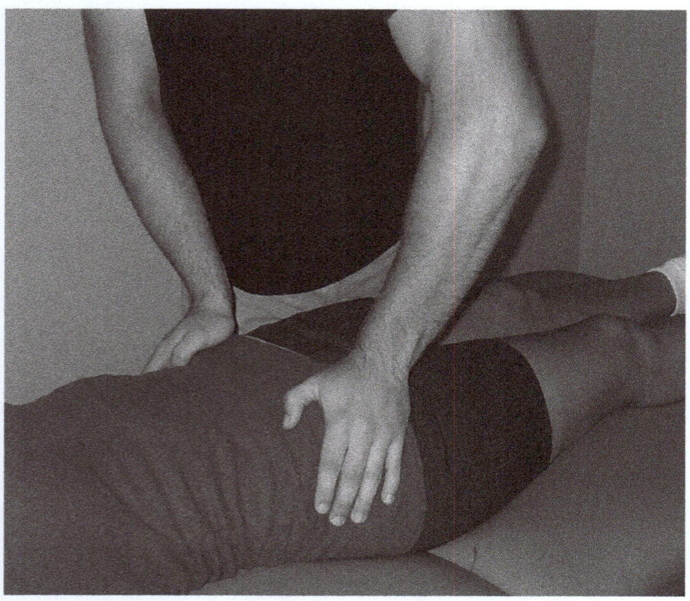

FIGURE 9.30 Shear test of sacroiliac joints

To rock the pelvis, keep the hands over the ASISs, with the heels of hands on ASIS to PSIS and the fingers over the lateral portion of the hip. With elbows still held flexed so the forearms are 30–45° (roughly angle of joint surfaces of sacrum and innominate), push one hand at a time in an alternating manner toward the table on an oblique angle. You are directing force toward the mid-line, but as if the target is two or three inches below the patient's sacrum.

You are looking for a little give in the joint; look for a little delay before you feel the alternate hip lift up or rock up into your hand. A blocked SI joint will cause you to feel the other side immediately lift up into the other hand.

Ruling out the knee joint (Figures 9.31–9.33)

This is best done in side-lying where the hip can be kept near neutral. It is best to have the hip slightly flexed, which should be a position of comfort. Otherwise, flexion of the knee could be compromised at end-range by the pull on the rectus femoris on the pelvis (through its attachment on the AIIS), causing movement of the hip via anterior hip rotation, which is equivalent to flexing the hip. As with all of the rule out testing, the patient often has to be non-acute to be able to position and test the joints above and below the area of the chief complaint.

An overview of range of motion testing for the hip is given in Box 9.4.

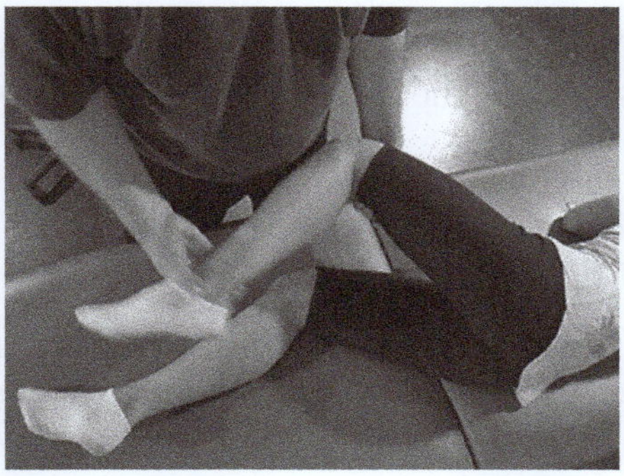

FIGURE 9.31 1. Positioning for testing knee

With the patient laying on the unaffected side, flex the hip and knee. Support the knee and ankle.

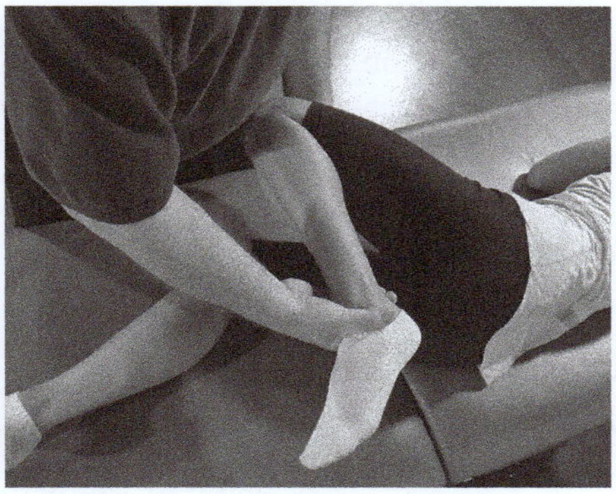

FIGURE 9.32 2. Full flexion of knee

Bring the patient's heel to the buttocks.

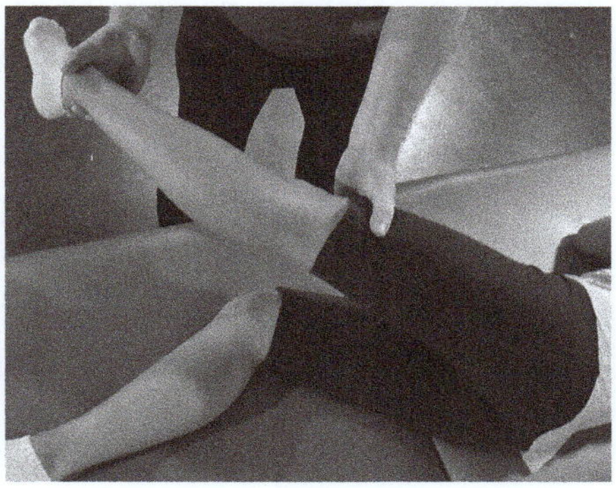

FIGURE 9.33 3. Extension of knee with over-pressure (O-P)

Bring knee into extension. If there is no pain, apply slight O-P.

Box 9.4 An overview of range of motion testing for the hip

There are six ranges of motion in the hip:

- flexion and extension
- abduction and adduction
- internal and external rotation.

Whenever possible have the patient perform these actions with the low back, hip, and pelvis in what is neutral or normal for them. Remember that some postural deviations – an anteriorly rotated hip, for example – already put the hip in slight flexion and it may appear that the patient has lost some ROM when, in fact, they may have not. Rather, any loss found may have more to do with changes in orientation of the bony structures of the joint than with soft tissue. You need to take this into consideration as you analyze the results of your testing. You must do more than just observe range of motion of the hip joint; you must also see the patient's hip motion within the context of its environment and its position relative to surrounding structures. That is, we must see the hip joint (local testing) within the global context (the whole body) as the patient presents to us that day. To reposition the joints and structures in order to measure the "true range of motion" for that joint specifically is to deal with a fictitious patient.

Furthermore, correcting the patient's posture or repositioning the hips in true neutral may cause pain or impairments that the patient has not experienced (as they are not moving from such a neutral position normally). Or, this re-positioning could prevent the patient from experiencing the pain or impairments they usually suffer.

Therefore, first have the patient perform the actions while in positions that at least approximate neutral. Then you can help the patient get into an even more neutral position and repeat them, if you feel that will give you better information. In this manner, you will have allowed the patient to perform actions that are less painful first and get better information about functions they can do, and then proceed to "truer" testing positions.

Range of motion testing (ROM)

Active free range of motion (AF-ROM)

The position of the patient during AF-ROM varies depending on the degree of discomfort that the patient is experiencing. The patient performs these tests while standing if they are suffering from only slight discomfort. Do the movements in prone and supine position if the patient is in mild to moderate discomfort or pain. If the patient is suffering with an acute, painful, unilateral impairment of the hip, position the patient side-lying with the unimpaired side down. Though you lose bilateral comparison at least some testing can be done. This latter position is used when we wish to avoid moving the patient at all from prone to supine positions as we proceed through the testing, where such movement will cause or exacerbate the pain and quickly bring ROM testing to an end as all and any movement may become painful.

The following is a suggestion for taking the patient's comfort into account when choosing the order in which to do ROM testing of the patient's hip. If the patient did AF-ROM standing then test PR-ROM with the patient supine and do all five PR-ROM motions before doing extension so that if turning causes the patient pain most of the testing will not have been compromised. However, if the patient did AF-ROM while lying prone on the table, then end AF-ROM with extension done in prone and begin PR-ROM with extension. Ordering your testing this way means that the patient needs to turn supine to prone and back to supine only once during all of AF- and PR-ROM testing.

In order to have the testing move along efficiently it may be helpful for the therapist to perform the requested movements along with the patient. Just verbally instructing the patient to move in certain ways often leads to having them re-do movements till they "get it right." This latter situation can make a patient feel flustered or irritated and thereby negatively impact the therapeutic relationship.

See also Box 9.5.

The following AF-ROM testing figures can be found over the next two pages.

AF-ROM of the hip: flexion and extension (Figures 9.34, 9.35)

Testing abduction standing/supine (Figures 9.36–9.38)

Testing adduction standing/supine AF adduction 30° (Figures 9.39–9.41)

Medial rotation and lateral rotation (Figures 9.42A, B and 9.43A, B)

When testing medial (internal) and lateral (external) rotation, have the patient standing to take the weight off the leg being tested and have them rotate the leg internally and then externally. If the patient is supine then these actions can be performed without weight-bearing.

If the patient flexes the hip (and knee) slightly they should gain more movement internally/medially and externally/laterally as the hip is closer to its resting position where there is more laxity in the capsule and ligaments. While in neutral (as in standing), the fibers of the capsule, which are in a spiral or twisted orientation, give only a moderate freedom of motion to the joint.

Note that a number of patients may be starting rotation with the hip already rotated somewhat either internally or externally. Therefore, first observe the resting position from which the hip is starting its movement. Ensure that the patient does not assist

Box 9.5 Joints working synergistically

While it is often true that patients will compensate for lack of range in one joint by moving more from joints above or below, we must not be so strict when doing AF-ROM testing as to count only movement from that joint alone, and then discount the movement in other joints.

Most joints in the body work synergistically, and nearby joints often need to move in order for the principal joint to have its full range. In the shoulder, for example, acceptable and normal glenohumeral motions can only occur if the acromioclavicular (AC) joint, sternoclavicular (SC) joint, and scapula all move in concert with the glenohumeral (GH) joint, and some motion from the thoracic spine. We are especially assessing the living body when doing AF-ROM, and not some anatomical piece of it all on its own, in isolation. In normal movement of the hip (acetabulofemoral joint) there needs to be small movements in the sacroiliac joints, in the pubic joint, and in the lower lumbar vertebrae (via the iliolumbar ligaments). The knee needs to flex if full hip flexion is to be seen.

We need to learn from experience what is acceptable as accessory motion in the surrounding tissues and learn when such motion is compensatory. We will see compensations more clearly when we are doing PR-ROM and then compare those motions to what was seen in AF-ROM.

PR-ROM, along with its over-pressure (O-P), can reveal loss of motion from joints and their supportive structures in isolation from the other joints and muscles and differentially assess how much loss is due to the joint itself (non-contractile tissues) in comparison (with AF and AR) to how much restriction or impairment is coming from contractile tissue.

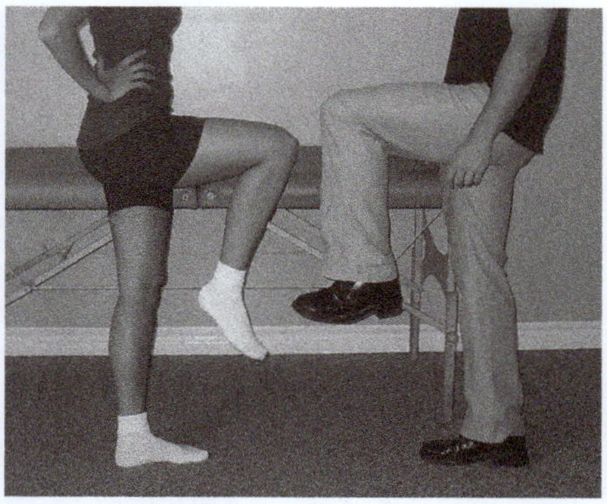

FIGURE 9.34 AF-ROM hip flexion 110–130°

The patient flexes the hip as far as possible. Make sure they do not bend forward in an attempt to bring knee closer to the body. This can also be done in supine or side-lying.

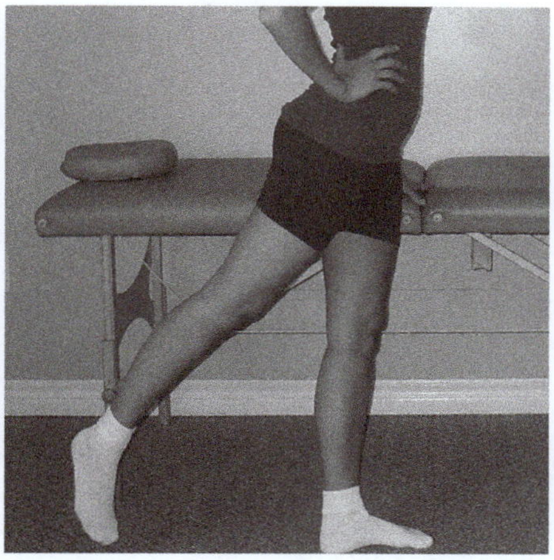

FIGURE 9.35 AF-ROM hip extension 10–20°

The patient extends the leg. Make sure extension is from the hip, and not from the lumbar region. In other words, note when extension of the hip has ended and further extension is then actually coming from extending the low back. This can also be done in prone or side-lying.

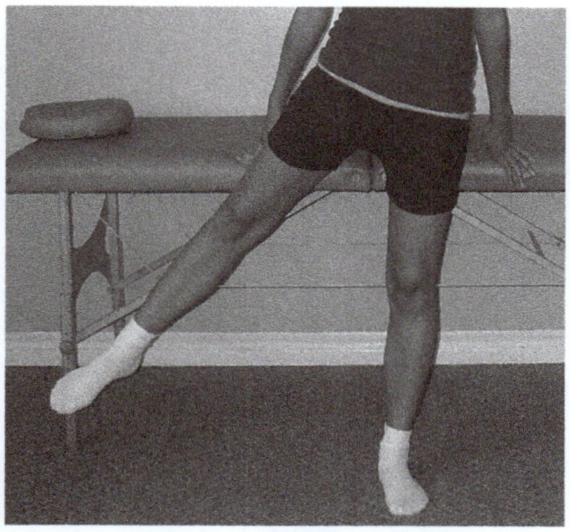

FIGURE 9.36 AF abduction 30–50°

Have the patient abduct the hip. Assist them in keeping balance. End-range is reached when the patient needs to side-bend away from leg being abducted.

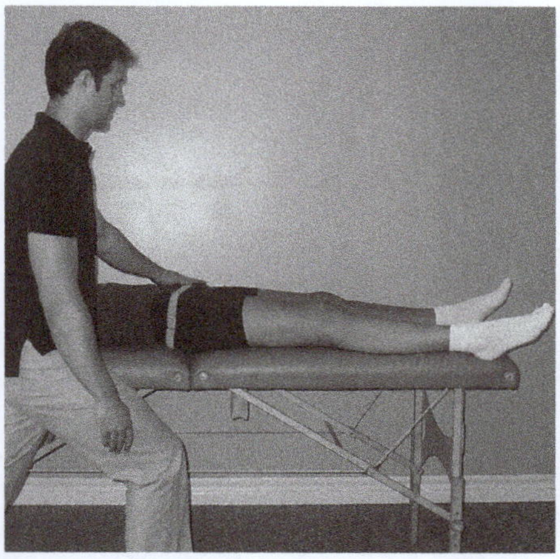

FIGURE 9.37 1. AF abduction 30–50° (supine)

Reach across to palpate the contralateral ASIS.

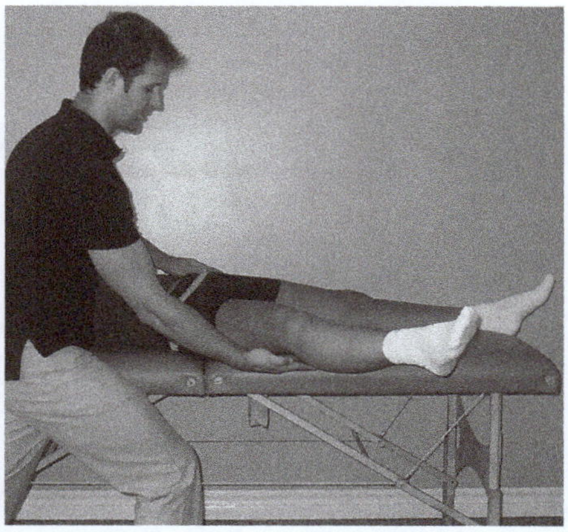

FIGURE 9.38 2. AF abduction (supine)

When the leg clears the table while abducting, support enough to negate gravity. This helps keep hip flexors from engaging and confusing results. Abduction is considered at end-range when you feel the contralateral ASIS start to move inferiorly.

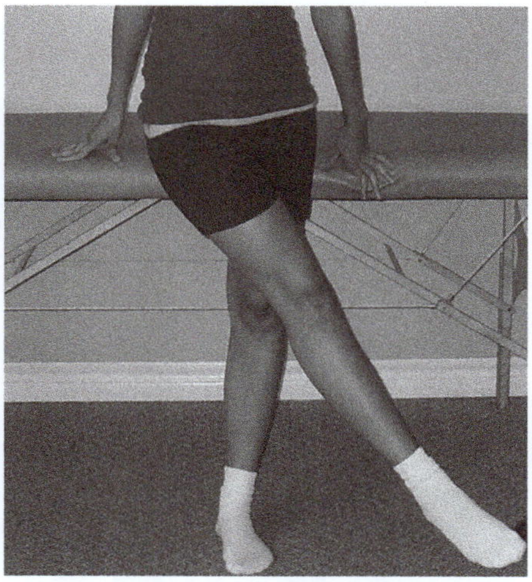

FIGURE 9.39 AF adduction 30°

When the patient adducts the hip while standing, the movement is called cross-adduction. This is when the patient flexes the hip being tested (and supported by the therapist) just enough to allow the leg being moved to pass in front of the other leg.

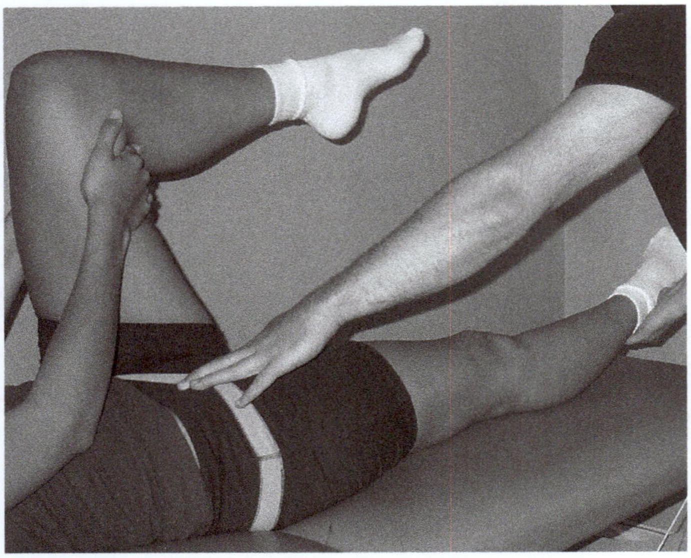

FIGURE 9.40 1. AF adduction

Palpate the ipsilateral ASIS. Have the patient flex the opposite hip and knee so they then can adduct past the midline. Have the patient first lift the leg just off the table and place the hand under the lower leg near the ankle to give a gentle support as the patient moves the leg.

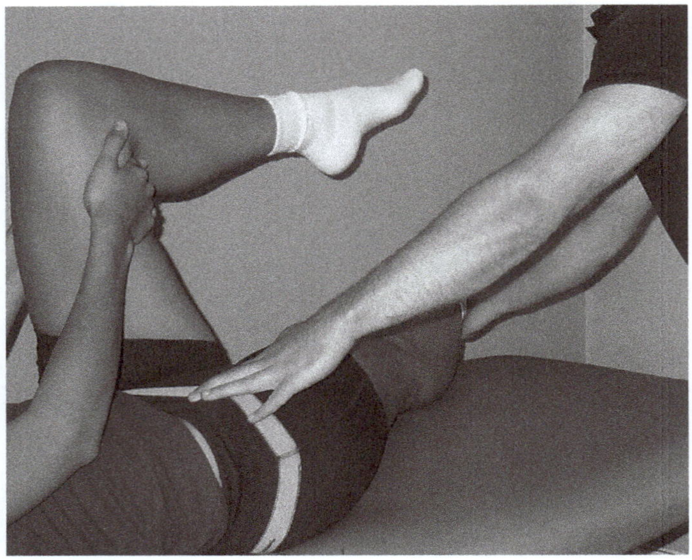

FIGURE 9.41 2. AF adduction

Tell the patient to relax and let you hold the foot off the table as they focus on actively adducting. When the ASIS begins to move inferiorly adduction is at end-range.

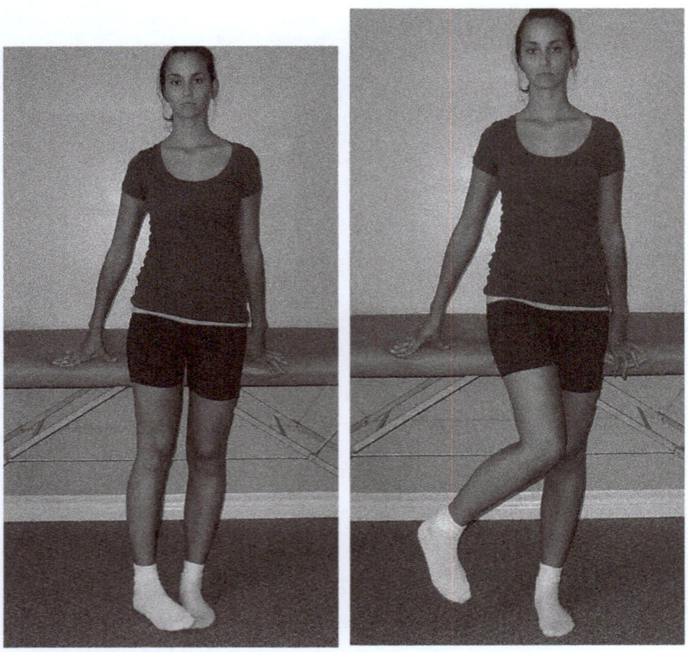

FIGURE 9.42A, B AF medial rotation: 30–40°

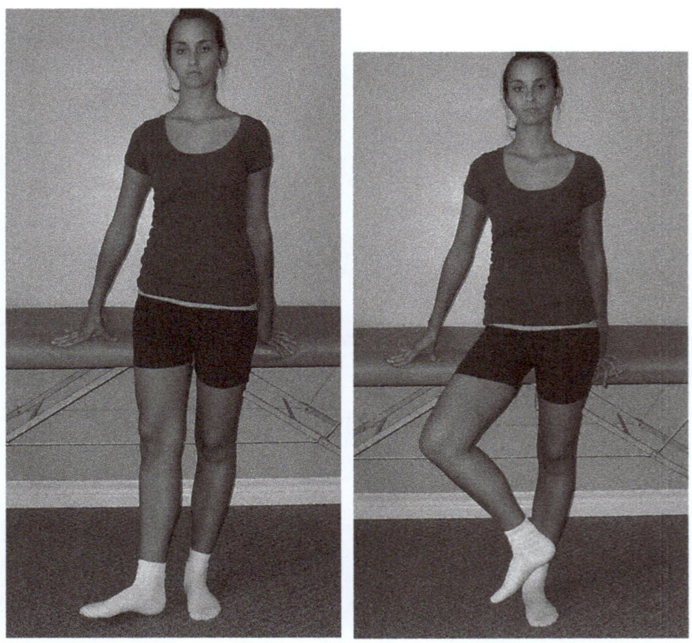

FIGURE 9.43A, B AF lateral rotation 40–60°

rotations by rotating the trunk. Remember that anteversion and retroversion of the hip will affect the amounts of lateral versus medial rotation you observe. Palpate the trochanters for some clues about this. A further clue that the patient may have an anteverted or retroverted hip is if the rotation one way seems limited while the other direction seems excessive.

Passive relaxed range of motion (PR-ROM) (Figures 9.44–9.49)

These are best done in supine and prone. They can be done side-lying for an acute (unilateral) impairment with the affected side up if it is the only position of comfort, though side-lying negates a bilateral comparison. When end-range is reached, and only if there is no pain, you may apply slight over-pressure (O-P) to determine the end-feel.

If cross-adduction is used (i.e., both legs are straight), you can stand and palpate as above. With the other hand under the ankle, lift the patient's leg just high enough so it can cross over the contralateral leg. Bring the leg into adduction. When the ASIS begins to move inferiorly, adduction is at end-range. However, having the moving leg also in slight flexion alters the result slightly by slacking the joint capsule.

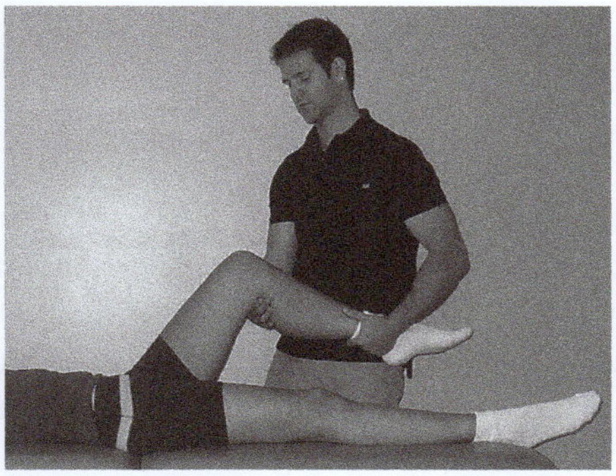

FIGURE 9.44 1. PR hip flexion
Raise the hip into flexion while flexing the knee for the patient to negate any muscular stretch from the hamstrings that may stop hip motion prematurely.

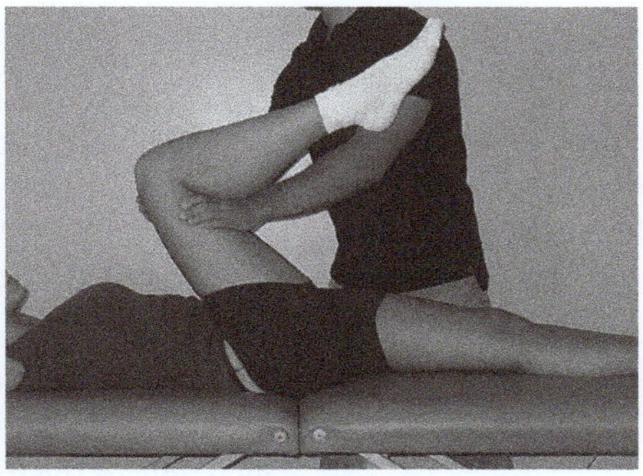

FIGURE 9.45 2. PR hip flexion with O-P
Apply O-P with the hand on the back of thigh so as not to put pressure through the knee joint. End-feel is tissue stretch or tissue approximation.

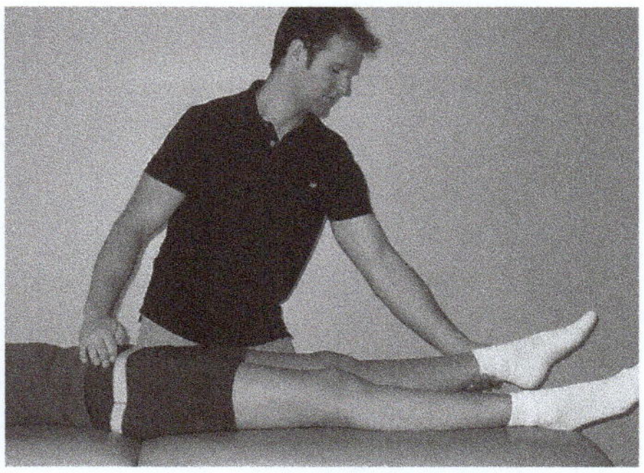

FIGURE 9.46 1. PR hip abduction
Hold the leg just above the ankle. With the other hand, reach across and palpate the patient's contralateral ASIS.

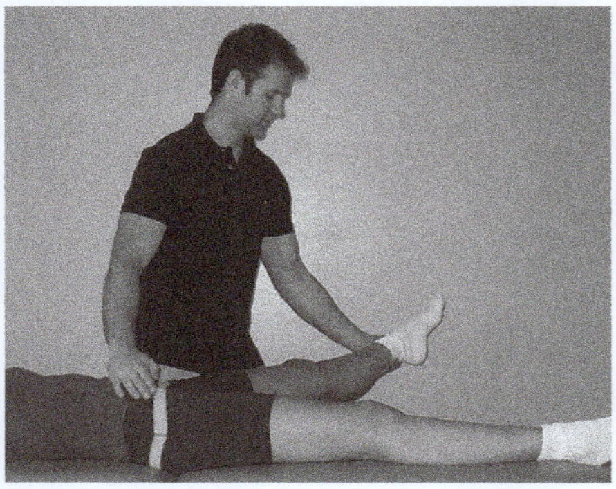

FIGURE 9.47 2. PR hip abduction and O-P
Slowly abduct the hip. End-range is when you feel the contralateral ASIS move. If movement is pain-free, then apply gentle O-P. End-feel is tissue stretch.

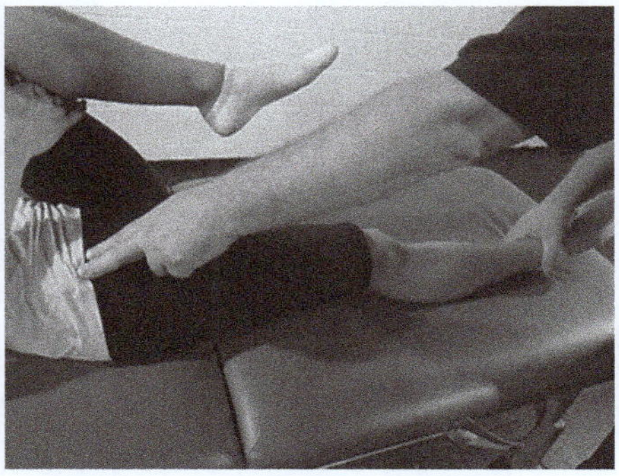

FIGURE 9.48 1. PR hip adduction
The patient holds the contralateral hip in flexion with the knee to the chest. Palpate the ipsilateral ASIS with one hand.

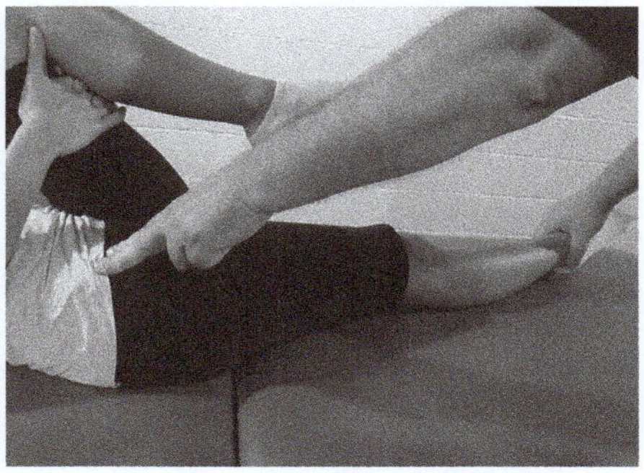

FIGURE 9.49 2. PR hip adduction and O-P
With the other hand, take the leg into adduction. If movement is pain-free, then apply gentle O-P. End-feel is tissue stretch.

External and internal rotation

There are several methods for assessing PR-ROM external and internal rotation in neutral.

Method 1 Testing internal and external rotation (Figures 9.50, 9.51)

Done in supine with the legs straight (neutral hip). Remember that in this position the natural tension in the twist of the hip joint capsule will resist large amounts of internal rotation, but on external rotation the capsule unwinds and permits a larger amount of movement.

REMINDER: You need to use your body-weight, along with broad contact, so that you do not just move soft tissue. On most people you will be able to sink down through the tissue and feel the femur and its movement. In this manner you can hook onto the side of the femur with the heel of the hand (with internal rotation) or with the finger pads (with external rotation). This may be a good method for a "quick test" but in acute or subacute impairment the movement of soft tissue can be a problem. Further, where the end of motion of the joint is and where the start of beginning O-P should occur can be very unclear.

Method 2 Testing internal and external rotation (Figures 9.52, 9.53)

Done with the patient prone and the leg being tested flexed at the knee. Note: To palpate end-range of motion you need to ensure that you are able to clearly feel the PSIS and not just the soft tissue over the pelvis. The soft tissue will begin to move along with the femur before the innominate will move. This movement of soft tissue alone is acceptable and not a sign of arriving at the joint's end-range. You need to be clearly feeling that the innominate is about to move (via the PSIS) in order to know you have reached end-range.

Method 3 Testing internal and external rotation (Figures 9.54–9.56)

Alternatively, you can flex the hip to about 60–90° and the knee to 90°. Use the lower leg to move the hip into lateral, then medial rotation. You will now see the maximum movement of the joint because of the laxity this position produces in the joint capsule. Therefore, be aware that you are not seeing the range available to the hip when it is weight-bearing.

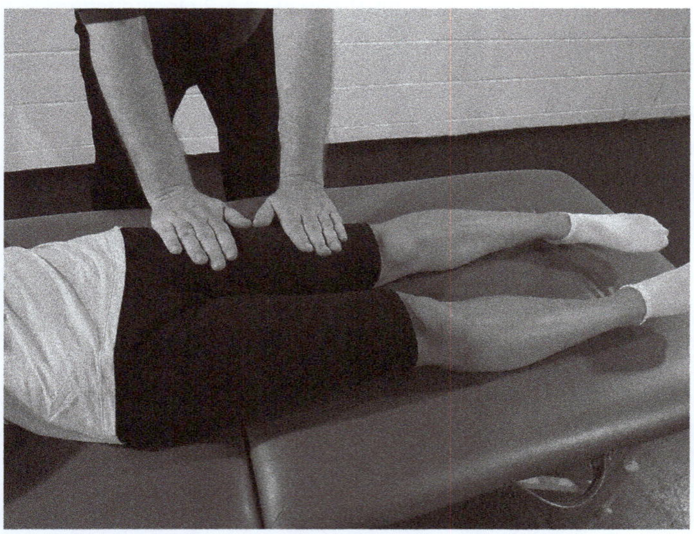

FIGURE 9.50 PR internal rotation of hip, method 1

If there is no complaint of pain in the quadriceps, you can place both hands on the anterior thigh and roll the patient's hip into medial rotation. Use the entire surface of the hands to move the thigh. Usually the therapist rolls the leg right into O-P. End-feel is firm capsular.

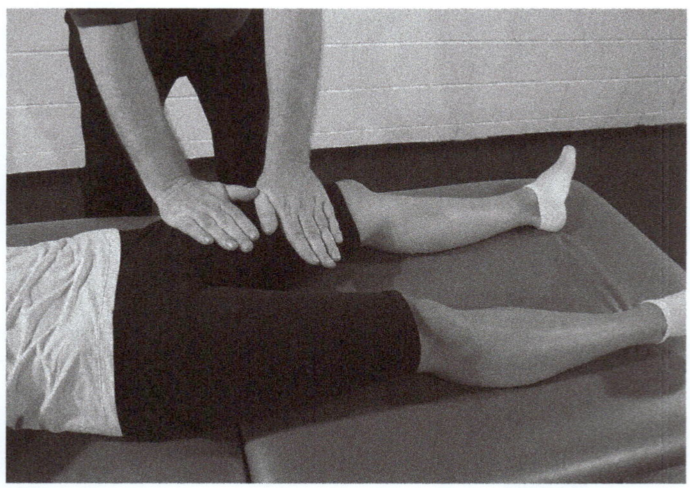

FIGURE 9.51 PR external rotation of hip, method 1

Then roll the hip into lateral rotation. Usually the therapist rolls the leg right into O-P. End-feel is firm capsular.

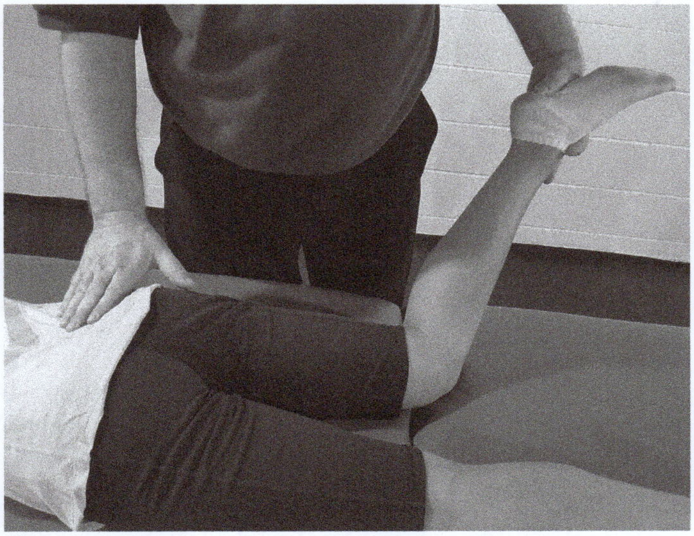

FIGURE 9.52 PR internal rotation of hip, method 2

Bend the knee, palpate over the PSIS of the hip on the side to be tested. Bring the ankle toward you to test internal rotation. When you feel the PSIS begin to move toward you end-range of the joint has been reached. If pain-free, then apply O-P. End-feel is capsular.

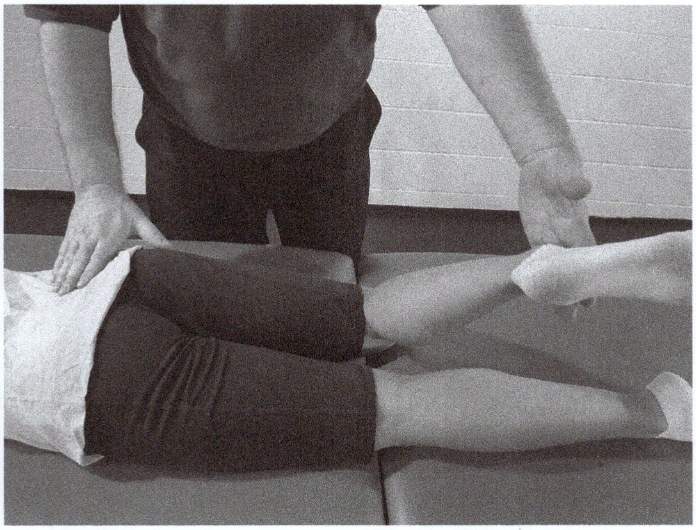

FIGURE 9.53 PR external rotation of hip, method 2

Return to neutral and then push the ankle away from you to test external rotation. When you feel the PSIS begin to move away, then you have reached the end-range of the joint. If pain-free, then apply O-P. End-feel is capsular.

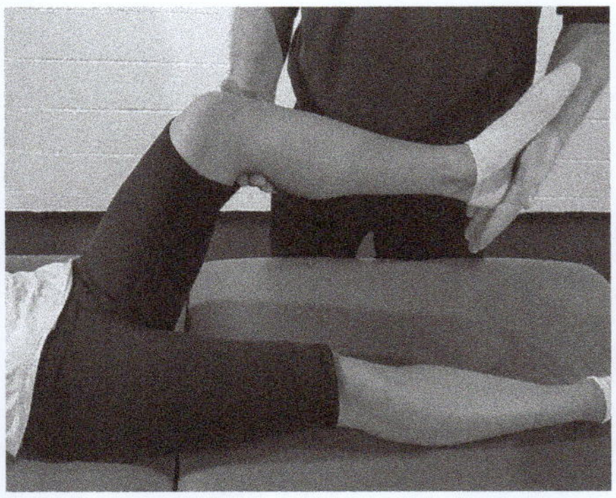

FIGURE 9.54 1. PR testing of hip rotations, method 3

Hold the patient's leg by the ankle and just below the knee.

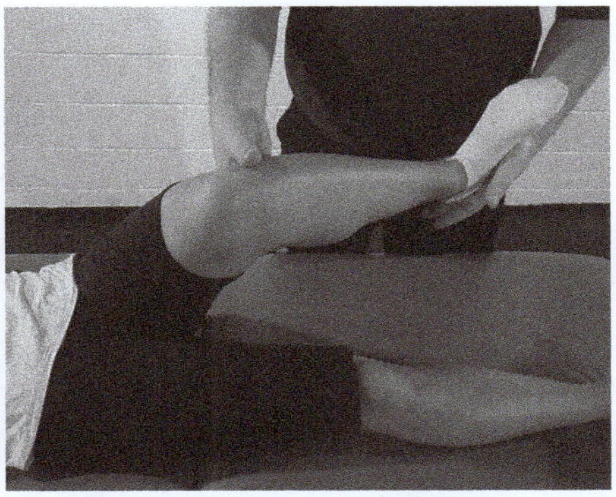

FIGURE 9.55 2. PR internal rotation of hip, method 3

Rotate the hip internally by moving the lower leg away from the mid-line. Apply O-P. If pain-free, then apply O-P. End-feel is capsular.

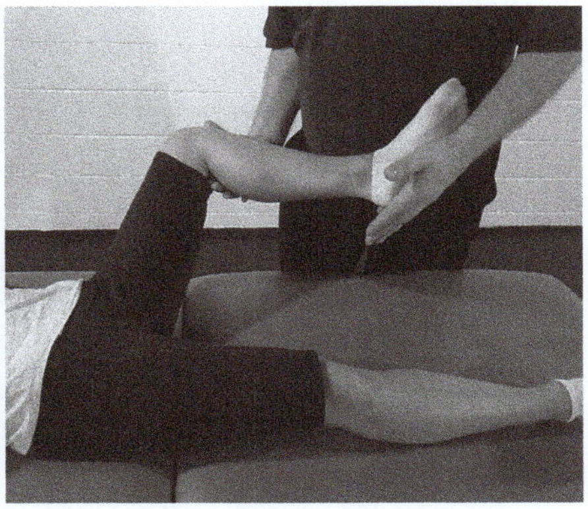

FIGURE 9.56 3. PR external rotation of hip, method 3

Rotate the hip externally/laterally by taking the ankle to the mid-line and letting the knee/thigh fall away from the mid-line. If pain-free, then apply O-P. End-feel is a capsular end-feel.

Hip extension (Figures 9.57, 9.58)

Extension will also occur in the low back if you do not hold the pelvis stable by having one hand over the sacrum. Apply a firm but gentle pressure. With the patient prone first flex the knee to 90°. Then lift the thigh off the table as follows: let the ankle rest against your shoulder, and lift the thigh with the hand cupped under the thigh just above the knee. Your free hand is placed over the sacrum and you simply lean on it to help hold the pelvis in place.

Carefully apply O-P, ensuring that there is little observable movement in the low back or rotation of the trunk, either of which would be signs that end-range has been exceeded. However, even without observable motion in the low back the joints may move enough for the patient to report pain in the lumbar spine and the sacroiliac joints if they are also impaired.

Passive testing by joint mobilization

Always try to use body-weight rather than pulling or pushing from the shoulders to move the limb. Remember the orientation of the acetabulum: facing laterally and slightly anteriorly and inferiorly. Ask about pain or any other symptoms and take note of both the quality and quantity of motion available in the joint. (*For more details and instruction see Part I, Chapter 3. Also, see the following for even more information and optional positioning of patient or limb, and variations or additional tests: Edmond 2006; Hertling & Kessler 2006; Kaltenborn 2006; Kisner & Colby 2012; Starkey & Brown 2015.*)

Traction/decompression of the hip (Figures 9.59–9.61)

Two versions of long axis tractioning of the hip in supine are presented here. Both versions traction the joint primarily inferiorly and slightly laterally. This will traction the head of the femur down off the superiorly oriented articular (horseshoe-shaped) surface of the acetabulum. The bulk of the weight from the trunk passes down through this surface onto the head of the femur.

A third version, done side-lying, may address the capsule more directly as it distracts the head of the femur perpendicular to the acetabulum.

NOTE: Though this side-lying version of tractioning the hip joint may be considered more involved than the long axis tractioning mentioned above, it is more specific to the joint capsule. Further, its line of pull is more perpendicular to the acetabulum than the long axis version.

Compression of the hip (Figures 9.62, 9.63)

If the therapist places his forearm, rather than his hand, over the greater trochanter they will be able to use their body-weight more easily and protect their wrist. However, be sure to use the soft tissue (muscle bellies of the flexors of the wrist and hand) portion of the forearm and not the bony edge of the ulna.

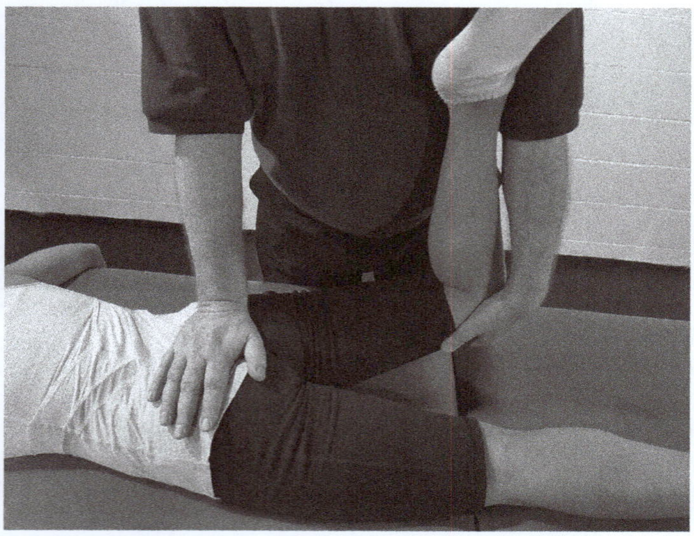

FIGURE 9.57 1. Hip extension

Ensure stabilization of the low back before proceeding with the test.

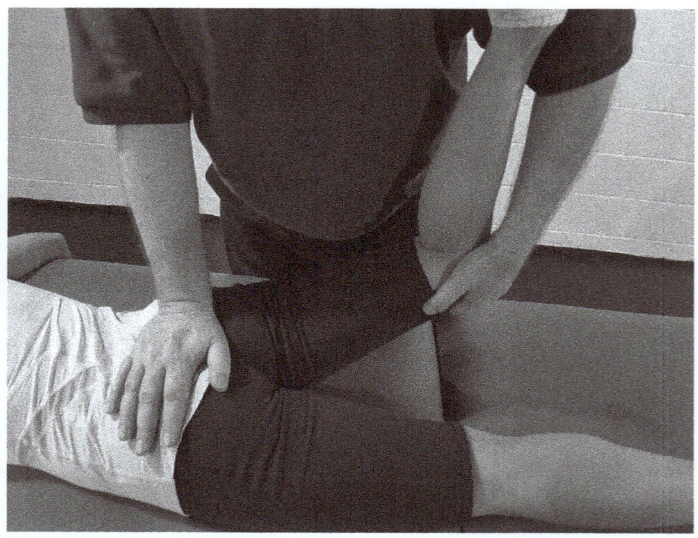

FIGURE 9.58 2. Hip extension with O-P

Apply O-P into hip extension. Ask about low back pain.

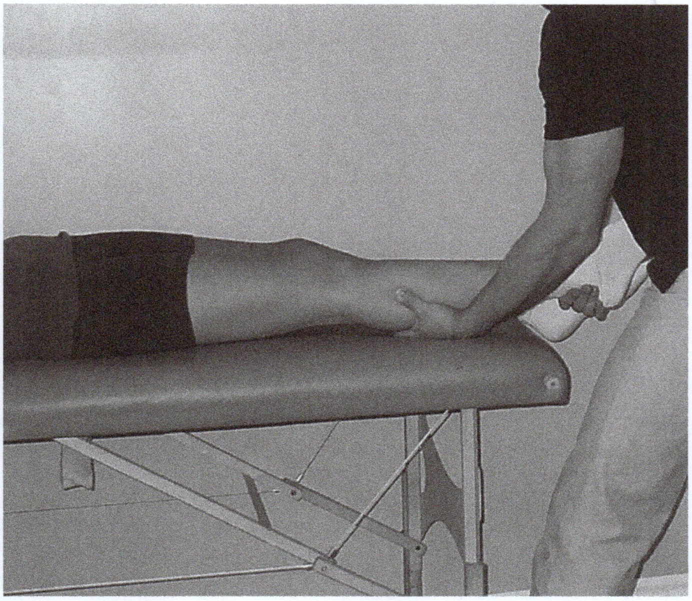

FIGURE 9.59 Classic long axis tractioning of hip

Cup the heel with one hand, and cup the heads of gastrocnemius just below the knee. Lean back pulling the whole leg inferiorly.

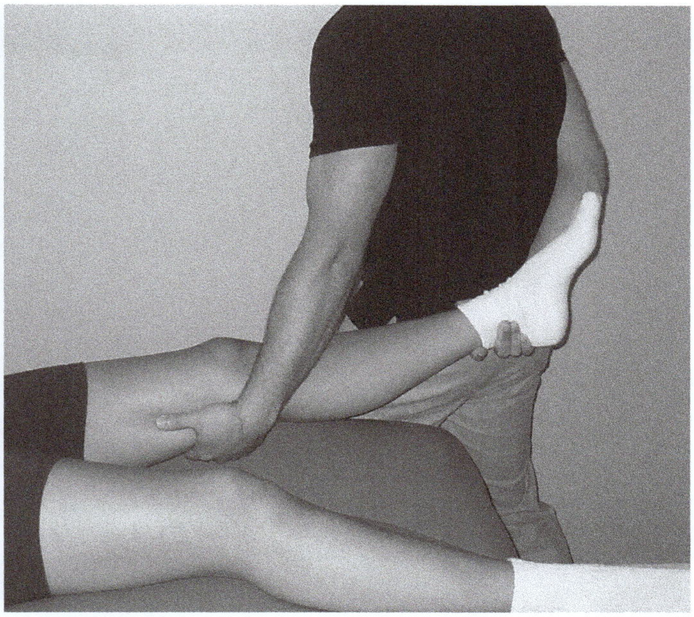

FIGURE 9.60 Alternative long axis tractioning of hip

Grasp the leg and hold with 15–30° of abduction and flexion, and let the leg externally rotate a bit as well. This creates the open packed position of the joint, a position of comfort for this joint. Traction the leg inferiorly. If the patient experiences any discomfort in the knee, place your superior hand under the thigh just above the knee. Use your body-weight to traction the patient's leg by simply transferring your weight to your back leg. This alternative method automatically positions the leg and hip in the open packed position.

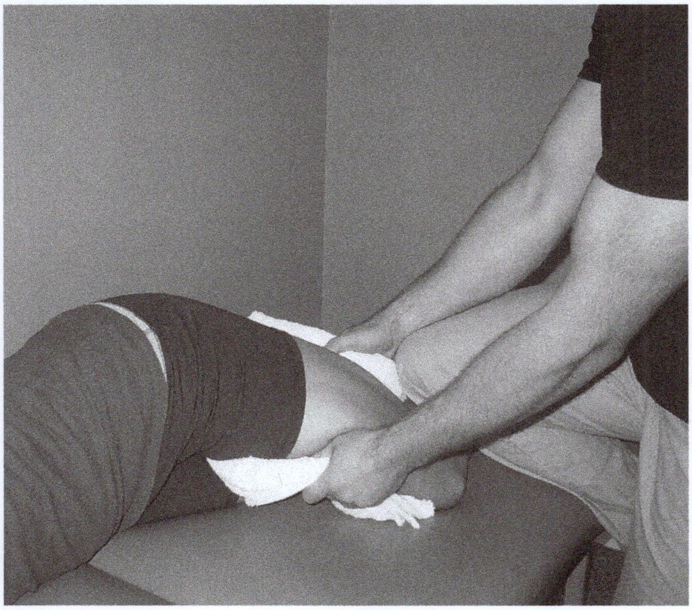

FIGURE 9.61 Hip distraction/decompression side-lying

With the patient side-lying, straighten the bottom leg and flex the upper leg so the knee rests on the table. Let the trunk roll slightly forward. Place a towel under the thigh to act as a sling for you to hang onto. Gently rest your knee on the distal thigh; you can place a folded towel over the patient's knee area to make this more comfortable. (We have not done the latter so that you can see positioning.) Now lean back, pulling on the towel to traction the hip. You need to stabilize (hold down) the knee otherwise it will lift off the table and the hip will be abducting without any significant distraction of the hip joint.

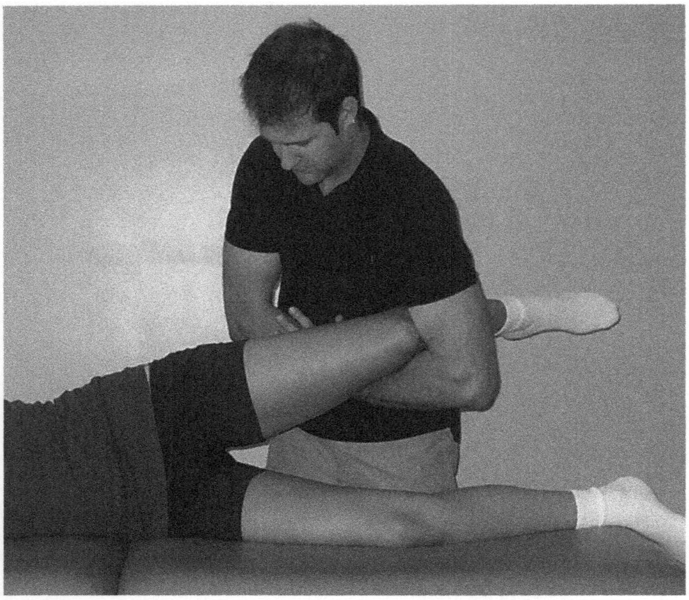

FIGURE 9.62 1. Positioning for compression of hip side-lying

Lift the patient's thigh into slight abduction, flexion, and external rotation. Hold this position with your forearm under the thigh.

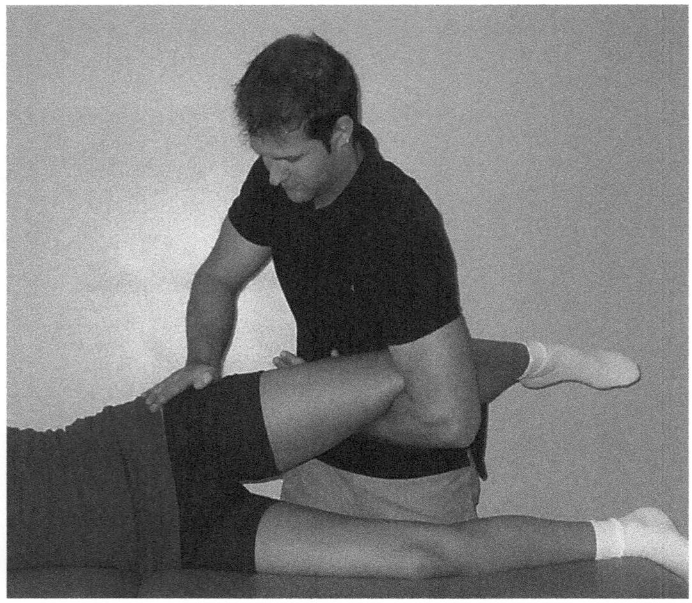

FIGURE 9.63 2. Compression of hip side-lying

Place the palm of the hand over the greater trochanter. Lean onto the trochanter to close pack or compress the joint.

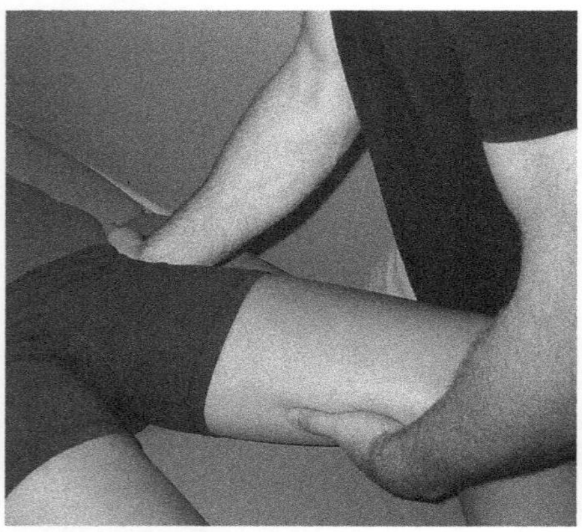

FIGURE 9.64 Posterior glide of hip in supine

Support under the distal portion of the thigh with one hand and let the hip and knee flex slightly. The heel of the foot is left on the table. Palpate for the greater trochanter and then place the thenar eminence of your hand on the anterior side. Lightly traction the leg and then lean onto the greater trochanter.

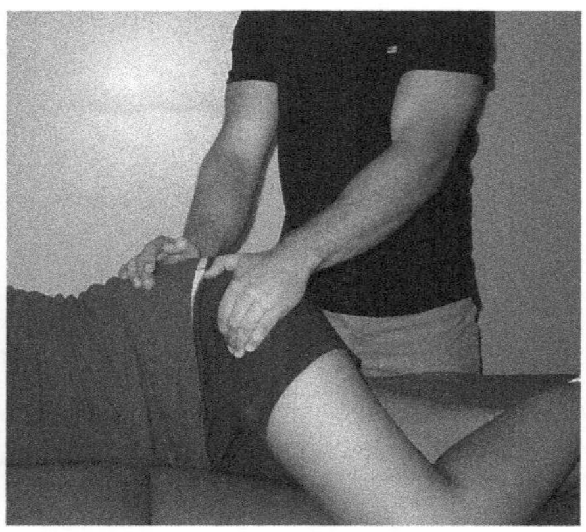

FIGURE 9.65 Posterior glide for hip side-lying

Stand behind the patient. Reverse hand positions: one hand stabilizing the hip over the PSIS and the other cupped over the anterior portion of the greater trochanter. Pull the trochanter toward you as you resist movement in the innominate at the PSIS.

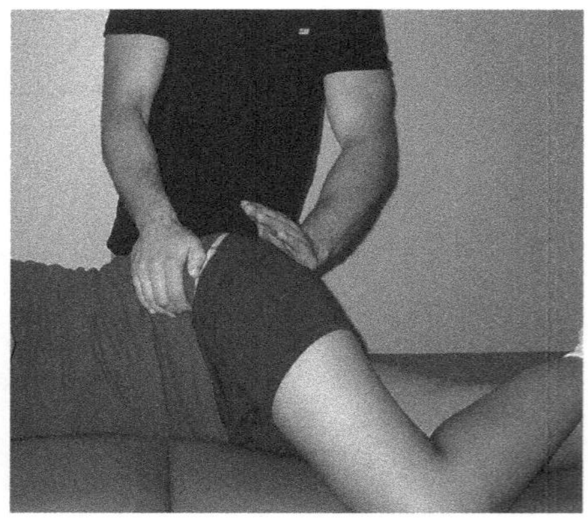

FIGURE 9.66 Anterior glide for hip side-lying

Have the patient's leg flexed forward at the hip and knee, with the lower leg straightened. With one hand, stabilize the hip with the fingers cupping the ASIS area of the innominate. Place the heel of your hand on the posterior area of the greater trochanter and push it forward.

Glides to hip joint can be seen above in Figures 9.64–9.66.

Active resisted range of motion (AR-ROM)

See Part I, Chapter 3 for a discussion of active resisted testing and what we learn from such testing, including a grading scale 0 to 5. (See Kendall et al. 2005 for a truly comprehensive exploration and instruction in muscle testing; see and compare: Dutton 2012; Hartley 2000b; Hertling & Kessler 2006; Magee 2014; Petty 2011.)

Perform active resisted testing with the patient supine/prone; or alternatively you may have them seated. If seated, have the patient sit with their arms crossed; otherwise, if their hands are on the table, they will often try to recruit the upper body to assist them. Remember the precautions for isometric testing:

- Perform all resistance testing at mid-range.
- Start with light exertion and slowly build up to full strength over five seconds, and then slowly reduce the exertion over five seconds.
- For thoroughness, hold at full strength if the patient can sustain this for at least five seconds.
- Use your body-weight to add resistance rather than pushing from your shoulder.
- When testing large or expectedly strong muscle, either sustain the exertion for longer (if the patient is holding strong) or repeat the test several times to fatigue a usually strong endurance muscle (e.g., the quadriceps or gastrocnemius).
- Finally, the testing is only considered specific to the contractile unit (and so differentiated from non-contractile joint structures) if it is truly isometric and no movement occurs at the joint.

The following AR-ROM testing is shown both in supine and seated positioning. The method you choose will depend on the patient's comfort and the positioning that feels safe and efficient for you. If you are concerned about the effect on an impaired low back, then have the patient crook-lying (if possible) to help prevent their low back muscles from any strain as they try to stabilize the area during testing. Further, if you are concerned that the patient will overpower you with their effort during testing you should position the patient so that they must resist your efforts.

AR-ROM hip flexion (Figures 9.67, 9.68A, B)

AR-ROM hip extension (Figures 9.69, 9.70)

External and internal rotation (Figures 9.71–9.74)

NOTE: External and internal rotation can only be effectively tested by resisting motion using the lower leg if the patient does

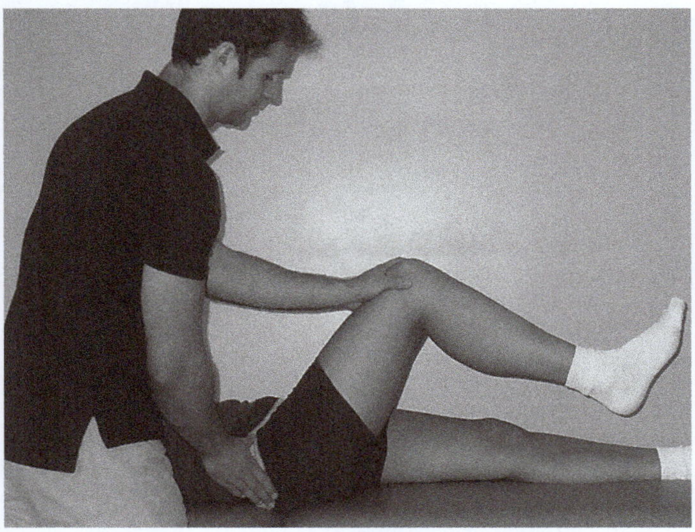

FIGURE 9.67 AR-ROM hip flexion in supine

Have the patient bend their hip 45° and knee at 90°. The patient should hold this and resist your effort to push their thigh back down. (The therapist in the illustration is not using two hands in order to show the area of applied resistance and how the patient is holding their leg.)

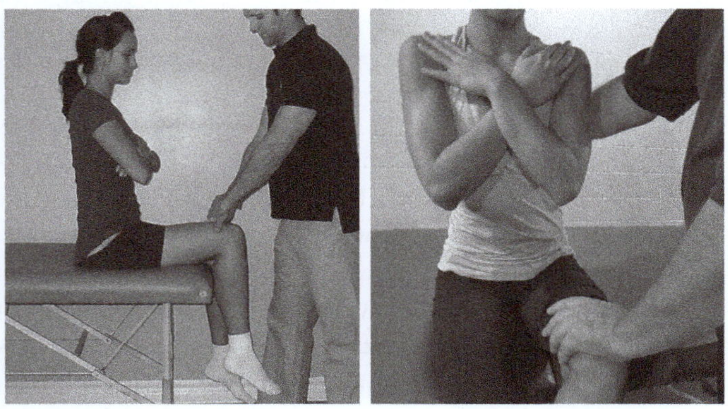

FIGURE 9.68A, B AR-ROM hip flexion seated

Patient sits with arms crossed, because if their hands are resting on the table they will recruit upper body strength to assist them. Have the patient lift the thigh off the table approximately 5–8 cm (2–3 inches) and hold the position as you push down. Make sure the patient is not leaning back. They often do so instinctively to prevent themselves from tipping forward. You may need to place a hand on their back which can help you gauge how much they are trying to assist by leaning back and also helps the patient to realize they are doing so.

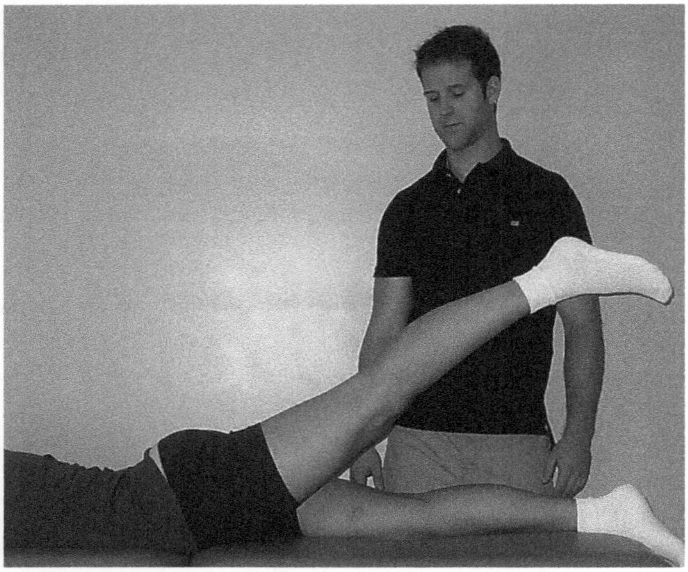

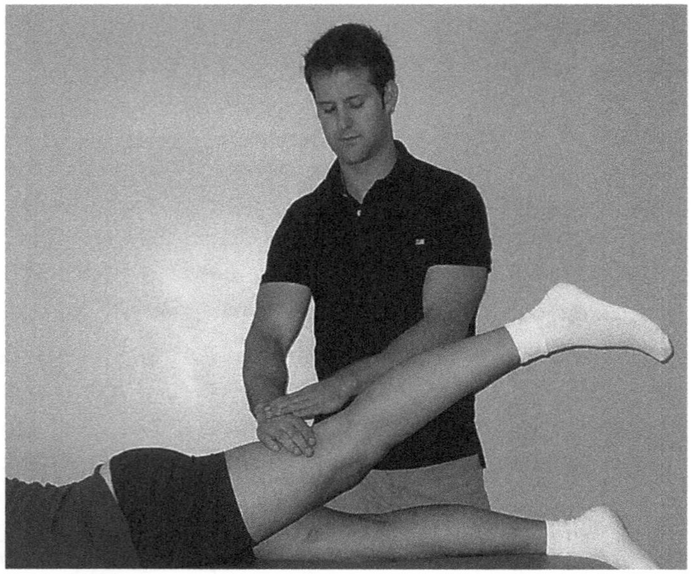

FIGURE 9.69 and Figure 9.70 AR-ROM testing of hip extension in prone

This test is done in two steps. 1. Have the patient extend their straight leg and hold it there. 2. If the patient can hold the leg in extension then apply pressure down toward the table, but do so just above the knee joint. These graduated steps help prevent many patients from being hurt doing the test. Only with a very strong patient would you then apply resistance on the lower leg, above the ankle.

not have an unstable or injured knee. To resist through the thigh will almost always result in the therapist only resisting the movement of muscle tissue, while the femur and the hip joint rotate beneath the tissue.

The following is done with the patient either supine (possibly crook-lying) or seated. It is important when using the lower leg to rotate the hip that the knee be kept in place. You may want to first show the patient the rotational motion that you want them to resist so they do not try to push the knee out (abducting the hip) or in (adducting the hip) while resisting rotation of the hip. Further, it is important to begin with a very light effort so that the patient both recruits all of the muscles needed to resist your effort, and also engages the appropriate muscles to stabilize the knee.

Abduction and adduction resistance testing (Figures 9.75, 9.76)

Alternative abduction and adduction resistance testing (Figures 9.77, 9.78)

An alternative test can be done with the supine patient only if the patient has no problems with their knees. The advantage of this version is that it is bilaterally testing. Since this uses a long lever

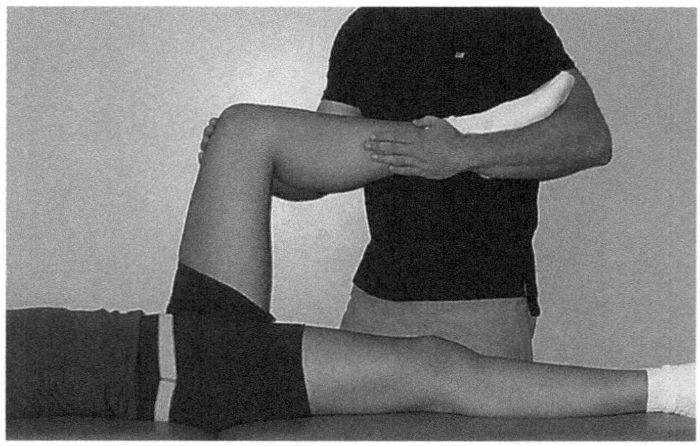

FIGURE 9.71 AR-ROM external rotation in supine

Place a supporting hand on the lateral side of the knee and the other hand and forearm on the medial side of the leg. Tell the patient you will start trying to take their foot away from the other leg, and so internally rotate their thigh with light pressure that will slowly increase. Ask the patient to match their resistance to your effort and try not to overpower you (which would also cause their hip to move).

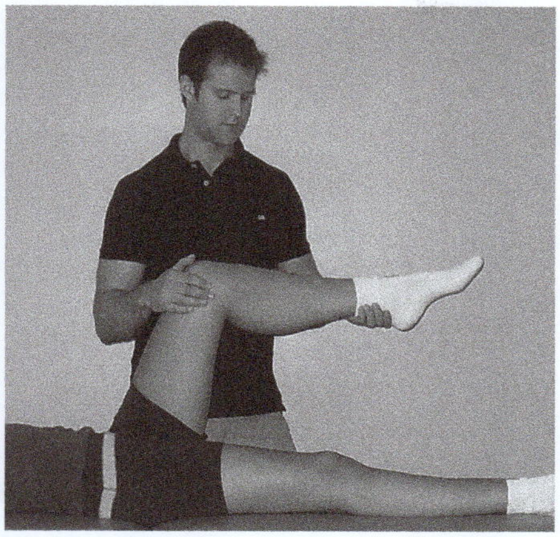

FIGURE 9.72 AR-ROM internal rotation in supine

To test internal rotation, place a supporting hand on the medial side of the knee. With your other hand, cup the ankle so the heel of your hand is on the lateral side of the tibia. Have the patient resist your effort to move the supported lower leg toward the unsupported leg and so try to externally rotate their thigh. Use caution, as mentioned above, when engaging the musculature.

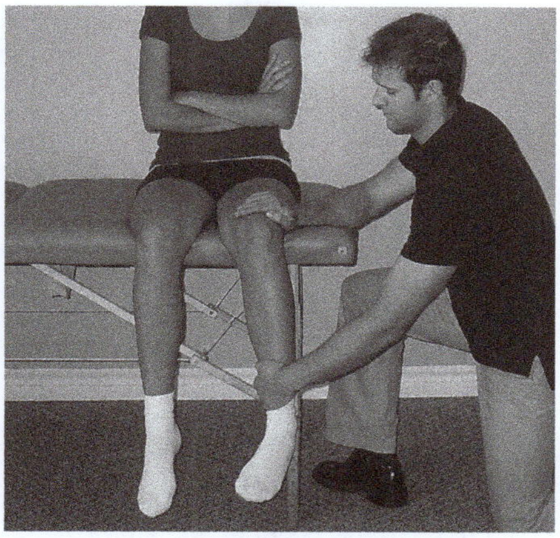

FIGURE 9.73 AR-ROM external rotation seated

Stabilize the patient's knee and grasp the ankle. The patient resists your effort to pull the lower leg toward you. Again, initial effort by the therapist should be light, building over five seconds to maximum.

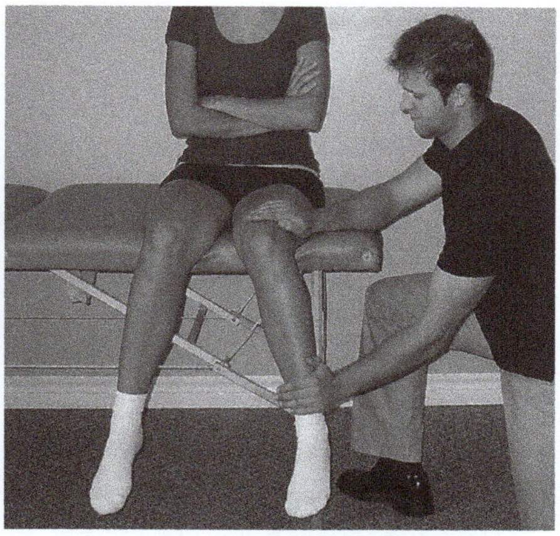

FIGURE 9.74 AR-ROM internal rotation seated

Stabilize the knee while the patient resists your effort to push the ankle toward the other leg.

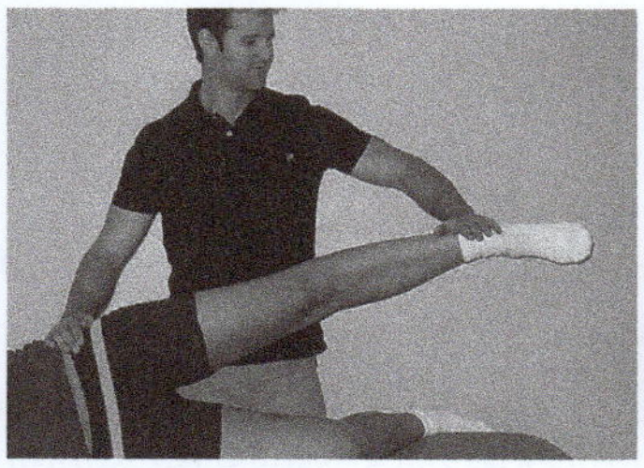

FIGURE 9.75 AR-ROM abduction of hip side-lying

The patient is side-lying with the downward leg bent, for stability. Lift the extended leg slightly into abduction and have the patient hold the position. If the patient can hold comfortably, then begin adding pressure.

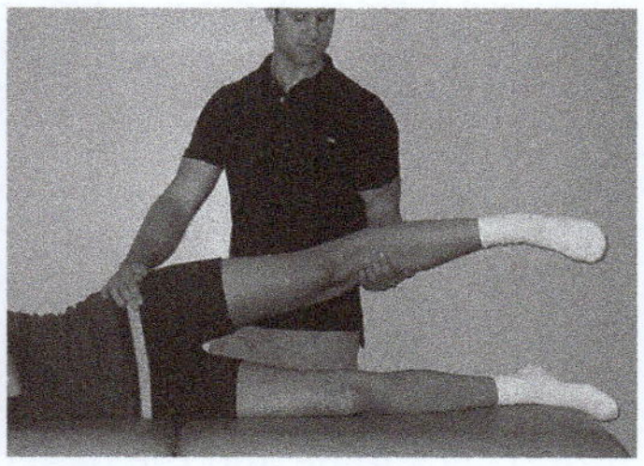

FIGURE 9.76 AR-ROM adduction of hip side-lying

With the patient in the same position (as for abduction) cup one hand under the leg just below the knee. Ask the patient to hold the position as you try to lift the leg. Alternatively, the patient can try to lower the leg.

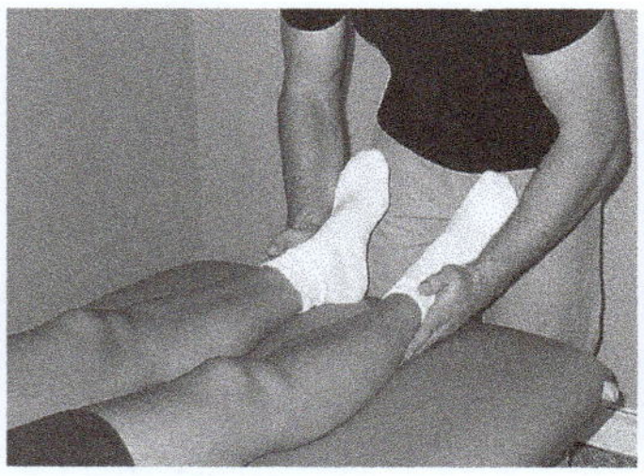

FIGURE 9.77 AR-ROM hip abduction in supine

For abduction, place a hand on the lateral distal portion of the leg just above the ankle and resist the patient's attempt to abduct.

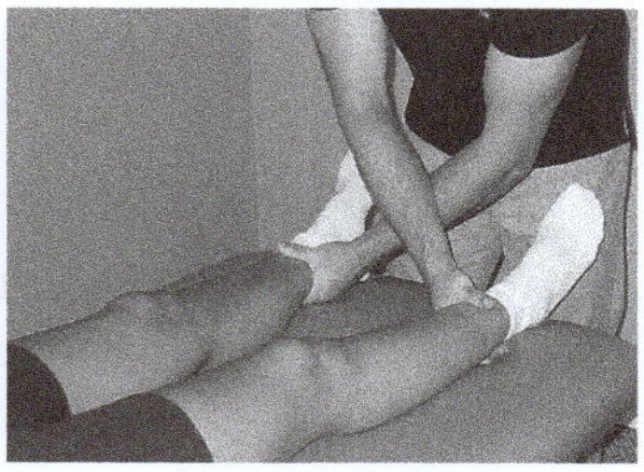

FIGURE 9.78 AR-ROM hip adduction in supine

For adduction, cross your forearms and place your hands on the medial portions of the patient's legs and resist the attempt to adduct.

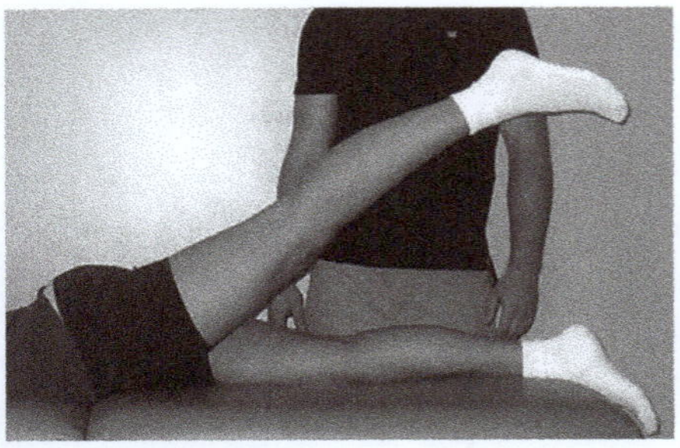

FIGURE 9.79 1. Initial testing gluteus maximus and hamstrings

Have the patient prone and lift the straight leg into extension. Have the patient hold position for a 5 to 10 seconds to see if they can do so.

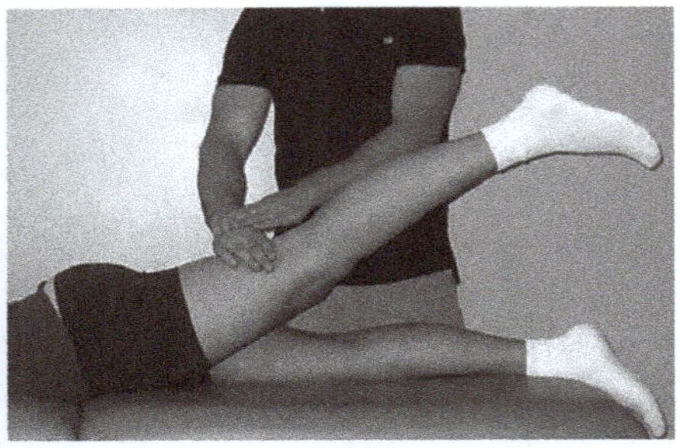

FIGURE 9.80 2. Testing gluteus maximus and hamstrings

If the patient can hold, then with your hand just above the back of the patient's knee, push the leg toward the table. This tests both muscles.

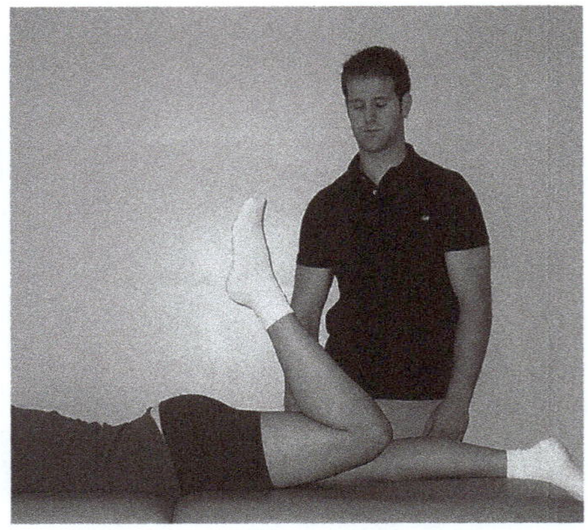

FIGURE 9.81 3. Focus on gluteus maximus alone

Flex the patient's knee to 90° and have them extend their hip. If the patient can hold this for several seconds then place your hand on the posterior thigh and push the thigh downward. You should expect a clear difference of strength now that the hamstrings have been made insufficient (too short to generate force).

approach, the therapist can easily resist the patient's attempt to do the motion.

Special tests

Differential muscle testing

The therapist uses differential muscle testing on muscles that have been implicated as impaired during AF-ROM or AR-ROM testing, or in which the patient's description of pain and/or dysfunction implicates the muscle. See Part I, Chapter 3. Positive signs for impairment are as for AR-ROM testing: pain and/or weakness (see Kendall et al. 2005).

For extension, differentiate between the gluteus maximus and the hamstrings. For hip flexion, differentiate between the iliopsoas and rectus femoris. Test separately the tensor fasciae latae, gluteus medius and minimus, medial and lateral hamstrings, and the sartorius specifically. It will require testing many different patients to get a feel for what is normal for various groups of people (e.g., athletes versus those who sit at a desk all day). Remember to ask about pain and/or weakness with each step in the process of differentiating. If you get a positive response then ask if this is the pain they presented with (i.e., their chief complaint).

Differentiating between gluteus maximus and hamstrings (Figures 9.79–9.81)

Differentiating between rectus femoris and iliopsoas

The test can be done supine or seated. If seated, patients should cross their arms across their chest to prevent compensating for weakness during testing by pushing off the table with their arms. If testing supine and the patient has low back issues, the supine position may be safer. In that case, have the untested side's hip and knee flexed (with foot on the table) (not done here in order to clearly show the testing procedure).

Seated testing (Figures 9.82, 9.83)

Supine testing (Figures 9.84, 9.85)

Alternative iliopsoas specific test (Figure 9.86)

This test is specific to the iliopsoas and is based on its ability to act as a hip flexor, an adductor, and an external rotator. The test is specific to the psoas because the psoas will be the only muscle that can, and must, exert itself to do all three actions at once. Therefore, it takes the greatest stress.

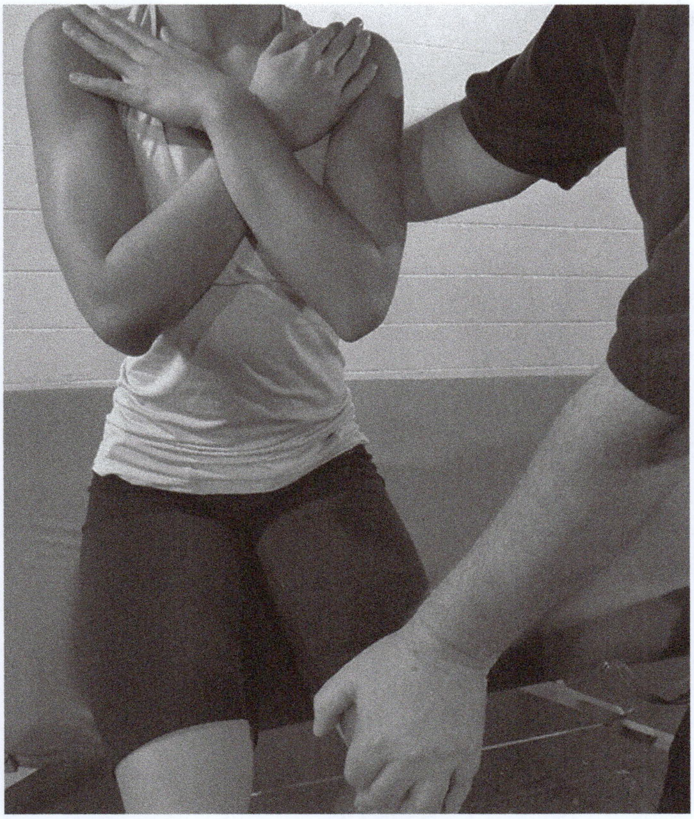

FIGURE 9.82 **1. Testing rectus femoris and iliopsoas together**

Have the patient try to lift their thigh off table as you resist. This tests hip flexors in general.

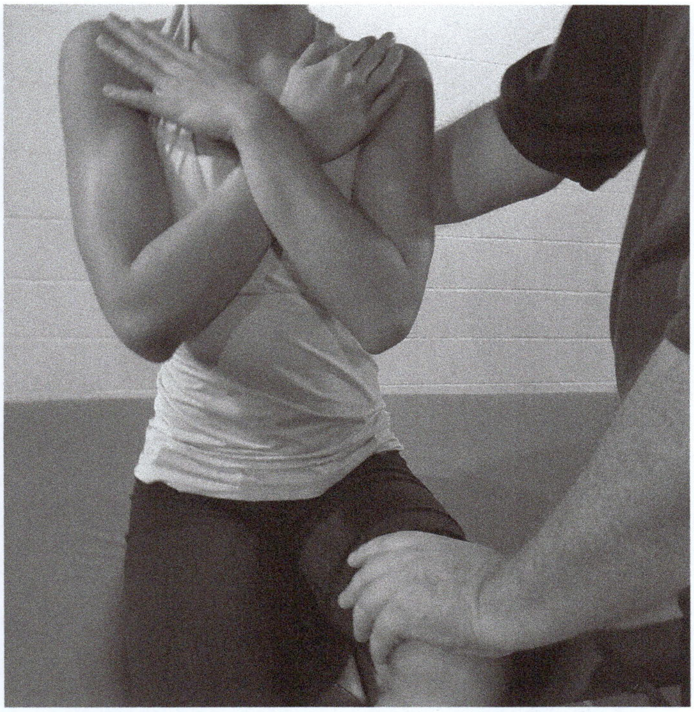

FIGURE 9.83 **2. Testing iliopsoas specifically**

By lifting the thigh off the table, rectus femoris (and other hip flexors attached on innominate) become too short and, hence, too weak to provide much resistance to hip flexion. The only muscle still able to provide significant resistance is iliopsoas. Compare with result from test 1.

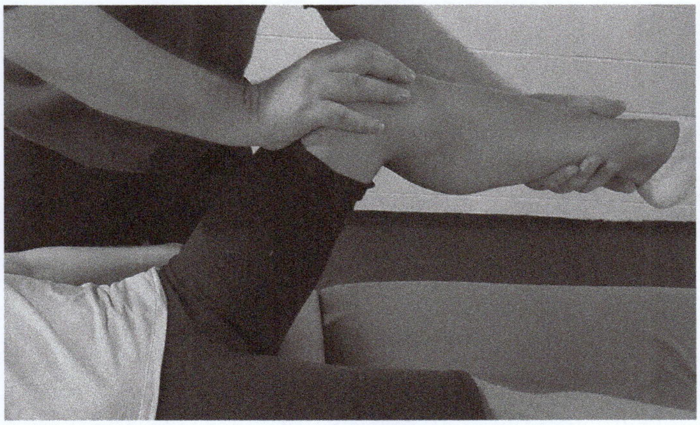

FIGURE 9.84 **1. Testing rectus femoris and iliopsoas together in supine**

Have the patient lift the foot off the table without flexing the hip as much as 90°. Ask the patient to resist your attempt to push the leg back into the table.

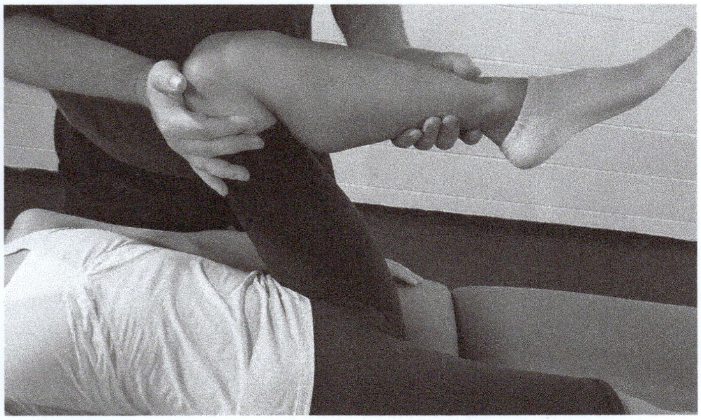

FIGURE 9.85 **2. Differentiating iliopsoas from rectus femoris in supine**

Have the patient flex the hip as high as they can. Press the thigh into extension as the patient resists. This stresses the iliopsoas primarily. Compare this result with test 1 above.

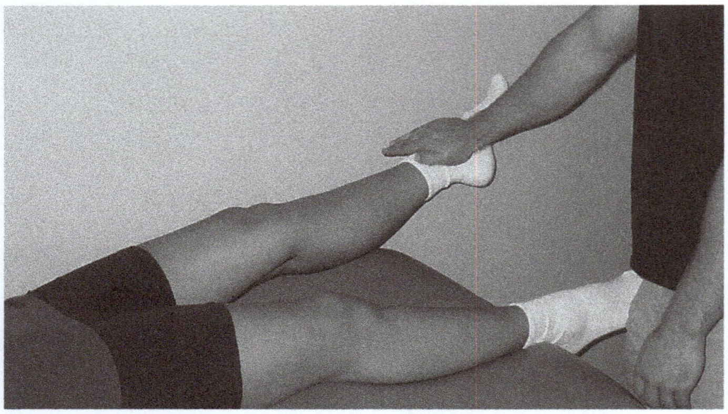

FIGURE 9.86 Specific iliopsoas test

With your assistance, have the patient slightly flex the hip to 20–30°, with the knee extended and the hip abducted approximately 10–20°. Externally rotate the leg. As a long lever, you may wish to first just have the patient hold the position for 5–10 seconds after you remove your assisting hand. To increase exertion, if needed, push down just above the ankle and slightly out into abduction as the patient tries to hold the leg in the air.

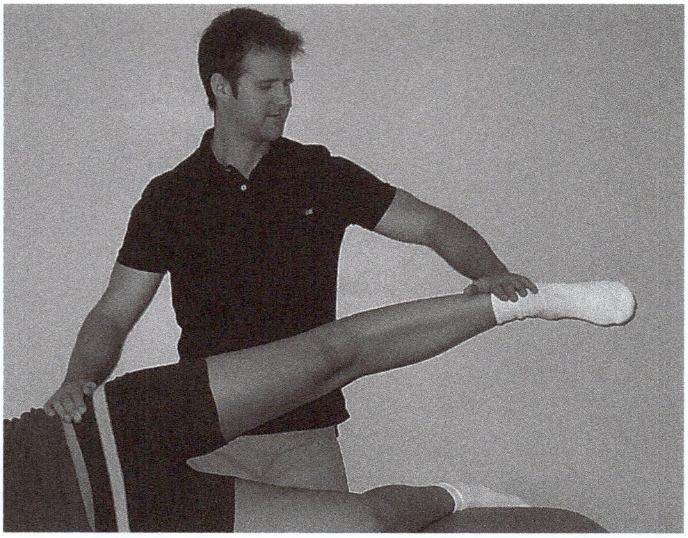

FIGURE 9.87 1. Test minimus and medius

Have the patient abduct the leg straight and hold and resist as you try to push it back toward the table. This tests both muscles.

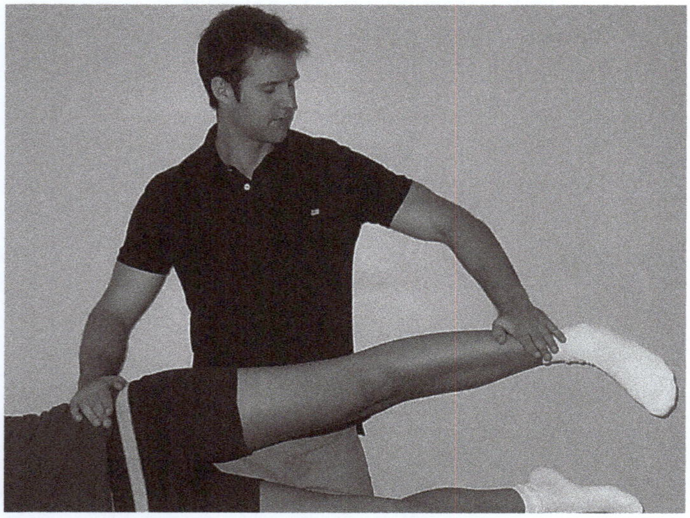

FIGURE 9.88 2. Test minimus specifically

To stress minimus more, slightly internally rotate the patient's whole leg and then push down and slightly toward extension.

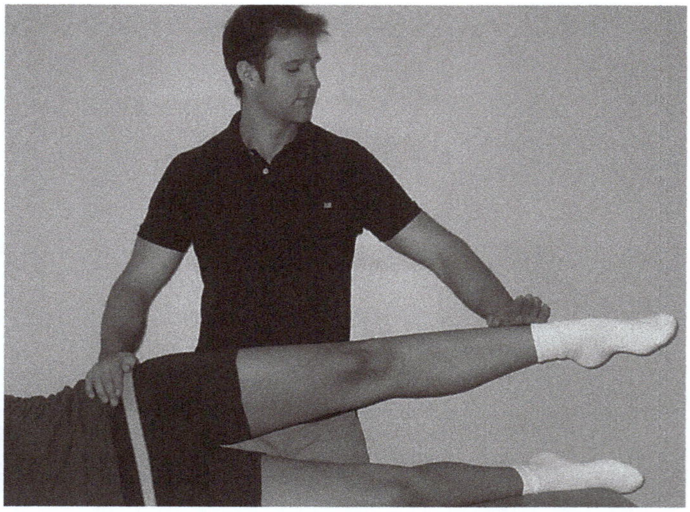

FIGURE 9.89 3. Stress medius specifically

To stress medius more, position as in the original test for both muscles but with slight external rotation to the leg, then push down and slightly into flexion. This stresses primarily posterior fibers of medius.

NOTE: The positioning seen in Figure 9.86 (Iliopsoas test) can be very useful when palpating the psoas. With the patient crook-lying, straighten the leg on the side to be tested. Palpate down through the lower abdomen over where the psoas should be. Holding the leg at the ankle, lift it off the table until the hip is flexed 20–30° and the knee extended. Slightly abduct the leg 10–20° and let it slightly externally rotate. Now, tell the patient you are going to remove your hand and they are to hold the leg in place. This will cause the psoas to push up into your palpating fingers. (Repetition of the patient holding this position with you palpating the psoas can also be a release technique for the muscle.)

Differential testing between gluteus minimus and gluteus medius (Figures 9.87–9.89)

Have the patient side-lying with the leg to be tested facing up and with the knee extended. The untested leg can be flexed at the hip and the knee to stabilize the patient.

Differential testing between hamstrings (Figures 9.90–9.92)

Compare the results and the patient's responses to questions about pain, and weakness or strain between all three testing positions as done in the order shown in Figures 9.90–9.92.

Specific test for tensor fasciae latae (TFL) (Figure 9.93)

The TFL muscle assists in flexing, abducting, and internally rotating the hip.

Specific test for sartorius (Figure 9.94)

When doing this test the patient is performing all of the actions that the sartorius muscle does: flexion, internal/medial rotation of the hip, and extension of the knee. During this test, the therapist is resisting flexion and internal rotation of the hip and flexion of the knee.

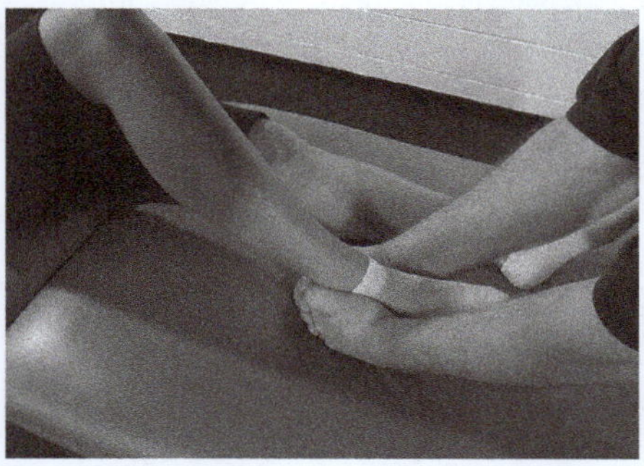

FIGURE 9.90 Testing hamstrings as a group

Interlace your fingers around the patient's ankle and lift the foot off the table about two inches. Ask the patient to try and bring the heel toward the buttocks. Resist the patient's attempt to flex the knee.

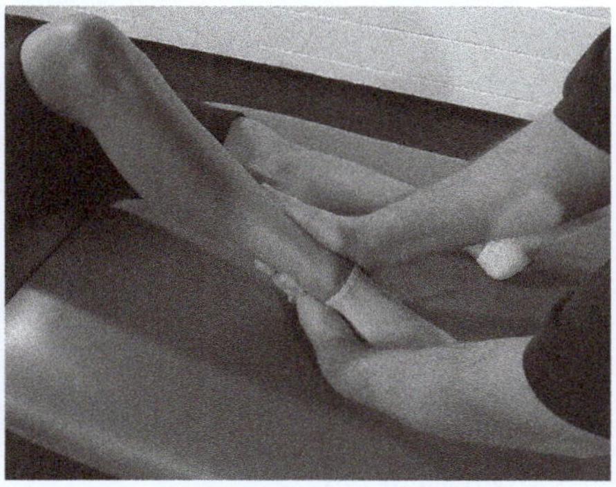

FIGURE 9.91 Testing biceps femoris hamstrings

To test the biceps femoris set of hamstrings externally rotate the lower leg (i.e., tibia) and foot. Grasp the heel and again lift the foot off the table about two inches. Tell the patient to pull the heel to the buttocks. Alternatively, you can ask the patient to hold the position as described above while you pull the heel toward you, trying to extend the knee.

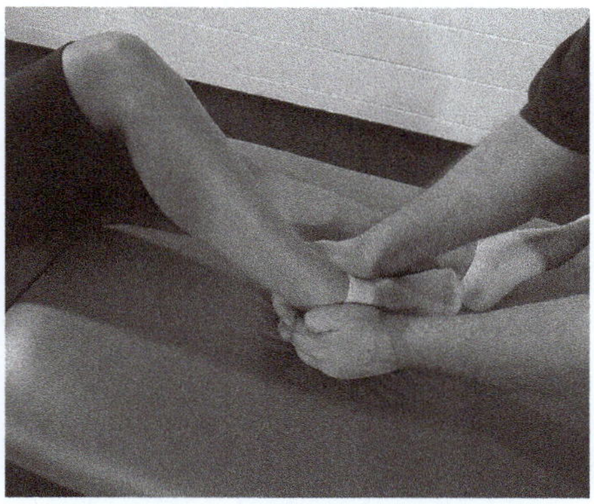

FIGURE 9.92 Testing semimembranosus/tendinosus

Test the semimembranosus and semitendinosus by internally rotating the lower leg then proceed as above.

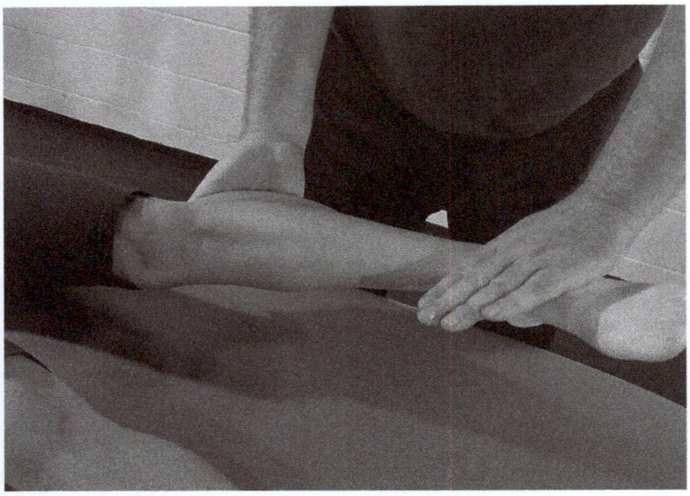

FIGURE 9.93 Testing tensor fasciae latae

Passively move the patient's lower limb so that you slightly flex the hip with the knee extended. Slightly abduct and internally rotate the leg. With one hand just above the knee on the superior-lateral surface of the thigh, push down diagonally toward the other leg, which is on the table (i.e., into extension and adduction).

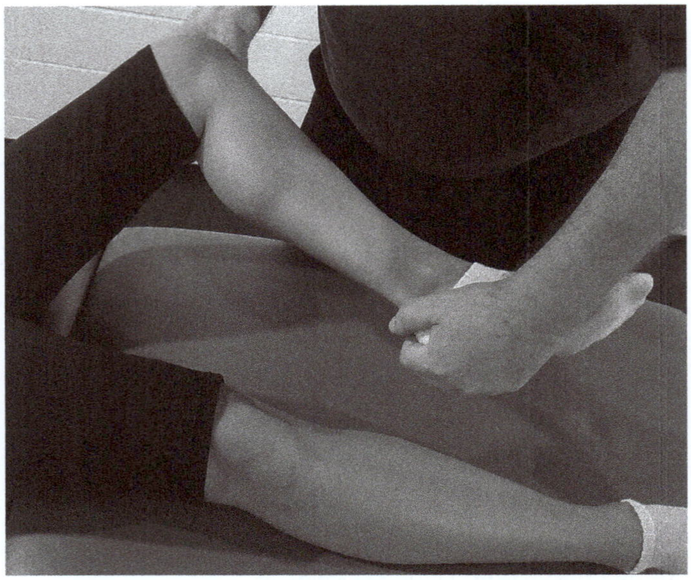

FIGURE 9.94 Testing sartorius

Passively place the patient's leg into a figure-4 position. Inform the patient that you are going to take the leg slightly back out of this position. Move the patient's leg into an open figure-4 (hip flexed at about 45°). Ask the patient to try to go back into a complete figure-4 position while you resist this effort.

Classic Thomas test (Figure 9.95)

This test was originally designed to test for a contracture of the psoas muscle. The classic or simple Thomas test is as follows:

The patient is lying supine on the table. Have the patient flex their knee to about 90° by sliding their heel along the table. Now, fully flex one hip until the lumbar spine loses its lordosis and is flat against the table. The therapist must sustain this flat back (i.e., reduce the lumbar lordosis and potential anterior pelvic tilt) by applying O-P on the untested hip as the patient is instructed to now extend the unsupported leg.

The test is positive for contracture if the extended thigh remains significantly off the table surface. Although a shortened psoas will not permit full extension of the leg, it will not appear as dramatic as a contracture. The test works because the pelvis is prevented from moving anteriorly by the therapist holding the untested leg in full hip flexion with the lumbar spine held flat against the table. If the therapist permits anterior rotation the test may appear negative.

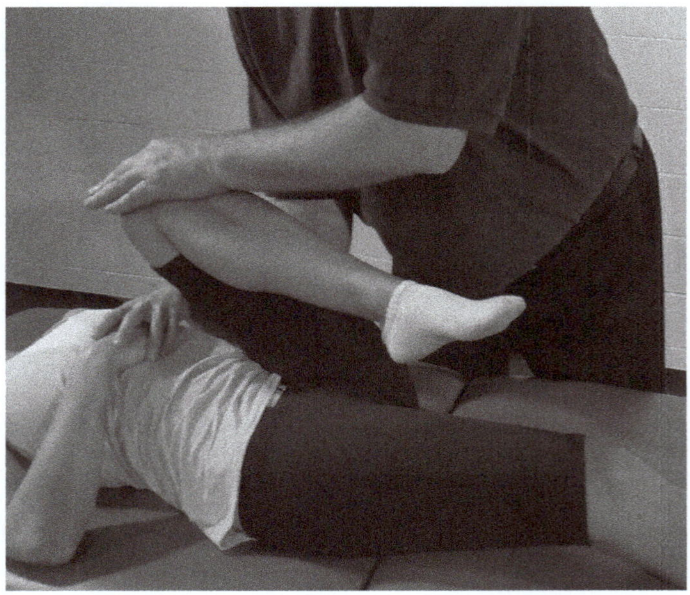

FIGURE 9.95 Classic Thomas test

Modified Thomas test (Figures 9.96–9.101)

This test can tell the therapist about the length of several muscles around the hip by changing the way the test is done slightly

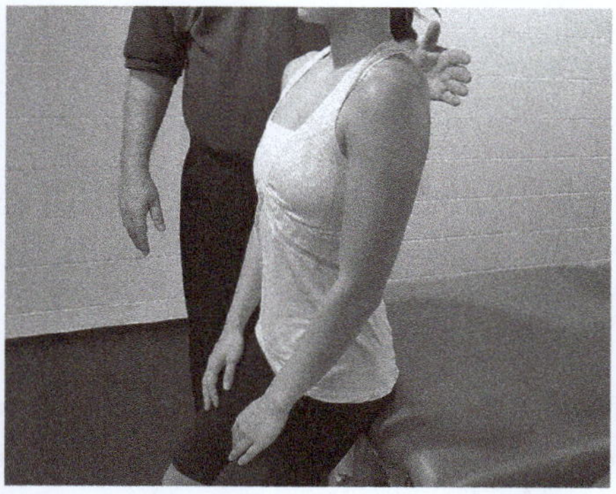

FIGURE 9.96 1. Positioning for modified Thomas test

Have the patient stand at the end of the table and then perch the buttocks on the edge of the table. Inform the patient that you want them to try and keep the arch in their low back to a minimum during the testing.

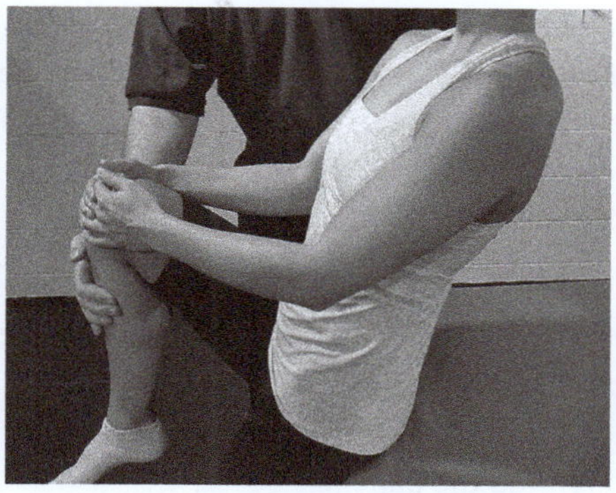

FIGURE 9.97 2. Positioning for modified Thomas test

Ask the patient to bring one knee to the chest and then lean backward onto the table.

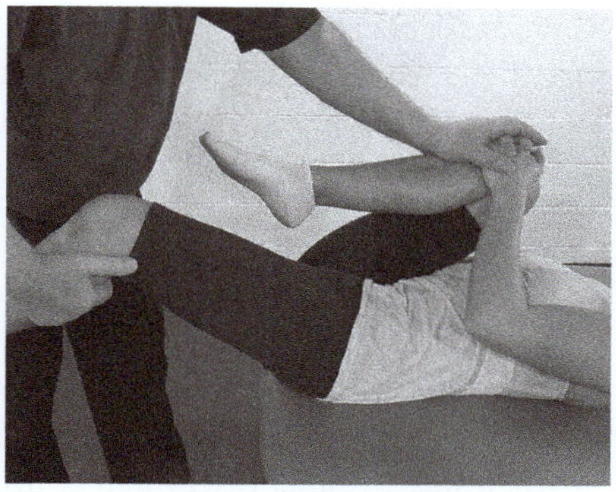

FIGURE 9.98 3. Positioning for modified Thomas test

Support and guide movement by supporting the patient's back with one hand and help raise the other extended leg as the patient lies back.

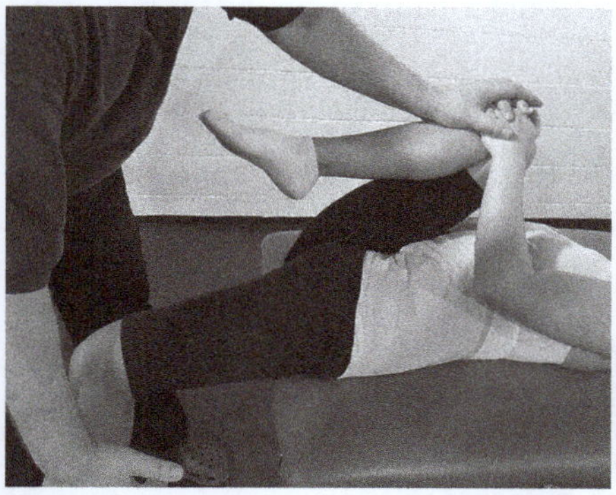

FIGURE 9.99 4. Positioning for modified Thomas test

Apply pressure to the patient's flexed knee to keep the low back relatively flat on the table. Be sure not to apply too much force so that the hip is actually posteriorly rotated. This can give false positive for psoas length. Observe the position of the free leg.

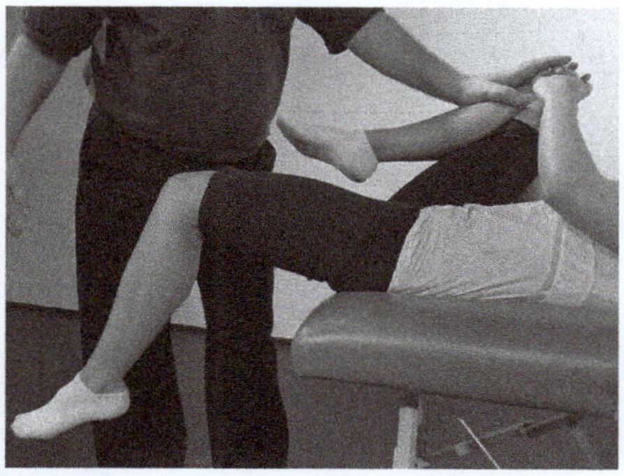

FIGURE 9.100 5. Example of contractured iliopsoas

The hip remains clearly flexed.

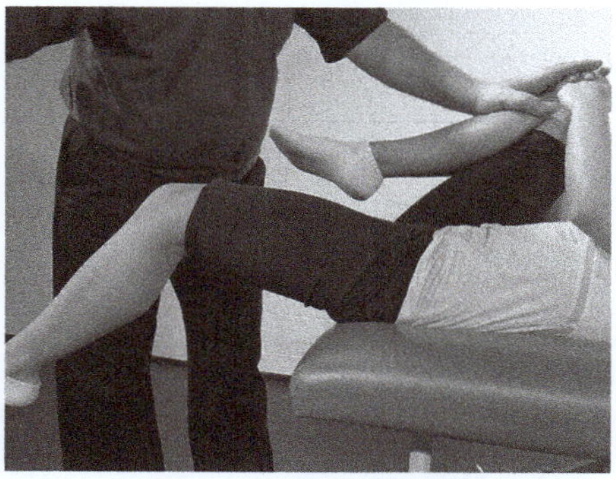

FIGURE 9.101 6. Example of tight and short rectus femoris

The knee is clearly extended if rectus femoris is short.

and by observing several potential movements or positions that the tested leg may display. In addition to hip flexors, we are also testing the adductors, abductors, and rotators (Hartley 2000b; Hertling & Kessler 2006). This test works well for chronic impairments, but its positioning is not suited to acute or even subacute stages of hip impairment.

Important note

Confirm all *apparent shortening of muscles* by applying a little O-P in the direction of the movement each muscle would allow if it was of normal length. The lower limb will spring back to the original starting position if it is really short or tight, and the patient may complain of pain or discomfort with the O-P, which is due to overstretching. We are talking about moving the limb only a couple of centimeters (roughly an inch), or less, just enough to increase tension on the muscle. If it really "wants" to be where it was positioned, it will bounce back there. However, if the patient was holding the limb there, then it will move to its real length. Therefore, this O-P procedure helps to ensure the accuracy of the testing.

However, do not further stretch any *apparently long muscles*! Rather, shorten the muscle slightly and see if it falls back to where it was. In either case, you may need to remind the patient to "relax and let go" if you suspect that they are still holding the limb tense or are actively moving the limb further than it would otherwise move.

These confirmations are necessary since the patient will often feel that they are in a precarious position, even though they are not. Therefore some holding, guarding, or other unintentional movements are to be expected when conducting this test.

Positive signs for other muscles (Figures 9.102, 9.103)

***Details and further actions to help clarify possible results of the Modified Thomas test*:**

- The thigh remains slightly flexed and not parallel to the table top (picture 5). This indicates a tight iliopsoas. Confirm with gentle O-P on the thigh by pressing it into further flexion. A firm, leathery feel (little or no give) implies contracture. Springiness implies hypertonus (tight and short).
- The knee does not flex to 100–110° (picture 6), but remains at a higher angle of 110–140°. This indicates a tight rectus femoris. Confirm with O-P applied to the leg near the ankle, flexing the knee.
- If the knee is flexed more than 90° (picture 7), then one can suspect a tight sartorius if the angle is 85–70°. Confirm with O-P by pulling (at the ankle) the knee slightly toward extension.
- If, as in picture 8, the leg has swung out laterally (more than the normal 10–15°), it may mean that the hip abductors, gluteus minimus and medius, including the TFL and ITB, are tight. Confirm with O-P into adduction.
- If the leg is positioned medially (less than 5° of abduction), it implies tight hip adductors. Confirm with O-P into abduction.
- If the thigh (and not just the lower leg/tibia) is rotated laterally, it implies tight lateral rotators including the piriformis. To confirm, roll the thigh toward medial rotation and see whether it comes back out into the laterally rotated position.
- If the thigh appears to be in neutral but the lower leg is excessively laterally rotated it implies: (1) tight biceps femoris

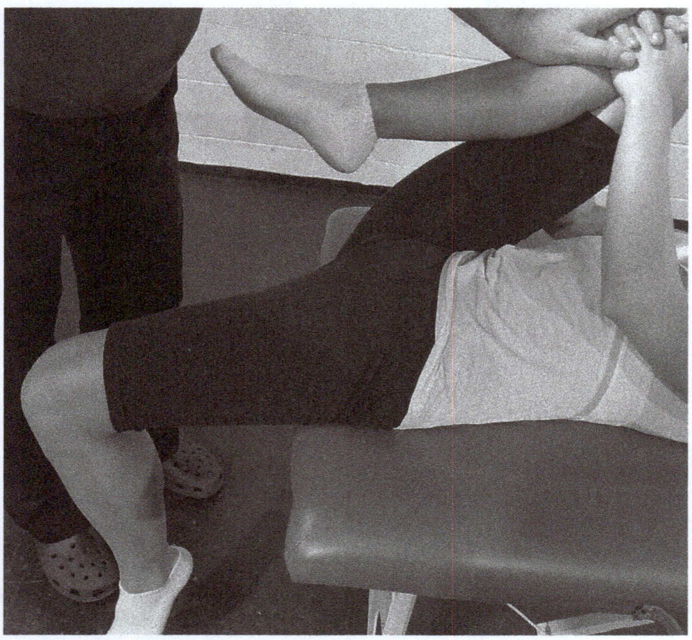

FIGURE 9.102 7. Example of tight and short sartorius

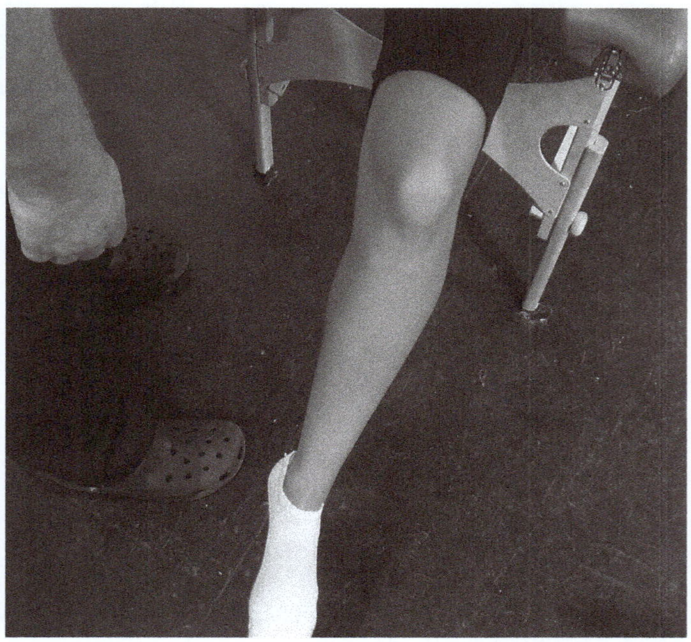

FIGURE 9.103 8. Neutral thigh with lateral tibial rotation

(especially if the thigh is also abducted); (2) a tight or contractured ITB; or (3) both. Confirm the first possibility with O-P of medial rotation to the tibia. To rule out ITB involvement, do the Ober's test below.

- On the other hand, if the tibia is medially rotated, it may imply there is a tight semimembranosus and semitendinosus, and/or popliteus.

Ober's test (iliotibial band test) (Figures 9.104–9.109)

This test was specifically designed to test for iliotibial band contracture. This is a much more difficult test to do than many orthopedic textbooks would have you believe. The most common cause of a false positive is the inferior movement of the pelvis due to the weight of the limb. The therapist has to be diligent in doing the test correctly, and strong enough to hold the pelvis from moving. Another reason for a false positive is improper positioning of the leg so that the iliotibial band has not moved over the greater trochanter. We will address both these concerns below.

The therapist now takes the hand closest to the patient's hip and places it firmly over the posteriolateral portion of the gluteus medius (just posterior and superior to the greater trochanter). You will need to apply a very firm support to stabilize the pelvis and prevent it from slipping inferiorly as you proceed with the test. Alternatively, you can use your forearm if it is carefully placed just under the iliac crest. Avoid making excessive contact (as best as possible) with the bulk of the gluteus maximus, the ITB and the TFL, otherwise you will shorten or put tension through the ITB. This would give a false positive result.

NOTE: If you choose to do the test using your forearm, be sure to apply your force through the fleshy anterior part of your forearm to avoid bone-on-bone contact (with the ilia), which will cause the patient pain. An advantage of the original Ober's test is that the flexion of the knee helps to decrease the weight of the leg as a whole and thus, makes it easier to stabilize the innominate.

If there is nerve pain or parathesia elicited during the test it may come from the femoral nerve, which can be placed on stretch when the knee is flexed (Magee 2014; Starkey & Brown 2015).

Modified Ober's test (straight leg)

The alternative version of the Ober's test is to repeat as above but with the knee extended. The straight leg should be able to lower at least to the height of the table with the ankle and

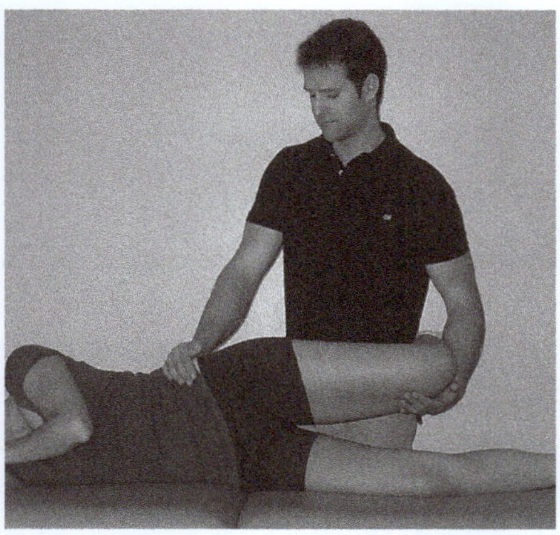

FIGURE 9.104 1. Original Ober's test

The therapist stands close to the table behind the side-lying patient who has been instructed to move close toward the edge of the table. Both hips and knees should be flexed: hips slightly (for patient stability) and knee to 90°. Support the patient's uppermost leg with your forearm with your hand under the medial side of the knee.

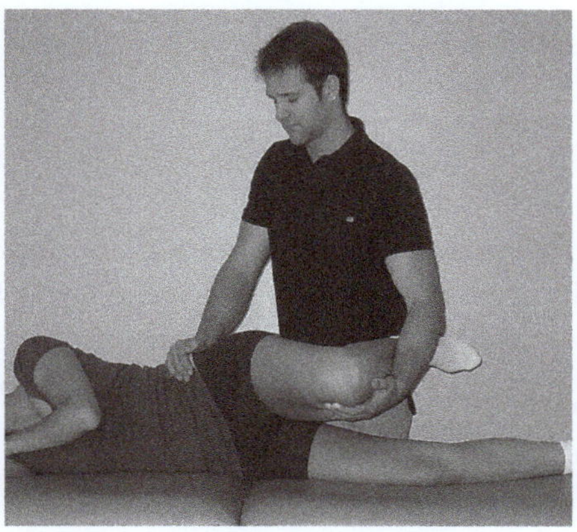

FIGURE 9.105 2. Original Ober's test

First move the hip forward into slightly more flexion.

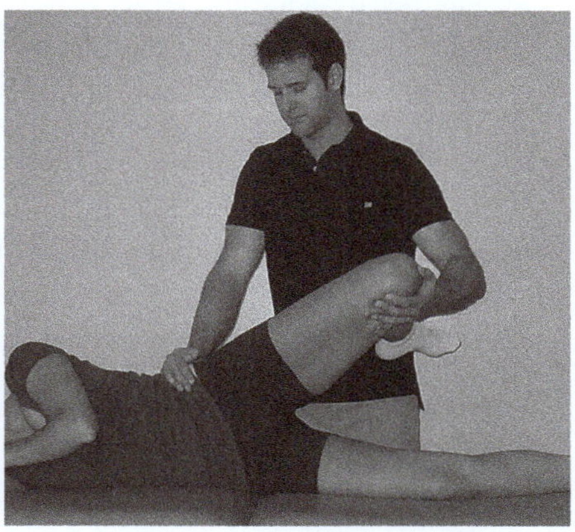

FIGURE 9.106 3. Original Ober's test

Now lift the limb up.

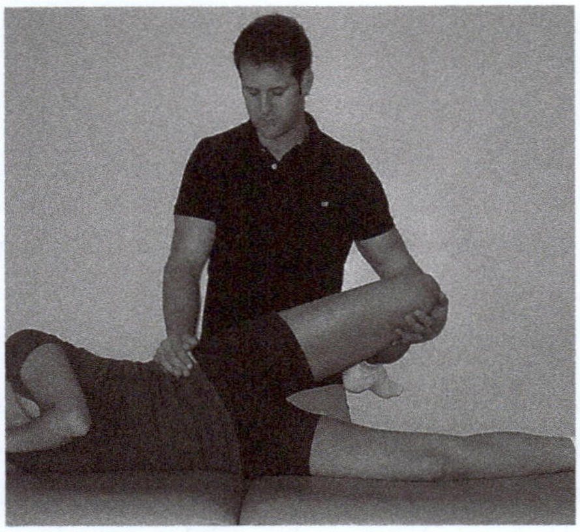

FIGURE 9.107 4. Original Ober's test
Then take it back into extension. This motion is a circumduction of the hip. This movement places the ITB on top of the greater trochanter. This is required for the test to work; otherwise you may get a false negative (length appearing normal). Having the ITB over the greater trochanter helps to ensure the ITB is not allowed to lengthen by being held either behind or in front of the trochanter. At this point, continue to hold the limb abducted.

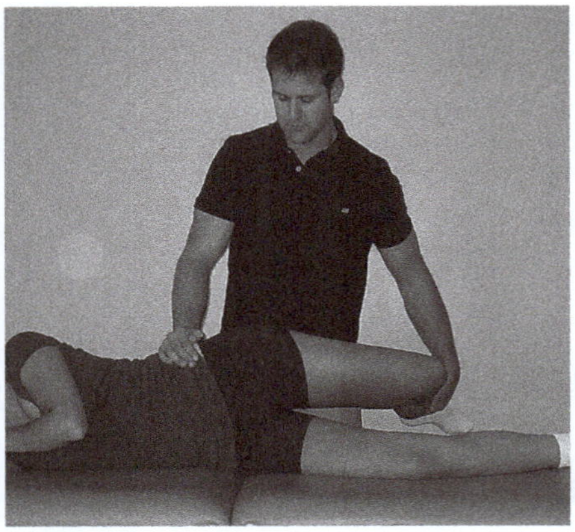

FIGURE 9.108 5. Original Ober's test
With the innominate stabilized, lower the limb to the table with the knee still bent. Ensure the thigh/femur does not externally or internally rotate as either rotation will slacken the ITB (which needs to remain over the greater trochanter). Use your hand on the lower leg to keep the femur in neutral position.

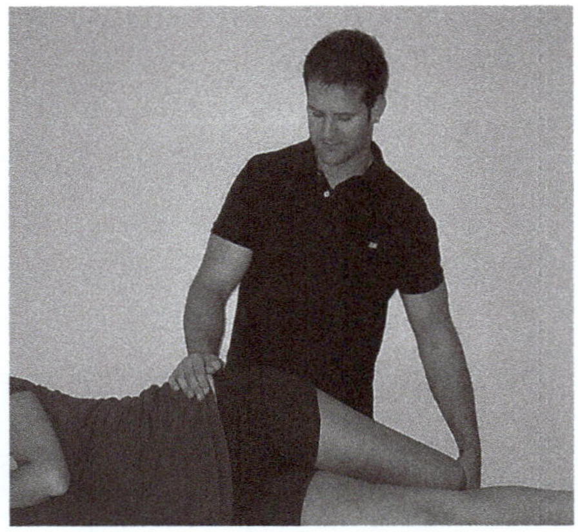

FIGURE 9.109 6. Original Ober's test
The test is negative if the knee can move down to the table or below. The test is positive if the leg remains horizontal (severe ITB contracture) or remains significantly off the table (moderate contracture). If the knee drops noticeably but is still quite a way from the table the ITB may be tight but not contractured.

foot even lower. If you positioned the patient close to you, as described above, and the whole limb is in some extension, then the lower leg should come down just off the table.

Be aware that a straight leg places weight further from the hip joint, and with such leverage, it will easily cause the superior innominate to move inferiorly. This results in a false negative. Also, the leverage in this position demands that the therapist has the weight and strength to resist the inferior motion of the hip in order to stabilize it. Without proper positioning of the forearm the test would render a false positive result. This modified version of the Ober's test is inordinately difficult, and this author suggests leaving it out of your hip-testing repertoire.

Piriformis length tests (Figure 9.110)

These two tests are variations on length tests for the piriformis. The first test shown is the one that is commonly used. It can be very specific in its stress to the piriformis as it reduces the impact of the other lateral rotators because of the positioning. The test transforms the piriformis into a medial/internal rotator when the hip is flexed to 90°. If the patient does not feel the stretch deep beneath the gluteus maximus you can presume it is close to normal length. However, gauging the length of the muscle can be a matter of interpretation. Hip joint pathologies may make this positioning difficult for the patient.

Alternate piriformis length test (Figures 9.111–9.115)

An advantage of this alternate version of the piriformis length test is that it allows for a more accurate measurement of the length of the muscle. It also allows for palpation of the muscle's tone.

Internally and externally rotate the hip while palpating deep to the gluteus maximus. The piriformis should be palpable as it tightens when you internally rotate the hip. A very hypertonic or spasming piriformis can be felt even when the hip is externally rotated (i.e., with the muscle shortened).

If the lower leg will not move significantly past 90° while internally rotating the hip, the piriformis is very short,

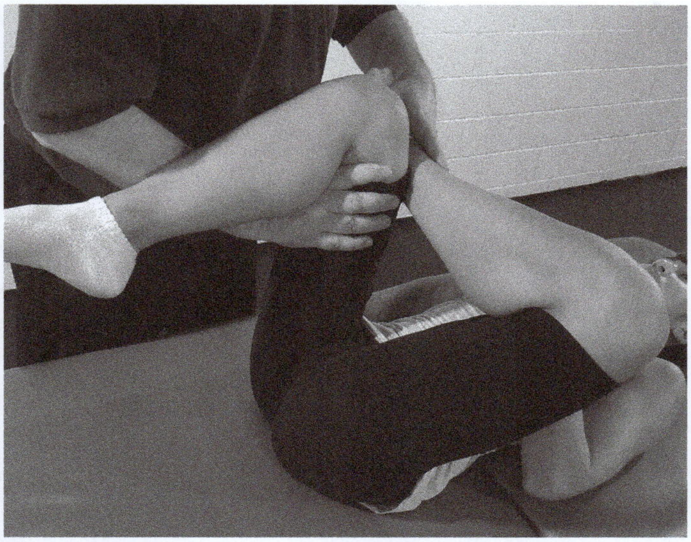

FIGURE 9.110 Common piriformis length test

The patient is in crook-lying position on the table with the ankle on the side to be tested placed on the opposite knee in a somewhat modified figure-4 position. Assist the patient in lifting the supporting leg into flexion, which will place a stretch on the piriformis.

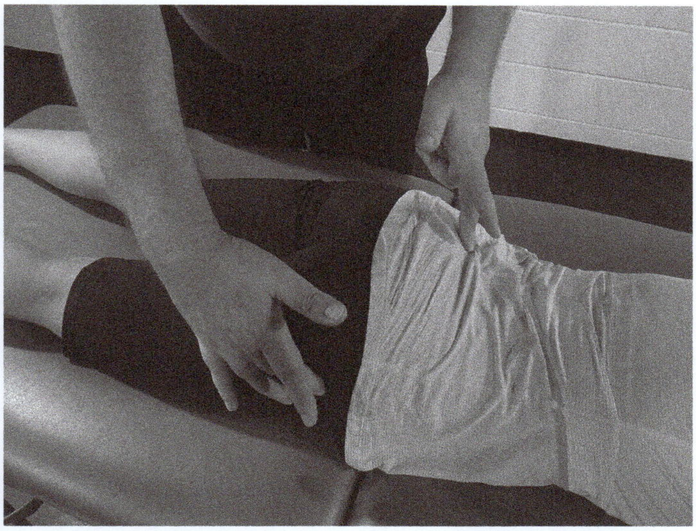

FIGURE 9.111 1. Landmarking for piriformis

Landmark the contralateral PSIS and ipsilateral greater trochanter.

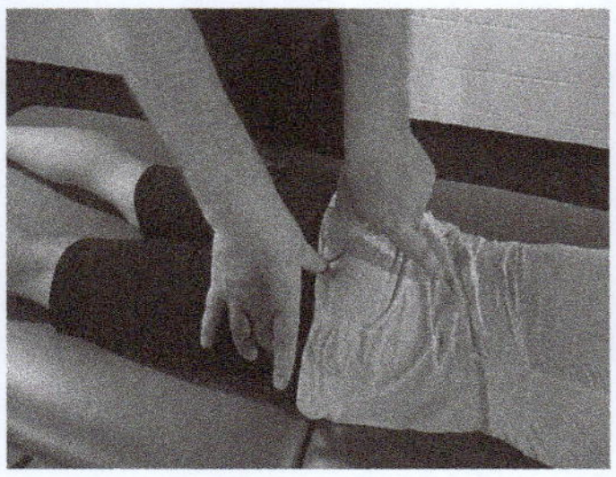

FIGURE 9.112 2. Locating piriformis

Bring the thumbs toward each other and press down into the gluteals. Deep muscle you will feel is the piriformis.

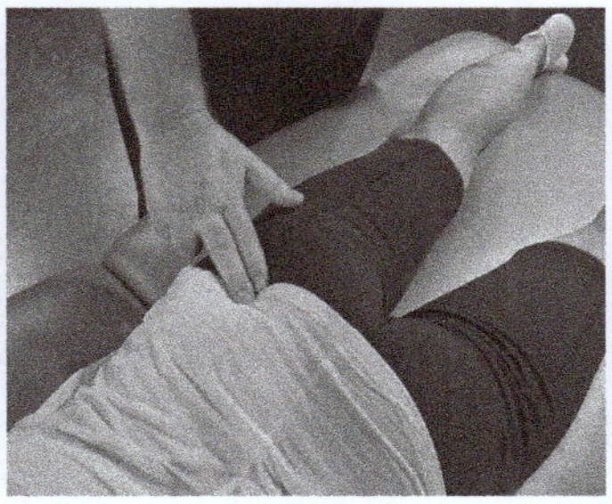

FIGURE 9.113 3. Palpating piriformis

Place the finger pads of one hand over the mid-point area.

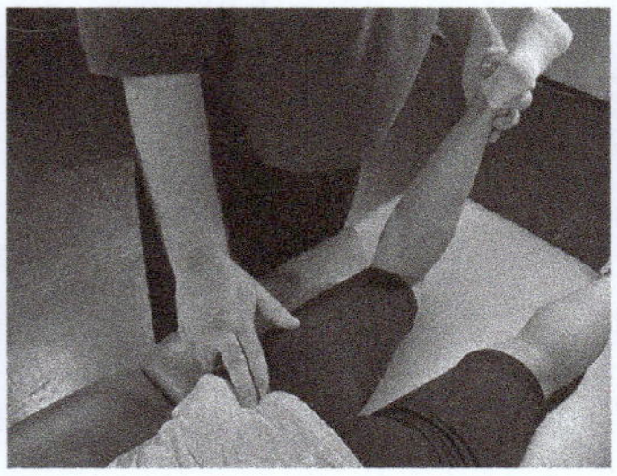

FIGURE 9.114 4. Motion palpation of piriformis

Flex the knee. Internally and externally rotate while palpating.

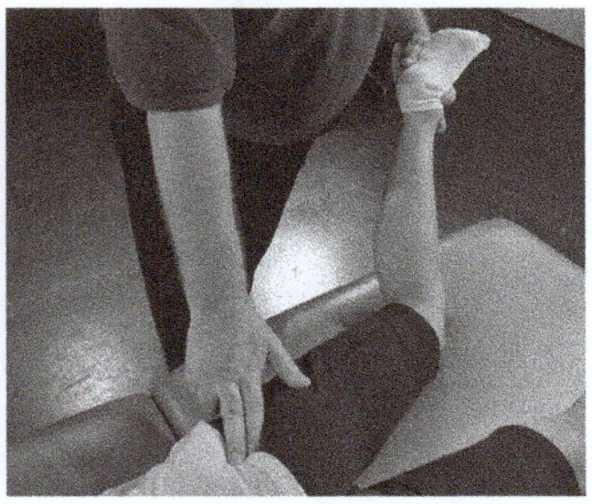

FIGURE 9.115 5. Measuring length of piriformis

Internally rotate the hip by pulling the ankle toward you.

hypertonic, or in spasm. This result should be palpable to the therapist. If this is not the case, there must be another reason for the restriction in internal rotation. Advanced osteoarthritis of the hip joint or swelling in the joint capsule are two examples of what can restrict internal rotation. On the other hand, if the leg moves significantly past 90°, to approximately 45°, it tells us that the length of the piriformis is normal, and a normal tone should be palpable to the therapist.

Trendelenburg's test (Figures 9.116, 9.117)

This is a functional test for the gluteus minimus and gluteus medius muscles. In order to test whether these hip abductors are

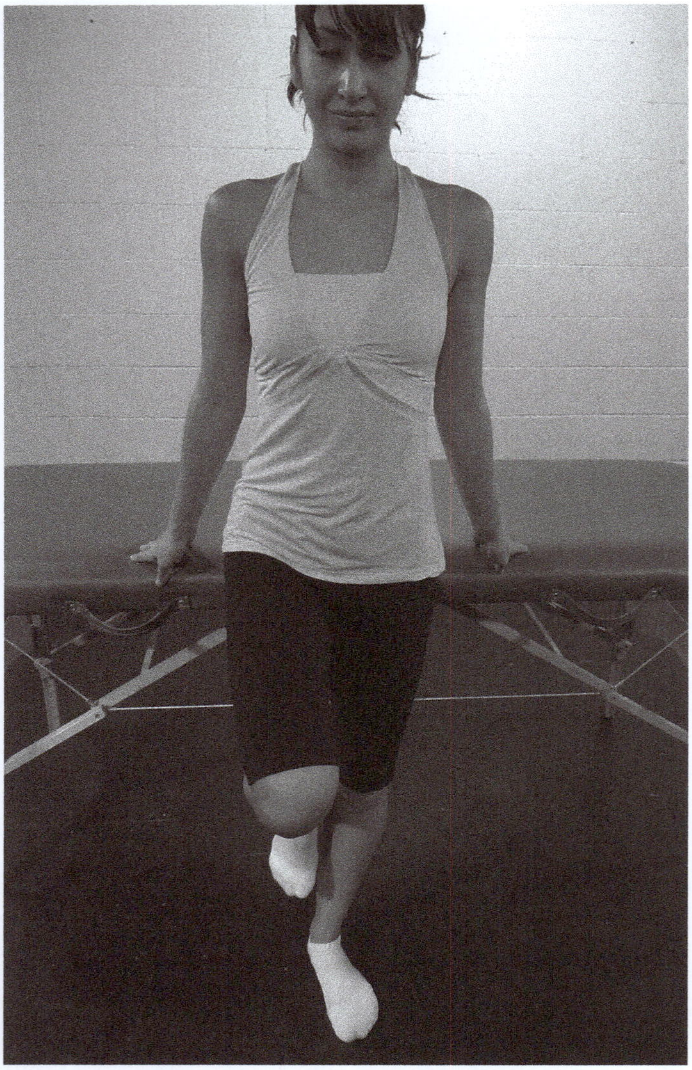

FIGURE 9.116 Negative Trendelenburg's test
Observe that the hip on the contralateral side remains slightly above that of the stance leg.

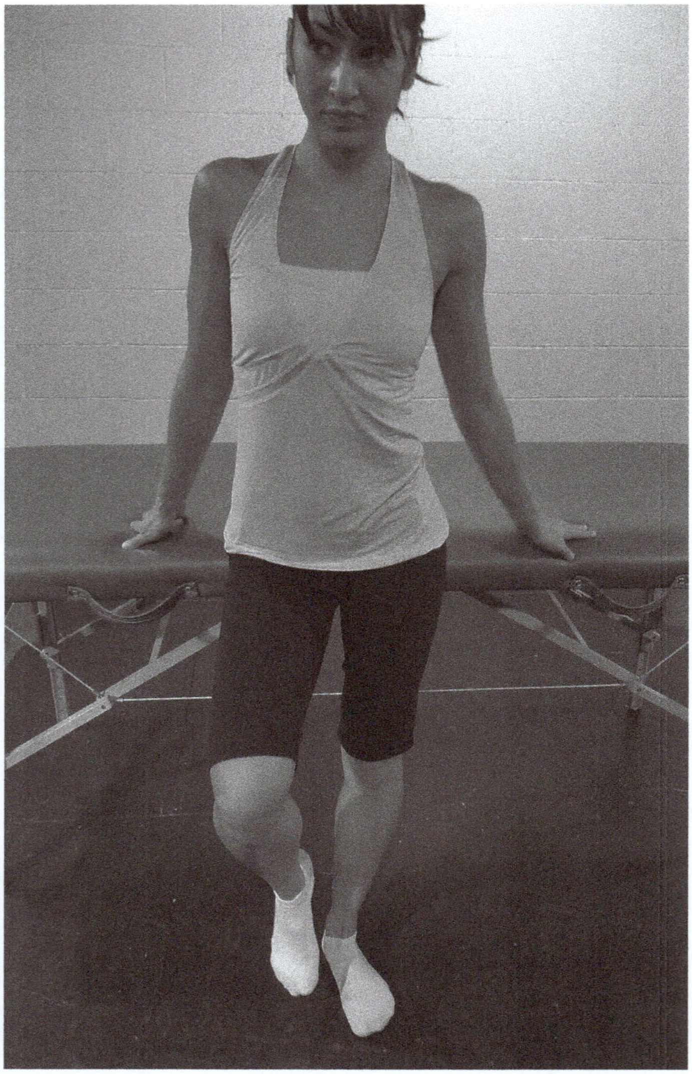

FIGURE 9.117 Positive Trendelenburg's test
Observe that the hip on the contralateral side is lower than that of the stance leg.

doing their job during the gait cycle, have the patient standing. You may assist the patient to keep their balance or allow them to lightly rest a hand on the table. They should not, of course, be placing any weight on the table when doing the test. Have the patient stand on one foot, with the other leg lifted slightly off the floor using a little hip and knee flexion. In this stance, the adductors of the weight-bearing leg are working to hold the hips level. It is normal for the contralateral hip to have a slight elevation compared to the hip of the stance leg. Therefore, a positive sign, implying inhibited or weak hip adductors, is the dropping of the hip on the unsupported side.

Scouring test (Figures 9.118–9.123)

This tests the articular surface of the head of the femur and the surface of the acetabulum. It is done by passively circumducting the hip joint, both clockwise and counter-clockwise, while compressing the joint surfaces together. Look for a smooth feeling of the joint surfaces moving on each other with no bumps or crepitus. A snap felt in the inguinal area may indicate a fibrosed iliopsoas-pelvic bone bursa (iliopectineal bursae); if painful this may be acute. The figures show the therapist moving the hip clockwise. Do two or three times in one direction, and then repeat in the other direction.

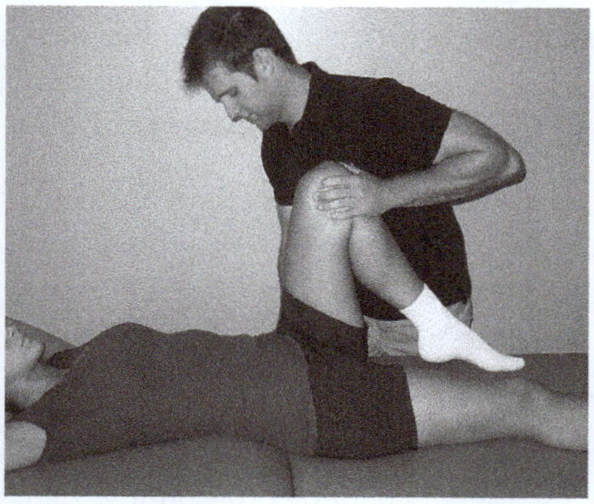

FIGURE 9.118 1. Start position

Bring the hip to 90° of flexion, with the femur perpendicular to the table (neither medially nor laterally rotated). Keep one hand on the patient's greater trochanter, pressing it toward the acetabulum.

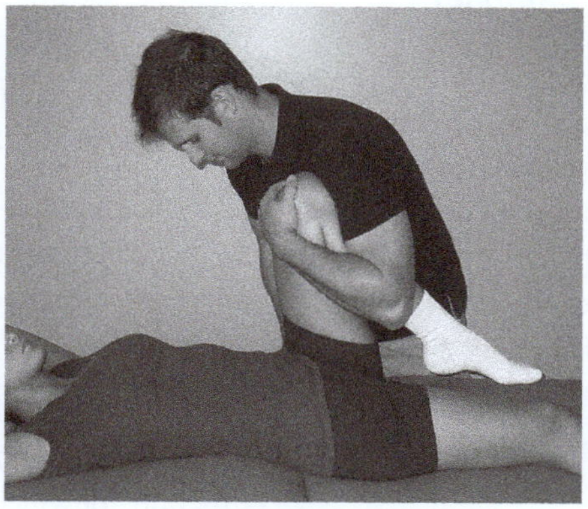

FIGURE 9.119 2. Medially rotating hip

Medially rotate the hip by gently pushing the knee toward the midline of the body with the hand on the knee. Begin fully flexing the hip, keeping pressure on the greater trochanter with the other hand, pushing it into the joint, compressing the joint as much as possible. Compression is to be kept throughout testing.

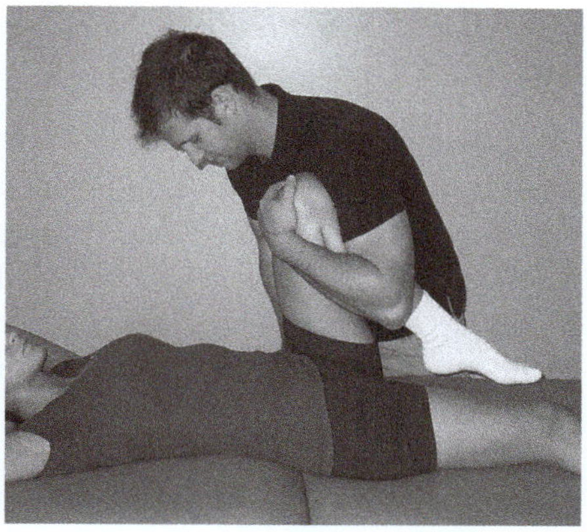

FIGURE 9.120 3. Moving hip into flexion

Begin swinging back to neutral (i.e., out of medial rotation) while you bring hip into full (pain-free) flexion.

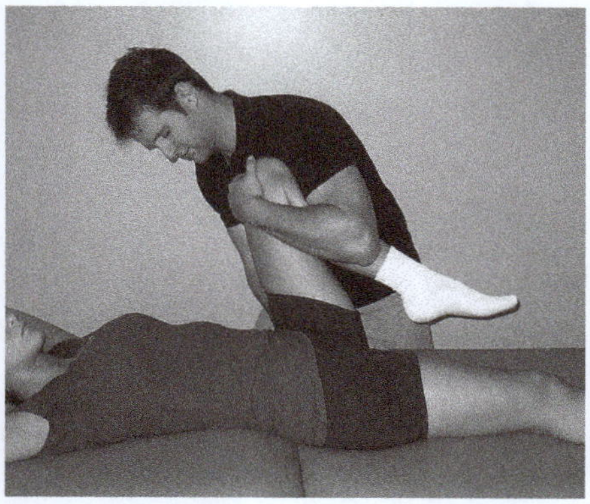

FIGURE 9.121 4. Laterally rotating hip

Bring hip out of full flexion and begin extension of the hip while also beginning to swing the knee out, laterally rotating the hip.

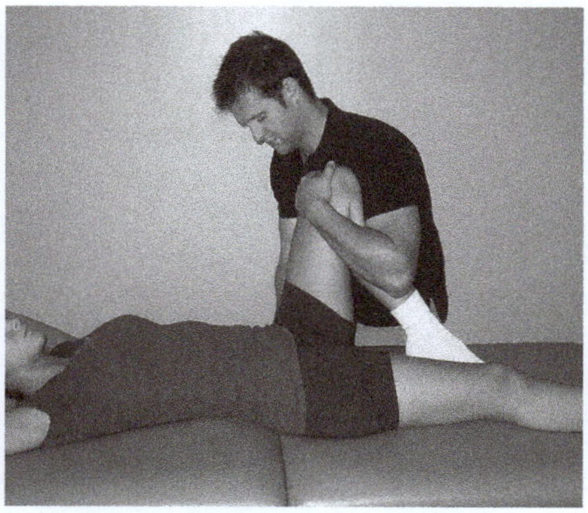

FIGURE 9.122 5. Extending hip

Continue to extend the hip and as you pass by 90° of flexion start taking the hip back out of lateral rotation and bringing it toward neutral.

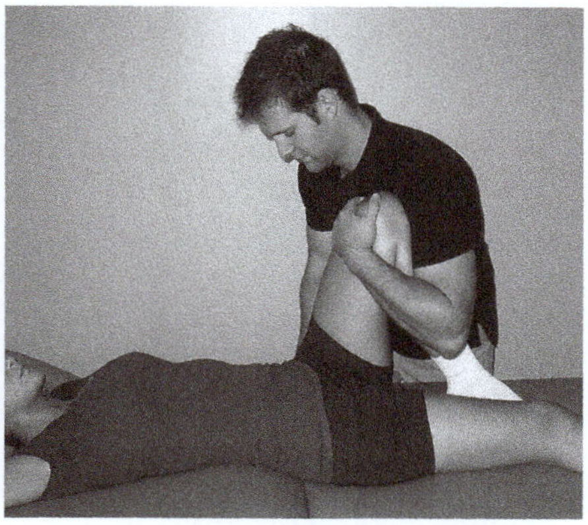

FIGURE 9.123 6. Return hip to start position

Return the hip to the starting position. Repeat circumduction three or four times in one direction, then in other.

FABER test (Flexion ABbduction External Rotation) or Patrick's test (Figure 9.124)

This test has been used specifically to check the length of the hip adductors (pectineus, adductor brevis and longus), for which it works well. Stabilize the patient's hips so that they do not roll. Either the ankle of the side to be tested is placed on the other thigh just proximal to the knee, or the sole of the foot is placed beside the other knee. For either position of the foot a negative test is when the patient's knee is able to rest close to the same plane as the one in which the ankle is lying. This implies that the adductors have excellent length. The higher the knee is off the table, the less abduction and external rotation is available at the hip, the tighter the adductors are considered to be and the more positive the test is considered for these muscles.

FABER test for joint provocation

Structures and tissues other than muscle can cause restrictions in range as well as pain. Therefore, this test may also be used as a provocation test to stress the hip joint structures (i.e., joint surfaces, capsule, and ligaments). It will, however, only provide very general information if positive, that there is a problem with hip function, but from what cause is still unknown (Magee 2014; Starkey & Brown 2015).

Impairment to the joint itself is said to be felt by the patient in the groin or inguinal area as pain or restriction in motion. Hip joint impairment is also seen by reduced range of motion, decreased abduction and external rotation (i.e., the capsular pattern of restriction).

It has also been used to test for ipsilateral sacroiliac joint dysfunction, for which it is also vague and inexact. The positive sign is pain felt usually in the ipsilateral SI joint area. If impairments exist in the joint, the type or manner is not revealed by this test, and if you try to now test the joint specifically (see Chapter 11), the pain caused by this provocation may well have compromised testing for that day. Hence, it is suggested that it not be used as a specific test for the SI joint. However, when it is used for testing muscle length or the hip joint, it can point to the possible involvement of the SI joint if the patient feels pain there. That then may be investigated later (often on a different day) with specific testing of the SI joint.

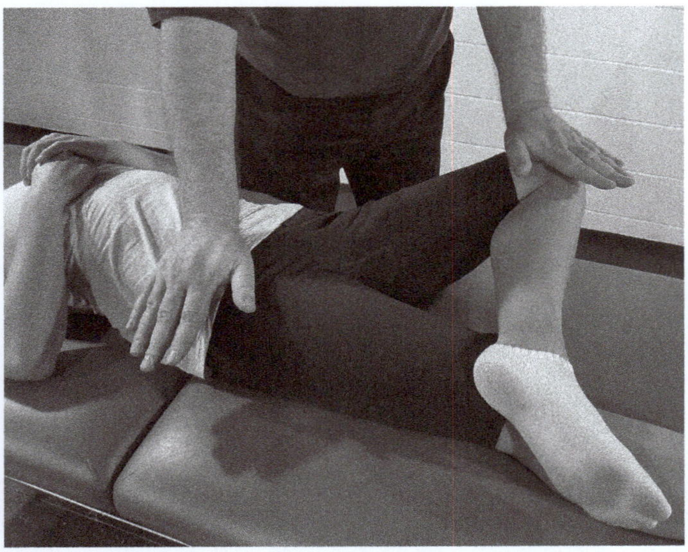

FIGURE 9.124 FABER test

Stand at the same side of the table as the leg being tested. Either place the ankle of the test leg just above the knee (patella), as shown here, or place sole of the foot up against the knee. Stabilize the hip by placing the palm of one hand over the contralateral ASIS. The knee of the test leg should be level with the anterior surface of the other leg's thigh if the adductors are of normal length. The shorter and more hypertonic the adductors, the higher the knee will be. Apply a gentle O-P on the medial thigh or knee of the test leg. See if tissues are springy, or leather-like (short, and possibly tender to stretch).

Ely's test (buttock sign) (Figure 9.125)

This test, also known as the "buttock sign," is for testing the length of the rectus femoris and/or its hypertonicity, which can have a direct effect on anterior rotation of the pelvis. The patient

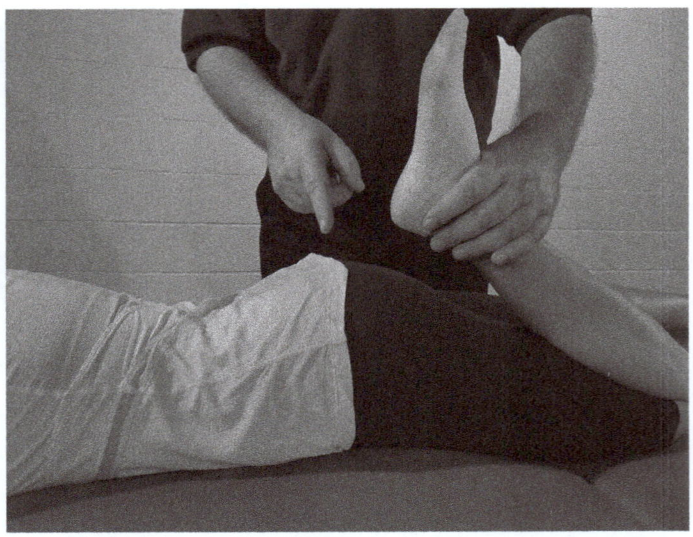

FIGURE 9.125 Ely's test

Take the patient's ankle toward the buttock. If rectus femoris is short the buttock will quickly lift before you get the knee flexed more than 90°. The patient may feel pain due to stretch at the muscle's origin at the anterior inferior iliac spine (AIIS).

is prone on the table. The therapist grasps the ankle and flexes the knee as the patient tries to remain passive. Flexing of the knee should be done slowly while you watch to see if the patient's buttock rises: this is the buttock sign. This is a result of the rising of the ischial tuberosity as the hip is rotated anteriorly. This movement is due to the flexing of the patient's hip by the stretch placed on the rectus femoris with the flexing of the knee. This causes the attachment on the anterior inferior iliac spine (AIIS) of the innominate to pull the hip into anterior rotation (since the thigh cannot move into flexion). However, if the patient suffers from low back pain this may prevent you from doing the test as it will extend the low back (as it flexes the hip) and provoke pain in the lumbar spine or sacroiliac joint areas.

Leg length discrepancy due to innominate rotation

The hips are a place where the body can compensate for impairments above and below them. Some of the compensations that can be found here are for leg length differences. One of the most common reasons for an apparent leg length difference is unilateral rotation of an innominate. As mentioned in the introductory material to this chapter, an anterior rotation of an innominate which moves the anterior superior iliac spine (ASIS) anteriorly and inferiorly on that side must also move the acetabulum anteriorly and inferiorly. The shift in the acetabulum makes the leg functionally longer. Conversely, a posteriorly rotated innominate with its ASIS moved superiorly and slightly posteriorly makes the leg functionally shorter (see Observations section earlier in this chapter).

The following testing – landmarking and the Stork test – is most useful when investigating leg length discrepancies where our postural findings for the pelvis are that the ASISs are not equal in height. One innominate's ASIS is lower, and its posterior superior iliac spine (PSIS) is correspondingly higher, than the other.

All else about the pelvis being equal, we can assume that one innominate is anteriorly rotated, or the other is posteriorly rotated (or that both of these opposite rotations are happening at the same time). With these tests we can determine which innominate is impaired and is the cause of a functional leg length discrepancy.

Landmarking for leg length discrepancy (Weber–Barstow maneuver) (Figures 9.126A, B, C, 9.127)

Possible findings

Straightforward findings for functional leg length differences:

- If you find that the longer leg's ASIS is inferior compared to the shorter leg's, and these differences seem roughly equal (i.e., the differences between each malleoli and between each

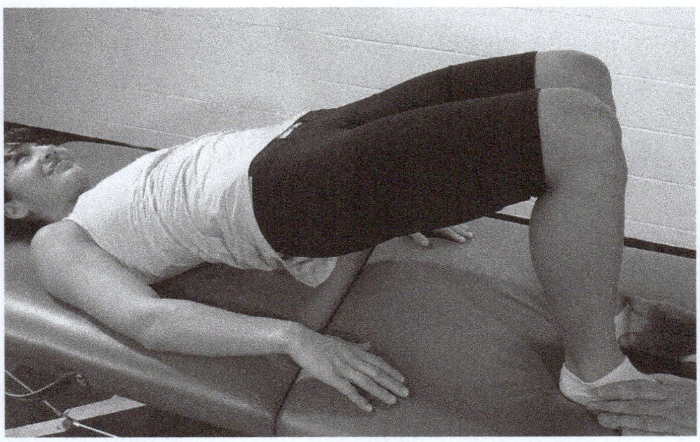

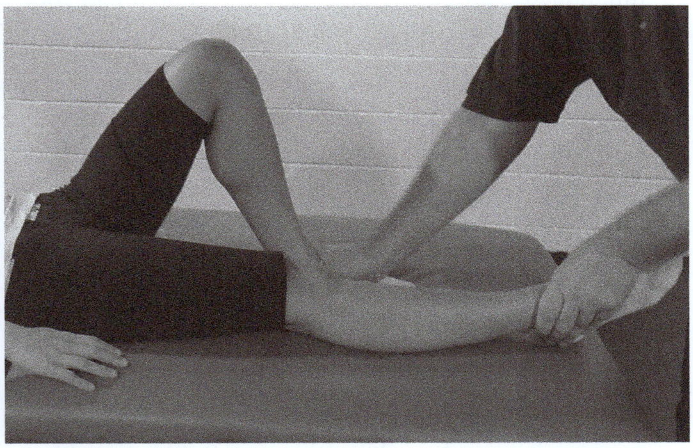

FIGURE 9.126A, B We need to first balance the pelvis

With the patient supine, the therapist stands at the end of the table at the patient's feet. Have the patient crook-lying. Instruct them to lift their buttocks off the table and then drop back to the table, letting everything relax. This will help to relax the musculature around the pelvis, enough so that only the truly impaired musculature is altering the balance of the pelvis. Most importantly, it helps to align the patient's limbs and trunk to their mid-line, so that your observations from landmarking are not misleading due to the patient unintentionally lying crooked on the table. Now, the therapist passively draws the legs one at a time out of crook-lying and into extension. Ensure the limbs are lined up with the rest of the body.

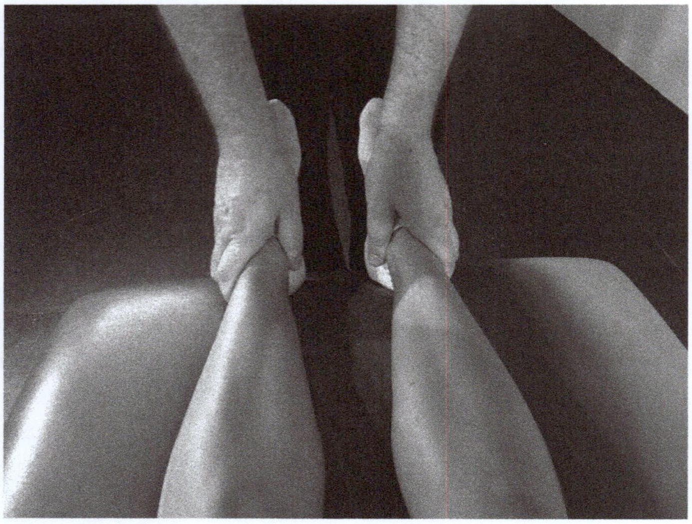

FIGURE 9.126C 1. Landmarking and comparing malleoli
Place a thumb under the most inferior part of each of the patient's medial malleoli and compare to see if one leg appears longer than the other.

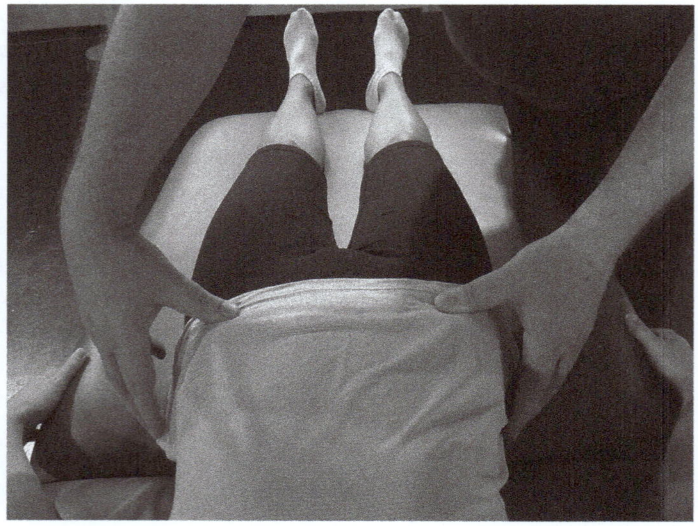

FIGURE 9.127 2. Landmarking and comparing ASISs
Even if malleoli appear relatively equal, go up and check ASISs by placing a thumb under each ASIS and noting if one appears higher than the other.

ASIS are roughly the same), then you can infer that the leg length discrepancy is due to a unilateral innominate rotation. This implies that the difference in leg length is probably functional, not structural, and is due to a rotation of the hip/innominate. However, is the longer leg's innominate rotated anteriorly or is the short leg's innominate rotated posteriorly?

To decide this, you need to perform the Stork test. This may tell you which innominate is impaired and being held in place. It is also wise to have already done a general postural assessment that has given you some basic information about the orientation of the pelvis/hips in general.

Stork test (Fowler's test/Gillet's test) (Figures 9.128, 9.129)

How motion palpation of innominate movement works:

1. The patient is standing arms' length distance from a wall. After you landmark the PSISs, the patient will flex one hip and knee to perform the test, often referred to as the "stork test" because of this stance on one leg.
2. The sacrum will be held in place by the stance leg as a result of force closure. This is the engagement of the musculature around the pelvis on the side of the stance leg which will close or fix that side's SI joint. While the other leg comes off the floor with the flexion of the hip and knee, the SI joint on that side unlocks and becomes capable of gapping. This laxity between the sacrum and the innominate permits that innominate to rotate posteriorly, if no impairment is present. This motion is seen by the PSIS on that side moving inferiorly as the patient flexes the hip while standing on one leg.
3. If there is impaired motion between the innominate and the sacrum, then the PSIS will not move inferiorly, but will remain at the same height or even move superiorly as the whole innominate will lift to compensate for the loss of movement within the joint (DeStefano 2011; Mitchell 2001).

Interpretation of stork test results

With respect to functionally longer and shorter legs we will find that:

- if the stork test is positive on the same side as the long leg, with the lower ASIS, then that innominate is considered anteriorly rotated, and the source of the leg length difference
- if the test is positive on the side that has the short leg, then that innominate is posteriorly rotated, and the source of the leg length difference.

Remember: It is possible that both are occurring. For a fuller discussion of this, see the discussion of postural observations in the introductory material of this chapter.

Note that not finding a positive result with this test does not mean that there is no rotation, posteriorly or anteriorly, to an innominate. The lack of result means that the rotation is not

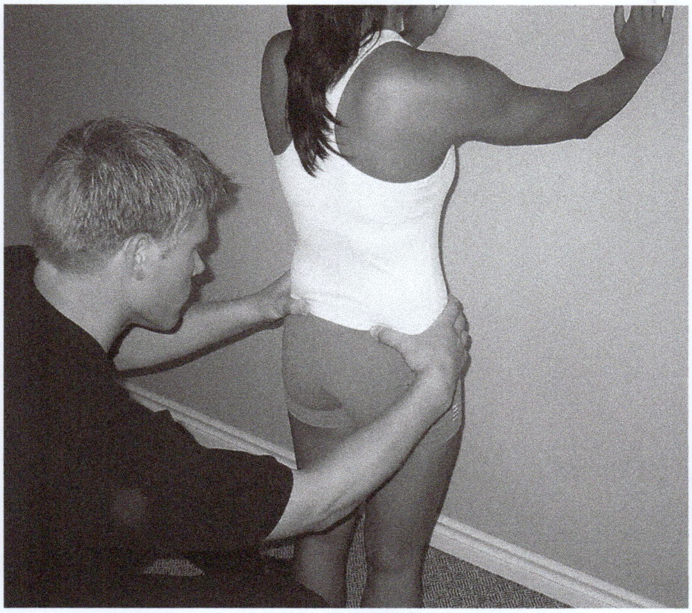

FIGURE 9.128 1. Landmark PSISs

Have the patient standing with the fingertips on the wall to retain balance during testing. Elbows should be slightly bent and the patient should not be leaning forward or backward. Palpate the PSISs with your thumbs. Make sure that your thumbs are tucked under the PSIS. This enables you to retain the landmark as the patient moves. Some therapists will slide the thumb on the side they are not going to be testing straight over to the mid-line and palpate S2. The advantage of having your reference thumb on the sacrum is that it is closer to the moving thumb and hopefully makes the result of the test clearer.

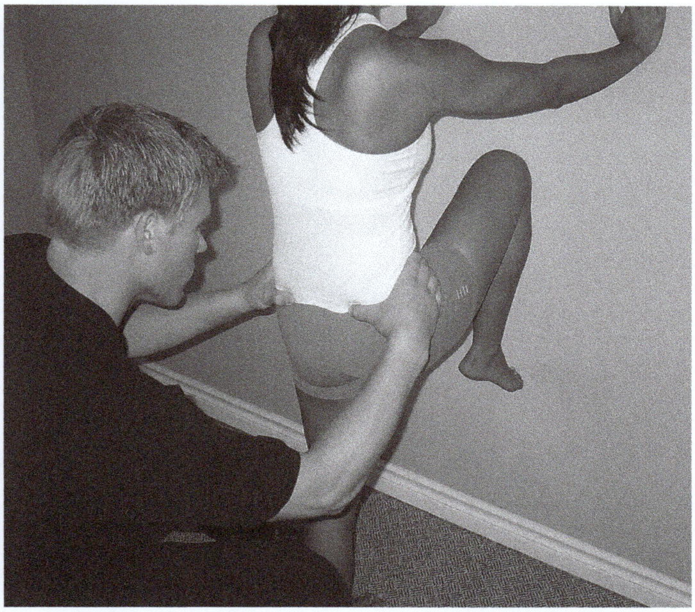

FIGURE 9.129 2. Continue to palpate as patient flexes hip

Have the patient flex the hip, bringing the knee up toward the ipsilateral shoulder. Ask the patient to bring the knee up as high as possible as you will often only feel and see distinct movement when the hip passes 90°. The PSIS should move inferiorly on this non-weight-bearing side with the flexed hip. A positive sign is that the PSIS will not move inferiorly, but may stay at the same level or actually rise as the patient "cheats" or compensates for lack of movement of the innominate by side-bending the lumbar spine and lifting the whole innominate. (**Note:** This patient's right PSIS has not moved lower and so we have a positive test. Further, the patient has used elevation and internal rotation of the hip to achieve flexion though the innominate is impaired.)

fixed in place or restricting movement of the innominate. There is no lesion, per se.

NOTE: Slightly more involved findings may occur when leg length differences may be structural.

- You may note that the malleoli are not equal, but the ASISs are! If both innominates are level, then the likelihood is that the leg that appears long may well be structurally longer. However, in such a case, the body often tries to accommodate this leg length discrepancy by anteriorly rotating the innominate of a short leg in order to lengthen it, and/or posteriorly rotate the innominate of a long leg in order to shorten it. This can result in equal malleoli with unlevel ASISs, or some version of this.

There are other possibilities that the therapist may encounter. Check your landmarking and re-do your testing. If the results still stand, then think through the anatomy and modes of compensation that may occur here. Patience and persistence will be rewarded with answers.

COMPREHENSIVE STRUCTURAL EXAMINATION OF THE SPINE AND PELVIS: CHAPTER OVERVIEW

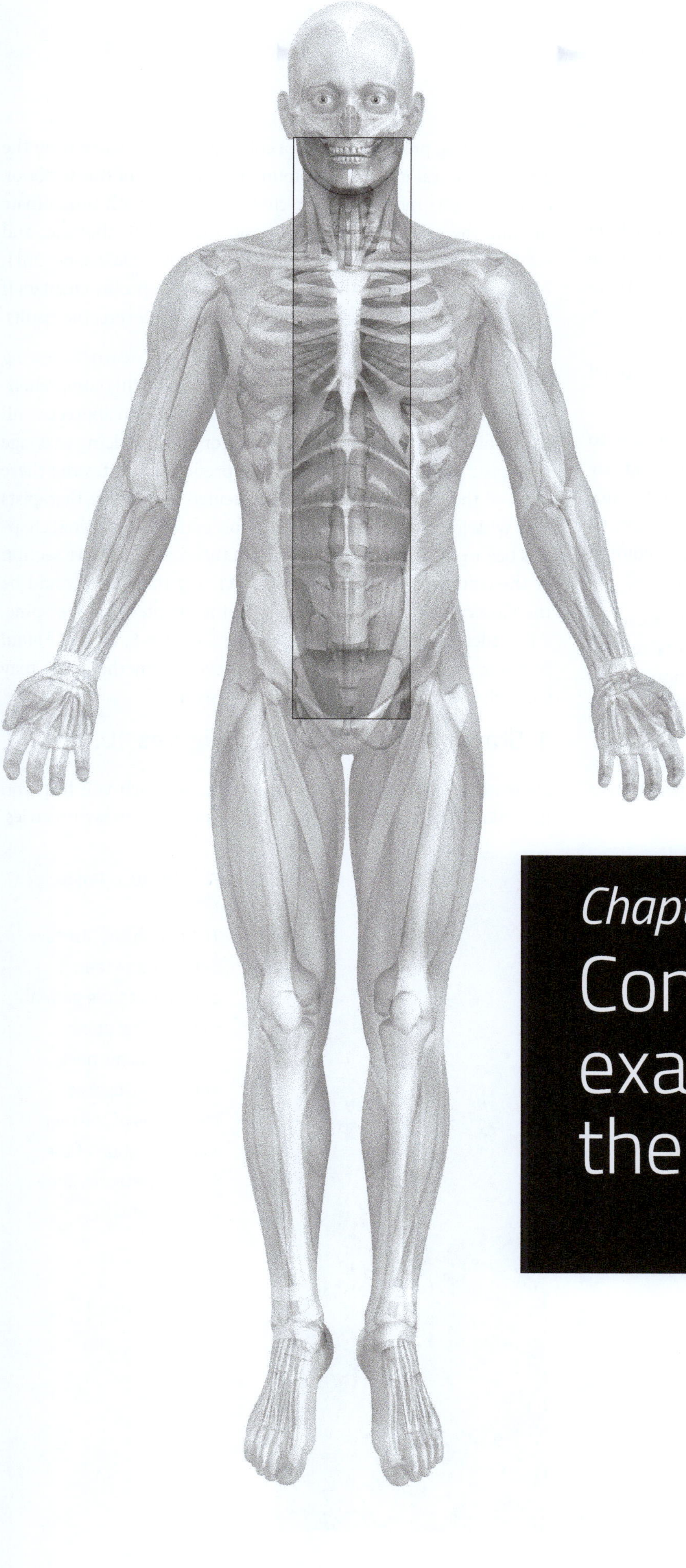

Chapter 10

Comprehensive examination of the spine

Comprehensive structural examination of the spine and pelvis

It should be understood that observation and landmarking during motion give us the best indicators as to which part of the spine has the greatest impairment. Further, including a general scan of the whole body and its posture guides us towards which other areas of the body may be contributing to spinal asymmetry or which areas of the body are compensating for spinal impairment.

This testing gives us clues as to which areas of the body need to be more fully examined. However, be careful about making any quick assumptions about what the results of this structural examination tell us. Results of this type of examination only give us very general impressions. Much more specific testing is required to find which tissues or structures are impaired and how.

Many of the elements presented in this general examination of the spine and pelvis are repeated in the chapters dealing specifically with the spine and pelvis. This presentation in this chapter has illustrations and some instruction to briefly demonstrate a global testing. Each of the chapters on the spine and the sacroiliac (Chapters 11–15) provides specific additional testing to follow up suspicions gleaned from the general examination as to areas requiring more testing.

The testing presented here is a collection of tests taken from the general postural examination found in Chapter 3 of this textbook and from tests included in the chapters dealing with innominate motion, the sacroiliac (SI) joints, and the lumbar, thoracic, and cervical spine (Chapters 9, 11–15) (Chila 2010; DeStefano 2011; Mitchell 2001, 2004, 2005). Refer to any of the specific chapters if you need more detail about how to do a test and interpret the results.

Students new to massage therapy are advised to learn the testing for the specific areas of the body prior to learning this comprehensive examination, otherwise they will not be able to appreciate all the information that can be gleaned from it. Practicing massage therapists can have varying levels of proficiency in testing these areas of the body in the manner presented here; some therapists may wish to review the testing protocols in the SI and spinal chapters before focusing on the material in this comprehensive section of the textbook. Of most use for practicing therapists would be the Clinical implications sections in the chapters on the spine. All readers may benefit from reading Chapter 6, Part I, *Spinal Motions: Structure and Function*. However, many therapists may feel well prepared to dive right into this section.

1. Standing postural views (Figures 10.1–10.4)

Shown here are the standing postural views which will help you in evaluating muscle balance and joint orientation asymmetries.

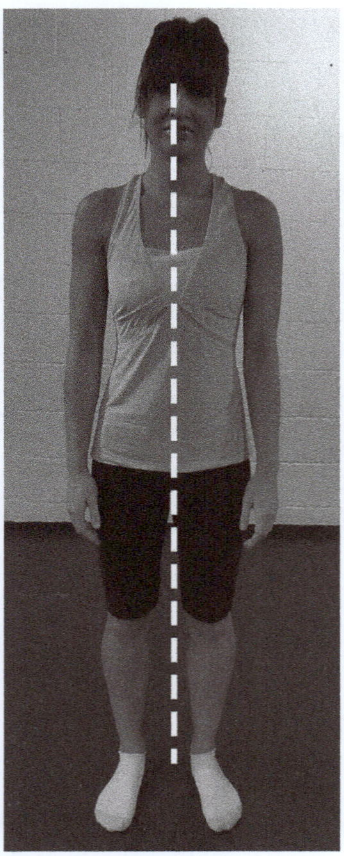

FIGURE 10.1 Frontal view

The plumb line begins at the feet (note the orientation of the feet and arches, etc.). It continues up between the knees, through the pubic symphysis, linea alba, middle chest (sternum), chin, nose, and eyes.

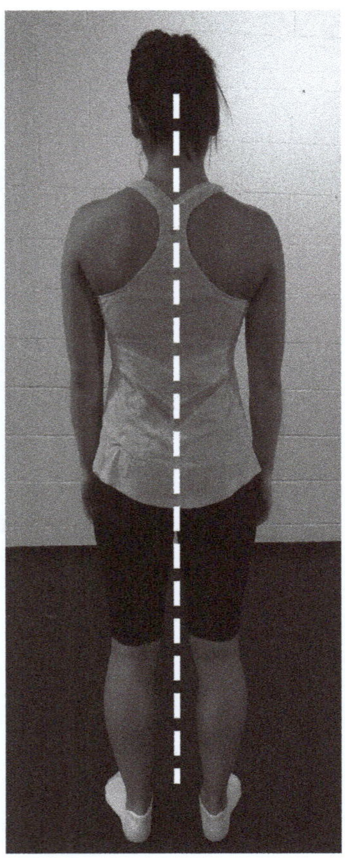

FIGURE 10.2 Posterior view

The plumb line starts between the feet; it continues to the gluteal cleft, lumbar spine, thoracic spine, neck, and head. Observe the arches of the feet, the orientation of the Achilles tendons, knee creases, etc.

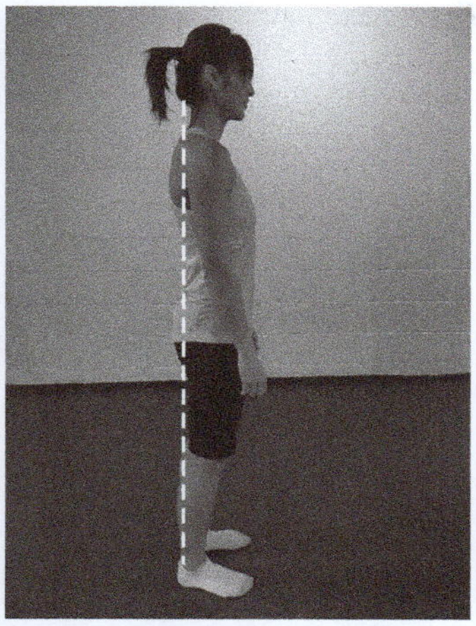

FIGURE 10.3 Lateral view (right)

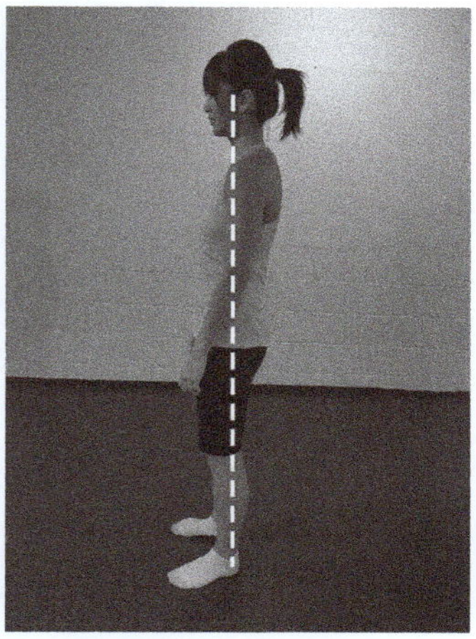

FIGURE 10.4 Lateral view (left)

The plumb line begins at the feet (slightly behind the lateral malleolus), continues through the knee (just behind the patella), through the greater trochanter, through the L3 vertebral body, through the mid-point of the glenohumeral joint and, finally, through the external auditory meatus.

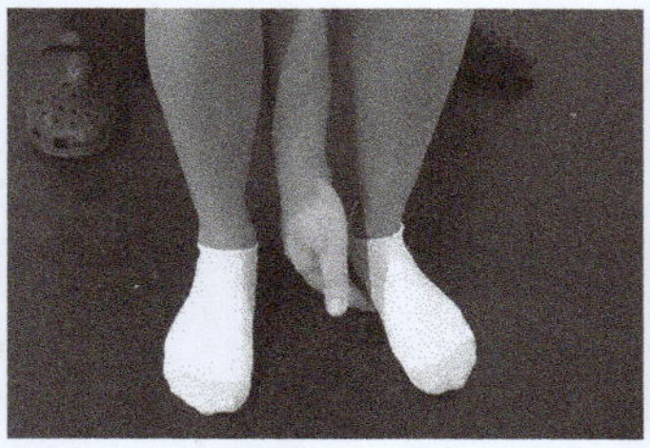

FIGURE 10.5

Arches.

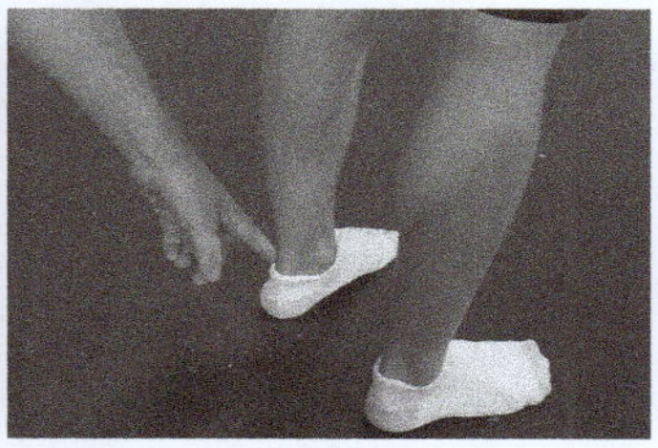

FIGURE 10.6

Achilles tendon.

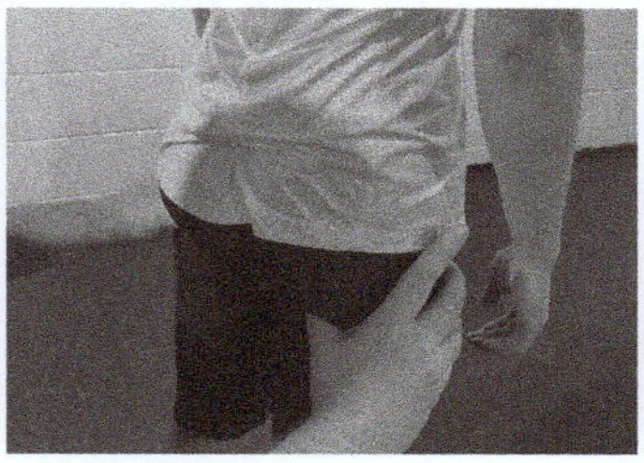

FIGURE 10.7

Ischial tuberosities.

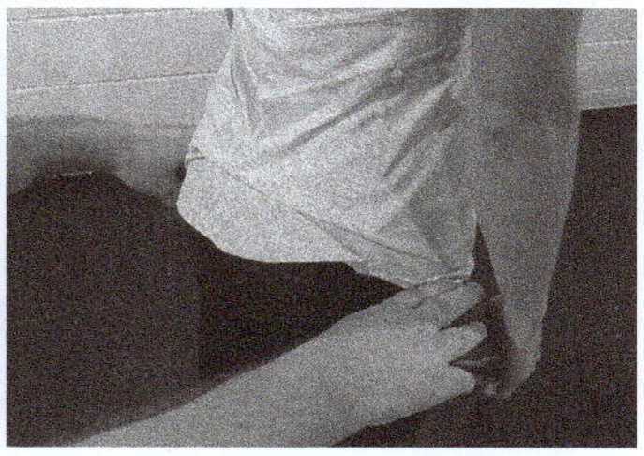

FIGURE 10.8

Greater trochanters.

A plumb line has been included to help you visualize asymmetries in bilateral landmarks. For more detail and information on the general postural examination and landmarking, see Chapter 5 in this book.

In the following views check the levels of the malleoli, patellas, trochanters, ASISs, iliac crests, acromions, mastoid processes, and eyes. Note any deviations at each level, to one side or other.

For the following two views check levels of the PSIS and ASIS (each side). Take note of the curves of the spine (hyperlordotic or hyperkyphotic). Is one foot/knee/hip/shoulder more forward than the other? For example: if the knee is not plumb, it may be flexed or hyperextended; if the greater trochanter is not plumb, the hip joint may be forward (extended) or back (flexed).

2. Checking symmetry of landmarks (Figures 10.5–10.12)

Landmark as follows: arches of the feet, Achilles tendon orientation, ischial tuberosities, trochanters, PSISs, iliac crest heights,

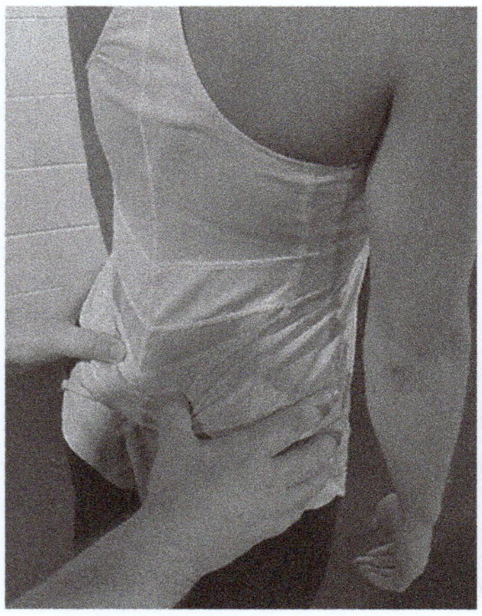

FIGURE 10.9

PSISs.

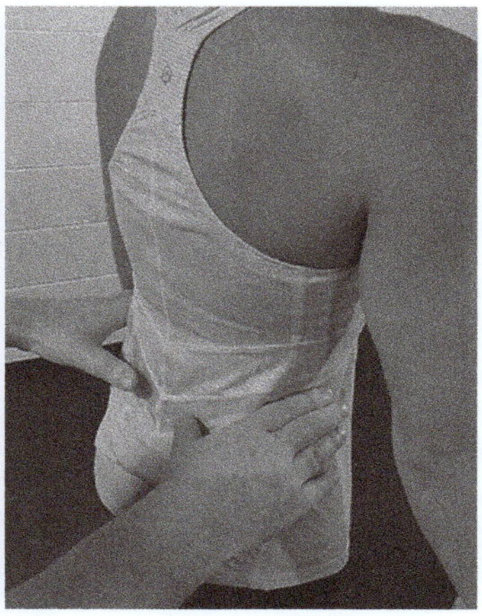

FIGURE 10.10

Iliac crests.

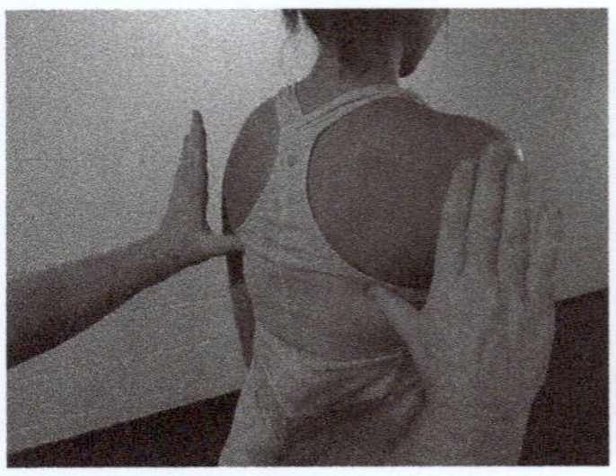

FIGURE 10.11
Scapulae.

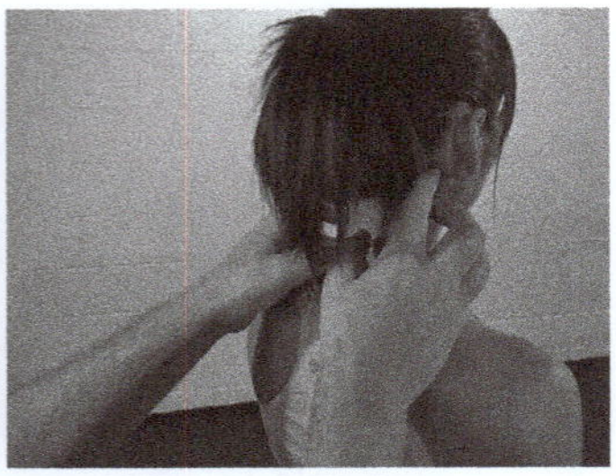

FIGURE 10.12
Mastoid processes.

(creases of) waist, inferior and superior angles of scapula, mastoid processes.

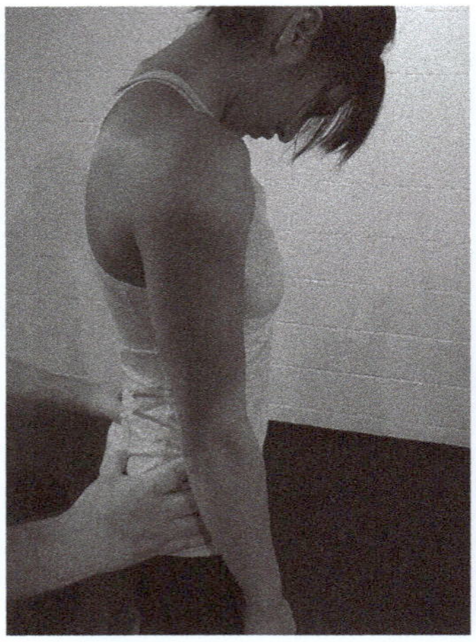

FIGURE 10.13
Start of flexion.

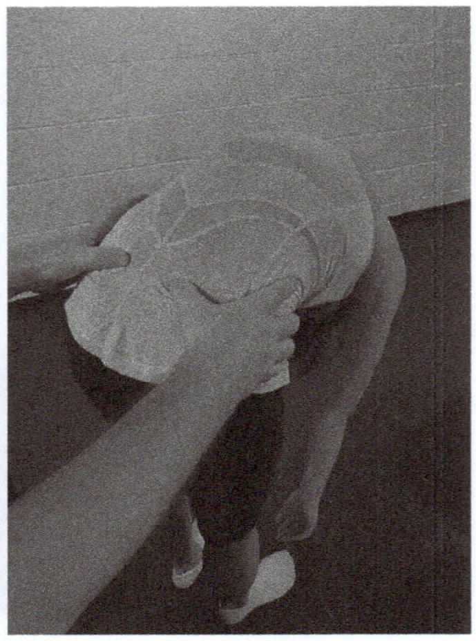

FIGURE 10.14
Full flexion.

3. Checking symmetry during AF-ROM (Figures 10.13–10.23)

Start off by landmarking the PSISs. First, have the patient bring their chin to their chest and then slowly roll down into lumbar flexion while noting the movement of the PSISs. This is the standing flexion test which we have already discussed in Chapter 9, on the hip and innominate. The PSIS that rises higher on flexion indicates either an innominate or a sacroiliac impairment.

Check the spine for flat spots, excessive curve, bulking of erector spinae, lateral curves, etc. Only then should the patient return to standing straight.

Ask the patient to look up to the ceiling (while leaving your hands on the patient's hips for their stability) and have them extend their back while observing changes to curves of the spine (lordosis-kyphosis).

Now, have the patient bring their ear to their shoulder, and then have them slide their hand down the side of their leg to their knee, observing how the spine curves from above during side-bending. Note the quality of the curves and the tissue changes. Check both sides.

Next, have the patient flex one knee while the other remains locked. Note the quality of lumbar side-bending and curve, as well as pelvic shifting. This tests influences from below on pelvic and lumbar orientation. Check both sides.

Finally, hold the patient's hip stable. Have the patient bring their chin over their shoulder and note head and cervical rotation; then have them bring that shoulder back toward you observing thoracic rotation. Note also the difference in the amount of resistance required at the hips to resist lower trunk rotation (ease versus effort).

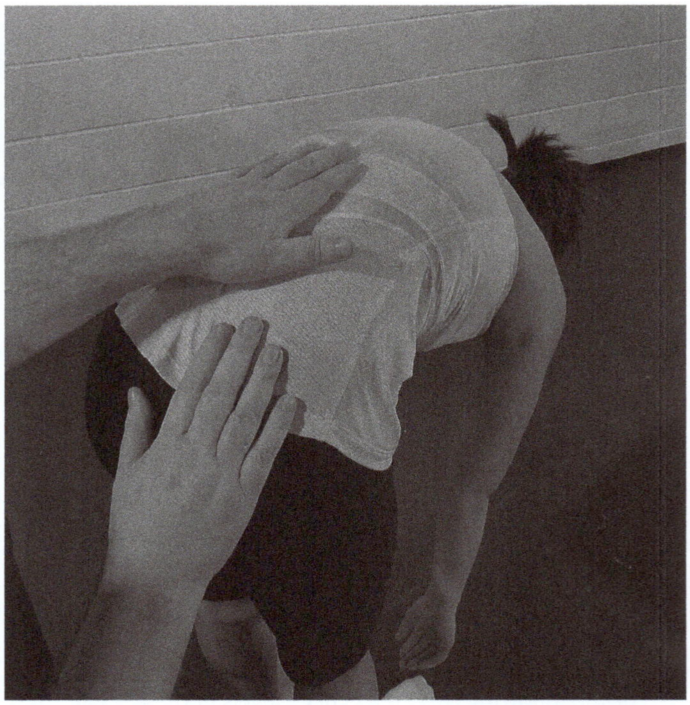

FIGURE 10.15
Check quality of curvature.

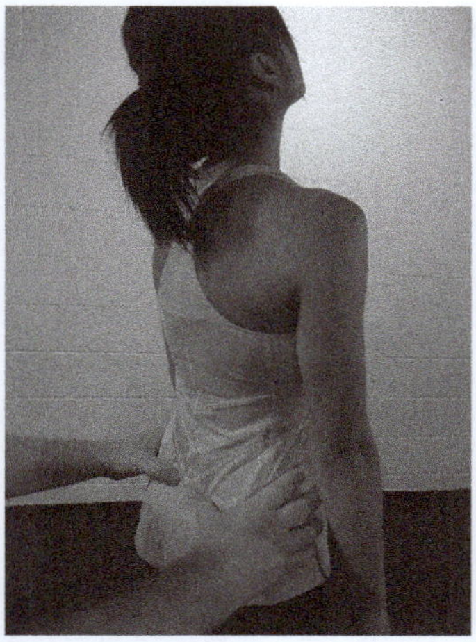

FIGURE 10.16

Patient looks up.

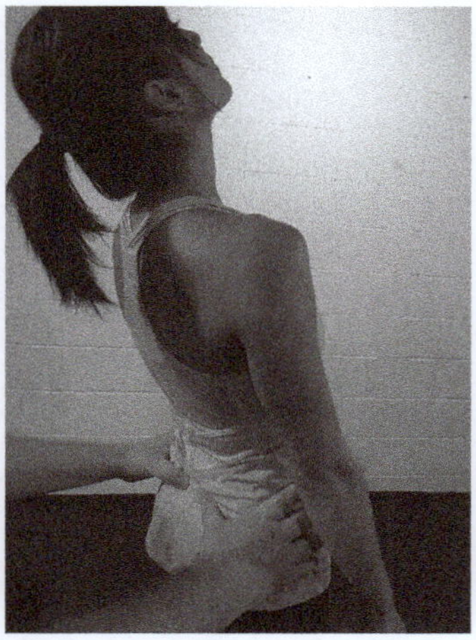

FIGURE 10.17

Then extends low back.

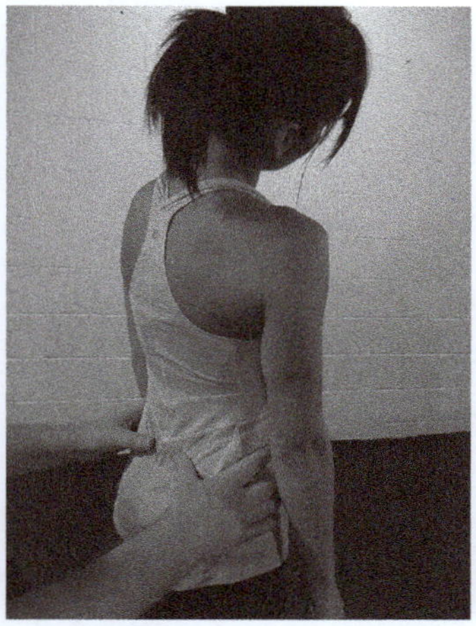

FIGURE 10.18

Ear to shoulder for cervical side-bending.

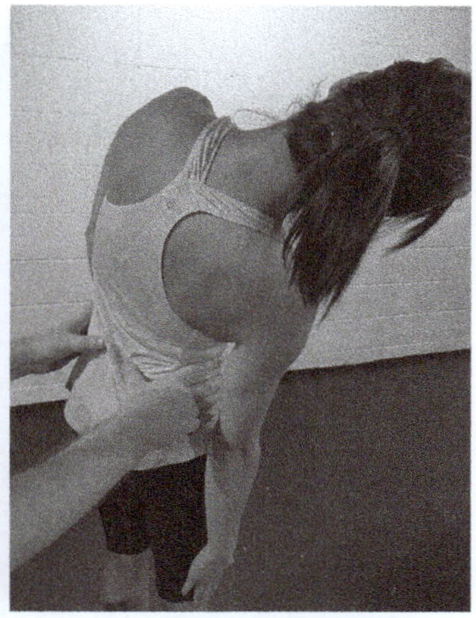

FIGURE 10.19

Reaching down side of leg to reveal thoracic and lumbar side-bending.

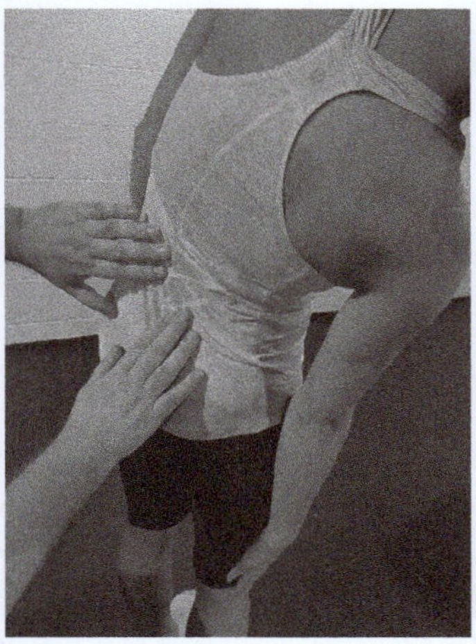

FIGURE 10.20

Observe curves and differences in tissue bulk.

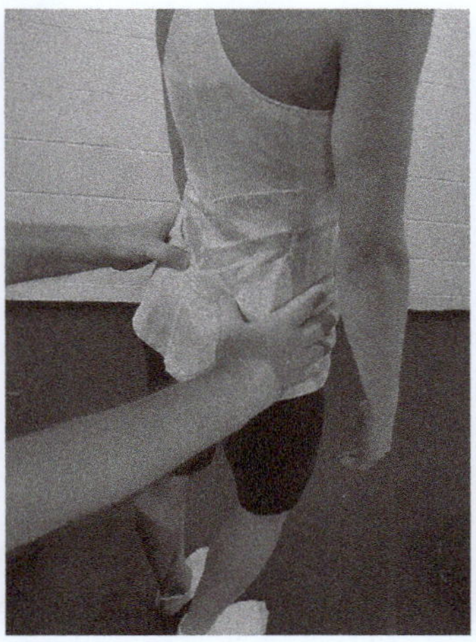

FIGURE 10.21

Flex one knee. Hold momentarily. Repeat on the other side.

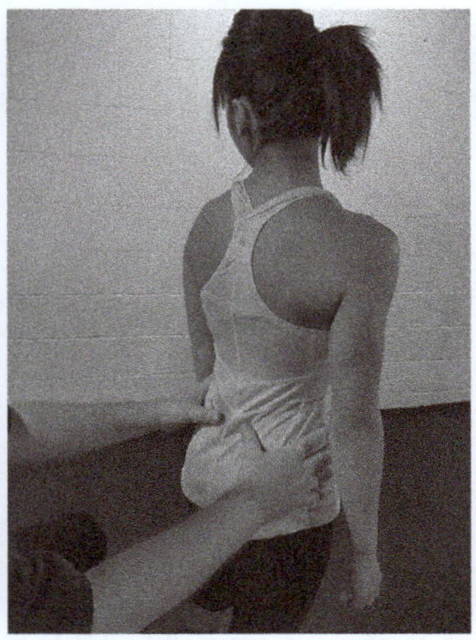

FIGURE 10.22

Rotate chin to shoulder.

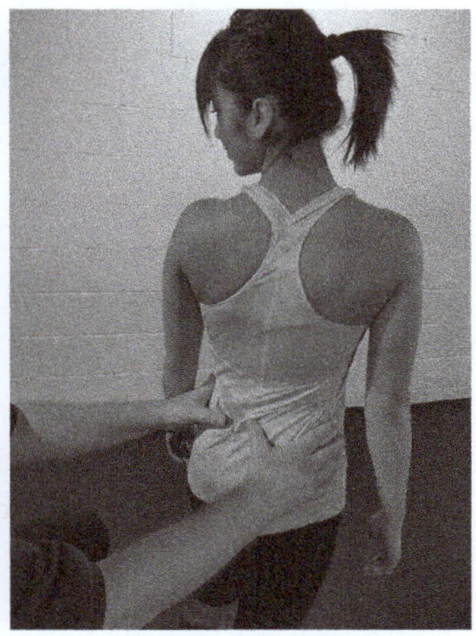

FIGURE 10.23

Push shoulder back.

4. Assessing postural stability (Figures 10.24, 10.25)

Challenge sagittal plane (anterior-posterior) stability (via manubrium and T2). This test requires gentle nudges. You want the patient to slightly rock back and forth. Observe which way they are willing to go and which way they resist. If the patient is willing to go one way and resists the other, they generally stand in the direction they are willing to rock. Challenge the coronal plane (side-bending) motion either by applying pressure on the acromions

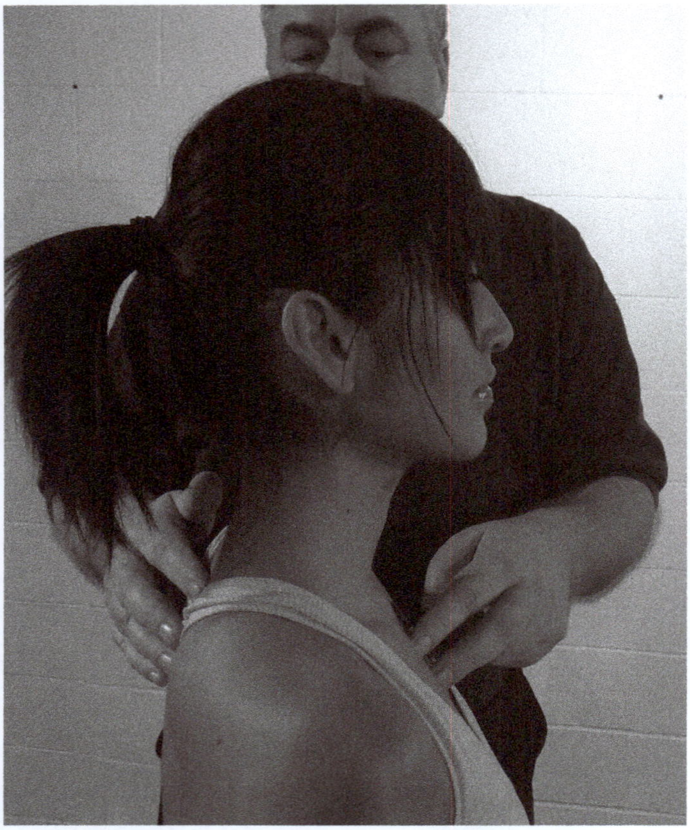

FIGURE 10.24

1. Gently push back and forth about a half an inch or so.

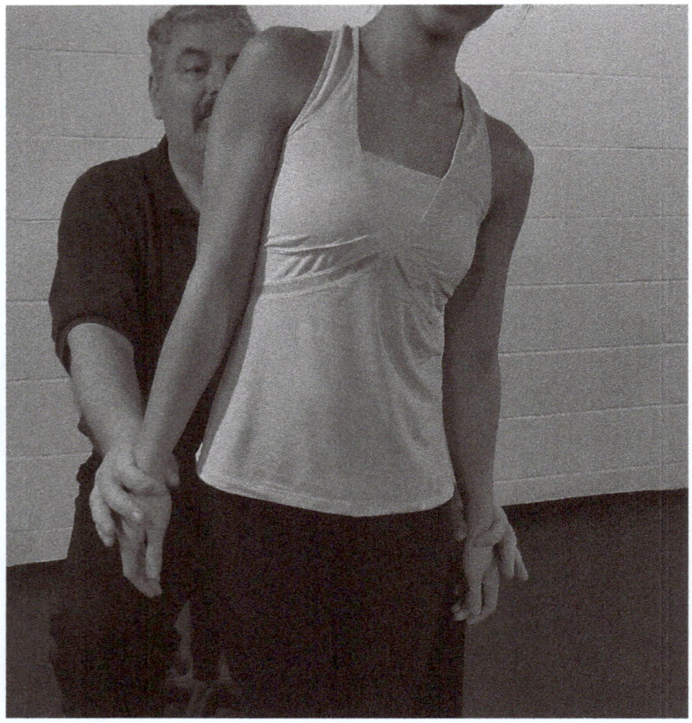

FIGURE 10.25

2. Gently tug on one wrist, then the other. Repeat the process two or three times.

or by an inferiorly directed tug on the wrists. The side to which the patient is more willing to side-bend is the side that the spine is bent toward.

5. Checking postural symmetries and AF-ROM while sitting (Figures 10.26, 10.27)

1. Re-check the iliac crest heights, the PSISs, the shoulder/scapula landmarks, the tissue bulk, etc. Observe all changes of orientation to landmarks, tissue changes, etc. during the following motions. Especially note changes in the symmetry of landmarks compared to the standing versions of these tests.

If there are no changes to the orientation of the landmarks, then the deviations noted while standing may be inherent in the pelvis and trunk. If the landmarks change orientation, then the lower body is impacting on the overall asymmetries seen in the pelvis and trunk.

2. **Seated flexion test.** While landmarking the PSISs, have the patient flex forward. Note asymmetry of motion. The PSIS on the impaired side of the sacroiliac joint will rise higher after flexing forward. This informs us that there is a possible impairment and on which side, but not what type of impairment (see the Chapter 11 for much more detail).

Have the seated patient also perform the three actions below, which duplicate some of the testing done in the standing postural exam. Compare the results found in the seated position with the findings from those motions when the patient was standing.

1. Side-bending: the patient, with elbows at 90°, brings the ear to the shoulder, then lowers the elbow toward the table. Observe side-bending of spine.
2. Rotation: the patient turns the chin toward the shoulder and at end-range, pushes the shoulder back.
3. Challenge to side-bending: push down alternately on each shoulder cap.

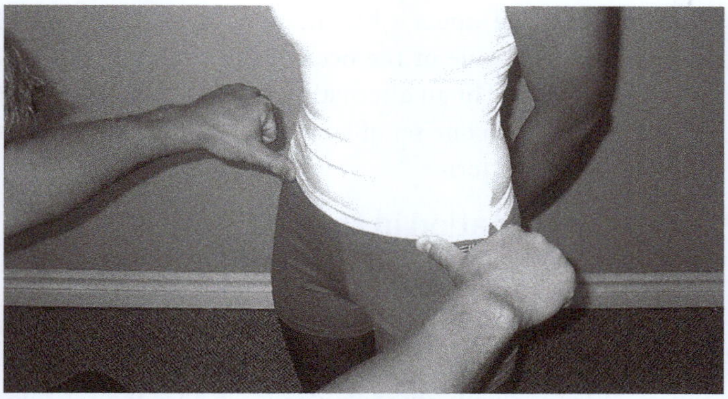

FIGURE 10.26

1. Palpate the PSISs to check if they are level.

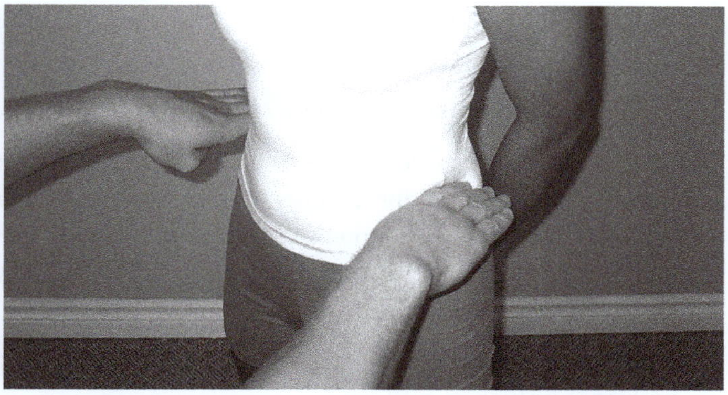

FIGURE 10.27

2. Then, have the patient flex forward while palpating the PSISs and re-check level.

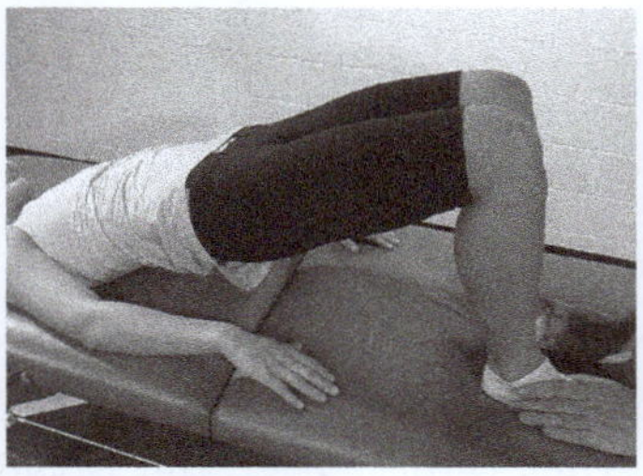

FIGURE 10.28

Crook-lying with hips raised.

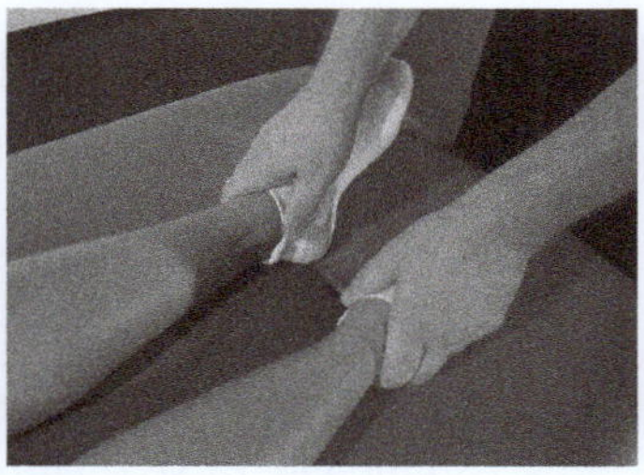

FIGURE 10.29

Thumbs need to be under the malleoli.

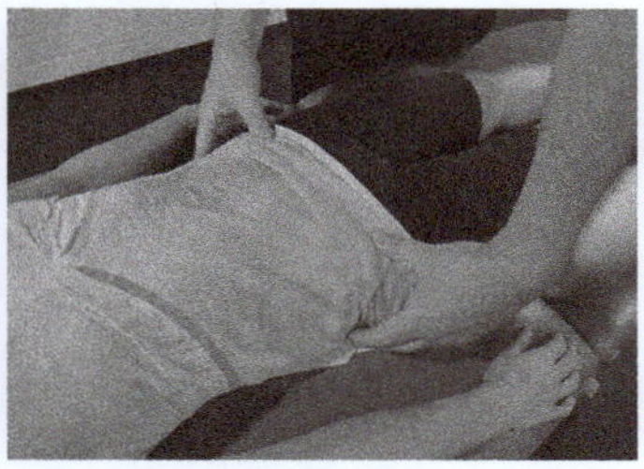

FIGURE 10.30

Level of ASISs horizontally.

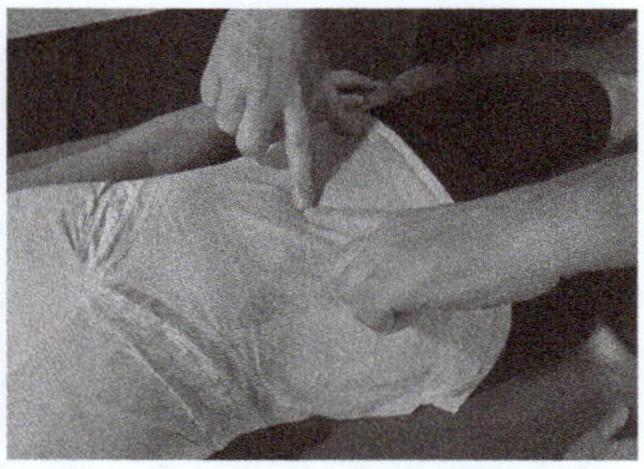

FIGURE 10.31

Checking for inflare/out-flare.

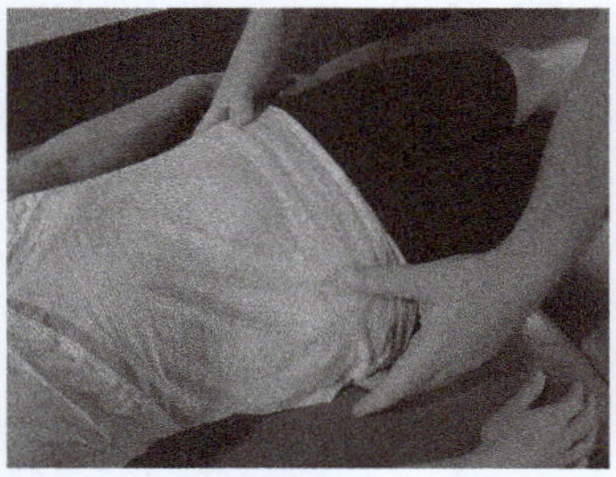

FIGURE 10.32

ASIS heights.

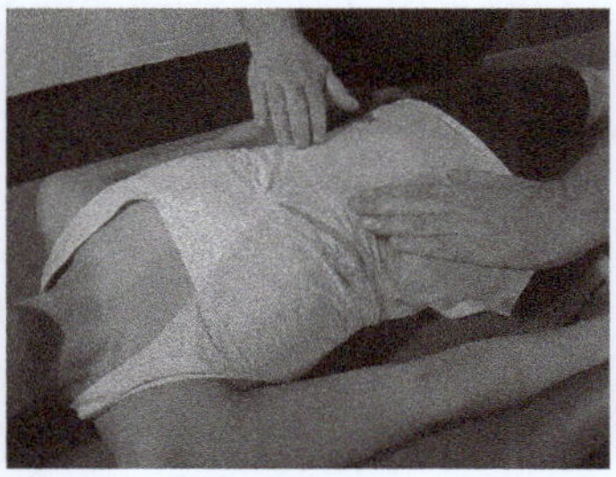

FIGURE 10.33

Lower rib heights.

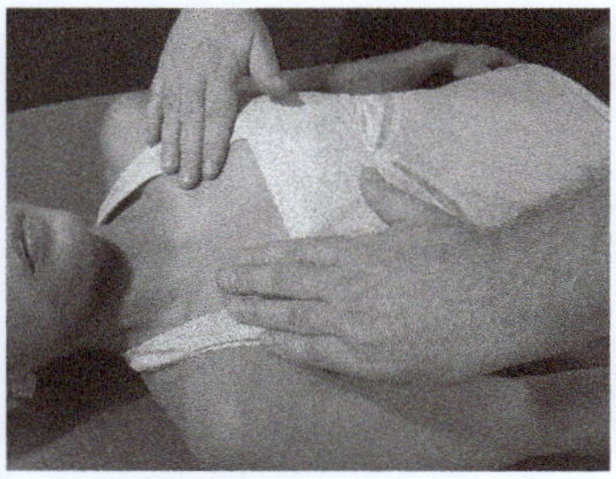

FIGURE 10.34

Upper rib heights.

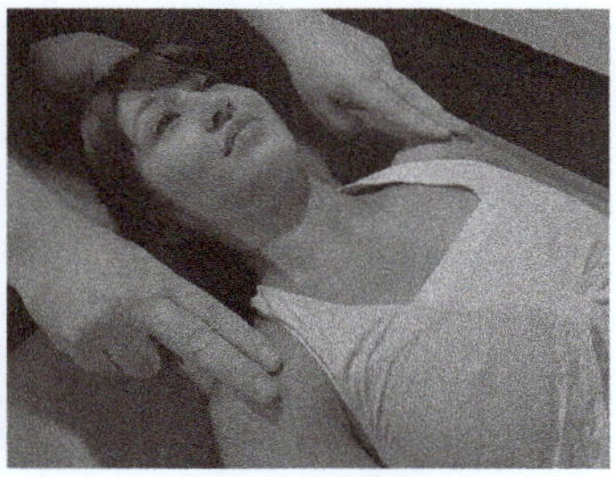

FIGURE 10.35

Anterior shoulder heights.

6. Checking postural symmetries while supine (Figures 10.28–10.36)

Assist the patient to lie in their natural orientation. Have the crook-lying patient lift their hips off the table and then let the hips drop back down to the table. The musculature around the pelvis will pull according to their current tautness (short or long) and as a result leave the patient supine according to their muscle balance. Passively pull each bent leg into extension. At this point check the malleoli for symmetry of leg length. Later you will compare those findings with ASIS levels.

With leg lengths noted, you can now check the patient's ASISs.

- With your thumbs under the ASISs, check to see if they are level in a superior-inferior direction (horizontally). In other words, is there unilateral innominate rotation? If there is this may be the cause of a leg length discrepancy, something fully discussed in the Chapter 9.
- Check the distance of the ASISs from the mid-line using umbilicus (inflare or outflare).

Next, you will proceed to check the trunk rotations (fascial examination). Compare the ASIS heights from the table, the lower ribcage, the upper ribs, the anterior shoulders, and the left and right side of the occiput. If there are rotations these should occur in an alternating fashion (e.g., left/right/left/right/left) from one set of landmarks to the next. This is a *compensating* pattern.

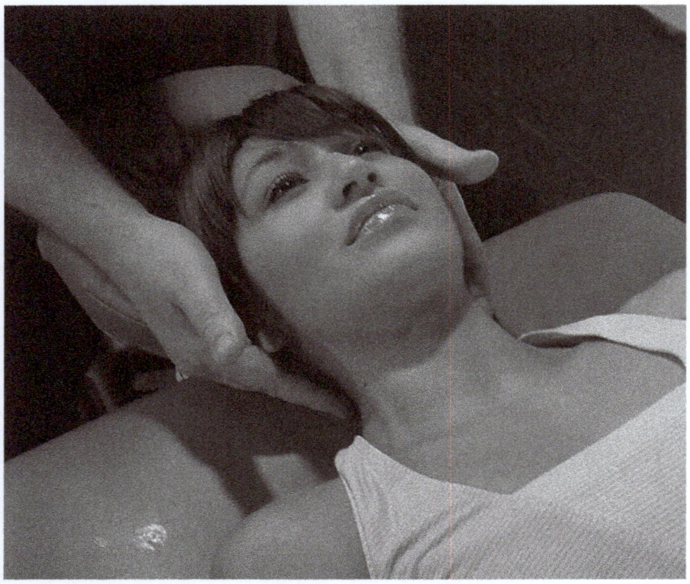

FIGURE 10.36

Occiput heights (can use mastoid processes).

7. Checking rotation in the body (Figures 10.37–10.40)

Good or bad, compensatory rotations exist in all of us. They can be due to many things, including something as simple as handedness. What is significant, however, is whether the rotations generally alternate from one level to the next. When examining for rotation in the trunk keep in mind that there are four transition zones of the spine to focus on (Chila 2010; DeStefano 2011; Mitchell 2001, 2004; Pope 2003):

1. lumbosacral junction: checked through ASISs
2. thoracolumbar junction: checked through lower thoracic ribs
3. cervicothoracic junction: checked through shoulder girdle
4. atlanto-occipital junction: checked through occiput.

If these rotations alternate from one junction to the next the patient is said to be *compensated*, i.e., has successfully managed to accommodate these rotations (in a vertical axis). This would imply successful accommodation of mild or minor asymmetries within the musculoskeletal system (for now, at least). If the rotations are not alternating, the patient is said to be *uncompensated*. This is usually found in patients with moderate to severe lesions or impairments which may or may not be trauma-based. Gordon Zink D.O. is the originator of these observations. In his clinical practice, mostly in hospitals, he noted that the uncompensated patient often suffered from some systemic, organ, or gland pathology while the compensated usually did not (Chila 2010). There is more on compensatory patterns in posture in Part 1, Chapter 5, *Postural Assessment and Gait.*

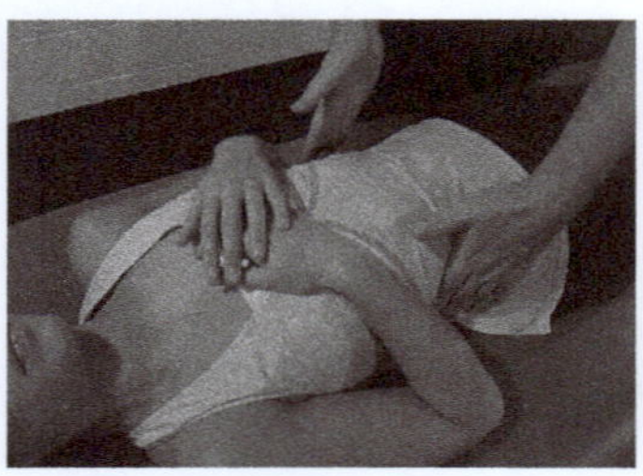

FIGURE 10.37

Waist.

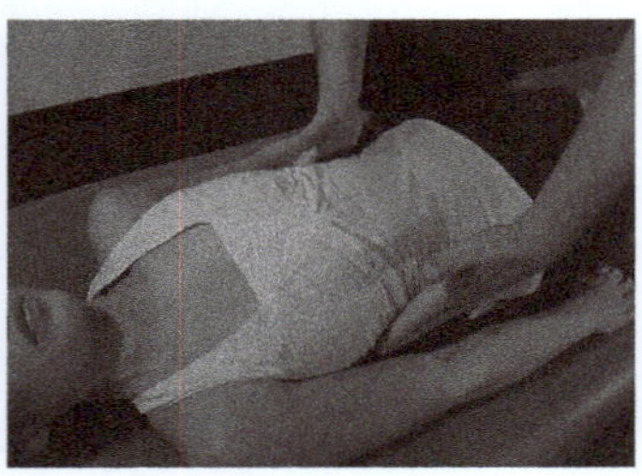

FIGURE 10.38

Lower ribs.

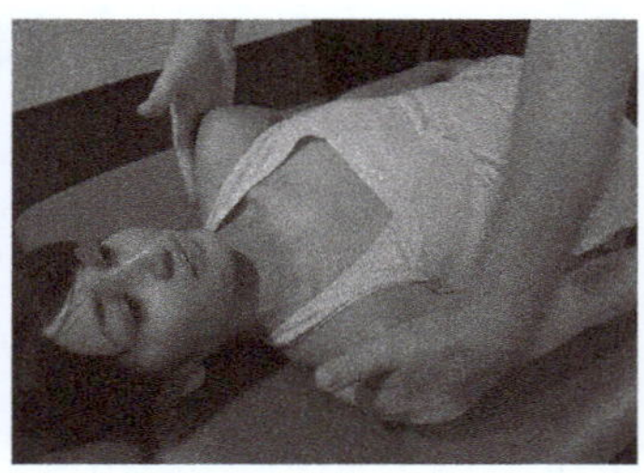

FIGURE 10.39

Shoulder girdle.

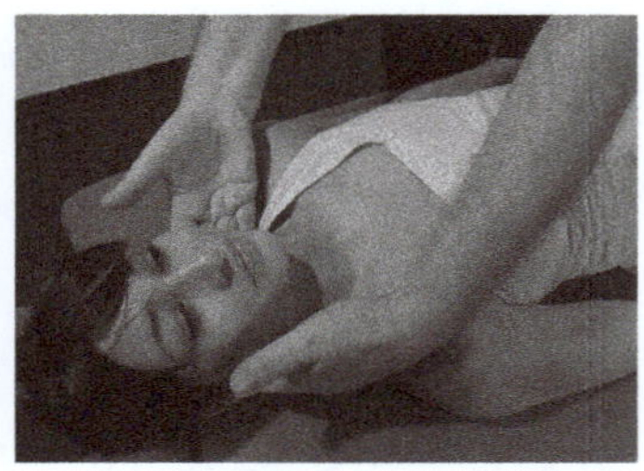

FIGURE 10.40

Cervical.

To assess motion at the spinal junctions we will check side-bending (ease/bind) at the waist, lower ribs, shoulder girdle and cervical spine. To determine how motion passes through the junctions we "push" these areas side to side, testing ease/bind at each level: waist (lumbosacral junction); lower ribs (thoracolumbar junction); shoulder girdle (cervicothoracic junction); neck (atlanto-occipital junction). The "pushing" should be gentle as you are only observing if the tissue is willing (ease) or unwilling (bind) to move in a specific way. This is a general mobility test for fascia, muscle, joint, etc. It will not reveal the reason for the bind but it may provide a clue to where more specific testing should take place.

8. Checking landmarks prone (Figures 10.41–10.46)

When, or if, specific testing has the patient prone, check the following: levels of plantar surface of heels; ischial tuberosities; PSISs (and height from table); lateral curves in spine; tissue bulk of erector spinae; and scapula orientation.

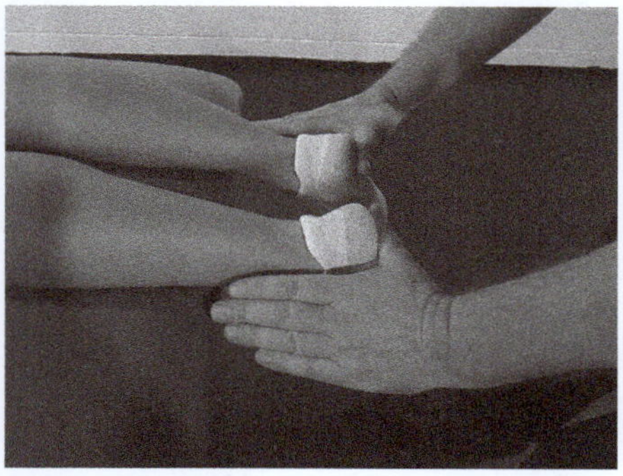

FIGURE 10.41

Heel levels.

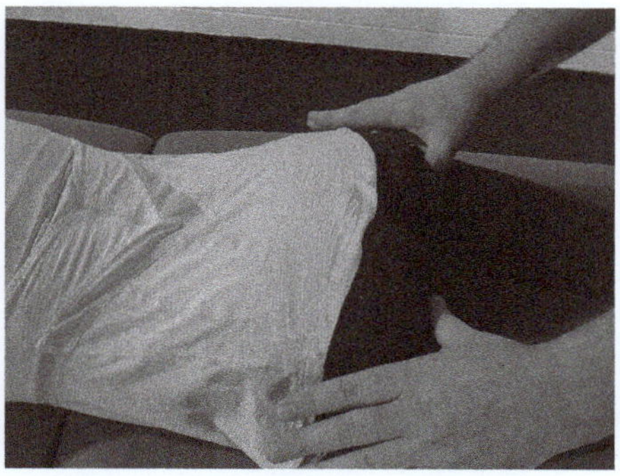

FIGURE 10.42

Ischial tuberosities.

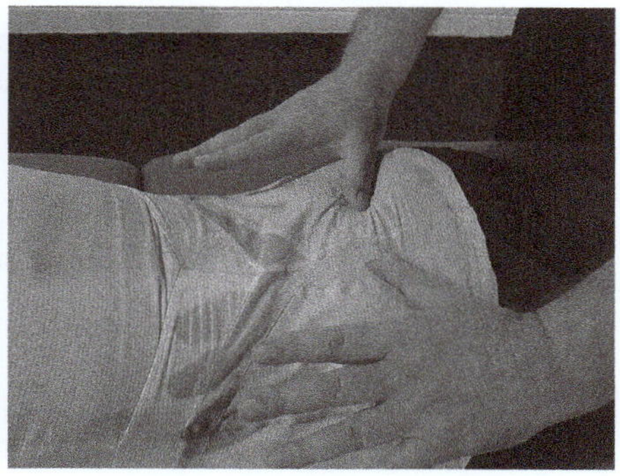

FIGURE 10.43

PSISs.

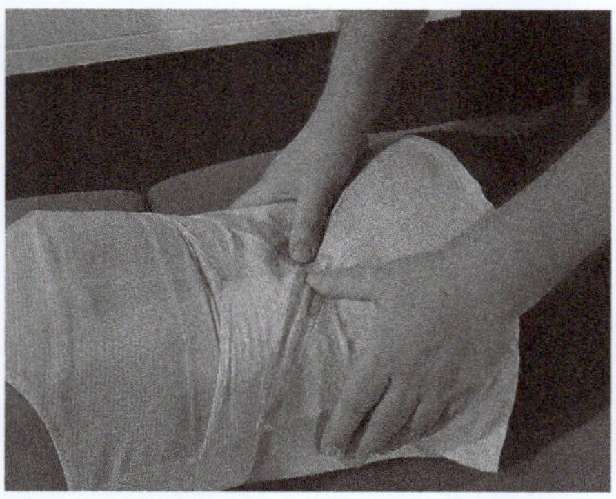

FIGURE 10.44

Lateral curves, etc.

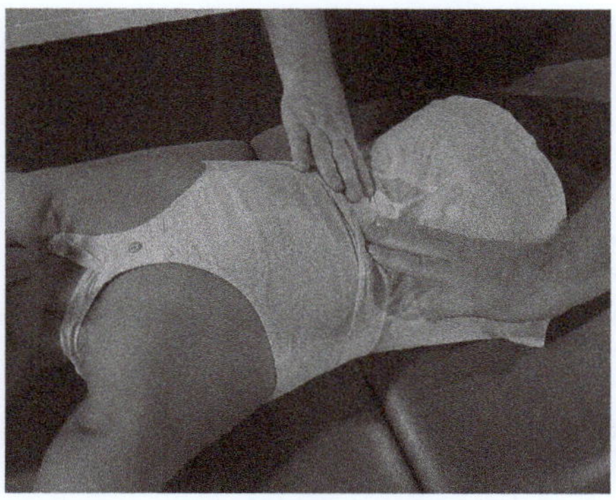

FIGURE 10.45

Tissue bulk of erectors.

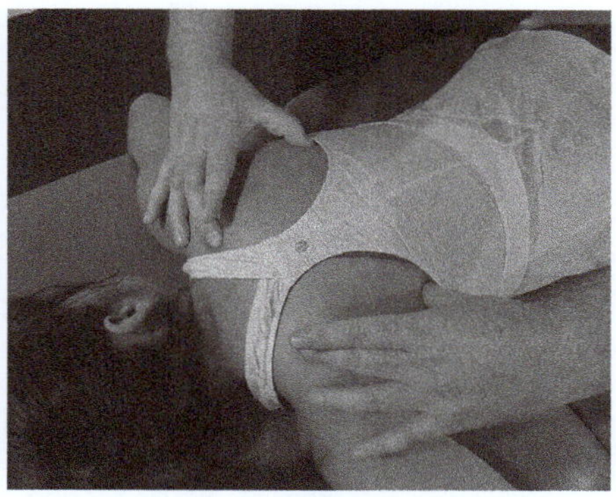

FIGURE 10.46

Scapular orientation.

SACROILIAC JOINT AND PELVIS: CHAPTER OVERVIEW

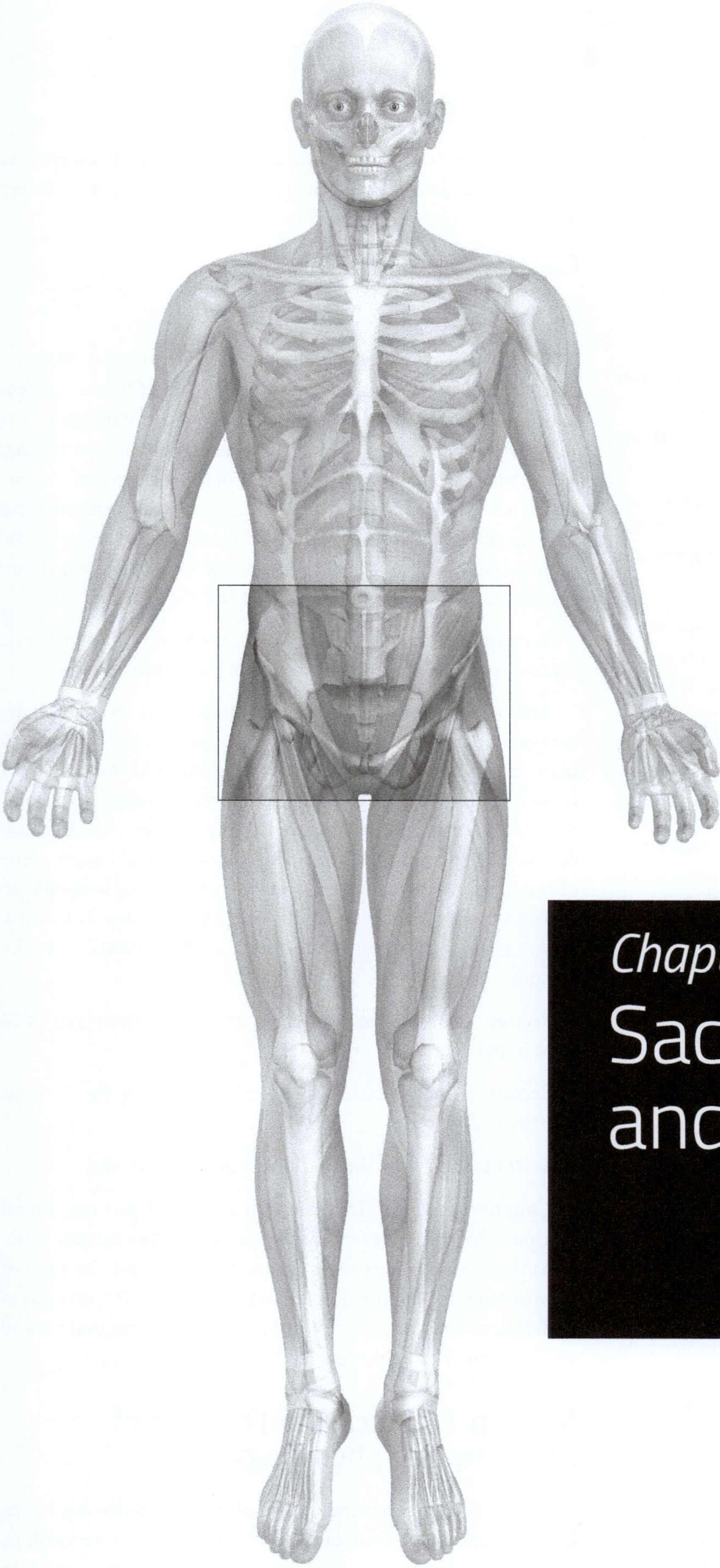

Chapter 11

Sacroiliac joint and pelvis

Note to the reader

This chapter is meant to expand the massage therapist's understanding of the function of the sacroiliac (SI) joints and how to assess them. Therefore, more information on anatomy and physiology (biomechanics) is given here than might otherwise seem reasonable in a guide to assessment.

See Chapter 10 for an outline of the comprehensive structural examination of the pelvis and spine. The comprehensive structural examination reproduced later in this chapter underlines those tests which, when positive, require more detailed testing of the innominates, the SI joints, or both. This chapter presents the detailed information and description of such specific testing, providing an overview of how testing should proceed in an organized and efficient manner.

Choosing the type and amount of information to be given in this chapter (and to a lesser degree, in all the chapters on the spine) has occupied many years of the author's thought. The basis for the choices presented has come from many years of study, instruction from others who were much more knowledgeable, and especially from my experiences teaching this topic to both students of massage therapy and practicing massage therapists.

As soft tissue therapists whose patients overwhelmingly come to us with back and neck pain and impairments to movement, I believe that we need to learn to appropriately and efficiently assess the synovial joints of the spine. How can we claim to be therapists if we cannot assess and treat the most common problems associated with back and neck pain?

As the base for the entire spine, the sacrum demands a firm understanding of its structure and function. Whatever is impaired or misaligned here will create impairments and dysfunctions throughout the upper body. Further, the motions, stresses, and strains coming from the lower body that try to pass through an impaired pelvis will be turned back onto the lower body, resulting in inevitable breakdown.

Though there are some orthopedic tests for innominate and sacroiliac impairments, they are not really of much use, except to provoke symptoms at the site of the impairment. They do not tell us about the nature of the impairment and so do not help us to develop a treatment plan. Further, if used prior to motion testing, which most of the chapter is devoted to, the provocation of pain or re-creation of the injury may well make motion testing impossible that day.

The orthopedic tests are presented primarily because of their traditional use, and because many other health care practitioners rely solely upon them. Understanding these tests assists us in communicating with other health care practitioners and in helping us understand the type of testing our patients may already have received prior to seeking our help.

Chapter organization

The chapter is organized into six sections:

Section 1 is an expanded clinical considerations of anatomy and physiology, containing definitions and brief biomechanical explanations of motions of the SI joint and the innominates. Sufficient information has been given to explain hands-on testing. More detail on gait and the movement of the sacrum and innominates is in the Chapter appendix. This material is extensive and may be difficult for some. Those who have a fair grasp of the material may wish to read only Sections 3, 5, and 6, which are specific to testing innominate motion and the SI joints.

Section 2 describes the types of innominate impairments. Once again, this provides mostly theory and information.

Section 3 focuses on testing for impairments to innominate motions or iliosacral dysfunctions. However, to test for innominate impairments we do need to understand SI joint motions (hence the importance of the information in Section 1). Therefore, included in this section are some palpatory exercises that double as basic sacral testing. Please note that although some of the information on the innominates and testing is similar to that in Chapter 9 it varies slightly (especially in depth) because we are viewing it specifically in terms of its relationship to the sacrum.

Section 4 focuses on describing more fully the types of SI joint impairments.

Section 5 then focuses on specific testing of the SI joint impairments.

Section 6 describes the traditional orthopedic tests.

Chapter appendix This contains details of gait and sacral motion, which provides many clues as to how the sacrum functions, how motion testing is meant to work, and the type of information that is gained. It is useful for therapists who need to understand how things work in order to be able to understand and learn the testing protocol.

Section 1: Clinical implications of anatomy and physiology

The following are some anatomical observations that have clinical implications. Understanding the functional relationships (physiology) between structures and tissues (anatomy) will help explain how structures of the pelvis, especially the sacroiliac and symphysis pubis joints, can be injured, and help us understand how orthopedic and motion tests work to provide the information that they do. It is suggested that the reader have an anatomy book at hand when reading, to more easily understand the information given (either a general musculoskeletal text or one that reviews in detail the anatomy of this specific area of the body). The information that has been summarized here has been chosen because of its direct relevance to orthopedic and motion testing and understanding of mechanical pathologies concerning the joints of the pelvis (see: Agur et al. 2014; Bogduk 2012; Chila 2010; DeStefano 2011; Dutton 2012; Hertling & Kessler 2006; Magee 2014; Mitchell 2001, 2005; Schuenke et al. 2014.)

The following key anatomical structures and tissues should be reviewed with a good anatomy text:

Sacroiliac joint Diarthrodial (synovial) joint between the sacrum and the ilia (innominate). Unusual in that the sacral portion is hyaline cartilage while the iliac side is fibrocartilage. In adults the surfaces are uneven, like hills and valleys, and interlock.

Symphysis pubis Cartilaginous joint.

Sacrococcygeal joint Usually fused in adults, uniting with the sacrum with a fibrocartilaginous disc.

Ligaments

- interosseous sacroiliac ligament (deepest, with transverse orientation)
- short and long sacroiliac ligaments (oblique fibers between the sacrum and innominates)
- long posterior sacroiliac ligament (fibers run almost vertically); part of the long dorsal ligament that has fibers running down from the lumbar aponeurosis, crossing the sacrotuberous ligament into the tendon of the hamstrings (van Wingerden et al. 1993)
- anterior sacroiliac ligaments
- sacrospinous ligaments
- sacrotuberous ligaments.

To do many of the testing procedures in this chapter you will need to be able to palpate or landmark the following:

Posterior structures (some shown in Figure 11.1)

- iliolumbar ligaments
- posterior superior iliac spine (PSIS)

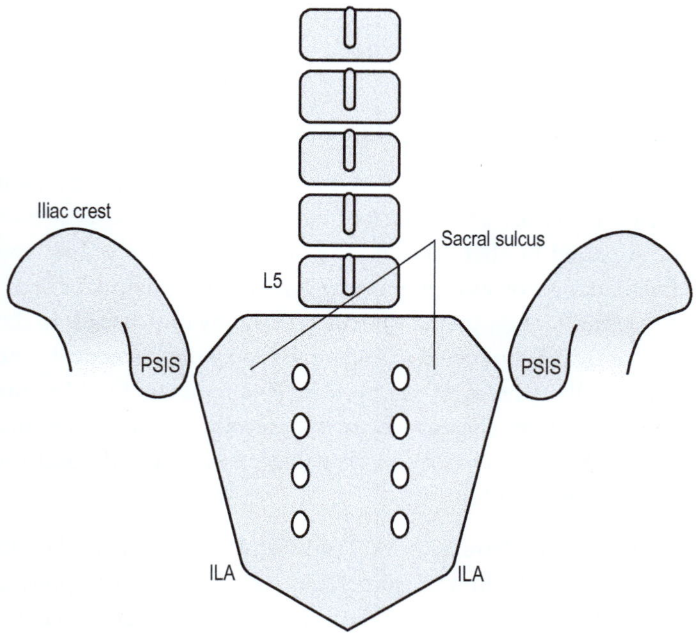

FIGURE 11.1

Posterior structures of the sacrum. ILA, inferior lateral angle; PSIS, posterior superior iliac spine.

- sacral base: superior portion of the sacrum on which L5 sits
- sacral sulcus: landmark the PSISs, which are at the level of S2, and palpate with the thumb just medial and slightly superior to the PSISs (approximately the S1 area). Needed to test for motion impairment to the SI joint
- SI joint line
- sacral crest: palpable crest down the center of the sacrum, to the sacral hiatus
- sacral hiatus
- inferior lateral angles (ILA): landmarking needed for testing of impaired motion to the SI joints
- ischial tuberosity.

Anterior structures

- iliac crest height
- anterior superior iliac spine (ASIS)
- anterior inferior iliac spine (AIIS)
- inguinal ligament

- symphysis pubis
- greater trochanter.

Sacroiliac joints and impairments

The SI joints are involved in many low back (lumbar) pain scenarios, either as a contributing factor or as a consequence of impaired lumbar motion. The SI joints are stressed by any imbalance of forces or impairments above in the trunk or head. Also, the SI joints are put under stress by any impairment to the hip, or forces conducted through the hip by impairments to the lower limbs. Therefore, we must be able to assess the SI joints sufficiently to be able to identify if these joints are impaired, and (if possible) how. Otherwise, we will not be able to fully address most low back or hip pain.

If the sacral base is unlevel (side-bent or torsioned), then to compensate, the lumbar spine must side-bend to the opposite side, which means a scoliosis is created. If the sacral base is tipped too far forward, then the lordosis of the lumbar spine is exaggerated due to the spine compensating; and if not tipped forward enough, then the lumbar lordosis is flattened. The consequences of this could be in the low back and/or anywhere else up the chain (i.e., up the spine): the thoracic spine and ribcage, the cervical spine and/or the occiput-C1 (occipital-atlanto joint). Of course, such changes to the SI joints will also affect innominate function, and the function of the lower extremities (Chila 2010; DeStefano 2011; Kapandji 2008; Mitchell 2001).

Within the curve of a scoliosis, the muscles on the concave side of the curve are usually short and tight, which can make them go into spasm, while the muscles on the convex side are lengthened and weakened and easily strained.

Of course, the SI joints can themselves be the cause of pain, whether sharp and intense or dull and achy, on-site or referred some distance. We will discuss how each type of impairment of the joint creates its specific pain once we have discussed the nature of the impairments that can occur and the findings of our testing.

NOTE: What follows is a detailed summary of the terminology, anatomy, and physiology (biomechanics) of the sacroiliac joints. Much of what is presented here is *a model* of sacroiliac motion that can assist the therapist in making clinical decisions. The rules of motion, etc., are *concepts*, not facts.

If you are familiar with this material, then you may wish to go directly to the testing protocols (see Sections 2, 3, and 4). If you are not familiar with this information, then please study it carefully and give yourself time to digest the material fully, to better understand what the testing seeks to find and how these tests accomplish this. (The principal sources of the information are: Bogduk 2012; Chila 2010; DeStefano 2011; Hertling and Kessler 2006; Kapandji 2008; Mitchell 2001, 2005).

Terminology and mechanics of sacral motion

- Physiological motion: these are motions that occur in a joint that constitute its normal functional movements. However, the joint can become restricted or fixed ("stuck") at the end-range of such a motion. These are referred to as *physiological impairments*.
- Non-physiological motion: these are motions that occur in a joint that are not normal for that joint or not in accordance with its anatomy and function/physiology. These usually result in impaired (dysfunctional) movements, also referred to as *non-physiological impairments*.

Movements of sacroiliac joints and their axes

- The SI joint is crescent-shaped. It has also been called *auricular* in shape, which means shaped somewhat like a human ear.
- No two SI joints are the same: no two people have the same shape or configuration of SI joints, and no single individual has two SI joints (left and right) with the same shape or configuration. Some joints may be shallower than most, or have an unusual auricular shape, for example. This variety in joint structure or configuration can help explain why some people seem prone to SI joint impairments while others are not, or why some individuals have a consistent recurring problem with one of their SI joints.
- The iliac portion of the SI joint surface is cartilaginous with a central crest running from the top to the bottom of the joint surface making this surface convex. This central crest stays roughly in the center of the joint surface and follows the crescent orientation of the articular surface. The apex of this convexity (its most prominent portion or bulge) is approximately at the level of S2 and is less prominent above and below that level. This is matched by a concavity in the sacral joint surfaces. Hence, we should not be surprised that the transverse axis on which the sacrum flexes and extends is at this S2 level where the ileum bulges the most into the sacrum.
- The sacral portion of the joint also has an irregularly shaped (wrinkled or corrugated) surface, but it has a central canal or groove, into which the ileum's joint surface fits. As mentioned above, the deepest portion of that concavity is at the S2 level of the sacrum.

- The joint surfaces are irregular with a wrinkled appearance, running roughly horizontally over the crest and canal, with the wrinkles matching on each side of the joint in such a manner that allows the two joint surfaces to mesh like a pair of gears.
- The sacral articular surface is made of hyaline cartilage. The ilia's articular surface is also hyaline in nature (histologically) but it is reinforced by dense bundles of collagen fibers that make it appear as if it is fibrocartilage.

The crescent-shaped surfaces of the SI joint permits some limited movement in a semicircular path. The appearance or placement of an axis during various movements of the sacrum may vary with each type of movement, due to the type and direction of forces exerted on the sacrum. Therefore, in general, flexion and extension move around a transverse axis at S2; however, the axis may slide about, shifting as the degree of sagittal movement increases from neutral. An alternating (moving from one side to the other) oblique axis is formed when we are walking. For more on this, see the information on gait later in this chapter.

Some points to consider

The amount of movement within the SI joints has been a contentious issue for over a century. That there is any functional movement at all in these joints has only recently (in the 1990s) been accepted by orthopedic professions such as physiotherapy and orthopedic physicians (Forst et al. 2006; Vleeming et al. 2012, 2013). The movements that have been traditionally spoken of (by osteopaths, etc.) are very small, and are considered to be less than a fraction of an inch (only a millimeter or two). Research has shown that the sacroiliac joint rotates only about 2° in the sagittal plane. During gait, for example, torsional forces go through these joints, where movements may be minimal but are nonetheless extremely important (Vleeming et al. 2012, 2013). Therefore, restriction on one side demands compensatory increase of motion in surrounding joints. Also, it may well be that often we are dealing with the result of tensile (tension) or compressive forces that are being exerted through the joint and its supportive structures, and the loss of potential movement for that joint translates into a rigidity that restricts certain pelvic or lumbar motions (Vleeming and Stoeckart 2007).

If there was no movement at all through the SI joints, and the pelvis was truly a fused-bone bowl, then the motions of gait would place such stress through this bowl that it would begin to fracture, and do so where the SI joints are located (Bogduk 2012). Therefore, movement must happen within the pelvis so that torsional and compressive forces can be accommodated. However, if the SI joints were held together by ligaments alone, "creep" (physiological changes in connective tissues due to sustained stress that causes them to lengthen) would cause the ligaments to quickly "fail" as support. Therefore, the study of movement in the SI joints needs to take the unique shape of the bones and joint surface anatomy into consideration to understand the ability of this joint to remain functional. For a discussion of this see below, "What stabilizes the SI joint?"

In light of this, let us propose that just as we can assess the mobility of synovial joints in the extremities according to the amount of potential joint space ("joint play") available to them (for accessory motions), we should in the same manner be thinking of assessment of the SI joints, assessing the "strain patterns" being placed through their structures, and not become fixated on whether or not there are gross movements taking place in sacroiliac joints.

With any region of the body we are not only concerned with a specific joint and its internal structures. We are also concerned with the effect that any restrictions or laxity in that joint may have on all the tissues and structures nearby, and even for those at some distance from that specific joint. Usually what we feel when testing a joint is which ranges of motion have a sense of "ease" and which have a feeling of "bind"; in which direction would the joint be willing to move and in which direction would it be unwilling to move? This is precisely the purpose of most SI joint palpation and testing.

Make no mistake, there is joint play available in the SI joints for the purposes of assessment and treatment. Motions can occur at these joints, and they can be moved both through trauma and through manipulation. All that is being proposed here is to also think of some of these dysfunctions described below as similar to losses of accessory motions in other synovial joints (see Joint mobilizations in Chapter 3), and not always as dysfunctions involving gross movement. Though small, the motions within the SI joints are essential for full function of the hips (especially during gait) and for the motions of the lumbar spine.

The model of SI joint motion outlined below is just that: a model. It is a model that helps explain what is palpated in the clinical setting. It is true that more could be happening than can be explained by this model, or the model may have difficulty explaining some clinical findings. But until we reach a point where we understand exactly all that is happening in the body (something that is not going to happen anytime soon, if ever), we have to work with models that help us to treat the impairments that patients present with. Certainly, these models can be questioned, scrutinized, and improved upon. But they should not be dismissed simply because they do not answer all questions or do not yet have "proof" of all their claims. As long as a model provides clinically observable beneficial results, and as long as no other explanation (model or metaphor) can do the job better, we are obligated to work with it. That is the meaning of the phrase "a working hypothesis" – the cornerstone of scientific enquiry.

Definitions of sacroiliac movements

Nutation (nodding)

Movement or positioning of the sacral base anteriorly and inferiorly with respect to the innominate. Sometimes called anterior nutation, or anterior rotation (flexion) of the sacral base. Nutation of the sacrum occurs when we are exhaling and our spine's lordosis and kyphosis exaggerate, when we stand up, and when we extend our lumbar spine. The term has also been used to describe movement or positioning of the innominate posteriorly with respect to the sacral base. To avoid confusion, we will use nutation for describing the position of the sacrum, and refer to the movement or positioning of the innominate as posterior rotation.

- During extension of the lumbar spine, the nucleus pulposus of the L5–S1 disc shifts forward, and pushes down on the anterior portion of the sacral base. The auricular (ear-shaped) surface of the joint directs the sacrum anteriorly and inferiorly. The sacrum flexes (nutates) when the lumbar spine extends.

Counternutation

Movement or positioning of the sacral base posteriorly and superiorly with respect to the innominate. Sometimes called posterior nutation, or posterior rotation (extension) of the sacral base. Counternutation occurs when we inhale and the spine lengthens, when we are sitting, or when we forward flex the lumbar spine. The term also describes movement or positioning of the innominate anteriorly with respect to the sacrum. Again, we will use counternutation for describing the position of the sacrum, and refer to the movement or positioning of the innominate as anterior rotation.

- During flexion of the lumbar spine the nucleus pulposus of the L5–S1 disc shifts backward, tipping the sacral base posteriorly while the flexing lumbar spine pulls the sacrum superiorly. The auricular surface of the joint directs the sacrum superiorly and posteriorly. The sacrum thus extends (counternutates) when the lumbar spine flexes.

Sacroiliac movement

Describes movement of the sacrum on a fixed innominate. The sacrum is moving in concert with the lumbar spine (and movements of the trunk). For example, when the spine rotates while the legs/innominates are not moving there are consequential movements in the sacrum.

Iliosacral movement

Describes movement of the innominate on the fixed sacrum. For example, when a lower limb is in motion (non-weight-bearing) causing movement of an innominate, the sacrum can be held fixed by the weight-bearing limb (by force closure of the SI joint, see below). To avoid confusion, we will usually speak of innominate motion/movements rather than iliosacral movement.

These last two definitions talk of a fixed sacrum or a fixed innominate, but this is to make the point clear about the meaning of the terms sacroiliac and iliosacral. Often neither is fixed and both are moving in concert, the sacrum mediating between the lumbar spine and the innominates. The terms are meant as referential, to help orient us when we are looking at the influences on the pelvic girdle and in the naming of impairment or dysfunctions (Box 11.1).

Sacroiliac impairments imply that the sacrum is the source of the dysfunction in the pelvis; that the sacrum has become fixed or hypomobile and will not move within the SI joint. If not for this, the innominates would be functioning normally (DeStefano 2011; Mitchell 2001, 2005).

Iliosacral impairment, or innominate impairment as it will be subsequently called, implies that the movement of the innominate is impaired. And while the sacrum may have some mild restriction of motion due to dysfunctional innominate motion, it is still capable of motion. If the innominate impairment is corrected, then the sacrum will function normally (DeStefano 2011; Mitchell 2005).

Pelvic tilt (innominate rotation)

(See Chapter 9 for more on this.)

- The innominates can bilaterally rotate anteriorly or posteriorly. These are pelvic tilts.
- They can also rotate unilaterally, anteriorly, or posteriorly. These are innominate rotations.
- Innominates move primarily in accordance with the lower extremities, while the spine usually drives the sacrum – hence, the trunk and lower body are said to meet at the SI joint.
- The pubic symphysis rotates during gait, with one pubic ramus rotating anteriorly as the other rotates posteriorly. These motions correlate to and match the innominates rotating anteriorly and posteriorly. Also, one ramus can translate

INSIGHTS

Box 11.1 The motion of walking comes to rest in the sacrum

Both iliosacral and sacroiliac motions are happening during walking:

- On heel-strike of the right foot, the right innominate rotates posteriorly (and with slight external rotation) and on toe-off, the left foot produces anterior rotation (with a slight internal rotation) of the left innominate. Thus, there is anterior and posterior rotation happening in the sagittal plane through a transverse axis, with the pelvis as a whole rotating slightly left on a vertical axis (in a transverse plane).
- Meanwhile, the trunk is rotating right with the left arm swinging forward and the right arm swinging back. Thus, the lumbar spine is rotating right (on a vertical axis through the horizontal plane) and side-bending slightly left (on an anterior-posterior axis through the coronal plane).
- Therefore, there is motion from above with trunk rotation and from below with innominate motion (via the legs). And, these motions are occurring all at once in several planes – and sometimes even in opposite directions – with all of these torsional forces meeting at the sacroiliac (SI) joints.
- In detail, the sacrum tries to accommodate all of this by moving in opposite directions:
  - The right sacral base (the right upper corner of the sacrum) moves forward/anteriorly and down (nutates) on the right innominate as it is posteriorly rotating.
  - The left sacral base tries to move ever so slightly posteriorly and superiorly (counternutates) on the left innominate that is rotating anteriorly. It is held almost still by the gluteus maximus, erector spinae, and quadratus lumborum (on the left). (See below, force closure.)
  - Since the sacrum has moved slightly inferiorly on the right, the sacral base as a whole is tilted to the right. Therefore, the lumbar spine compensates by side-bending to the left. (Otherwise our trunk and especially the shoulders would sway wildly to the right and then have to sway to the left as the legs change position.)
  - Because the right corner of the sacral base is anterior and inferior while the left is held in neutral (or very slightly posterior and superior) the anterior surface of the sacrum is turned to the left. Yet, the lumbar spine (side-bent left) is rotated right. (**Note:** It has to turn this way because the right posteriorly rotated innominate's iliolumbar ligaments attached to L4's and L5's transverse processes (TVPs) pull/turn the lumbar spine to the right.)

Therefore, as the sacrum is generally moving in the opposite direction to the motions of both the lumbar spine and the innominates it acts somewhat like a gyroscope, coordinating all of the forces that pass through it, keeping us upright as we move. By moving opposite to the structures around it, the sacrum becomes the center of motion during walking. And, like the hub of motion, the sacrum itself moves hardly at all.

(shear) superiorly or interiorly when under strain, as in jumping from a height and landing on one leg. Problems with shears (upslip/downslip) lead to problems with rotation, which will affect motion in the pelvis as a whole.

What stabilizes the sacroiliac joints?

A great source of information, with extensive references to research, about the structure of the sacroiliac joint, its function, and supportive structures can be found in Vleeming et al. (2012).

Stability by joint shape/structure

1. The upper portion of the SI joint (just above S2, at S1) is wider posteriorly than anteriorly.

   Thus, the joint surfaces are beveled. This restricts the superior portion from tipping too far forward (from nutating more) between the innominates. The innominate has a matching bevel. The lower portion (below S2) is wider anteriorly than posteriorly. This, in turn, prevents the lower portion of the sacrum from moving too far backward, again preventing excessive movement of the sacral base forward into nutation.

   The beveling especially provides stability to the spine when we are standing; specifically, preventing the sacrum from sliding forward out from between the innominates and causing excessive extension (hyperlordosis) of the lumbar spine. Thus, the sacrum can only move within the confines of the shape of the joint surfaces. This beveling works best to prevent the motion of nutation when standing still. However, during gait, with the gapping of the joints, some motion into nutation is possible (Kapandji 2008; Mitchell 2001).

2. The sacral joint surface is somewhat concave, while the surface of the innominate is somewhat convex. Also, each surface is

uneven – hills and valleys fitting into near matching hills and valleys, or fitting together like a set of gears. This helps, along with point number 1, to restrict excessive motion.

Ligaments

The posterior sacroiliac ligaments are thicker and stronger than the anterior. The deep ligaments run short and oblique, and as they become more superficial they move laterally and they become longer and more vertical. The lateral portion of the posterior ligaments, at this point referred to as the long dorsal ligament, blends with the sacrotuberous and sacrospinalis ligaments.

The anterior sacroiliac ligaments are much thinner and weaker than the posterior ligaments. The sacrum, therefore, is principally suspended between the innominates by the posterior ligaments.

However, no matter how tight these ligaments are, they cannot prevent all movement at the SI joints. The only way to absolutely prevent any movement is to fuse all of these joints together with bone, and this would have to be considered pathological in nature.

Muscles, ligaments, and the sacroiliac joint: movement and stability

Fibers from the erector spinae and multifidus meld with the posterior ligaments and into the long dorsal ligament. The superior fibers from the tendon of the biceps femoris hamstring are (usually) continuous with the sacrotuberous and in turn, the long dorsal ligament (Bogduk 2012; Vleeming et al. 2012).

As Vleeming et al. (1996) succinctly wrote:

> The long dorsal sacroiliac ligament has close anatomical relations with the erector spinae muscle, the posterior layer of the thoracolumbar fascia, and a specific part of the sacrotuberous ligament (tuberoiliac ligament). Functionally, it is an important link between legs, spine, and arms. The ligament is tensed when the sacroiliac joints are counter-nutated and slackened when nutated. The reverse holds for the sacrotuberous ligament. Slackening of the long dorsal sacroiliac ligament can be counterbalanced by both the sacrotuberous ligament and the erector muscle. Pain localized within the boundaries of the long ligament could indicate among other things a spinal condition with sustained counter-nutation of the sacroiliac joints. In diagnosing patients with a specific low back pain or peripartum pelvic pain, the long dorsal sacroiliac ligament should not be neglected. Even in cases of arthrodesis of the sacroiliac joints, tension in the long ligament can still be altered by different structures.

The gluteus maximus also uses these ligaments for part of its attachment. Further, the piriformis has some fibers that originate on the sacrotuberous ligament. The coccygeus and levator ani (which are part of the pelvic diaphragm) attach to the sacrospinalis ligament. These muscular attachments can increase the tension on these ligaments when they contract, or lessen the tension if they relax. In turn, misalignment of the sacrum, and the concomitant tension (or lack of) on these ligaments, can affect the tone and function of any and all of these muscles, which could lead to what has been called pelvic pain syndrome.

We should mention that the iliacus has fibers onto the anterior ligaments of the sacrum as well as the lower portion of the anterior body of the sacrum.

There are no prime movers of the SI joint. The sacrum moves and responds to the motion in the innominates and the lumbar spine, along with mass action of muscles that attach to the hip and pelvis. Or to put it another way: the movement of the spine from above (motion through L5) and movement from the hips through the innominates puts torsional (twisting) forces through the SI joints, causing the sacrum to oscillate (squirm or twist) between the innominates. Therefore, muscles are considered to only indirectly move the SI joint. However, they may have a more direct effect on fixing or holding still some parts of the sacrum; for example, muscles such as the piriformis, gluteus maximus, multifidus, hamstrings, etc.

All the muscles that move the hip joint pass their forces into the innominate bones and by the deformation of the innominates (inflares, outflares, etc., and by their anterior and posterior rotations), these muscles pass their forces into the SI joints.

Such deformations of the living (i.e., soft and pliable) bone of the innominate can occur from the rectus femoris, sartorius, tensor fasciae latae, iliotibial band; from the quadratus lumborum, the iliacus, and the obliques and transverse abdominal muscles.

For example:

1. The rectus abdominis directly affects the movements and stabilization of the symphysis pubis (rotation and translation/shearing) in concert with the adductor muscles attached to the pubic ramus.
2. The principal hip flexors (the iliopsoas and the rectus femoris) are the principal culprits in bilateral, or unilateral, anterior rotation of the innominate.

3. The further contribution of the iliacus and sartorius to anterior rotation also causes the innominate to flare inward as it anteriorly rotates.
4. The tensor fasciae latae, along with the iliotibial band and gluteus minimus and medius, promotes outflares of the innominate.

Form (static) closure and force closure

All of this brings us to what has been called form or static closure and force closure of the SI joints (DeStefano 2011; Dutton 2012; Mitchell 2001, 2005; Snijders et al. 1993).

Form closure refers to how the shape of the bones, joints, and ligaments hold the SI joint closed, i.e., stable. This was described at the beginning of this section in "What stabilizes the SI joint."

Force closure refers to the tightening of the ligaments and hence, the SI joint by the contraction of the gluteus maximus (especially), piriformis, biceps femoris, and from above multifidus and erector spinae (directly), and the muscles that exert forces through the thoracolumbar aponeurosis (such as the latissimus dorsi).

Force closure can be used by the body to fix one of the SI joints while leaving the other more free to move, as happens during walking. Thus, one SI joint can become an axis of movement for the sacrum. Or, force closure can be engaged to bilaterally fix the SI joints during times of exertion (which leads to locking of the SI joints) such as when lifting heavy loads; or it can be used to stabilize a hypermobile joint as protective spasming (often referred to as holding and guarding).

Findings within the general examination of the spine and pelvis that warrant further testing

This section reiterates some of the comprehensive examination of the spine from Chapter 10. The purpose here is to point out what findings from a general/comprehensive examination should prompt the examiner to follow up with further specific testing of the sacroiliac joints.

The observations below that are underlined require further testing if several of them are found to be positive. Generally, a positive observation shows asymmetry with respect to landmarks. A motion test is positive if restriction or asymmetry in the motion of a joint is found. Even if the therapist is sure that the SI joints or the innominates are impaired, they should perform the following comprehensive structural examination prior to specific testing. Doing so may reveal how innominate or SI joint impairments are affecting the rest of the body. You will then have done a truly comprehensive examination.

Standing postural views: front, side, back:

1. Look for relationships with gravity line: static plumb line vertical and horizontal landmarks.
2. Note asymmetries and deviations.

Sitting behind the standing patient:

1. Landmark levels of the arches of the feet, ischial tuberosities, trochanters, PSISs, iliac crest heights, (creases of) waist, inferior and superior angles of the scapula, mastoid processes.
2. Return to the PSISs. While landmarking the PSISs have the patient bring the chin to the chest, then roll down to lumbar flexion, noting movement of the PSISs (standing flexion test). Check the spine for flat spots, excessive curve, bulking of the erector spinae, then have the patient return to standing straight. Have the patient extend the back while observing changes to the curves of the spine (lordosis-kyphosis).
3. Have the patient bring the ear to the shoulder; then have them slide their hand down the side of the leg to the knee, observing how the spine curves during side-bending (from above). Check both sides.
4. Have the patient flex one knee while the other remains "locked" – note lumbar side-bending (from below). Check both sides.
5. Hold the patient's hip stable. Have the patient bring their chin over a shoulder and note head and cervical rotation; then have them bring that shoulder back toward you – observing thoracic rotation. Note also the difference in the amount of resistance required at the hips to resist lower trunk rotation (ease versus effort).
6. Challenge sagittal plane (anterior-posterior) stability (via the manubrium and T2).
7. Challenge coronal plane (side-bending) motion, either by pressure on the acromions or an inferiorly directed tug on the wrists.

Have patient sit:

1. Re-check the iliac crest heights, PSISs, shoulder/scapula landmarks, tissue bulk, etc. Observe all changes of orientation to landmarks, tissue changes, etc., during the following motion.
2. Seated flexion test: while landmarking the PSISs, have the patient flex forward. Check for asymmetry of tissue bulk on either side of the spine.

3. Side-bending: with the elbow at 90°, the patient brings the ear to the shoulder, then lowers it toward the table.
4. Challenge to side-bending: push down alternately on each shoulder cap.
5. Rotation: turn the chin toward the shoulder and at end-range, push the shoulder back.

Patient supine (after traction of legs or other corrections to patient's orientation):

1. Note medial malleoli levels.
2. Check the ASISs
   - level (possible innominate rotation)
   - height from the table (possible pelvic rotation)
   - distance from the mid-line (possible inflare/outflare).
3. Check rotations (fascial exam). Compare the height from the table of hips (ASISs, as above), lower ribcage, upper ribs, anterior shoulders, L and R occiput, i.e., from the table compared to the norm and compared bilaterally; and then compare directions of rotation from one set of landmarks to the next.
4. Tests side-bending comparing ease/bind: at waist (lumbar), mid-ribs (thoracic), and neck (cervical).

When/if specific testing has the patient prone, check the following:

1. Levels of plantar surface of heels, ischial tuberosities, PSISs (and height from table), and the lateral curves in spine, tissue bulk of erector spinae, and scapula orientation.

If the tests underlined above were positive, then a more thorough examination of either the innominates or the SI joints is needed. The tests mentioned specifically (underlined), and all of the further specific testing for the region, are explained and shown in this chapter.

Ideal testing order

Ideally, the iliosacral and sacroiliac joints would be tested at the same time, but to simplify instruction, they will be presented in this chapter separately. Once the student is comfortable with both sets of tests, they can be combined in the ideal fashion as follows:

1. Testing for postural asymmetries: do a standing postural examination.
2. Test for motion impairment of the innominates (iliosacral) using the stork test or its alternative, the standing flexion test.
3. Seated flexion test: do this to check for sacroiliac motion impairment.

If we have a positive stork test but a negative seated flexion test, we need to do the following specific innominate testing:

- Identify the orientation of the innominate that the stork test revealed as lesioned.
- Note the effect on leg length, if any.
- Pelvic challenge for pubic symphysis impairments.
- Passive palpation of sacral motion (four-point palpation of respiratory motion and/or sacral springing and/or gapping of the SI joint).

If we have a positive seated flexion test, we would still do the innominate testing as above and add to that SI joint testing as follows:

- Palpation of six-point landmarking.
- Prone extension test (Sphinx test) to identify the nature of the lesion.

Testing order for instruction purposes

We will now proceed to Section 2, to discuss innominate motions and their impairments. Following that we discuss the testing for those impairments to innominate motion in Section 3. We will then go through the causes and types of sacroiliac impairments in Section 4, and then the testing protocol for SI joint impairments to motion in Section 5.

Section 2: Innominate motions and impairments

We need a few more definitions of the terms used in characterizing normal physiological motions of the innominate versus impaired motion (see: DeStefano 2011; Hertling & Kessler 2006; Mitchell 2001, 2005).

Movements of the lumbopelvic girdle

The innominates go through predictable movements during flexion and extension of the spine and hence, through nutation or counternutation of the sacrum:

- When the spine is extended, the sacrum nutates by sliding inferiorly and anteriorly. This results in a narrowing of the space between the PSISs. This means that the PSISs have moved slightly toward each other, which is matched by the ASISs moving apart. Further, the ischial tuberosities move slightly apart. (Each ischial tuberosity motion matches or complements the motion of the ipsilateral ASIS.) These innominate movements are known as an outflare, a gapping force through the pubic symphysis.

- As the spine flexes the sacrum counternutates, sliding superiorly and posteriorly. This results in a widening of the space between the PSISs. This means that the PSISs have moved slightly apart, while the ASISs move toward each other. Further, the ischial tuberosities move slightly toward each other. These motions are collectively known as an inflare, which places a compressive force through the pubic symphysis.

When testing for inflares and outflares (described below), the principal references are the ASISs. However, when inflares or outflares are suspected, other landmarks, such as the PSIS and the ischial tuberosities, should also be investigated. For brevity, we will often refer only to the position of the ASIS, but the other landmarks are implied.

Outflare

When the lumbar spine is extended – and the sacrum nutates – we have a bilateral outflare. Or when a single innominate is posteriorly rotated, the ASIS on that side may move away from the mid-line (a unilateral outflare). This outflare (or external rotation) of the innominate means that the position of the acetabulum has changed, and the hip joint will be also externally rotated. However, the hip joint may compensate with internal rotation.

It is also possible that the innominate can be pulled to an outflare position by muscular and fascial forces, without necessarily rotating the innominate posteriorly. Remember that living bone is pliable and plastic. Some of the most common culprits here are the tensor fasciae latae, the iliotibial band, and gluteus minimus.

Inflare

When the spine is flexed, and the sacrum counternutates and the ASISs move toward each other, we have a bilateral inflare. A unilateral inflare can occur when a single innominate is anteriorly rotated (the ASIS on that side moves toward the mid-line). However, the anterior portion of the innominate can be pulled toward the mid-line without the presence of anterior rotation. As with outflares, it is usually muscular and connective tissue force that causes the inflare, via the iliacus, internal obliques, sartorius and a contracturing inguinal ligament.

Upslip (superior shear)

If the ASIS, PSIS, and the ischial tuberosity on the same innominate are all higher than the contralateral innominate, then we have what is called an "upslip" of the innominate on the sacrum. This is the result of a shearing of SI joints and the pubic symphysis. Another palpable observation is that the greater trochanter on the side of the upslip should be higher than its opposite. (If the femur and tibia are truly equal in length, the leg on the side of the upslip will likely look shorter.) There would be a shearing taking place at the pubic symphysis. Therefore, if palpated, the pubic bone would also be found to be higher on the side with the upslip (Figure 11.2).

It follows that there is the possibility of a "downslip", or inferior shear, the opposite of an upslip. A downslip would usually immediately self-correct upon weight-bearing. However, even if corrected by weight-bearing, the sacral joints and the pubic symphysis may not all necessarily correct automatically. One or more joints may be held misaligned due to a persistent muscle imbalance caused by the original shearing. If the downslip does not correct on its own, it may imply a dislocation of the SI joints and pubic symphysis, and would present as severely painful. Refer out to primary physician.

NOTE: If on palpating and landmarking you find that the PSIS and ASIS are higher on one side, but the ischial tuberosity is level or even lower than the contralateral ischial tuberosity, then the patient may have what is referred to as a "hemipelvis" (Figure 11.3). This means that one innominate as a whole is actually larger than the other. This can occur in any paired bones of the body. It can even happen to vertebrae, which can be thicker, for example, on the left side and thinner on the other, creating a wedge-shaped vertebra. This is often seen in a structural scoliosis.

Physiological motions of the innominates during gait gait (Box 11.2)

Unilateral anterior rotation of the innominate

The ASIS on the innominate that is anteriorly rotated is lower when compared to the contralateral ASIS. Also, the PSIS will

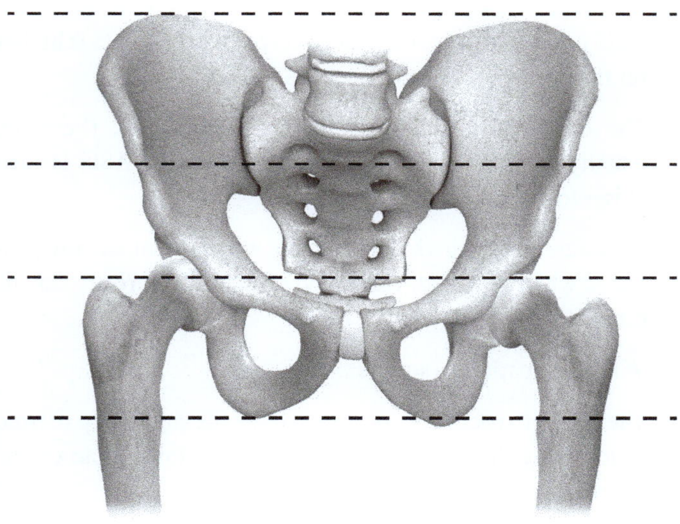

FIGURE 11.2
Upslip on right side.

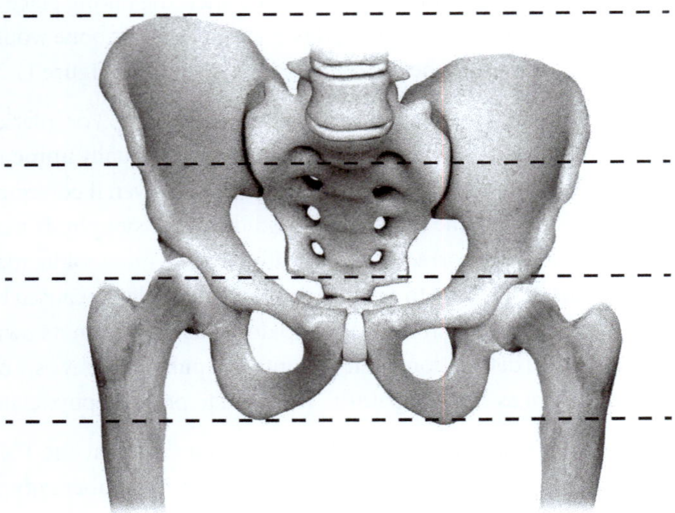

FIGURE 11.3

Hemipelvis.

be higher on the side that is rotated anteriorly, compared to the other side. This occurs naturally during gait when that foot is toeing-off (and the hip is in extension).

When one innominate rotates anteriorly, the acetabulum and the head of the femur on that side also move anteriorly and inferiorly compared to the other hip. This then makes that leg "functionally" longer than the non-rotated side.

When the innominate is held anteriorly rotated, the palpatory findings would be as follows:

- ASIS is lower on one side and its corresponding PSIS is higher on that innominate as well.
- The unilaterally anteriorly rotated innominate, therefore, usually assumes an inflared position, and the ASIS is then closer to the mid-line.
- This innominate's ischial tuberosity may present slightly posterior when palpated, compared with the tuberosity on the other side.

When the patient is supine:

- The greater trochanter on the side of the anteriorly rotated innominate should also palpate as slightly lower than on the other side.
- That side's pubic ramus may be rotated inferiorly at the pubic symphysis (see Pubic symphysis impairments later in this section).

INSIGHTS

Box 11.2 Further postural implications

With a functionally longer leg present (on the right, for example), the hips may shift toward the shorter leg (in this example, the left leg). This, in turn, leads to the upper body side-bending over that shorter leg, which makes the shorter leg the principal weight-bearing leg. When the patient begins to favor using this shorter leg to bear the bulk of the weight of the body, it causes this stress load to slowly but surely rotate the innominate on that side posteriorly. The mechanism for this is that the "short leg" compensates by extending the hip to try and lengthen itself. This moves the acetabulum forward, and the forces running down to the hip and up from the ground through the leg push the innominate into posterior rotation. However, the hips may not shift away from the long leg, but rather the upper body may bend over the long leg. Thus, the long leg becomes favored in weight-bearing. Either of these situations could have consequences for both sacroiliac (SI) joints and the joints of the lumbar spine, and beyond.

When the innominate becomes fixed anteriorly (usually from muscle imbalance, such as tight hip flexors), then other structures of the leg on that side may compensate for the added length (rotation of femur, or tibia, valgus knee, and/or pronation of foot, etc.). A functionally longer leg can, therefore, have the same consequences on posture that a "structurally long leg" would have. Therefore, for example, the patient may present with medial knee pain that could be due to an anterior innominate with a valgus compensation at the knee (see Chapter 9 for more on this).

- The leg on the anteriorly rotated innominate can appear longer and palpation at the malleoli will reveal this (if the bones of the leg are relatively equal in length on both sides).

REMEMBER: If a longer leg is observed, and the difference is only functional, the difference between the heights of the malleoli should match the difference in height between the two ASISs.

Unilateral posterior rotation

The ASIS on this side is higher and the PSIS will be lower. This occurs naturally during gait when that foot is in heel strike position (and the leg is in flexion). The leg on this side will become shorter and if the innominate becomes fixed posteriorly (usually from muscle imbalance), then the leg on that side will remain functionally shortened. The body may then compensate for that functionally shortened length by externally rotating the femur and internally rotating the tibia (resulting in a varus knee), and further, supination of the foot may occur; all of which help to make that short leg longer.

When the innominate is held posteriorly rotated, the palpatory findings would be as follows:

- ASIS is higher on one side, and its corresponding PSIS is lower on that innominate as well.
- The unilaterally posteriorly rotated innominate, therefore, usually assumes an outflared position, seen by the ASIS farther from the mid-line.
- As well, this innominate's ischial tuberosity may be palpated as slightly anterior compared to the other side.
- With the patient supine:
- The greater trochanter on the side of the posteriorly rotated innominate should palpate slightly higher than it does on the other side.
- That side's pubic ramus may be rotated superiorly at the pubic symphysis (see Pubic symphysis impairments, below).
- The leg on the rotated innominate can appear shorter, and palpation at the malleoli will reveal this (if the bones of the leg are relatively equal in length on both sides).

REMEMBER: If a shorter leg is observed and the difference is only functional, the difference between the heights of the malleoli should match the difference in height between the two innominate's ASISs. These functionally longer/shorter legs can, in turn, unlevel the sacral base and lead to compensatory changes in the spine (such as scoliosis) and hence, predispose the patient to impairments of the spinal and/or sacral joints.

Bilateral anterior rotation of innominates (anteriorly tilted pelvis)

This is when both ASISs are lower than the PSISs (when compared bilaterally) by an angle of more than 15° from level when viewed from the side. Such malpositioning of the pelvis is usually due to muscle imbalance, especially short hip flexors. This will result in an increased lumbar lordosis (hyperlordosis) which will put increased strain on the intervertebral joints (discs, vertebral bodies, facet joints, ligaments, etc.). The anterior tilt also moves the lumbar spine out of neutral position: the joints of the spine and the SI joints will behave as if the person is bent backward into extension at the low back. This predisposes all these joints to more readily become injured and impaired. With respect to the sacrum, this anterior tilt causes it to go into nutation and resist returning to neutral. Therefore, during walking the SI joints will lose some of their mobility.

Note that even though both ASISs are lower and the pelvis can be defined as an anteriorly tilted pelvis, one innominate may still be more rotated than the other – and so there can be an accompanying unilateral anterior rotation impairment occurring as well.

Bilateral posterior rotation of innominates (posteriorly tilted pelvis)

Both ASISs are level with, or even higher than, the PSISs when observed from a lateral angle. This causes a decrease in the lumbar lordosis or "flat back." The sacrum is pulled into a counternutated position. This positioning of the structure of the lumbar spine and sacrum will impact on the function of the associated joints, affecting the health of the intervertebral discs and making the SI joints prone to impaired motion. One of the most consequential effects of this is loss of the natural spring that belongs to the regularly curved lumbar spine: movements coming up from the ground are now more jarring through the spine. Again, note that one innominate may be more posteriorly rotated than the other.

Pubic symphysis impairments

Any shift in innominate positioning will impact on the pubic symphysis joint. Even if this joint is the axis of movement, there will be rotational stress within the cartilaginous disc (often drawing the pubic rami toward each other, i.e., compressing the joint).

Superior/inferior shears

These impairments have one pubic ramus shifted higher or lower than the other. Often, they are accompanied by unilateral rotations of the innominate on that side. Hence, a unilaterally posterior innominate could have its pubic ramus elevated or sheared superiorly, while a unilaterally anterior innominate may have an inferior shear of its ramus. Note that this is not automatically the case.

The pliability of the bones which comprise the pelvic bowl can allow for the possibility of unilateral rotations of an innominate without a shear occurring. The rotation of the innominate (depending on the conditions of the muscles and connective tissues involved) could occur on an axis that is close to, or even in, the symphysis pubis. The cartilaginous disc may then have rotational stress through it but not shear forces specifically, e.g., one ramus may appear sheared when it is in fact rotated.

Compressed pubic symphysis

The cartilaginous disc can be placed under compressive forces in a number of circumstances, and this could be sustained by muscle imbalance and/or connective tissue shortening. The compression could be seen along with a bilateral inflare of the innominates, with a bilateral counternutation impairment of the sacrum, trauma, or even from sustained rotational forces from unilateral innominate anterior rotation impairment.

Gapped pubic symphysis

A decompression or gapping between the ramus of the pelvis can occur with nutation impairments of the sacrum, bilateral outflares, or trauma. One of the most common occurrences happens for women during the birthing process with the widening of the birth canal. The pubic symphysis may not automatically return to its normal position post-partum. This can result in a pain in the area, and is also commonly involved in "back-labour" pain, since such gapping is concurrent with sacral misalignment post-partum.

- Any of these impairments could be a hidden or uninvestigated source of persistent pelvic pain.
- Always check, by palpation, the obliques and rectus abdominis muscles for balance of tone.

Symptoms of innominate impairments

With respect to pain, the impairments mentioned above fall into two basic categories. Innominate rotations, unilateral or bilateral, along with inflares and outflares, do not usually generate specific pain patterns but are themselves asymptomatic. Pain is the consequence for related structures above and below that will present as painful: sacroiliac, lumbar, symphysis pubis, hip, or farther afield, in pain or impairment to the knee, ankle, thoracic, or cervical areas.

This fact speaks to the need for the pelvis to always remain an area of investigation when treating almost any musculoskeletal dysfunction or impairment. The pelvis often displays the effects of impairments in any area of the body and can, in turn, be one of the predisposing factors in mechanical impairments throughout the body. It is suggested that once you have assessed a specific impairment that a patient presents with, first address the immediate concerns and later perform what we have called the comprehensive structural examination of the pelvis and spine.

Pubic symphysis impairments and innominate shears often present with some local pain: groin pain, iliosacral pain, and the like. Altered gait patterns will accompany innominate impairments. They may be obvious or quite subtle: asymmetry seen in stride, hip motion (side to side and/or superior-inferior), heel strike or toe-off, upper body motions, etc.

Case history questioning

Investigation for sacroiliac or iliosacral dysfunctions should certainly be done if the patient points to the area around a sacroiliac joint. Note that patients may come in complaining of "low-back pain" or "hip pain" but when asked to point to or draw a boundary around where they feel the pain they may point to the sacroiliac joint(s) area. This is one example of the need to always have the patient point to where they feel the pain or impairment!

Investigation of this area may be warranted if the patient mentions falling, especially if landing on a hip or buttock. Sometimes, the patient may speak of *almost* falling, "but I managed to avoid doing so;" nevertheless, they came away from the incident with low back or hip pain. It can happen that a near accident can leave the patient in worse condition than if they had actually fallen. The powerful hip muscles – adductors, abductors, rotators, flexors and extensors – can exert great force that may strain them and disarticulate the joints of the pelvis and lumbar spine.

Low back pain or impairment during pregnancy, especially in the third trimester, may warrant some investigation of the sacroiliac area. Post-partum low back pain should certainly include investigation of the pelvis: sacroiliac joint and symphysis pubis impairments may be occurring/developing during labor as these joint surfaces "open up" as the infant's head engages and passes through the birth canal. The joint surfaces may not always return to their original orientation. The contractions during labor, especially during the last stages of birthing, along with the musculature used to "push" may pull the bony articulations of the pelvis asymmetrically. A strong clue for the need to investigate the pelvic joints for impairments is when the mother talks about "back labor" during delivery and persistent symptoms of this post-partum.

Section 3: Testing for innominate impairments

Assessing the nature of the impairment to the innominate requires careful postural landmarking and palpation skills. The motion tests that follow are simply AF-ROM or PR-ROM movements done while palpating specific landmarks and noting motion or lack of motion in specific structures. To confirm an assessment of innominate impairment, we need to gather information from three sources:

- We need to observe the position of the innominates, relative to one another and to the surrounding structures. This is done by palpating and landmarking while observing the patient's posture. We are specifically looking for asymmetries in the landmarks of the pelvis. This gives us the orientation of the various bones that comprise the pelvis.
- We will challenge the structure to move in a specific way and observe if it does or does not do so. This is sometimes referred to as motion palpation. Motion palpation is simply moving the joint either by the therapist (PR-ROM) or by having the patient perform a specific AF-ROM while the therapist palpates specific landmarks. We will employ the stork test for this to observe innominate motion.
- Lastly, we will palpate to see if normal physiological motion is present in the SI joint, which tells us if there is sacroiliac involvement. If there is, we will need to pursue specific SI joint testing as outlined in Section 5 of this chapter.

NOTE: If there is a sacroiliac dysfunction that is causing the innominate impairment that has been found (i.e., if the sacroiliac impairment is primary and the innominate dysfunction secondary), then treatment of that innominate will either not produce a healing response, or the correction will not hold, and the impairment will soon return.

After gathering the three types of information listed above, we will be able to make a judgment about which impairment to innominate function is present. However, we need to do some further testing to clarify the specific muscles and tissues that are involved and how they may contribute to, or be a consequence of, impaired innominate function. Therefore, we add a fourth source of information.

We will carry out some differential muscle length and strength testing around the pelvis and lumbar spine. Taken with the postural information noted already and specific information about what is tight or taut, short or long, hypertonic or hypotonic, it will allow us to understand the specific muscle imbalances and possible connective tissue involvement contributing to the impairment of innominate functions. (In this chapter, we will review tests presented in Chapters 9 and 12).

Only when the therapist knows the position of the innominates, how they are moving or impaired, how the soft tissues are involved, and the effect this may be having on the SI joints, can the therapist consider truly appropriate treatment approaches and have some hope for their effectiveness.

NOTE: Once we have discussed and explained the testing, we will provide a brief synopsis of the findings specific for the various impairments possible for innominate motion and function.

Observation and inspection

Standing postural exam (Figure 11.4A, B)

IMPORTANT: Have the patient stand in a natural pose.

To assist in this, instruct the patient to look up slightly (i.e., you do not want them watching their feet) and ask them to take a couple of steps, while staying in place. Do not correct feet positions, head positions, etc. You are trying to have them stand as they naturally do (or as near to natural as possible in a clinical setting). The views observed are frontal, lateral (both sides), and posterior (see Chapter 5 for more detail and images).

NOTE: Much of this information from the standing postural examination is needed to compare with supine and prone examinations, so we are not misled by what we see when the patient is on the table in those positions.

- Note the upper body's general orientation, especially rotations and side-bending of the shoulders or spine.
- Note the lower body's general orientation, hips, thighs, knees, tibias, ankles and feet. Note if the hips are shifted right or left over a leg, proportions (tissue bulk), and orientation of the thigh and lower leg (rotations throughout the course of the limbs down to the feet, varus or valgus of knees or ankles, arches of the feet).

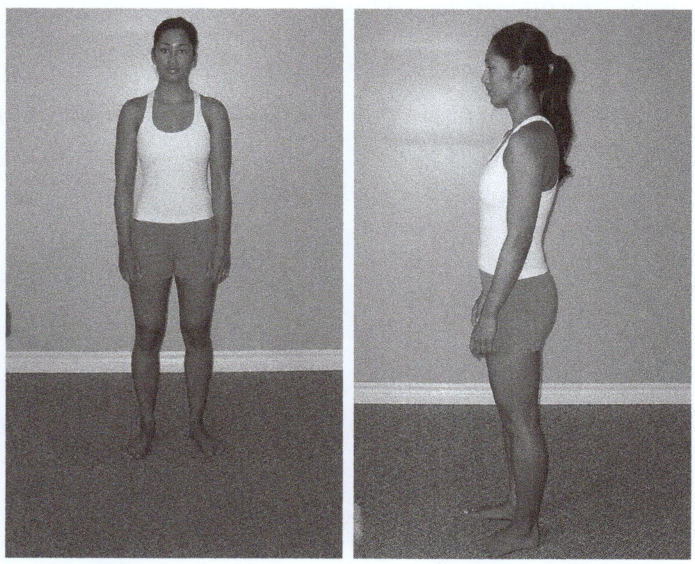

FIGURE 11.4A, B

Standing postural exam.

Be specific and exact with the following:

- Check iliac crest and greater trochanter heights.
- Record ASIS and PSIS heights from the anterior, posterior, and lateral views. Compare heights of the ischial tuberosities.
- Note pelvic obliquity – change in height of one hip compared to the other.
- Note if the pelvis appears rotated around a vertical axis, in other words, does one ASIS (hip pointer) appear more anterior (in the coronal plane), and whether the ASISs are level with each other.
- Observe if the patient has shifted their pelvis to one side over a leg (which then usually becomes the principal weight-bearing leg).
- Note whether the patient has a hyperlordosis or a hypolordosis of the lumbar spine. Observe whether the lumbar spine seems rotated and/or side-bent.
- Observe whether there is an anterior pelvic tilt (usually with a hyperlordosis) or posterior pelvic tilt (usually with a flat back/hypolordosis). Check line from PSIS to ASIS. Normal tilt is from 5° to 15°. (Women tend to have slightly more of a tilt than men.) Check both sides in order to evaluate if one innominate is more anterior than the other (Figure 11.5A, B).

Take all of the information you have accumulated to this point and from that, create a description or mental picture of the relative positions of one innominate to the other, and then to the structures above and below.

Anterior pelvic tilt with hyperlordosis (Figure 11.6)

A bilateral anterior pelvic tilt is a good example of the most common muscle imbalances found in the clinical setting (see Chapter 12 for more examples).

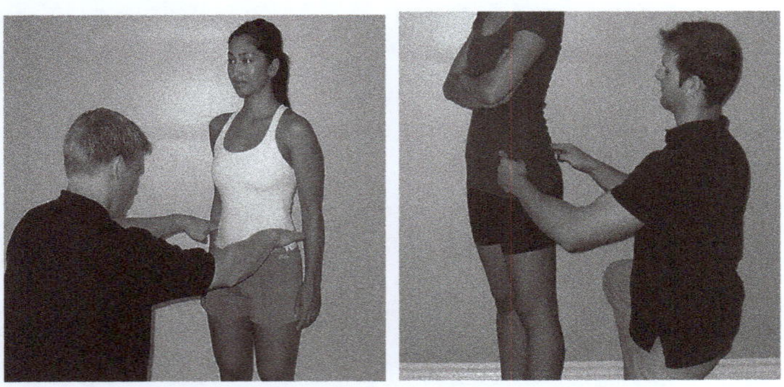

FIGURE 11.5A, B

Observe whether there is an anterior pelvic tilt or posterior pelvic tilt. Check line from PSIS to ASIS.

Normalizing the hips prior to supine postural exam is described in Box 11.3.

Testing for leg length discrepancy

After straightening the supine patient on the table (see Box 11.3), or if they are able, do the *Weber–Barstow maneuver* by having the patient lift their hips off the table momentarily (for details see Chapter 9), then proceed to do the following:

Compare any differences between the levels of the malleoli and the ASISs (Figures 11.7 and 11.8): do they roughly match? For example, if the right malleolus was an inch lower than the left, is the right ASIS also lower?

Signs of innominate rotations (using examples)

Having had a positive stork test on the right (see stork test that follows this section for details):

- Right malleolus lower than left; matched by right ASIS lower than left. Implies right innominate is anteriorly rotated, the right leg will act as if long.

Having had a positive stork test on the left:

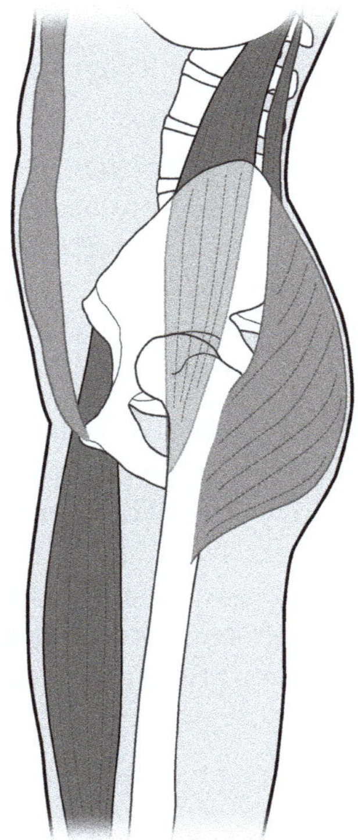

FIGURE 11.6 Anterior pelvic tilt with hyperlordosis

Tight and facilitated muscles:

Lumbar erectors, QL, iliopsoas, piriformis, rectus femoris, TFL, thigh adductors.

Taut hamstrings:

Taut means lengthened, but hypertonic. They are "stretched" or lengthened by being the only muscle holding the pelvis from rotating further anteriorly and over time, contracture to this length.

Weak and inhibited muscles:

Rectus abdominis, transversus abdominis, gluteals, vastus medialis, vastus lateralis.

INSIGHTS

Box 11.3 Supine postural exam

It is best to normalize the hips prior to landmarking and palpating structures around the pelvis and hip as the patient may not be lying straight on the table. Do the following, if the patient is able (see postural assessment photos in Chapter 5 and Figures 5.34 and 5.35).

Have the patient crook-lying (supine with hips and knees bent). This position is usually comfortable for the patient. Have them lift their pelvis off the table a few inches for just a few seconds and then instruct them to let their hips drop back down to the table. Have them relax and let you move their legs. Proceed to extend the legs one at a time. The active lifting of the pelvis off the table engages the musculature in and around the pelvis which will pull the hips into what is the normal position for that patient.

Once the patient lets the hips drop back to the table, the musculature can relax and the patient should then allow the therapist to passively straighten the legs. This has the effect of aligning the patient into what is the neutral position for them, so that you can more accurately palpate for asymmetries that are actually present in the body, and not be misled by those that are just an accident of how the patient happens to be lying on your table at that moment.

NOTE: This normalizing of the hips is useful prior to any testing that takes place with the patient in supine, since it usually places the patient in a position where the musculature and joints want to hold their hips and pelvis. Hence, the tension being placed through specific structures during testing will more accurately test those structures for impairments.

- Conversely, the left malleolus is higher than the right and the left ASIS is higher than the right. Implies the left innominate is posteriorly rotated.

Other possibilities include the following:

- The right malleolus is lower but the right ASIS is level with the left or even higher. The suspicion is that the right leg has a bony length difference, where the femur or tibia on the right is actually longer than its paired bone on the left. Also, a hemipelvis (where the whole pelvis on one side is larger) could produce a longer leg. You could have no positive stork test, or you could have a positive on either side. Actual bony leg length differences can produce a variety of impairments in the pelvis, not to mention the legs themselves.

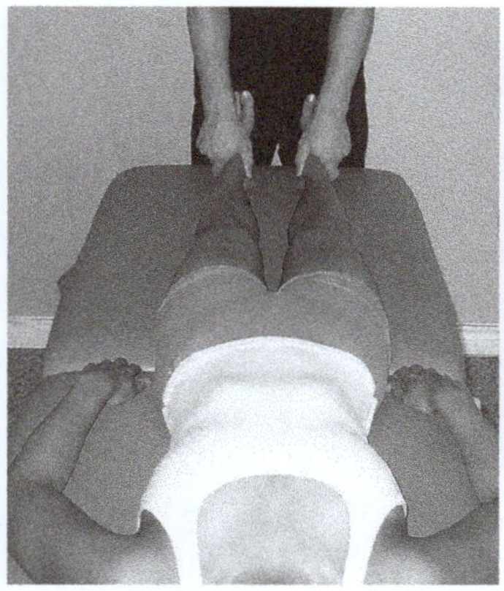

FIGURE 11.7 1. Note medial malleoli levels

Landmark the malleoli at their inferior border (underneath the malleoli). Compare levels.

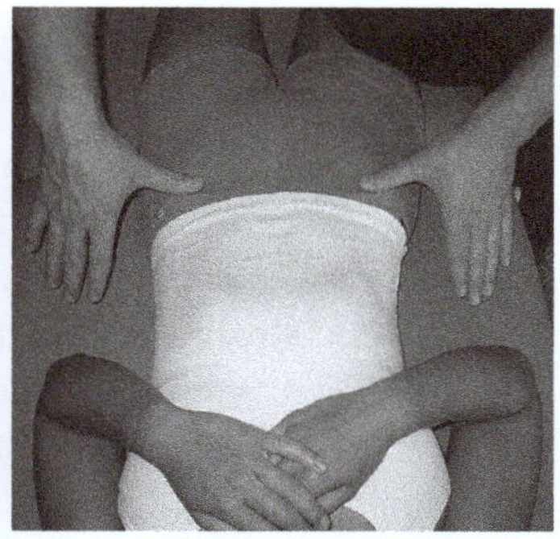

FIGURE 11.8 2. Check ASISs

Landmark underneath the ASISs for the horizontal level. Compare with the malleoli.

A shoe lift may be the appropriate answer for patients with an anatomically short leg, and they should be referred to a podiatrist. But there may well be other issues or impairments that also need to be addressed. Temporary palliative relief can be given until the patient gets a corrective lift or, once they have a corrective lift, chronic changes, compensations, and persistent impairments from the leg length discrepancy may well need to be addressed by the massage therapist in an effort to help the body readjust to a newly leveled leg/pelvis condition. Refer the patient out to their physician or podiatrist for a diagnosis and fitting of a lift.

Other observations to be made while the patient is supine are: (1) compare the heights of the ASISs from table (pelvic rotation to the right or left); (2) compare the distance of the ASISs from the mid-line (inflare/outflare).

Box 11.4 contains information on patterns associated with a functional long or short leg on the right and left side.

Assessing for inflares and outflares (Figure 11.9)

REMEMBER: An inflare is when the ASIS on one side is closer to the mid-line of the body, and usually accompanies an anteriorly rotated innominate. Conversely, an outflare is when the ASIS is further from the mid-line, commonly found with a posteriorly rotated innominate. How can we tell which of the two is occurring? It is the innominate which will have a positive stork test, described later.

Box 11.4 Functional long/short leg

Remember that the functional long leg or the functional short leg can be on either side. However, clinical experience shows that most right-handed people whose lead foot is also on the right will tend to have an anterior innominate on the right. When a right lead foot person has the long leg on the left (or short on right) they often have more acute symptoms in the lumbopelvic girdle. Left-lead-foot persons, however, do not share the reverse pattern as they live in a right-handed/footed world where they are forced to be more ambidextrous. How do you know which is a lead foot for a specific person? Ask them which foot they would use to kick a soccer ball that was rolling by.

NOTE: Even though a person has a rotated innominate on one side (example, seen supine), they could have had a negative stork test. This negative test is due to a muscle imbalance, but the innominate, as part of an iliosacral joint, still retains its mobility. Changing the imbalance by correcting a low back or hip joint impairment results in the innominate usually being re-balanced automatically. However, always check to see if this has occurred. For more on rotated innominates, see Chapter 9.

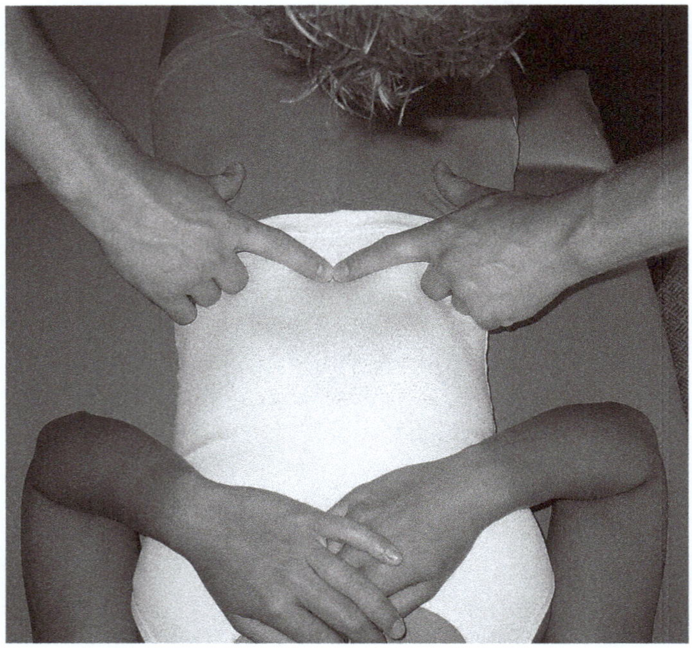

FIGURE 11.9 Checking for inflares and outflares

Landmarks the ASISs and take the index finger tips to the umbilicus. Compare the distance of the ASISs from the mid-line.

Placing innominate orientation in the context of the trunk and the head

With the testing that follows, you can collect, through your clinical experiences, many insights into the numerous correlations of tissues and structures of the pelvis, spine, shoulder girdle and heel.

Check rotations (fascial exam) with the patient supine:

- Compare the heights from the table of the hips (ASISs, as above), then the lower ribcage, upper ribs, anterior shoulders, left and right occiputs. Compare the heights from the table to normal and to the other bilaterally, and then compare the directions of rotation from one set of landmarks to the next.

A compensatory pattern would have the hips rotated in one direction, with the lumbar spine rotated in the opposite direction continuing in an alternating pattern all the way to the head. This compensatory (alternating) pattern was seen by Gordon Zink D.O. (Chila 2010; DeStefano 2011; Mitchell 2005; Pope 2003) in clinical situations where the patient usually suffered only minor to moderate impairments amenable to treatment. He observed, however, that a non-compensatory (non-alternating) pattern often accompanied more serious impairments (especially from trauma) and/or that the patient suffered from some pathology/illness (Chila 2010; DeStefano 2011; Mitchell 2005; Pope 2003).

Compare the above rotations with these side-bending patterns, done while gently pushing the following areas of the body side to side, comparing ease and bind:

- at the waist (lumbars)
- mid-ribs (thoracic)
- neck (cervicals).

Motion palpation of innominates

Two tests, the stork test and the standing flexion test, are presented next for the sake of thoroughness. The stork test is preferred by the author because it removes hamstring tautness that could hide positive results which may occur during the standing flexion test. This second test can be used as an alternative if the patient has difficulty performing the stork test, i.e., has problems standing on one leg (Chila 2010; DeStefano 2011; Hertling & Kessler 2006; Magee 2014; Mitchell 2001, 2005; Starkey & Brown 2015).

A positive motion test only tells us which side has impaired function. Which type of innominate impairment there is depends on the postural palpatory findings, as described above.

Stork test (Gillet's test/Piedallu's sign) (Figures 11.10, 11.11)

This test works by fixing the sacrum and moving the innominate. The SI joint can be thought of as functioning as a clutch: when a leg is weight-bearing, the SI joint on that side closes or becomes fixed or more stable (see force closure, earlier in this chapter). Meanwhile, the non-weight-bearing side gaps slightly and is left free to permit a small amount of movement, allowing the innominate on that side to rotate anteriorly or posteriorly.

Have the patient standing at arm's distance from a wall. They should have their fingertips or hands on the wall to retain their balance during the testing. The elbows should be slightly bent and the patient should not be leaning forward or backward. Palpate the PSISs. Have the patient then flex their hip as you continue to palpate PSISs, bringing their knee up toward their shoulder. It is important to ask the patient to bring the knee up as high as possible because, even though you will feel movement and can get a result with modest flexion of the hip, you will always get a significantly clearer result when the hip passes 90°. Normally, the PSIS should move down on the non-weight-bearing side.

The positive sign is the PSIS not moving inferiorly, but staying at the same level or even moving slightly superiorly. Some therapists will landmark as follows: palpate one PSIS with one thumb, and palpate S2 (approximately) with the other thumb. Have the patient then flex their hip on the side of the PSIS you are palpating.

Errors in testing can occur with having the patient doing the test with only one hand resting on your table or the back of a chair. This can invalidate the test, as the patient is then more likely to side-bend the low back when lifting one or the other leg. They will certainly not move symmetrically one side to the other. This can also occur if the patient is standing at 90° to the wall and is using only one hand to stabilize themselves. If balancing with unilateral support, the average patient will inevitably side-bend quite a lot to keep their balance, and may do so more on one side than the other.

To repeat, if all is functioning well during the testing the PSIS on the flexed hip side will move slightly inferiorly. However, if the PSIS does not move inferiorly, and even moves superiorly, then the test is positive. This implies impaired motion between the innominate and the sacrum on that side.

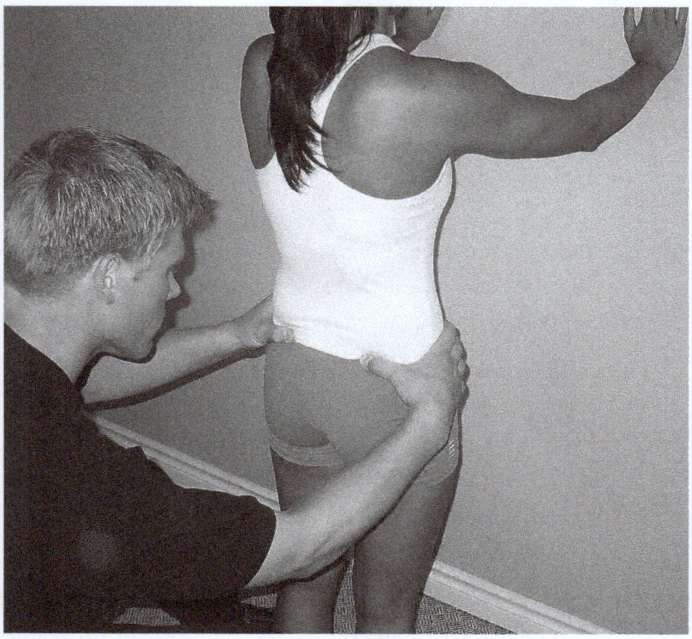

FIGURE 11.10 1. Positioning for stork test

Landmark the PSISs while the patient stands arm's distance from the wall.

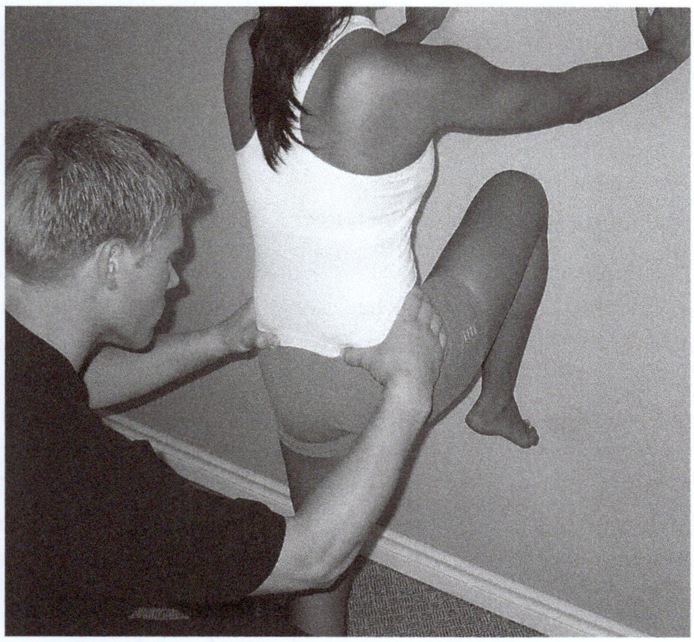

FIGURE 11.11 2. Performing stork test

Palpate the landmarks with hip flexion, first one leg, then the other.

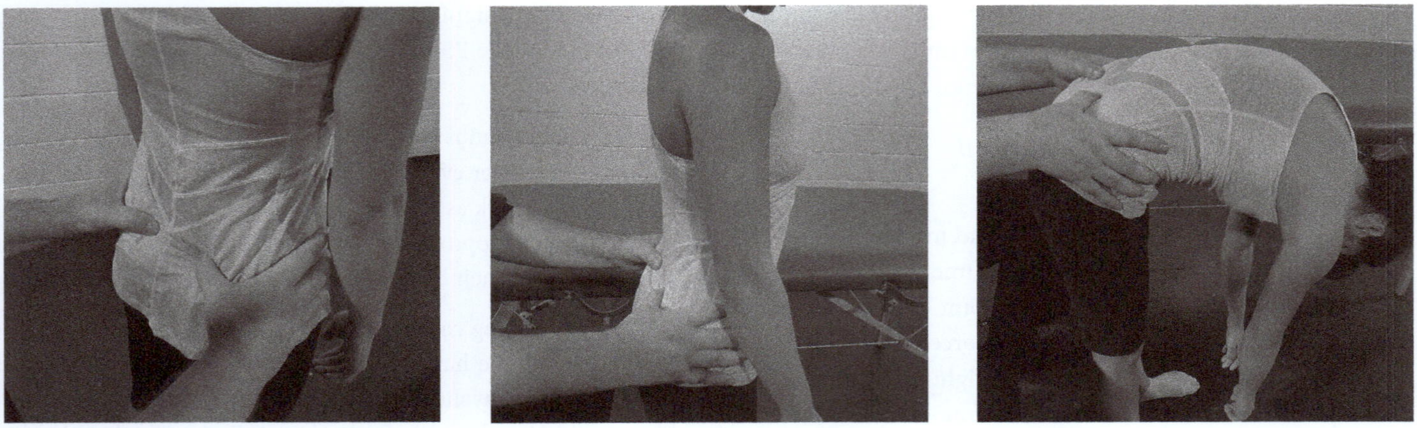

FIGURE 11.12A–C Standing flexion test

Landmark PSISs and have the patient bend forward: first tucking the chin in, then slumping the thoracic spine, then flexing the lumbar spine until bending from the hips.

Standing flexion test (Figures 11.12–11.14)

This test is primarily used as a test for innominate dysfunctions. It is presented here because of its common usage. However, note the reservations about this test mentioned above and those mentioned below. We are looking for similar movements of the PSISs as in the stork test.

When one side "rides higher" that side is the side of the dysfunction, but it can indicate impairment either to the innominate or to the sacrum. However, one could generalize about the results of testing and postulate that a positive sign for an impairment of innominate motion (an iliosacral dysfunction) is when a PSIS very quickly moves superiorly, relative to the other side, at the beginning of forward flexion (DeStefano 2011; Mitchell 2001).

However, it can be a positive sign for a hypomobile SI joint (a sacroiliac dysfunction) when, near the end of forward flexion, the PSIS "suddenly" rides high in comparison to the other PSIS. This implies that the innominate on the side that rides up is being dragged along by the sacrum as it counternutates, moving posteriorly and superiorly (DeStefano 2011; Mitchell 2001, 2005). This will be discussed more fully in Sections 4 and 5 (along with the seated flexion test, which would be done after the standing flexion test to clarify if we have an iliosacral or a sacroiliac impairment).

Standing leg extension test (testing for innominate anterior rotation problems) (Figure 11.15A, B)

Many see this as a redundant test, but it may well be wise to use it when clarification of results from either the stork test or standing flexion test is needed. Some feel that it will accurately

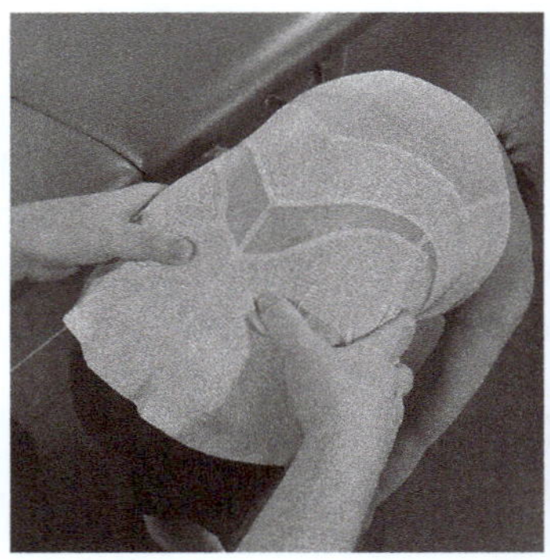

FIGURE 11.13 Negative standing flexion test

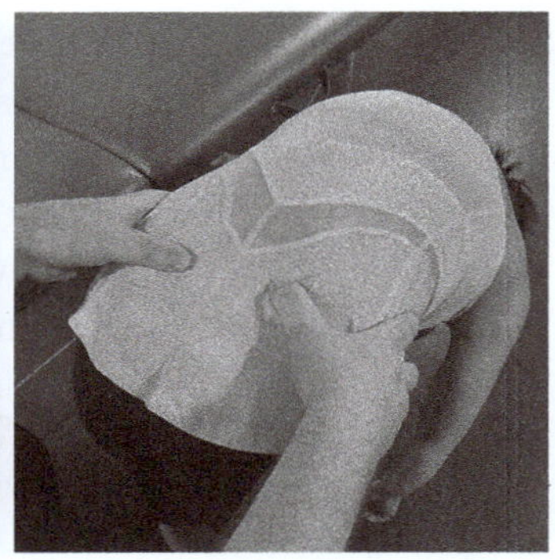

FIGURE 11.14 Positive standing flexion test

reveal when the innominate is fixed in a posteriorly rotated position. Its biggest drawback is that it will extend the lumbar spine, which if impaired, may exacerbate low back issues when testing.

Have the patient standing arm's distance from a wall. They should have their hands on the wall to maintain their balance during the testing. Palpate the PSISs with your thumbs. Have the patient extend a leg while you sit or kneel off to one side. Ensure that your dominant eye is the eye closest to the midline of the patient's back.

You watch to see if the PSIS will rise, i.e., will the testing side of the pelvis anteriorly rotate. If there is no motion or the results are not clear have the patient first flex the knee and then extend the hip (in case a hypertonic/spasming and short hamstring is preventing movement). A positive test is when the PSIS on the side of the extending leg does not rise up, which means that the innominate is held in posterior rotation.

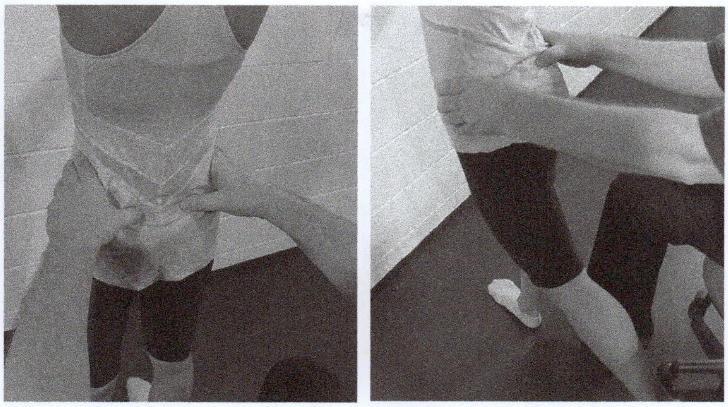

FIGURE 11.15A, B Standing extension test

Position the patient as in the stork test. Landmark and follow the PSISs as the leg is extended.

We now have enough information to conclude whether we have impaired innominate function and on which side. Positive test results at this point allow us to focus on the innominate and its supportive tissues as a source of the impairments. However, as yet we cannot conclude that there are no impairments to the sacroiliac joints.

If the patient is able and willing then we proceed to see if there is any accompanying sacroiliac malfunction.

Palpation exercises and inspection palpation of sacral motion on the innominate

The following tests can be used to locate impaired motion between the sacrum and the innominate but also can be very instructive palpation exercises for those studying sacroiliac motion, assessment, and treatment.

This testing is done after completing the palpation and landmarking along with the stork test so that we can see if impairment of innominate motion is accompanied by impaired SI joint motion. (Note, however, that the SI joint may be fine, but we can still have an innominate impairment.)

The following are used both as palpation exercises to increase sensitivity to motion at the SI joint and also as testing procedures for confirming sacroiliac motion impairments (Chila 2010; DeStefano 2011; Hartley 2000b; Magee 2014). These palpations can become testing procedures only once the therapist becomes familiar with the feel of the normal motion and "springiness" of the SI joints. Doing these palpations with a variety of patients is the only way to develop this sensitivity. In many ways these palpations can be considered a form of joint mobilization of the sacroiliac joints.

Four-point test (Figure 11.16, 11.17)

With the patient prone, place the finger pads of the thumbs over the inferior lateral angles (ILAs) and the index finger pads over the sacral sulcus (S1 area). Palpate the motion of the sacrum as the patient breathes. As the patient takes in a very deep breath, the sacral base should go posterior while ILAs go anterior. This is counternutation. The lumbar spine also flattens somewhat. Then, as the patient forcibly exhales, the sacral base should go anterior, and ILAs go posterior: the sacrum goes into nutation, and the lumbar lordosis increases. Have the patient exaggerate their breathing through three or four cycles. Now, tell the patient to start breathing normally, and continue to palpate. Usually, after a few normal breaths, the patient further relaxes and their breath goes quieter and more shallow. See if you can still palpate this much more subtle movement. This four-point test is to help confirm impairment of movement between the innominate and the sacrum.

Once this is practiced for a while, the therapist can begin to practice palpating the motions during the patient's breathing by lightly placing the whole of their hand lightly on the patient's sacrum. Place the thenar eminences of the hand on the two ILAs, with the palm of the hand over most of the body of the sacrum, and the tips of the fingers (depending on the size of the therapist's hand) extended over onto the lumbar spine. Keep the elbow bent and loose, and have the shoulder relaxed. When we feel that one side is not moving, or not moving as well as the other, then we may have impaired motion at that SI joint.

This advanced version of the four-point test (Figure 11.17) is used instead of the preliminary version once you have

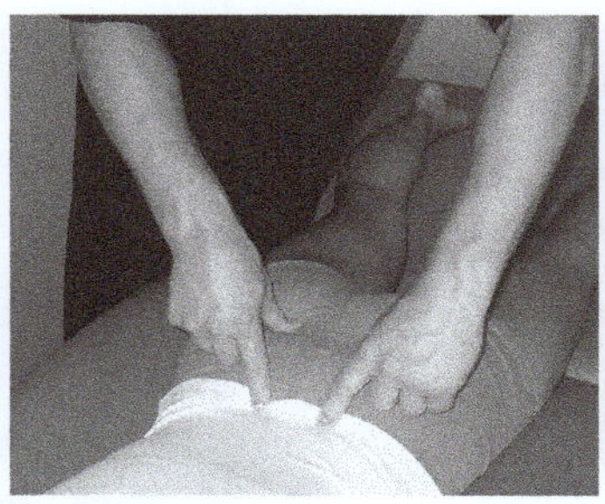

FIGURE 11.16 Four-point test of sacral motion

Place thumbs on ILAs, index fingers at sacral sulcus. Have patient take several deep breaths. Palpate for restriction and symmetry of motion.

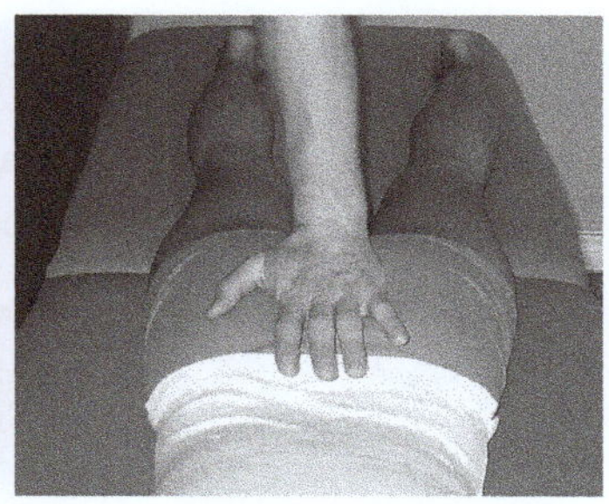

FIGURE 11.17

Advanced version of the four-point test. Palpate for restriction and asymmetry of motion.

gained the skill of palpating the rocking of the sacrum into nutation and into counternutation. You can always return to the earlier version if you have difficulty palpating motion with a particular patient. (Osteopaths often refer to this test as the rock test.)

The next two exercises also increase the therapist's palpatory and landmarking skills. Though presented here as palpatory exercises to practice, they can also be used to further investigate and so clarify if there is a problem with the SI joint. ***NOTE:*** The tests combined can also become a possible treatment modality for sacroiliac dysfunction. Gapping the joint can provide enough laxity so that appropriate springing of the ILAs or of the sacral base can move the sacrum back into neutral.

Spring test (Figure 11.18A, B)

Spring the ILA anteriorly (i.e., push anteriorly on the ILA in a slow, rhythmic on/off manner) while palpating first the ipsilateral and then the contralateral sulcus, for the sacral base to counternutate. In other words: while springing the right ILA, palpate the right sacral sulcus for movement; then palpate the left sulcus and look for movement while you continue to spring the right ILA. As you push down on the ILA, you should feel the sacral base (at the sacral sulcus) move posteriorly (or up into your palpating finger). Now, spring the left ILA and palpate the left sacral sulcus; then the right sulcus. Finding one side of the sacral base not moving implies impaired function at that SI joint. This more "aggressive" test can be used if the four-point test does not present a clear result.

Gapping test (Figure 11.19A, B)

Flex the knee and internally rotate the femur while palpating for motion between the sacrum and the innominate (at SI joint line). You are palpating to see when the innominate begins moving away from the sacrum before being pulled along by its ligamentous and muscular ties with the innominate. This is referred to as gapping the SI joint. Slow, incremental motion (external rotation of hip) is needed to feel the gapping. Once found, gently rock back and forth from internal to external rotation, feeling the quality and quantity of motion available within the gap. This is the same as laxity or potential joint space available in any synovial joint.

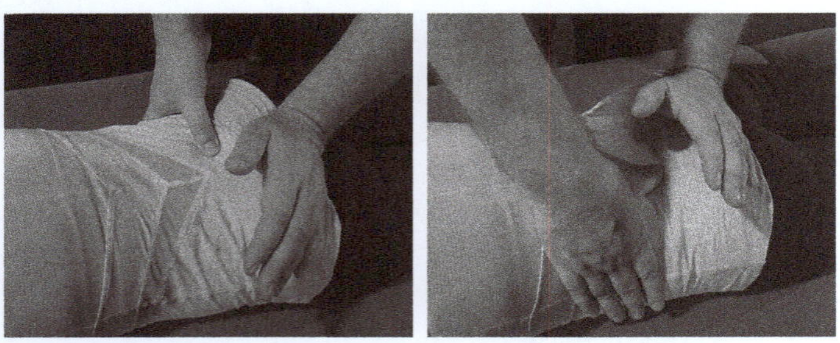

FIGURE 11.18A, B Spring test of sacrum

Press down on the ILA and palpate at both sacral sulcus areas. Change ILA and repeat.

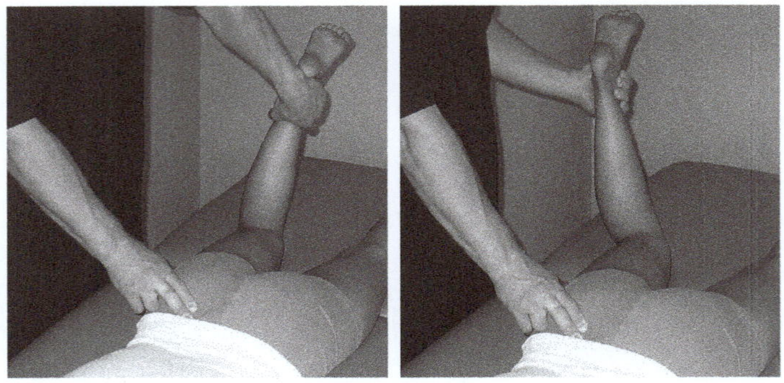

FIGURE 11.19A, B Gapping sacroliliac joint

Palpate the SI joint line. Have the hip in slight external rotation. Pull the ankle toward you slowly. Stop when you feel the innominate begin to move but the sacrum has not yet moved.

An inability to gap the joint – to always have the sacrum move immediately along with the innominate – implies restriction of motion in that SI joint.

Gapping is very subtle movement. The SI joint will gap with very little internal rotation (5–10°). Perform the test in a slow motion. Start with the hip in external rotation (10°), slowly move to neutral, then into internal rotation. This lets you find the soft gap point easily and gently oscillate the innominate laterally away from the sacrum. This is referred to as joint mobilization, increasing the joint play or gapping within the joint.

If the patient has knee problems preventing you from using the leg for internally rotating the innominate, place a pillow above the ankle and the palm of the movement hand over the greater trochanter. Push trochanter toward the table to have the femur and the innominate internally rotate.

Pelvic challenge for pubic symphysis impairments (Figures 11.20, 11.21)

This test uses the adductors and abductors of the hip to provoke symptoms. It is used when the therapist does not palpate and evaluate positions of pubic rami at the pubic symphysis. Any shift in innominate positioning will have to impact on the pubic symphysis joint: even if this joint is the axis of movement, there

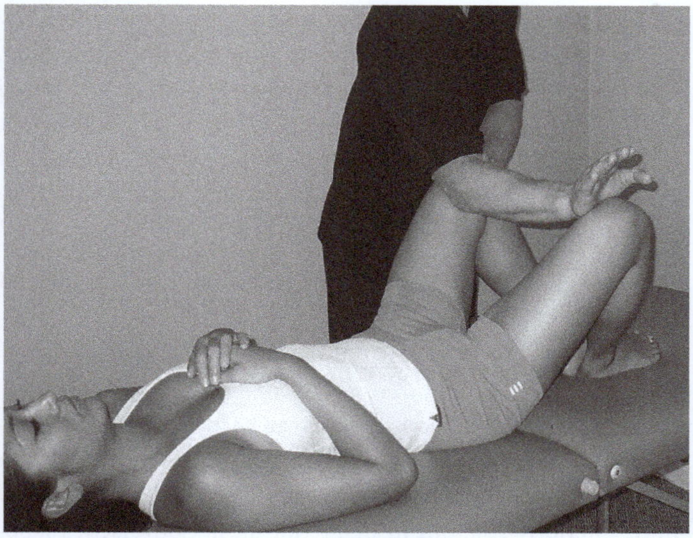

FIGURE 11.20 Part 1 of pelvic challenge

The patient tries to bring the knees together, starting with minimal effort, building to full effort. This test stresses the adductor muscles that attach to the pubic rami, and will stress the joint by gapping it. If the joint is misaligned or impaired, this test will usually generate pain.

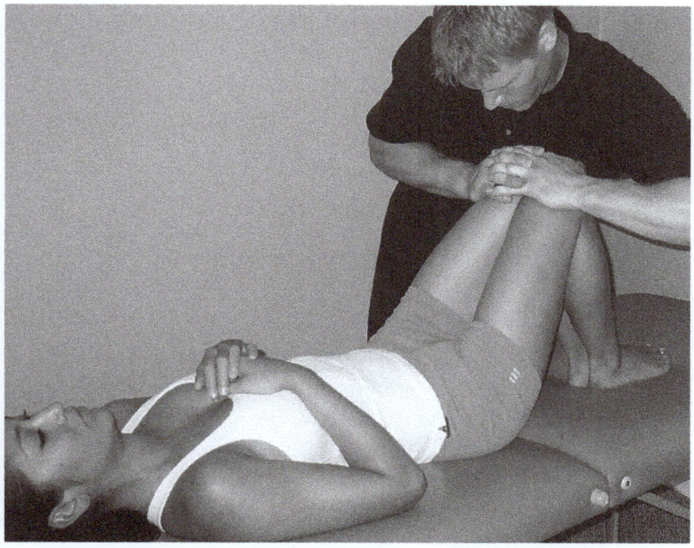

FIGURE 11.21 Part 2 of pelvic challenge

The therapist holds the patient's knees together as the patient tries to draw the knees apart. The patient should start with minimal effort, slowly building to full effort. This test stresses the symphysis pubis by compressing it. This action also gaps the posterior SI joints; therefore, pain felt at these joints means they must be evaluated, if that has not already been done.

will be rotational stress within the cartilaginous disc (often drawing the pubic rami toward each other, i.e., compressing the joint).

With the patient supine, have them bend their knees. Tell them to keep their feet together but let their knees fall apart. Place your forearm between their knees, with the thenar eminences on the medial side of the knee farthest from you and your elbow on the medial side of the knee closest to you. Instruct the patient to try to bring their knees back together with minimal strength, and slowly increase the effort until they are using full strength. Remind them, however, to stop if and when they feel any pain. Pain at the pubic symphysis area is a positive sign.

Interpreting the results of motion testing and palpatory findings (see also Box 11.5)

Unilateral anterior rotation of the innominate

- Positive (+) stork test (notes impaired side).
- ASIS lower on impaired side, and medial[1]; PSIS higher on impaired side and lateral[2].
- Possible confirming four-point test (4-PtT) for decreased (↓) SI joint motion[3].
- Leg will appear longer on impaired side.

Box 11.5 Testing to examine strength/length of muscles around hip and innominates

- If we have impairments to an innominate, we must check the muscle length of the principal muscles in and around the hip and innominates to clarify the innominate dysfunctions. This is especially important, as muscle imbalance is the most common cause of impairments to innominate positioning and motion.
- **Modified Thomas test** Can tell about the length of several muscles around the hip by changing the way the test is done slightly and by observing several potential movements or positions that the tested leg may display.
- **Differential muscle tests** Strength testing of gluteus medius and minimus (painful SI joint may reflexively inhibit the ipsilateral gluteus medius), gluteus maximus, tensor fasciae latae, lateral rotators, especially palpating the piriformis, erector spinae, quadratus lumborum, psoas, and abdominals.
- For more on these tests, see Section 6.

Unilateral posterior rotation of the innominate

- + Stork test.
- ASIS higher on impaired side and lateral[4]; PSIS lower on impaired side and medial.
- Possible confirming 4-PtT for ↓ SI joint motion.
- Leg will appear shorter on impaired side.

Unilateral inflare

- Possible + stork test, or it may be inconclusive.
- ASIS more medial on impaired side.
- Possible confirming 4-PtT for ↓ SI joint motion.
- Leg may present as internally rotated on impaired side, but neither significantly longer nor shorter.

Unilateral outflare

- Possible + stork test (or it may be inconclusive).
- ASIS more lateral on impaired side.
- Possible confirming 4PtT for ↓ sacroiliac joint motion.
- Leg may present as externally rotated on impaired side, but neither significantly longer nor shorter.

Superior shear of innominate

- + Stork test.
- ASIS, PSIS, pubic ramus, ischial tuberosity all higher on impaired side.
- Possible confirming 4-PtT for ↓ SI joint motion.
- Leg may present shorter on impaired side (greater trochanter higher on impaired side).

Inferior shear of innominate

- + Stork test.
- ASIS, PSIS, ischial tuberosity all lower on impaired side.
- Possible confirming 4-PtT for ↓ SI joint motion.
- Leg may present as longer on impaired side (greater trochanter lower on impaired side).

NOTES

1. Likely, but not necessarily, an inflare of the innominate.
2. PSIS may or may not shift laterally – does so if there is an inflare present.
3. Remember: the function of the SI joint may be affected by the malpositioning of the innominate when it is impaired. This speaks to the possible compensatory problems resulting from impaired innominate function and misalignment. But the presence of an innominate impairment does not in itself mean that there necessarily is a sacroiliac dysfunction (like those discussed in Section 4).
4. Again, as with anterior rotated innominate, likely, but not necessarily so.

Strain to the symphysis pubis

Shears through the pubic symphysis can be found in a full innominate shear. At the symphysis pubis, they can also arise when an innominate rotates anteriorly. The pubic bone on that side may move inferiorly, resulting in an inferior shear. Conversely, a superior shear follows a posterior rotation of the innominate. If sustained, this can put a strain on the cartilaginous joint. Inferior and superior shears can also come from muscle imbalances such as unilateral adductor or abdominal muscle spasms or shortness. The joint can also be gapped when the innominates are in an outflare position, unilaterally or bilaterally; or the joint can be compressed by an inflare.

Section 4: Introduction to sacral dysfunctions

Gait: the innominates and sacroiliac joints

What follows is meant to be just enough to help us to understand the dysfunctions outlined below. For a more detailed look at what is thought to be happening to the sacrum, innominates, and muscles during gait, see the Chapter appendix. The detail in the appendix can give many valuable palpatory clues by describing and explaining:

- which muscles are contracting when we walk or run (or go into spasm)
- which positions the sacral base will be in during certain phases of the gait cycle and hence, its position in certain dysfunctions
- which position the lumbar spine may present in.

Oblique axes (Figure 11.22)

The oblique axes are named for their superior pole. The left oblique axis runs from the left sacral sulcus (or superior joint surface of the left SI joint) to the right inferior joint surface (the R inferior pole above the inferior lateral angle, or ILA).

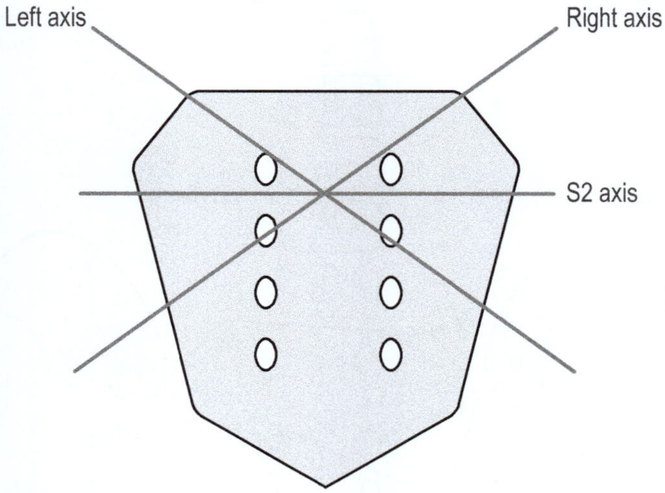

FIGURE 11.22

These axes are in use when walking or running. During gait, the innominates rotate posteriorly when a leg goes forward into heel strike and anteriorly when a leg extends in toe-off. This creates torsional forces through the sacrum. A "torsion" motion means that we are speaking about movement around an oblique axis.

The right oblique axis runs from the right sacral sulcus area to the left inferior joint surface (the L inferior pole).

Normal physiological motions of the sacrum during gait

During gait, the normal motion is for one side of the sacral base to nutate over or around an oblique axis during heel strike while the other side (toeing off) remains basically neutral (Mitchell 2001).

For example, on a right heel strike, the right sacral base nutates (nods) around an oblique axis running from the upper portion of the left joint to the lower portion of the right joint. This is accompanied by the left ILA moving posteriorly. This is to say that the right sacral base nutates as it rolls over the axis that runs from the upper left to lower right. Therefore, the anterior surface of the sacrum turns slightly to face the left. This action, and positioning of the sacrum at this point in the gait cycle, is called a Left on Left (L on L): it describes the condition of the anterior surface of the sacrum turning to face the left on a left oblique axis.

Of course, the reverse positioning occurs when the left foot is at the heel strike position. Now, it is the left sacral base that nutates around a right oblique axis that runs from the upper right to the lower left of the SI joint. The nutating of the left sacral base, in turn, causes the right ILA to move posteriorly. Therefore, the anterior surface of the sacrum is now described as turning to the right on a right axis. The short form for this is a Right on Right motion of the sacrum (R on R).

Impairments to the SI joint, in brief

The following impairments to the SI joint are only brief definitions and descriptions. What is given below is just enough information to allow you to proceed to testing.

Physiological motions where the sacrum can become fixed

These are impairments where the sacrum has become fixed ("stuck") in a position that it undergoes in normal (physiological) movement of the sacroiliac joint. For more detail on these, see the Chapter appendix.

Impaired nutation on oblique axis (torsions) (Figures 11.23, 11.24)

NOTE: With everything being equal, the lumbar spine needs to side-bend toward the side of the sacral base which is higher, to compensate for the unleveling of the sacral base. Therefore, the lumbar spine and lower thoracic side-bends left while it rotates right. An error around establishing the direction of side-bending occurs when a therapist only palpates the L5 transverse processes (TVPs). It would seem that L5, during an L on L, would side-bend right as the right TVP of L5 is lower than its left. However, L5 is tilted to the right, as is the sacral base, but it is still participating in the left side-bending of the lumbar spine.

Impaired motion on transverse axis

- **Bilateral nutation dysfunction** The sacrum is "stuck" in nutation bilaterally on a transverse axis at S2. Usually due to excessive extension of the lumbar spine. Can be found in chronically hyperlordotic patients.
- **Bilateral counternutation dysfunction** The sacrum is stuck in counternutation on a transverse axis bilaterally. Usually due to excessive flexion of the lumbar spine. Not common, but possible. A chronic flat-back could contribute to this.

Non-physiological motions where the sacrum can become fixed

These are impairments where the sacrum has become fixed ("stuck") in a position that is not normal (non-physiological) movement of the sacroiliac joint. These usually occur when:

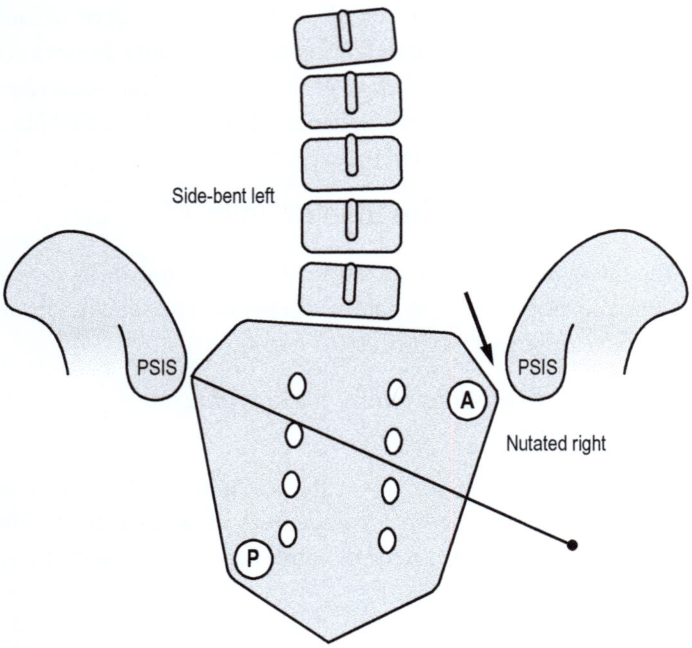

FIGURE 11.23 Left facing sacrum on left oblique axis (L on L impairment)

A, anterior/deeper; P, posterior/higher.

- The right sacral base is stuck forward and inferior in nutation on a left oblique axis. This leaves the ILA on the left more posterior than the one on the right.
- This leaves the anterior surface of the sacrum facing left.
- Hence, the left facing sacrum is fixed in place on a left oblique axis: an L on L dysfunction.
- This is the most commonly occurring torsional impairment found.

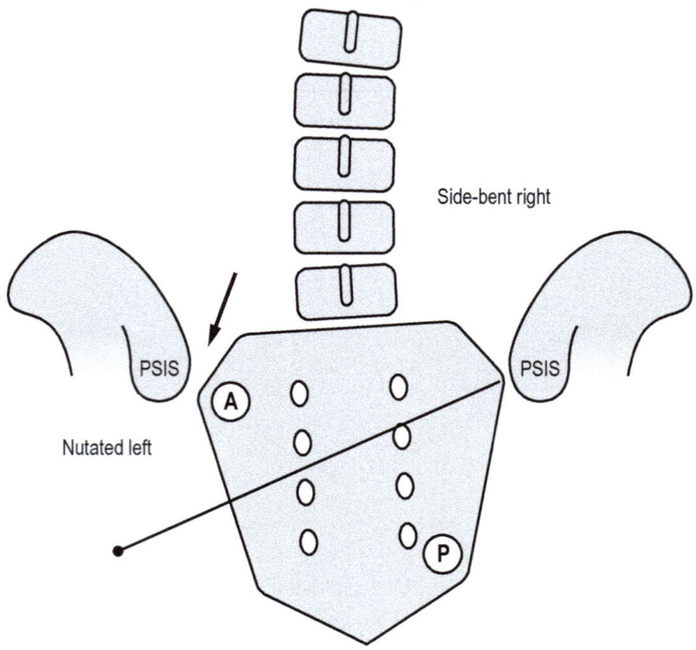

FIGURE 11.24 Right facing sacrum on right oblique axis (R on R impairment)

The left sacral base is stuck forward and inferior in nutation on a right oblique axis. The right ILA is more posterior than the left.

- This leaves the anterior surface of the sacrum facing right.
- Hence, it is a R on R dysfunction.
- The lumbar spine side-bends over the origin of the right axis and rotates left.

(1) the lumbar spine is flexed or extended and then side-bending and rotation occurs, driving the sacrum into a position from which it cannot return, even when the patient returns to an upright position; (2) malpositioning of the innominates exacerbates the above forces, driving the sacrum from below. For more detail on these, see Chapter appendix.

Non-physiological impairments occurring on oblique axis: torsions

These usually occur in a lift-and-twist injury, i.e., when the spine is in flexion or extension. They can be the source of the problem when a patient says, "I bent over, but could not straighten up."

Posterior rotation (counternutation) on oblique axis (Figures 11.25, 11.26)

Torsional lesions, in general

Review all four torsional lesion diagrams. ***NOTE:*** (1) The axis (the superior pole for which it is named) is always on the opposite side of the lesion; (2) the piriformis that establishes the lower pole of the axis is always on the same side of the lesion, therefore, you should expect, in general, that the lesioned side's piriformis is short, tight (if chronic), and tender; (3) if there is no innominate dysfunction and the bones of the pelvis and legs are symmetrical, then the lumbar spine should be side-bent toward the higher side of the sacral tilt (in the sagittal plane). Nonetheless, never assume that this must always, and absolutely, be the case. The body is wonderful, but can work in mysterious ways!

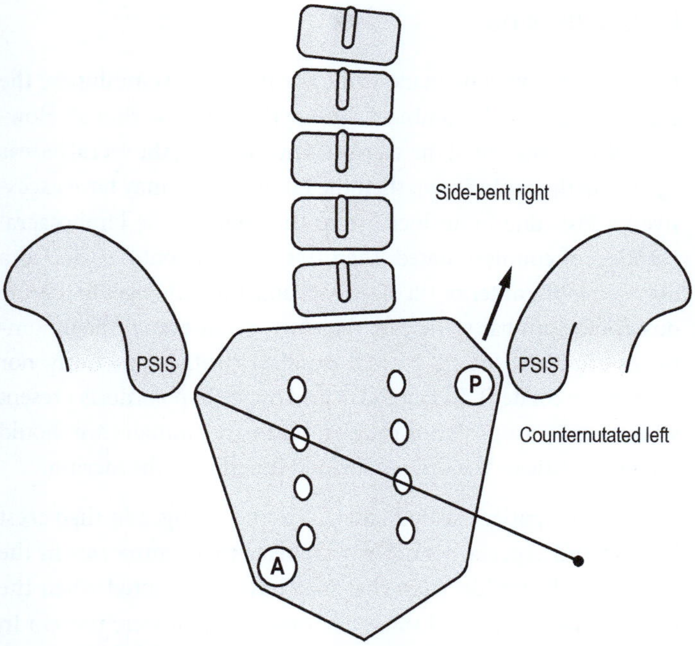

FIGURE 11.25 Right rotation on left oblique axis (R on L)

- The right sacral base comes back (and slightly superiorly) in counternutation while on a left axis; the sacral sulcus on the right will feel shallow compared to the left side, while the left ILA will be more anterior than the right one.
- This leaves the anterior surface of the sacrum facing right.
- Hence, the R on L designation for this dysfunction.
- The lower spine in general side-bends to the right side, over the high side of the sacral base.

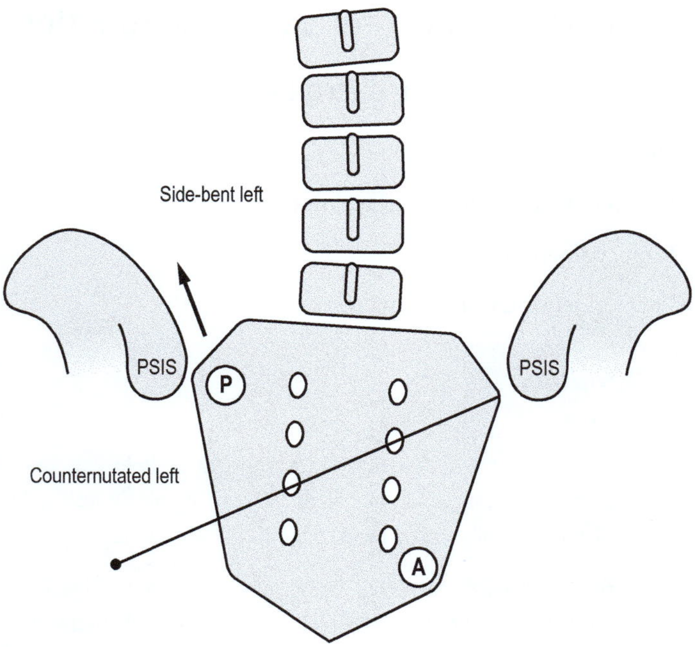

FIGURE 11.26 Left rotation on right oblique axis (L on R).

- The left sacral base counternutates while on a right axis. The right ILA goes deeper/anteriorly.
- This leaves the sacrum facing left.
- Hence, we have an L on R dysfunction.
- Therefore, the lumbar spine and lower thoracic side-bends left, while it rotates right.

Other non-physiological impairments of the sacroiliac joints

There are non-physiological impairments that do not occur on an oblique axis, such as: shears of the SI joint or side-bending of the sacrum. This type of lesion can come from trauma and injuries due to forces acting on the body from without. They can also arise from lift-and-twist injuries or any injury that involves muscular exertion in and around the pelvis. They have also been referred to as a unilaterally flexed/extended sacrum (Box 11.6), and we will use the latter names as well to avoid confusion with innominate shears and side-bending of the spine.

Palpatory landmarks

A unilaterally flexed or extended sacrum is a not uncommon lesion to be found in the clinical setting and has the following palpatory landmarks:

- *Unilaterally flexed sacrum*: when compared with the unlesioned side, the lesioned side's sacral base is found to be anterior and inferior as if in nutation, or in other words found to be in flexion. However, the lesioned side's ILA is also found to be anterior and distinctly inferior.
- *Unilaterally extended sacrum*: when compared with the unlesioned side, the lesioned side's sacral base is found to be posterior and superior as if in counternutation, or, in other words, found to be in extension. However, the lesioned side's ILA is also found to be posterior and distinctly superior.

What will help determine if we have a unilaterally flexed sacrum or a unilaterally extended sacrum is seeing which side is impaired when motion testing the SI joints. The test to find the lesioned side is discussed in the next section.

Translations (dislocations): anterior/posterior

These imply that the whole sacrum is pushed, either anteriorly or posteriorly. Hence, they are given the designation here of dislocation. Extreme pain and loss of mobility would be present.

Section 5: Testing for sacral dysfunctions

Protocol for testing sacroiliac joints

Observations

Seated flexion test of sacroiliac joint

Prone palpation

Prone extension test (Sphinx test)

> ***INSIGHTS***
> **Box 11.6**
>
> The following three descriptions are meant to help you see what may be happening at the sacroiliac (SI) joint when we have a unilaterally flexed or extended sacrum.
>
> - Both the sacral base and the inferior lateral angle (ILA) on one side (unilaterally) are found to be either shifted anteriorly and inferiorly or shifted posteriorly and superiorly on the lesioned side's innominate. This has been called a shear.
> - It is sometimes referred to as a side-bent sacrum. It is as if the sacrum got there by rotating around an anterior-posterior axis that is somewhere in the middle of the sacrum and around which the sacrum has been forced to move.
> - Yet, it can also be imagined that the sacrum has been forcibly rotated around a vertical axis running down the middle of the sacrum. We can imagine one side of the sacrum rotating anteriorly: the sacral base moves anteriorly and inferiorly while its matching ILA is forced to move anteriorly and inferiorly as well.

Observations

Postural observations made while the patient is standing are the same as those for innominate dysfunctions (see Section 3). However, please note that if the sacrum is nutated (i.e., the sacral base is tipped further anteriorly), then the lumbar spine may have excessive lordosis due to an increase in the angle of the lumbosacral junction; if counternutated, then less lordosis could be due to a decrease in the anterior tilt of the sacrum. These changes to the lordosis of the lumbar spine can, therefore, occur even if the innominates appear to be in normal position (neither anteriorly nor posteriorly rotated). In fact, if we find hyper/hypolordosis present with no anterior/posterior rotation of the innominates we should always investigate the orientation and function of the sacrum.

With the patient seated, check for any changes in iliac crest heights and especially note any changes to asymmetries in the lumbar and shoulder area that may have been noted when the patient was standing. If those asymmetries that were present in the trunk when standing disappear or change when the patient sits, then we can assume that these postural deviations are from asymmetries in the lower limbs and from the asymmetrical position of the pelvis when standing. Note that the lumbopelvic girdle may compensate for lower limb asymmetries, yet it is free of serious impairments. If this is the case, the pelvic landmarks should level when the patient sits.

Seated flexion testing of sacroiliac joint (Figures 11.27–11.29)

Fixing the innominate and moving the sacrum

The patient is sitting on a stool; this fixes the innominates by the patient having the weight of their trunk on their ischial tuber-

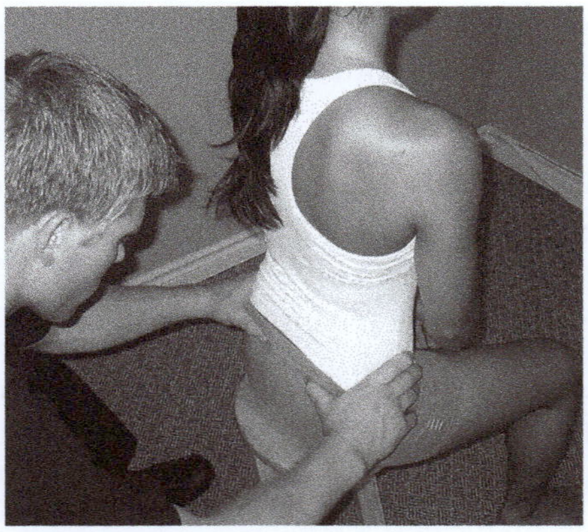

FIGURE 11.27 Starting seated flexion test

Palpate the PSISs.

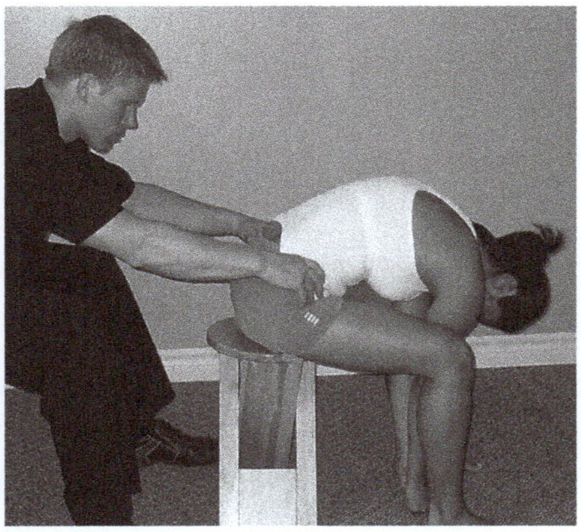

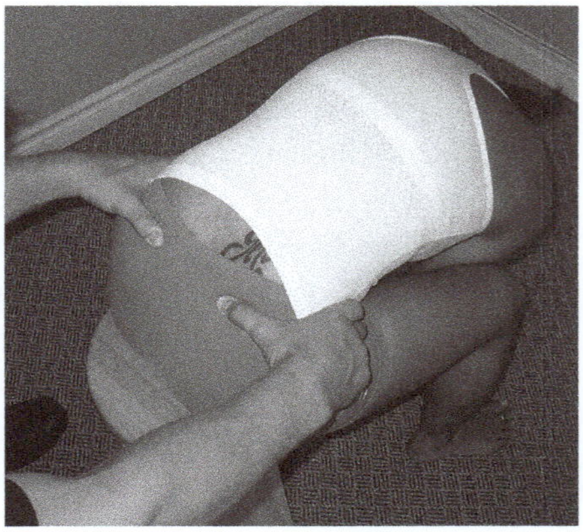

FIGURE 11.28, 11.29 Performing and completing seated flexion test

Have the patient bend forward and observe symmetry of the PSISs.

osities. Palpate both PSISs, and have the patient bend forward to the point that their head is between their knees or as close to this as is possible for them. A positive sign for a hypomobile SI joint is when a PSIS will start in neutral, then, near the end of forward flexion, ride higher in comparison to the other PSIS. This implies that the innominate on the side that rides up is being dragged along by the sacrum as it counternutates and moves superiorly and posteriorly. For some therapists the test is best done with the eyes closed as the movement may be easier to perceive with palpation than visually – but use sight to confirm the difference between the start position and the end position.

Again, as with the standing tests, the seated flexion test has only shown us which side is impaired, but not what the nature of that impairment is. Clarification comes with the tests that follow.

Prone palpation of sacrum

Six-point landmarking of the sacrum (Figures 11.30–11.32)

Bilaterally palpate and compare the symmetry of:

1. The depth of the sacral sulcus.
2. Whether the ILAs are level with each other or whether one seems more anterior/posterior to the other.
3. Landmark the inferior borders of the ILAs. Note if one is superior/inferior to the other.

Steps 1 and 2 give information important to impairments that involve an oblique axis. Steps 1, 2, and 3 are necessary in determining the possibility of sacral shears or a unilaterally flexed/extended sacrum.

The palpations described in Section 3 of this chapter (innominate impairments) should also be done at this time, namely the four-point test, springing test, and gapping test. See that section for instruction.

Ask yourself as you palpate:

- Symmetry or asymmetry?
- Is the motion free?
- Is there restriction on one side?
- Is there restriction on both sides?

Prone extension (Sphinx) test (Figures 11.33–11.35)

This test is meant to differentiate and ascertain if the sacrum is fixed in a nutated or counternutated torsion. The test works with impairments of the SI joint that involve an oblique axis. Once fixation is known, then joint play or other techniques can be applied after the soft tissue has been prepared.

REMEMBER: Extension of the spine is expected to produce nutation of the sacrum. Hence, the sacral base should flex forward/nutate – go deeper during this test.

Palpate with thumbs deep to the sacral sulcus area on both sides (S1 area, just medial and superiorly to the PSIS). Note if one side feels deeper, or do they feel of equal depth. Once you have decided this, have the patient extend their back and rest their chin on their elbows. Tell the patient to relax their abdomen and let it sink into the table to slacken the connective tissue and musculature. Now, palpate the depth of each sulcus area and compare with your previous results.

You can continue to palpate the sulcus and have the patient return to the starting position, and observe results

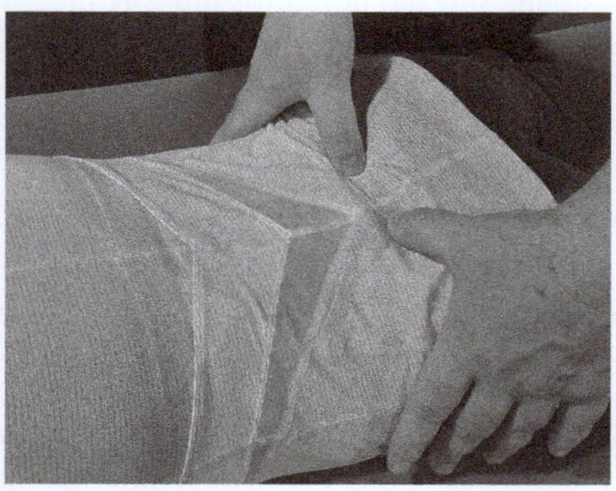

FIGURE 11.30 Six-point landmarks of sacrum

1. Check the symmetry of the sacral sulcus.

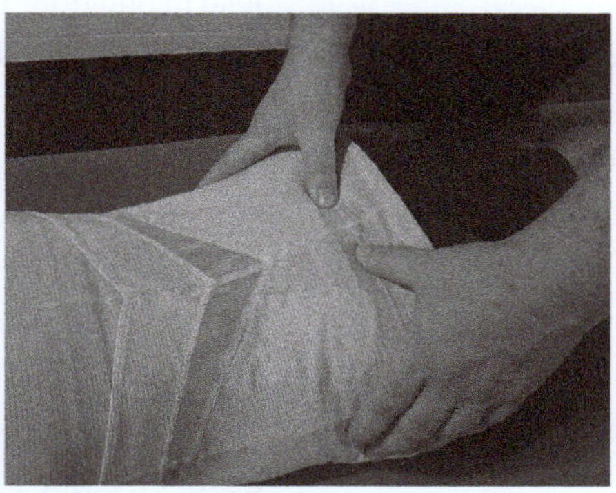

FIGURE 11.31

2. Check the symmetry of the ILAs.

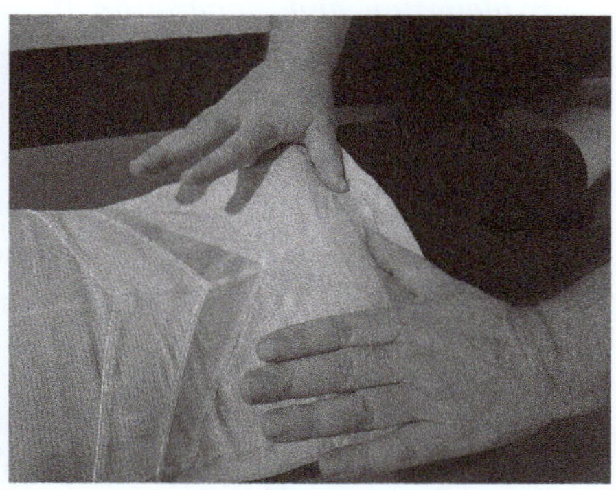

FIGURE 11.32

3. Check the symmetry of the inferior border.

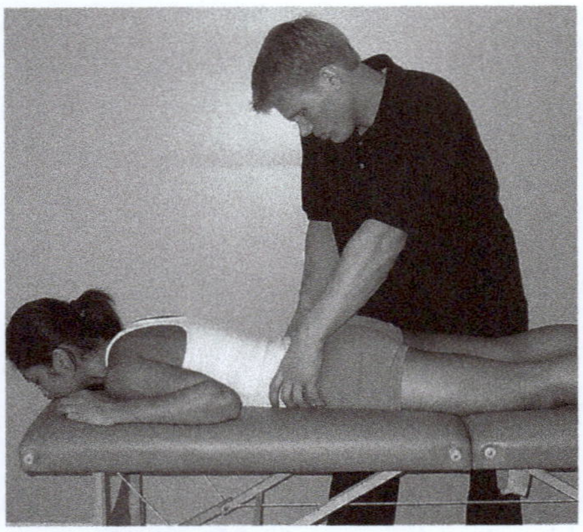

FIGURE 11.33 1. Sphinx test starting position and landmarking

Palpate the sulci depths for symmetry.

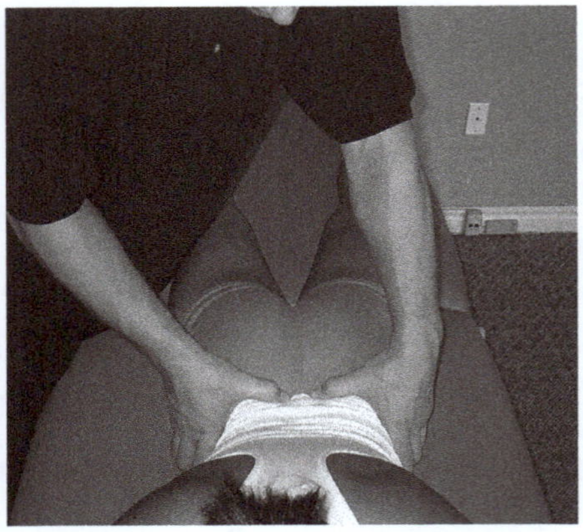

FIGURE 11.34 2. Landmarking sulcus detail

Note symmetry of depth.

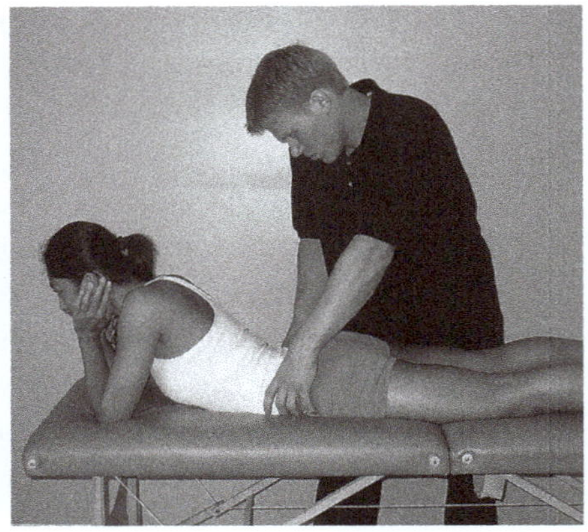

FIGURE 11.35 3. Final position of Sphinx test

Re-evaluate depths for symmetry.

of this. Have the patient again go into the Sphinx position while still palpating, to help confirm findings.

If all was normal, and there is no sacroiliac lesion, you should feel that the sacral base felt of equal depth when the patient was prone and both may now feel deeper but still of equal depth. This means that the sacral base has nutated bilaterally. The depth of the two sulci remains symmetrical. In turn, the inferior lateral angles (ILAs) will have both moved posteriorly.

If the test is positive, you may note the following:

- Asymmetry in neutral which remains or increases in hyperextension, implying a counternutation lesion on the shallow side.

Explanation and elaboration If the two sacral sulci feel unequal in neutral and remain or become more unequal in hyperextension, then the side that does not go deeper is said to be stuck in a counternutated position. In counternutated or non-physiological torsions, the two sides remain unequal, both in prone and in hyperextension, and the asymmetry may even increase between the two sides. This is said to be a non-physiological lesion.

In other words One may find that one side feels slightly deeper when the patient is lying prone (in neutral), and then that side goes even deeper (anterior) on extension. This means that side is moving and is functioning. The side that stays shallow or posterior is stuck counternutated and cannot move into nutation (i.e., move deeper). In counternutated torsions, the two sides often become even more unequal.

Or you may note the following:

- Asymmetry in neutral which is replaced by symmetry when hyperextended; this implies a nutation lesion and is on the side that was originally deeper when the patient was lying in neutral.

Explanation and elaboration The side that seemed shallow in prone seems to now go deeper as the spine extends. In hyperextension, the two sulci are now equal in depth. This means the side that felt shallow while the patient lay prone in neutral but which in hyperextension became as deep as the other sulcus is the side of the sacral base that has moved, and so is functional. In this situation, the two sulci have become symmetrical. The lesioned side in this case is the side that felt deep originally – it is being held in nutation. This lesioned side did not move, but was already held in nutation. This is said to be a physiological lesion because nutation is a common action for the sacral base.

In other words If one side had felt deeper, and after hyperextension the other side came down to its level (moved deeper), then the side that had always felt deep is held anteriorly in nutation. In forward (physiological) torsions, the two sides become equal in extension and the asymmetry disappears.

In general, we can say that, during the Sphinx test, changes in depth on a side means that the side that changes is moving – it is functioning normally.

However, if you find:

No change noted in the prone extension test, or it is unclear, compare palpatory findings of landmarking. You could have a lesion that does not involve an oblique angle, such as a unilaterally flexed or extended sacrum. Or you have an iliosacral lesion but not a sacroiliac lesion. Re-test for innominate impairment and correct any impairment found. Then, re-do the seated flexion test.

A summary of potential findings during Sphinx testing is given in Table 11.1.

Summary of possible palpatory findings during testing for sacral torsions

A summary of findings for sacral torsions is given in Box 11.7.

Presentation of pain experienced by patient with torsion lesions

Nutation lesions

Often (but not always), with a unilaterally nutated sacral impairment, the patient may present with the lesioned side seemingly symptom free but the opposite SI joint and involved musculature can be inflamed and hypertonic. This may be due to the fact that: (1) although a nutation lesion is restricted, this will often be a physiological position and; (2) the contralateral side has followed the general rule (that loss of motion in one joint is compensated for by hypermobility in the corresponding/associated joints) and so the contralateral SI joint may be a hypermobile joint. This can lead to joint capsule and ligamentous inflammation, along with hypertonicity of the muscles associated with that joint.

As a result, a patient may present with pain in the area of the left SI joint but on testing, you find the lesioned joint is the right SI joint and that is held in nutation. The left SI joint must still be treated for inflammation and hypertonicity of the musculature but the problem will continue to recur until that right SI joint is returned to proper function. In this situation, the patient often reports that continuous or long periods of activity bring on the symptoms (on the non-lesioned side), but that rest can help.

Counternutation lesions

The patient usually experiences pain immediately or soon after the lesion occurs. The pain can be intense and debilitating, depending on the degree of displacement of the joint surfaces.

TABLE 11.1
Summary of findings during Sphinx testing

Prone flat (neutral): starting position	Prone extended (Sphinx): finished position of test	Motion	Lesion
Sulci are level = of equal depth = symmetrical	Both feel deeper = symmetrical	Both sides moved = symmetrical motion	No lesion = normal motion
Sulci are level = equal depth = symmetrical	One side deeper = asymmetrical	Deeper side (is the one that that moved) – created asymmetry	Side that stayed shallow in extension is counternutated (minor torsional lesion)
Sulcus unlevel = one side deep, one shallow = asymmetrical	Deeper side goes deeper = more asymmetrical	Deeper side moved deeper = asymmetry increased	Shallow side counternutated. (moderate to severe torsional lesion)
Sulcus unlevel = one side slightly deeper than the other = asymmetry	Both sides go deeper and become equal in depth = become symmetrical	Both sides moved, but the shallow side moved more = asymmetrical motion	The originally deeper side is nutated (mild torsional lesion)
Sulcus unlevel = one side deep, one shallow = asymmetrical	Shallow side goes deep = sulci become symmetrical	Shallow side moved - creating symmetry	The originally deeper side is nutated (moderate to severe torsion)
Sulcus unlevel = one side deep, one shallow = asymmetrical	Remains unchanged = same asymmetry	N/A	Non-torsional lesion

As a non-physiological lesion, the joint and its supportive structures and muscles have been forced into a position that the body recognizes as "not right." Further, it is common for the lumbar spine's mechanics to be altered, and so quickly contribute to the impaired function and pain experienced in the low back and pelvis.

Box 11.7 Summary of findings for sacral torsions

Physiological torsions (L on L; R on R)

- Seated flexion test + on side of lesion.
- Palpation: sacral sulcus deep on lesioned side; contralateral inferior lateral angle (ILA) posterior (inspection palpation: confirms restricted motion on side of lesion).
- Prone extension test: lesioned side feels deeper initially, and on extension both sides become symmetrical.
- Some further palpatory findings that may be found with physiological torsions; with respect to the lesioned side:
- The contralateral inferior lateral angle will be moved posteriorly, making that sacrotuberous ligament taut and probably tender if the lesion is chronic.
- The ipsilateral piriformis will be tight/tender (as it holds the axis in place).
- The contralateral quadratus lumborum (QL) will be tight/short (as that is the side to which the lumbar spine will bend).

Non-physiological torsions (L on R; R on L)

- Seated flexion test + on side of lesion.
- Palpation: sacral sulcus shallow on lesioned side; contralateral ILA anterior (inspection palpation: confirms restricted motion on side of lesion).
- Prone extension test: lesioned side feels shallow, and on extension both sides become even more asymmetrical.
- Some further palpatory findings that may be found with non-physiological torsions; with respect to the lesioned side:
- The contralateral inferior lateral angle will be moved anteriorly, thus slackening the contralateral sacrotuberous ligament.
- The ipsilateral piriformis will be tight/tender (as it holds the axis in place).
- The ipsilateral QL will be tight/short (as that is the side to which the lumbar spine will bend).

The patient will almost always report that they could not straighten up at the time, and they still may not be able to. The patient's posture is almost always twisted as the body tries to stand and move while still trying to minimize stress through the injured tissues and joints. They will have pain (perhaps intense) walking, standing, and sitting, and often find only minor relief with lying down.

Sacral shears: summary of findings

The clinical presentation of a patient with a sacral shear dysfunction often follows no specific patterns of impairment. However, in general, shears are painful, from a dull ache to a sharp stinging pain on movement. Yet which movements are most painful or relieving varies from individual to individual. A summary is presented in Box 11.8.

Bilaterally nutated or counternutated sacrum

There is no specific testing for bilateral nutation or counternutation other than landmarking and inspection palpation. If the

Box 11.8 Summary of findings for sacral shears

Unilaterally extended (counternutated) sacrum

- Seated flexion test positive (gives side of lesion).
- Inspection palpation (six-point): lesioned side posterior at both sacral base and inferior lateral angle (ILA), and ILA is superior on that side.

Four-point test palpation confirms + on lesioned side for motion restriction.

- Prone extension test negative (no change in asymmetry).

Unilaterally flexed (nutated) sacrum

- Seated flexion test positive (gives side of lesion).
- Palpation (six-point): lesioned side anterior (deeper) at both sacral base and ipsilateral ILA, and that ILA is also inferior (as compared to the opposite side).

Passive sacral palpation confirms + on lesioned side for motion restriction.

- Prone extension test negative (i.e., no change in asymmetry).

sacrum is nutated the lumbar spine may have excessive lordosis due to an increase in the angle of the lumbosacral junction; if counternutated, then there will be less lordosis than normal due to a decrease in the lumbosacral junction. There is not sufficient anterior or posterior tilt to the innominates to explain the excessive or lessened lordosis.

Results of the seated flexion test may appear inconclusive. All the motion palpation exercises (four-point test, springing test, and gapping test) would show restriction of motion in both SI joints bilaterally.

With the prone extension test, both sides remain shallow (counternutated) or palpate equally deep both prior to extending and then after extending.

With bilateral nutation, the patient will have full lumbar extension (which requires nutation) but be restricted in flexion, which requires the sacrum to counternutate. The patient will usually present with a lumbar hyperlordosis.

With bilateral counternutation the patient will have full lumbar flexion (which requires counternutation) and be restricted in extension, which requires the sacrum to nutate. The patient will tend to present with a "flat back" (hypolordosis of the lumbar spine).

Box 11.9 Summary of findings

Bilaterally counternutated sacrum

- Seated flexion test inconclusive.
- Palpation: sacral sulci palpate as shallow and all landmarks are symmetrical.
- Inspection palpation: all show bilateral restriction in motion.
- Prone extension test: depth palpated at sulcus appears equal prior to and after extension (i.e., remain shallow).

Bilaterally nutated sacrum

- Seated flexion test inconclusive.
- Palpation: sacral sulci palpate as deep and all landmarks are symmetrical.
- Inspection palpation: all show bilateral restriction in motion.
- Prone extension test: depth palpated at sulcus appears equal prior to and after extension (i.e., remain deep).

Bilaterally nutated or counternutated sacrum: summary of findings

A summary of findings concerning a bilaterally nutated or counternutated sacrum is presented in Box 11.9.

Section 6: Orthopedic assessment of sacroiliac joints and pelvis

The following information comes from the classic orthopedic tradition, which has historically been very poor in being able to present a detailed assessment of the nature of the impairment to sacral functions. Therefore, while it is intended to fill out the understanding of testing available concerning sacroiliac and iliosacral dysfunctions, most of the information gathered by such testing is not helpful in locating and understanding (or modeling) actual impairments other than possible reproduction of pain.

Since most orthopedic tests are designed to provoke the symptoms of impaired function and pain, they can, when dealing with the SI joints, sometimes do more harm than good. Also, with some of the special orthopedic tests that have been traditionally used we often only find the structures that the patient has already pointed out as being painful. The principal exception to the failing of orthopedic testing can be found through differential muscle testing. When done after all other palpatory or motion testing, very pertinent information is gained concerning muscle function and length.

Nonetheless, muscle testing, and especially differential muscle testing, is always of great value whenever this is possible with the patient. After all, most pelvic impairments are sourced in or sustained by muscle imbalances. As with most muscle testing, it is contraindicated with acute impairments of the sacroiliac joint. However, in chronic conditions and especially after successful treatment of a sacroiliac impairment it is invaluable for investigating muscle impairments or imbalances that may either have predisposed the joint to become impaired or are now the result of an impairment.

Rule outs

Lumbar spine

This is not actually possible to rule out with active free range of motion testing because of its connection with the SI joint via the sacro-lumbar joints and iliosacral ligaments.

The therapist may wish to do the following joint mobilizations to assess joint play, or palpation:

- anterior glide to lumbar vertebrae
- lateral pressure to spinous processes (inducing rotation into the vertebrae)
- palpation of transverse process of lumbar vertebra
- palpation of PSISs
- fascia/musculature (note scoliosis if present and changes when standing, sitting, and supine).

Hip

Rule out the hip by medial rotation and over-pressure (O-P), and then flexion with O-P (though the latter may not be possible with a SI joint injury/dysfunction). Therefore, the therapist may wish to do the following palpation or assessment of joint play:

- joint play to the hip may be possible – anterior, posterior glides and distraction
- palpation of ASIS, AIIS, PSIS
- ischial tuberosities
- sacrotuberous ligament
- fascia and musculature.

Differential muscle testing (Figures 11.36–11.50)

This is of immense use when seeking to understand the musculature involved with innominate dysfunctions.

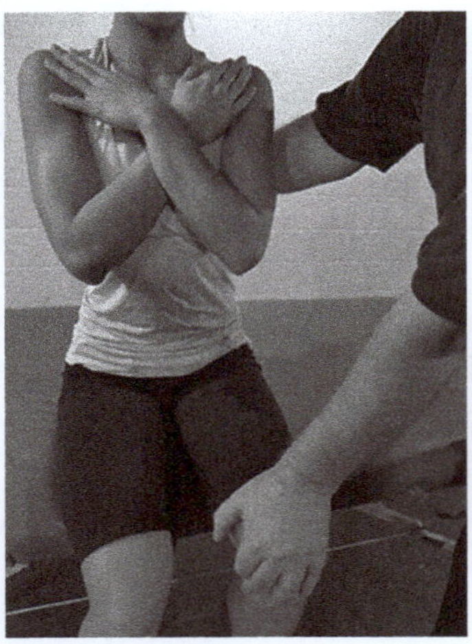

FIGURE 11.36 1. Testing hip flexors

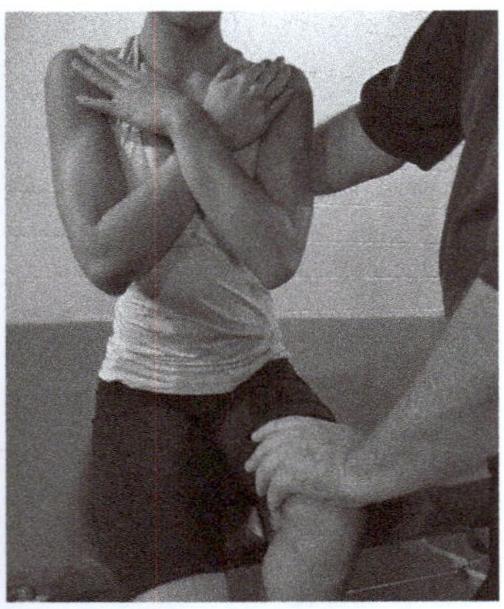

FIGURE 11.37 2. Testing psoas specifically

Have the thigh off the table, then have the patient flex the hip as high as is comfortable.

Strength testing Gluteus medius (***NOTE:*** a painful SI joint may reflexively inhibit the ipsilateral gluteus medius) and gluteus minimus, gluteus maximus, tensor fasciae latae, lateral rotators, especially palpating the piriformis, erector spinae, quadratus lumborum, psoas, and abdominals.

To differentiate between the hip flexor muscles Have the patient seated. They should cross their arms across their chest to prevent compensating for weakness during testing. Have the patient lift the leg just off the table, flexing the hip slightly more, and have them hold this position. Push down on the leg just above the knee (Figure 11.36). To remove the rectus femoris from the picture and focus on the psoas, have the patient flex the hip as high as they can actively do so. Now, press down as the patient resists (Figure 11.37). This stresses primarily the psoas.

Alternate test for psoas (Figures 11.38, 11.39)

Testing the tensor fasciae latae (TFL) (Figure 11.40) Passively move the patient's leg so that you slightly flex the hip with the

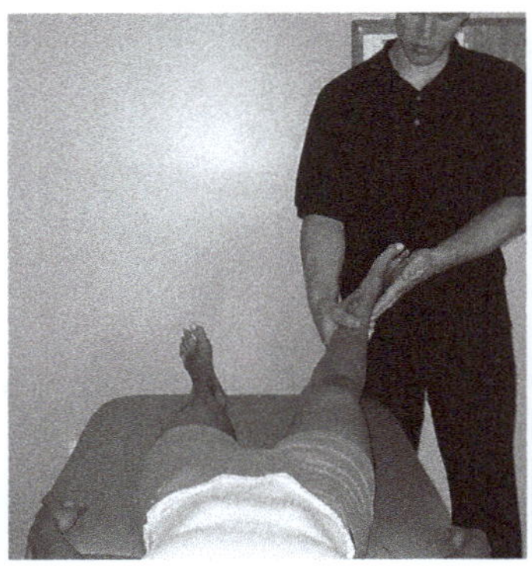

FIGURE 11.38 1. Positioning for psoas test

Passively move the patient's leg so that you slightly flex the hip with the knee extended. Slightly abduct the leg about 15° and then externally rotate the leg and hip.

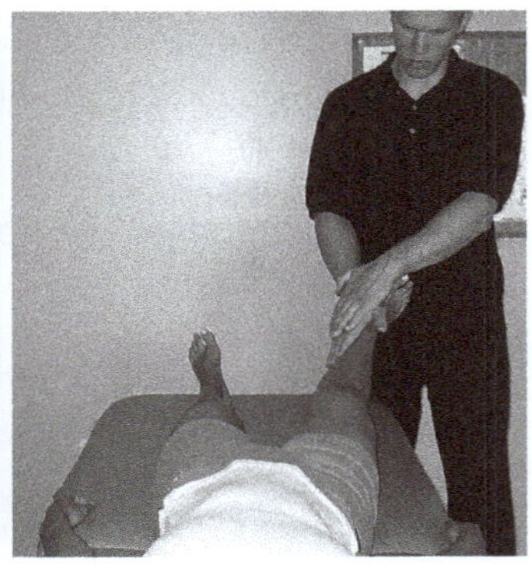

FIGURE 11.39 2. Testing with gravity and applying pressure

First tell the patient that they are to hold their leg in this position and that you are going to stop supporting the leg. Take your hands away (just a few inches/cm) and see if they can hold. If they can hold, then again support the leg and position hands so as to be able to push gently down and slightly out into abduction. Ask patient to resist.

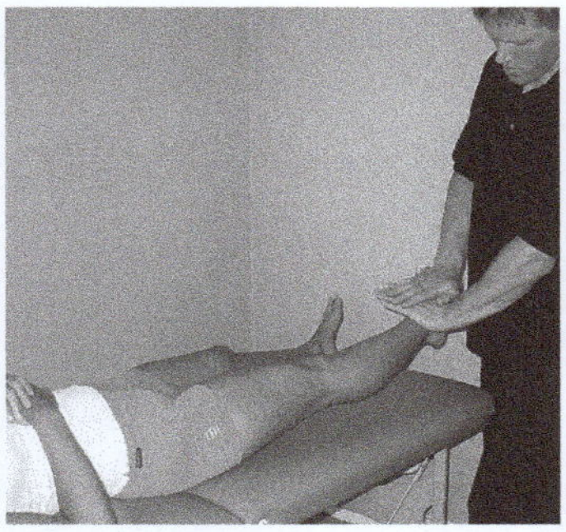

FIGURE 11.40 Testing tensor fasciae latae

Push the elevated leg toward the other leg, which is on the table.

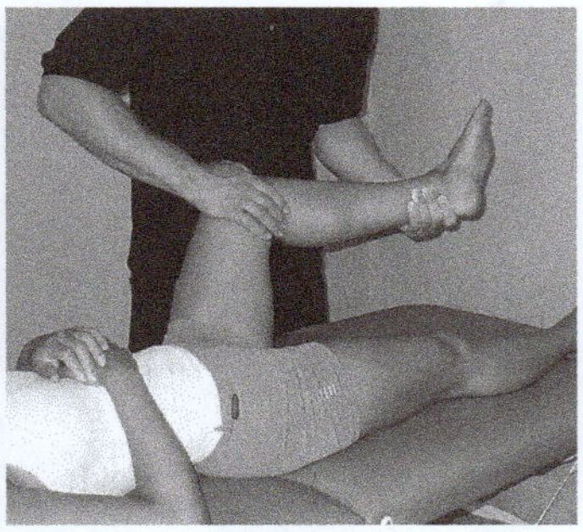

FIGURE 11.41 Testing sartorius

Resist the patient's attempt to take the left ankle to the contralateral knee.

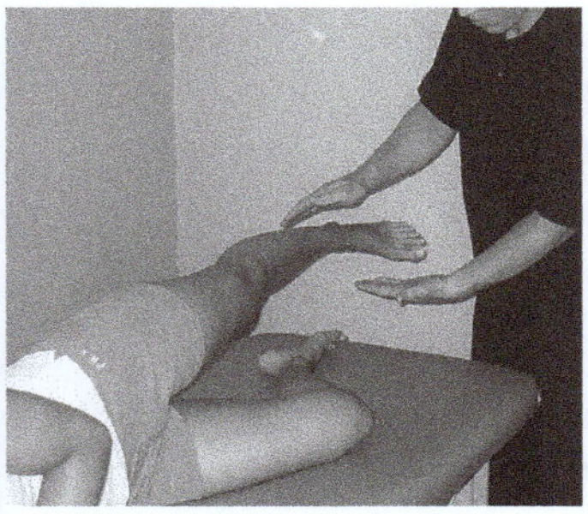

FIGURE 11.42 1. Hip abductors (general) positioning

Ensure the patient can hold the position without the hip rotating.

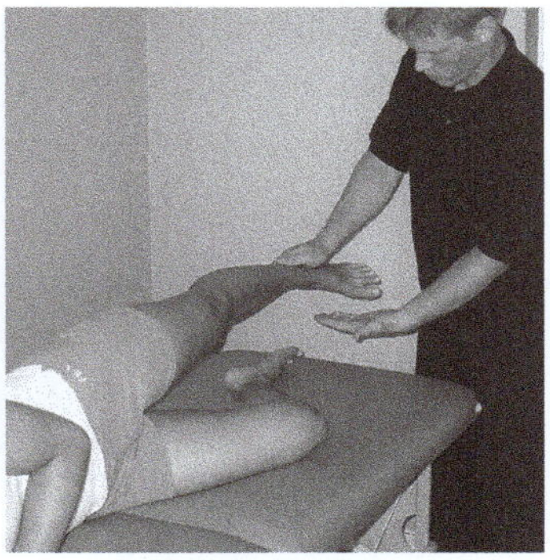

FIGURE 11.43 2. Apply resistance to all abductors

Apply resistance straight downward.

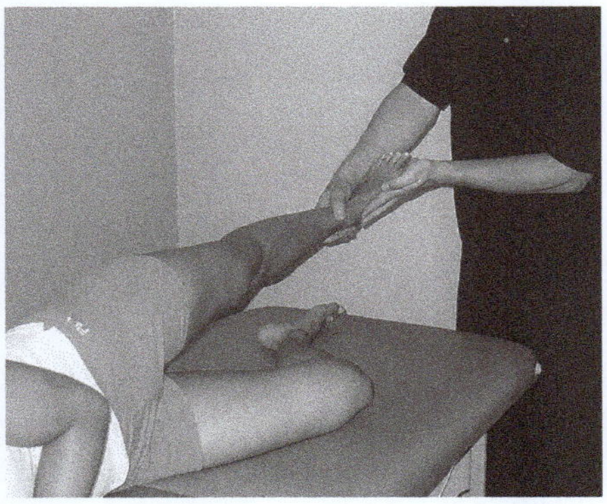

FIGURE 11.44 1. Positioning to stress gluteus medius

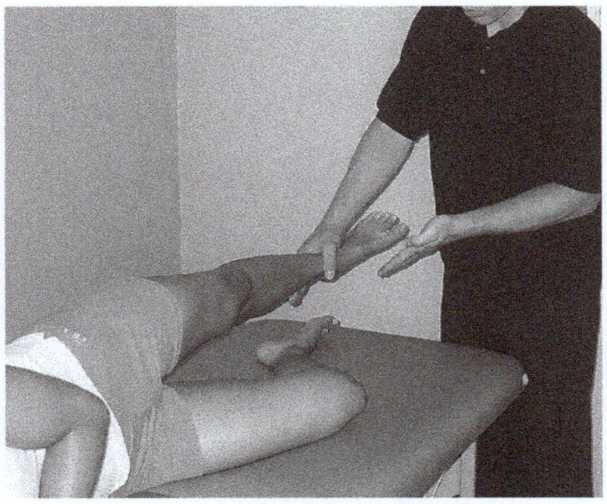

FIGURE 11.45 2. Apply resistance

To stress medius more, slightly externally rotate the leg, push down and slightly into flexion.

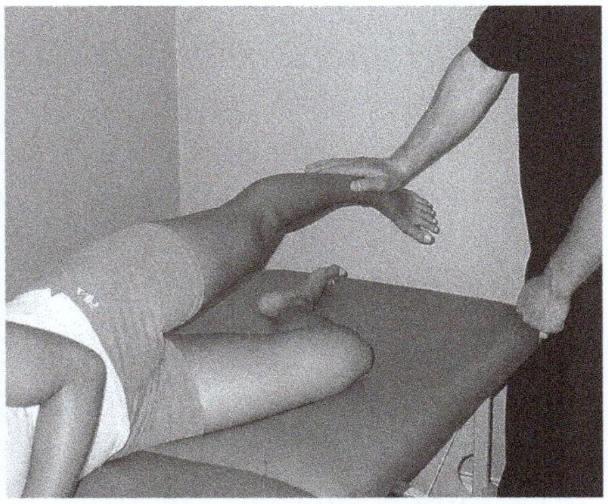

FIGURE 11.46 To stress gluteus minimus

Slightly internally rotate the leg and push down and slightly toward extension.

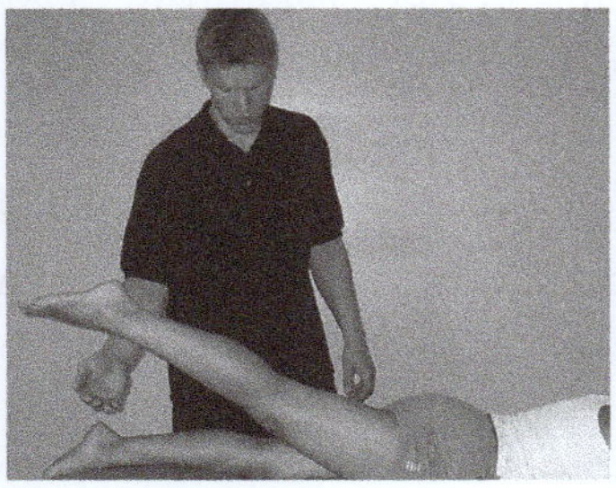

FIGURE 11.47 1. Holding extensors against gravity

The patient extends and holds the leg in extension.

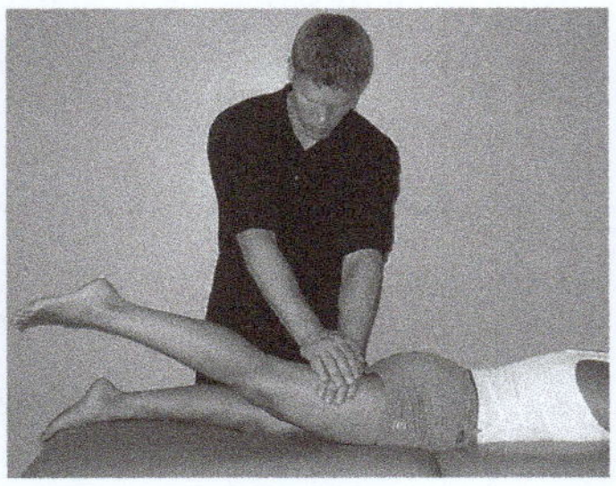

FIGURE 11.48 2. Applying resistance

Apply increasing pressure just below gluteals.

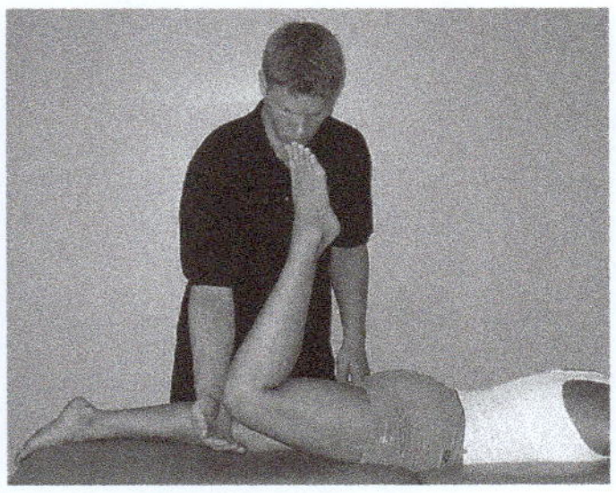

FIGURE 11.49 1. Holding gluteus maximus against gravity

Knee flexed, hip extended.

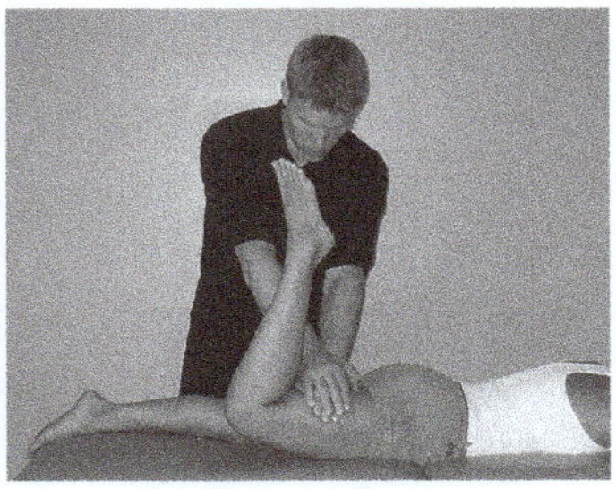

FIGURE 11.50 2. Applying resistance

Apply increasing pressure toward the table.

knee extended. Slightly abduct the leg about 15° and then internally rotate the leg and hip. To test the TFL, push down diagonally and medially toward the other leg.

To test the sartorius muscle (Figure 11.41) Passively position the patient's leg into an open Figure 4. Instruct the patient to try and take their ankle and place it on their other knee, i.e., the patient tries to assume, or complete the move toward, a Figure 4 position. The therapist resists this attempt by the patient to achieve a Figure 4.

To differentiate between the gluteus minimus and medius Figures 11.42 and 11.43 show how to test all hip abductors. Have the patient side-lying with the leg to be tested up. Figures 11.44-11.46 show how to differentiate gluteus medius and minimus. For medius, have the patient slightly externally rotate the hip and leg, then press down and slightly forward. For minimus, internally rotate, and press down and slightly into extension.

To differentiate between the gluteus maximus and the hamstrings (Figure 11.47–11.50) Have the patient prone, and passively lift the straight leg into extension. Have the patient hold this position for a moment to see if they can hold against gravity alone and then push the leg toward the table with your hand on the thigh. This tests both muscles.

To focus on the gluteus maximus, position as above but bend/flex the patient's knee to 90°, and then push the thigh down to the table, with your hand just above the back of the knee. Expect to feel a distinct difference in strength when the hamstrings are removed (made insufficient).

Special tests

The orthopedic tests on the following pages are designed to locate the source of pain or discomfort arising from joint surfaces or ligaments.

Compression/approximation test (Figure 11.51)

Before starting this side-lying compression test, use the back of your hand to palpate the SI joint margins and the lumbosacral junction, checking for heat (inflammation). The back of the hand is much more sensitive to temperature than the finger pads or the palm. Use light pressure to check for tenderness and bogginess (edema).

The compression test is designed to test the joint surfaces of the SI joint. It should be performed first when done in conjunction with the following two tests for sacral ligaments. We need first to know if the joint surfaces are involved in a patient's dysfunction/pain so that the latter two tests are not compromised. Although the gapping test and the pelvic shear test primarily test ligaments, they will also involve aspects of the joint surfaces.

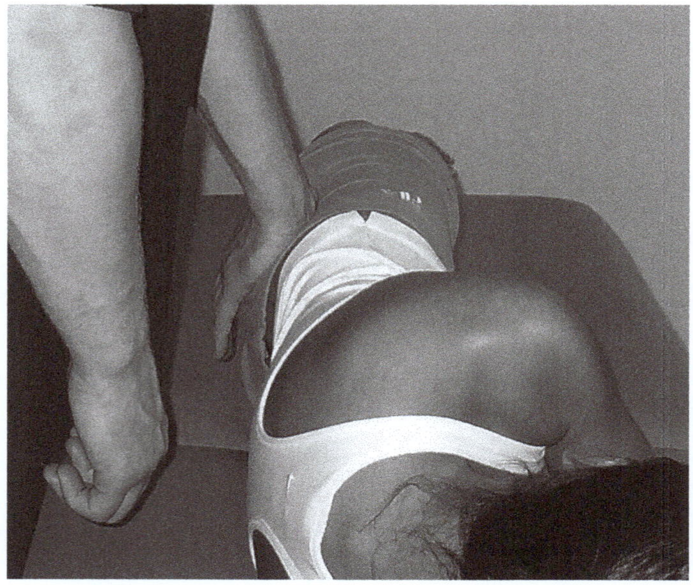

FIGURE 11.51 Compression test of sacroiliac joints
The patient is side-lying. Landmark over the iliac fossa and apply pressure straight down into the table. Make sure your hands are not too far anterior (near ASIS), otherwise force will not be through joint surfaces, but may gap the SI joint.

If your table is well-padded, it may be best to repeat the test with the patient side-lying on the other side, as the cushioning may not make the test bilateral (as it would be on a firm surface). The positive sign is pain felt along the joint margin. A positive sign here may well compromise the next two tests.

Two tests for anterior/posterior rotation of innominate (Figure 11.52–11.54)

The following two tests are based on the assumption that taking an anteriorly or posteriorly rotated innominate further into its rotation will stress sacroiliac ligaments and generate pain. These tests will involve many tissues and structures, so their specificity is questionable.

Since the patient will now be supine, and with gravity and weight-bearing removed as factors, it is a good idea to again palpate/landmark and record iliac crest heights, ASIS heights and distance from the mid-line, and leg length symmetry (see Chapter 9 for a quick test). Here, we have the opportunity to observe if chronic muscle shortening/imbalances or fascial restrictions, etc., are holding the body in patterns or positions.

Posterior displacement test

This test involves posteriorly rotating the innominate on the sacrum to its end-range. While standing at the level of the supine patient's hips, flex the patient's uppermost knee and hip. Make sure you hold the hip in flexion with the hand that is stabilizing the thigh on the posterior portion of the thigh, and not over the knee. Place your other hand under the gluteals so that your wrist is just superior to the ischial tuberosity. While you push the patient's thigh into more flexion, the wrist pulls the ischial tuberosity up and toward you (into anterior rotation), all of which helps to rotate the innominate posteriorly. The positive sign is pain, or an increase in discomfort, along the joint margin (or an increase in referred pain). This is taken to imply that the innominate is already posteriorly rotated, and trying to force it further produces the increase in symptoms.

Anterior displacement test

This test involves anteriorly rotating the innominate on the sacrum to its end-range. While standing at the affected side, flex the knee to 90° and cup your hand under the patient's knee while your other hand rests on the sacrum, fixing it in place. You need to place your body-weight onto the sacrum so that it does not pull the low back into extension. Now, lift the knee off the table, forcing the ipsilateral innominate into anterior rotation.

The positive sign is pain, or an increase in discomfort, along the joint margin (or an increase in referred pain). This implies that the innominate is already anteriorly rotated, and trying to force it further produces the increase in symptoms.

If placing the patient prone for the first time, then check to see if the PSISs are level. Note tension and tenderness in the sacrotuberous ligaments. If the patient has a unilateral anterior rotation of an innominate, the ipsilateral sacrotuberous ligament will be lax compared to the more tense (and possibly tender) contralateral ligament.

FABER test (Patrick's test/Figure 4 test) (Figure 11.55)

This test is for hip and sacroiliac pathologies. It is a good test for the length of the adductors but does not clarify the nature of the pathology of the hip or SI joints. Hence as a test for sacroiliac lesion it only reproduces the pain the patient has already told you about, and then only occasionally. FABER is an acronym for Flexion-ABduction-External Rotation: the very movements of performing the test.

With the patient supine and the therapist standing on the side to be tested, place the patient's ipsilateral ankle on their contralateral knee (by flexing, abducting, and externally rotating the hip). Stabilize the opposite hip at the ASIS while you press on the medial thigh just above the knee, and attempt to abduct and externally rotate the hip even further. The positive sign is pain in the sacroiliac region. The positive sign for the abductors or for hip joint problems is pain and restriction of movement into abduction and external rotation. Abductor pain is usually felt at the medial thigh and/or on the pubic ramus. Hip joint pain can show as deep inguinal pain which is just anterior to the joint surfaces and capsule.

Ganslen's test (Figure 11.56)

NOTE: The following is this author's opinion about this test. *This is a test that should not be done. It can place a lot of force through the SI joint and it is possible that it could make some lesions even worse. It may even produce a lesion where there was none before, either an innominate or a sacroiliac lesion. If this test is used, the nature of the lesion is not revealed and the potential for recreating pain in a lesioned joint is high, which then interferes with doing further testing. It is a commonly mentioned test in orthopedic texts, and is described here only to make you acquainted*

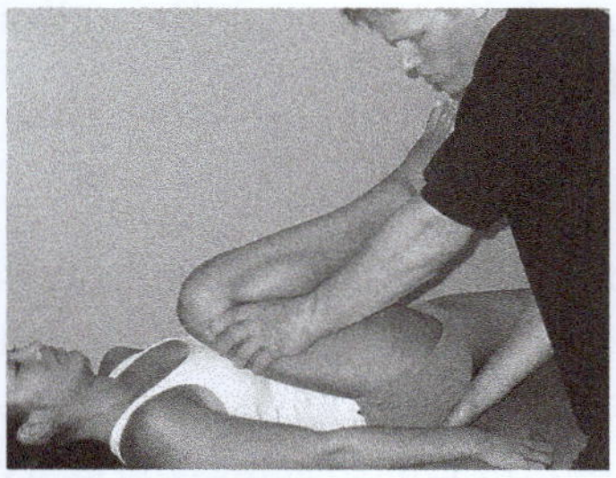

FIGURE 11.52 Posterior displacement test

Push the patient's knee toward their shoulder and pull the ischial tuberosity anteriorly.

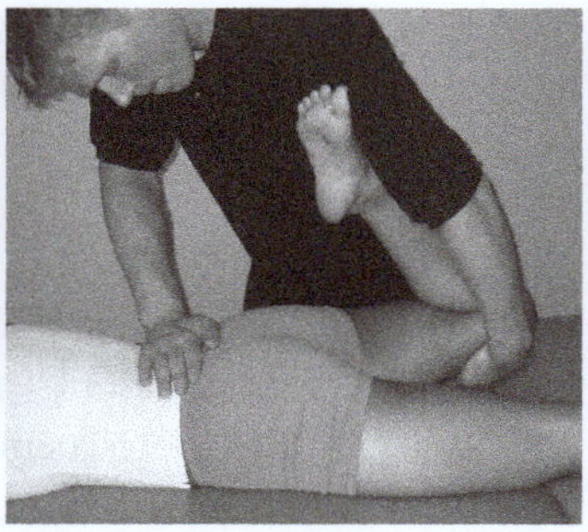

FIGURE 11.53 Anterior displacement test start

Stabilize the sacrum.

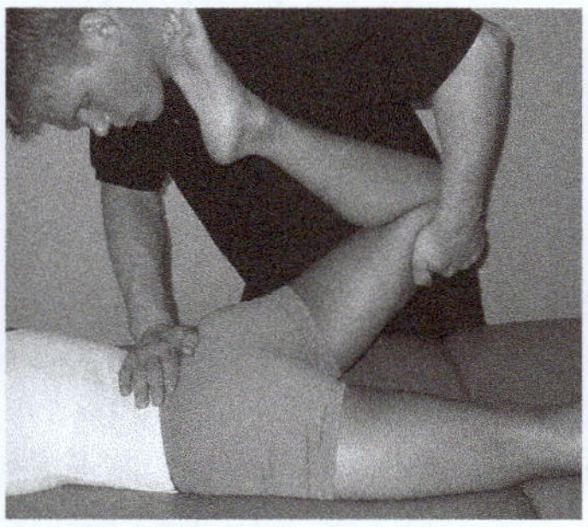

FIGURE 11.54 Anterior displacement test completed

Then lift patient's knee off the table.

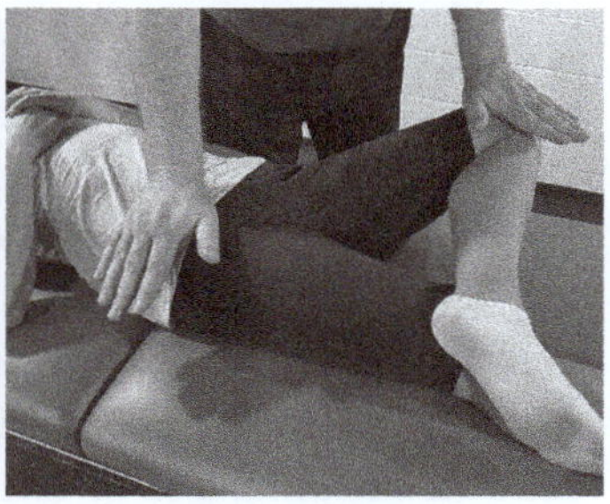

FIGURE 11.55 FABER test

Apply downward pressure to the knee.

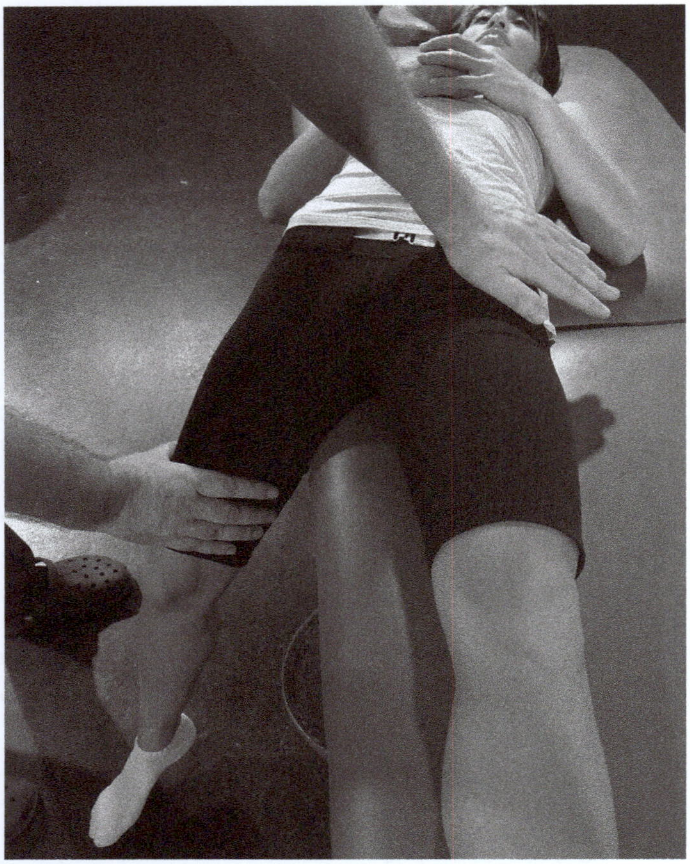

FIGURE 11.56 Ganslen's test

Push thigh toward ground.

with it, as a patient may describe this test as having been done to them previously by another health care provider.

The patient is placed supine and asked to come close to the side of the table. Both knees are taken to the patient's chest. Slightly turn the patient so their hip closest to you is off the table while the trunk of their body is still fully on the table. Extend the leg of the hip closest to you and so posteriorly rotate the innominate fully. The leverage generated by the extended leg creates a large stress through the hip and SI joint, which makes the test potentially unsafe for the injured patient. Like many other low back and pelvic orthopedic tests, this test is safer on the uninjured or unimpaired patient. For the injured or impaired patient, such testing may make the situation worse and so be contraindicated. The test can also be done with the patient side-lying, with the therapist taking the leg of the side being tested into extension.

Chapter appendix

Gait and sacral motion

Following is a summary of a model of how the sacrum moves during gait; a theoretical model of sacral motion during gait. That motion occurs is not in doubt, but the details have been, and will continue to be, debated for some time. What follows is this author's understanding, derived from many hundreds of hours, over many years, of reading, thinking, puzzling, and re-thinking about this topic. Any faults and misunderstandings that there may be here are the responsibility of this author alone. Nonetheless, thinking through the structure and function of the pelvis as it is involved in motion, in gait for example, has been immensely valuable in understanding how the sacroiliac joints not only function, but how they get into trouble, and further, help one understand the information provided by palpation and testing.

Walking, gait, as a normal motion for the human body, is referred to as *physiological motion*: how it is meant to function during gait. This section is useful in introducing further terminology and understanding of sacral motions for those who wish to pursue a deeper understanding of sacral dysfunctions. It is not intended as introductory material as it requires a good understanding of the anatomy of the pelvis and lumbar spine. Still, with patience, one can come to an understanding of the model in a manner that greatly aids one in appreciating the complexity, yet simplicity, of the design of this structure. It is a clear example of how structure enables function, and function shapes structure.

Each section uses the same example of right heel strike with left toe-off. It is repeated several times while going through different tissues and structures to demonstrate the numerous interactions and interconnections of the hips, pelvis, sacrum and spine – their joints, musculature, ligaments – and how all of these work seamlessly as a whole.

Walking/running

1. As the right heel is about to strike: the right innominate is posteriorly rotated, outflares, and drops slightly. The left innominate is anteriorly rotated, inflares, and is slightly elevated as the left foot is toeing off. The lumbar spine (and hence the whole trunk) is side-bent over the higher left innominate to help keep the center of gravity closer to the mid-line.
2. Right piriformis contracts, contributing to a left oblique axis by fixing the right ILA (inferior lateral angle). The right

sacrotuberous ligament tightens as the ischial tuberosity moves anteriorly. At this point, the right gluteus maximus is relaxed (allowing the right SI joint to open or gap – the right beveled edge of the sacrum is now able to move forward and be pushed forward by the PSIS area as it moves in medially).

3. The left leg is extended, the left gluteus maximus is contracting/tight (force closure of the left SI joint), the left piriformis is relaxed, and the left sacrotuberous goes lax as the left ischial tuberosity has moved posteriorly. This allows the left ILA to move posteriorly.
4. Hence, left oblique axis is established: this means the left sacral base (the superior pole) is fixed by the left gluteus maximus and hamstring tightness; and the right inferior pole and ILA are fixed by a tight sacrotuberous ligament and right piriformis. However, the right sacral base (superior pole) can still move, as can the left ILA with the slack left piriformis and sacrotuberous ligament.
5. With right heel strike, the left arm is forward, i.e., the trunk (and lumbar spine) is rotated to the right (side-bent left). Following mechanics of the sacrum, the right sacral base nutates/flexes around the left oblique axis, so that the anterior surface of the sacrum faces left. (Left facing on a left axis = left on left.) This means the right sacral base is moving anteriorly and inferiorly into nutation.

Therefore, the right sacral base has taken advantage of the situation described above in 4 and moved forward following the joint's semicircular shape and is also pulled down along the joint's semicircular surface by the right piriformis contracting. This inferior-anterior motion of the sacrum is assisted by the posteriorly rotating ilium/innominate. Because of the left oblique axis and the nutating right sacral base, the left ILA moves posteriorly.

NOTE: The spine sitting on the sacral base turns right, pulled by the right iliolumbar ligament, which is attached to the posterior rotated right innominate and the transverse process (TVP) on the right side of L5 (and also sometimes L4). There is more in the next section on how the iliolumbar ligaments guide the motion of L5.

The lumbar spine also side-bends left, compensating for the right tilt or lowering of the sacral base along with the dropping of the right hip (on heel strike) and the higher left innominate (at toe-off).

- The side-bending of the lumbar spine is assisted by the tightening of the left QL muscle, which is also involved in "hiking" the left hip as the left leg prepares for toe-off.
- As the left leg prepares to move from toe-off toward the swing phase of gait, the left QL tightens further to hold up the left hip as it begins its swing. This increases the side-bending to the left of the lumbar spine until mid-stance, where the right sacral base reaches maximum nutation. Then, the left QL begins to loosen/eccentrically contract until it lets go at left heel strike, where the oblique axis now changes over to a right oblique axis.
- While the left QL was tightening so were the right gluteus medius and gluteus minimus. They have the job of holding up the left hip as the left leg swings through and in turn, they pull/shift the hip laterally to the right, moving the center of balance over the right leg, which is the leg assuming the weight of the body.

ADDITIONAL NOTE: Though mentioned briefly above and below in this summary, the importance of the upper body in gait is immense. For example, arm motions via the latissimus dorsi are transferred through the thoracolumbar fascia and distributed into the quadratus lumborum, the erector spinae muscles, and the innominates themselves via the attachment of the thoracolumbar fascia on the bone. Motion from this thoracolumbar fascia is also transmitted to the long dorsal ligament, into the posterior sacroiliac ligaments, sacrotuberous ligaments, and down into the biceps femoris muscles. However, space does not permit exploring this fully here.

Gait: torsional movements – normal physiological motion (Figure 11.57)

- *Left on Left* = Right sacral base nutates (goes forward and inferior) and hence, the anterior surface of the sacrum turns to face the Left on a L oblique axis (while leaving the left SI joint in neutral).
- *Right on Right* = L sacral base nutates (forward and inferior) and hence, the anterior surface of the sacrum turns to face the R on a right oblique axis (leaving right SI joint in neutral).

Rules of movement for the sacrum and L5

Physiological motions

The vertebral segments of the lumbar spine work as a group, according to Fryette (Chila 2010; Mitchell 2001), and when the

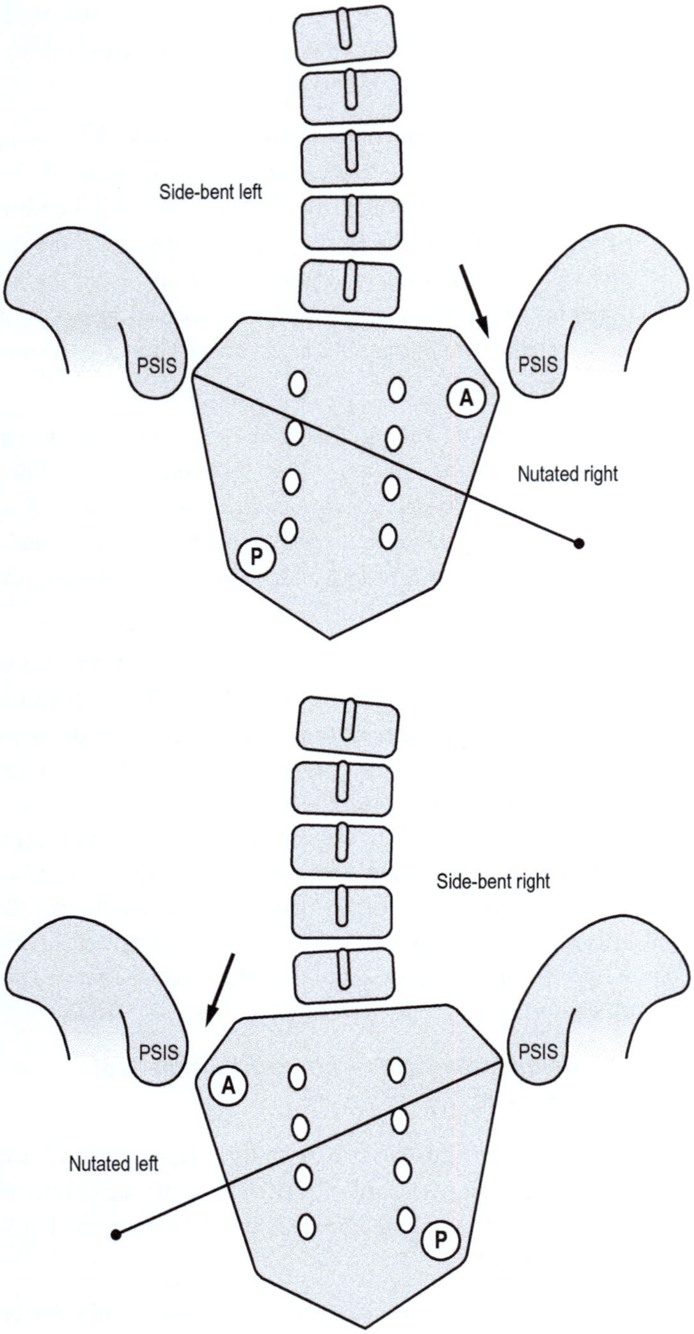

FIGURE 11.57
Torsional movements in normal physiological motion.

spine is in neutral (neither flexed nor extended) they side-bend one way as they rotate to the opposite side (see Chapter 12). However, in neutral during motion between L5 and the sacrum, if L5 side-bends left and rotates right the sacrum will side-bend right and rotate left. The sacral movements as a whole will go in the opposite direction to L5 during physiological motion.

This occurs for many reasons, but can be understood if we look at some of the ligaments involved in the sacrum and the lumbar spine that help guide these movements. We will use the example above talking about right heel strike.

On right heel strike, the right innominate rotates slightly posteriorly. Moving posteriorly, the right iliolumbar ligament attached to L5 *pulls* on the transverse process of L5 and makes it turn to face right. Meanwhile, the left iliolumbar ligament to L5 is made slack by the left innominate moving anteriorly. This *allows* L5 to rotate right.

Meanwhile, the sacrum has nutated on the right, which makes the sacrum turn and face left (as seen above). We noted that the posteriorly rotated right innominate has its ischial tuberosity move anteriorly, which tightens the sacrotuberous ligament. This pulls on the right ILA of the sacrum, moving it anteriorly and slightly inferiorly (as the sacrum follows the semicircular course of its joint with the ilium), therefore also helping to nutate that right sacral base. The left sacrotuberous ligament loosens tension as the left ischial tuberosity moves posteriorly, with the left innominate rotating anteriorly (on toe-off). This allows the left ILA to move posteriorly, which it needs to do if the right sacral base is to be able to tip forward over a left oblique axis, as it does in right nutation.

One of the things we can see from this is that the lumbar spine will tend to side-bend to the side of the oblique axis (i.e., its superior pole or origin).

Side-bending of the lumbar spine, sacral motion, and scoliosis

The lumbar spine compensates for the now unleveled sacral base (by side-bending) in the opposite direction to the position of the sacrum. This is the origin of most functional or adaptive scoliosis in the spine. Note that the thoracic spine, etc., will in turn compensate for the motions below it and so we often have an S curve in the spine as a whole.

This reciprocal motion between L5 and the sacrum is happening when we are walking or running. We can conclude that L5 moves in the opposite direction to the sacrum during physiological motions, whether the lumbar spine is flexing (sacrum bilaterally counternutating) or extending (sacrum bilaterally nutating) over a transverse axis. And as we have seen, L5 also moves opposite to the motion of the sacrum during gait; (on right heel strike the lumbar spine rotates to the right while the sacrum turns to the left). Therefore, any impairment to motion between L5 and S1 will eventually impact on gait and any changes to gait (from a sprained ankle, for example) can impact on L5 and S1's motion relationship.

LUMBAR SPINE: CHAPTER OVERVIEW

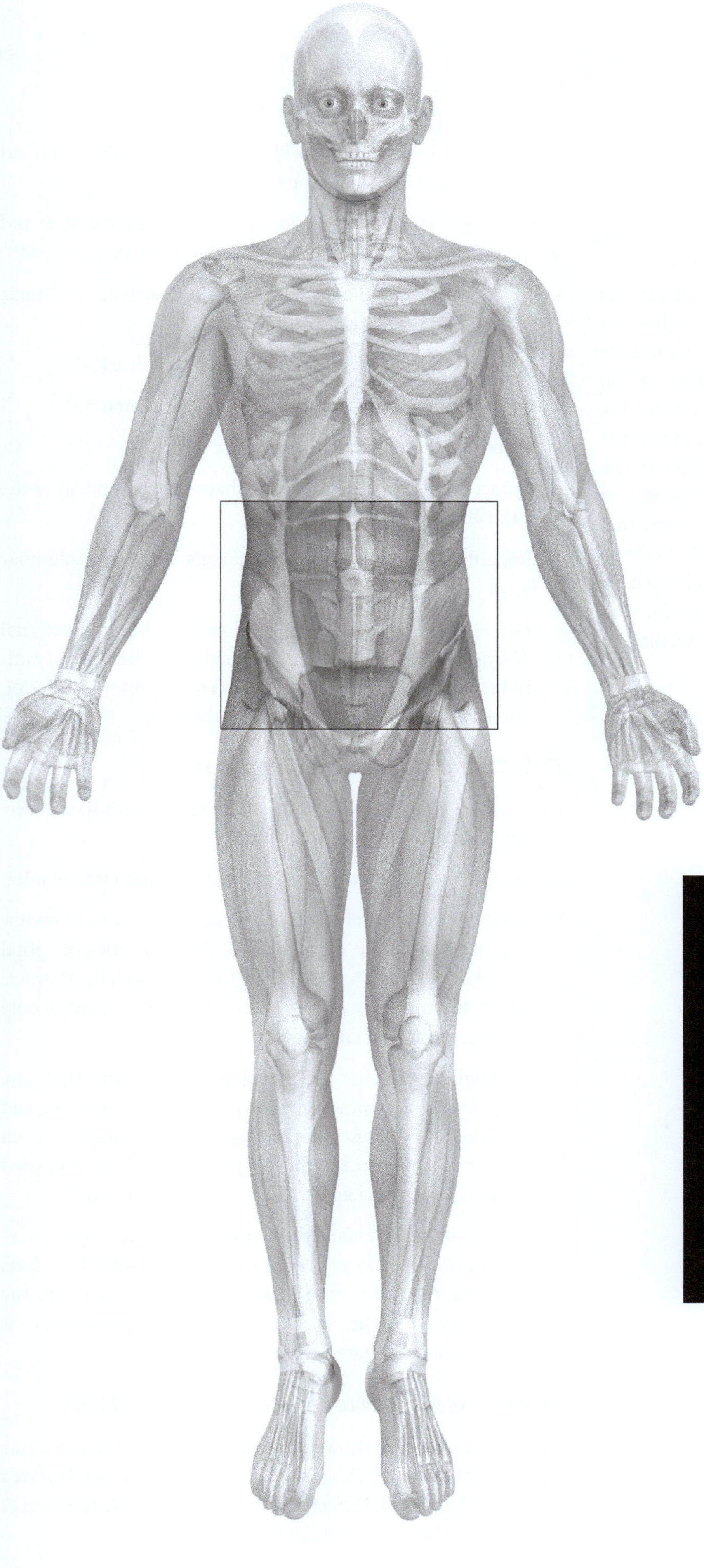

Chapter 12

Lumbar spine

Chapter 12

Clinical implications of anatomy and physiology

The following are some anatomical observations that have clinical implications. Understanding the functional relationships (physiology) between structures and tissues (anatomy) will help explain how structures of the lumbar spine can be injured, and also help us understand how orthopedic and motion tests work to provide the information that they do. Please review the anatomy of the joints and muscles involved in the function of the low back. It is suggested that the reader have an anatomy book at hand to more easily understand the information given in this section (either a general musculoskeletal text or one that reviews anatomy in detail of this specific area of the body). The information that has been summarized here has been chosen because of its direct relevance to orthopedic testing and understanding of mechanical pathologies of the lumbar spine (Agur et al. 2014; Bogduk 2012; Chila 2010; DeStefano 2011; Dutton 2012; Hertling & Kessler 2006; Levangie & Norkin 2011; Magee 2014; Maitland 2001; Mitchell 2001, 2005; Schuenke et al. 2014).

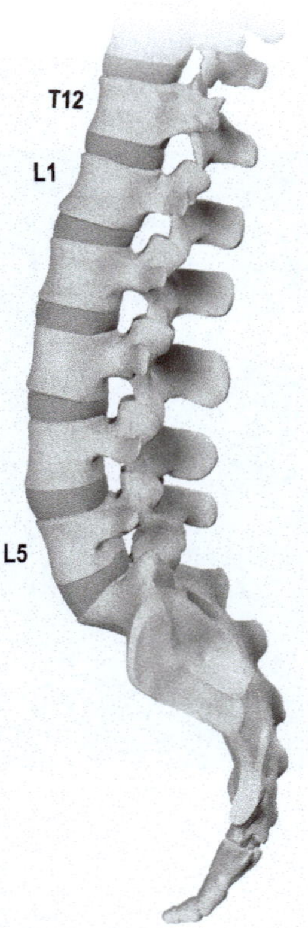

FIGURE 12.1

Lumbar spine.

Please review the following joints, tissues and the origins and insertions of the musculature involved along with their actions:

- lumbar vertebrae, the parts of a lumbar vertebra, and their relation to one another (Figure 12.1)
- supportive ligaments and the intervertebral disc (IVD)
- facet (zygapophyseal) joints (noting their orientation)
- lumbosacral junction
- thoracolumbar junction and the shape and placement of the 12th rib
- iliolumbar and lumbosacral ligaments and thoracolumbar fascia
- musculature: psoas, rectus abdominis, internal/external obliques, transverse abdominis; quadratus lumborum, multifidus, rotatores, latissimus dorsi; serratus posterior inferior, iliocostalis lumborum, longissimus thoracis.

Definitions and clinical considerations

- A motion segment of the spine is defined as two adjacent vertebrae and the joints between them.
- The commonly used term for zygapophyseal joint is facet joint.
- Group and segmental facet joint motions: we need to review what are commonly referred to as Fryette's rules of spinal motion. These rules (or "concepts") apply to both the thoracic and the lumbar spine. Before we do, however, we need to note a couple of observations.
  - Spinal movements are coupled. This means that any motion of the spine impacts on any other motion, and further, that some motions generally accompany each other. With respect to the last point, it has been proposed that side-bending and rotation are always coupled.
  - The motions are named from the perspective of the vertebra above, with reference to the one below. Therefore, to state that a vertebra is side-bent and rotated is to say that relative to the vertebrae below the vertebrae above is side-bent and rotated.

Fryette's rules of spinal motion (Figures 12.2, 12.3)

These rules have been shown to be valid (as a model) for motions in the lumbar spine (Bogduk 2012). (For more on Fryette's rules see: Chila 2010; DeStefano 2011; Dutton 2012; Hertling & Kessler 2006; Mitchell 2001, 2005.)

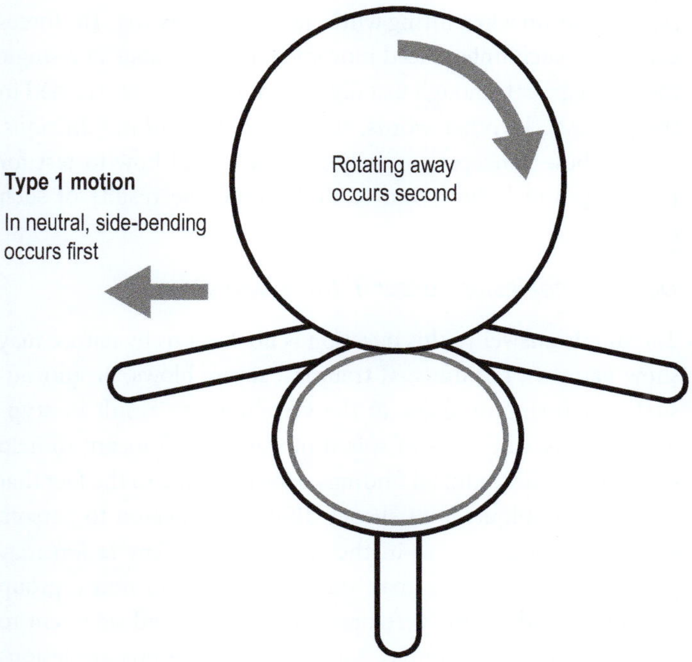

FIGURE 12.2 Fryette's rules of motion
Type I motion.

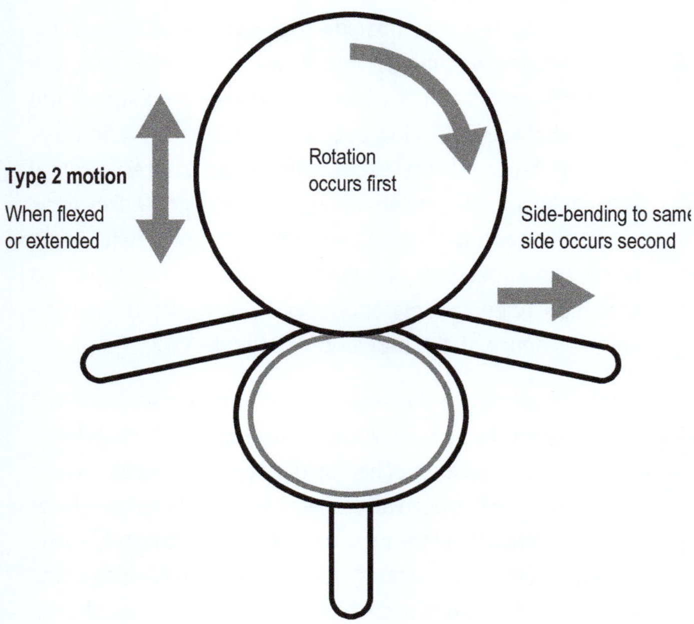

FIGURE 12.3 Fryette's rules of motion
Type II motion.

Fryette's first rule of spinal movements (Figure 12.2)

When moving from neutral the spine side-bends first and then rotates in the *opposite* direction.

The acronym NSR, which stands for neutral, side-bent, and rotated, is commonly used in describing or noting spinal motions.

- Neutral here means the spine is neither flexed nor extended. It is in a normal lordosis posture.
- The first letter in a notation based on Fryette's rules always refers to movement in the sagittal plane (flexion and extension).
- Side-bending occurs in the frontal or coronal plane.
- Rotation happens in the transverse plane.
- When speaking of motions in neutral, side-bending occurs before rotation.
- Notation follows the order of movement between side-bending and rotation when the spine is in neutral.

Since the motions are opposite to each other, specific instances can be notated as such: NSrRl, which means that when a spine is in neutral the superior vertebra in a motion segment is side-bent to the right while rotated to the left. NSlRr, therefore, means the reverse. Many osteopaths will contract this type of notation further. For example, NSRl indicates the spine is in neutral and therefore, the side-bending must be to the right since the vertebra is rotated left. In this text we will, however, keep the longer version for the sake of clarity, and for those using this notation for the first time. Further, using the fuller notation recognizes that the vertebrae may *not* always follow Fryette's rules.

Kapandji says the following to explain how this coupled movement in opposite directions occurs:

> This automatic rotation of the vertebrae ... *[When side-bending/lateral flexion occurs]* ... depends on two mechanisms : compression of intervertebral discs and the stretching of ligaments. The effect of disc compression is easily displayed on a simple mechanical model ... If the model is flexed to one side, contralateral rotation of the vertebrae is shown by the displacement of the various segments off the central line. Lateral flexion increases the internal pressure of the disc on the side of movement; as the disc is wedge-shaped its compressed substance tends to escape toward the zone of lower pressure, to rotation, i.e., contralaterally ... Conversely, lateral flexion stretches the contralateral ligaments, which tend to move toward the mid-line so as to minimize their lengths ... It is remarkable that these two processes are synergistic and in their own way contribute to rotation of the vertebrae. (Kapandji 2008)

Fryette's second rule of spinal movements (Figure 12.3)

When the spine is non-neutral (when in flexion or extension), rotation happens first and then side-bending occurs, both in the *same* direction. This is denoted as FRS or ERS r or l. There is only one direction that needs noting since rotation and side-bending usually occur to the same side in this situation. For example: FRSl means the superior vertebra is flexed, rotated and side-bent to the left. When the spine is working normally or unimpaired, rotation precedes side-bending and this is reflected in the notation.

Impairments are more likely to happen if the order of vertebral motion is not synchronized. For example, if the spine is in neutral and the patient side-bends and rotates, and this is *followed by flexion or extension*, the chances for an impairment or dysfunction increase substantially. Knowing that the order of movements increases the odds of injury happening helps the therapist understand how the patient became lesioned when the patient describes how the injury occurred.

Fryette's third rule of spinal movements

Introducing motion to a vertebral joint in one plane automatically reduces its mobility in the other two planes.

This rule is fairly self-evident. It is important, however, for understanding how injuries occur. When the patient's spine is moved following the second rule (FRSl, for example), as the vertebrae are flexed some degree of motion is no longer available for side-bending and rotation. However, if the person then moves the spine into extremes in any other plane, that also increases the chances of injury occurring. If while flexed the person then side-bends and rotates (using all planes) then the chance of injury now becomes highly probable. Add in some extra weight and injury will be hard to avoid (this is the classic "lift and twist" low back injury). If the IVD and facet joints are driven too far and with too much load then injuries to these joint structures, to the ligaments, and to the (intrinsic and extrinsic) lumbar muscles of the spine are likely to occur.

Fryette's first rule is often referred to as *Type I motion*. In turn, impairments involving this type of motion are *Type I dysfunctions* and usually occur as a group (as in a scoliosis, for example). Therefore, they are referred to as a *group* (or *neutral*) *dysfunction*, where several vertebrae side-bend one way and rotate in the opposite direction. This information will help explain how we can motion test for this type of spinal lesion.

The second rule covers *Type II motion*. Therefore, *type II dysfunctions* follow their motion pattern, with the spine already flexed or extended. They usually occur in isolation, as a single segment strain when lifting while flexed and twisting. The forces exerted in such unbalanced movement can summate at a single motion segment (though usually several muscles are strained in the process). In other words, they are *segmental dysfunctions*. Again, these concepts can help us understand how to test for these types of lesions, and to understand the results of such testing.

Do all spinal lesions occur in these ways?

The simple answer to this question is no. Lesions by nature may show patterns, but unusual traumas, severe blows, or an unusual structuring or shape to the vertebrae can result in atypical patterns. The rules of spinal movement are meant to help explain common clinical findings. However, due to the fact that everyone is unique, joint shapes differ from person to person, even from joint to joint in the same person. Any lesion may present as unique. You may, on a rare occasion find a group dysfunction where the vertebrae seem rotated and side-bent to the same side, for example. After all, many lesions are lesions because things have gone wrong. Thus, we need to know how to accurately palpate and test the joints of the spine and, more

INSIGHTS

Box 12.1 Why are we using so much from the osteopathic tradition?

Ever since the 1930s, when James Cyriax championed and espoused the view that most low back pain, especially chronic low back pain, was due to disc injury and dysfunction, the orthopedic profession has focused on disc herniation as the most probable cause of low back pain. While the new and revolutionary findings in the 1920s and 1930s that intervertebral discs could herniate and prolapse, etc., was a great discovery, it has proven to have been unwarranted to credit it with being the cause of most back pain. In fact, it is now thought that "no more than 12 percent of patients with low back pain had any clinical evidence of disc herniation" (Bogduk 2012).

Further, the presence of herniation does not necessarily mean it is the cause of the pain. However, owing in part to Cyriax's influence and the acceptance of his books on assessment as classics in the field, there has been a decreased interest in exploring facet joint dysfunctions and their role in back pain. Fortunately, many osteopaths (and chiropractors) never bought into the idea of the dominance of disc dysfunction as the principal cause of back pain. Osteopaths in particular developed and refined techniques to test and explore facet joint function and dysfunction that are especially accessible to massage therapists.

importantly, not make assumptions about how it should be and thus forgo specific testing. We need to be open-minded enough so as to be prepared to find the unexpected.

Box 12.1 examines the ways we look at low back pain

The lumbar intervertebral disc (IVD) (Figure 12.4)

The lumbar intervertebral disc (IVD) is a polyaxial joint. It is capable of accommodating any direction of motion, including shear forces and compression. The ball-shaped nucleus pulposus at the interior of the IVD is a gel that helps accommodate the compressive forces exerted on the disc. It remains gel-like until middle age, when it becomes fibrosed. The disc is made up of cartilaginous layers, known as annular fibers, with diagonal fiber directions that vary in their direction layer to layer. This variation within the cartilaginous layers and the nucleus pulposus gives greater resistance to the various forces that the disc undergoes. However, if the layers are continually, or forcibly, put under stress, their integrity can begin to break down. Then the gel-state nucleus will begin to push its way outward through these breaks in the annular fibers and force the layers in front of it to bulge.

In the lumbar spine, the nucleus is not in the center of the disc, but is slightly posterior in order to better accommodate the compressive force when the spine is in neutral. In other words, because the lumbar posterior (lordotic) curve puts more mechanical stress on the posterior portion of the disc, the nucleus being slightly posterior to center provides better support.

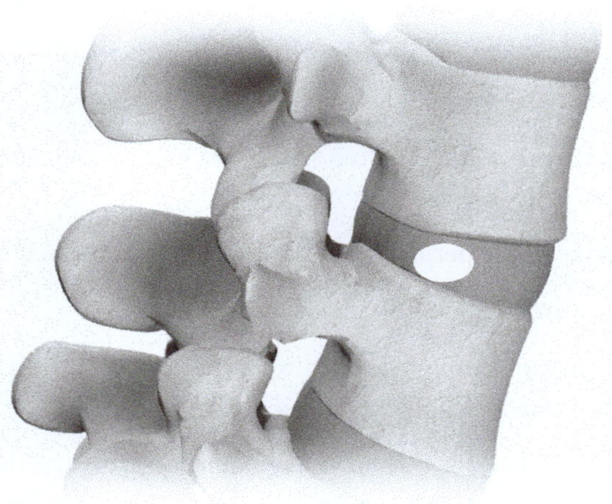

FIGURE 12.4

The lumbar intervertebral disc.

However, with flexion of the lumbar spine the compression of the anterior portion of the disc pushes the nucleus even more posteriorly. If the posterior cartilaginous layers are weakening then the nucleus will begin to shift even more posteriorly, causing the weakened layers to bulge. The posterior longitudinal ligament (which is quite narrow at the lumbar spine) often helps sustain the integrity of the most posterior fibers of the disc and so the bulging nucleus often rolls out around this ligament and moves to the side, moving in a posterior lateral direction. This puts it on a collision course with the neural foramen and the spinal nerve at that level.

Causes of low back pain

This is a highly controversial subject where there is much theory about clinical presentation. But research to date has often been inconclusive in establishing the exact mechanisms of pain from the variety of tissues implicated. Chronic low back pain is even more controversial. Research using nerve blocks cannot always isolate their effect to just one specific tissue in the lumbar spine, and the same can be said for injecting an irritating solution into the tissues (Bogduk 2012). With imaging techniques we can see a great deal but slight tears in facet joint capsules, for example, are still difficult to find. Further, just because we see an abnormality does not mean it is the cause of the patient's pain. We will briefly touch on the controversy with respect to "discogenic" (intervertebral disc or IVD-sourced) pain (Magee 2014).

With respect to other tissues as sources of pain, we will list the usual suspects. Even though some may remain unproven as causes, we do this because they have not yet been disproved to be sources of pain. This is because current testing procedures cannot always isolate them sufficiently or it could be unethical to create the lesion in a subject in order to investigate it.

The intervertebral disc and chronic low back pain

The IVD was for some time considered aneural, and this idea persisted until recently even though it has been known to be otherwise by some. However, there is no evidence that this limited innervation is sufficient to be involved in low-back pain (Bogduk 2012). In the past, therefore, it was thought that the pain experienced by the patient was not from the disc itself but rather from the tissues the bulging (herniating) or prolapsing disc pushed on (usually ligament, and sometimes nerve). While it is possible that a bulging disc may put enough pressure on soft tissue to cause pain note that the herniation may often protrude in a direction where it does not impinge on any pain-sensitive structure and can be completely asymptomatic.

Levels of degenerative disc disease (DDD)

- *Herniated disc*: a bulging disc (that could possibly press on ligaments or nerves nearby) that has lost its height, usually meant to imply a slight bulging all around the disc.
- *Prolapsed disc*: the nucleus pulposus begins moving through the torn layers of the disc. This has the disc bulge in a very specific direction.
- *Sequestered*: a portion of the nucleus is extruded out of the disc. As this material is thought to have no self-marker, the body attacks it as foreign with an immune and inflammatory response. If part of the nucleus enters the spinal canal the inflammation results in extreme pain and the nerves at that level (and above and below) often become dysfunctional (resulting in numbness/weakness) until the inflammation resolves.

As mentioned, herniated discs pressing on nerve roots as a cause of pain experienced *in the low back* specifically is not substantiated by research. Compression of lumbar nerve roots produces numbness and tingling into the buttocks and lower limb, but not in the low back. Research has not shown that either compression or the tractioning of nerve roots on its own causes local pain, or even referral into the lower limb, though it may cause numbness or paresthesia (Bogduk 2012).

One mechanism by which herniated or prolapsed discs could cause pain would be the resultant loss of disc height. The consequence of this loss of height is that facet joints that would normally have a slight gap or joint space between the articular surfaces when the lumbar spine is in neutral could now become closed and weight-bearing. This stress to the articular structures can, for example, result in an inflamed joint and/or stress fractures in the pars articularis (spondylolysis), which can produce pain felt locally. This scenario can occur over time. On the other hand, a sudden loss of disc height due to a traumatic injury to the disc would not only affect facets joints but also create a situation of joint instability in that spinal motion segment. The ligamentous and joint capsules associated with that joint are suddenly too lax to stabilize and properly guide movement on-site. The body's response to this instability is to induce protective muscle spasming to "hold and guard" the area, thereby restricting all movement in that motion segment. This muscle spasming will quickly set up the conditions for pain in the area.

One source of chronic low back pain being proposed is still thought to come from the IVD and is known as *discogenic pain*. It is now thought to be the result of what is being called IDD, which stands for *internal disc disruption* (Bogduk 2012). This is considered a "focal disorder" within the disc, rather than the type of general degeneration seen in a herniated disc. (However, a herniation may be one of the end stages possible for this condition.) What is being proposed is that the IVD endplate suffers injury which precipitates a cascade of metabolic changes in the nuclear and cartilaginous matrix that changes the quality of the material that constitutes an IVD. If the IVD endplate does not heal successfully this may result in an inflammatory process (possibly chronic) which is capable of producing pain.

Endplate fractures can be produced through the compressive forces that a motion segment goes through, especially from repetitive action or from the spine being compromised (such as being flexed and rotated) when these forces are applied. This occurs when the spine is not in strict neutral position as in standing straight. Side-bending and rotation will increase the likelihood of increased stress through these endplates; but the stress will dramatically increase if the spine is also in flexion or extension with side-bending and rotation added.

Further, such disruption to the integrity of the endplate will affect the nutrition, etc., available to the IVD. This restriction of nutrition available from the vertebral body for the IVD would play a large role in the degeneration of the IVD. This could be one source of degenerative disc disease (Bogduk 2012).

Suspected sources of intermittent and chronic low back pain

Vertebrae

- Bone pain, which is often sharp and bright when acute, and a deep ache otherwise.
- Injury to the periosteum (via abrasion or muscular tension).
- Fractures, whether hairline or crushing.
- *Kissing spines*, where two spinous processes impact each other on extensions causing a bony lesion.
- Lamina impact due to hyperextension causing an inferior facet process to impact on the lamina of the vertebrae below.
- Spondylolysis: a fracturing of one or both pars interarticularis (they need not always be painful, however). Spondylolisthesis, which is the slipping forward of the vertebral body due to spondylolysis, may not itself be painful, but the tension placed on other tissues could be painful along with the resultant muscle guarding of the area.

Muscle

- Pain: in acute injury a sharp pain is felt which, as it resolves (or when chronic), becomes a deep ache with indistinct borders.
- Sprain: when a muscle has been stretched while contracting enough to cause injury. In the low back, this is most often caused by trying to lift too heavy a weight or a large and awkward object. Sudden stretch usually causes injury at the musculotendinous junction. Sustained stretch (from overloading) usually causes injury throughout the muscle and, if overload is great enough, then
  - a rupture or avulsion could occur.
- Repetitive strain: can cause micro tearing of muscular tissues, often resulting in tendinopathies.
- Spasm: where the pain is considered from ischemia and/or irritation from retained metabolites.
- Trigger points: these are considered a common cause of local and/or referred pain.

Thoracolumbar fascia

- Can either exhibit the burning, stinging pain of connective tissue injury, or (as the thoracolumbar fascia is part of the various muscle compartments of the low back musculature) it could produce the muscle pain of a deep ache and sense of weakness common to compartment syndromes (Willard et al. 2012).

Ligamentous strain

- Usually felt as a deep, achy pain but the iliolumbar ligaments, for example, can produce a sharp pain on stretch (during motion) or palpation.

Dura mater

- Possible source of sharp pain when tension is placed through the tissue due to it being adhered to vertebral bone.

Zygapophyseal or facet joints

- Either sharp, piercing pain when acute or a deep ache when chronic. This could be due to joint surface injury, loose body, joint capsule tear, or pinching of inner joint structures. Lumbar facet joint pain can be local or can refer down into the buttock and even the leg (Bogduk 2012).

Sacroiliac joint

Pain can be local, over the joints, and/or refer into the lower limb (see Chapter 11 for more on this).

INSIGHTS

Box 12.2 Are X-rays, CT or MRIs really better than hands-on testing?

Often, in the face of technology, health professionals have acquiesced to employing or relying on a machine for orthopedic assessment. Are not X-rays, CT scans, or MRIs a truly objective base for judgments about soft tissue pain and dysfunction? The short answer is yes and no.

For acute trauma-based injury the answer may be yes; for cancer and other diseases it is yes. For chronic or recurring injury to the low back the answer is actually no. In a 1998 article summarizing his work in *Scientific American*, Dr Richard A. Deyo brought together some interesting studies about assessment when addressing low back pain (Deyo 1998, 2002; Deyo et al. 2009; Weinstein et al. 2006). In one article he concluded that "at least for adults under age 50, X-rays added little diagnostic value to office examinations" (Deyo 1998). Further, referring to epidemiological research, it was revealed that "many conditions of the spine that often received blame for pain were actually unrelated to the symptoms and multiple studies determined that many spine abnormalities were as common in asymptomatic patients as in those with pain. X-rays can, therefore, be quite misleading;" and lastly, "even highly experienced radiologists interpret the same X-rays differently, leading to uncertainty and even inappropriate treatment" (Deyo 1998; see also Deyo 2002; Deyo et al. 2009).

Though hands-on assessments by various health care professionals of the same patient can also produce a variety of conclusions, the point is that X-rays are no more objective and, other than in trauma or pathological disease scenarios, they add nothing to case history taking and manual assessment skills.

Nor are the newer imaging methods such as CT scans and MRIs any better for soft tissue injuries. In one study looking at pain-free individuals under 60 years of age who never had a history of either back pain or sciatica, "MRI found them [herniated discs] in one fifth of pain-free subjects ... Half that group had a bulging disc, a less severe condition also often blamed ... Of adults older than 60, more than a third have a herniated disc, visible with MRI, nearly 80 percent have a bulging disc and nearly everyone shows some age-related disc degeneration." Another study found two-thirds of pain-free individuals had disc abnormalities. "Detecting a herniated disc on an imaging test, therefore, proves only one thing conclusively: the patient has a herniated disc" (Deyo 1998).

Visceral referral

Kidney disease or injury is felt as low back pain. Pain is usually felt superficially over the kidney, from T10 to just under T12, and the kidney can refer and feel as flank pain. (See Part I, Chapter 4 for this and other organs that refer into the low back.)

Box 12.2 compares hands-on testing and imaging modalities in the assessment of low back pain and other disorders.

Introduction to facet joint dysfunction and pain

The assessment of facet joint dysfunction in cases of low back pain is a specific area of assessment that many massage therapists often leave to other health care professionals. As low back pain is one of the most common of the musculoskeletal dysfunctions that send sufferers to seek treatment from massage therapists, our lack of knowledge and skill in assessing these joints brings into question how helpful we are when treating such patients. This lack of knowledge limits us in the use and application of techniques we have been taught or have at our disposal. We are often unsure of how to apply the techniques safely and effectively because the nature of the impairment is not clear enough for us. Therefore, assessment of the facet joints of the spine is included in this text.

When health care professionals attempt to locate the sources of low back pain, the statistical average is very poor: at best the causes will be found only 20 percent of the time (Hertling & Kessler 2006).

Almost any motion of the lumbar spine is controlled by the interplay of the shape of the osseous structures, along with the anatomy and physiology of the discs, facets, ligaments, muscles, and fascia. These somatic structures, including radicular (nerve root) or other neural structures, can rarely be dysfunctional individually without some of the other tissues being injured. This, in turn, causes local musculature neuroreflexive stimulation to splint the area. Impaired motion in spinal segments can lead to decreased blood flow in the area which, in turn, creates acidosis, leading to an inflammatory response by tissues in the area. Tissue health (articular, muscular, vascular, and neural) can be compromised.

Group impairments

We need all the tools we can possibly have at our disposal when assessing low back pain, precisely because of the interrelationships that all of these joints and tissues have. For example, an unlevelled base (say, from a leg length discrepancy or a unilaterally rotated pelvis) will cause the spine to curve in compensation so that the trunk can remain perpendicular. It is a functional scoliosis, one that may well disappear as the person assumes different positions. It will no longer exist if the underlying causes are removed. However, if this curve persists then muscles, joint capsules, and other supportive tissues may over time shorten or fibrose and create a group dysfunction in the lumbar spine (a persistent scoliotic curve). Such a situation may result from unilateral chronically short muscles, such as the quadratus lumborum or the deep layer of intrinsic back muscles (rotatores, etc.) that side-bend and rotate and fix the vertebrae into the rotoscoliotic curve. Conversely, if the scoliotic curve in the spine is a compensation for another structure, such as the pelvis and sacrum being on a tilt, then the short muscles and tissues are a result of the scoliosis. They can be the result of a structural or biomechanical asymmetry somewhere else in the body.

Unlike a functional scoliosis, the group dysfunction does not disappear when the patient changes position. It has progressed to being a dysfunction that is now self-sustaining. It remains observable through flexion and extension, and is itself responsible for measurable losses of range of motion in the lumbar spine. The group dysfunction now can be a precipitating cause for further changes in function of the low back, thoracic spine, or pelvis. As mentioned, loss of motion of the spinal components within this group dysfunction eventually leads to poor tissue heath and impaired function of the involved tissues. Nonetheless, these group dysfunctions often have precipitating causes which need to be corrected (like a unilateral pelvic tilt) before the dysfunction can be addressed (e.g., by lengthening a quadratus lumborum (QL) and appropriate rotatories, etc.) in a manner that will sustain the correction.

Segmental impairments

The second type of facet dysfunction is a segmental dysfunction. This refers to a dysfunction that only occurs between two vertebrae, to a vertebral motion segment. In this situation a facet joint of the spine does not open as it should or will not close as it should. The suspicion is that these impairments arise from strains to the spine when it is not in a neutral position, that they occur when the spine is already flexed or extended and then has rotation or side-bending movements added on. Therefore, they are often call non-neutral dysfunctions (on this subject and the text below see Bogduk 2012; Chila 2010; DeStefano 2011; Kapandji 2008; Magee 2014; Mitchell 2001, 2005).

When the spine is flexed all the involved facet joints open. As rotation and side-bending are now introduced to one side the facet joints approximate (close) on that side. On the contralateral side the facet joints grow further apart, and may even exceed the normal anatomical limit for that joint.

The joint capsule and supportive ligaments, along with the deep fourth layer intrinsic muscles on that hyperflexed side get stretched and potentially strained, especially if an excessive load or tension is now placed on them. If such a joint cannot return to neutral when the rest of the spine does, then that joint is said to have a flexed-rotated-side-bent (FRS) dysfunction. This FRS remains even when the spine is extended. On the other hand, those approximated joints (referred to in the beginning of the above example) are actually prevented from hyper-movements and thus, avoid injury.

In any case, the likelihood is that the motion segment at the apex of the side-bending (lateral curve) would be the one most strained and therefore, where the lesion will occur. Now the motion segments above and below the apex of the lateral curve move in the same manner but to a lesser extent, often protecting them from lesioning. These lesions usually occur at one motion segment rather than in a group, and hence the term segmental dysfunction.

The L5 vertebra is a very common segmental lesion site. The principal reason for this is that L5 sits on the sacrum (i.e., it is part of the lumbosacral junction). As a result, there are unique stressors placed through L5. Besides the forces spoken of above that can occur when the spine is flexed and then has rotation and side-being occurring, there is in addition further movement generated in L5–S1(and often L4–5) because of connections to the innominates via the iliolumbar ligaments. Thus, how the feet and hence the hips are oriented can add even greater stress to the L5–S1 motion segment.

The other possibility for the occurrence of a segmental dysfunction is when the spine is bent back into extension and then rotation and side-bending are added. In this situation, both facet joints of a motion segment have been closed. Then, on the side to which rotation and side-bending occurs, more closure is demanded by those additional actions; the joint structures and ligaments are hyper-compressed This could result in injury to the joint. Further, the fourth layer muscles were forced to contract while in a shortened position; in other words, the muscles already shortened by extension are then called on to contract even more to perform side-bending and rotation. This is the classic recipe for strain and/or muscle spasming, which is what could hold the joint closed.

Again, the lesioning usually occurs at the apex of the curve, where the forces are most intense. Therefore, with an extension impairment the lesion occurs on the side where rotation and side-bending occurs. This is an extension-rotation-side-bending (ERS) dysfunction. One side of a motion segment remains in the ERS position when the spine returns to neutral, and even when the spine flexes.

With excessive extension, the intrinsic structures of the joints (fat pads, joint folds, meniscoid pads, etc.) could get jammed between the surfaces. With excessive flexion, these same structures could get dragged out of place (overstretched and displaced). In either case, a sharp or intense pain occurs that in turn causes a neuroreflexive reaction in the spinal muscles so that they spasm or tighten in a manner that does not allow the joint to move away from its position. The patient may feel this pain as a pinch or piercing type of pain (like a pin prick) that may stay, become intermittent (i.e., provoked only by movement) or fade.

The hypomobile ("stuck") joint as either FRS or ERS then has consequences for the motion segment of the spine of which it is a part. Also, the segments above and below must compensate. Therefore, a common occurrence found during testing is of a group dysfunction above the segmental dysfunction. For example, having a L4–5 segmental dysfunction that tilts/unlevels L4 (when the spine is in neutral) then requires the spine above to compensate by having a group of vertebrae (e.g., L3 up to T11) side-bend back toward the mid-line. Since this is occurring while the spine is in neutral the rotation in this group is to the opposite side. This compensation is the body's attempt to return the trunk to a posturally balanced position. The longer the segmental dysfunction remains, the more likely it is the compensatory curve will fibrose and/or have associated muscles spasming, which then produces a group dysfunction.

Further, the structures and joints below will be affected whenever motion comes from above (as in lifting an arm and rotating the thoracic spine). The motion from above may often cause pain at the level of the segmental dysfunction. The lesion will distort the motion as it tries to pass down through the dysfunctional segment and not allow the lower structures and tissues to appropriately compensate. Therefore, even a single segmental lesion is not just a small or focused issue but one that spreads its effects beyond itself. The longer the lesion exists, the more far-reaching and numerous the effects.

NOTE: The following common short forms for parts of a vertebra are used throughout the text:

- SP, spinous process
- TVP, transverse process.

Active ranges of motion of the lumbar spine

Flexion: 40–60°

Extension: 20–35°

Side-bending: 15–20°

Rotation: 3–18°

(This last is difficult to measure, as it may depend on the pliability of the IVD and coupled-motion. It is also difficult to define: are we adding up the range of motion till each facet joint closes? Or are we including "living motion," i.e., the motion segments, including rotational torsion occurring within the IVD (Kapandji 2008; Bogduk 2012)?)

See the Appendices at the end of the book for charts and tables on muscles (muscle origin, insertion, innervation, action and synergists), joints (actions, ranges, muscles used, tissues stretched and compressed); another table on capsular patterns (of restriction, open packed/resting positions and close packed positions); and several charts on neurological testing where any such testing would involve this chapter's region.

The testing protocol (Box 12.3) begins with the case history.

Box 12.3 Protocol

Case history (specific questions)

Observations

Rule outs

Active free range of motion (AF-ROM)

Passive relaxed range of motion (PR-ROM)

Resisted isometric testing and strength testing

Special tests

Case history (specific questions)

- Is this a result of a fall or accident?
- Is this a result of any strain to the low back? Such as lifting or carrying; or an awkward movement?
- Do you ever experience pain in the low-back with coughing or sneezing? With bowel movements?
- What positions are you most often in during the day (such as sitting, standing, or performing repetitive movements for extended periods of time)?
- Is the pain local or does it travel?
- Does your low-back feel weak? Occasionally or constantly? Suddenly or gradually? Do you ever feel weakness in the legs?
- Have you had any pain in either or both legs? [Pain in both legs can be a red flag, especially if it is accompanied by weakness. Refer the patient to their physician, who can then explore the possibility of spinal canal stenosis.]
- Is there any feeling of numbness, tingling, or weakness in the legs? [If the patient gives any indication of neurological impairment by their description of their pain or symptoms, you will need to do a neurological examination. Further, always refer the patient back to their physician if they have not already discussed these symptoms with their doctor.]
- What activities of daily living is this (impairment) affecting?
- Do you have any diagnosis of arthritis in the spine? Disc herniation? By X-ray, MRI?
- Is the pain related to pregnancy or post-partum?

Observations

Look for bruising, lacerations, redness or blanching of the skin. Note lordosis of the lumbar spine and if there are any apparent deviations of the spinal column. Check the level between the PSIS and ASIS on each side. An anterior tilt of 5–15° is normal. It is necessary here to look carefully at the whole hip-pelvis-lumbar complex. Most of this, and what follows, would have already been done during the comprehensive examination of the spine.

REMEMBER: Observing includes palpation. While observing, perform light palpation to assess tissue texture changes to the skin and connective tissue, to the joint capsules and, of course, to the musculature. Look for any of the following autonomic responses in the skin (which may occur over the site of an impairment): enlarged pores, dimpling or orange-peel texture, excessive moisture or dryness of the skin, and trophic changes to the skin such as thickening or thinning.

Look for the classic signs of inflammation in an acute injury, the "*four Ts*": *temperature* (heat, and redness), *tissue texture* (due to autonomic responses), tone (hypertonicity or laxity) and *tenderness* (acute sensitivity, bright or sharp local pain). Check the temperature with the back of your hand (it is more sensitive than the fingertips or palm). A chronic injury usually displays the following: coolness, blanching of the skin and, sometimes, bogginess (chronic edema), all of which are due to decreased blood flow. Muscle is often hypertonic, which contributes to the decrease in circulation of blood and drainage of lymph. Pain is often less localized, and feels deeper and duller. The patient will commonly refer to pain in the chronic situation as an ache. Also, the trophic changes to the skin are more apparent in the chronic situation since sufficient time has elapsed for physiological changes to have taken place to the dermal and subdermal layers as well as the glands of the skin.

Comprehensive examination of the spine

This testing protocol is usually done when the therapist wants to perform a more detailed postural examination (static and dynamic) of the patient. If several of the tests underlined below are found to be positive, then a more thorough examination of the lumbar spine needs to be performed, such as is presented in the rest of this chapter. Pain, asymmetries, and other impairments on-site at the lumbar spine area can occur with standing, sitting, or with motion from above or below; if present they demand further investigation. For more detailed information and pictures, see Chapter 10.

Standing postural views: front, side, back:

1. Looking for relationships with gravity line: with a plumb line, check vertical landmarks, observe horizontal landmarks (again, see introductory remarks on spinal assessment for details).
2. Note asymmetries and tissue texture changes.

Sitting behind the patient: note asymmetries and any restrictions to range of motion:

1. Landmark the levels of arches of the feet, ischial tuberosities, trochanters, PSISs, iliac crest heights, (creases of) waist, inferior and superior angles of scapulae, mastoid processes.
2. Return to the PSISs. While landmarking the PSISs have the patient bring the chin to the chest, then slowly roll down to lumbar flexion while noting the movement of the PSISs (standing flexion test). Check the spine for flat spots, excessive curve, bulking of erector spinae, lateral curves, and the like. Have the patient return to standing straight. Ask the patient to look up to the ceiling (while you leave your hands on the patient's hips for stability) and extend their back while observing changes to curves of the spine (lordosis-kyphosis).
3. Have the patient bring the ear to the shoulder; then have them slide the hand on the same side down the side of the leg to the knee, observing how the spine curves during side-bending (from above). Check both sides.
4. Have the patient flex one knee while the other remains locked; note lumbar side-bending (from below). Check both sides.
5. Hold the hip stable. Have the patient bring their chin over a shoulder and note head/cervical rotation; then have them bring the shoulder back toward you, observing thoracic rotation. Note the amount of resistance required at the hips to resist lower trunk rotation (ease versus effort).
6. Challenge sagittal plane (anterior-posterior) stability (via the manubrium and T2).
7. Challenge side-bending, either by pressure on the acromions or an inferiorly directed tug on the wrists.

Have the patient sit:

1. Re-check the iliac crest heights, PSISs, shoulder/scapula landmarks, tissue bulk, etc. Observe all changes of orientation to landmarks, tissue changes, etc., during the following motion:
2. Seated flexion test: while landmarking the PSISs, have the patient flex forward. Check for asymmetry of tissue bulk on either side of spine.
3. Side-bending: with the elbow flexed at 90°, the patient brings the ear to the shoulder, then lowers the shoulder toward the table.
4. Rotation: turn the chin toward the shoulder and, at end-range, push the shoulder back.
5. Challenge to side-bending: push down alternately on each shoulder cap.

Patient supine (after traction of legs or other corrections to patient's orientation):

1. Note medial malleoli levels.
2. Check the ASISs:
   - level (innominate rotation)
   - height from the table (pelvic rotation)
   - distance from the mid-line (inflare/outflare).
3. Check rotations (fascial exam). Compare the height from table of the hips (ASISs, as above), lower ribcage, upper ribs, anterior shoulders, L and R occiput, i.e., the height from table compared to the norm and compared one to the other bilaterally, and then compare directions of rotation from one set of landmarks to the next.
4. Push the following side to side comparing ease/bind (testing side-bending): at waist (lumbars), mid-ribs (thoracic), and neck (cervicals).

When, or if, specific testing has the patient prone check the following:

1. Levels of the plantar surface of the heels, ischial tuberosities, PSISs (and height from the table); and the lateral curves in the spine, tissue bulk of the erector spinae, and scapulae orientation.

Key observations during postural assessment (Figures 12.5–12.7)

You may have made these observations during a comprehensive examination of the spine, but if you did not do the examination then do the following.

It is important that the patient stands in a natural pose. To assist in this, instruct the patient to look up slightly (you do not want them watching their feet, etc.) and take a couple of steps, while staying in place. Neither you nor the patient are to correct feet positions, head positions, etc. You are trying to have them stand as they naturally do, or as close to natural as is possible, even though they are in a clinical setting.

Take note that much of this information is needed to compare with the supine and prone examination so that we are not misled by what we see when the patient is on the table in those positions.

- Pay attention to the general orientation of the upper body, especially rotations and side-bending of the shoulders or spine.
- Note the general orientation of the hips, thighs, knees, tibias, ankles, and feet. Look to see if the hips are shifted right or left over a leg; compare the proportions (tissue bulk) and orientation of the thigh and lower leg (rotations throughout the course of the limb down to the feet, varus or valgus of knees or ankles, arches of the feet, to name some examples).

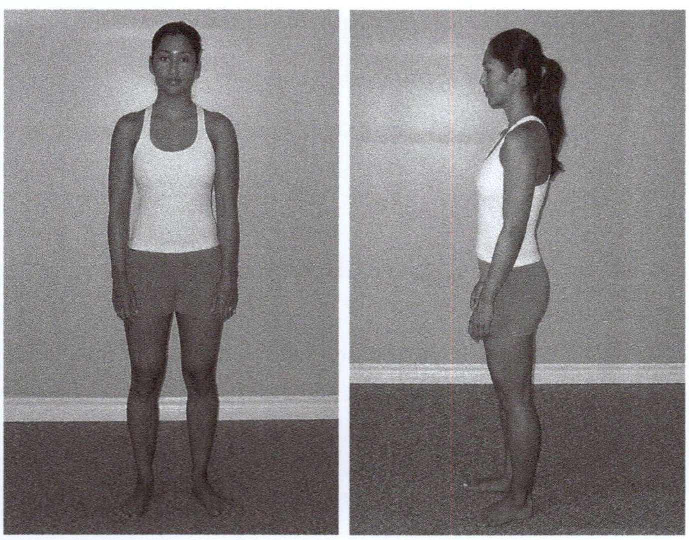

FIGURE 12.5A, B Postural assessment

Front and side views.

Be specific and exact with the following:

- Check iliac crest and greater trochanter heights (Figure 12.6).
- Record ASIS and PSIS heights from the anterior, posterior, and lateral views (Figure 12.7). Compare heights of the ischial tuberosities.

Pelvic obliquity and tilts

After completing your postural assessment you may have noticed some pelvic obliquity, a change in height of one hip compared to the other, creating a horizontal tilt to the sacral base. This is usually due to a unilateral anterior or posterior rotation of the innominate affecting leg length (i.e., functional leg length difference), but it can also be the result of (the more rare) true leg length difference due to differences in the length of the long bones of the lower limbs.

Make a note of the following:

- whether the pelvis is rotated around a vertical axis. In other words, does one ASIS appear more anterior than the other (in the coronal plane), and whether the ASISs are level with each other
- if the patient has shifted their pelvis to one side over a leg (which then usually becomes the principal weight-bearing leg)
- whether the patient has a hyperlordosis or a hypolordosis of the lumbar spine. Check to see if the patient has an anterior or posterior pelvic tilt and how that relates to the anterior curve (lordosis) of the lumbar spine. Observe whether the lumbar spine seems rotated and/or side-bent.

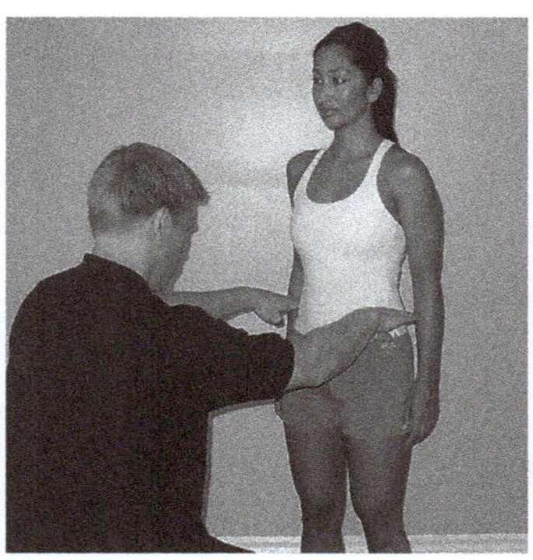

FIGURE 12.6

Check iliac crest heights.

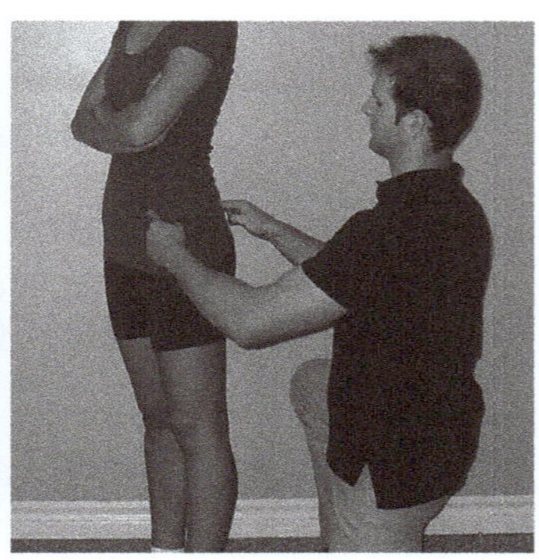

FIGURE 12.7

Check ASIS and PSIS relationship.

Common postures and how they affect the lower back (Figures 12.8–12.12)

(For more details on types of postures and the impairments they present with see: Janda & Jull 1987; Kendall et al. 2005; Magee 2014.)

In the *normal posture* (Fig. 12.8) the ear sits roughly over the shoulder, the shoulder sits over the trochanter and the gravity line runs just behind the patella and just in front of the malleoli. The spine has its proper elongated S-shape that provides a spring to cushion the joints and structures of the spine. The line of gravity (plumb line) runs through the body of vertebra L3.

In *sway back (forward hip) posture* (Figure 12.9), sway refers to the tendency of a person with this posture to sway back and forth (i.e., anteriorly and posteriorly). The reason for this is that with the hips thrust forward, their weight will shift onto the toes and this easily creates a feeling of imbalance so the musculature of the legs and hips will alternate in tension, causing the person to sway back to front as they remain perched on their toes (Kendall et al. 2005) The lumbar spine is extended (hyperlordotic) at the lowest lumbar vertebrae, which are sitting on posteriorly rotated hips. The hip joint is in extension, as are the knees. (The thoracic kyphosis and cervical lordosis are also exaggerated.) The first one or two lumbar vertebrae and lower thoracic vertebrae are often flattened and resist motion. This adds to the compressive force on the lowest hyperextended lumbars.

Muscles creating sway back posture:

- *Tight and hypertonic muscles*: lumbar erectors, quadratus lumborum; hamstrings and gluteus maximus (for the knees: vastus medialis, vastus lateralis, vastus intermedius).
- *Weak and inhibited muscles*: abdominals, except for internal oblique which may be hypertonic, iliopsoas, rectus femoris.

The *military posture* (Figure 12.10) is named for the classic "head up, stomach in, and chest out" position of a soldier at attention. It requires the person to extend their low back (increasing lumbar lordosis) while lengthening or flattening the thoracic kyphosis as the shoulders are retracted. Often the chin is lifted, extending the upper cervical spine. Note that the line of gravity runs slightly behind L3's vertebral body.

Muscles creating the military posture:

- The low back and mid-back erectors are short and tense, abdominals are tense, rhomboids and lower trapezius are short and tense. The suboccipitals are short and tense, along

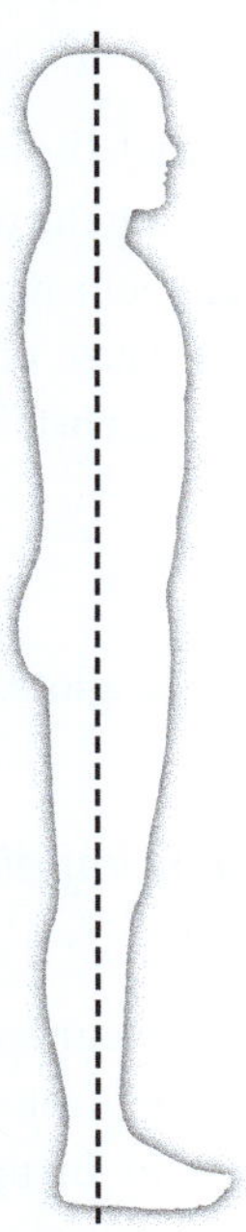

FIGURE 12.8
Normal posture.

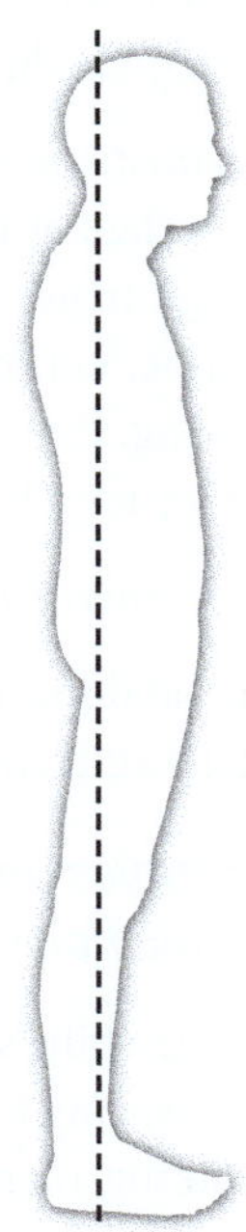

FIGURE 12.9
Sway back (forward hip) posture.

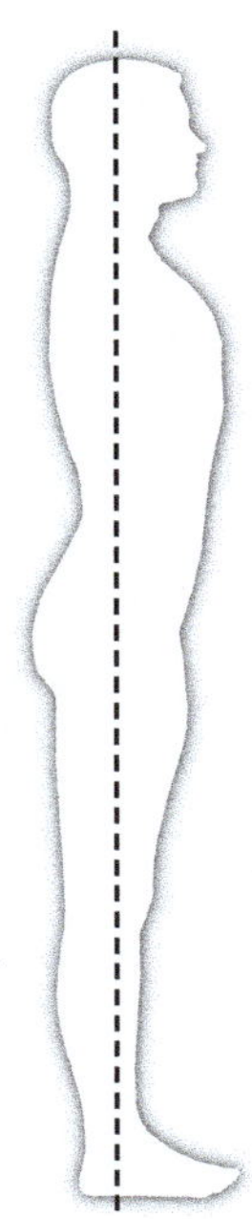

FIGURE 12.10
Military posture.

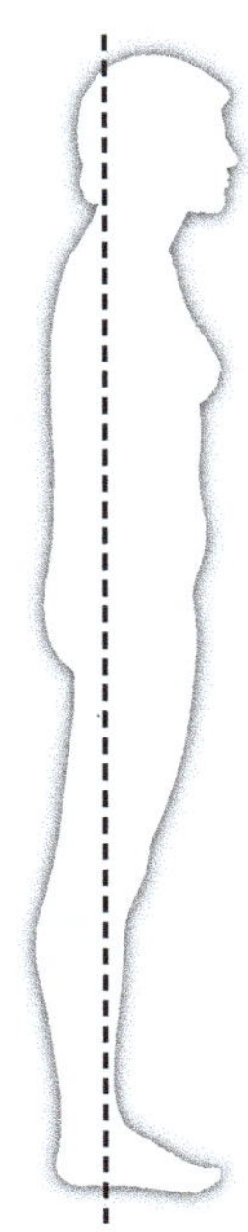

FIGURE 12.11
Flat back posture.

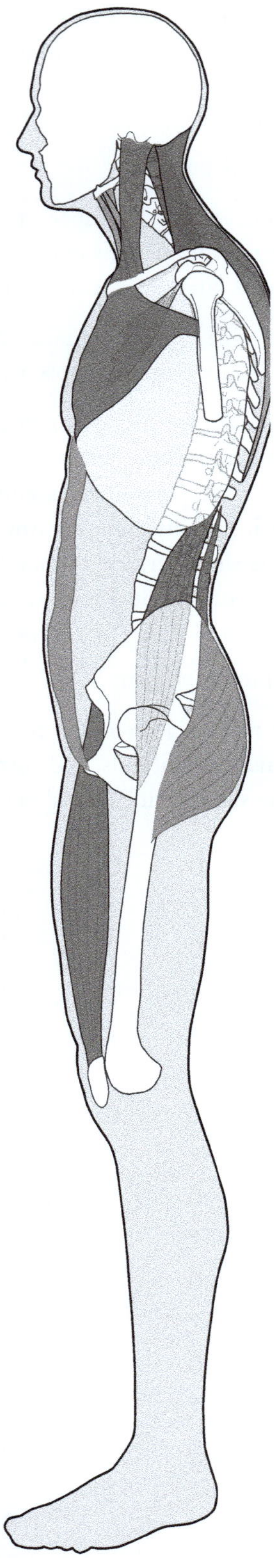

FIGURE 12.12

Hyperlordotic posture (lower cross syndrome).

with the scalenes (holding the first two ribs up). The pectoral muscles are also short and tense (lifting the ribs and sternum while lowering the clavicle onto the ribs underneath it).

In the *flat back posture* (Figure 12.11) the lumbar spine curve is decreased/flattened. As a result, the body compensates for this by throwing the head forward (upper thoracic hyperkyphosis and upper cervical hyperlordosis).

Often, the whole body tilts forward which results in the toes grabbing the ground and the toe flexors therefore contributing to a pes cavus (high arch) in the foot.

As a result of the flat back posture the pelvis-lumbar complex has:

- lumbar spine flexed, stretched low back erectors
- posterior pelvic tilt with extension of hip joint, tight, short hamstrings, short abdominals and lengthened rectus femoris and iliopsoas.

Hyperlordotic posture (lower cross syndrome) (Figure 12.12)

The *hyperlordotic posture* (Figure 12.12) is associated with a bilateral anterior pelvic tilt, which is a common muscle imbalance found in the clinical setting.

Tight and facilitated muscles:

- Lumbar erectors, QL, iliopsoas, piriformis, rectus femoris, TFL, thigh adductors.
- Taut hamstrings (lengthened but hypertonic): the hamstrings are stretched by being a muscle group holding the pelvis from rotating further anteriorly (along with gluteous medius) and, over time, contracture to this length. Because of this contracturing, they will appear short (loss of extensibility) when tested for length.

Weak and inhibited muscles:

- Rectus abdominis, transversus abdominis, gluteals, vastus medialis and lateralis of the quadriceps.

Lumbar curves and L3: the source of many impairments and dysfunction within the lumbar spine

The lumbar spine's normal lordosis (anterior curve) is meant to act as a spring to cushion the forces coming from below (as when walking or running) or from above (as in upper body movements and carrying or lifting). This springiness comes from the shock-absorbing qualities of the intervertebral discs (IVDs). This works well when the spine is generally in a neutral position. In neutral the plumb line, or line of gravity, runs through the vertebral body of L3, which is also the apex of the normal lumbar lordosis (Bogduk 2012; Mitchell 2001).

However, in most of the postural variations (from neutral), the lumbar curve is held out of line, or repositioned with respect to the line of gravity. This means that the direction of forces on L3 (and the rest of the lumbar spine's vertebrae and IVDs) are altered. While the lumbar spine is accepting and capable of handling such repositioning for brief moments, the spine is not capable of handling this for long periods of time. Changing the lines of force and tension, etc., inevitably will result in changes to structure and function of the tissues of the spine.

The IVDs, the facet joints, the bony structures and the ligaments are all put under long-term tensile and compressive stresses that will inevitably affect those structures physiologically and structurally. Changes to the orientation (or structure) of the lumbar spine's curvature will inevitably change how it functions. Changing how the spine functions for extended periods of time will in turn begin to change the very structure of each of the components listed above. Such changes are the primary causes of degenerative disc disease (DDD; disc degeneration, herniation, vertebral body osteophyte formations, etc.) and degenerative joint disease (DJD; e.g., facet joint osteophyte formations, ligamentous stretching or shortening, synovial joint surface osteoarthritic changes, etc.). Most of these changes, after prolonged postural deviation, are permanent (or only minimally reversible or repairable), even if the normal curve is returned to neutral.

Some examples of lumbar curve impairments and their effects include:

- During hyperlordosis, L3 is shifted in front of the line of gravity. The more L3 moves forward of the gravity line (as in excessive hyperlordosis, e.g., in a sway back), the greater are these excessive forces on the posterior portion of the IVD, resulting in degeneration (cracking and tearing) of the annular fibers. In fact, the nucleus pulposus, which was centered under the lines of force running through L3 (by being slightly posterior within lumbar IVDs), is now being shifted forward of the line of gravity, etc. It now can actually become a fulcrum increasing the amount of compressive forces in the posterior portion of the IVD and the tensile (stretching) forces in the anterior portion of the IVD, much in the same way as shifting more weight to one side of a seesaw (teeter-totter). Osteophytes will begin to form anteriorly in order to try to hold or reinforce the stretching annular fibers, and also posteriorly to reinforce the posterior annular fibers from being crushed and broken down.
- Further, this shift of force or weight may make the facet joints become weight-bearing. This will speed up osteoarthritic changes in these joints. The pars articularis will also receive excessive force and may crack. Ligaments around the facet joint become shortened and so can no longer appropriately guide the movements of the facet joints nor properly stabilize the joints at their end-range. This permits excessive side-bending and rotation within the lumbar spine. All of this can also threaten impingement of nerve roots by decreasing the size of the neural foramen.
- A scoliosis (rotoscoliosis) is a lateral curve; a side-bending and rotation in the spine. In the lumbar spine L3 shifts away from the side to which the spine is bent. As a sustained orientation (posture) of the spine, changes (as in hyperlordosis) to the forces running through the lumbar spine (from above and below) will occur. However, with a scoliosis, the compression happens on the concave side, and the increased tensile forces happen on the convex side. With the addition of rotation (that happens in a scoliosis) the compressive forces are increased within both the disc and the facet joints on the concave side.
- During hypolordosis, L3 may remain somewhat in the line of gravity. However, the flatness of the lumbar spine (from its flexed position, relative to the pelvis) is what changes the lines of force running through the IVD in this case. Now compression occurs in the anterior portion of the disc and tensile in the posterior portion of the disc. The facet joints are gapped excessively, and can no longer momentarily help with weight-bearing during extension of the lumbar spine, nor appropriately guide motions within each spinal motion segment. Stretch (tensile) forces occur to the posterior ligaments and facet joint capsules. The stretch of ligaments around the facet joints will cause these ligaments and joint capsules to undergo excessive tensile force on flexion, rotation, and side-bending: either as individual motions, or especially during a combined motion of all three. Thus, making it easier to strain and tear these ligaments, especially if the person is carrying or lifting something.

Due to these changes in the curve of the lumbar spine, we can clearly see how the possibility of injury to the structures of the vertebrae will increase as the deviation of L3 (and all vertebrae) increases from a neutral position. These postural deviations may well play a part in the predisposing factors (or even causes) of most lumbar spine impairments and dysfunctions.

Rule outs

This can be difficult to do for the lumbar spine as many actions above or below it may induce movement in the lumbar spine. (Hartley 2000b)

The hip Ruled out by flexion and medial rotation, both with over-pressure (O-P). These two actions will stress enough of the ligaments, muscles and the joint capsule to rule out hip pathologies.

Thoracic spine Have the patient seated with their lumbar spine supported (either using a chair with good lumbar support, or with the patient seated on a stool with their low back against the therapist's massage table, if the respective heights work for this). Have the patient reach up and place their hands around their cervical spine to minimize movement here. They should bring the elbows close together in front in order to help lock the cervical joints.

Test flexion of the thoracic spine by asking the patient to slump forward while keeping their low back against the support, thereby, moving only the thoracic spine. If there is no pain, then apply a slight O-P at T1 directly downward (not forward, or the lumbar spine will be flexed). Most of the pressure will be absorbed by the flexed thoracic spine rather than travel down into the lumbar area.

Side-bending, rotation, and extension are then each done. However, no O-P is used as the force will inevitable be transferred through the lumbar vertebrae. When the patient performs side-bending and rotation, the therapist should place a hand under the patient's 12th rib and instruct them to bend over their hand or rotate just their ribcage to the left. Giving the patient's body this sensory input helps them to possibly separate thoracic side flexion/rotation from lumbar side flexion/rotation.

Landmarking for the patient like this also helps the therapist to both stabilize the lumbar spine and helps the therapist to feel when movement is about to go down into the lumbar spine and they can then instruct the patient to stop and go no further. You must give clear instructions about keeping the lumbar spine still against its support and about moving very slowly.

Range of motion testing (ROM)

Exceptions for range of motion (ROM) testing and use of motion palpation testing

Though many manual therapists would perform motion palpation after a postural assessment and before, or even instead of, ROM testing, we will place the instruction on motion palpation immediately after AF-ROM. This is done for the purposes of learning. In many ways, AF-ROM is already included in motion palpation. It is also shown before PR-ROM, because of PR-ROM's difficulty and also its lack of specificity in the lumbar spine.

We would skip PR-ROM generally (except for joint mobilization/play assessment) for the reasons given. However, as PR-ROM has been used extensively in orthopedic practice (rather than the performing of motion palpation), we will fully describe it. So, too, for AR-ROM. Note though that when you do use this testing it is recommended that the patient never be in an acute condition. A chronic condition may lend itself to such testing once you have some idea about the sources of pain and other impairments. Then you can make an informed clinical judgment about the use of these tests. It is this author's opinion that they are suitable for assessing a relatively pain-free individual who has shown restricted range of motion and/or deconditioning. In that situation they give valuable information about how to advise the patient about remedial exercises to help strengthen or increase mobility in the low back. Therefore, PR-ROM and/or AR-ROM are of use after the initial assessment has been done, and in the course of treatment and reassessment.

Joint mobilization techniques can be specific to each motion segment in the spine and the author strongly recommends you learn these for all areas of the spine; but, again, only after motion palpation has been performed. Besides giving some information about the joints of the spine, they can also be valuable treatment techniques. If a joint mobilization movement is done gently (in grade I or II), absolutely pain-free, and by repeating each movement several times, spinal joints can be mobilized. This is often referred to as an oscillatory technique. Further, by activating the proprioceptive receptors, oscillation has been shown to be an effective pain-reduction manipulation, as well as a muscle relaxation (or inhibitory) technique.

Lastly, as testing of the lumbar spine takes on its own unique protocol, we are also going to add into AF-ROM testing some movements that are often placed under the section of special tests. Also, remember that many suggestions that are presented in AF-ROM may only be valid for an orthopedic style of testing, rather than a "mixed" form of testing, as described above.

Active free range of motion (AF-ROM) (Box 12.4)

If possible, have the patient's skin bare over the lumbar spine when doing range of motion testing.

Be sure to pay close attention to the various joints of the lumbar spine and how they move in relation to each other. Have the patient do the following actions and see if they reach normal degrees of movement. Note any pain or limitation of their range.

> ***INSIGHTS***
>
> **Box 12.4 Use of over-pressure during AF-ROM**
>
> Suggested only when motion palpation has already been done, or is not to be done.
>
> If the patient experiences no pain or recurrence of their symptoms while performing each of the following movements, you may, at the end of range of each movement, apply a gentle over-pressure (O-P) to clarify the end-feel. In this way you can get some information that is usually obtained only during PR-ROM testing. Remember: never do O-P with extension of the spine.
>
> When applying O-P, be careful with the amount of pressure you use: do not forget that the weight of the upper body exerts a lot of strain on joints and their supportive tissues. Before using O-P, try having the patient hold their position at their end-range for 10 or 15 seconds to see if that provokes the return of their symptoms. Or, you may have the patient repeat the movement to end-range several times in an attempt to reproduce their chief complaint. If there is no recurrence of their symptoms, then you may wish to apply O-P. You may choose to first complete all of the motion palpation testing before having the patient perform these motions one more time and adding the O-P.
>
> The usual end-feel is firm and springy. Though rarely encountered, you may find a bony end-feel if there has been ossification of the supportive ligaments between vertebrae. This finding requires you to avoid any testing that would reach or exceed this end-range. Suggest the patient sees their physician for an X-ray. Any throbbing pain felt with O-P should also be investigated by a physician as it may signify a pathological condition.

AF-ROM flexion (Figures 12.13, 12.14)

Many patients with restricted movement in their lumbar spine will compensate with excessive hip or thoracic flexion that hides or compensates their loss of range in the spine. A clear sign of lack of range is noting that the lordotic curve does not flatten out or reverse slightly, as it normally should. Take care to record if there are any flat areas (hypomobility) over one or more segments of the lumbar spine. Note as well if there is any excessive movement (hypermobility) between two or more vertebrae, which will often appear as a sharp angle.

The best way to tell if the movement is within normal range is to measure from T12 to S1 before and at the end-range of forward flexion to see if there is an increase of 2 to 3 inches. You may initially place the index finger of one hand on their T12 and another on S1 before they bend forward and take note if this distance increases roughly that amount. ***NOTE:*** Hypermobility would result in a measurement increase of 4 inches or more. However, there are some people who can even place their hands on the ground and still retain their lumbar curve. They actually have excessive range in hip flexion. Gymnasts and dancers are two examples of patients who may well show this ability.

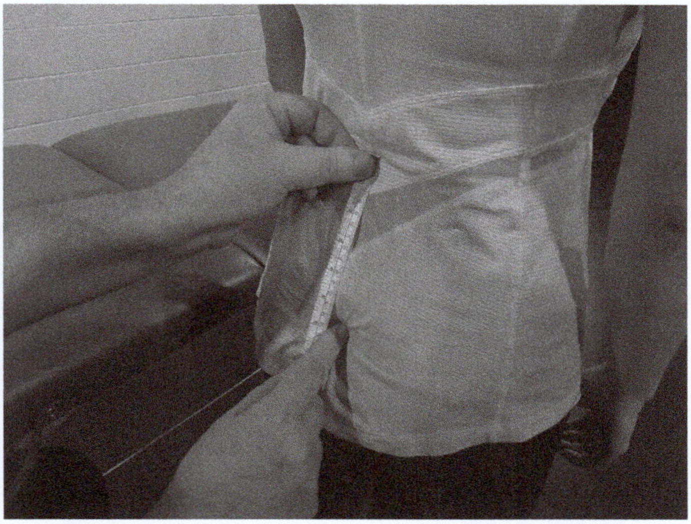

FIGURE 12.13 1. Measuring flexion (40–60°)

Landmarking in preparation for lumbar flexion.

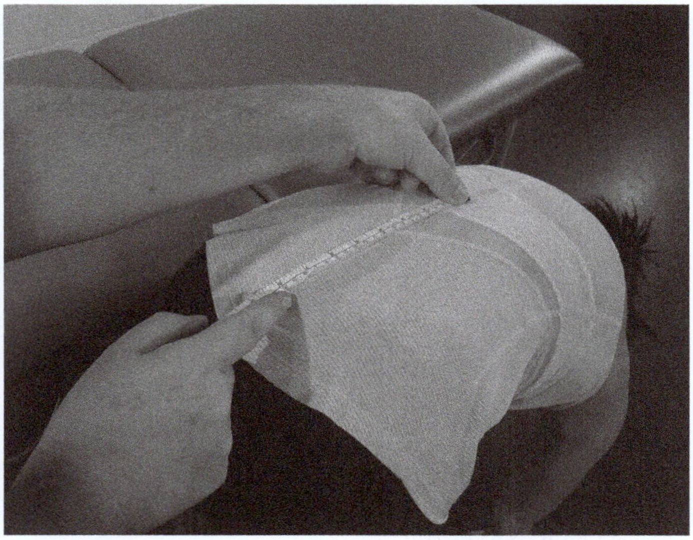

FIGURE 12.14 2. Measuring flexion

Measuring at end-range.

With the patient flexed forward, note if there is any appearance of increased bulk on one side of the lumbar spine. This implies a neutral group dysfunction (a fixed scoliosis). The increase in bulk occurs when the spine is rotated to one side. The transverse processes (TVPs) rotate toward one side and are, therefore, closer to the surface on that side. This results in the TVPs lifting up the tissue that overlies them creating a look of increased bulk. Often, this is mistaken as hypertonic muscle (which also can appear more prominent or larger in bulk).

An increase in bulk on one side due to rotation becomes even more apparent or exaggerated upon flexion of the spine. Therefore, following Fryette, the spine is most likely rotated toward that side and side-bent the other way. This will need to be confirmed with motion testing. You may notice that the patient can side-bend further to one side than the other. Often, the side to which they can side-bend more is on the concave side of a scoliotic curve, on the side to which that portion of the spine is already bent. The person will usually have restriction side-bending to the opposite side (the convex side). This is a good example of how organized testing creates a picture of what is going on with the structures being assessed.

NOTE: The following are suspicions of what may be happening, and are not meant to be taken as conclusive. They are rules of thumb that can point to what structures or tissues need further testing or closer attention. Remember, when you ask a patient where they feel the pain, also ask them if they can point to the pain with one finger. This often denotes a superficial and/or acute injury. On the other hand, if they need to point out an enlarged area, this often implies a deeper or more chronic injury.

Further, always be sure to inquire about the quality or type of pain the patient is experiencing as this can give valuable clues in differentiating the tissue(s) involved in the injury. See below for some details on the type of pain and what type of tissue may be the cause. See also the introduction to the text for a general discussion of this matter.

The patient may deviate to one side as they bend forward (or extend for that matter) and this may be due to a number of things:

- unilaterally tight muscles or contracture of supportive connective tissue
- facet joint dysfunction
- a hip joint lesion or pelvic muscle (e.g., piriformis) tightness
- avoidance of pain (avoiding using or placing compression or tension on injured tissues).

Pain on flexion

Pain felt in the lumbar area during flexion will often be due to injured tissue being stretched when reaching the patient's end of range of motion.

- The muscles of the erector spinae group: the posterior longitudinal ligament, ligamentum flavum, inter- and supraspinous ligaments, along with the iliolumbar ligaments, facet joint capsules and thoracolumbar fascia (Bogduk 2012; Vleeming et al. 2012).
- Non-contractile pain is best discerned by location of the pain: often ligamentous pain in the spine results in tenderness felt through the spinous process when palpated and challenged with firm pressure (i.e., felt in the bone it is directly or indirectly attached to). Strains of interspinous ligaments have been shown to be a source of low-back pain and can refer into the lower limbs (Bogduk 2012).
- Facet joint pain is often local and, when it spreads or radiates, it often does so to local tissue. In general, the referral region of a facet joint is oval in shape, spanning a joint or so above and below. The joint capsule itself remains the focus of sharp and bright pain when palpated (which, to avoid irritating the tissue, should only be done once all other testing has been completed).
- Thoracolumbar fascia creates a burning pain from the top of the iliac crest to the spine and up toward the muscle body of the latissimus dorsi (Vleeming et al. 2012).

If the patient reports radiating or neurological pain traveling down the posterior portion of the thigh or leg that returns (or increases) during forward flexion, we may be looking at nerve root compression. This can be happening at the nerve root or further along the course of the peripheral nerve. These will be differentially tested for in the section on special tests.

With respect to disc herniation as a possible cause of radicular pain: forward flexion increases pressure on the anterior portion of the IVDs which in turn causes the nucleus pulposus at the center of the disc to move posteriorly. If there is a weakness or loss of integrity of the annular fibers of the disc, the nucleus can cause the fibers to bulge and press on a nerve root.

If more than one or two nerve roots are affected (i.e., pain runs through two or more dermatomal areas), then we may be looking at a cauda equina syndrome where pressure is being put on several nerve roots that make up the cauda equina as it passes by the lesioned area. This could be done by a severe prolapsed disc pushing through the posterior longitudinal ligament and into the spinal canal. This can affect one or both legs.

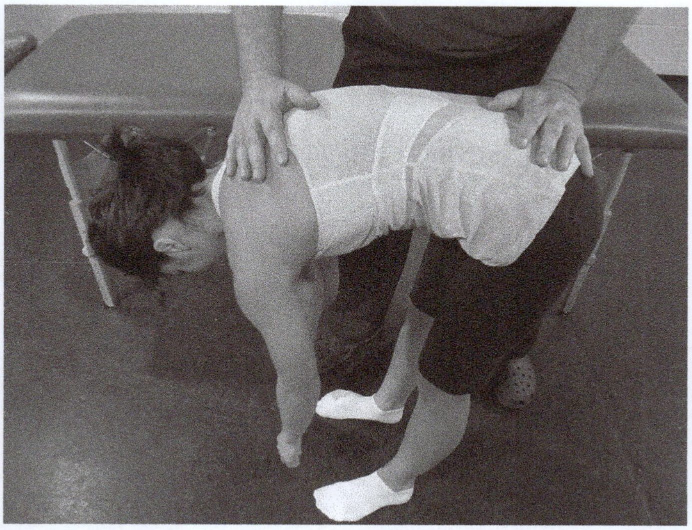

FIGURE 12.15 Applying O-P to flexed lumbar spine

Support the patient over the sacral area so that they do not tip forward as you apply O-P.

NOTE: This is a red flag, and the patient should be instructed to seek medical attention as soon as possible. However, the bulging disc does not always press on a nerve root and, by pushing on the posterior longitudinal ligament or any ligament in the area, can cause pain to be felt locally.

If pain decreases with forward flexion, we may be looking at facet joint dysfunction or spasming muscle. With forward flexion, the facet joints are opened, and this often gives relief from pain arising from compressed joints and their structures. Also, a slight stretch to hypertonic muscles often brings relief. However, if the joint capsule is swollen, then there could be an increase in pain as the already stretched (swollen) capsule is stretched even more. Palpating the joint capsule (when all other testing is done!) could be informative.

AF-ROM flexion with overpressure (Figure 12.15)

If and when you elect to apply over-pressure (O-P) to the lumbar spine during AF-ROM, do so only if the patient has no pain on forward flexion. Make sure the patient is not moved by the pressure and feels secure. Applying slight O-P at this time can, to some degree, simulate passive testing.

When the patient returns to an upright position, you should note the return of the patient's lordosis beginning around the last 45° of extension. If pain occurs when returning from the fully flexed position, we could be looking at possible strain to:

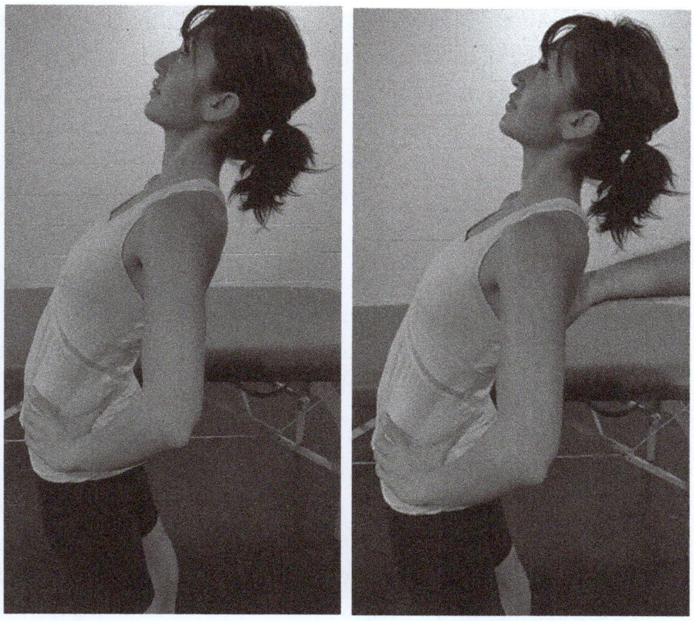

FIGURE 12.16A, B Extension (20–35°)

The patient rests the hands on the hips before starting. To provide more stability, support their mid-back with your hand.

- the erector spinae group of muscles, if the pain is felt close to the spine, and/or
- the more lateral muscles, such as the quadratus lumborum (pain superior to iliac crest) or the gluteus maximus (pain inferior to the iliac crest).

AF-ROM extension (Figure 12.16A, B)

If the patient appears frail or is having difficulty with their balance you may still want to provide the added support of your hand on their mid-back when they are against the table. Reinforce your instruction by reminding the patient to only go as far as they feel they are able.

Pain on extension

Possible explanations: pain is caused by compression of posterior tissue or structures, the stretch of inflamed or irritated tissues, or the spasming of shortened muscles. Structures and tissues that are provoked with extension are:

- Facet joints: extension is the close packed position for these joints. Injuries to intrinsic joint tissues and the joint surface will, therefore, be provoked as the patient goes into extension.
- Stretch of an irritated anterior longitudinal ligament: this is felt as an indistinct (deep, dull) pain that will, of course, not be found with palpation.

- Pain from stretched abdominal muscles, which will be working eccentrically to control extension of the spine. The patient can generally point to the area and will usually report a sudden pain. Remember the trigger point (TrP) referral patterns for abdominal muscles (especially the obliques) as some referrals are felt down into the groin area (Travell & Simons 1992).
- Spasming of the quadratus lumborum and/or the multifidi muscles, along with the long extensor muscles of the back. The patient should be able to help you with recognizing this when you ask about the quality of the pain.

Relief of pain, especially of referred pain, can occur in extension, often when the patient's pain is the result of a compressed nerve root. When the patient extends there is pressure on the nucleus pulposus to move anteriorly and thereby decrease any pressure placed on the nerve root. Many patients will tell you that they purposely go into extension in order to get relief from their low back nerve root pain. Physiotherapists often give patients repeated extension as a remedial exercise to help relieve their mild to moderate nerve root compression pain ("McKenzie exercises"). Though the referred pain may lessen, the patient may still experience local pain due to the splinting musculature.

If a patient with chronic low back pain reports that after sitting they tend to arch their back when they first stand up then you should investigate whether the patient has a short psoas (see modified Thomas test later in this chapter). The patient may even tell you that without doing this hyperextension they feel that they will not be able to stand up straight. The shortened iliopsoas muscles will tighten even more as they sit and, when they stand, they have to stretch the muscle to become fully erect. However, this patient will almost always present with an anterior pelvic tilt because in fact the innominates do not want to rotate posteriorly back to neutral due to these tight hip flexors. Further, the shortened iliopsoas itself pulls anteriorly on the lumbar spine.

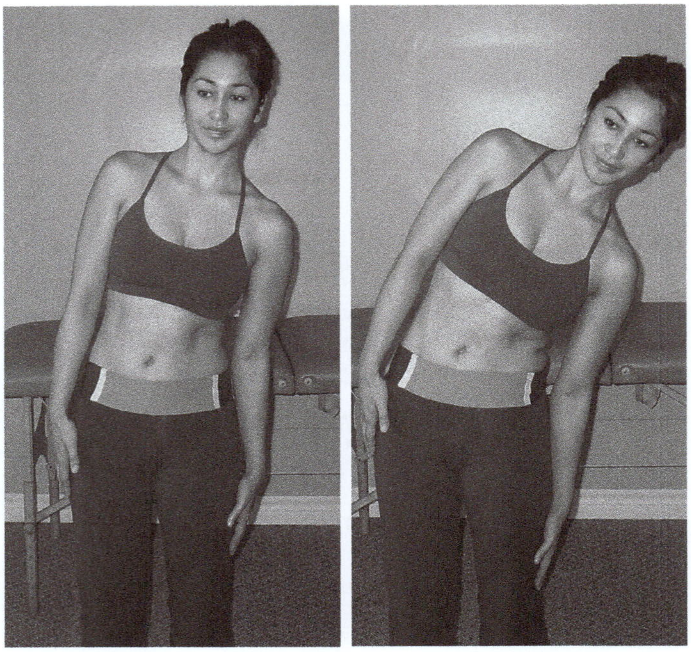

FIGURE 12.17A, B Side-bending (15–20°)

The patient runs the hand down the lateral side of the leg toward the knee.

AF-ROM side-bending (Figure 12.17A, B)

Ask the patient to run their hand down the lateral side of their leg. If you notice them compensating by adding forward flexion or extension to the movement, ask them to do the action again without this movement, if possible. You can compare bilaterally by noting how close their hand comes to their knee on each side. But, more importantly, observe from behind the quality of the lumbar spine as it curves laterally with the motion. It should be a smooth, even curve. Note if there are two or more vertebrae where little or no movement is occurring (i.e., are straight or hypomobile) while above and/or below show a sudden or sharp bend or angulation (i.e., have excessive movement between the hypomobile vertebrae and the one above and/or below). Compare the quality of the curve bilaterally. Note also if the patient shifts their hip laterally when they side-bend.

When a scoliosis is present in the low back, the patient will generally be free to side-bend to the side that the spine is already side-bent toward (i.e., to the concave side), and the curve may look normal. However, when they try to side-bend to the opposite side, you will usually see that portion of the spine has much less curvature, even appearing straight. This is the convex side of the curve.

A scoliosis is named for the convex side and for the vertebrae at the apex of the curve. For example, L2 scoliosis on the right means the convexity is on the right (the concavity on the left), and the L2 vertebra is the furthest vertebra from the mid-line. Also, it is normal to record the extent of the curve, so, following our example above, it may be reported that the scoliosis is: L2 scoliosis R, T12–L4. In other words, L2 is the apex of a convexity on the right, and the convexity runs from T12 down to L4.

Pain on side-bending

Pain felt laterally on the side stretched can come from stretched external or internal obliques, transverse abdominis, or their supportive connective tissue. If the pain is felt between ribs it may well be intercostal muscles. A strained QL being stretched will provoke posterior low back pain, as can a stretched erector spinae (with the pain felt closer to the spine). Pain that feels as though it goes up into the posterior ribs is often the iliocostalis of the erector spinae group, while pain that radiates up toward the shoulder can be from the latissimus dorsi.

If there is an increase in referred pain into dermatomally specific areas of the contralateral lower limb (the one the patient is bending away from), then the patient may have an IVD herniation or prolapse.

Pain on the side the patient is bent toward can come from the compression of external and internal obliques or transverse abdominis, or their supportive connective tissue. If the pain is felt between ribs, it may be intercostal muscles. Compression of the quadratus lumborum and erector spinae can also produce pain (via spasming, as they shorten with use). As well, pain can come from ipsilateral facet joint surfaces or the joint capsule if inflammation is present. If the dermatomal pain is into the ipsilateral side, then it may be due to osteophytes around the facet joint compressing the nerve as it leaves the neural foramen. Or the size of the neural foramen may be affected for other reasons, as in loss of disc height.

Neurological symptoms may decrease on the side the patient is bent toward if side-bending causes the nucleus pulposus to be pushed back toward the center of a herniated disc. This appears as a decrease of symptoms that begins distally and, with repetition of side-bending, progresses back up the posterior aspect of the leg until the pain becomes centralized in and around the lumbar spine. If the patient now does several extensions of the spine this centralized pain itself may decrease and even disappear. If these actions have been successful in decreasing the radiation of pain, and even the centralization of the pain, then you have both tested for and given a remedial exercise for disc herniation.

AF-ROM side-bending with over-pressure (Figure 12.18)

If you elect to apply O-P to the lumbar spine during AF-ROM, do so only if the patient has no pain on side-bending. Make sure the patient is not moved by the pressure and feels secure. Applying a small O-P at this time can, to some degree, simulate passive testing.

Pain experienced while applying O-P on the compressed side usually means a joint lesion (either facet or intervertebral) or that there is a muscle spasm occurring in a shortened muscle. Pain on the lengthened side often comes from stretching of a muscle, ligament, or joint capsule.

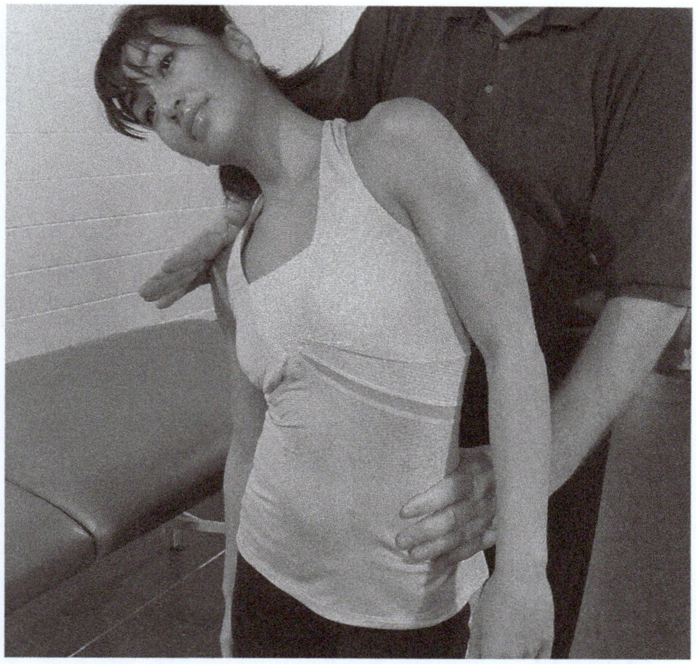

FIGURE 12.18 Applying O-P to lumbar spine side-bending

Stabilize the patient by placing your hand on the opposite hip while applying gentle O-P by pressing down on the patient's shoulder on the side being tested.

Hip drop test (Figures 12.19, 12.20)

An alternative test for side-bending of the lumbar spine is the hip drop test. This test is considered more specific to the lumbar spine itself, as the side-bending test (above) will be influenced by curvatures or rib dysfunctions happening in the thoracic spine. The therapist may be especially misled if they were not paying close attention to the curving of the lumbar spine but only noting how far down the leg the patient could reach (Hertling & Kessler 2006; Magee 2014; Mitchell 2001).

You can try to get more dropping of the hip by asking the patient to lift their heel off the floor and letting their knee flex a little more.

The test is positive for restriction in side-bending (away from the dropped hip) when either:

- the hip will not drop, or
- it does so, but there is no gentle curve observable in the lumbar spine. Rather, movement comes from above, in the thoracic spine. This is often observed as the patient drops the contralateral shoulder because the side-bending is occurring in the thoracic spine.

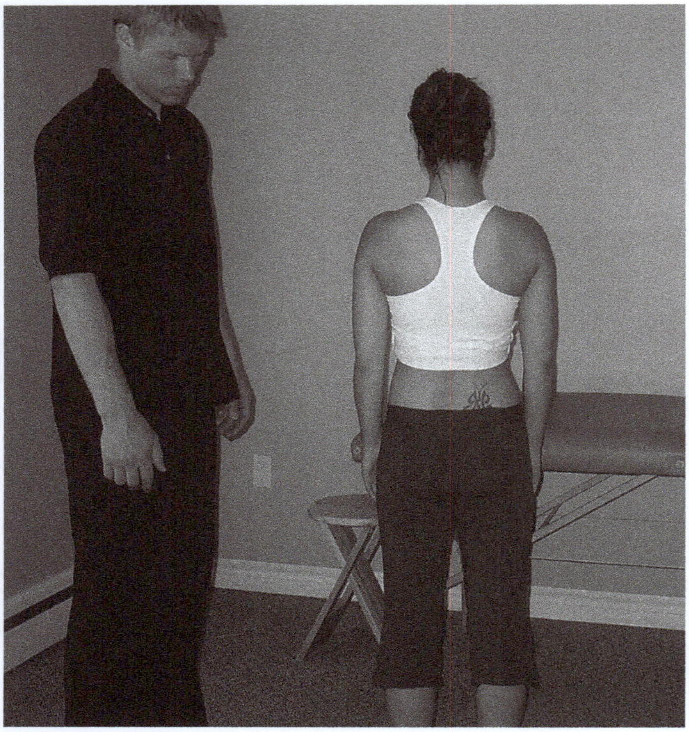

FIGURE 12.19 1. Hip drop test

Standing in a natural pose.

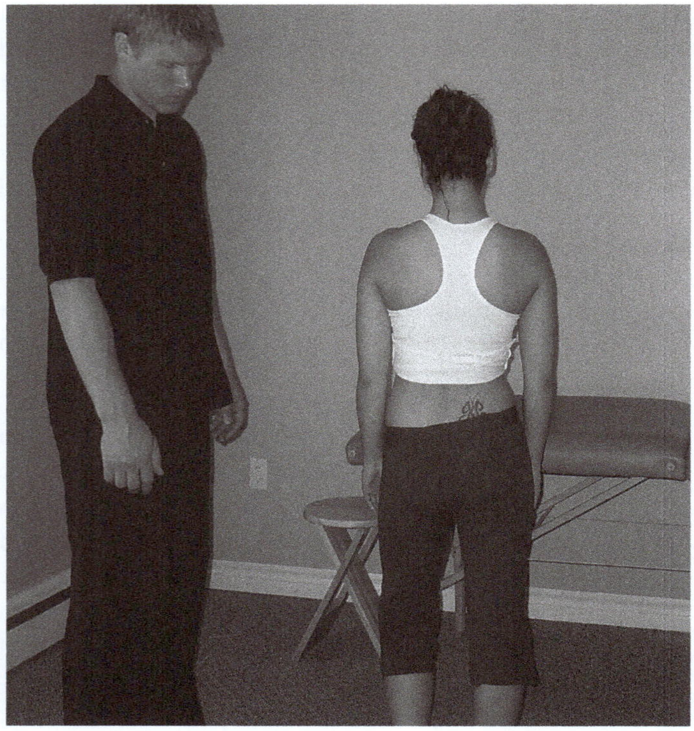

FIGURE 12.20 2. Hip drop test

The patient bends one knee and then lets the hip drop.

The negative sign (normal motion) is the dropping of the iliac crest by 20–25° when compared to the opposite iliac crest.

Lumbar spine rotation (Figures 12.21, 12.22)

This test shows the relationship between hip motions (as in walking) and the required lumbar spine motion needed for walking.

Have the patient cross their arms across their chest to ensure that they do not use their arms with their hands on the table to push their rotation farther than their trunk musculature could achieve on its own. The end range of motion is noted when the patient's contralateral knee moves forward. The therapist may want to place their thigh against this knee to note when end range is reached.

The therapist may have their hands on the patient's shoulder caps before the rotation so that they are in a position to apply over-pressure without having to reach afterwards. However, during rotation ensure you are neither resisting nor assisting the patient's movements.

Due to the orientation of the facet joints in the lumbar spine, they are the primary restriction to rotation. After 1° or so of rotation a lumbar vertebra's facet joint surface comes into contact with its partner. The cartilaginous surfaces within these may compress (and give off water) to gain another degree or so, at most. (Upon returning to neutral and the removal of compression, the joint cartilage will reabsorb the fluid from the joint space.) A little more movement may yet still occur as the force of rotation running through the closed and compressed facet joint will now transfer into rotation through the IVD, possibly gaining another degree or more. (Since rotation beyond normal range can be harmful to the cartilaginous layers of the lumbar disc if done in flexion or extension, a natural structural restriction of rotation in the lumbar spine makes sense; see Bogduk 2012.)

It is difficult to note just lumbar spine rotation and not be misled by the rotation that occurs throughout the whole spine. After doing the test as above and noting symptoms, etc., you may want to do the test from behind the patient and palpate the spinous processes of the lumbar vertebrae to note any movement from one vertebra to the next over several repetitions of movement side to side. Do this only if it does not cause pain or excessive discomfort to the patient.

As with side-bending, if some of the vertebrae are fixed in rotation (and side-bending), then the patient can usually rotate

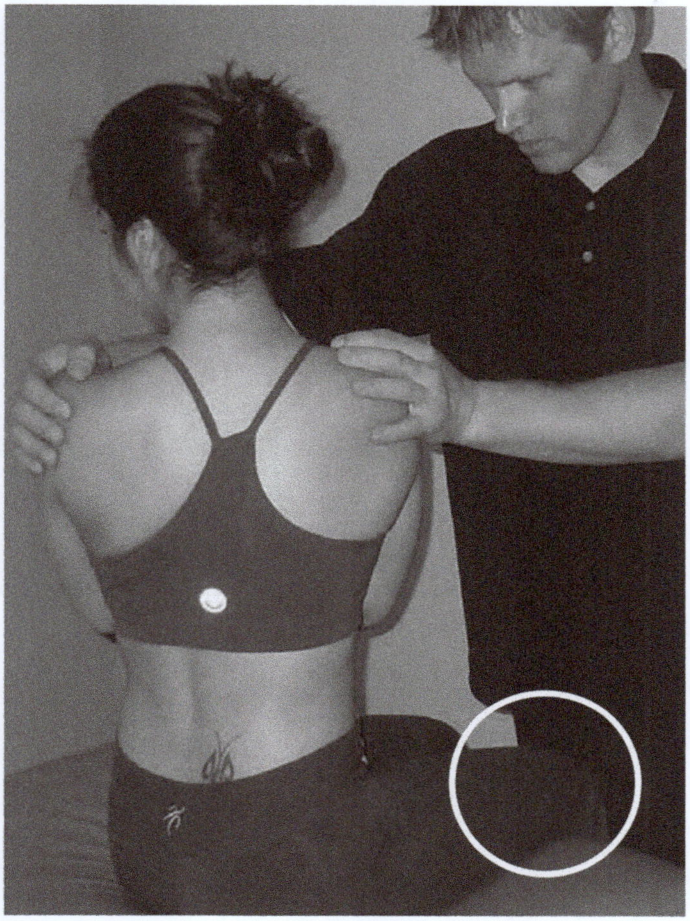

FIGURE 12.21 Lumbar rotation (3–18°)

This is best tested with the patient seated to reduce movement of the pelvis and lower limbs so as to focus on movement in the spine. The therapist places their thigh against the contralateral knee to note end of range.

quite well in that direction, while they will show restriction in the other direction.

Ipsilateral pain can also come from compression of injured, inflamed or irritated facet joint surfaces or joint capsules. The pain may also come from compression of the iliolumbar/sacral ligaments or thoracolumbar fascia. Shortened muscles that are irritated or injured may spasm.

Contralateral pain can come from a stretch of structures or tissues such as those just mentioned. Relief may come to an injured facet joint surface(s) when the patient rotates away and opens the joint. However, the joint capsule may then cause pain when it is stretched, if there is inflammation in the joint and it is edematous.

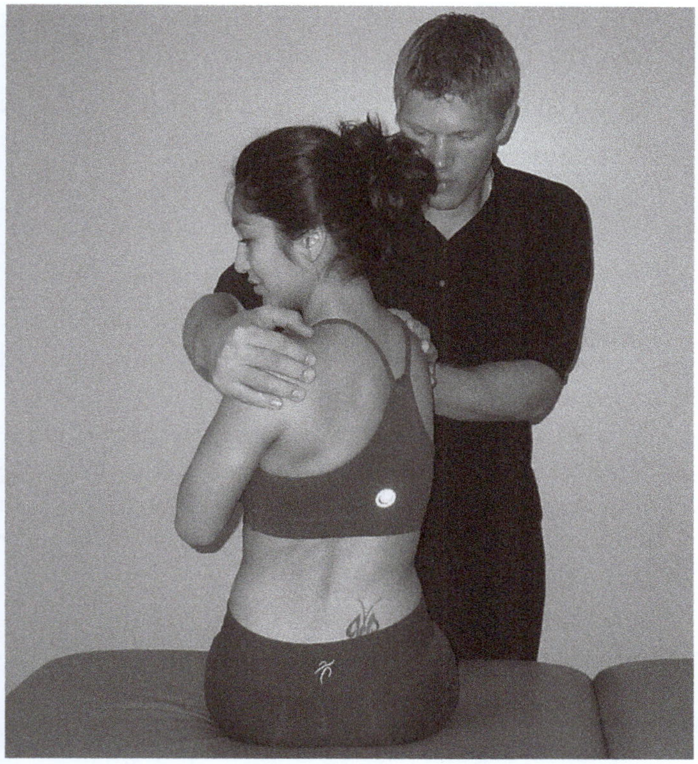

FIGURE 12.22 Over-pressure to lumbar rotation.

While blocking the contralateral knee, apply O-P to rotation.

Blocking the knee from moving forward stabilizes the pelvis. This ensures O-P is applied through the joints of the spine and is not moving into the pelvis and lower limbs. Remember to apply O-P only if the patient reports no pain up to and including the end of their AF-ROM. O-P in rotation often clarifies vague sensations that the patient might report with just active free movement alone.

Motion testing for facet joint dysfunctions in the lumbar spine

This testing is done by observation and motion palpation (Chila 2010; DeStefano 2011; Mitchell 2001, 2005):

- We are looking for symmetry/asymmetry in vertebral alignment, both static and in motion.
- We are looking for restriction of motion, or even hypermobility.
- We are looking for tenderness or any reproduction of the patient's complaints or impairments.
- We do this by noting whether the TVPs appear to be more prominent on one side of the spine than the other. If a group of vertebrae is rotated to one side, the TVPs moving poste-

riorly lift the tissue above them, giving the appearance of more bulk to the tissue on that side of the spine.

- We may note a group of TVPs on one side, and should see some side-bending (scoliosis) toward the opposite side of the prominent TVPs, or we may note a single prominent TVP.
- We can look at the spine standing, seated, or prone.

What are we looking for and feeling as we palpate?

You are not trying to palpate through the tissue for the TVPs, as at this level of the spine the thickness of the erector spinae and connective tissue would make them difficult to discern, especially at the L4 and L5 levels. Rather, having landmarked where they are, you should note the tissue thickness or bulk over the TVPs and compare side to side. Therefore, strictly speaking, you are palpating the hardness that belongs to the bony TVPs *under* the tissue that overlays them.

- When several vertebrae rotate to one side, as in a group dysfunction or scoliosis, there is bulkiness on the side of the spine to which they are rotated.
- When an individual vertebra is rotated, as in a segmental dysfunction, then you will usually not see any extra bulk on that side, but will palpate as a specific firm or hard spot.
- However, neither type of dysfunction may be very clear when the patient is in neutral, especially for the therapist who is just beginning this type of assessment.
- Palpating and observing in flexion and extension usually exaggerates the feel and appearance of this bulkiness.

We will first describe seated palpation for facet impairments in neutral, in flexion, and then in extension. After that we will describe an alternate palpation in extension done while the patient is prone. (*The prone position is initially the easiest to palpate.*)

Palpating in neutral (Figures 12.23, 12.24)

Have the patient seated and sit or kneel behind them. The patient should be sitting up straight but relaxed. Landmark the disc space between L4 and L5. To do this, find the highest points of the iliac crest on each hip and draw a line with your fingers from each toward the spine and you will arrive at the approximate level of the IVD between L4 and L5. Palpate down to the L5 spinous process (SP) – this can be tricky to locate at first as it is deep and surrounded by tissue. Alternatively, the TVP for L5 will be located just below the level of the inferior pole of L4's spinous process (the lowest point of the SP). Now move out about an inch or so from that and you are over the TVPs of L5. The very tips could be even further out, depending on the size of the patient.

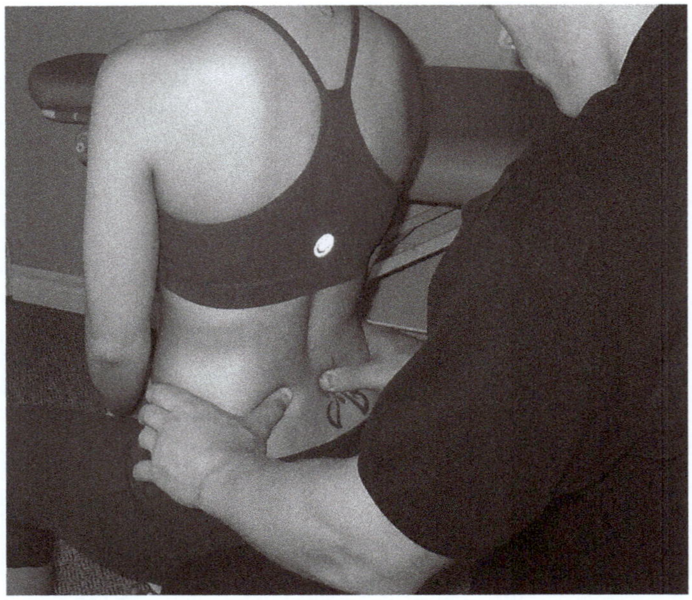

FIGURE 12.23 1. Landmarking for space between L4 and L5

Alternatively, to find L4's TVP, palpate the lowest point of L3 and then move out about an inch, and just slightly down. You can continue in this manner to find each vertebra's TVPs and therefore L1's TVP is at the level of T12's lowest point on its SP.

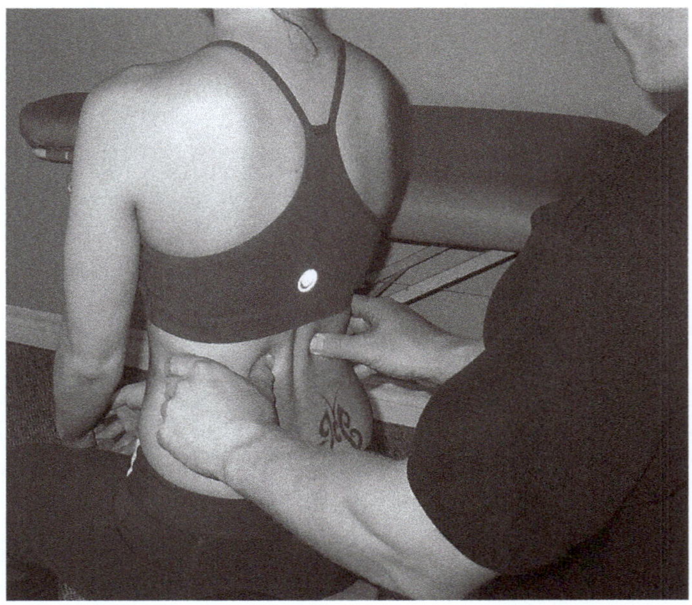

FIGURE 12.24 2. Palpating lumbar TVPs

Palpate up from L5 to L1 (or higher).

Continue to palpate each set of lumbar TVPs, working your way up to L1. We are palpating to see if any vertebrae are rotated, as mentioned previously. When a vertebra rotates toward one side, the TVP on that side has to move posteriorly, lifting the tissue and making that side have more bulk than the other side (or at least feel like a specific "hard spot"). At the same time, the other TVP of that same vertebra must go deep/move anteriorly as the vertebra rotates away from that side (making the tissue on that side of the spine appear less bulky, or producing a "hollow spot"). For example: if L2's right TVP feels deep while its left feels shallow, then that segment is rotated to the left. Therefore, if we find asymmetry of depth of TVP from side to side we have found a possible impairment in the lumbar spine.

The basic rules for motion testing in the spine are summarized in Box 12.5.

Box 12.5 Basic rules and findings of motion testing in the spine

1. **Observing and palpating an increased bulk on one side, over several vertebral levels, indicates a scoliosis:**

A fixed scoliosis remains in both flexion and extension, and can look exaggerated, especially on flexion.

- The side of increased bulk is the side to which the vertebrae are rotated.
- Therefore, as a group dysfunction, the vertebrae are side-bent to the opposite side.

2. **When palpating a flexed spine, you find extension lesions:**
   - A TVP's inability to flex open will create a palpable bump.
   - The extension lesion is on the side you feel the bump/TVP; when felt during flexion (and maybe in neutral). However, you will not feel it during extension.
3. **When palpating an extended spine, you find flexion lesions:**
   - A TVPs inability to extend and close will create a palpable bump; but only on extension (or, maybe in neutral). It disappears on flexion.
   - However, the flexion lesion is on the opposite side to the palpable bump/TVP.

Palpating in flexion and extension (Figures 12.25–12.29)

Have the patient flex forward, dropping their arms toward the floor between their legs, as they sit with feet apart. Before palpating, first just observe the patient's lumbar and lower thoracic spines. You are looking for any asymmetries, color changes or unusual tissue appearance. Look especially to see if there is more bulk on one side of the spine compared to the other. Do you notice any curve or deviation to the spinal segments? Now, palpate for these, along with additionally noting the temperature of the tissues and any excess moisture (or dryness).

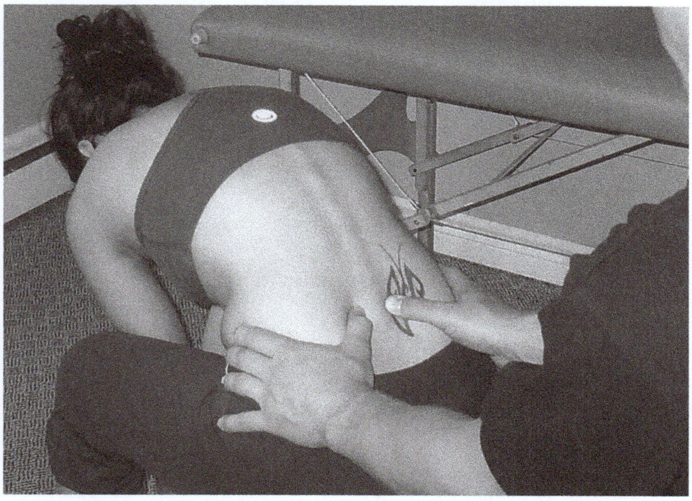

FIGURE 12.25 **1. Palpating lumbar TVPs in flexion**

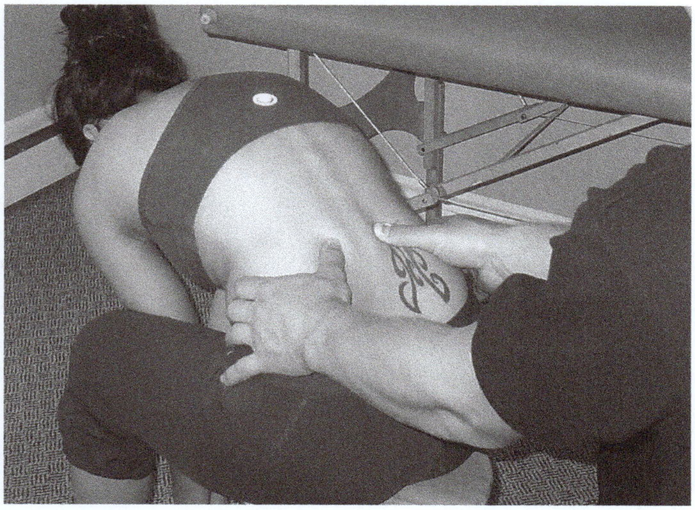

FIGURE 12.26 **2. Palpating up to L1**

Palpate each lumbar vertebra's TVPs, looking for asymmetries felt as a bump or firmness.

INSIGHTS

Box 12.6 Seated flexion

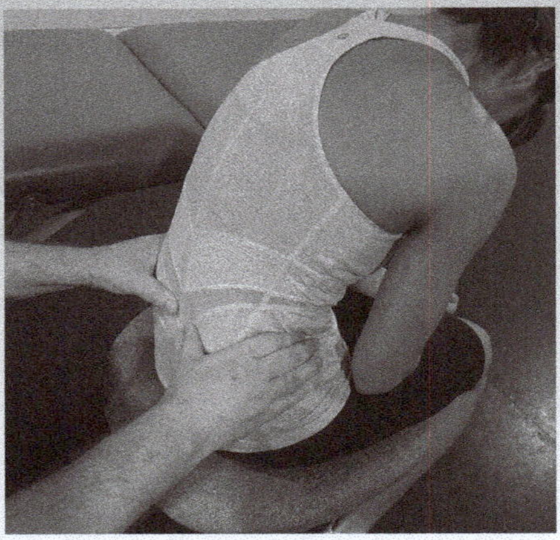

FIGURE 12.27

Testing in seated forward flexion.

Many experienced therapists only need the patient to slump forward. Just ask the patient to pull their stomach in and slump slightly forward. This movement can flex the lumbar spine sufficiently for testing purposes. You need to be aware, however, that some hyperlordotic lumbar spines may have greatly reduced forward flexion and so can still sustain a lordosis and prevent accurate testing. If this is noted, then full forward flexion of the spine may be needed to force the lumbar spine to move into flexion as much as possible for testing. Therefore, to help those who are just learning these skills, and to avoid offering too many alternatives and confusing the issue, we have chosen to do the full seated flexion motion.

Repeat the palpation with all of the lumbar spine's TVPs as was done in neutral – from L5 to L1 (or higher). Note when and where you feel (and see) the TVPs that are rotated. Note if it is a group of vertebrae or an individual vertebra, and at what level. Compare your findings with what you found when palpating in neutral.

To gain experience and develop your palpation skills you can palpate L5's TVPs while the patient is in neutral (upright) and remain palpating as they bend forward. Have them come back upright to neutral while you continue to palpate at that level. Then go up to the TVPs of L4 and repeat as above, palpating while the patient flexes and returns to neutral. Do for all five lumbar vertebrae. This is similar to palpating the PSISs of the

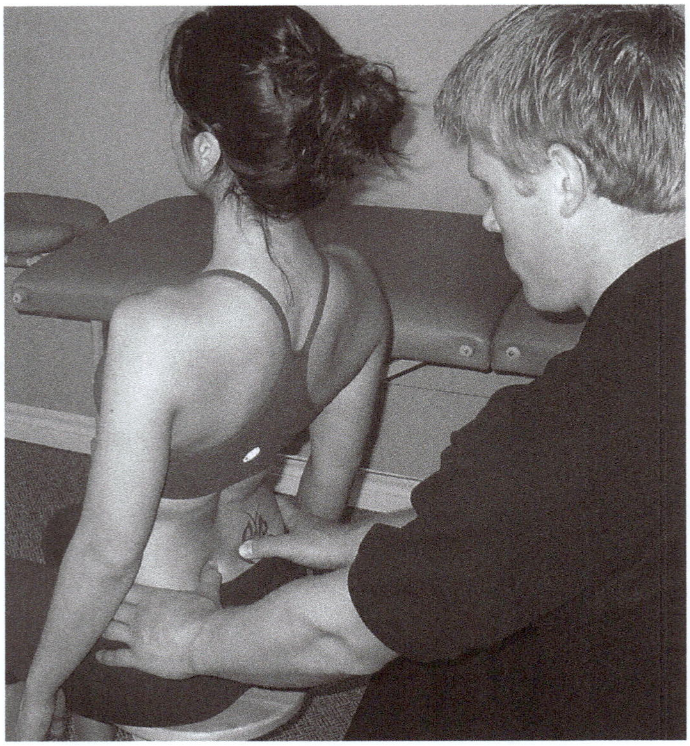

FIGURES 12.28 1. Palpating L5 in extension

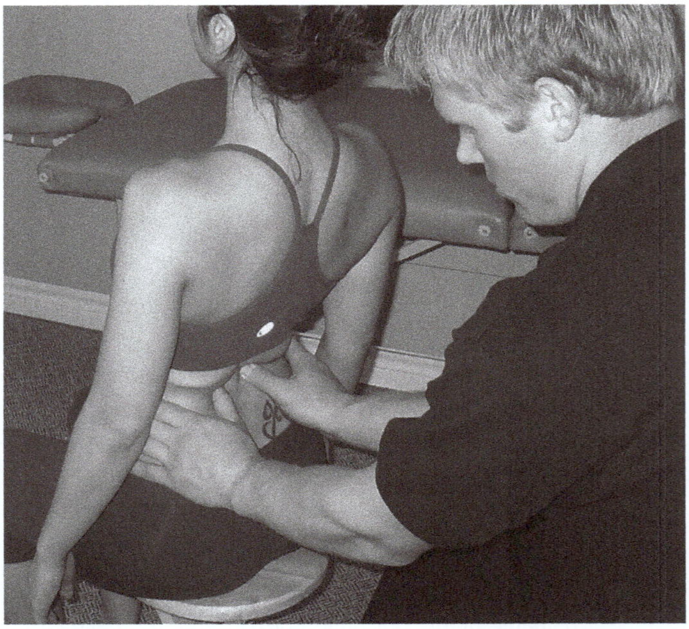

FIGURE 12.29 2. Palpating up to L1

Landmark L5 and have the patient extend. Palpate each pair of TVPs up to L1 for symmetry.

hip while the patient does a seated or standing flexion test (see Chapters 9 and 11).

The reason for palpating all levels while the patient remains flexed (or extended) is to speed up the testing and to avoid aggravating the patient's condition by repetitive motion.

Seated flexion is discussed further in Box 12.6.

Return to palpating the TVPs of L5. Now, have the patient extend their low back by telling them to stick out their stomach (sometimes called the "beer belly" position). Repeat your palpation as above. Compare your results with both the neutral and the flexed positions.

Findings, explanations, and examples

Group dysfunctions are noticed by the increased bulk appearing on one side over several segments. Such a dysfunction will remain palpable, and even visible, whether the patient is in neutral, flexed, or extended. As the side that feels thicker or looks bulkier is the side to which the vertebrae are rotated, following the rules of movement in the spine, they are side-bent toward the other side. For example, if we find that the spine has more bulk on the right than on the left at several levels of vertebrae, then it is side-bent toward the left (NSʟRʀ = Neutral, Side-bent left and Rotated right). ***NOTE:*** Often this extra bulk on one side is interpreted by therapists as being hypertonic muscle rather than a possible rotation in the spine.

Curvatures of the spine may often arise as compensation for adaptation to muscle imbalances and/or of the unleveling of vertebrae (or the sacral base). However, many curvatures disappear with a change in the positioning of the patient, such as from standing to sitting or from the spine in neutral to flexion or extension. If the curve changes, then it is not a dysfunction in itself, but the consequences or compensation of a problem above and below. However, a rotoscoliosis (a fixed curvature) needs to meet the following criteria:

- A group of three or more segments are rotated and side-bent.
- Restriction of motion is greater (more obvious) in side-bending and rotation, rather than in flexion or extension.
- Side-bending is in one direction, and rotation in the other.
- The segments never become completely symmetrical in flexion or extension (though asymmetries usually become exaggerated with flexion). However, the curvature and rotation may diminish with side-bending or with rotation (DeStefano 2011).

Segmental dysfunctions will be felt as an asymmetry at one level only. Though it may have been noted in neutral, it shows itself even more distinctly either in flexion or extension, but not in both. The criteria for a segmental dysfunction are:

- Occurs in a single motion segment.
- Often due to trauma or strain/sprain from improper movement patterns.
- Lesions happen within flexion or extension when there is side-bending and rotation (which will occur to the same side).
- Restriction and pain can be found in multiple ranges of motion.

In testing motion palpation in flexion and extension:

- A flexion restriction will become symmetrical (disappear) in forward flexion, since the impaired joint is already flexed. However, it becomes but more asymmetrical in extension. This is because it is being held open/flexed, and cannot close.
- An extension restriction will become more symmetrical in extension, since it is already extended, but more asymmetrical in flexion. This is because it is being held closed/extended and cannot open.

For example: L4 appears in neutral to be asymmetrical, that is, the TVP is palpably more pronounced on the right (and deeper on the left) when compared both bilaterally and to the TVPs above and below (which appear symmetrical). We then know that L4 is rotated right (on L5). If it is true that this is the only vertebra that is asymmetrical, then (following the rules of Fryette) it is likely to be side-bent to that side as well. What we do not know is whether the right facet is being held closed, or if the left facet is being held open.

Let us look at two cases for the previous example. Remember that the TVP was found to be prominent on the right side.

First case

When the patient now flexes and the vertebra palpates as symmetrical (or at least more symmetrical), we know that both facets between L4 and L5 will open. On the other hand, if it becomes even more asymmetrical when the patient goes into extension (the right TVP is even more prominent), then we know that L4–5's left facet joint will not close/extend. Therefore, L4 is being held flexed on the left, and side-bent and rotated right. L4 is FRSr.

- When it is being held flexed (an FRS lesion), the dysfunctional facet is on the opposite side to the prominent TVP.

Second case

If L4's TVPs become more symmetrical on extension, then we know both facet joints will close (or extend). If they become more asymmetrical on flexion (the right TVP is even more prominent), then we know that the right facet joint between L4 and L5 is being held (is "stuck") in extension, held closed. L4 is side-bent and rotated to the right because the right facet joint is being held closed in extension. L4 is ERSr.

- When it is held extended (ERS), the dysfunctional joint is on the same side to which the superior vertebra is side-bent and rotated (in this case, on the right).

NOTE: In both scenarios given above, the vertebra is being held side-bent and rotated to the right. In either situation, while the spine is in neutral, the vertebra (i.e., its TVPs) will palpate the same with the right TVP prominent. Therefore, the only way to distinguish between the impairment being on the left (held flexed) or on the right (held extended) is by motion palpation.

As a final note on motion palpation, the author would like to point out the following: once we understand how all segments are functioning, and the orientation or position this results in, we can then begin to imagine how other tissues involved in the spine (and beyond) are acting or responding to that situation. Reviewing the section on lumbar curves and L3 earlier in this chapter can further help you visualize what may well be going wrong and causing the patient's chief complaint.

The fixation, in either case, is most likely due to either spasming (possibly even fibrosed) fourth layer muscles, or to some impairment intrinsic to the joint (such as fibrosis of a joint capsule, swelling in the capsule, or a trapped meniscal/fat pad).

Palpatory findings and what they imply are in Table 12.1.

Alternative motion palpation testing for extension in prone

The testing of extension while seated requires excellent palpation skills and, just like learning to palpate any particular tissue, palpating TVPs takes practice. Though even the newly trained therapist can easily see group dysfunctions, individual or segmental dysfunctions can take time to discern clearly. Initially, you may wish to start testing these structures using the seated position for testing in flexion (as described previously) and the prone positions described below to test in extension. Even experienced therapists may continue using the seated and the prone positions to test the lumbar spine because of their accuracy, and because they can also simultaneously check the SI joints using this pair of positions. *It is often wise to check the sacrum when testing the lumbar spine, and vice versa, because of their obvious interconnections and interaction. Dysfunction of one usually results in dysfunction of the other (see Chapter 11).*

TABLE 12.1
Palpatory findings

In neutral	In flexion	In extension	Dysfunction
TVP prominent right	More asymmetrical	Symmetrical[1]	Impaired facet joint is extended on the right [ERSR][2]
TVP prominent right	Symmetrical	More asymmetrical	Impaired facet joint is flexed on the left [FRSR]
TVP prominent left	More asymmetrical	Symmetrical	Impaired facet joint is extended on the left [ERSL]
TVP prominent left	Symmetrical	More asymmetrical	Impaired facet joint is flexed on the right [FRSL]

Notes

1. All of the boxes with "symmetrical" could just as well be written as "more symmetrical," especially as that matches many clinical findings. However, we have chosen to leave that adjective out here so as to simplify the chart: "more symmetrical" and "more asymmetrical" simply look too similar and this could cause confusion.
2. ERSr means that the vertebra is being held Extended and is Rotated and Side-bent to the right. Therefore, the vertebra is being held extended on the right side. FRSr means that the vertebra is being held Flexed while Rotated and Side-bent to the right. Therefore, the vertebra is rotated and side-bent to the right but the vertebra is being held flexed on the left side.

TVP, transverse process.

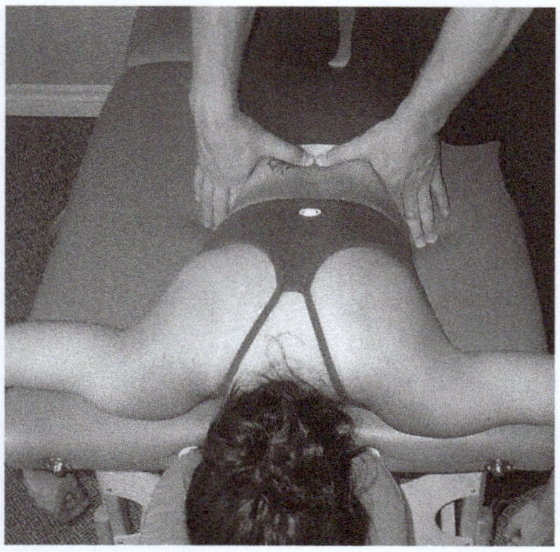

FIGURE 12.30 1. Landmarking

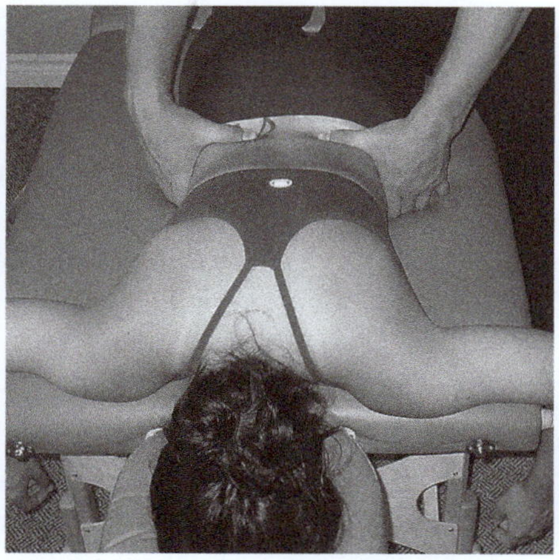

FIGURE 12.31 2. Palpating L5 TVPs.

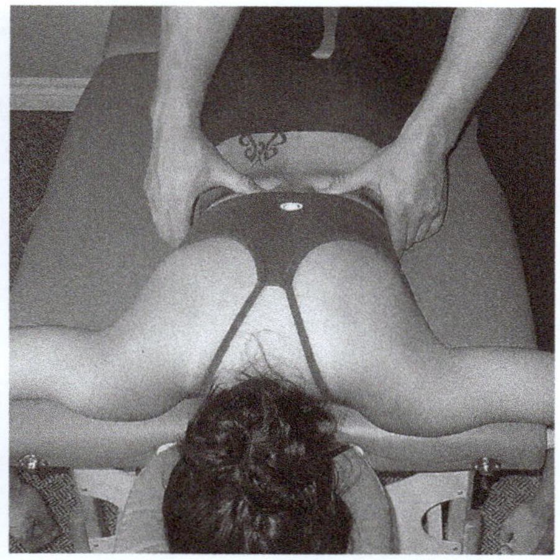

FIGURE 12.32 3. Palpating LI TVPs.

First landmark and find L4–5 disc space. Drop to L5 TVPs and begin noting symmetry. Continue up to L1.

Prone palpation of TVP symmetries (Figures 12.30–12.34)

With the patient prone, place your thumbs or fingers over the TVPs of L5. This is done by coming in from the iliac crests to the L4–5 disc space, going up to the inferior tip of L4's SP and out roughly an inch. Note any asymmetry and then proceed to move up the lumbar spine checking at each vertebra's TVPs for symmetry. This provides us with an assessment of the lumbar spine in neutral and, hence, our baseline to compare with the results from the previous seated flexion test and the prone extension test that follows.

In order to palpate in extension, have the patient come up onto their elbows (they can place their chin in their hands) and tell them to relax their abdominal muscles and let their belly relax on the table. This is sometimes referred to as "the Sphinx position" (Figures 12.33, 12.34) Many consider this a hyperextended position that can clearly show how the lumbar spine is responding to extension. Therefore, this positioning yields the clearest results when palpating in extension.

Again, starting at L5 palpate each pair of TVPs all the way up to L1 (or T12). Compare your findings from this position with what was found in neutral and in forward flexion. Interpret your results according to Table 12.1. Also, ask the patient if they experience any pain or other symptoms when in this position, as it would give information similar to PR-ROM testing.

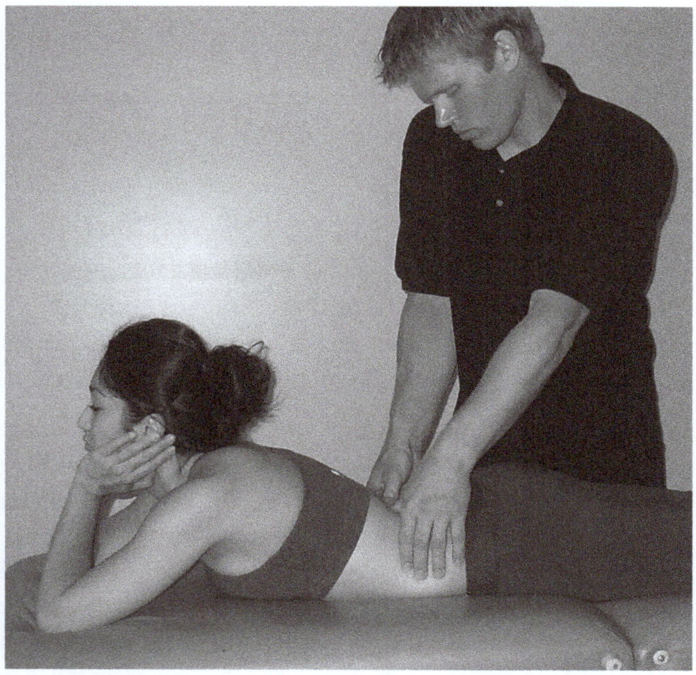

FIGURE 12.33 1. Palpation in Sphinx position

A common clinical finding: the disappearing scoliosis

If a scoliosis that was apparent on standing disappears on sitting or when the patient lies prone, then the scoliosis may well be due to the spine sitting on an unlevel base. The curve present in the spine while

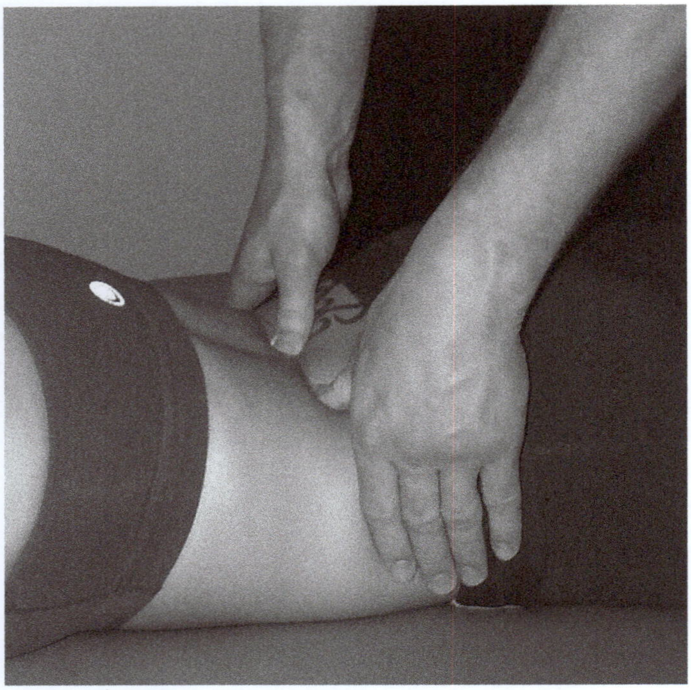

FIGURE 12.34 2. Detail of palpation

Check symmetry of paired TVPs from L5 to L1. Compare to findings found in neutral and in flexion.

the patient is standing in neutral is there because it is compensating. Such an unlevel sacral base could be due to a SI joint impairment, innominate impairment, structural or functional leg length discrepancy (or there only when seated), a hemi-pelvis, etc. There is some asymmetry somewhere down the chain provoking this curve.

A closely related cause for a disappearing spinal curve is a muscle imbalance on one side of the spine that is pulling and/or rotating a portion of the spine. As muscle imbalance is one of the most common causes of postural imbalances (unleveling of structures), close inspection of the structures above and below the curve will probably reveal some asymmetry that corresponds to the curvature present in the spine. Changes in position will affect muscle length or tone that can have the curve disappear or become exaggerated in certain positions, or when the body changes from weight-bearing to resting positions. Therefore, we should think of muscle imbalance and postural or structural imbalances as interdependent causes of asymmetries and deformations found in the body.

Such curvatures are not always generated by an unlevel base, but can also be brought about in the spine by structures above or at the same level. The principal culprit here would be the shoulder girdle. For example, on the dominant hand side of the body (let us say the right), that shoulder is often more protracted than the non-dominant side. This rotates the shoulder girdle to the left.

This shoulder girdle rotation is matched by rotation in the upper thoracic spine, which will also be to the left. Following Fryette's rules of spinal motion, rotation (in our example, to the left) through a group of vertebrae will be accompanied by side-bending in the opposite direction (in this case, to the right). This permits the right shoulder to drop. Or, to avoid getting caught up in arguments about which is cause and which is effect, we might just want to say the thoracic curve accompanies the dropping of the right shoulder. This is another common clinical finding. This thoracic curve may require the lumbar spine (and hips) to further compensate the rotations and curvatures from above.

Another example of change generated from above would be when there is impaired motion at the occipitoatlantal (OA) joint. An impairment here can tip the head to one side and the cervical spine may compensate by side-bending in the other direction (to keep the head/eyes level). This cervical curve can, in turn, be matched by a gentle thoracic spine curve to bring the upper thorax and head to balance over the center of gravity. And so on down the spine.

Lumbar curves and segmental dysfunctions

The following may be confusing to those new to assessing segmental and group dysfunction. If that is the case, you may want to leave it until a later time when you have had some experience using the testing.

Group curves can be due to sitting atop a vertebra that has a segmental dysfunction. Since a segmental dysfunction is rotated and side-bent to the same side, it creates a sufficient unleveling to require a compensating curve in the vertebrae above.

When a curve disappears in either flexion or extension (but not both) we have been given a clue as to what type of segmental dysfunction may be present.

If the curve only disappears in flexion, a segmental dysfunction is possible at the bottom of the curve seen in neutral. Why? Because, in flexion, all the facets can apparently open, and therefore, the previously unlevel segment will become level. Hence, there is no need for a compensating curve above it. Therefore:

- look for flexion lesion by testing in extension
- look for a single prominent TVP, or
- if the scoliosis returns on extension, then the lowest of the vertebrae TVPs of the scoliosis may well be part of the superior vertebra of a lesioned motion segment that is FRS. Correcting that lesion could also make the scoliosis disappear altogether.

If the curve disappears only in extension segmental dysfunction is possible because this means all facets can close, leveling the impaired segment, and disappearance of the curve above it. Therefore:

- look for extension lesion in flexion
- look for a prominent TVP, or
- if the scoliosis returns on flexion, then the lowest of the vertebrae TVPs of the scoliosis may well be part of the superior vertebra of a lesioned motion segment that is ERS. Correcting that lesion would also make the scoliosis disappear altogether.

Passive relaxed range of motion (PR-ROM)

As mentioned, passive relaxed movements of the lumbar spine are awkward at best, and usually more difficult and uncomfortable for the patient than warranted by the quality of information obtained. O-P findings can be gathered during AF-ROM when the patient is at (pain-free) end-range, as described earlier. For these reasons it is suggested that therapists forego passive movements of the lumbar spine until all other testing has been done.

On the other hand the patient may be too apprehensive or in too much pain to move enough during AF-ROM, yet may be willing to be moved passively. This is especially true if active movement requires use of injured muscles. Therefore, some PR-ROM of the lumbar spine may be useful with respect to general spinal and ligamentous mobility.

Further, besides relying on the patient's subjective reporting concerning pain, you can be feeling for when certain groups of muscles engage in protective spasming. This will provide more specific information than that found in AF-ROM about what further testing may be most informative.

Passive motions of the lumbar spine (Figures 12.35–12.37)

With the patient side-lying, have them bend their knees to roughly 90°, with the hips around 45° of flexion. Palpate the lumbar spine with your fingers spread out over the lumbar spine. Using your thigh, push the hips up to 90° of flexion as you palpate the spine. Low back muscles may twitch, or even spasm, as you do so. If you slow the movement or stop it altogether, do the muscles let go? As you further flex the hips past 90°, the innominates will begin to rotate posteriorly. This is usually taken as the end of "easy" lumbar flexion. The sacrum should counternutate, making the sacrum feel fuller. Continuing further would be applying O-P to the spine.

Return the hips to 90°. Lift the ankles upwards, palpating the side-bending of the lumbars (Figure 12.36).

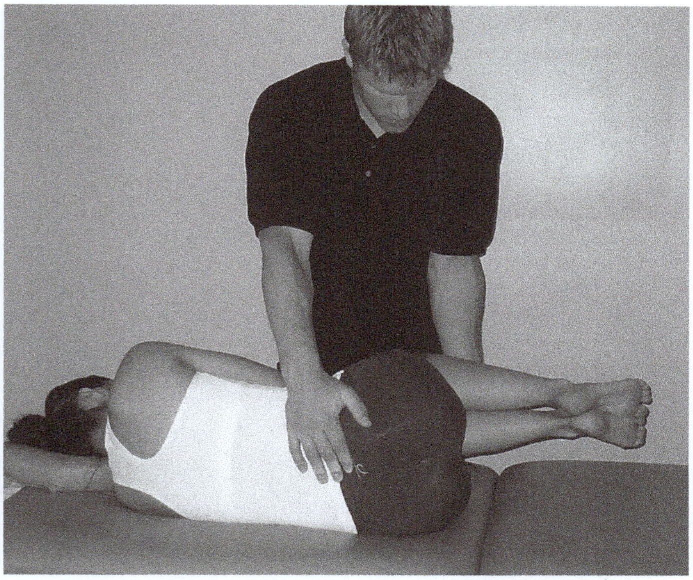

FIGURE 12.35 Passive flexion of lumbar spine

With the patient sidel-lying and the knees and hips at 45° of flexion, palpate over the lumbar spine and innominate (ilium). Using your thigh, push the hips up to 90° or more of flexion feeling for the flattening of the spine. When only the innominates move that is the limit of lumbar flexion.

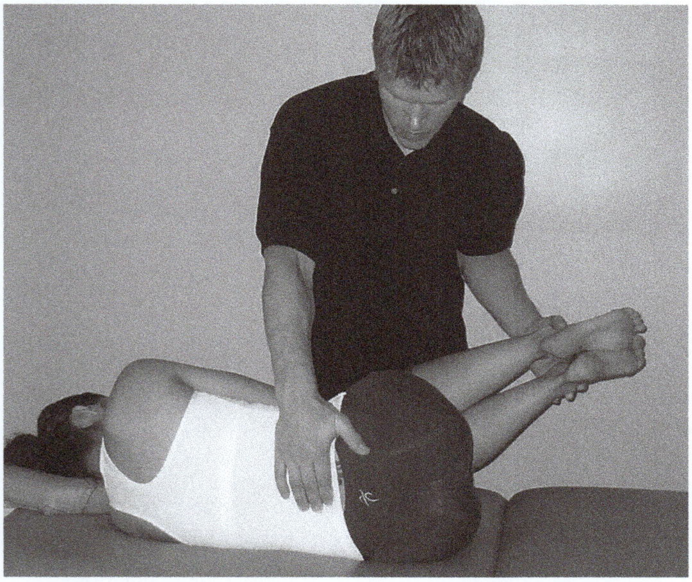

FIGURE 12.36 Side-bending of lumbar spine

Return the hips to 90°. Lift the ankles toward the ceiling to side-bend the lumbar spine.

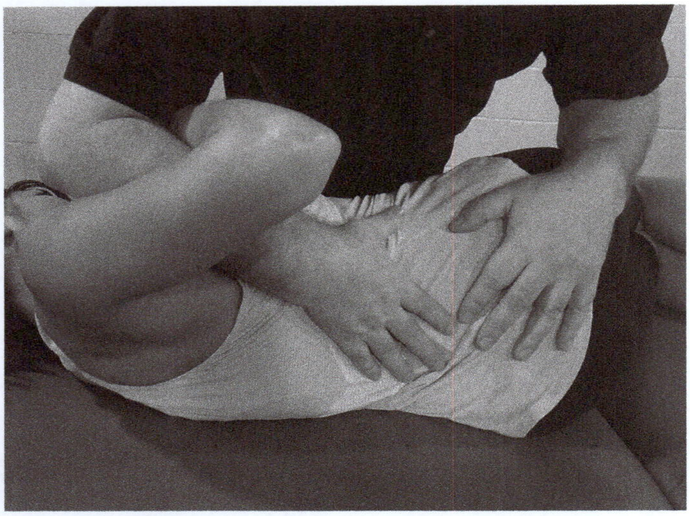

FIGURE 12.37 Rotating lumbar spine

Push the shoulder posteriorly while palpating the lumbar spine. Do this slowly to clearly see how well rotation is happening, and/or whether pain is produced.

Change hands for palpating Figure 12.37. Slip your arm under the patient's arm and position your forearm against their anterior shoulder. You can now rotate the spine from the top down, from the thoracic into the lumbar vertebrae. Remember that there is only slight rotation available in the lumbar spine! Rotation here can stress the facet joint's articular surfaces as they compress against each other as rotation passes through its level.

Passive motions of the lumbar spine done seated (Figures 12.38–12.41)

The patient is seated on a stool with feet on the floor. Have them "sit up straight," re-creating the lumbar lordosis that is normal for them. Have the patient cross their arms so their hands are touching the front of their shoulders, arms against their chest. Reach across and cup the patient's elbow. Instruct the patient to relax and let you support their upper body and allow you to move them, without them helping. Each range of motion can be repeated several times, allowing the patient to relax and permit you to move them without helping. The range of motions follow in sequence, one after the other, without the therapist having to change much in the way of supporting the patient's trunk.

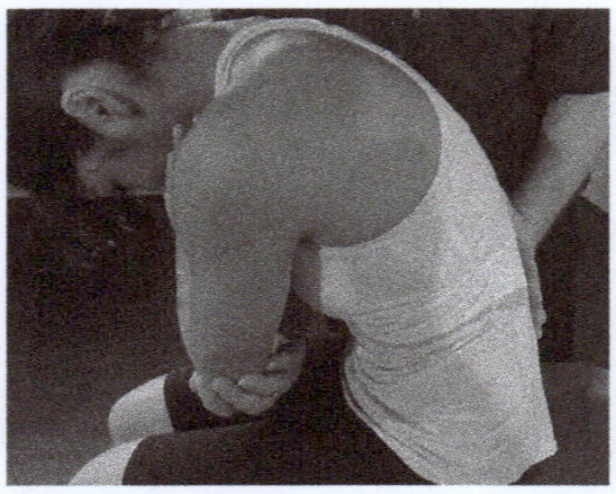

FIGURE 12.38 Passive flexion of lumbar spine

Lower the patient's arms letting them slump forward. Palpate over the lumbar spine. Lift them back to the starting position, continuing to palpate.

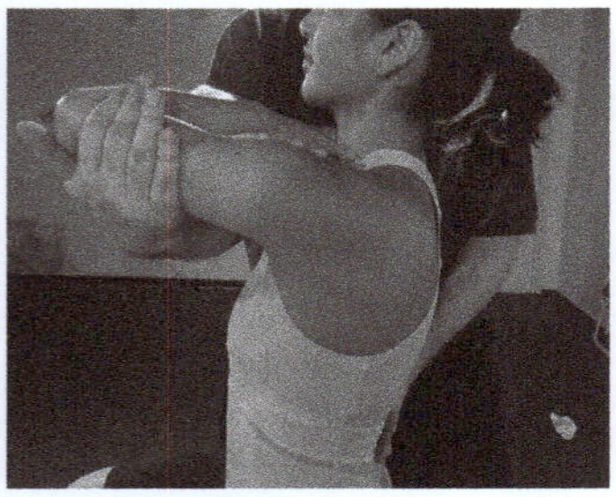

FIGURE 12.39 Passive extension of lumbar spine

Lift the patient's arms to about 50–60°. While still cupping their elbow shift your forearm so that it now supports the elbow closest to you. Lift the arms up in an arc to extend their spine while palpating. Return to the starting position, continuing to palpate.

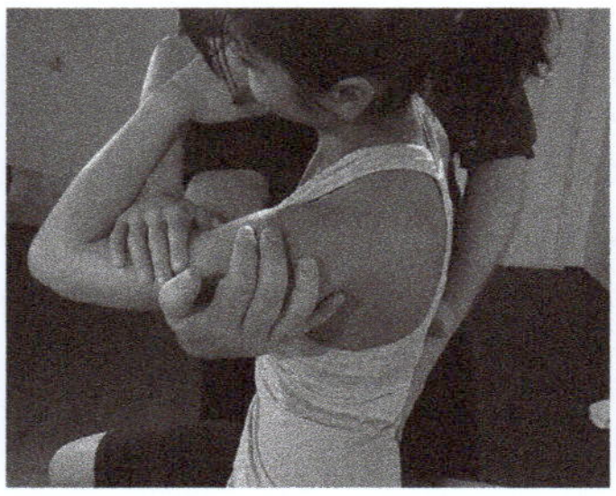

FIGURE 12.40 Passive side-bending of lumbar spine

In the starting position, the therapist slides their hand up the patient's opposite arm until they are holding the middle or upper area of the patient's arm and the therapist's forearm is still under the elbow closest to them. Pull the far shoulder down while you raise and tilt your forearm. Return to the starting position, continuing to palpate the lumbar spine.

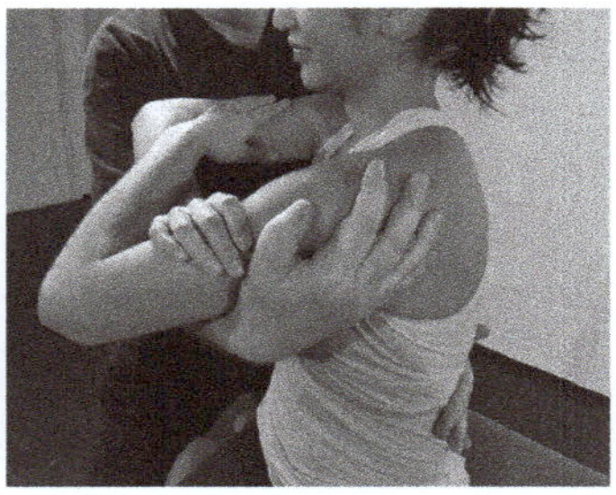

FIGURE 12.41 Passive rotation of lumbar spine

Having returned to neutral, with hands in the same position, pull the opposite shoulder toward you, rotating the patient's trunk.

NOTE: The suggestion here is to test side-bending on one side and immediately test rotation on that side as well. Then, move to the other side and repeat the two tests in the other direction. This will save time and thus avoid having the patient hold the position for too long. It will also feel more fluid and more organized to the patient, rather than shifting back and forth from side to side.

Box 12.7 describes assessment of the lumbopelvic motion in supine (see Figures 12.42, 12.43).

Passive range of motion: joint mobilization of the lumbar spine

Specific joint mobilization techniques for the lumbar spine should be done only after motion testing for facet joint

INSIGHTS

Box 12.7 Assessing lumbopelvic motion in supine

You can perform passive movements that would, for example, move the lumbar spine, pelvis/SI joints and hip in order to see how the lumbar lesion is affecting this whole pelvic area. Like joint mobilization, the following motion palpation can be pain relieving and free up minor restrictions in the hip.

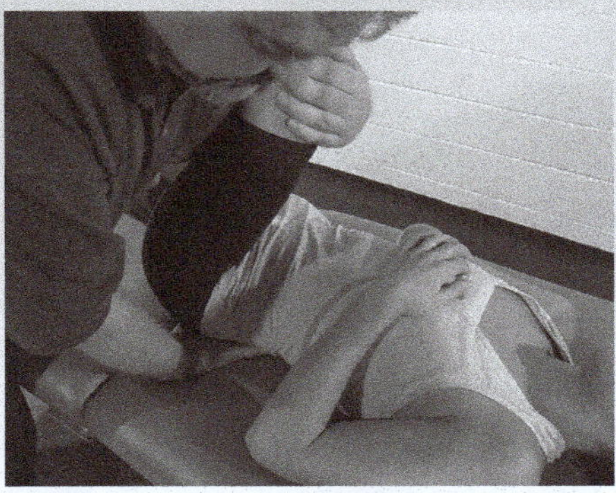

FIGURES 12.42

1. Assessing lumbopelvic motion in supine.

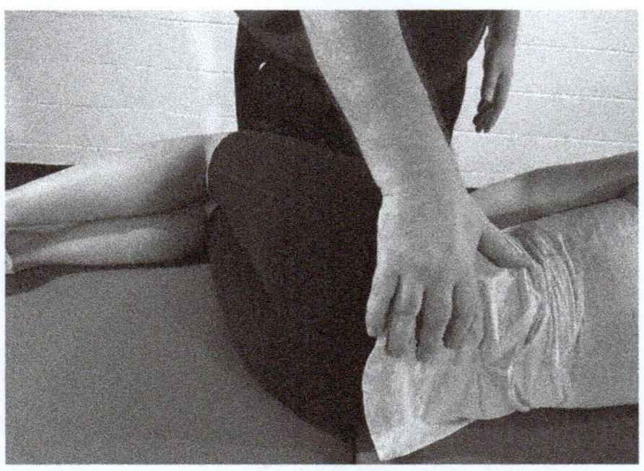

FIGURES 12.43

2. Hand position.

In the supine position, place the fingers of one hand under L5, the PSIS and the SI joint on that side in order to palpate these structures (see Figure 12.43 for hand placement). To slide your hand into place, you can take the leg with the flexed knee and push it away from you, lifting that side's pelvis enough to gently get your hand in place. Bring the hip into 90° of flexion to start (Figure 12.42); push the hip into more flexion, and then less, oscillating the patient's hip through the range of "easy" flexion available while you palpate. Move slowly. Do not forcibly move through any restrictions encountered. The more you do the rotations or oscillations, the more the joint will free up. Note the innominate motion, sacral motion, and the movement in L5. Keep your attention on one of these at a time; do not try to feel all three at once, at least not until you are proficient.

Still palpating, and with the hip at around 90°, now push the legs medially-laterally back and forth (within pain-free range). This will adduct and abduct the hip, rotate the lumbar spine, and alternately gap and compress the SI joint on that side. Do not try to feel all of these at once, but pay attention to each, one at a time.

NOTE: By going slowly and keeping the palpating hand relaxed, you can begin to feel and distinguish more of what is occurring at these joints, and with their supportive tissues.

There are numerous variations of this motion palpation: some therapists will perform a circumduction motion, thereby doing flexion-extension and adduction-abduction in a continuous circumduction. Variations can include having the patient in prone (knee at 90°, hip neutral, and using the lower leg to circumduct) while palpating as above. Even side-lying can be used. With experience, all of these can provide you with a vast amount of information, especially about the lumbopelvic-hip complex.

dysfunction has been completed, because these techniques could produce discomfort or pain when the low back is injured or impaired that would then compromise such testing.

Try to keep your hands relaxed as you apply pressure. The pressure should come from your body-weight rather than from muscular exertion. In other words, lean into your hands once they are positioned, rather than push into the patient's tissue.

Before engaging in any joint mobilizations tell the patient that they must immediately report any pain or other sensations felt either on-site or at a distance. If they have any response immediately remove your pressure. Discuss with your patient what they felt and then decide on how to proceed and/or if you need to refer out. Stress to the patient that they need to relax and not resist your pressure. If the patient cannot do this, then it is suggested you forgo testing with joint mobilization.

If all is moving as it should you should feel a slight springiness as you push. The patient should feel no pain. If there is pain or discomfort, but movement (springiness) nonetheless, then there may be soft tissue injury (ligament, joint capsule, or intrinsic muscles of the spine) or osteoarthritic changes within the joints. If there is restriction or resistance to movement, there will be a hard feeling under the mobilizing hand. Any movement felt is then often palpated or sensed above or below the restricted site. The patient may or may not feel pain or discomfort. This may indicate a locked motion segment, held fixed by spasming muscles and/or facet joint swelling, for example.

Always try to use body-weight rather than pulling or pushing from the shoulders to move the limb. Ask about pain or any other symptoms and take note of both the quality and quantity of motion available in the joint. (For more details and instruction see Part I, Chapter 3. Also, see the following for even more information and optional positioning of patient or limb, and variations or additional tests: Edmond 2006; Hertling & Kessler 2006; Kisner & Colby 2012; Starkey & Brown 2015.)

Posterior-anterior (P-A) glide (ventral glide) (Figure 12.44) This translation of the vertebra anteriorly is used to test flexion and extension of the lumbar spine. Though thumbs can be used, it is better to use the heel of the hand over the spinous processes (SPs). This is easier on your hands and also gives a broader pressure, which is usually tolerated better by the patient. The classic way of performing this is to landmark and apply the pressure via the pisiform area of the hand.

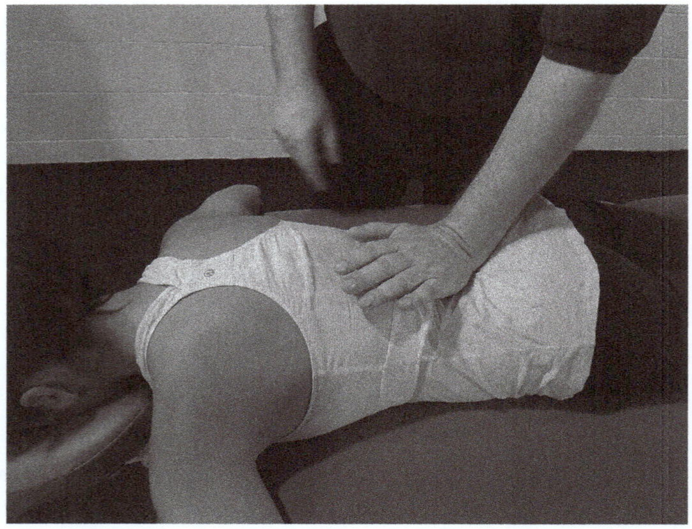

FIGURES 12.44 P-A glide to lumbar spine

Lean onto spinal process gently, and only as pain-free with increasing weight, and then slowly lean back, reducing pressure.

The patient is positioned prone. If hyperlordotic, place a pillow under their abdomen to reduce lordosis. Landmark the SP of the vertebra you wish to challenge. Using your body-weight, lean onto the SP. Do not move quickly, but rather increase the pressure over two or three seconds, and then hold for two or three more seconds. Release the pressure over the same span of time.

Rotation of vertebra (Figures 12.45–12.47) Example: to rotate L1 vertebra to the left.

1. Landmark the right TVP of L1.
2. Landmark the TVP of L2 and on the side opposite to the mobilizing thumb (i.e., on the side to which you are going to rotate L1). Thus, your mobilizing thumb is on the right TVP of L1 and your stabilizing hand's thumb is over the left TVP of L2.
3. Press anteriorly (down) on L1's right TVP while you resist L2's left TVP from moving posteriorly (i.e., you are resisting L2 from "lifting," thus preventing it rotating along with L1). Use your body-weight rather than pushing with the arms. Start with very gentle pressure and if pain-free slowly add a little more weight. *Do not force* a vertebra to move or rotate. Remember, you are looking for only small movements with a hard springy feel.

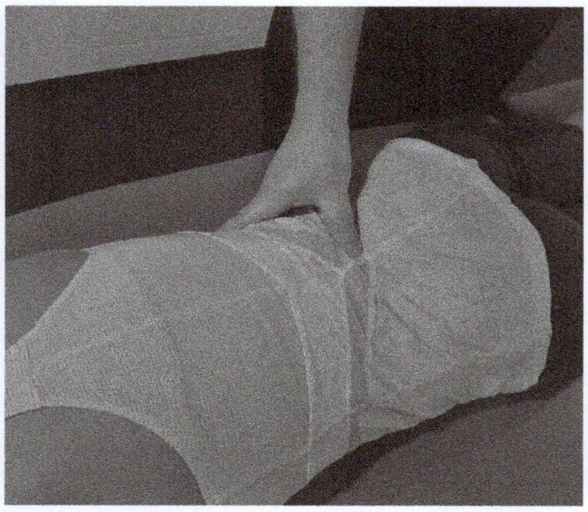

FIGURE 12.45 1. Rotation (TVP) landmarking

Landmark TVP to move.

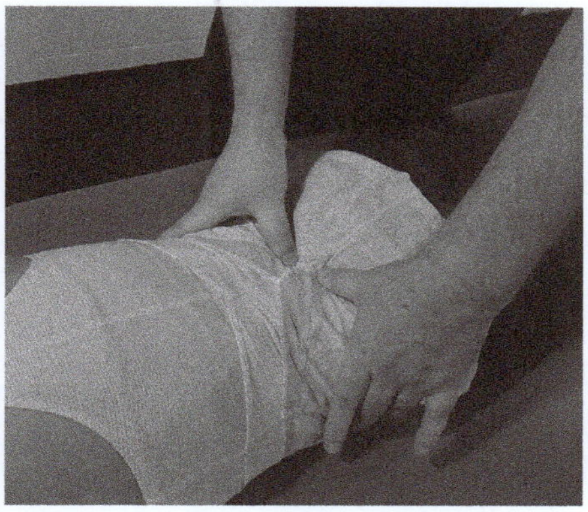

FIGURE 12.46 2. Landmarking for stabilization

Landmark TVP to resist.

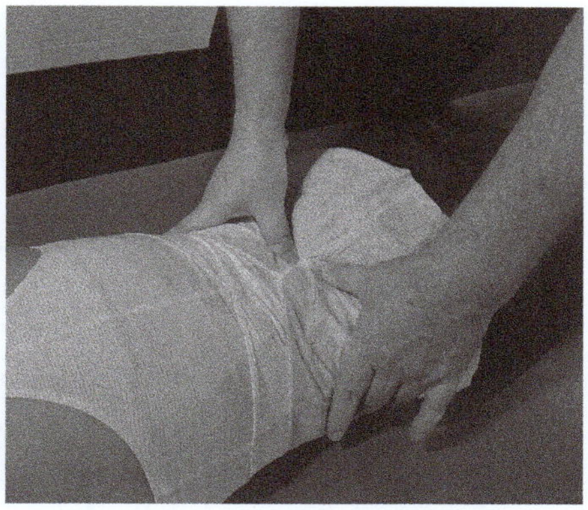

FIGURE 12.47 3. Mobilization

Press down anteriorly on one side.

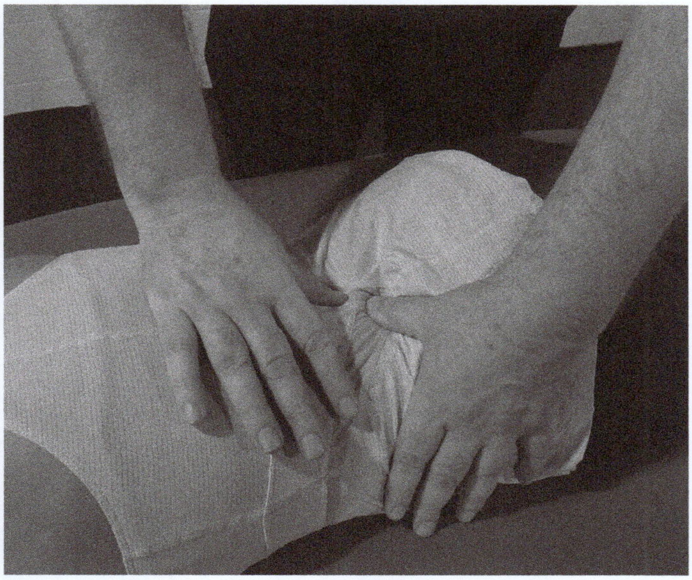

FIGURE 12.48 Lateral challenge lumbar vertebra via SP

Using the thumb, press into each SP. Note resistance and the patient's feedback on pain/tenderness.

It is best to start at L1 and work your way down the lumbar spine. If you started at L5, for example, when you move L5 (stabilizing the opposite sacral base) then L4, 3, 2, and 1 will also rotate to some degree, compromising your results. Because you are testing the lumbar spine by starting at L1, it is not crucial if the thoracic vertebrae move (though they are generally stabilized by their rib attachments). Therefore, working down from L1 will differentially test the lumbar vertebrae.

Lateral translation using lateral challenge (Figure 12.48) Engage the lateral area of the spinous process (SP) and push laterally into the SP. Be sure your contact is fully on the SP. You must get deep enough into the tissue beside the SP so you can place the side of your thumb or finger pad up against the laminar groove, or as close as possible. If not, you may end up applying a diagonal pressure on the SP. Start at L1 and work your way down to L5, if you can go that far. It is not uncommon when working with patients who are hyperlordotic, have spasming erector spinae muscles, or who have more tissue around the lumbar spine, to find it difficult to have good access to the side of the SP. To stabilize the vertebra below, place a thumb on that SP, but on the opposite side, to prevent movement through it. Placing a pillow under the abdomen may relax the patient's musculature.

RED FLAGS: SPs are notoriously tender and often compromise this test. The tenderness can be due to excessive tension placed on the periosteum by various hypertonic muscles and strained ligaments. However, fractures (pars articularis, for example), tumors/neoplasms, various bone diseases or infections, etc., can also cause tenderness at the SP. Run through some of the pertinent case history questions, especially those around pain. Any excessive tenderness requires a referral out to the patient's physician or local emergency department.

Box 12.8 looks further at lateral challenge.

INSIGHTS

Box 12.8 Lateral challenge: rotation, side-bending, or translation?

This classic maneuver has been used to test side-bending of a motion segment, and also to test rotation. However, it is more specific to translation of a vertebra. Translation is a lateral movement of one joint surface in relation to the other, which, in synovial joints, is considered an accessory movement rather than the normal physiological motion of the joint. In the lumbar spine, Fryette's rules of motion tell us that when the spine is in neutral the motion segment side-bends and rotates in opposite directions. For example, if L2–3 begins to side-bend left, it will rotate right. Further, Fryette postulates that side-bending will begin first (with the spine in neutral), and then rotation will start. Using our example of left side-bending of L2 (on L3), let us walk through and explain how translation ends up happening, rather than the coupled movements of side-bending and rotation:

- Lateral pressure is applied to the left side of L2's spinous process (SP), pushing it toward the right.
- L2 begins to side-bend left (on L3).
- Because of this, L2 should attempt to rotate to the right. However, this makes a demand for L2's SP to move left.
- But, the lateral pressure to the SP being applied (toward the right) will prevent this.
- Therefore, the facet joint surface of L2 (inferiorly between L2 and L3) will have to translate or glide to the right.

Granted, there may well be some attempt for the facet joints (superiorly and inferiorly) on the left to slightly close and those on the right to slightly open, but whatever side-bending does occur due to the lateral challenge is not accompanied by rotation and so the motion is not physiological, i.e., normal.

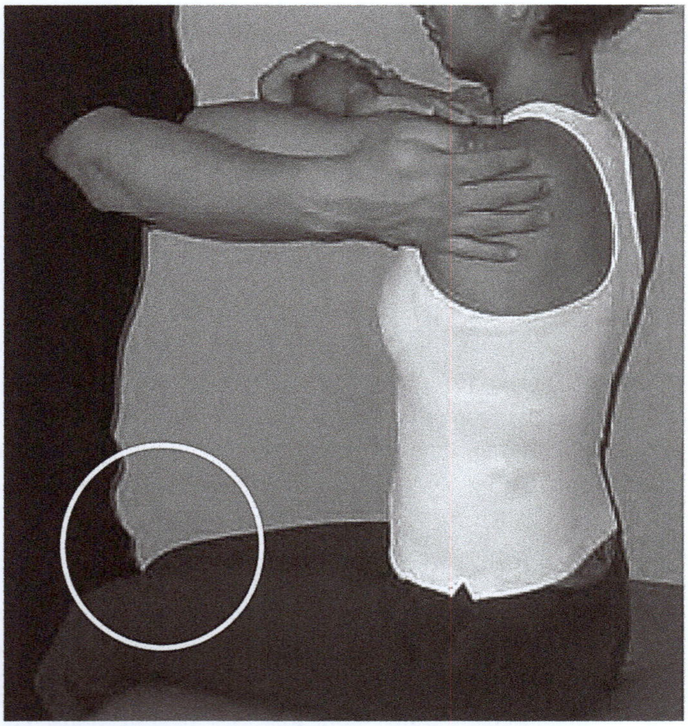

FIGURE 12.49 Rotation

The patient is seated. Stabilize the patient's knee with your thigh on the opposite side to the one they will be rotating. Have your other leg extended behind you for stability. Resist both movement of the shoulder that comes toward you and the shoulder moving away. As with active free movement of rotation, have the patient cross the arms with the hands on the shoulders. This tests ipsilateral deep rotators, internal oblique, and contralateral external oblique.

Resisted isometric testing and strength testing (Figures 12.49–12.53)

Resisted testing, like passive testing, can be difficult and hazardous for the patient (and also for the therapist) when testing the musculature around the lumbar spine. Commonly, when performing some of the strength testing of the low back, we not only allow movement but use the amount of movement the patient has as the means to grade the strength of the musculature being tested. Obviously, if the patient is in pain or suffering neurological symptoms that suggest the possibility of any degree of disc herniation we should forgo these tests. Even if the patient is presently asymptomatic, the following should be done with extreme caution. It is better to skip one or more of the following than risk reinjuring the patient.

These tests can be performed more easily with patients who have had an injury in the past but are now well into recovery from low back injury or strain. The testing then become helpful in gauging how much deconditioning (weakness, etc.) the otherwise healthy individual is suffering from. This information helps the therapist to design an appropriate remedial and strengthening exercise program. It is also useful when assessing issues with those who are engaged in a sport or demanding physical activity, who wish to improve performance, or who have minor impairments occurring without a clear cause.

NOTE: The test can be misleading because the low back musculature may be strong but weak mid- and upper back muscles may not allow the patient to raise the chest off the table (Hartley 2000b; Kendall et al. 2005). If there is facet joint irritation or previous back injury the patient may be too apprehensive to perform the test.

Take note if the patient rotates the body when the shoulder clears the table. If the abdominal external obliques are stronger, their chest rotates toward the table. If the internal obliques are stronger, they will rotate toward the ceiling. If the muscles of the back, the latissimus dorsi, quadratus lumborum, sacrospinalis, and other long erectors of the spine are stronger, then the patient will extend the back as their shoulder comes off the table.

If you suspect a disc lesion, you should be cautious with this test, as it increases the pressure of the disc onto other structures (longitudinal ligaments and nerve roots, for example).

Special tests

Differential muscle testing

In addition to the previous AR-ROM tests when appropriate it would be wise to test the length and strength of the ilipsoas and rectus femoris, as these hip flexors directly affect the orientation of the lumbar spine by their effect on anterior pelvic tilt (and increased lumbar lordosis). Further, the attachment of the psoas to the lumbar spine can also be a source of low back pain when this muscle is strained. We should also test the gluteals and hamstrings. Again, these can only be tested adequately and safely as long as the patient is not in an acute situation. Use caution. See Chapter 9 for instructions on testing.

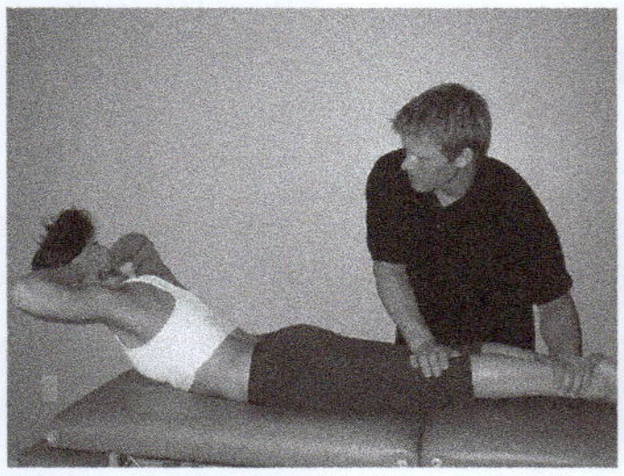

FIGURE 12.50 Extension

With the patient lying prone, stabilize the legs so as to allow the patient stability to raise the trunk off the table. Grasp both lower legs just above the ankles. Ask the patient to place the hands behind the neck and try to lift the chest off the table. If they can lift up until the xiphoid process clears the table, and can hold the position for count of five, this is graded as excellent. If they cannot hold the xiphoid off table, this is good.

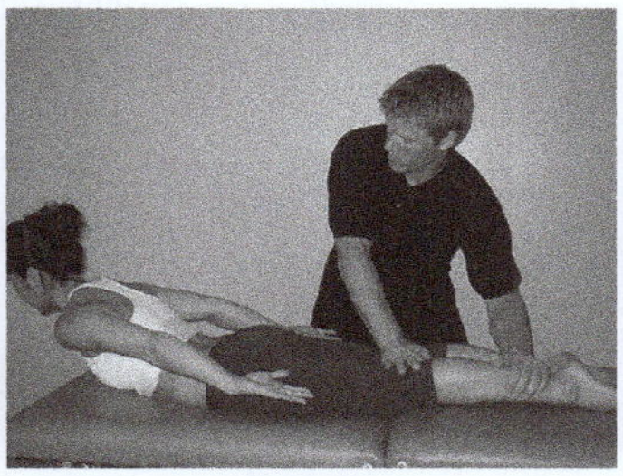

FIGURE 12.51 Modified extension test

If the actions in Figure 12.49 and 12.50 are too hard, have the patient place the arms at the side. If they can lift the xiphoid process off the table, this is a fair response. If they cannot hold the xiphoid process for a count of five, or raise it off the table, the grade is poor. We are testing the extensors of the back, latissimus dorsi, quadratus lumborum, and trapezium.

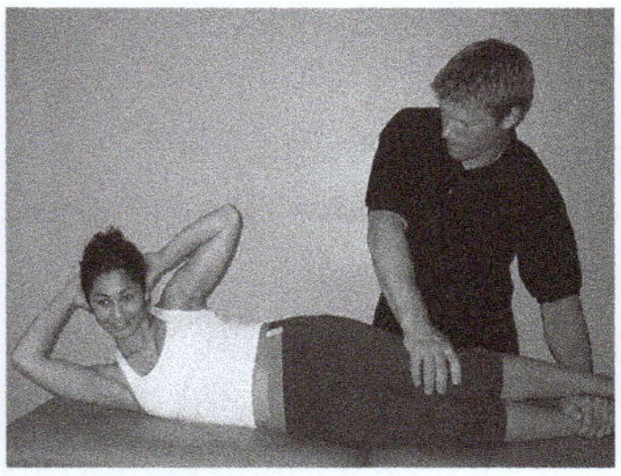

FIGURE 12.52 Side-bending/lateral flexion

Have the patient side-lying, and again stabilize their lower legs. With the hands behind the head, have the patient try to raise the shoulder and upper chest off the table and hold. This is *excellent*. Able to lift the shoulder only is *good*. Unable to hold the shoulder up is *fair*. If patient is unable to lift the shoulder, strength is considered *poor*.

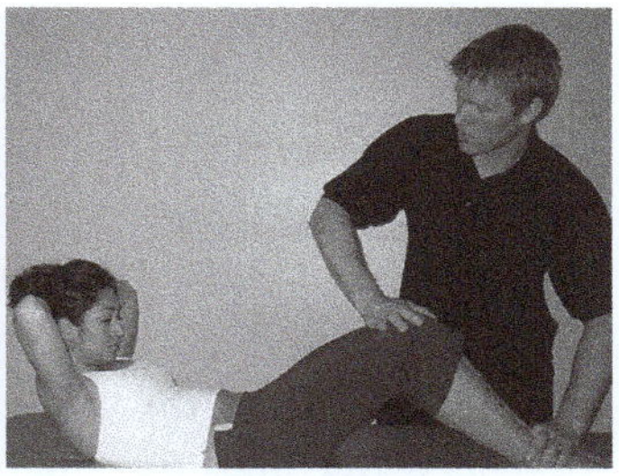

FIGURE 12.53 Forward flexion

With the patient lying supine with the knees bent, stabilize their legs. Have the patient do a curl, lifting the shoulder blades off the table, and hold this position for a count of five. This is considered *excellent*. Unable to hold for the entire count of five is *good*. Able to hold only with the hands at the side is *fair*. Unable to hold with the hands at the side is *poor*.

Note on orthopedic testing of the lumbar spine

The following orthopedic tests are designed to test specific structures in and around the lumbar spine and pelvis. The first group is for the lumbar spine and tests neurological structures. These tests are designed to simulate the movements that neurological tissues and their supportive structures can go through, but in a controlled manner so as to see what movements and what structures provoke the patient's chief complaint. The second group of tests applies to joint dysfunction. (See and compare: Dutton 2012; Evans 2009; Hammer 2007; Hartley 2000b; Hertling & Kessler 2006; Hoppenfeld 1976; Kisner & Colby 2012; Magee 2014; Palmer & Epler 1998.)

General neurological tests (Group 1)

Note that most of the neurological tests given here were designed to confirm that a disc herniation or prolapse is present and is the source of the neurological symptoms. We do know that though this is a possibility, there are also other sources of compression or irritation that can be the cause of neurological symptoms. Examples include: (1) compression by a spasming piriformis (piriformis syndrome); and (2) compression (or irritation) caused by osteophyte growth around facet joints either narrowing the neural foramen or projecting out into the foramen and causing mechanical irritation to the nerve root as it moves in and out of the neural foramen with movements of the lumbar spine and lower limbs. Further, neurological symptoms in the anterior and lateral thigh can be from compression of the femoral nerve (meralgia paresthetica, aka lateral femoral cutaneous nerve entrapment by the inguinal ligament).

Except for the straight leg raise (SLR) and the slump test, most of the special tests of the lumbar spine described in group 1 either lack evidence from research or the evidence is inconclusive about their validity. One need only note that Magee (2014) rates most of these tests as questionable concerning their reliability. Starkey and Brown (2015) do not rate them much higher.

Straight leg raise (SLR) test for neurological signs (Lasegue's sign/test)

We will present three variations of this test. Each test can accommodate the needs of patients who are suffering from varying degrees of neurological symptoms in the lower limb and/or low back.

CAUTION: The straightened leg needs to be lifted slowly and the patient needs to be instructed to tell you immediately when they feel their symptoms returning, especially if these are neurological symptoms. If the leg is lifted quickly and a nerve is trapped and tethered along its course, then tearing of axons can take place (Kapandji 2008).

By passively placing a stretch on the sciatic nerve (including its distal peroneal and tibial nerve branches) we can provoke the symptoms caused by a disc herniation or prolapse (or any space occupying lesion) that is pressing on one or more of the nerve roots which contribute to the sciatic nerve. However, other reasons for entrapment and compression can be engaged to produce positive signs for an SLR test. Some of these include a spasming piriformis and entrapment (tethering) in connective tissue (such as in the hamstring area). Further, more than one site could contribute to the overall lesion.

Straight leg raise (Figures 12.54–12.57)

This test is made up of *progressive movements* used to pinpoint the source of the patient's chief complaint. The positive neurological sign is the reproduction of the patient's neurological symptoms: pain, numbness, and tingling down the back of the leg. These signs can arise from as little movement as 10°, and on up to 70°. After 70° the sciatic nerve is not stretched further, and local low back pain past 70° is most often due to lumbar spine structures or the sacroiliac joint (Hertling & Kessler 2006; Magee 2014).

The last stage of the test, forward flexion of the cervical spine, may be positive for meningeal irritation if the patient reports

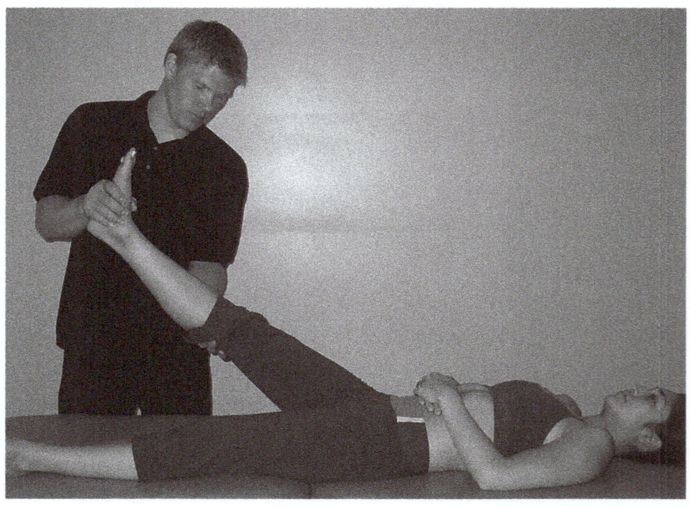

FIGURE 12.54 First stage: straight leg raise part A

The patient lies supine, as relaxed as possible. Have the patient's leg slightly adducted and allow it to be medially rotated if it rests that way. Lift the straight leg slowly until the patient reports pain or tightness in back of the leg.

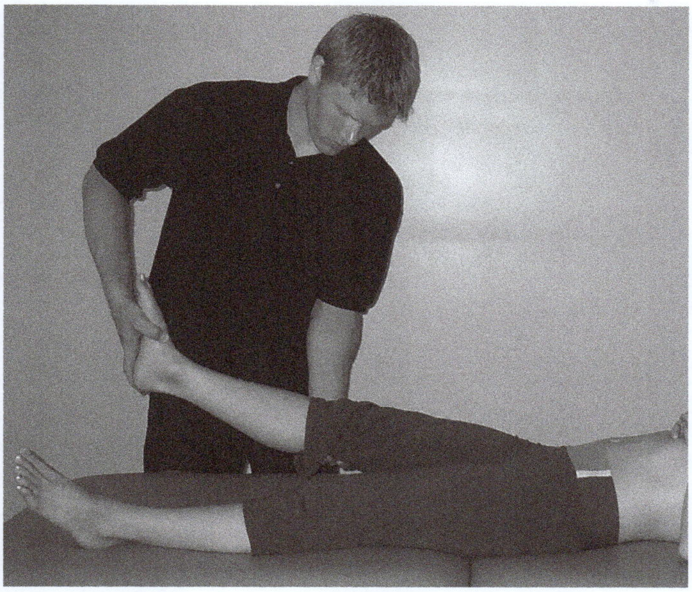

FIGURE 12.55 **First stage: straight leg raise part B**

Now, lower the leg until the symptoms are gone.

symptoms of pain or restriction only in the upper back or cervical spine (usually accompanied by an increase in head pain). If the patient has these symptoms, then stop lumbar testing. This testing is referred to by several names: Sotto-Hall or Brudzinski's sign or Kernig's sign, etc. (see Magee 2014).

The cervical flexion part of the test is meant to test for meningeal irritation. Therefore, if the patient complains of head, cervical, or upper thoracic pain you should return the patient to the neutral supine position. Then, test specifically for meningeal irritation. Have the patient lying supine and ask them to forward flex their cervical spine by trying to bring their chin to their chest.

During forward flexion of the cervical spine, the patient suffering from acute meningeal irritation would reflexively flex the hip and knees in an involuntary attempt to release the tension off the meninges. If the patient suffers from meningitis, they may not be able to dorsiflex the head at all, or only with great pain in the neck and head. Any of these results constitutes a ***red flag*** and requires immediate referral to a physician, or better yet, a hospital emergency department.

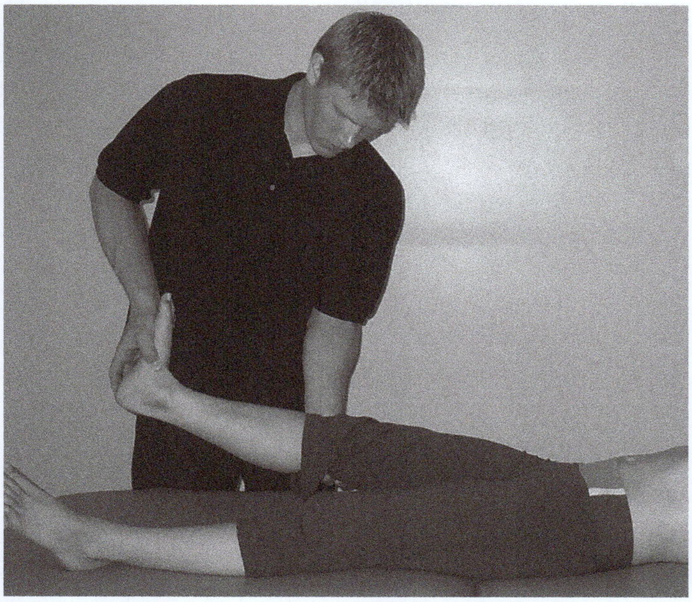

FIGURE 12.56 **Second stage: dorsiflexion of foot**

The patient's foot is passively dorsiflexed, placing more stretch via the tibial nerve. If the patient's symptoms return the test is positive. This dorsiflexion of the foot is sometimes called Bragard's test.

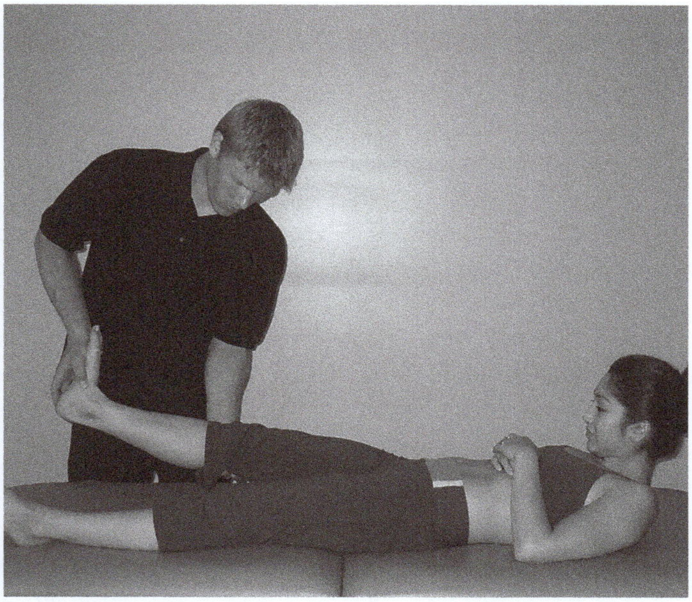

FIGURE 12.57 **Third stage: cervical flexion**

Perform *only* if the second stage does not reproduce symptoms. The patient actively forward flexes the head while you sustain dorsiflexion of the foot. Forward flexion places a stress through the dura mater and down through the sciatic nerve.

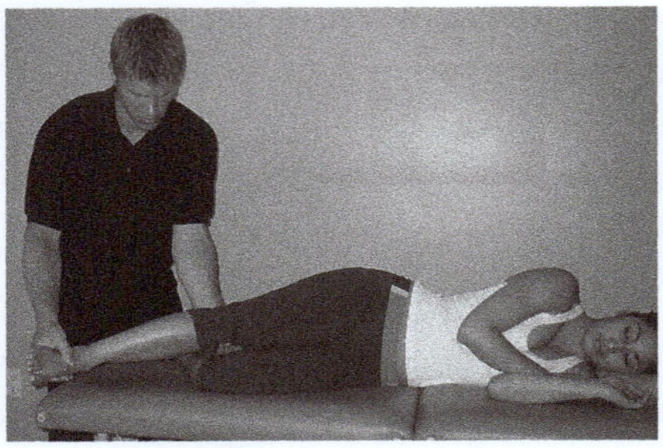

FIGURE 12.58 Side-lying SLR

Flex the hip until there is reproduction of the symptoms, then take back into extension until symptoms subside.

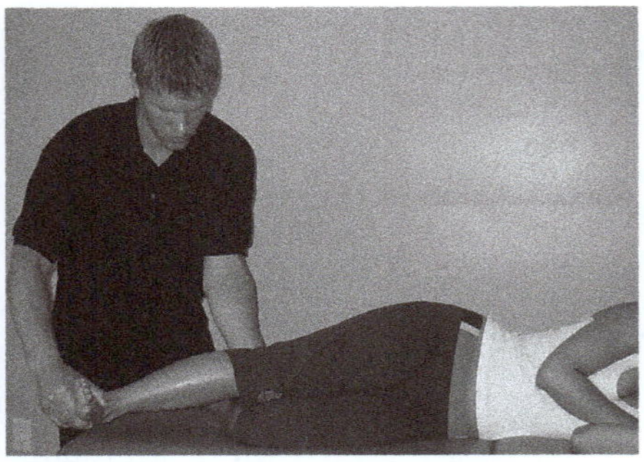

FIGURE 12.59 Dorsiflex foot

Dorsiflex the foot and ask the patient if symptoms have returned. If so, it is a positive test.

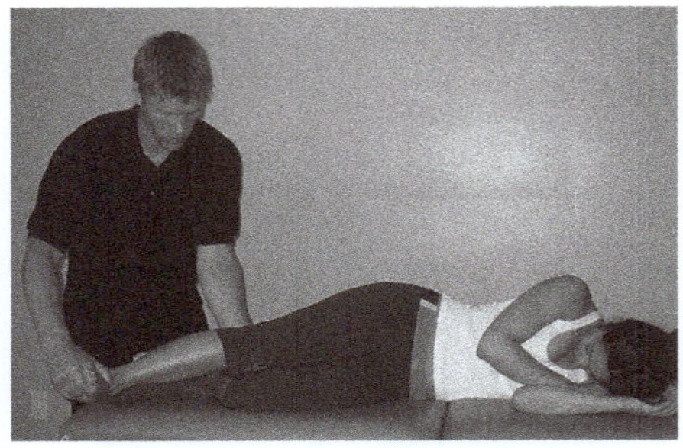

FIGURE 12.60 Cervical flexion

If symptoms did not return with dorsiflexion then ask the patient to flex the neck, chin to chest. If symptoms return then it is positive; if not, then the test is negative.

The therapist may observe what has been called the *Cox sign* when beginning the SLR: the patient will lift the hip off the table within the first 30° of the SLR in order to avoid hip and lumbar flexion. This reflexive response is attributed to a prolapsed disc in the lumbar spine protruding into the neural foramen (Evans 2009).

Alternate straight leg raise (SLR) (Figure 12.58–12.60)

This straight leg raise for neurological signs could be modified for the patient who cannot lie supine on the table with the legs extended. This is common for the patient who suffers from low back pain. Have the patient start side-lying, with the knees bent comfortably. Straighten the uppermost leg so it is in neutral (as if standing). While supporting the weight of the whole leg, slowly raise it by flexing the hip while keeping the knee extended. Do so until the patient experiences either a return of symptoms, or reaches their end-range for hip flexion. If the patient's symptoms return, proceed as above; back off the stretch, and then dorsiflex the foot. If the symptoms do not yet appear then add cervical flexion.

As in the standard supine SLR test, if flexion of the neck creates pain in the neck or head then stop this test. Perform testing for meningeal irritation, which can be found in the cervical chapter. *If positive it is a red flag for immediate medical attention.*

Well leg raise

This test is performed on the leg that does not have any neurological symptoms down its posterior aspect (i.e., the unaffected leg). It is the same as the previous SLR test, only done on the unaffected leg, which is what the therapist should already have tested (i.e., by first testing the unaffected side, and only then testing the affected side). It will be positive if it reproduces the patient's neurological signs and symptoms *down the patient's affected leg* (though often with less intensity than the SLR on the affected leg). This positive sign points to a severe space-occupying lesion (e.g., disc herniation) that is pressing on the nerve root(s) governing the affected limb.

The test works because the SLR, doing one leg at a time, causes some rotation in the lumbar spine. This rotation will shift a severely herniated disc (or any other large tissue such as a tumor) via the stretch on the dura mater toward the opposite side, increasing the space-occupying lesion's pressure on the contralateral nerve root. Usually, the unaffected leg needs to be lifted farther than the affected leg to get a positive sign, because sufficient rotation of the lumbar spine needs to occur (Magee 2014). Often there is no dorsiflexion of the foot or neck flexion added, but it should be done nonetheless. This demonstrates to the patient what may be done on the affected side.

Slump test (Figures 12.61–12.65)

A variation of the SLR test for neurological signs. This version of testing for "space occupying lesions" (i.e., disc herniations impacting on nerve roots) may be the best test when patients also have pain in the low back or hip, or sciatic symptoms that include muscle weakness in the leg. It does not require the patient to get on and off the table and lie down supine or side-lying. While often described as beginning with the patient high-sitting (in other words, sitting on the table) it can be just as effectively done with the patient in a chair or on a stool. Once the patient is sitting, do the following:

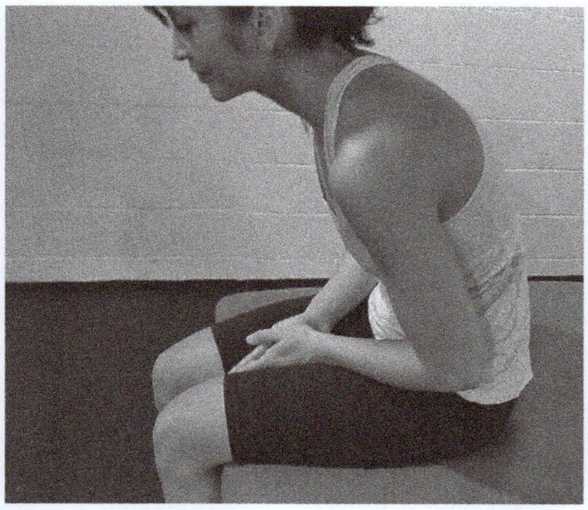

FIGURE 12.61 Slump test step 1

Have the patient slump forward (i.e., flex the lumbar and thoracic spine without bending forward from hip).

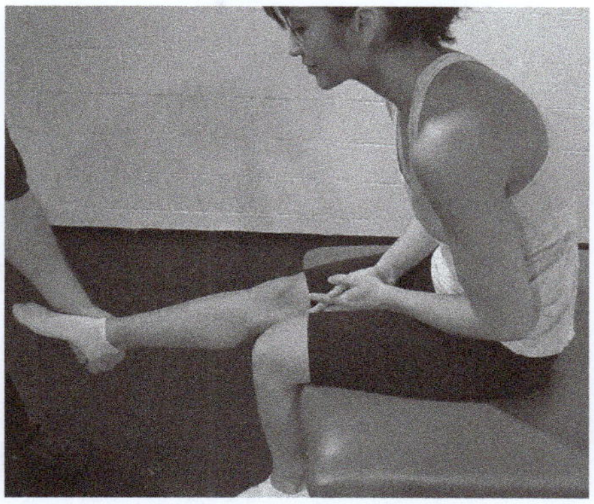

FIGURE 12.62 Slump test step 2

Now, raise their leg (extend the knee) until either the patient's symptoms return or they reach end-range.

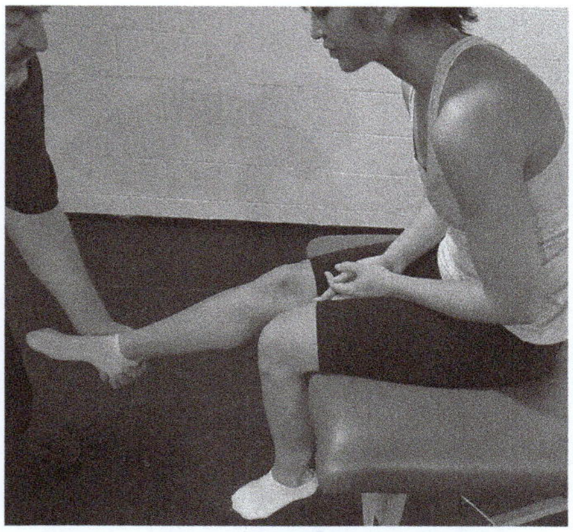

FIGURE 12.63 Slump test step 3

If symptoms return, flex the knee slightly until the symptoms disappear.

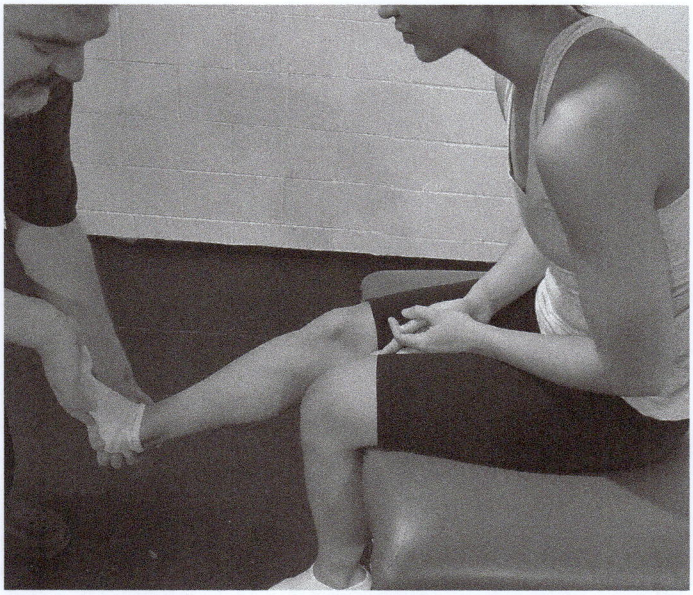

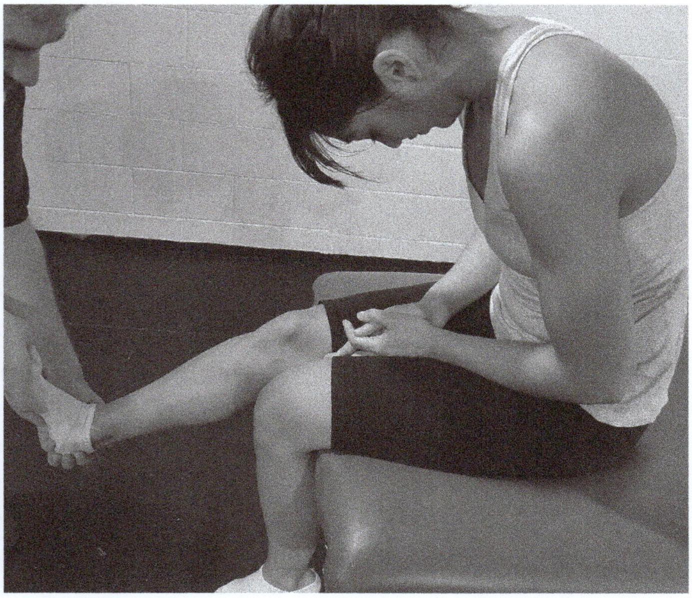

FIGURES 12.64, 12.65 Slump test step 4

Dorsiflex the foot. If that does not reproduce the symptoms, then ask the patient to drop the chin to the chest.

As mentioned previously, the SI joints may complain during the SLR, anywhere between 0° and 70°. If acute, this will occur early during the SLR, but the pain is felt at the SI joint area. However, SI joint pain *can* refer down the posterior leg and mimic sciatic pain. It is generally accepted as a rule of thumb that after 70° of hip flexion there is no more tension placed on the sciatic nerve or the SI joints and thus pain felt at the low back past 70° is due to musculature in the area pointed to/reported by the patient.

Bowstring sign (Figures 12.66, 12.67)

If the straight leg raise test is positive, then irritation and inflammation of the sciatic nerve is probable. The sciatic nerve may be directly palpated in the popliteal fossa of the knee. Having

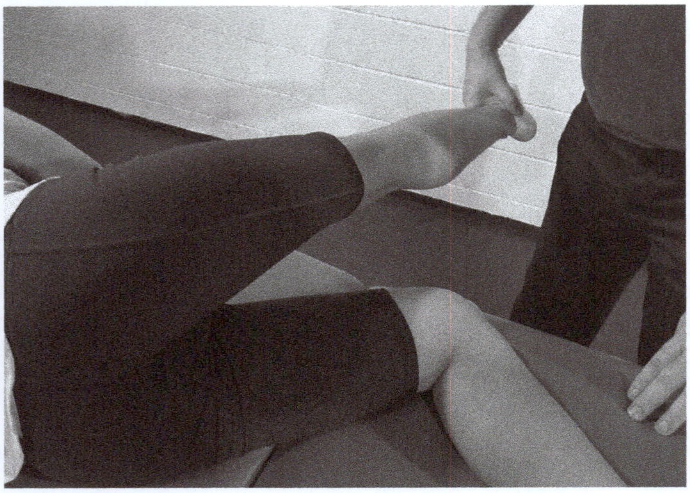

FIGURE 12.66 Bowstring sign step 1

Perform SLR until symptoms occur, then bend knee until symptoms disappear.

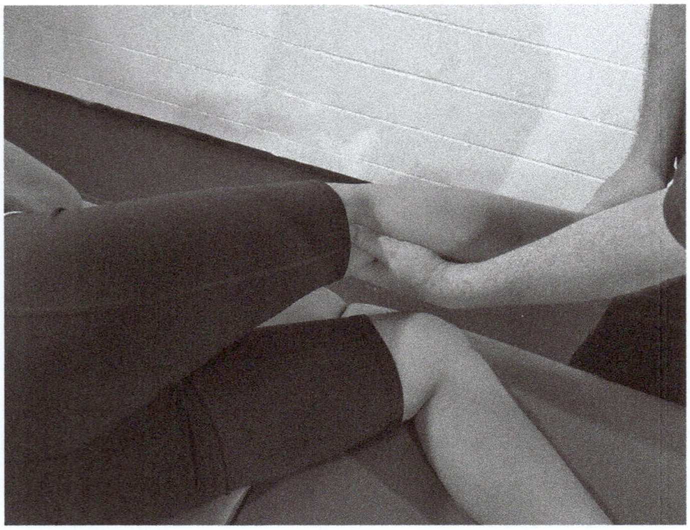

FIGURE 12.67 Bowstring sign step 2

Palpate for and strum sciatic nerve.

pressure on, or a *strumming* across, the nerve will cause symptoms to be felt locally and usually will refer up and down the leg from the part of the nerve being irritated by the palpation. In order for this test to be positive, the sciatic nerve needs to be inflamed and the neurolemma swollen down to or near to the section of the nerve that is to be strummed. Therefore, this will only occur if sciatic nerve irritation (at the low back) has been there for some time.

With the patient still supine (or side-lying or high-sitting), passively raise the leg until pain or paresthesia is felt down the back of the leg. Now, flex the knee slightly (removing the symptoms) and place the ankle between your arm and trunk in order to support the leg. Palpate with your thumb just medially to the tendon of the biceps femoris in the popliteal fossa. If the inflammation has been chronic, the nerve itself can be palpated, feeling like a braided cord. If not, pressure applied or a strumming action on the fossa will bring on the symptoms. The positive sign is a return of the patient's neurological signs and symptoms, and the therapist may be able to feel the swollen irritated nerve. It is shown here (Figures 12.66, 12.67) in side-lying in order to be able to show the area of the popliteal fossa "strummed."

Valsalva's test (Figure 12.68)

This test works by increasing the intrathecal pressure in the spinal cord, the positive sign of pain or paresthesia will be felt locally in the spine or felt traveling down into the legs if there

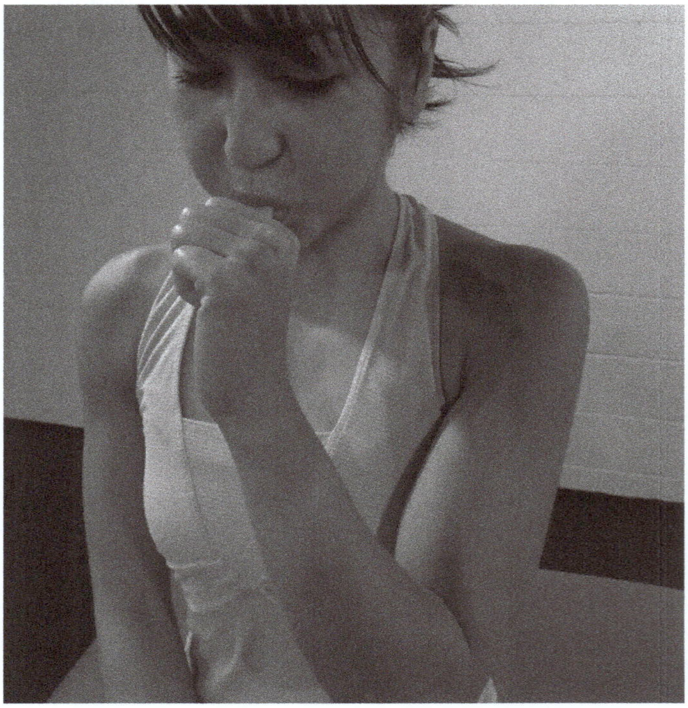

FIGURE 12.68

Valsalva's test. Have the patient take a deep breath and hold while bearing down as if having a bowel movement. Alternatively, have them place the tip of the thumb in the mouth and pretend they are blowing up a balloon.

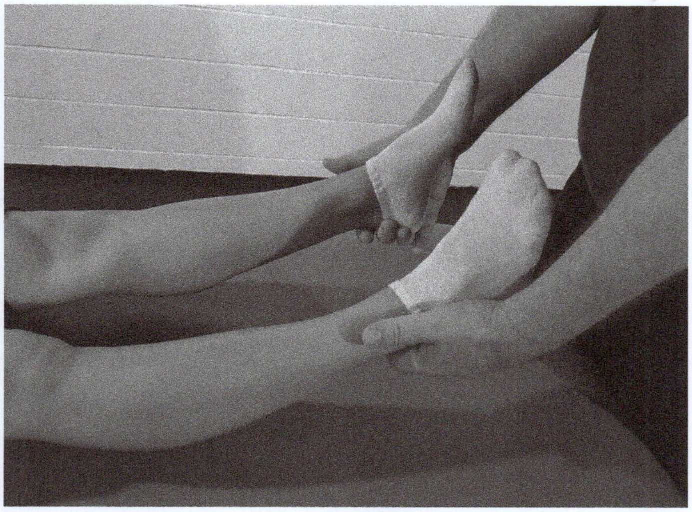

FIGURE 12.69 Hoover's test

With the patient supine, the therapist takes each of the patient's heels in the palm of a hand. Ask the patient to raise each of their legs, one at a time. The therapist notes if they can feel the patient trying to lift the affected leg.

is a space-occupying lesion such as a tumor, herniated disc, or osteophytes.

Hoover's test (Figure 12.69)

This test is designed to see if the patient is malingering or exaggerating their complaint of low back pain. You ask the supine patient to lift each straight leg, one at a time, while you hold the heels of their feet in the palm of your hands. When the patient tries to raise one leg, you should feel a downward pressure in the palm of your hand holding the opposite leg. This pressure comes from the patient's exertion, their effort. If you do not feel such pressure, then the test is positive: the patient is not really trying to lift their leg.

Neurological testing (Group 2)

If a patient tests positive for any neurological test, they should be referred to their doctor. It would be wise for you to write a note that the patient can take with them explaining what testing done during the neurological assessment was positive, and for what levels, so that their physician knows what testing to do to try and replicate your results.

Myotome testing for the lumbar spine

The patient must use their full strength in neurological tests, or when doing strength testing for that matter, otherwise they may inadvertently mislead the therapist about the true strength of a muscle. If you ask for only half of their strength when testing, the patient will often only be able to gauge that by the resistance they feel being applied. Hence, they may use 50 percent of their strength on the uninjured side of their body being tested first, and 70 percent on the other; pushing against the therapist's resistance until both sides feel the same. The patient is not trying to trick the therapist; they will believe they have applied the same force because it felt the same.

Using half-strength has traditionally been cited as a means to prevent further injury. However, if the testing is performed correctly, then this rule is unnecessary. As in AR-ROM testing, during myotome testing the patient should be instructed to begin their effort or resistance with minimal effort and take a good five seconds to build up to maximum strength. If the therapist is applying the effort for the patient to resist, they need to follow the same rules by slowly building up to maximal effort. This gradual increase in effort can, in fact, be more protective to re-injury than giving the patient some specific level of strength to use during testing. The therapist may also wish to count out loud to help reinforce how long it takes to get to maximal effort.

Another rule of myotome testing is that the maximum effort by the patient is sustained for at least five seconds. This is done because a muscle suffering from a minor or moderate neurological deficit may still be able to generate a normal maximal effort for a second or two, but then will noticeably begin to lose strength. The patient is further instructed to stop and slowly decrease their effort as soon as there is any pain or reoccurrence of symptoms.

Scale for isometric strength testing of myotomes

Record the results of testing by placing the numerical value of your finding over 5, for example:

4/5 R Myo L2, or record as Good R Myo L2.

5 = Normal: Full strength available with strong resistance applied.

4 = Good: Can resist with only slight resistance applied.

3 = Fair: Can only resist the affect of gravity alone.

2 = Poor: Cannot resist gravity but can move the limb in the horizontal plane.

1 = Trace: No movement, only "flickering" of muscle present.

0 = Zero: No trace, no flickering, flaccid.

Kendall et al. (2005) also suggest that negative and positive signs can be added to the number or term applied to the finding

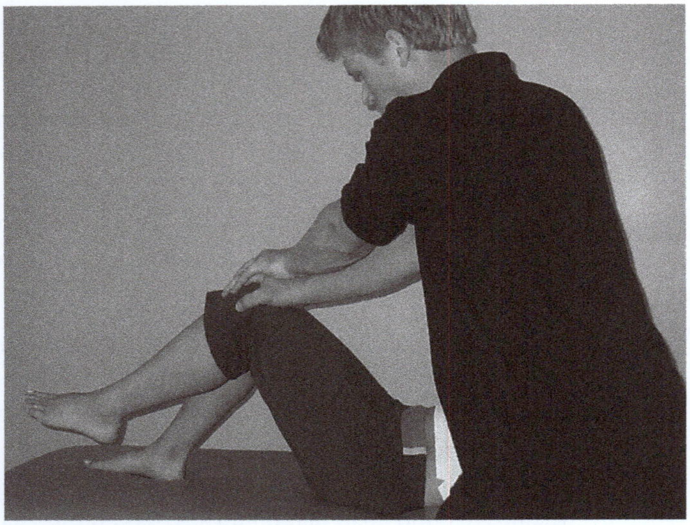

FIGURE 12.70 L2 resisted hip flexion (iliopsoas)

Have the patient lift the foot a couple of inches off the table. Place both your hands on the patient's knee. Have them try to flex their hip while you provide resistance. Or, tell the patient to hold the position while you slowly build up your force and try to push their foot back down to the table. Remember to ease off slowly, and to do so if the patient begins to allow movement during testing (i.e., if you are overpowering them).

in order to "fine tune" them to the variety of functionality observed in clinical settings. For example: 4+/5 R Myo L2, or record as Good + R Myo L2.

To start myotome testing for the lumbar spine and lower extremities, have the patient supine with their knees bent and feet flat on the table. The bent knees are necessary for the patient who suffers from low back pain to be comfortable, and to reduce the chance of re-injury. Testing from a seated position can increase the chance of re-injury and also increases the instances of the patient recruiting other muscles, limbs, or their weight (by leaning backwards) during testing.

The supine position described above is also helpful in reducing the apprehension of pain that may otherwise prevent the patient from using their full strength during testing. It is the starting position for each of the following tests, so there is no need for the patient to change position.

Myotome testing (Figures 12.70–12.76)

These tests should be done with the therapist resisting the patient's movement or, better still, with the patient holding their position while the therapist applies force. *Note that there is no L1 myotome.*

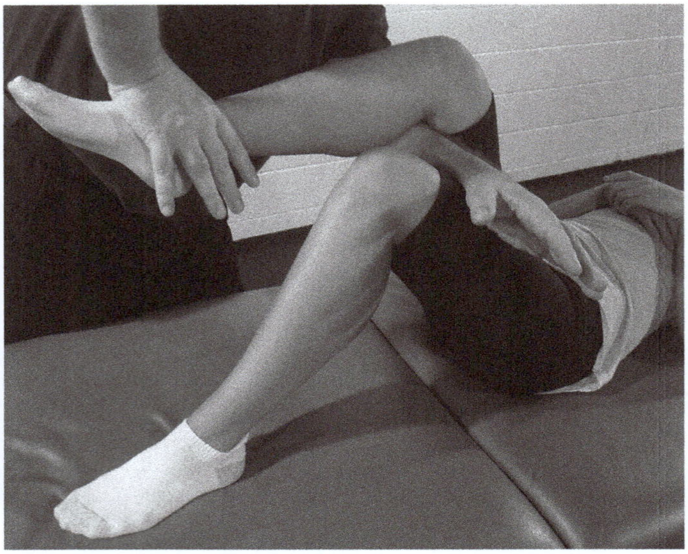

FIGURE 12.71 L3 knee extension (quadriceps)

Reach under the knee of the leg to be tested with the arm closest to the patient's head and place the proximal part of your wrist on the patient's far knee. Lift the leg slightly until your forearm is parallel to the table and their leg is draped over your forearm. The knee should remain flexed to roughly 80–90°. With your other hand on their ankle, turn your body until it faces the patient's upper body so you are in a position of mechanical advantage to resist their attempt to extend their knee. Be sure to keep your wrist neither flexed nor extended while you resist knee extension. Again, you may wish to have the patient hold and resist while you push.

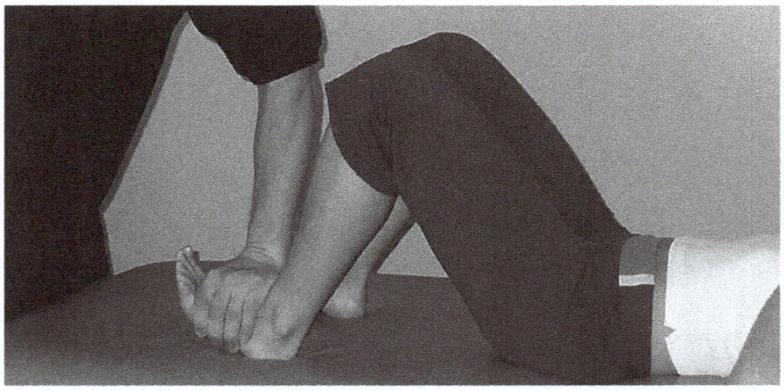

FIGURE 12.72 L4 ankle dorsiflexion (tibialis anterior)

Stabilize the lower leg with one hand by pushing the heel into the table, while you place the ankle/foot in neutral (roughly having the ankle in 90° as if standing), and have the patient hold the position while you try to bring the sole of their foot to the table.

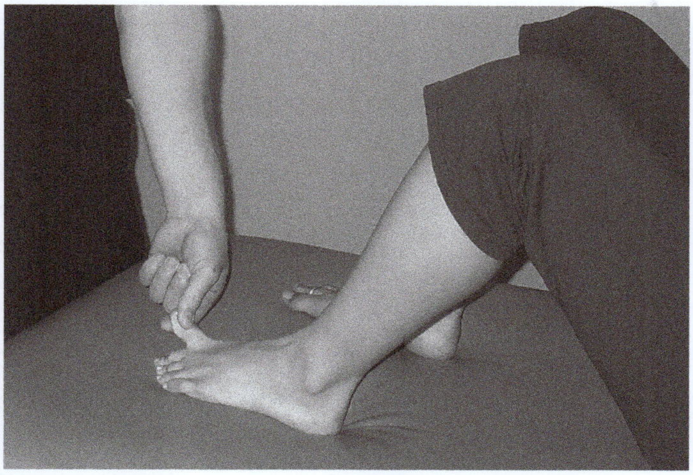

FIGURE 12.73 L5 extension of the big toe (extensor hallucis longus)

Stabilize across the metatarsal with one hand, with the ankle/foot in a neutral position, and either ask the patient to raise their big toe toward their head, or if necessary lift it for them. (Many patients have trouble consciously doing this so, to save time, you may wish to assist by lifting for them.) Have them hold this while you try to flex the joint.

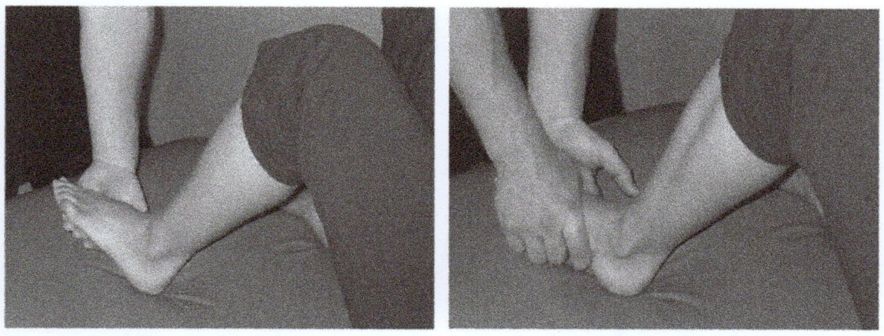

FIGURES 12.74, 12.75 S1 ankle eversion (peroneus/fibularis longus and brevis)

With the patient's ankle in neutral have them evert the foot, or bring the outside of the foot up toward their knee. Again, have them try to hold the position while you try to bring the foot into inversion. S1 can also be tested with the patient prone by having them extending the hip, but this may put too much stress on the lumbar spine. Figure 12.74 shows the position of the foot. Figure 12.75 shows the position of the therapist's hands for testing.

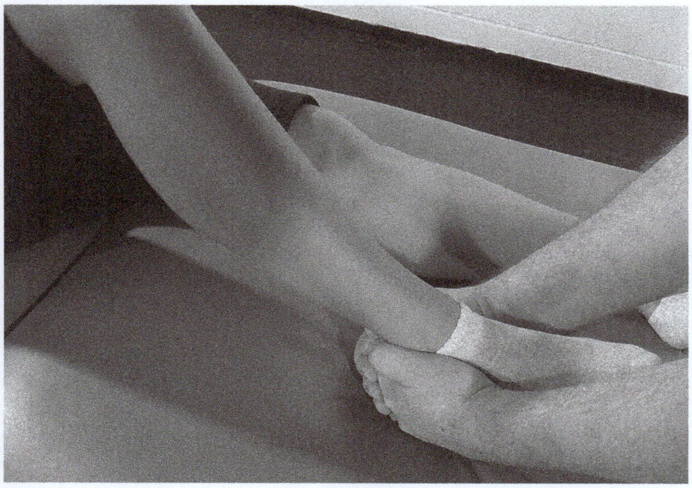

FIGURE 12.76 S1 and S2 knee flexion (hamstrings)

While standing at the end of the table, clasp both hands around the patient's ankle (and heel if possible). Lift the foot off the table and resist their attempt to bring the ankle toward the buttock. Or, they can resist your attempt to extend the knee. ***Note:** if test of ankle eversion or S1 was negative, but there is a positive while testing knee flexion (S1 and S2), then S2 is the affected myotome.*

Dermatome testing (Figures 12.77–12.84)

Initially, the therapist may wish to do some quick testing for sensory nerve enervation dysfunctions relating to sensory nerve roots. This can be done with the patient supine or standing. Test bilaterally at the same time. To do so, brush with the finger pads or the back of your fingers several times in the mid-section of each of the lower dermatomes, asking the patient if they notice any difference from one side to the other. Often, a delayed response or uncertainty on the patient's part can be considered a possible positive sign (of a mild problem). If you wish, you can repeat this with deep touch, hot and then cold, two-point discrimination and vibration.

For a map of dermatomes of the lower body, see Figure 12.77. The areas to brush correspond to the generally undisputed areas of the various dermatome maps that have been developed over the last hundred years or so. Further, dermatomes by nature overlap to some degree in everyone. Therefore, the suggestion here is to test the central areas of each dermatome.

As can be seen from a dermatome map, the dermatome areas in the lower body run a spiral pattern. In the instructions below for these dermatomes we describe the starting point from which to start the brushing and where to end. Therefore, assume

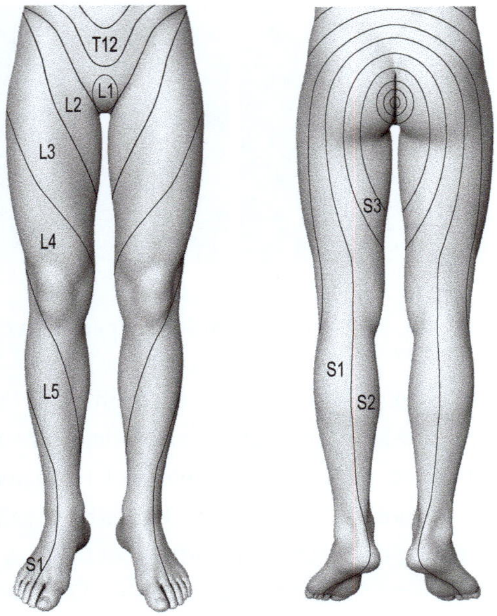

FIGURE 12.77

Dermatome map of the lower body.

a spiral motion (in a lateral to medial direction) should be followed between the two while testing.

NOTE: If two or more dermatomes are affected, the patient may be suffering from compression of the cauda equina; in other words, a compression within the spinal canal. A compression of the cauda equina can also cause bilateral loss, as can any reason for spinal stenosis. This is a ***red flag*** and the patient should be told to see a physician promptly.

Remember that peripheral nerves also suffer from compression syndromes and dysfunction. You should compare your dermatome findings, especially if the results are not clear, with the map of peripheral nerve sensory innervation in Figure 12.84.

To record your findings: *L3 dermatome +*. If you have tested various levels *and kinds of sensations*, then write that in after: *L3 dermatome + light touch and vibration.*

Compare your sensory testing with the peripheral sensory nerve map in Figure 12.84, in case your findings more accurately match a peripheral nerve rather than a nerve root's dermatome pattern. You can use the brushing technique for testing peripheral nerve areas as well as for dermatomes.

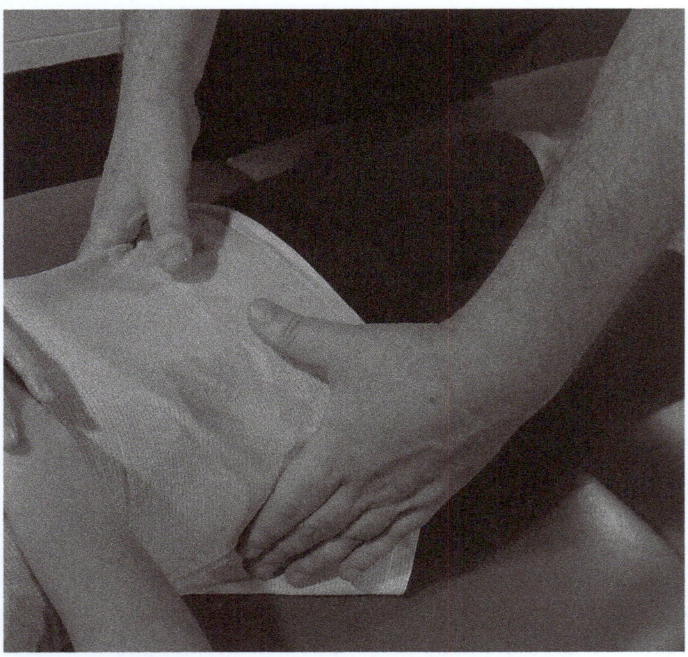

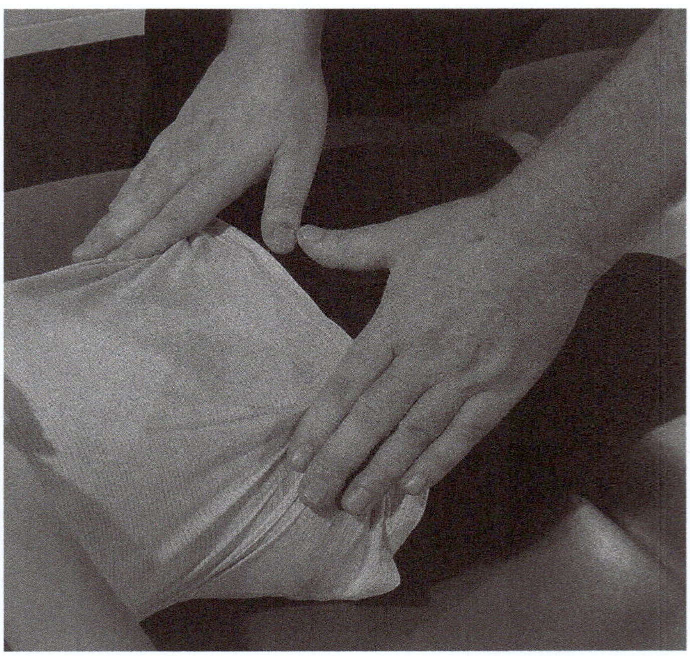

FIGURE 12.78A, B L1 dermatome testing

Begin just above the highest part of the iliac crest and following along the curve of the crest, brush down to the ASIS.

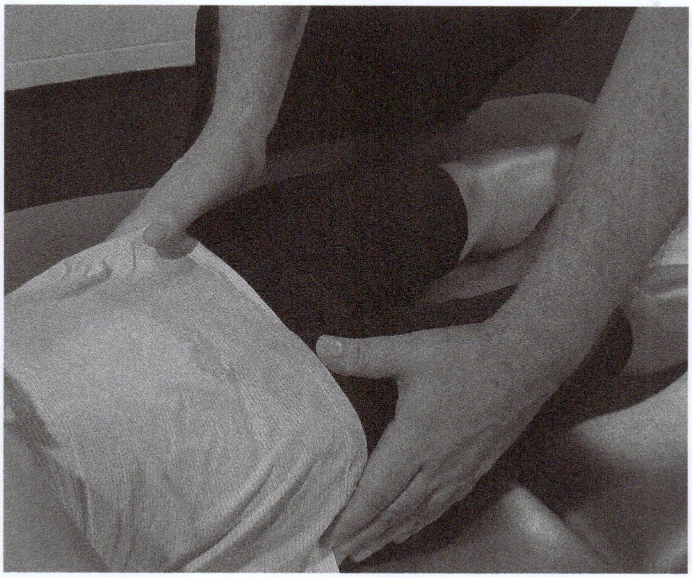

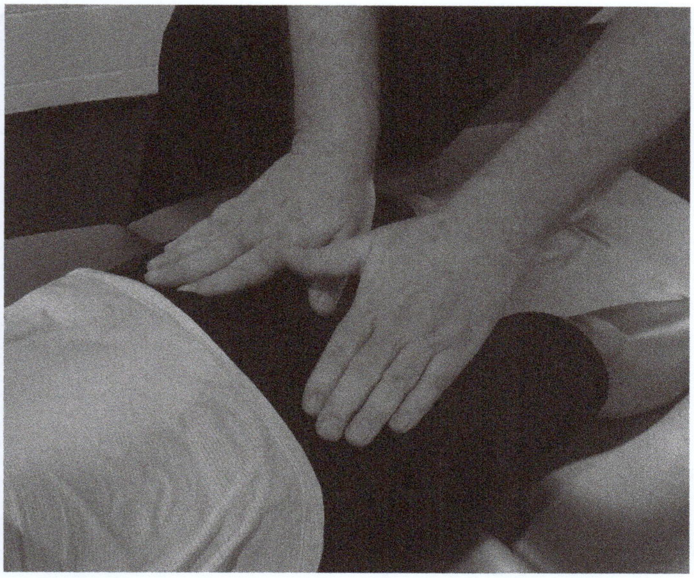

FIGURE 12.79A, B L2 dermatome testing

Begin over the gluteus minimus area (lateral area of the ilium) and brush down and over to the top of the thigh just below the inguinal line.

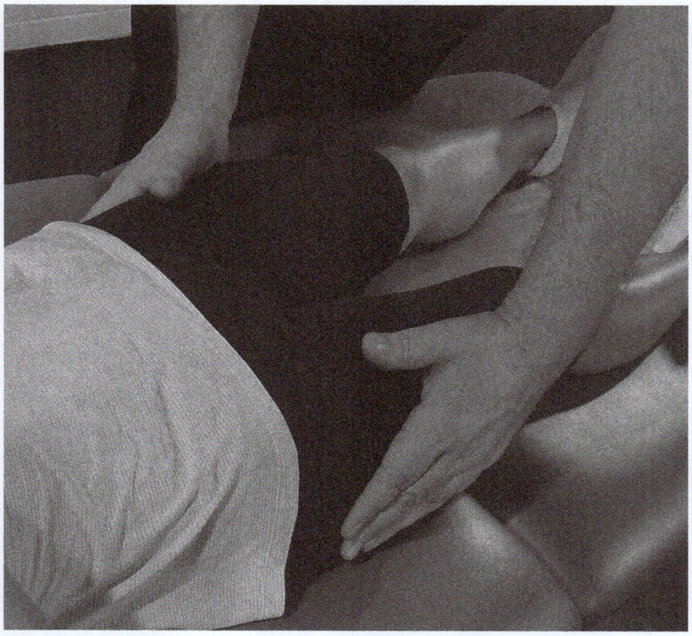

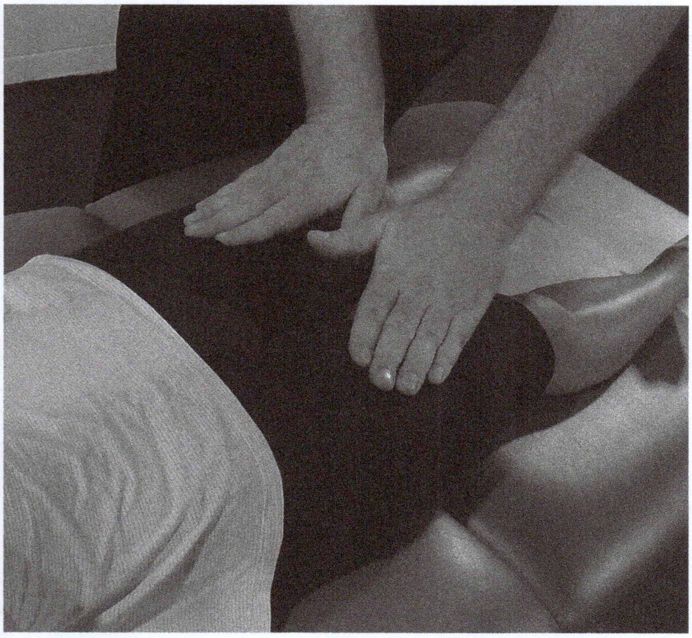

FIGURE 12.80A, B L3 dermatome testing

Begin just under the greater trochanter and brush down in a spiral and over the anterior mid-thigh area.

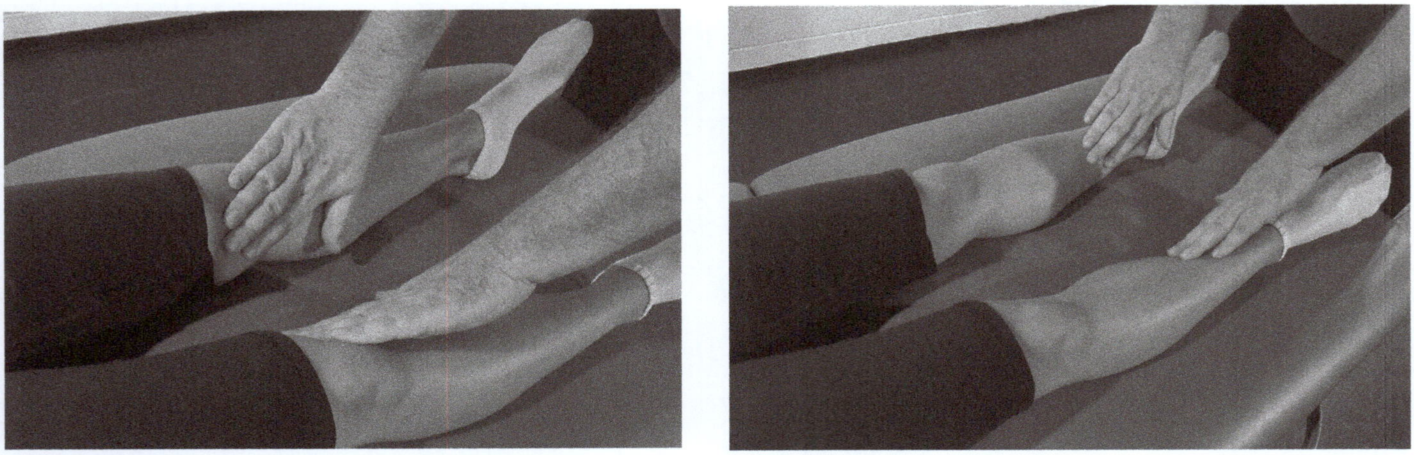

FIGURE 12.81A, B L4 dermatome testing

Begin just below the medial kneecap and brush down onto the medial lower leg. Stop a few inches above the medial malleoli.

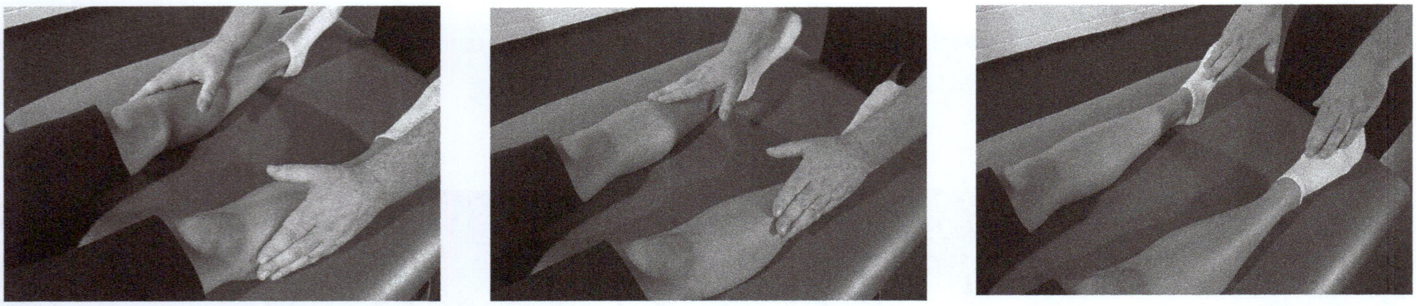

FIGURE 12.82A, B, C L5 dermatome testing

Begin over the anterior lateral lower leg (three inches below the knee), moving diagonally down to the anterior-medial part of the foot below, finishing by running along the medial side of the first metatarsal and big toe to its end.

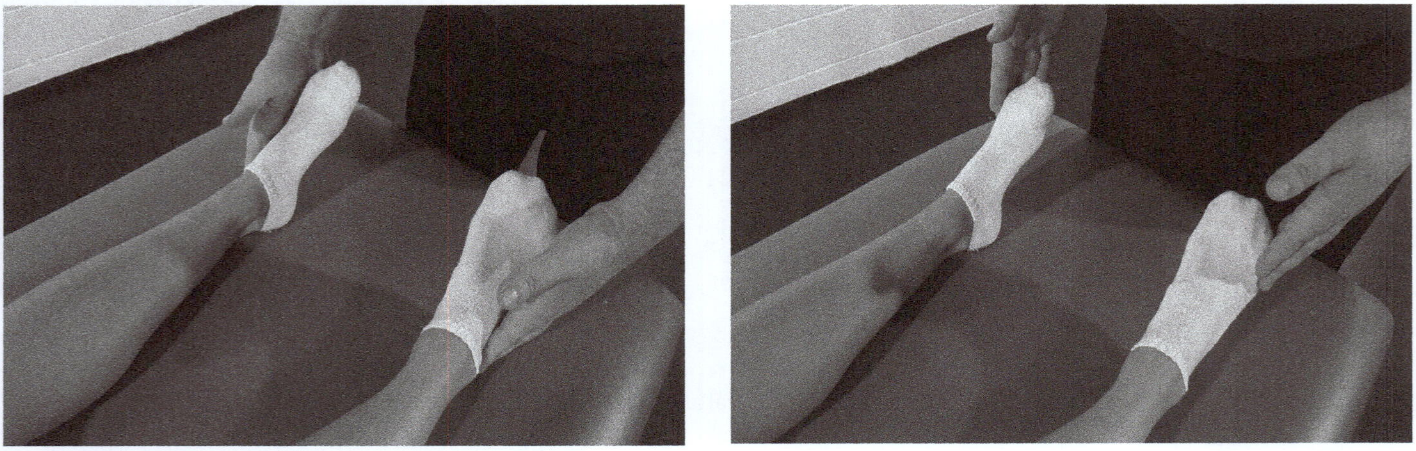

FIGURE 12.83A, B S1 dermatome testing

Begin at the lateral side of the foot, at the end of little toe, and brush back to the lateral side of the heel of the foot.

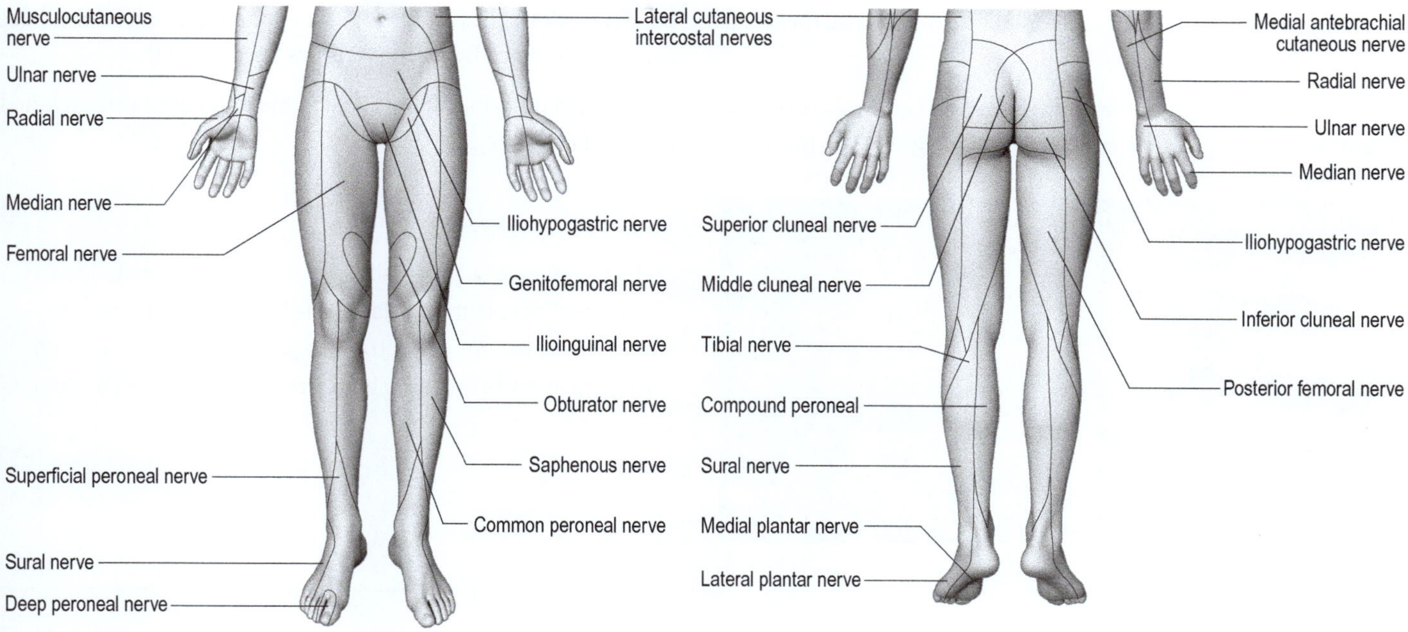

FIGURE 12.84

Peripheral nerve map of the lower body.

Deep tendon reflexes (DTR) (Figures 12.85, 12.86)

Rather than the classic strike or two with a reflex hammer (a *quick test*), it is wise to test each DTR on each side of the body with seven to 10 strikes to see if there is a progressive lessening of the response. This decreasing response is a positive sign of neurological impairment. The obvious positive sign for this is a difference bilaterally. You can have a decreased or absent reflex on one side as a positive sign, or you could have a hyper-reflexive response on one side as a positive sign.

However, if you get little or no response from both sides, that is what is normal for that person and is not a positive sign. The lack of response is due to the fact that we are using a stretch reflex to test innervation. If the muscle is long, or low in tone, the response could be minimal or absent.

With the Achilles tendon, the therapist can increase the likelihood of a stretch reflex response by placing one hand under the patient's foot and slightly dorsiflexing the foot. Do both tests with the patient seated on the table so that their feet are off the floor.

Reflex grading scale

4 = Hyper-reflexive. Pathology implied.

3 = Greater than normal response. May be pathological if unilateral; if bilateral, it may be due to hypertonicity of the musculature involved in the reflex.

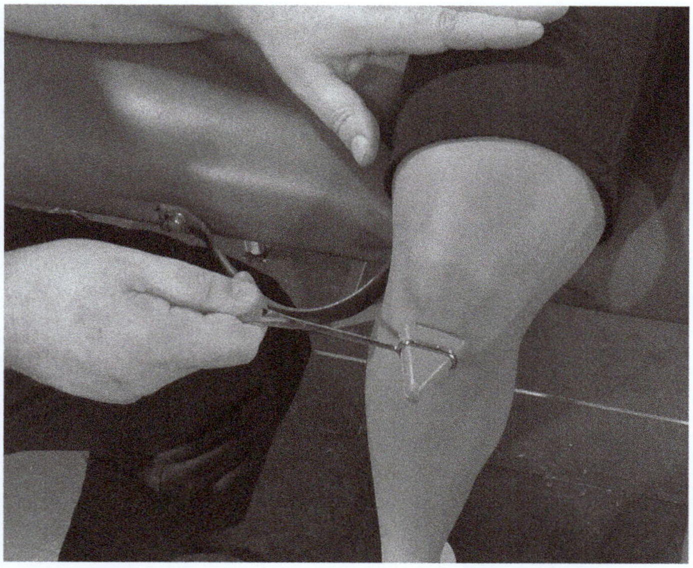

FIGURE 12.85 L3–4 DTR

Test by striking the infrapatellar tendon and comparing knee jerk bilaterally.

2 = Normal response.

1 = Hyporeflexive. Pathology may be present if response is unilateral; if bilateral it may be due to hypotonicity or deconditioning.

0 = No response. Pathological if unilateral; if bilateral, the test is considered negative.

To record your findings, place the numerical equivalent over 4. Examples: 0/4 DTR R L4 equals number 0 grade for the right patella tendon reflex; 3/4 DTR R S1 equals a finding of number 3 grading on the right for the Achilles tendon DTR.

Box 12.9 describes some classic tests that have been excluded, and explains why.

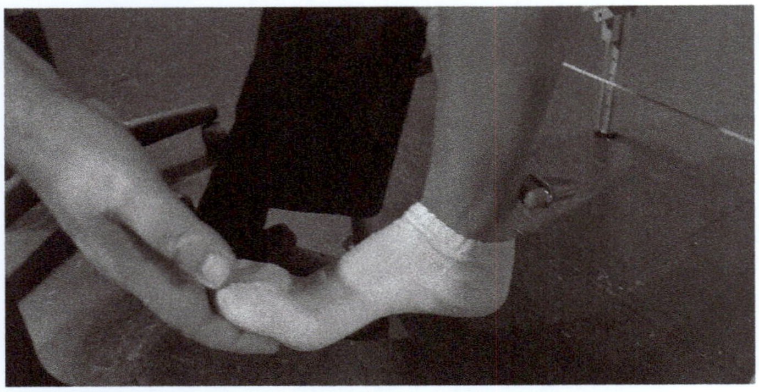

FIGURE 12.86 S1 DTR

Hold the foot in slight dorsiflexion. Test the Achilles tendon and watch for plantar flexion. If the foot plantar flexes but very slowly returns to neutral, the patient should be referred to a physician as they may be suffering from hypothyroidism.

Box 12.9 Excluded classic tests

These classic tests have been excluded from the testing protocol for this chapter because of their lack of specificity or their over-provocation of tissues:

Femoral nerve stretch (Nachlas' test)

With the patient prone, bring their heel to their buttock. For further provocation, passively extend the thigh with the knee still fully flexed. Reproduction of pain or paresthesia over the L2 and L3 dermatome area may indicate a lesion of or irritation to the femoral nerve.

The positive sign is a **bright shooting pain** down the front of the leg, possibly accompanied by pain in the low back around the L3–4 vertebral area. However, these positive signs could also be imitated by a contractured rectus femoris – sharp burning pain. Also this test can cause the taut rectus femoris to anteriorly rotate the innominate (hip), which will increase lumbar lordosis and irritate inflamed facet joints or short muscles that may spasm, all causing low back pain.

Quadrant test (Kemp's test)

The test can be highly provocative. It may tell you what action (or one of the actions) that could be producing the symptoms but as so many tissues are involved in the maneuver it is not highly specific.

Have the standing patient place their ipsilateral hand on the back of the leg being tested. This is side-flexion with extension. Have them slowly slide the hand down the back of the leg as far as they can. Ask the patient to tell you when they feel any discomfort or pain, or if they have a recurrence of any neurological signs or symptoms. This combined movement is usually referred to as the quadrant test for the lumbar spine. It is used to provoke neurological signs and symptoms due to neural foramen narrowing.

With the patient standing, have them place their ipsilateral hand on the back of the leg being tested. This is side-flexion with extension. Have them slowly slide the hand down the back of the leg as far as they can. Ask the patient to tell you when they feel any discomfort or pain, or if they have a recurrence of any neurological signs or symptoms. This combined movement is usually referred to as the quadrant test for the lumbar spine. It is used to provoke neurological signs and symptoms due to neural foramen narrowing.

This movement provides greater provocation of nerve root compression by decreasing the intervertebral foramen of the lumbar spine on the side to which the patient bends. The test also puts maximal stress on the facet joints by placing them in their close packed position. Facet joint pain may be site-specific to the facet provoked, or may radiate around the joint.

Localized pain and pain referred to other sites on the same side may also come from an injured muscle being placed in a shortened position and then spasming, from low back erectors to the piriformis. Further, piriformis trigger points are capable of mimicking sciatica with its referral pattern. However, the piriformis can also be responsible for the compression of the sciatic nerve. Pain can also come from pressure placed on inflamed iliolumbar ligaments or from compression of the joint surfaces of the sacroiliac joint. The latter can mimic neurological pain in the gluteal-hip region. Pain from the side not being tested usually comes from tissue being stretched.

Milgram's test

This test is designed to test the joints of the lumbar spine. However, patients with low back pain will not be able to do the test or would refuse out of apprehension.

The patient is supine; they raise both heels off the table three or four inches and hold the position for 30 seconds or until there is positive sign of the recurrence of the symptoms. The test is better not used because of the stress and loading it can place on the low back. Yet it was designed to be used if you suspect disc herniation or severe muscle strain! This would not just add insult to injury, but assault to injury if the patient had a prolapsed disc.

THORACIC SPINE AND RIBS: CHAPTER OVERVIEW

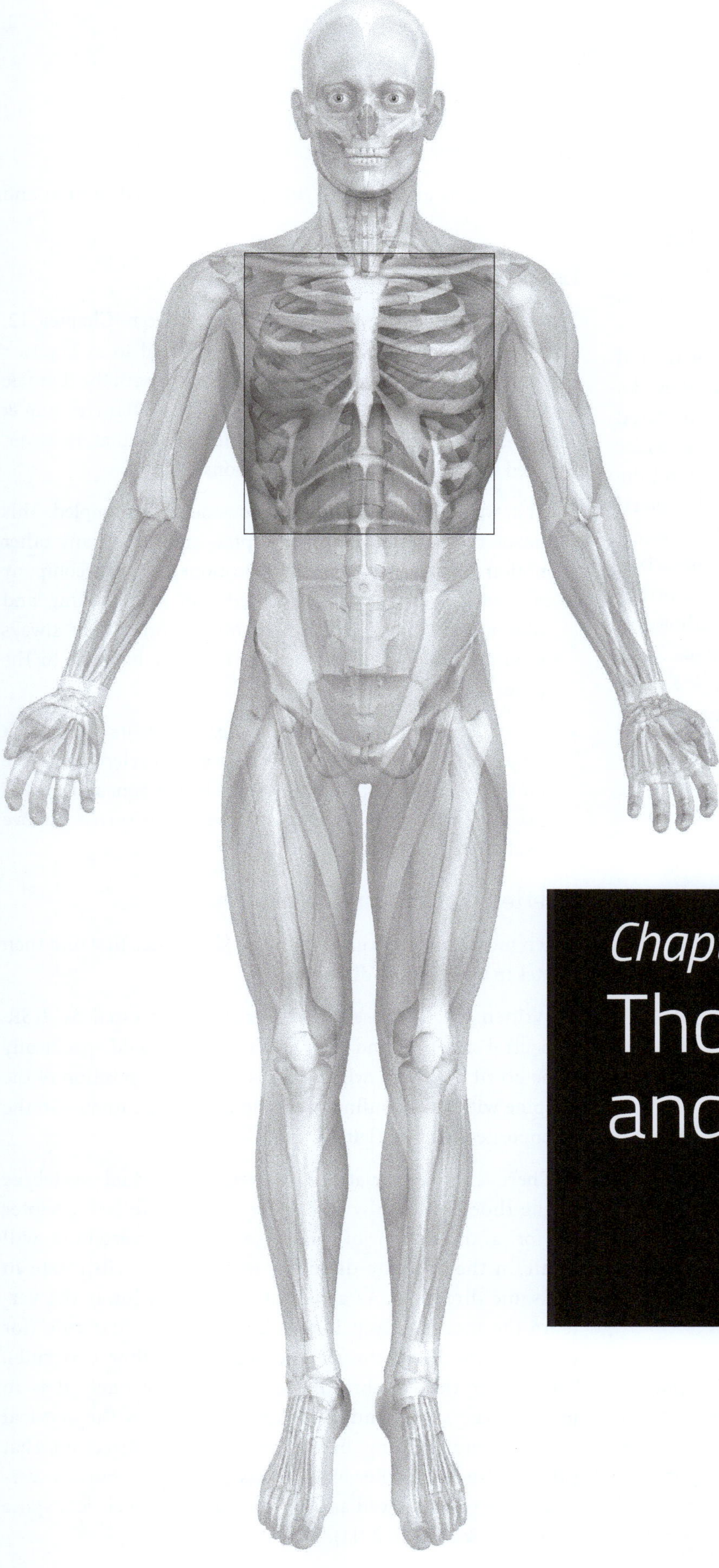

Chapter 13

Thoracic spine and ribs

Clinical implications of anatomy and physiology

This section presents some anatomical observations that have clinical implications. Understanding the functional relationships (physiology) between structures and tissues (anatomy) will help explain how structures of the thoracic spine and ribs can be injured, and help us understand how orthopedic and motion tests work to provide the information that they do. Please review the anatomy of the joints and muscles involved in the function of the thorax. It is suggested that the reader have an anatomy book at hand to more easily understand the information given below (either a general musculoskeletal book or a text that reviews anatomy in detail of this specific area of the body). The information that has been summarized here has been chosen because of its direct relevance to orthopedic testing and understanding of mechanical pathologies of the thoracic spine and ribs (Agur et al. 2014; Bogduk 2012; Chila 2010; DeStefano 2011; Dutton 2012; Hertling & Kessler 2006; Levangie & Norkin 2011; Magee 2014; Maitland 2001; Mitchell 2004, 2005; Schuenke et al. 2014).

Review the following anatomy:

- thoracic vertebrae shape and variations
- intervertebral discs and joints
- rib shape and variations
- rib joints
- ligaments
- musculature
- intercostal nerves
- arteries veins and lymphatic vessels.

Active range of motion for the thoracic spine

Flexion = 20–45°

Extension = 25–40°

Side-bending = 20–40°

Rotation = 40–55°

See the Appendices for charts and tables on muscles (muscle origin insertion innervation action and synergists), joints (actions ranges muscles used tissues stretched and compressed), a table on capsular patterns (of restriction, open packed/resting positions and close packed positions) and several charts on neurological testing where any such testing would involve this chapter's region.

Definitions for spinal motions

For definitions and detailed discussion on spinal motion and references see Chapter 12.

Group and segmental facet joint motions

Presented here is *a brief review* gleaned from Chapter 12. We need to review what is commonly referred to as Fryette's rules of spinal movements. These rules apply to both the thoracic and the lumbar spine (Chila 2010; DeStefano 2011; Hertling & Kessler 2006; Mitchell 2004, 2005). Before we do that, however, we need to make a couple of observations.

- First: we must note that spinal movements are coupled. This means that any motion of the spine impacts on any other motion, and further, that some motions always accompany each other. It has been proposed that side-bending and rotation are always coupled. In other words, they always occur together whenever one or the other happens in the spine.
- Second: any motion in Fryette's rules derives its name from the perspective of the vertebrae above with reference to the one below. Therefore, to say a vertebra is side-bent and rotated is to say that relative to the vertebra below the vertebra above is side-bent and rotated.

Fryette's first rule of spinal movements

When moving from neutral the spine side-bends first and then rotates in the opposite direction.

- Written out in short form the rule is expressed as: NSR, neutral side-bent and then rotation. This would specifically be noted as: NSrRl, which stands for neutral position of the spine with side-bending to the right and then rotated in the opposite direction (left).

There can be variations between individual vertebrae in the thoracic spine with respect to this rule (see Chapter 12 for a discussion of this issue). Some vertebrae will rotate in the opposite direction while others will rotate in the same direction. As a rule of thumb, the lower the vertebra the more likely it is to follow Fryette's first rule (for example, the lumbar vertebrae generally follow this rule). The higher the vertebra, however, the more likely it is to move in the same manner as the vertebrae in the cervical spine, where rotating occurs in the same direction that side-bending does. Because of this the upper thoracic vertebrae are often viewed as an extension of the cervical spine (Levangie & Norkin 2011).

Fryette's second rule of spinal movements

When the spine is already non-neutral, i.e., when in flexion or extension rotation happens first and then side-bending both in the same direction.

- Written out in short form as FRSr (flexion) or ERSr (extension).

Fryette's third rule of spinal movements

Introducing motion to a vertebral joint in one plane automatically reduces its mobility in the other two planes.

Motion impairments

The first rule is often referred to as type I motion. When *type I impairments* occur and follow this NSR motion pattern they usually occur as a group, as in a scoliosis, for example. In other words, they are a *group dysfunction* where the vertebrae side-bend one way and rotate in the opposite direction. Group dysfunction is the term we will usually employ in this text.

The second rule is type II motion. When *type II impairments* occur and follow this motion pattern with the spine already flexed or extended they usually occur in isolation (single segment strains that happen with lifting and twisting as an example). They are *segmental dysfunctions,* where in each affected motion segment the superior vertebra side-bends and rotates to the same side. Segmental dysfunction is the term we will usually employ in this text.

Thoracic intervertebral disc (IVD)

A polyaxial joint accommodates any direction of motion including shear forces and compression. The ball-shaped nucleus pulposus inside of the IVD is a gel that helps accommodate the compressive forces exerted on the disc. It remains gel-like until middle age, when it becomes fibrosed.

The cartilaginous layers or annular fibers surround the nucleus like the layers of an onion.

The fibers of these layers are oriented in alternating diagonal directions with the occasional layer running up and down. This orientation gives the IVD integrity as it undergoes a wide variety of motions available to it.

- The nucleus pulposus is not compressible. In other words, it cannot be made smaller, though it can change shape if the annular fibers around it give way. The nucleus acts as the pivot around which the motions that occur in a motion segment happen.
- The annular fibers are compressible. The liquid in them can be shifted around the layers. As a motion segment side-bends to the left, for example, the annular fibers on the left compress and lose height while the fibers on the right increase in height by taking on the water/matrix squeezed out of the compressed portion. The superior vertebra tips to the left over the nucleus-pivot like a see-saw.

Note, however, if the cartilaginous layers are continually or forcibly put under stress their integrity can begin to break down. Then the gel-state nucleus will begin to push its way outward. The bulge created is often referred to as a herniated disc (literally a disc with a hernia). If the nucleus pulposus breaks out of its restraining annular fibers then we call it a disc prolapse, where the disc has a loss of height.

In the thoracic spine, the nucleus is roughly in the center of the disc (unlike the posteriorly positioned lumbar nucleus) in order to better accommodate the compressive force when the spine is in neutral. Because the motion of the thoracic spine is limited in scope due to the ribs it is very rare for one of its discs to herniate. Herniation would require the thoracic spine to undergo a severe traumatic event. For more on herniated and prolapsed IVD see Chapter 12.

Rule of threes for landmarking and palpating the thoracic spine

The spinous process (SP) of a thoracic vertebra can be quite long and at certain levels on a severe downward angle. Therefore, when we palpate a thoracic SP it can be quite difficult to locate the corresponding transverse process (TVP) for that specific vertebra. This rule is a mnemonic that helps us to remember the relationship between the SP of the vertebrae and the position of that vertebra's TVP. It is called "the rule of threes" because the thoracic spine is divided into four divisions of three vertebrae each (Mitchell 2004) (Figure 13.1 and Table 13.1).

REMEMBER: This rule of threes provides approximations of where to find the vertebra's TVP relative to its SP (Table 13.1). Only T1, T4, and T7 would most accurately be described by the rules that apply to their groups. The two immediately below each of these will vary slightly (and become increasing closer to the next rule). The last group of three each correspond pretty well with their rule, which is that T10 is most like the third group, T11 is like the second group, and T1 is like the first group.

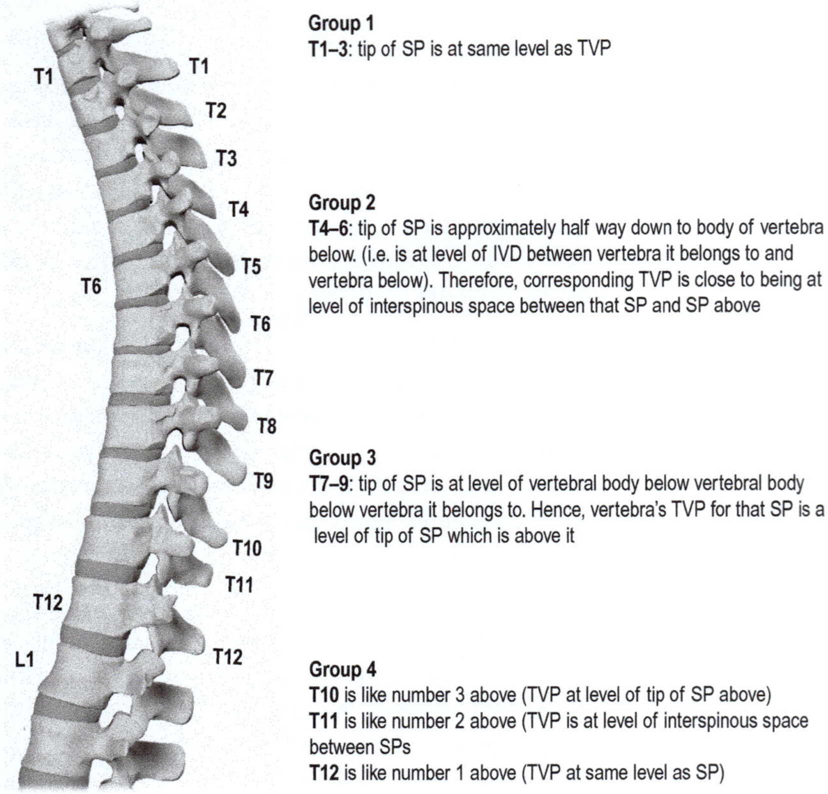

FIGURE 13.1 The thoracic spine. SP, spinous process; TVP; transverse process; IVD, intervertebral disc

TABLE 13.1
The rule of threes

Rule #	Vertebra	Location of TVP
1	T1, T2, T3, also T12	TVP at same level as tip of SP
2	T4, T5, T6, also T11	TVP at level of interspinous space
3	T7, T8, T9, also T10	TVP at level of SP of vertebra above

TVP, transverse process; SP, spinous process.

Comprehensive examination

This testing protocol is usually done when the therapist wants to perform a more detailed postural examination (static and dynamic) of the patient. If several of the tests underlined below are found to be positive, then a more thorough examination of the thoracic spine needs to be performed such as the one presented in the rest of this chapter. Pain asymmetries and other impairments on-site at the thoracic spine area can occur with standing, sitting or with motion from above or below, and also demand further investigation as either precipitating factors or consequence. For more detailed information and pictures see Chapter 10.

Standing postural views: front, side, side and back

1. Looking for relationships with gravity line: with plumb line check vertical landmarks, observe horizontal landmarks. Note asymmetries and tissue texture changes.

Sitting behind the patient note asymmetries and any restrictions to range of motion:

1. Landmark levels of arches of the feet, ischial tuberosities, trochanters, PSISs, iliac crest heights, (creases of) waist, inferior and superior angles of scapula, mastoid processes.
2. Return to PSISs. While landmarking PSISs have the patient bring the chin to the chest then slowly roll down to lumbar flexion while noting movement of the PSISs (standing flexion test). Then check the spine for flat spots, excessive curve, bulking of erector spinae, lateral curves, and the like. Then have the patient return to standing straight. Ask patient to look up to the ceiling (while you leave your hands on the patient's hips for their stability) and have the patient extend their back while observing changes to curves of the spine (lordosis-kyphosis).
3. Have the patient bring the ear to the shoulder; then have them slide the hand down the side of the leg to the knee,

observing how the spine curves during side-bending (from above). Check both sides.

4. Have the patient flex one knee while the other remains locked and note lumbar side-bending (from below). Check both sides.
5. Hold the patient's hip stable. Have the patient bring their chin over a shoulder and note head and cervical rotation; then have them bring that shoulder back toward you while observing thoracic rotation. Note also the difference in the amount of resistance required at the hips to resist lower trunk rotation (ease versus effort).
6. Challenge sagittal plane stability by a light push anterior-posterior via the manubrium and T2.
7. Challenge coronal plane (side-bending) motion either by pressure on the acromions or inferiorly directed tug on the wrists.

Have the patient sitting:

1. Re-check iliac crest heights, PSISs, shoulder/scapula landmarks, tissue bulk, etc. Observe all changes of orientation to landmarks, tissue changes etc. during the following:
2. Seated flexion test. While landmarking PSISs have the patient flex forward. Check for asymmetry of tissue bulk on either side of spine.
3. Side-bending. With the elbow at 90°, the patient brings the ear to the shoulder then lowers the trunk toward the table.
4. Rotation. Turn the chin toward the shoulder and at end-range push the shoulder back.
5. Challenge to side-bending. Push down alternately on each shoulder cap.

Patient supine: (after traction of legs or other corrections to the patient's orientation)

1. Note medial malleoli levels.
2. Check ASISs
   - level (for innominate rotation)
   - heights from table (for pelvic rotation)
   - distance from mid-line (for inflare/out-flare).
3. Check rotations (fascial exam). Compare heights from table of hips (ASISs, as earlier), lower ribcage, upper ribs, anterior shoulders and L and R occiput
   - i.e. height from table compared to norm and compared one to the other bilaterally and then compare directions of rotation from one set of landmarks to the next.
4. Push the following side-to-side comparing ease/bind (testing side-bending): at waist (lumbars), *mid-ribs* and neck (cervicals).

When or if specific testing has the patient prone check the following:

1. Levels of plantar surface of heels, ischial tuberosities, PSISs (and height from table) and the *lateral curves in spine, tissue bulk of erector spinae and scapula orientation.*

The testing protocol (Box 13.1) begins with the case history.

Box 13.1 Protocol

Case history

Observations

Active free range of motion (AF-ROM)

Passive relaxed range of motion (PR-ROM)

Active resisted range of motion (AR-ROM)

General testing of the ribs

Case history (specific questions)

- Any sudden sharp pain in the thoracic area with specific movements (or activities)?
- Is this a result of a fall or accident?
- Is this a result of any strain such as from lifting or carrying; or an awkward movement?
- What activities of daily living is this (impairment) affecting?
- Do you ever experience pain in the mid-back with coughing or sneezing? With bowel movements?
- What positions are you most often in during the day? Such as sitting standing or performing repetitive movements for extended periods of time?
- Is the pain local or does it travel?
- Does your mid-back feel weak or fatigued? Do you experience an achiness that does not alter with movement? – However, some momentary relief while in flexion?
- Have you recently had a cold, flu, bronchitis, or any chest congestion? Any long bouts of sneezing or coughing prior to your symptoms?

- Do you have any diagnosis of arthritis in the spine? Disc herniation? By X-ray, MRI?
- Ask the patient if they have noticed any sharp pain in the spine or ribcage when they might have taken a deep breath. If they have – or even if they have not – the therapist should ask them to do so now. Instruct them to do so slowly and to stop if they experience pain. If the patient complains of a sharp pain upon deep inhalation this may be an indication of a subluxed rib. Ask the patient if they can describe where they feel the pain (which side approximate spot on the spine etc.). The therapist should gently palpate over the junction between the thoracic vertebrae and ribs in the general area the patient reported and have the patient say when the exact spot (if possible) is reached.

Observations

See the postural assessment material in Part I, Chapter 5 for details concerning specific postural patterns and tissues involved. Some of this material is presented in Chapter 12 as well.

Light inspection palpation

Assess tissue texture changes to skin and connective tissue of the back. The appearance and feel of tissue texture changes can imply joint impairments under their presence, or at the spinal root level (via the sympathetic ganglion) that innervates the dermal area where these tissue texture changes occur. Check for heat or coolness over joints and musculature. Look for bruising, lacerations, redness or blanching of the skin. Also, look for any sign of autonomic or sympathetic responses such as areas of the skin showing a pilomotor response ("goose bumps"), patches of skin that differ in dryness or where the skin's pores look different than the rest of the back (larger or smaller).

NOTE: Use light palpation at this time, as techniques such as skin rolling may cause pain and interfere with testing results. Many of the palpable skin changes come from altered neurovascular perfusion to the tissue. A common reason for this is an altered sympathetic response to impairments in the joints and tissues associated with that area.

Standing postural examination

It is very important to have the patient stand in a natural pose. To assist in this, ask the patient to look up slightly (i.e., you do not want them watching their feet), and have them take a couple of steps while staying in place. Tell the patient to try not to correct feet positions, head positions, etc. You are trying to have them stand as they naturally do, or as close to natural as possble given that they are in a clinical setting. Recognize that much of this standing postural information is needed to compare with supine and prone examinations, so that we are not misled by what we see or do not see when the patient is on the table.

Note the following:

- orientation of the upper body, especially rotations and side-bending of the shoulders or spine
- orientation of the hips, thighs, knees, tibias, ankles, and feet. Looking to see if the hips are shifted right or left over a leg, proportions (tissue bulk) and orientation of the thigh and lower leg. Some examples include: rotations throughout the course of the limb down to the feet, varus or valgus of knees or ankles and arches of the feet.

Be very specific and exact with the following:

- Check iliac crest and greater trochanter heights.
- Record ASIS and PSIS heights from the anterior, posterior, and lateral views. Compare heights of the ischial tuberosities.
- Note pelvic obliquity. This is the change in height of one hip compared to the other, which may be due to a unilateral anterior or posterior rotation of the innominate, for example.
- Note whether the pelvis appears rotated around a vertical axis. In other words, does one ASIS (hip pointer) appear more anterior than the other (in the coronal plane), whether the ASISs are level with each other or not.
- Note whether one shoulder is higher, and so too for the scapula (by landmarking with inferior angle).
- Note if one shoulder is more forward. The lower shoulder usually is, and is often closer to the mid-line.
- *Note if the upper thoracic cage is rotated.* Usually the lower and forward shoulder points to rotation toward the other side, but check! If the patient is compensating, then this rotation may be opposite to any hip rotation. If not compensating, then it may be rotated to the same side as the hip.
- Observe if the patient has shifted the pelvis to one side over a leg, which then usually becomes the principal weight-bearing leg.
- Note any lateral curves in the spine (scoliosis).
- Note whether the patient has a hyperlordosis or a hypolordosis of the lumbar spine, or of the cervical spine. Observe whether the lumbar spine seems rotated and/or side-bent.
- Note whether the thoracic spine is hypokyphotic or hyperkyphotic (Box 13.2).

Box 13.2 Observations made of a forward head posture and hyperkyphosis (Figure 13.2)

Hyperkyphosis in the thoracic spine means the upper and mid-thoracic spine is more flexed than normal while the lower thoracic segments are more extended. The increased flexion in the upper and mid-thoracic spine stretches the musculature on the back at these levels making them long and therefore weaker/inhibited.

In turn the upper and middle ribs are depressed leaving the rib-cage fixed and held as if the person is always exhaling, thereby decreasing lung capacity. This shortens the pectoralis major and minor, pulling the shoulders forward with the scapula protracted.

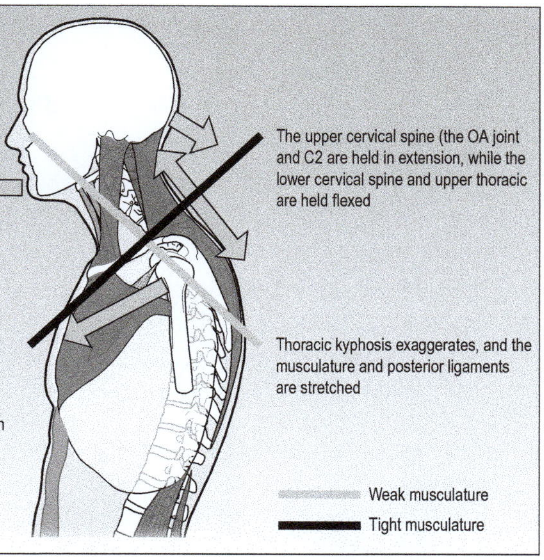

- Note if there is notable asymmetry to the look and shape of the ribs.
- Note the shape and orientation of the thoracic cage. Does the ribcage look inflated or inhaled (as if the patient is holding their breath), or does it look exhaled (as if the patient had completely breathed out and is holding that position)? Is there any abnormal shape to the ribcage?

From your observations consider if you have found any possible causes or suspicions for the patient's chief complaints. Did you find any postural or other structural faults that may predispose the patient to further impairments (not yet present)? Some of this can be answered by deciding which muscles may be short and tight, and which may be long and weak. Other possibilities may be found by asking: which joints may be under extra tensile or compressive stress? Are any ribs (and hence the lungs) being compromised, and is the neurovascular flow to the upper extremities (or anywhere else) possibly being compressed?

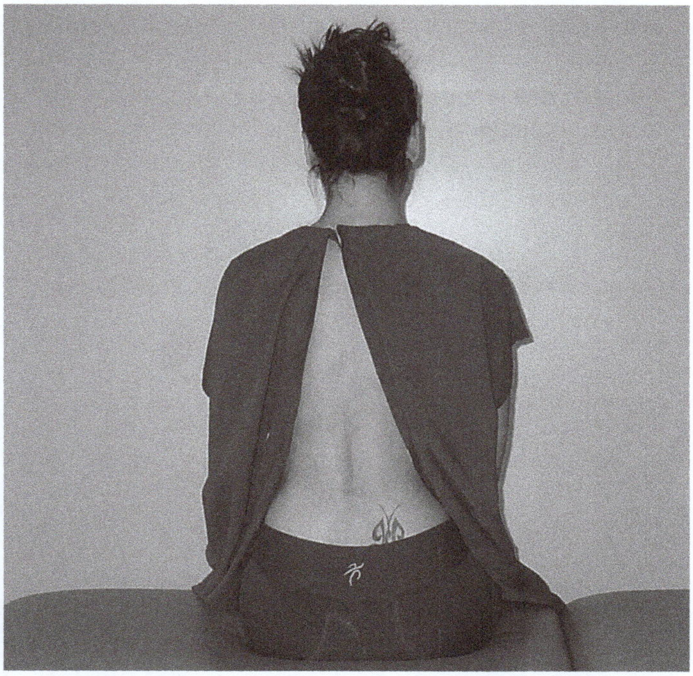

FIGURE 13.3 Observing the T-spine

The patient can be seated during testing to reduce motion that could come from hips and lower body. The therapist may wish to use a gown that opens in the back to clearly see the contours of the spine, ribs, and muscles.

Range of motion testing (ROM)

Have the patient seated if possible when testing ROM. This helps reduce the amount of motion that could come from the hips and the lower body. Try to have as much of the spine visible as is practical.

Chapter 12 has a more detailed list of tissues that may be revealed as involved in the patient's pain or impairment by testing different ranges of motion whether in AF- or PR-ROM testing.

During AF-ROM and PR-ROM we will often be palpating the spine and usually in the area over the TVPs. As the spine is made up of many joints we need to evaluate each level and each side if we are going to adequately test how these joints are functioning.

> *INSIGHTS*
>
> **Box 13.3 Isolating the thoracic spine from the rest of the spine: what to do?**
>
> You can have the patient clasp their hands behind their head or more specifically, behind their neck. This is done in order to help stabilize the cervical spine and reduce movement there. Of course this position requires the use of most of the shoulder musculature, which is going to impact on the thoracic spine and will skew results. If this proves uncomfortable for the patient then have them cross their arms in front.
>
> Because of problems in isolating the thoracic spine it could be argued that it may be best to avoid trying. Therefore, natural movements through anatomical planes may be the most informative. Again, as with all areas of the spine the interrelatedness of joints and tissues makes it impractical to localize all tension and motion to just one specific area. You will have to rely on your clinical judgment and experience in choosing how to do your testing. How the patient presents and what stage of treatment they are at can provide clues about what would be best for testing the thoracic spine, even if only for that specific appointment.
>
> We will present the testing with various options to give some idea about the spectrum of ways to do ROM testing in the thoracic spine.

The observations of general motions described next in AF-ROM are used to highlight areas that need the more focused testing of motion-palpation.

Observing the T-spine during testing (Figure 13.3)

Further information about observing the thoracic spine can be found in Box 13.3.

Active free range of motion (AF-ROM)

General flexion and extension of the thoracic spine (Figures 13.4–13.7)

Once you have observed the general presentation of the thoracic spine in neutral have the patient forward flex the thoracic spine, or rather, have them slump forward in order to have most of the motion come from the thoracic spine. At this time, you may want the patient to hold this position if it is pain-free while you palpate the SPs to see if they have opened up and/or are tender.

As all the vertebrae function together some thoracic motion is going to go into the lumbar and/or cervical portions of the spine. Therefore, in side-bending (aka *lateral flexion*) we would not say that the thoracic portion of the spine has reached its limit of side-bending as soon as the lumbar spine began to move. The intervertebral discs are slightly compressible and for them to reach their maximum contribution to side-bending the whole trunk must be involved. So too for the discs' contribution to rotation which is involved in side-bending, even if minimal.

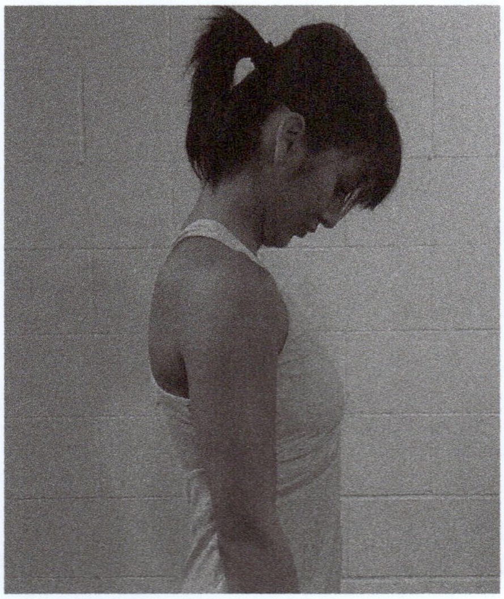

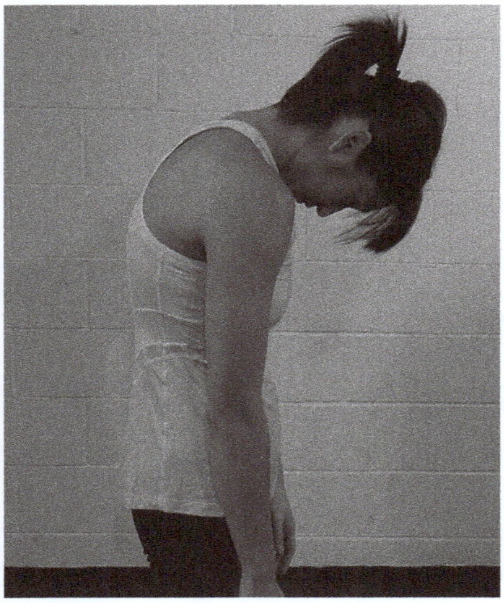

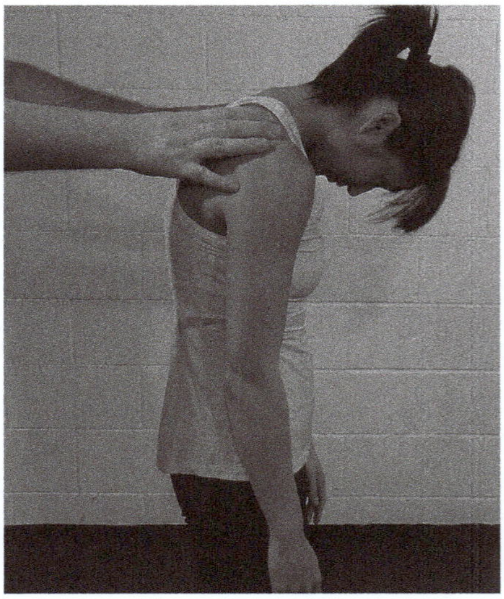

FIGURE 13.4–13.6 Flexion of thoracic spine

Ask the patient to bring the chin to the chest and then to slump forward. Palpate over flat spots or excessively flexed areas. If standing, the patient should be instructed not to bend forward from the hip.

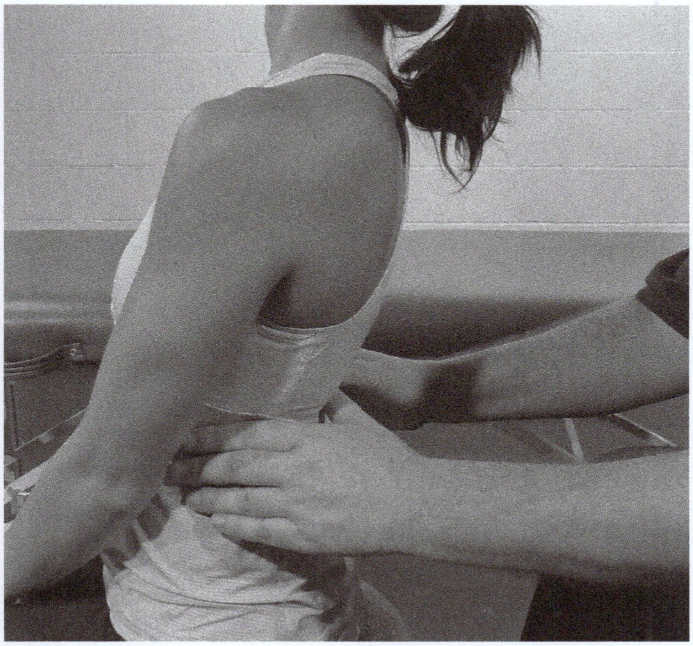

FIGURE 13.7 Extension of thoracic spine

Have the patient arch the back. Make sure the patient does not extend from the hips as they will unavoidably extend the lumbar spine while trying to reach end-range of thoracic extension. Ask the patient to avoid extending the head. In other words, ask them not to look up as they arch the middle of the back.

Note: *Never* apply over-pressure to the extended spine.

The point here is that we need to keep our focus on the thoracic spine so that we are not misled by unavoidable movements of lumbar or cervical vertebrae. To watch carefully for when movement begins and ends in the thoracic spine (and further motion is coming only from below it, for example) it may help during AF-ROM to place the index finger of one hand on T1 and the index finger of the other hand on T12 as an aid to focus specifically on the thoracic spine's movements or restrictions.

If there is no pain or reproduction of any impairment, then the therapist may choose to apply gentle over-pressure (O-P) towards flexion. If so, then the end-feel can be noted now. In other words, PR-ROM need not be repeated later. (See Part I, Chapter 3 concerning range of motion testing; see also Chapter 12, Lumbar spine, for a fuller discussion about the use of over-pressure.)

Scoliosis

If the patient has a lateral curve (scoliosis) in the thoracic spine that is seen in neutral and this curve does not substantially change during flexion or extension then a group dysfunction or scoliosis exists. The patient may well not report any pain or increase in discomfort stemming from motion through a scoliosis but a loss of range mostly seen in side-bending or rotation can be observed.

In a scoliosis of the thoracic spine the side the vertebrae are rotated towards will cause the tissue/muscle above their TVPs to be lifted. In neutral, this is observed as one side of the spine having more bulk. When the patient bends forward this look of bulk will be further exaggerated by the rotated ribs of those vertebrae creating the appearance of a "hump" on one side of the spine. Since group dysfunctions follow the rule of side-bending to one side and rotating to the other the thoracic spine will be side-bent or curved to the opposite side to which we see the hump. If this humping is on the right, for example, then we can infer that the thoracic spine at those levels is rotated right and side-bent (concave) left *if that portion of the thoracic spine is following Fryette's rules.* Confirmation may come (as to whether they are following the rule or not) when the therapist compares the quality of motion as the patient side-bends to one side and then the other.

Remember that we name a scoliosis for the side of the convexity. Therefore, in the example used we say that the patient has a scoliosis on the right. We record the curve by naming it for the apex of the curve. If the scoliosis is to the right and the middle of the curve (which should be the point farthest from the mid-line of the body) is at T5 then we have the notation C curve R T5. If we have an S curve which means that we have a compensatory curve present, then we note for example:

S curve – Superior C R T5, inferior C L T9.

A segmental dysfunction between two adjacent vertebrae may not be as directly observable by eye with flexion and extension of the thoracic spine. However, restrictions of motion and possibly pain may be indicators of the presence of such dysfunctions. Motion palpation which will be done shortly will find these segmental dysfunctions.

Side-bending motion in the thoracic spine (Figure 13.8A, B)

The therapist is looking for the symmetry of motion, etc., and observing the quality and quantity of the curve this motion makes in the thoracic spine compared bilaterally.

If the patient has a scoliosis they can often bend freely to the concave side and the curve may look normal. However, there will be restriction bending to the other (convex) side and the curve generated may have straight portions with the possibility

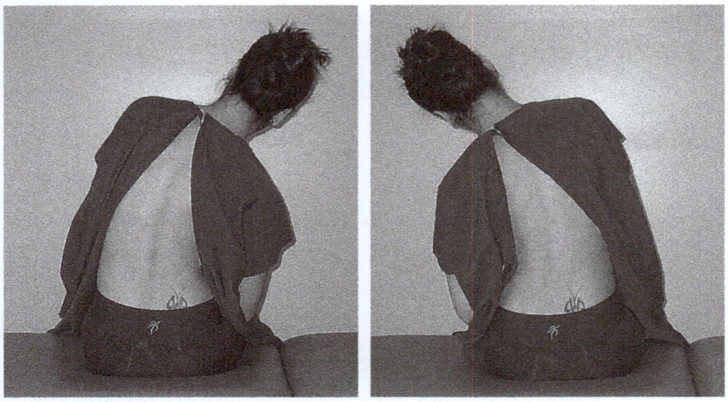

FIGURE 13.8A, B Side-bending of thoracic spine

Have patient side-bend right and left. Note quality of curve and quantity of movement.

of acute angulations above or below those. These sudden angulations or hypermobile joints are compensating for hypomobile joints (seen in straight portions). This implies a chronic curve because the hypermobility to compensate for loss of motion elsewhere usually takes time to develop.

Rotation of thoracic spine (Figure 13.9)

Stand in front of the patient and ask them to rotate to one side and hold and then to the other. They should have their arms crossed in front of them. With the arms crossed they are less likely to use their hands on the table to push themselves further into rotation. Further, when for example the patient is going to be asked to turn to the left the therapist should block the patient's right knee with one of their legs to prevent movement in the hips giving the appearance of more trunk rotation than is actually available.

Over-pressure (O-P) in AF-ROM side-bending and rotation

When the patient has reached their end-range for PR-ROM side-bending (or rotation) have them hold that momentarily as you ask them about pain or recurrence of their chief complaint. If there is no pain, then apply O-P. With O-P in rotation keep the knee blocked so that the O-P does not pass down into the pelvis but stays specific to the thoracic spine. Again, ask the patient about pain.

Passive relaxed range of motion (PR-ROM) of the thoracic spine (Figures 13.10–13.16)

Have the patient high-sitting at the end of the treatment table or on a stool. Ask the patient to cross their arms in front of their chest, placing their fingers on the opposite shoulder. When

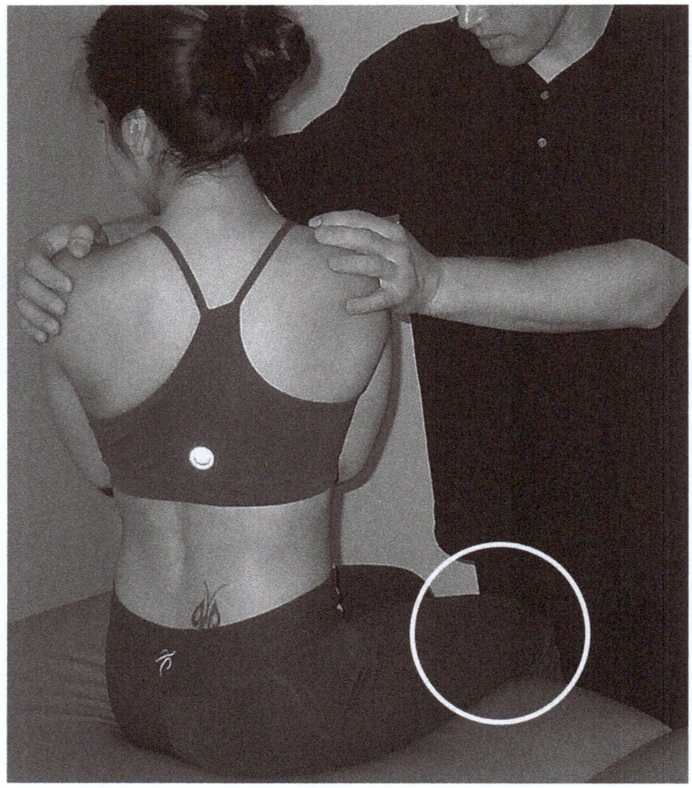

FIGURE 13.9 Rotation of thoracic spine

This ROM is best tested with patient seated to reduce movement of the pelvis and lower limbs so as to focus on movement in the spine. The therapist places their thigh against the patient's contralateral knee to note end-range (i.e., as the hips begin to move the patient's knee will be pushing forward).

end-range has been reached and only if there is no pain apply slight O-P to determine the joint's end-feel. There is no O-P done on extension of the thoracic spine.

Over-pressure (O-P) with side-bending and rotation

When the patient has been taken to their end-range for PR-ROM side-bending (or rotation) have them hold that momentarily as you ask them about pain or recurrence of their chief complaint. If there is no pain, then apply O-P. Keep the knee blocked so that the O-P does not pass down into the pelvis but stays specific to the thoracic spine. Again, ask the patient about pain. Repeat in the other direction.

Testing end-range of rib motion (Figures 13.17, 13.18)

This is a *quick test* to see if a rib dysfunction may be the cause of an apparent lesion in the thoracic spine; or to see the degree of impairment to rib motion due to a lesion in the thoracic spine.

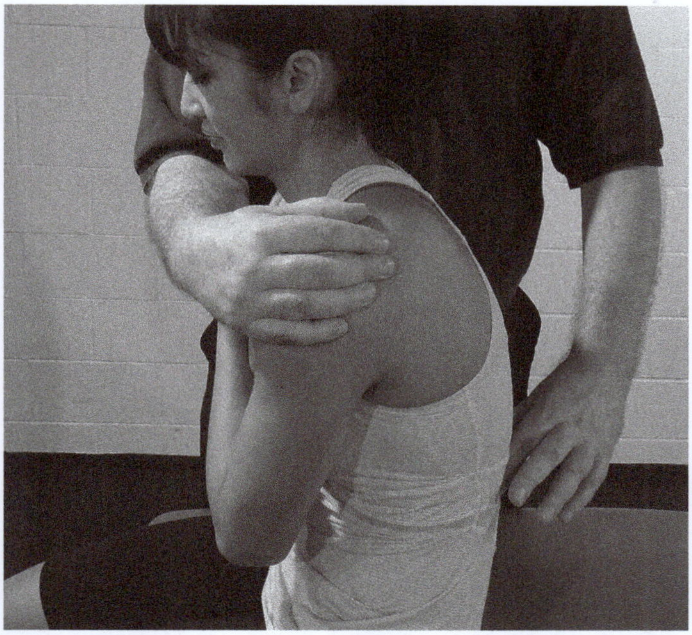

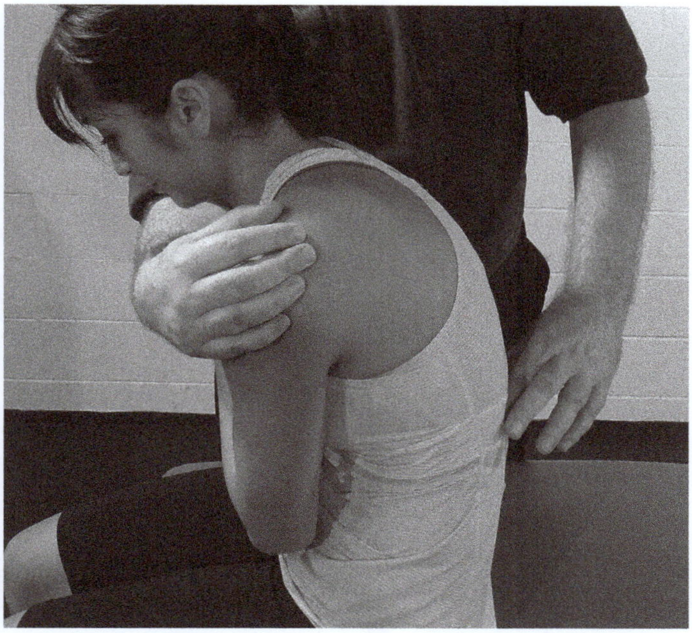

FIGURES 13.10, 13.11 PR flexion of thoracic spine

Reach across and place a hand on the far shoulder. Place the other hand on the upper thoracics. The patient relaxes, slumps forward, and lets you take their weight. Forward flex the thoracic spine until you note flexion is going through the lumbar spine.

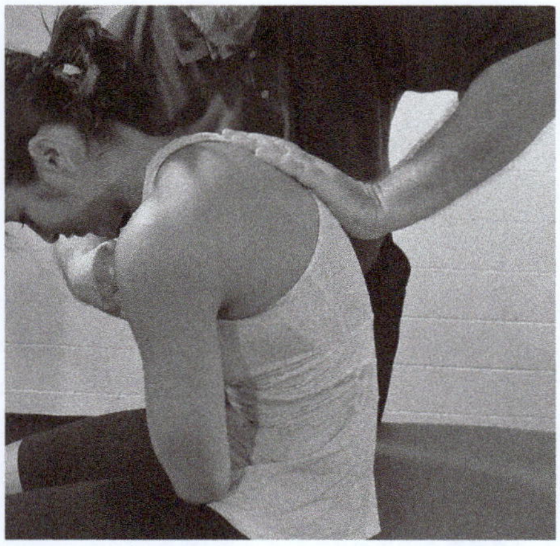

FIGURE 13.12 O-P flexed thoracic spine

Stabilize across the patient's clavicles while you press down through the upper thoracic vertebrae.

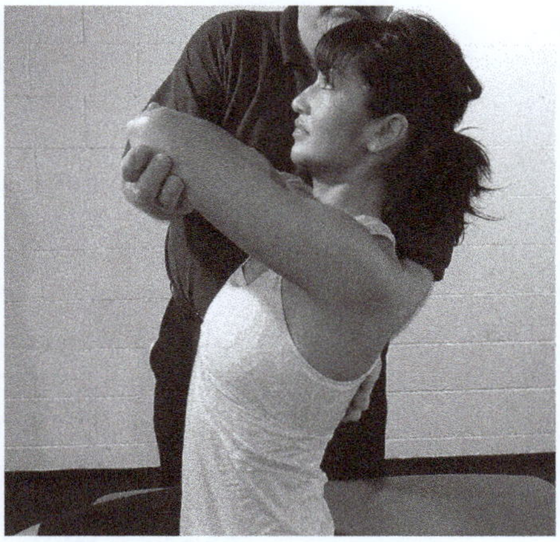

FIGURE 13.13 PR-ROM extension of thoracic spine

Bring the flexed patient to neutral. Reach underneath crossed arms and lift, placing the patient into extension.

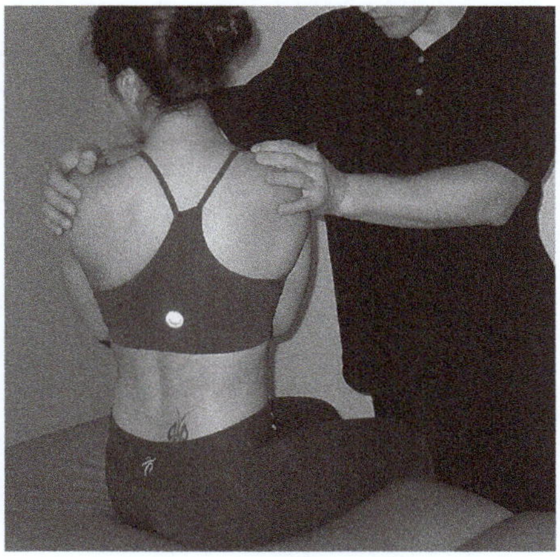

FIGURE 13.14 PR rotation of thoracic spine

Block the patient's knee with your leg. Rotate the patient to the other side. The knee pushing forward marks end-range. Block the other knee and rotate the opposite way. In this picture, the right knee is blocked with patient rotating left.

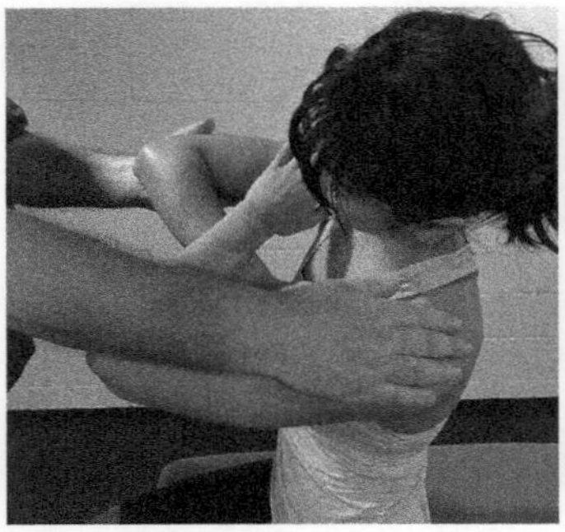

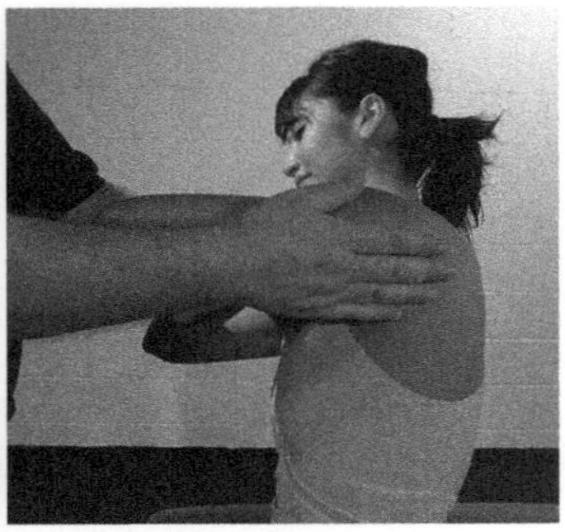

FIGURES 13.15, 13.16 PR-ROM side-bending thoracic spine
Stand in front of/behind the patient. Push down on one shoulder while you lift the contralateral side's arm.

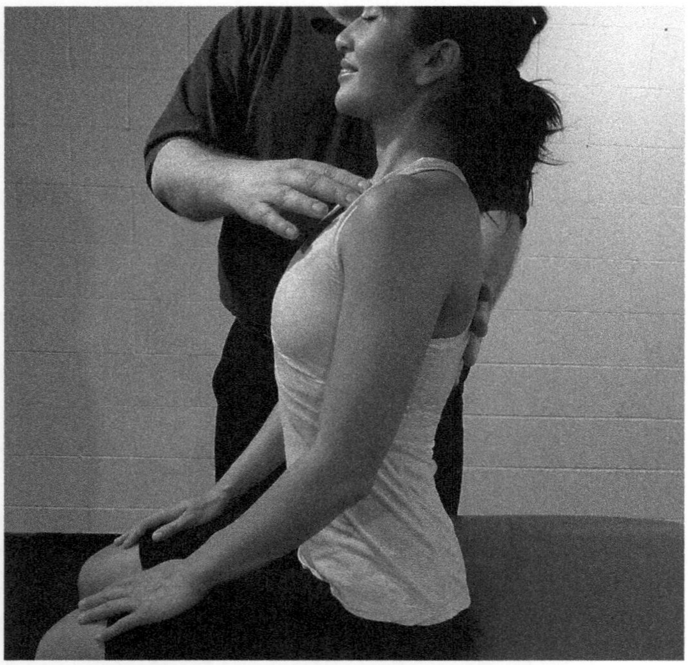

FIGURE 13.17 Full inhalation of breath
Have the seated patient slowly take in as deep a breath as they can and hold it for count of 5.

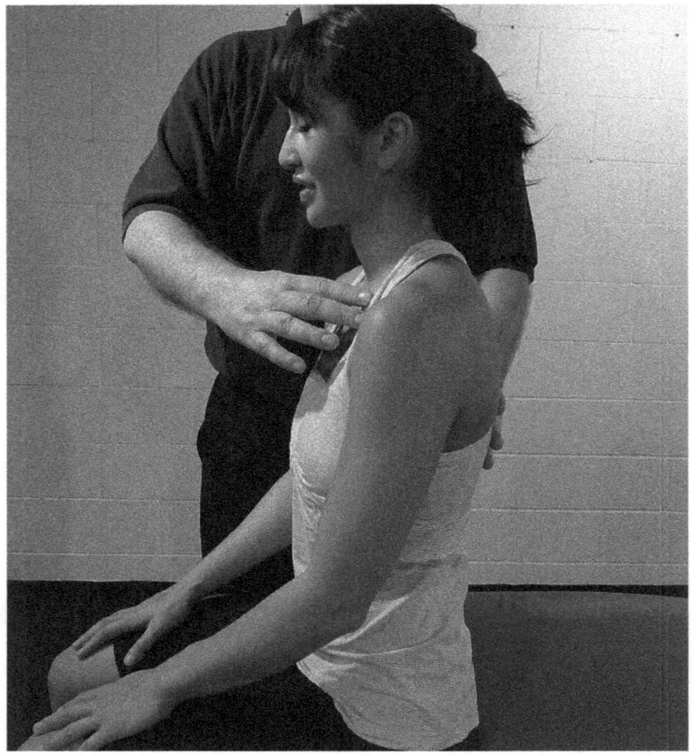

FIGURE 13.18 Full exhalation of breath
The patient exhales completely, emptying the lungs and compressing the abdomen, holding for count of 5.

After each of the tests ask the patient (as two separate questions) about: (1) the recurrence of their presenting complaint and (2) if there is any new complaint. If the patient complains of a sharp pain upon deep inhalation this may be an indication of a subluxed rib.

If the patient has good thoracic spine motion and rib motion you should notice that the curve of thoracic spine (and of the lumbar and cervical) flatten and lengthen on the in-breath and increase on the out-breath.

The therapist has two fingers on either side of the sternomanubrial joint, palpating the rise of the sternum on the in-breath and its fall on the out-breath. (This tests also the available motion of the sternomanubrial joint, but more on that later when discussing more specific testing of rib motion later in this chapter.)

Motion palpation of the thoracic spine

This would be the appropriate point in the protocol of assessing the thoracic spine to perform motion testing of the thoracic vertebrae for specific impairments to motion. The following joint mobilization testing for available joint play in the thoracic spine can often provoke sufficient pain or discomfort when performed on impaired motion segments. If that is the case, or suspected to be the case, then motion palpation testing will then be compromised. Therefore, do motion palpation first, then joint mobilization.

Further, caution should be taken here as many massage therapy programs may consider this testing (which can also be a treatment modality) as an advanced technique. Hence, it will be up to instructors to decide when or if this material will be taught in an assessment class. If the reader is a practicing massage therapist but has not had instruction in this material, they should seek out specific training from a qualified instructor. The author strongly urges the reader not to use this as a self-instruction manual for joint mobilization.

The material presented here is sufficient if studied with a qualified instructor, or as review for a practicing massage therapist who has had previous training in these joint mobilization techniques.

Joint mobilization of the thoracic spine

Specific joint mobilization techniques for the thoracic spine should be done only after any of the previous testing has been completed because these techniques can produce discomfort or pain that would then comprise such testing. Try to keep your hands relaxed as you apply pressure which comes from your body-weight rather than from muscular exertion. In other words, lean into your hands once they are positioned rather than pushing into the patient's tissue. Pressure *always* starts very light and gradually increases, just enough to feel the springy end-feel. *Always* keep communicating with the patient about what they are feeling, at every step: on landmarking, placement of hands, initial gentle pressure, during increasing pressure, at end-feel *and* on slow release and then after removing contact.

If all is moving as it should then you should feel a slight springiness as you lean. The patient should feel no pain. If there is pain or discomfort but movement (springiness) nonetheless, then there may be soft tissue injury (ligament joint capsule or intrinsic muscles of the spine) or osteoarthritic changes within the joints. If there is restriction or resistance to movement, there is a hard feeling under the mobilizing hand. Any movement felt is then often palpated or sensed above or below the restricted site. With restrictions to motion the patient may or may not feel pain or discomfort.

Ask about pain or any other symptoms and take note of both the quality and quantity of motion available in the joint. (For more details and instruction see Part I Chapter 3. Also, see the following for even more information and optional positioning of patient or limb and variations or additional tests: Starkey and Brown 2015; Kisner & Colby 2012; Edmond 2006; Hertling & Kessler 2006.)

Important: Before engaging in any joint mobilizations inform the patient that they need to immediately report any pain or other sensations felt either on-site or at a distance. If they have any such response then immediately start to remove your pressure (slowly, no sudden removal). Discuss with your patient what they felt and from this discussion decide how to proceed and/or if you need to refer out.

Joint mobilization of thoracic spine: flexion and extension

Anterior glide (ventral glide) (Figure 13.19)

Though thumbs can be used it is better to use the heel of the hand over the spinous processes (SPs). Use of the heel of the hand is easier on the therapist's hands and it gives a broader pressure which is usually tolerated better by the patient. The classic way of using the heel of the hand is to landmark and put the pressure through the pisiform.

The patient is positioned prone. Start at L1 to begin testing flexion of the thoracic spine. Landmark the spinous process of the vertebra that you are going to challenge. (Remember the rule of threes for locating the appropriate SP.) Using your body-weight lean onto the SP. *Do not move quickly* but rather increase the pressure over two or three seconds and then hold for two or three more seconds. Release the pressure over the same span of time.

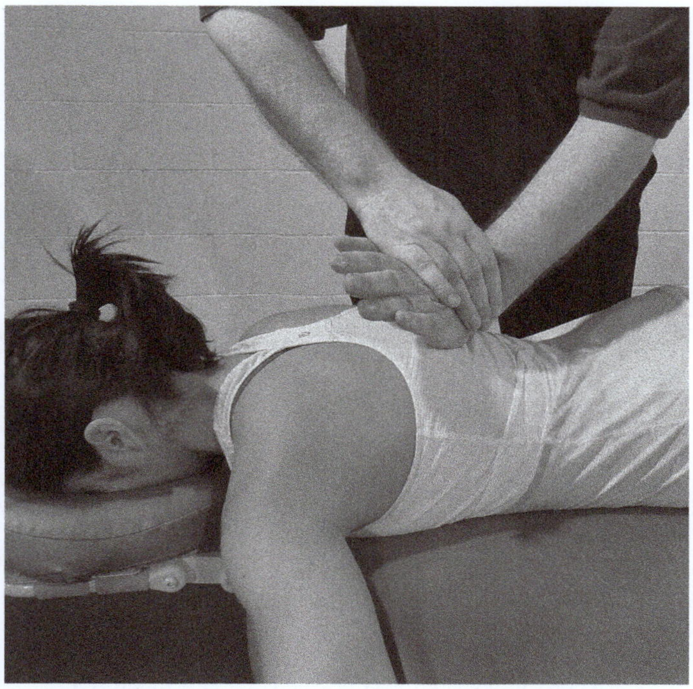

FIGURE 13.19 Thoracic joint mobilization for flexion and extension

Landmark SP of vertebra and apply downward (anterior) pressure via hypothenar eminence.

As most of the thoracic vertebrae have downward sloping SPs we are testing both extension and flexion of different motion segments. When pressure is applied we get more of a backward rotation of the vertebra than a straightforward motion because of the SP being lower than the vertebral body. Therefore, extension occurs between the vertebra below the vertebra being mobilized while flexion occurs between the vertebra mobilized and the vertebra above. For this reason, always begin your testing at L1 so that T12 is pushed into flexion on L1; and when pressing on T12 it will go into extension on L1 while T11 goes into flexion (Edmond 2006).

Rotation of thoracic vertebra by joint mobilization

With your thumb landmark the TVP belonging to the vertebra you wish to rotate. For example, landmark the right TVP of the vertebrae you wish to rotate to the left. Remember the rules of three! We are using the TVP to generate the motion of rotation as (1) it gives us a longer lever than the SP can, and (2) it is easier to block the motion of the vertebra below.

Testing rotation of several segments (Figures 13.20–13.22)

Described below is a general testing of a group of several vertebrae, though only the TVP of one receives the mobilizing force. In other words, applying pressure anteriorly over a TVP should cause that vertebra to rotate toward the opposite side. Pushing down on the left TVP of T6, for example, will encourage it to rotate to the right. Of course, the numerous interconnections

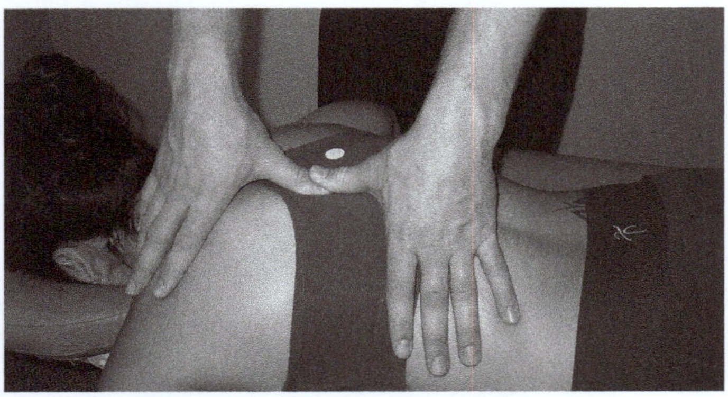

FIGURE 13.20 Group testing for rotation

Place one thumb over the lateral end of a TVP. Reinforce with the other thumb. Apply pressure downward (i.e., anteriorly). You should notice a springy feel as pressure is applied. If not, a hard rubbery resistance implies that one or several segments are restricted. As you proceed down one side the extent of restriction to rotation can be found.

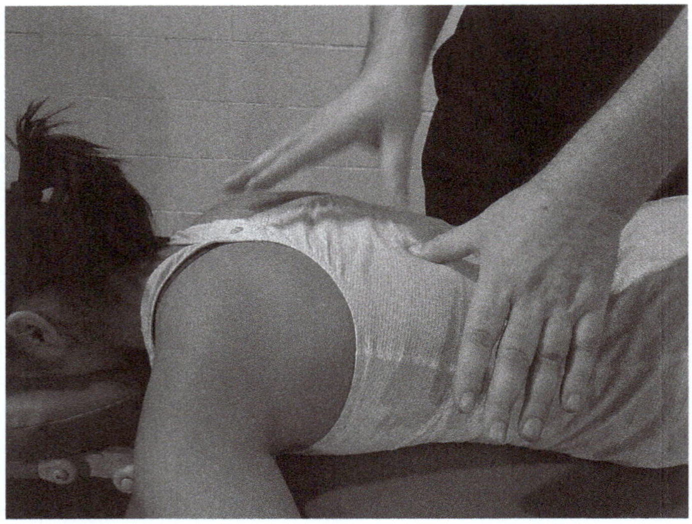

FIGURE 13.21 Landmarking TVPs for testing rotation within a motion segment

Palpate the TVP of the vertebra to be moved and the TVP of the vertebra below that is to be stabilized. In order to stabilize the inferior vertebra pressure will be applied anteriorly (down) on its TVP as soon as it attempts to move posteriorly.

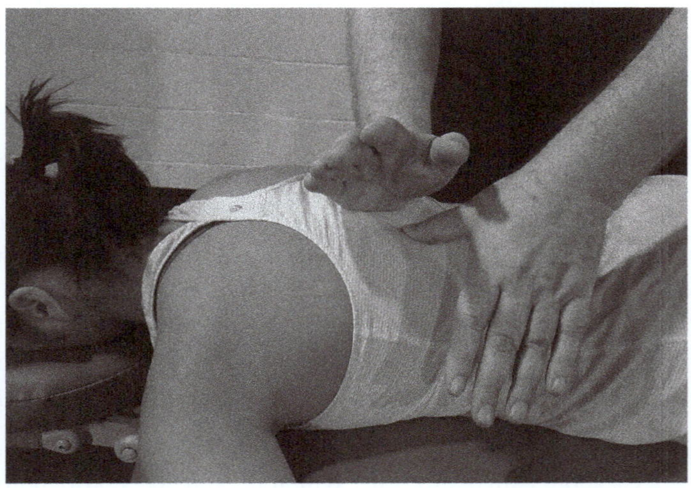

FIGURE 13.22 Rotating vertebra by joint mobilization

Press down (anteriorly) with your mobilizing hand while stabilizing the lower vertebra's TVP. Apply pressure slowly, starting very light. If rotation is available in this segment there should be a very slight and brief delay before the inferior vertebra begins to try and move in concert with its superior partner.

between vertebrae will transmit this force through one vertebra into those adjacent, above and below. A slight springiness should be felt as the mobilizing force is applied. However, if the rotation is restricted over several adjoining vertebrae there will be no sense of springiness.

Testing rotation within a single motion segment:

Now landmark the TVP of the vertebra below and on the side opposite to the mobilizing hand. For example, if you are trying to rotate T5 to the right your mobilizing hand is on the right TVP of T5 and your stabilizing hand's thumb is over the left TVP of T6. You press anteriorly (down) on T5's right TVP while you resist T6's left TVP moving posteriorly (resist T6 from rotating along with T5).

Always start a full investigation of the thoracic spine at T1 stabilizing T2's TVP/vertebra. For as T1 rotates it will want to rotate the vertebrae below it. However, stabilizing T2 also prevents the thoracic vertebra below T2 from moving. For example, when you arrive at the point to mobilize T5 and stabilize T6, vertebrae above T5 will rotate along with it while those below T6 should not move.

If the superior vertebrae cannot rotate without the inferior vertebrae moving, then rotation is not available in that motion segment.

Joint mobilization testing side-bending of thoracic vertebrae

Since we cannot get a finger on the superior or inferior aspect of a TVP it is difficult to mobilize a motion segment into side-bending. Pressing on a SP will more likely cause rotation than side-bending. *However*, since rotation and side-bending are coupled motions in the thoracic spine we are also testing side-bending when we test rotation. Remember that when you test rotation to the left you are testing side-bending to the right, according to Fryette's model; this is truer of the mid to lower thoracic spine while less so when testing the uppermost thoracic vertebrae.

Lateral translation (Figures 13.23–13.27)

There is some "translation-motion" between the vertebrae in a motion segment in all ranges of motion of the spine. The term "translation" describes when one of the vertebral bodies of a motion segment glides side-to-side over the one below. Therefore, an anterior glide (as discussed above) is a translatory motion occurring in flexion. Some translation also happens in side-bending, hence, lateral translation

When flexing or side-bending the strain of shear forces within the intervertebral disc can be at their highest, potentially damaging the integrity of the intervertebral disc (Costi et al. 2007). The amount of strain generated by the lateral glide as described below is far below those levels.

To try and achieve lateral translation or lateral glide the following needs to be done:

- Engaging the lateral area of the spinous process (SP) and pushing laterally into the SP. Be sure that your contact on the SP is fully on the lateral side of the SP.

To avoid over-using thumbs, it may be possible to use the pisiform area of the heel of the hand to apply lateral pressure. Let the hypothenar eminence sink between the lateral side of the SP and the paraspinals. You need to get deep enough into the tissue

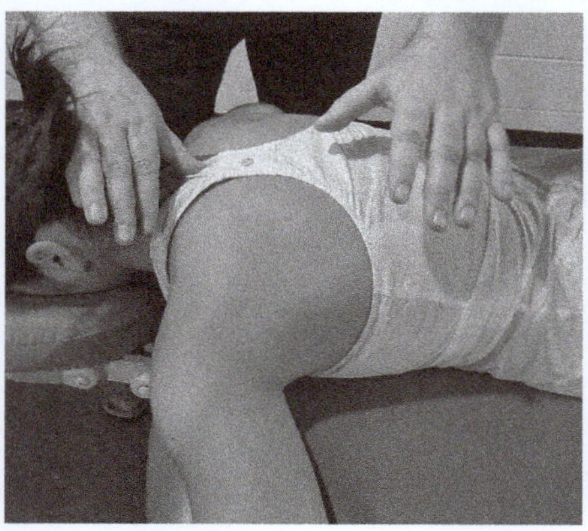

FIGURE 13.23 1. Lateral challenge of thoracic spine

Engage the side of the SP of the upper vertebra. Start at T1.

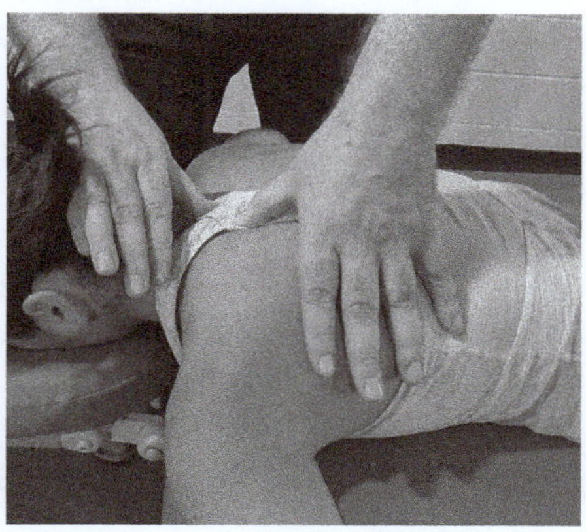

FIGURE 13.24 2. Lateral challenge of thoracic spine

Stabilize the lower vertebra's SP on the opposite side.

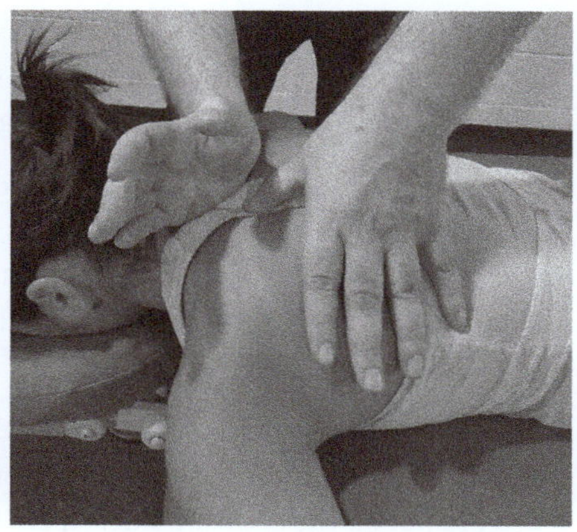

FIGURE 13.25 3. Lateral challenge of thoracic spine

Push laterally with the motion hand.

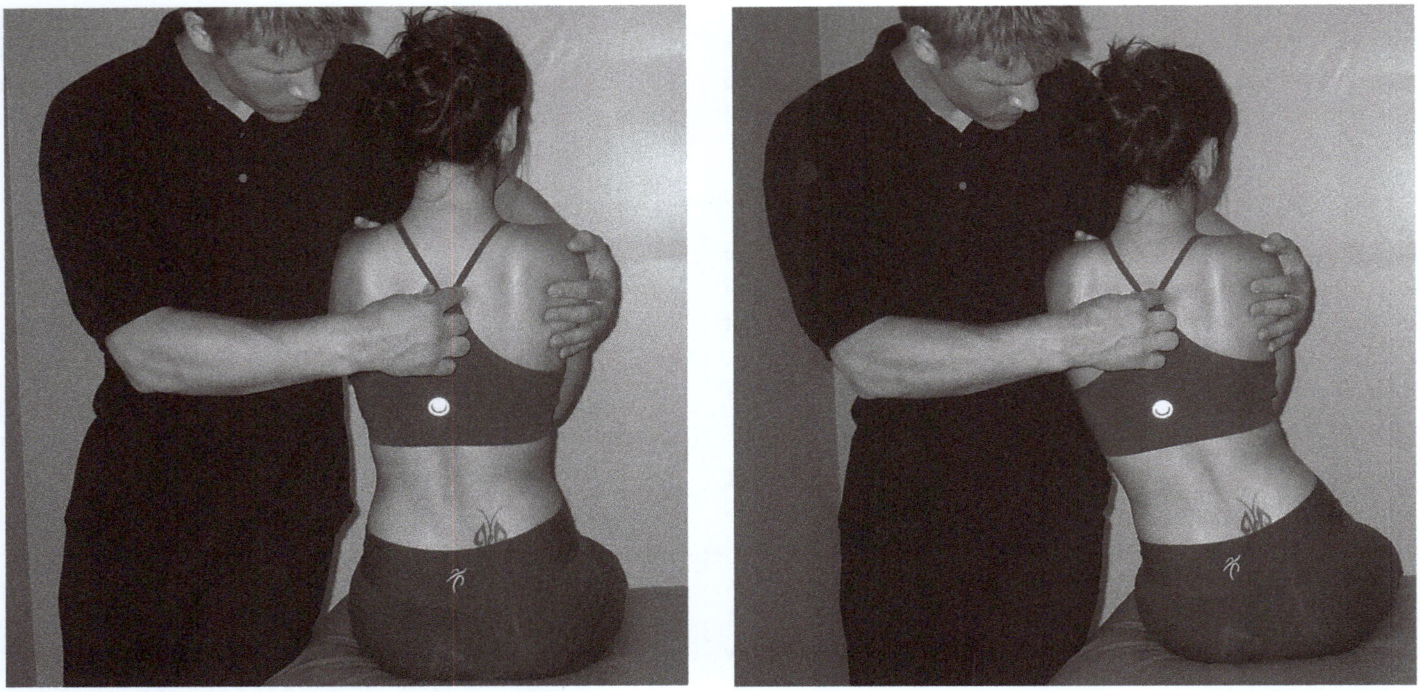

FIGURE 13.26 1. Positioning

FIGURE 13.27 2. Lateral glide

Have the patient high sitting on the end of the table. Have them cross their arms in front of them. Reach across and cup your hand over the uppermost part of their shoulder, and with the other palpate individual segments via their spinous process. Draw the patient towards you as you palpate. Return them to neutral, and move down one vertebrae at a time, repeating the side-bending and translation. Repeat on the other side.

beside the SP so that you are against the laminar or vertebral groove, or as close as possible, in order to get sufficient lateral glide or translation. If not, then you may end up applying a diagonal pressure on the SP. You can try using your thumb if need be.

Start at T1 and work your way down to T12. It is not uncommon when working with patients who are hyperkyphotic or hypokyphotic to have spasming paraspinal muscles. Translations or glides, if done slowly and carefully, can often reduce the tone of these muscles.

To stabilize the vertebra below the one you are about to translate place a thumb on the lateral side of the SP of the inferior vertebra but on the opposite side. Apply just enough pressure to resist any movement occurring in this lower vertebra.

The testing described above is not always easy to do. Issues such as hypertrophic tissues in the lamina groove may prevent getting the depth required to properly orienting the motion hand, or the pressure applied to the SP provokes discomfort or pain.

Alternative challenging of lateral translation (Figures 13.26, 13.27)

The following passive motion testing allows for palpating individual segments of the thoracic spine as they translate side to side. We are using side-bending to challenge lateral translation. This test is, strictly speaking, a PR-ROM form of testing. It has been placed here in order to further both our testing and our understanding of translation, the glide available between segments.

Active resisted range of motion (AR-ROM)

We can attempt to test a few groups of muscles responsible for motion in the thoracic spine but we will not be able isolate the testing to just to the thoracic spine. As you ask about pain weakness or other symptoms remember that almost all of the large musculature either comes up from the iliac crest or lumbar region or down from the shoulders and cervical areas.

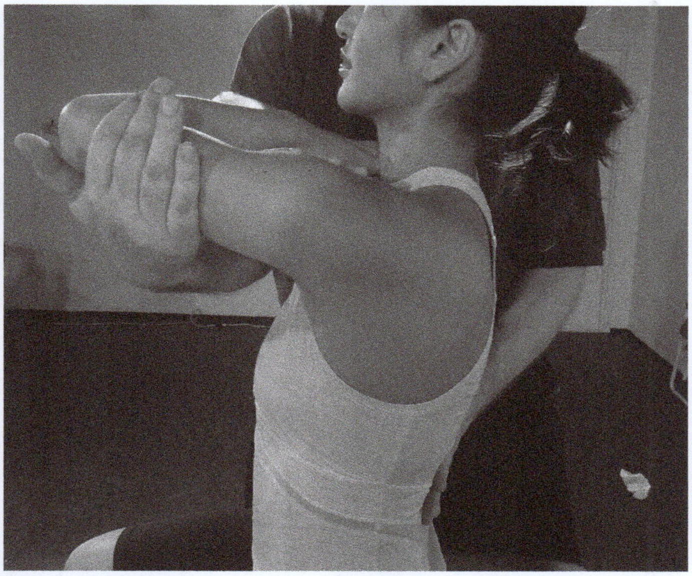

FIGURE 13.28 AR-ROM thoracic flexion

Ask the patient to slump forward as you resist.

There are numerous small muscles or muscles that tend to be de-conditioned in many people in the thoracic area. Therefore, make sure to reinforce to the patient that they need to start any effort with a minimum of strength and slowly increase their effort to maximum full strength. They must slowly relax when they are instructed to do so. Remind them that many times these smaller or weaker muscles can spasm upon exertions that are not often performed in everyday life.

Forward flexion (Figures 13.28, 13.29): Have the patient high-sitting on the table and have them cross their arms in front of them, holding them up. Hold the patient's forearms near their elbows. Instruct the patient to slightly slouch or slump forward just enough to slightly exaggerate their thoracic kyphosis. Try to ensure that they have not bent forward from the hips.

Even though the patient will be using their shoulder muscles to help in pushing against you, if they cannot stabilize (due to pain or weakness) the thoracic area the strain employed by the test will provoke symptoms there. Therefore, this testing is not true strength testing of the thoracic spine musculature but by the patient's response to the test they can help you locate painful tissues.

If the patient feels pain, weakness, or any symptom in the thoracic spine or rib area you should try to locate the area by palpation at the time before moving on to the next test.

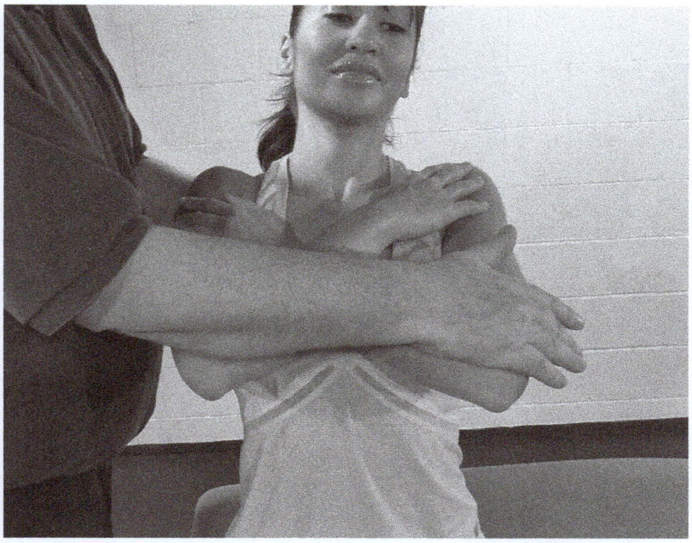

FIGURE 13.29 AR-ROM thoracic extension

Ask the patient to flatten the back as you resist motion through their crossed arms.

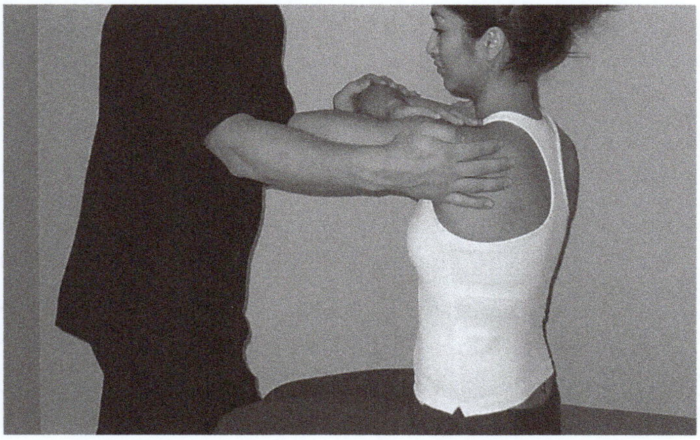

FIGURE 13.30 AR-ROM thoracic rotation

Resist the patient's attempt to rotate to the left. Reverse your hand and bracing positions to test rotation in the other direction.

AR-ROM thoracic rotation (Figure 13.30)

For this testing have the patient seated with their arms crossed in front of them. The therapist applies resistance through the patient's elbow and shoulder. For example, if the patient is going to try to turn left then the therapist resists at the right elbow and behind the left shoulder. Further brace the patient's (right) knee

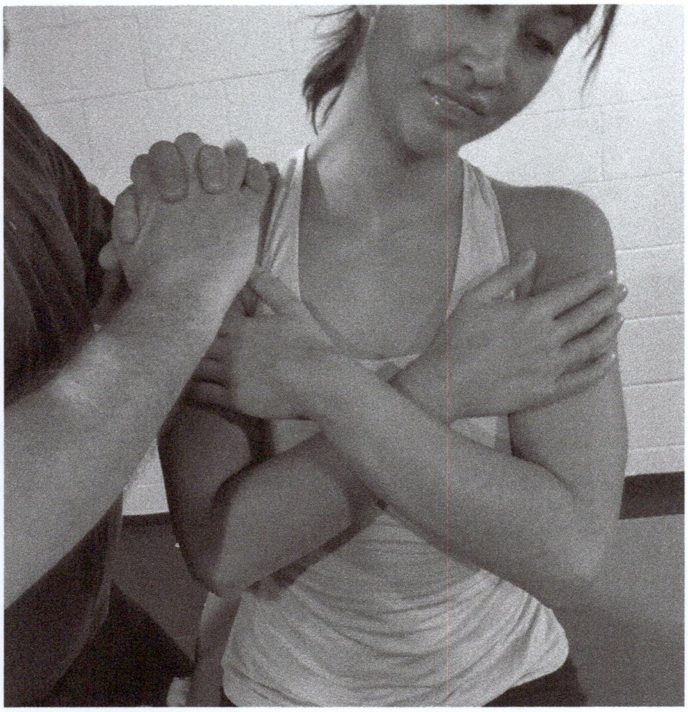

FIGURE 13.31 AR-ROM thoracic side-bending

Stand on one side of the patient. Clasp your hands together and place them over the top of the patient's shoulder. Ask the patient to try to side-bend away from you.

with your left thigh. Reverse your resistance and bracing to test rotation in the other direction (in this example toward the right).

AR-ROM thoracic side-bending (Figure 13.31): When testing for side-bending be sure to position yourself as close to the patient as possible to provide the best leverage for maximum resistance and your own safety.

Palpation of the ligaments of the thoracic spine (Figures 13.32A, B, 13.33)

We have access only to the supraspinous and interspinous ligaments. Pain originating from ligaments is not only felt locally but can refer away from the spine and out around to the lateral ribcage. One of the most serious consequences of any strained ligament (and its associated ligaments and tissues) is when it is over-stretched and becomes lengthened. This creates instability in the associated motion segments which threatens the neural structures of the spine. Associated muscles will then spasm to splint the area. This ligamentous laxity is one of the reasons why a patient's musculature around the spine will continually re-tighten after (or between) each treatment. We may well have restored too much motion to an unstable segment which requires the musculature to spasm once excessive motion again happens through the segment.

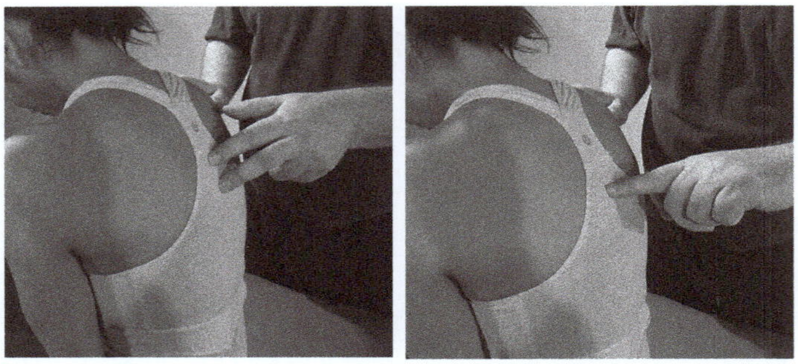

FIGURE 13.32A, B Palpating supraspinous ligaments

The patient slumps forward to open up SPs. Palpate over the SPs and between them.

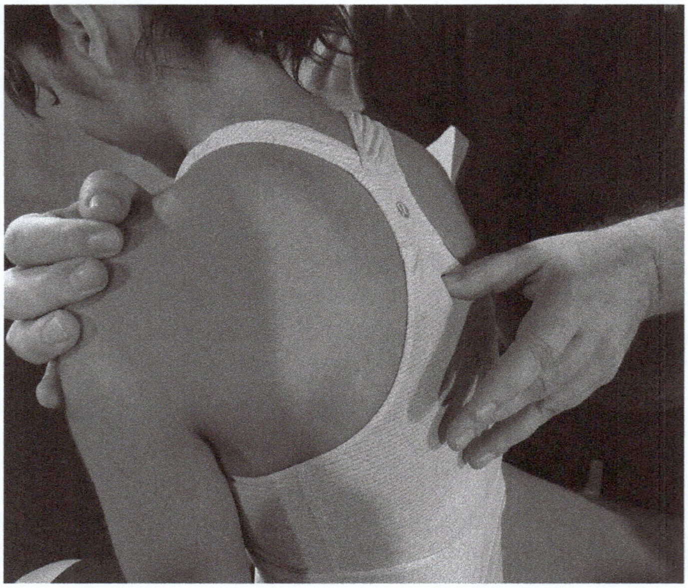

FIGURE 13.33 Palpating interspinous ligaments

The patient is still slumped forward. Press into the interspinous region from an oblique angle.

Have the patient seated with the thoracic spine slightly flexed. The flexion is required because the thoracic spinous processes have a tendency to lie almost on top of each other and therefore it is hard to palpate between them. Note any interspinous spaces that seem too far apart compared to the ones immediately above and below. Compare only above and below as those vertebrae and their SP shapes are most similar. Further if when slumped forward you still find the interspace between two adjacent vertebrae not opened then you need to investigate that motion segment for a flexion dysfunction.

Supraspinous ligaments are palpated running right along the very end or tip of the SPs. They will not only be sensitive in between spinous processes but also often along the tips of the spinous processes.

Thoracic spine neurological symptoms

Each dermatome corresponding to a spinal nerve root follows a rib around to the front of the body. For the levels and the skin that they innervate see the dermatome map of the upper body at the end of this chapter (Figure 13.73). In general, T2 to T11's intercostal nerves innervate the area only between the appropriate ribs.

Autonomic nervous system (ANS)

Sympathetic symptoms in the extremities can come from specific areas of the thoracic spine. The upper limbs are innervated by sympathetic ganglion at the level of T5 to T7. The lower extremities are innervated by sympathetic ganglion at the level of T10 to L2.

Table 13.2 is a chart of the various organs and areas of the body and the levels of the sympathetic ganglion that are responsible for their sympathetic nervous system innervation. Many schools of manual therapies (the most well-known being chiropractic and osteopathy) believe that lesions at specific spinal segments (from which the innervation of the corresponding sympathetic ganglion originates) can adversely affect that flow of neural information and as a consequence affect the corresponding tissues and viscera associated with those ganglion.

TABLE 13.2
Organs and areas of the body and their sympathetic nervous system innervation

ANS area of effect and visceral organs	Spinal cord level
Head and neck	T1–4
Heart	T1–5
Respiratory system	T2–7
Arms	T5–7
Upper gastrointestinal tract Stomach Liver Gall bladder Spleen Portions of pancreas and duodenum	T5–9
Middle gastrointestinal tract Portions of pancreas and duodenum Jejunum Ileum Ascending colon Proximal 2/3 transverse colon	T9–12
Lower gastrointestinal tract Distal 1/3 transverse colon Descending colon Sigmoid colon Rectum	T12–L2
Kidneys	T11–L1
Adrenal medulla	T10
Upper ureters	T10–L1
Lower ureters	L1–2
Bladder	T11–12
Gonads	T10=L2
Uterus and cervix	T10–L2
Legs	T10–L2
Erectile tissue of penis and clitoris	T11–L2

ANS, autonomic nervous system.

Motion palpation of the upper thoracic spine

For a more detailed explanation of motion testing and how to interpret your findings see the explanation in Chapter 12 (with examples) under motion testing of the lumbar spine. Nonetheless there is a lot of information throughout this section here for many therapists to be able to understand and employ this testing.

Ideally, this testing would take place prior to joint mobilization testing and AR-ROM since those forms of testing can induce pain or discomfort that could skew the results of motion testing if done right after them. However, we have placed it here so that the traditional flow of range of motion instruction remains.

This testing is done by observation and motion palpation (Chila 2010; DeStefano 2011; Mitchell 2004):

- We are looking for symmetry/asymmetry in vertebral alignment, both static and in motion.
- Looking for restriction of motion, or hypermobility.
- Looking for tenderness or any reproduction of the patient's complaints or impairments.
- We do this by noting whether the TVPs appear to be more prominent on one side of the spine than the other. If a group of vertebrae is rotated to one side the TVPs moving posteriorly

lift the tissue above them giving the appearance of more bulk to the tissue on that side of the spine.

- We may note a group of TVPs on one side and should see some side-bending (scoliosis) toward the opposite side of the prominent TVPs (a *group dysfunction*); or we may note a single prominent TVP, a *segmental dysfunction*.
- We can look at the spine standing, seated, or prone.

What are we looking for and feeling as we palpate?

You are not trying to palpate through the tissue for the TVPs as at this level of the spine the thickness of the erector spinae and connective tissue would make them difficult to discern especially at the L4 and L5 levels. Rather, having landmarked where they are, you should note the tissue thickness or bulk over the TVPs and compare this side to side. Strictly speaking, you are palpating the hardness that belongs to the bony TVPs under the tissue that overlies them.

- When several vertebrae rotate to one side as in a group dysfunction or scoliosis there is bulkiness on the side of the spine to which they are rotated.
- When an individual vertebra is rotated as in a segmental dysfunction then you will usually not see any extra bulk on that side but will palpate as a specific firm or hard spot.
- Both types of dysfunction, however, may be unclear when the patient is in neutral, especially for the therapist who is just beginning this type of assessment.
- Palpating and observing in flexion and extension usually exaggerates the feel and appearance of this bulkiness.

In general, we are searching for not just where the symptoms are but also for the source of what provokes them, what impedes or alters motion in the thoracic spine.

A summary of the rules and findings for motion testing in the spine can be found in Box 13.4.

Box 13.4 Summary of rules and findings for motion testing in the spine

1. Observing and palpating an increased bulk on one side over several vertebral levels indicates a scoliosis.
   - A scoliosis remains both in flexion and extension and is exaggerated in flexion.
   - The side of increased bulk is the side to which the vertebrae are rotated. The ribs tend to make this hump even more prominent.
   - Therefore, the vertebrae are usually side-bent to the opposite side.
2. When palpating a **flexed spine**, you find **extension lesions**.
   - A TVP's inability to flex open will create a palpable bump.
   - The extension lesion is on the side you feel the bump/TVP.
3. When palpating an **extended spine** you find **flexion lesions**.
   - A TVP's inability to extend and close will create a palpable bump.
   - However, the flexion lesion is on the opposite side to the palpable bump/TVP.

Motion palpation of the upper thoracics

You will be using forward flexion and extension of the cervical spine to observe and palpate the motion of spinal segments of the upper thoracic spine from T1 to T5 or T6. Motion of the cervical spine is used because the first several thoracic vertebrae will move in concert with the lower cervical segments. After flexing the cervical spine (chin to chest) have the patient then flex the upper thoracic spine (more of a "slump"). After extension of the cervical spine the patient is asked to extend the upper thoracic spine. Instruct the patient to move slowly; you may wish to place a hand on their forehead to guide the speed of their actions.

You will be looking at symmetry of motion restrictions at particular levels, noting any tissue texture abnormalities while you ask the patient about tenderness or pain. This testing is focused on finding and assessing impairments of segmental dysfunctions.

The patient should have relative freedom of PR-ROM of the cervical spine (in flexion and extension) which is pain-free or at least which exhibits only very minor discomfort on movement. Many therapists test for rotation of a single vertebra by observing the position of the spinous processes (SPs). However, SPs are notorious for being misshapen or bent and therefore, are not reliable indicators of whether or not a specific vertebra is rotated. Further, it will not by itself tell us the nature of the impairment. The inconsistencies of orientation of the SPs therefore require that we should motion test all vertebrae in those portions of the spine that are implicated in impairments.

First palpate the symmetry or lack of symmetry in the upper thoracic spine while the patient sits in neutral. Place a thumb and fingertip over the area of the first thoracic vertebra's TVPs. Note that each pair of TVPs are generally short. However, the ribs attached to the TVP will also be moving. Palpate your way

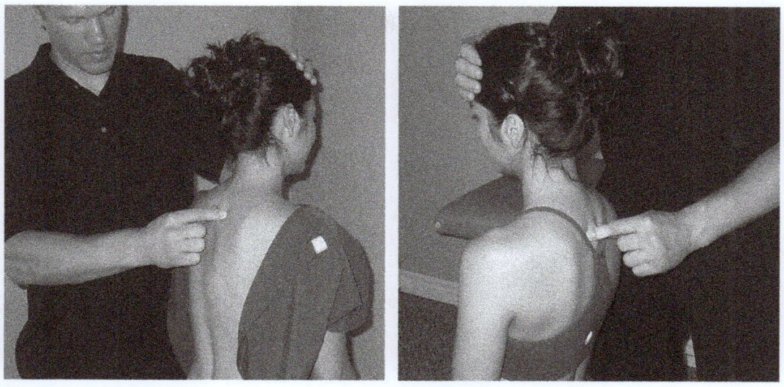

FIGURES 13.34, 13.35 1. Palpation of upper thoracics in neutral

In neutral (starting position) check for asymmetries.

down, vertebra by vertebra. Regarding segmental dysfunctions, note if one TVP feels shallow (closer to the surface of the skin) or deeper than its opposite and those above and below it.

NOTE: With slight or mild lesions or dysfunctions of a motion segment it may be difficult to palpate a difference side to side with the patient in neutral. So, if for other reasons (such as case history patient pointing to a specific joint, etc.) you suspect any specific vertebral level you should still test all of the thoracic and lower cervical vertebrae from the top down when motion testing. Pain from facet joints can be site-specific if acute, but they can also refer one or two levels up and down. They can also refer a distance such as out to the scapulae, for example.

Remember that when we are palpating a pair of TVPs of a specific vertebra during motion testing we are testing the *motion segment* which is made up of that vertebra and the one directly below it. When a facet joint of a motion segment has impaired motion (with a segmental impairment) the superior vertebra will not move symmetrically. It will side-bend and rotate (same side) left or right depending on which of the joints is affected or what position it is being held in.

Two ways to palpate upper thoracics (Figures 13.34–13.39)

There are two ways to palpate the upper thoracic vertebrae. One way is to palpate all of the vertebrae as a group, in three steps: when the spine is in neutral, when the patient is flexed, and when the spine is extended. This is the best way to conduct an assessment of vertebral dysfunction of the upper thoracics.

A second, alternative method is to palpate each vertebra individually as you have the patient move from neutral into flexion then into extension and then back to neutral. Then proceed to

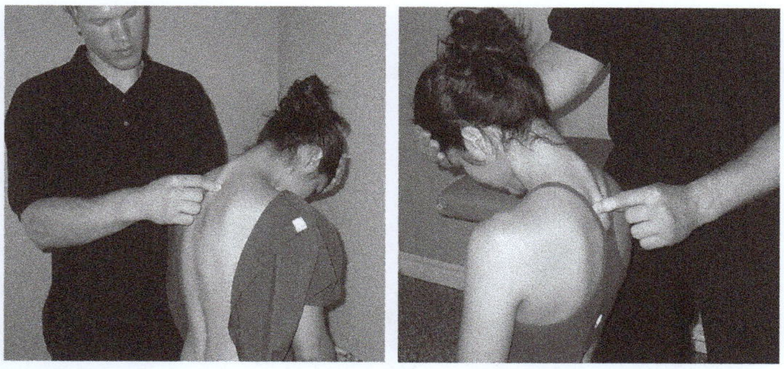

FIGURES 13.36, 13.37 2. Palpation of upper thoracics in flexion

Have the patient forward flex the head first tucking the chin in then lowering it to the chest. Slump the upper thoracics. Does any asymmetry disappear or does it become more pronounced?

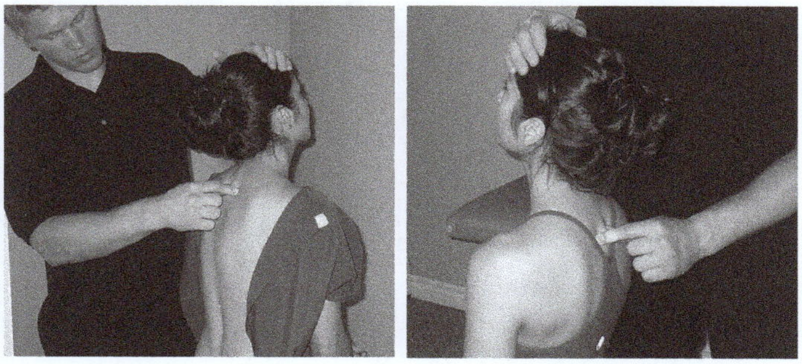

FIGURES 13.38, 13.39 3. Palpation of upper thoracics in extension

While palpating have the patient extend the head, then flatten the upper thoracics. Note if any asymmetry disappears or becomes more pronounced.

do the same with the next vertebra. This version is best used once impairments are found (from the testing mentioned above) and the therapist wishes to more fully palpate the involved structures.

Examples of palpating through clothing and with the patient wearing a medical examination gown are demonstrated.

Note that in the examples above the therapist's fingers are close to the spinous processes. The TVPs here are not as long as lower down in the spine. The therapist is feeling for one transverse process becoming more or less prominent in flexion or extension. Further, if palpating each vertebra moving through flexion and extension then the therapist may also feel rotations or "wobbles"

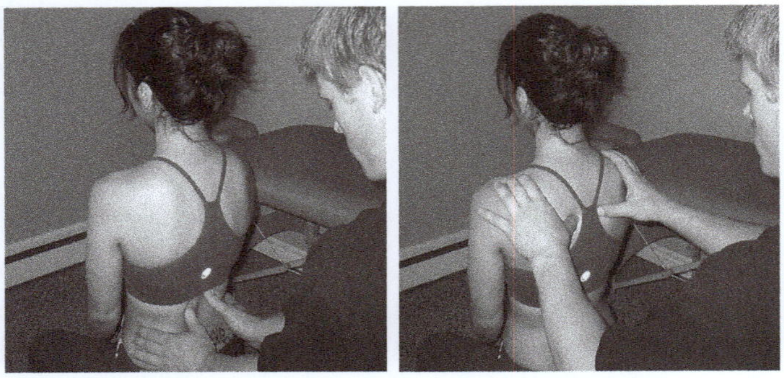

FIGURE 13.40A, B 1. Palpating in neutral

The therapist may wish to begin at the lumbar spine and proceed up into the thoracic spine.

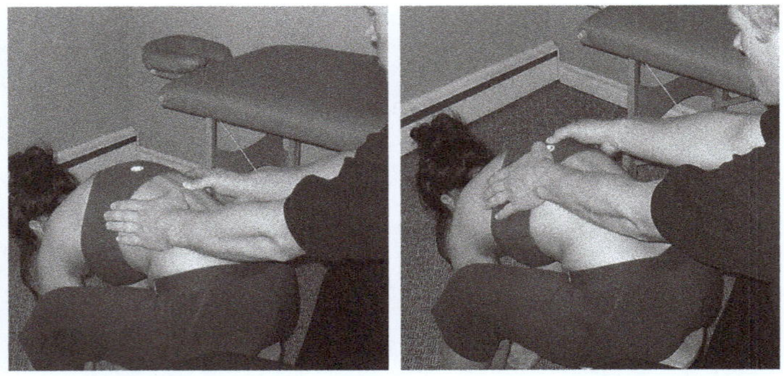

FIGURE 13.41A, B 2. Palpating in flexion

With the patient bent forward palpate over the TVPs to check for asymmetries.

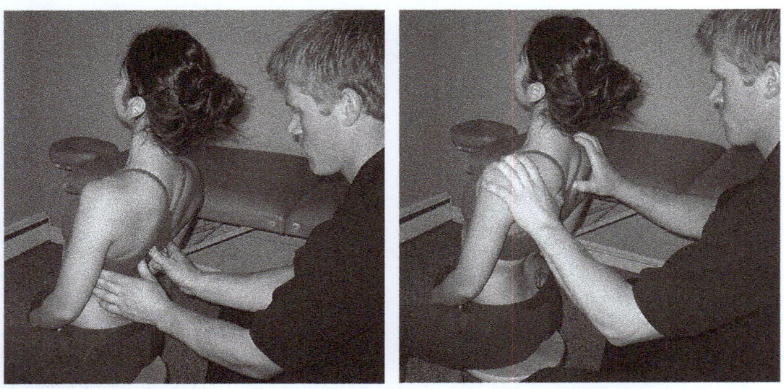

FIGURE 13.42A, B 3. Palpating in extension

Have the patient extend the spine by asking them to push their abdomen forward and then arch back. Ask them to keep looking forward.

in the SPs that sometimes can be felt when an impaired vertebra moves between the end-ranges of flexion and extension.

Testing of the mid and lower thoracic spine (Figures 13.40, 13.41, 13.42)

With the patient sitting upright and the spine in neutral palpate each vertebra's TVPs. If the patient is sitting on the table stabilize them for testing by having their feet on a chair or stool. This helps the patient keep their balance and allows them to relax the muscles of the back. Begin the testing by asking the patient to flex the spine in its entirety. Full flexion is used to test the mid- or lower thoracic spine, and the lumbar spine can also be included to make the testing more thorough.

If you wish to include the upper thoracic spine assessment and make this a full thoracic assessment then just perform the testing much as above: prior to full flexion first have the patient "slump" forward flexing the upper thoracics, and after palpating each vertebra's TVP position then have the patient fully flex the whole spine. The same too for testing in extension: flattening the upper thoracics, palpate upper TVPs and then going into a fuller extension of the whole spine, palpating the lower thoracic TVPs. This may avoid excessive movement to injured, impaired, or inflamed tissues.

When the patient is in flexion and then extension:

- You can landmark specific areas of concern and check those first if you initially want to stay focused on those segments.
- Remember to always re-check the whole area for minor to moderate lesions that may not be clearly evident while the patient was in neutral.

Gradations of asymmetry

If during flexion or extension the asymmetry becomes apparent for the first time this indicates a minor lesion. If it remains the same, it is a moderate lesion. If it becomes more asymmetrical it indicates the presence of a severe lesion.

Review of findings and what they mean

When flexing the spine, we are testing the motion segment to see if it is able to flex. If we find increased asymmetry, then we have discovered a joint that is being held extended. Remember that *testing in flexion finds extension lesions.*

- The joint fixed in extension acts as a pivot around which the vertebra rotates. The joint that can flex will have its TVP move even further anteriorly as it rotates around the fixed extended joint. This pushes that fixed side's TVP even further posteriorly making it even more distinct.

When extending the spine, we are testing to see if the motion segment is able to extend. If we find increased asymmetry, then we have found a joint that is being held flexed. Remember that *testing in extension finds flexion lesions.*

- The joint fixed in flexion acts as a pivot around which the vertebra rotates. The joint has its TVP already slightly anterior making the other side's TVP slightly posterior. As the spine extends the fixed side's TVP cannot move posteriorly. However, the joint that is able to extend will have its TVP come even further posteriorly while the fixed side's moves anteriorly.

Palpation of a segmental flexion lesion (Figures 13.43–13.45)

The flexion lesion is on the left. In other words, the left facet will not close. This causes the vertebral segment to rotate and side-bend to the right when the spine is in neutral or when it is extended. This lesioned segment will, however, become (more) symmetrical when the segment is flexed as the right facet is functioning normally and is able to flex and extend.

Remember that the lesion is named for the position it forces the superior vertebra of a motion segment to become fixated in. Therefore, in this example the left facet of the superior vertebra is held in flexion which in turn holds the vertebra side-bent and rotated toward the right: FRSr.

Palpation of a segmental extension lesion (Figures 13.46–13.48)

The extension lesion is on the right. In other words, the right facet will not open. This causes the vertebral segment to rotate and side-bend to the right when the spine is in neutral or when flexed. This lesioned segment will, however, become (more) symmetrical when the segment is extended as the left facet is functioning normally; it is able to flex and extend.

Summary of findings

A summary of findings can be found in Table 13.3.

NOTE: All the boxes in the table with "symmetrical" could just as well be written as "more symmetrical" as that matches many clinical findings. However, we have chosen to leave that out here so as to simplify the chart. "More symmetrical" and "more asymmetrical" are simply too similar in appearance and this could cause confusion.

REMINDER: The notations are to record the position of the superior vertebra on the one below. They do not overtly tell us which side the lesion is on. However, if it is a flexion lesion (FRS) the lesion is always on the side opposite the one to which the superior vertebrae is rotated and side-bent. An extension lesion (ERS) is always on the side to which the vertebra is side-bent and rotated.

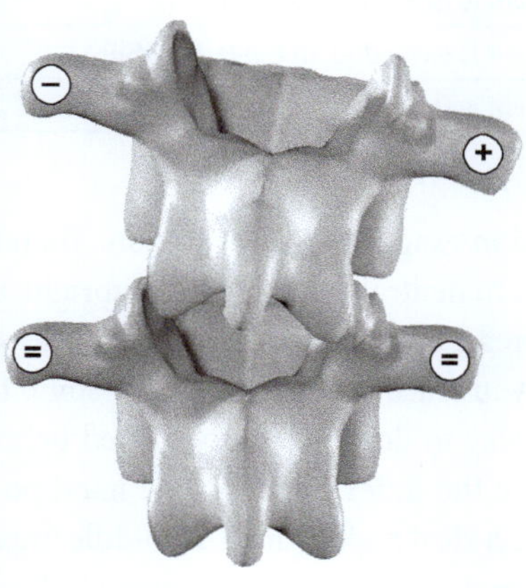

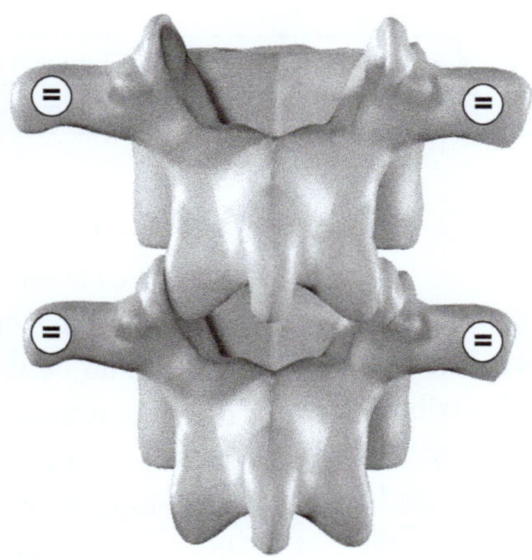

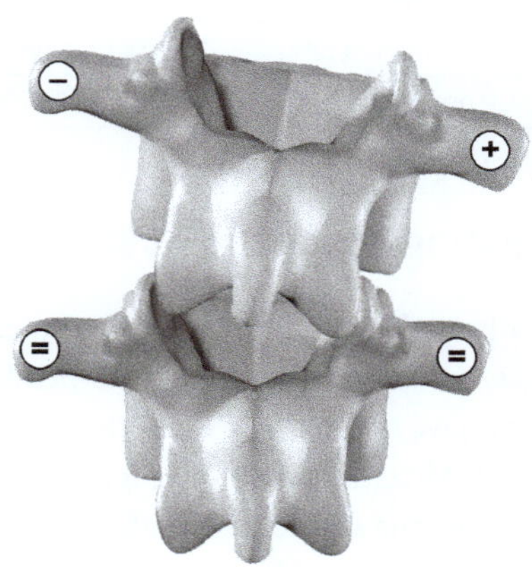

Legend: = equal; – deeper/anterior; + prominent/posterior

FIGURE 13.43 Palpation in neutral

Right TVP prominent when the spine is in neutral position.

FIGURE 13.44 Patient flexes forward

TVPs now equal.

FIGURE 13.45 Palpation in extension

Right TVP (even more) prominent. Flexion lesion is on the left side: FRSr. Left facet will not extend/close.

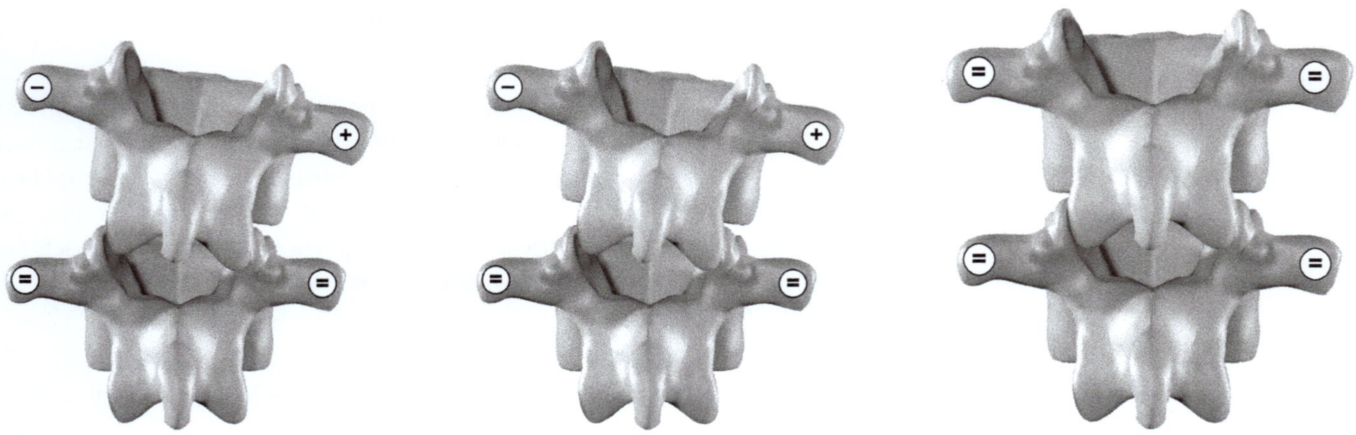

Legend: = equal; – deeper/anterior; + prominent/posterior

FIGURE 13.46 Palpation in neutral

Right TVP is prominent when the spine is in neutral position.

FIGURE 13.47 Patient flexes forward

Right TVP (even more) prominent. Extension lesion is on the right side: ERSr. The right facet will not flex/open.

FIGURE 13.48 Patient extends spine

TVPs now equal.

Table 13.3 Summary of findings

In neutral	In flexion	In extension	Dysfunction
TVP prominent right	More asymmetrical	Symmetrical	Impaired facet joint is extended on the right (ERSr)
TVP prominent right	Symmetrical	More asymmetrical	Impaired facet joint is flexed on the left (FRSr)
TVP prominent left	More asymmetrical	Symmetrical	Impaired facet joint is extended on the left (ERSl)
TVP prominent left	Symmetrical	More asymmetrical	Impaired facet joint is flexed on the right (FRSl)

TVP, transverse process.

Testing for group dysfunctions

To help determine group impairments, most commonly scoliosis, we investigate using side-bending. But first, the therapist may have noticed that when the patient was in full flexion (either in ROM testing, or testing for segmental dysfunctions) the rib-cage on one side looked higher. A layperson's term might be that it looks "humped" on one side. This hump is created by the ribs being elevated on that side; and they are elevated because several of the vertebrae they are attached to are rotated to that side. This implies a group dysfunction: several vertebrae are being held in lateral-flexion (side-bent) in one direction while rotated in the other direction. (See Fryette's first rule of spinal motion at the beginning of this chapter.)

For example, if when the patient has fully flexed their spine and the right side of the thoracic cage is elevated ("humped") over the space of several vertebrae, we can conclude that those vertebrae are rotated to the right (lifting their ribs) and will be side-bent to the left. Flexion exaggerates the rotation. Therefore, when the patient's spine is in neutral, when they are upright, such a humping may not be present. However, the curve of the scoliosis should be visible if you trace the outline of the spine from top to bottom. The best way to do this is to be seated behind a standing patient and place the index finger of one hand on one side of spine, up into the cervical region, and the middle finger of the same hand on the other side. Trace down the spine (following the laminae groove) noticing any deviations side to side.

By landmarking when the curvature begins and where is ends try to determine which vertebra is the furthest from the mid-line. That vertebra is the *apex of the curve*. When finding a curve in the thoracic spine it is not uncommon to find a curve in the other direction below in the lumbar and/or in the cervical spine. If there is a curve in the lumbar spine area then the curve above in the thoracic's is often seen as a compensating curve for the one below. In turn, a cervical curve above is most likely compensating for the thoracic curve.

If there is only one curve it is referred to as a C-curve. If there are two curves, one compensating for the other, this is called an S-curve. Sometime a scoliosis will be named for its apex and the vertebrae involved, T6 R, T11–T4. The vertebrae are side-bent left, rotated right with T6 the furthest from the mid-line. Others may simply say T11-T4 L: side-bent left from T11–T4.

You should have the patient re-do AF-ROM side-bending, to each side, and clarify where the curves are, their extent and the apex; see if there are curves above or below; which motions are restricted and/or produce discomfort, etc.

Seated lateral translation (Figure 13.49–13.52)

The following testing is valuable at any number of places within the assessment of the thoracic spine including at the end of AF- or PR-ROM testing, and after motion palpation for flexion and extension (finding facet lesions). It is also a great palpation exercise for students.

This motion testing can be used to observe how individual or small groups of segments respond to side-bending. This may be helpful to further explore the mechanics of the thoracic spine, especially if the nature of the impairment(s) remains hidden. It can reveal individual segment impaired motion (i.e., that there is a problem but not necessarily what that problem is). Also, it is useful in investigating group dysfunctions.

Further if you are exploring the possibility of impaired rib motion this test can help you see how the rib is affecting and being affected by the tissues and structures around it. Simply modify the palpating position by moving your fingers out over the ribs (note whether they open or close). It also provides valuable regional information regarding thoracic spine motion in relation to the shoulder girdle or cervical spine. Use whenever your clinical judgment sees fit.

By shifting into the table the therapist causes the patient's thoracic spine to shift or "translate" along with the therapist. In the picture above the patient's thoracic spine is now side-bent left.

Standing "passive" side-bending (Figures 13.53, 13.54)

Though less specific for palpating specific vertebrae, this is a good way to palpate general motion of segments while observing

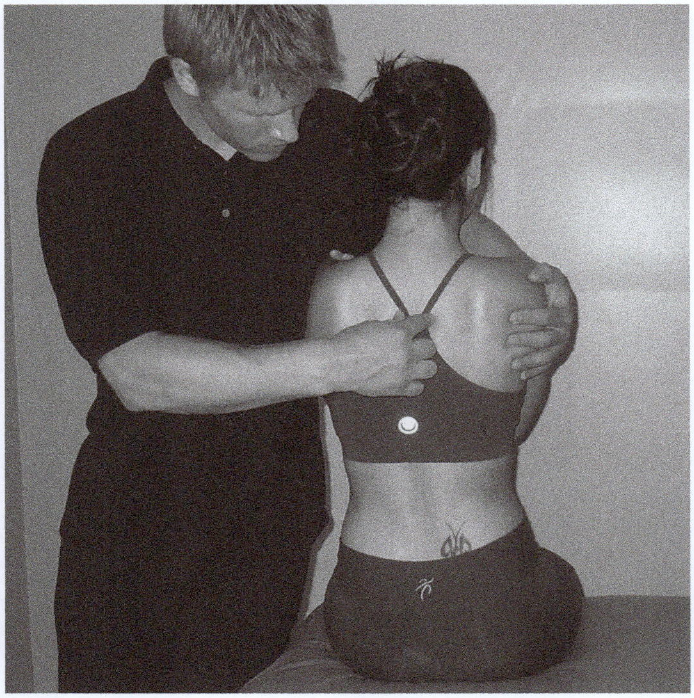

FIGURE 13.49 1. Starting position lateral translation

The patient is seated at end of the table with arms crossed. Support the shoulder with your trunk as you palpate a pair of TVPs. The other hand holds the far shoulder. Ask the patient to relax and let you move them.

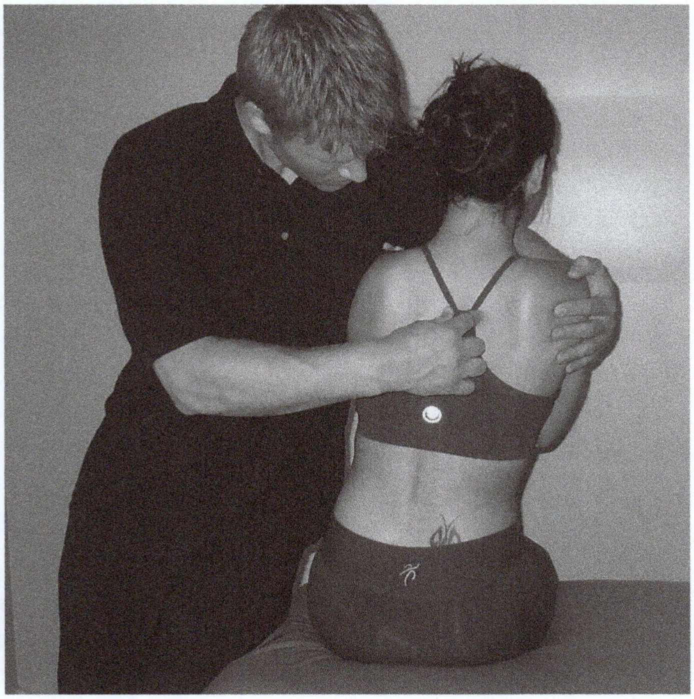

FIGURE 13.50 2. Shift right side-bend left

Shift your body into the table while continuing to support the patient with the hand and the body, pushing their shoulders along with you. All the while palpate motion of the vertebra. You need to keep the patient's shoulders level with table.

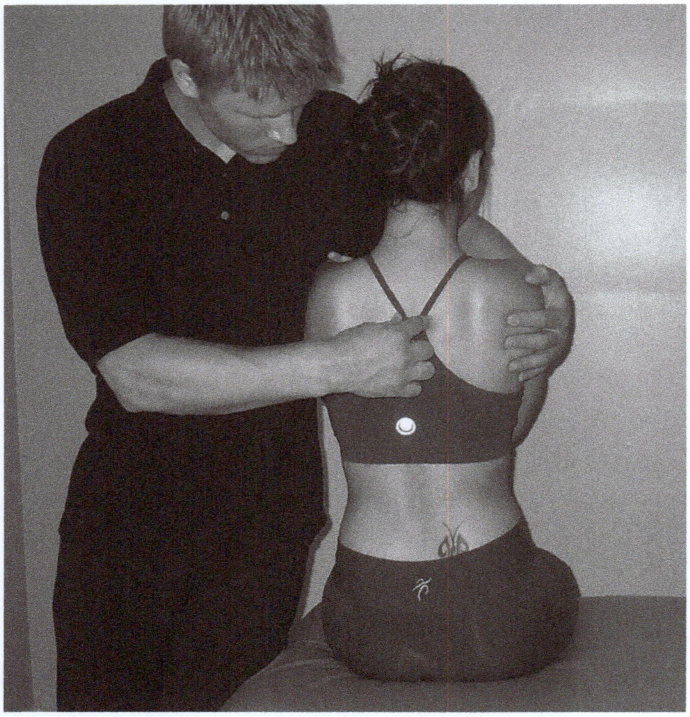

FIGURE 13.51 **3. Return to neutral**

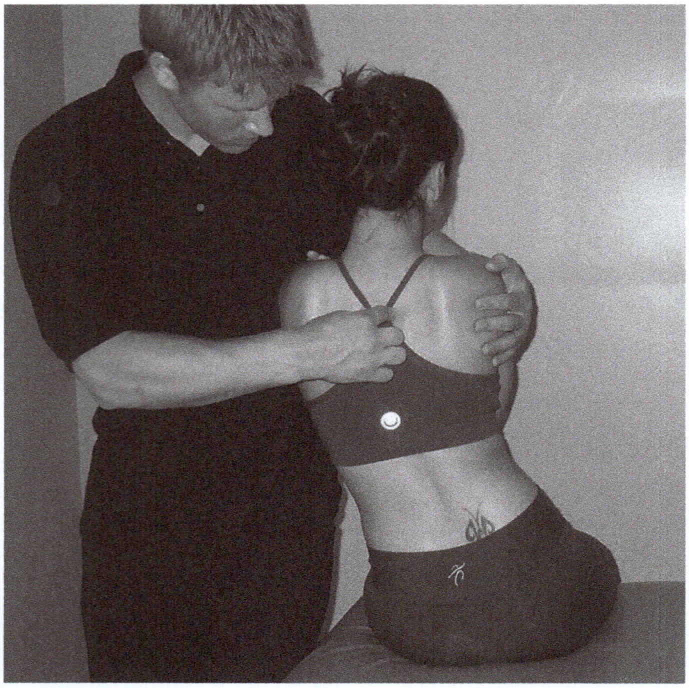

FIGURE 13.52 **4. Shift left, side-bend right**

Then without changing level palpated lean away from the table, pulling the patient's shoulders with you. The thoracic spine is now side-bent right.

group movement, especially when investigating scoliotic curves in the spine. You can see which way the spine likes to bend (concave side of a scoliosis) and which way it does not want to bend (convex side).

The patient stands with their back to you as you sit on a stool. Ask the patient to place their feet together. Place the medial portion of your knees on either side of the patient's legs. Use a gentle but firm pressure; just enough to stabilize the patient and make them feel secure. Place the fingers of one hand over a pair of TVPs. Lightly grasp one of the patient's wrists. Explain to the patient that you are going to gently pull their arm and you want them to relax and let themselves side-bend. (*In Figure 13.54 the therapist is off to one side to show palpation during movement.*)

Give the wrist a gentle and slow, even pull down to the floor about an inch or so. Palpate the quality of the motion and observe the quality of the curve generated. Repeat over the levels you wish to investigate. If you use the method to get a general feel and observation of the motion of side-bending of the trunk (and influence on the shoulders, etc.) you can skip every other level, and so cover the whole thoracic spine in six or seven rocking motions to the side. If you are doing a focused assessment of side-bending in the thoracic spine proper, then check every level. Repeat on the other side.

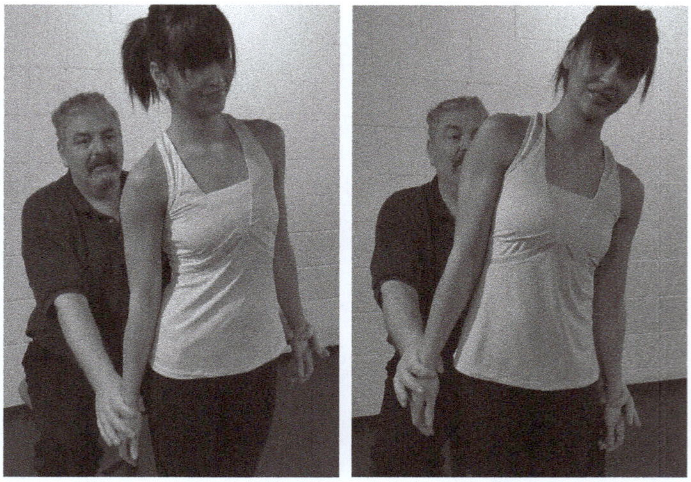

FIGURE 13.53A, B **Standing side-bending of thoracic spine**

Grasp the wrist and ask the patient to let you move them. Pull down on the arm while observing curves in the spine. Repeat two or three times to determine to which side movement is easier. This tells you which direction the spine is bent in.

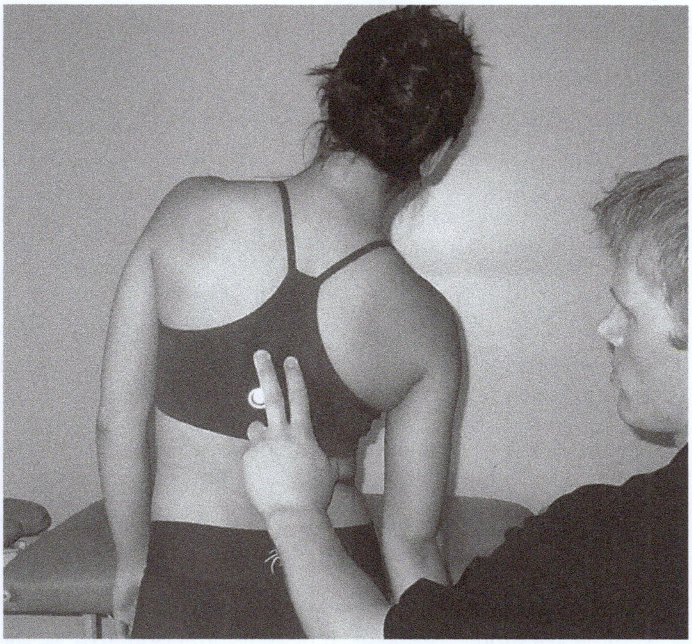

FIGURE 13.54 Motion palpation of segments during side-bending

Now the therapist can add palpation of specific segments to side-bending, looking for hypertonic paraspinal muscles at specific levels. (The therapist is gently pulling down on the right wrist.)

Introduction to the ribs

Testing rib function requires basic understanding of rib anatomy and how ribs move and function.

In this section, we will often include the palpation/testing when we give the structure and function of ribs within their classic categorization. Refer to an anatomical text for details of the musculature and especially for the joints involved. (Agur et al. 2014; Chila 2010; DeStefano 2011; Dutton 2012; Hertling & Kessler 2006; Kapandji 2008; Levangie & Norkin 2011; Magee 2014; Maitland 2001; Mitchell 2004; Schuenke et al. 2014.)

The testing presented here assumes that the basic thoracic spine ROM has been done.

Musculature

The diaphragm is the principal muscle used for inhalation. Some have included portions of the external intercostals and the scalenes as also involved in quiet inhalation (Levangie & Norkin 2011).

The following muscles can be employed for forced inhalation:

- Scalenes: lifts ribs 1 and 2 which are described as moving superiorly and inferiorly.
- Sternocleidomastoid: raises the sternum which expands the ribcage anterior-posteriorly.
- Pectoralis minor: lifts ribs 2 to 5 anteriorly and superiorly.
- Pectoralis major: assists in lifting the sternum.
- Serratus anterior: with the scapula stabilized the serratus anterior lifts the middle ribs (4–8/9) opening all of them up (ribs 1–8/9) laterally as it does so.
- Levatores costarum (which are posteriorly from C7 to T1 from vertebra above to rib below): assist in forced inspiration.
- External intercostals: anterior portions ("parasternal") thought to lift the ribs on inhalation.

Forced exhalation is principally done by the abdominal group of muscles:

- internal and external intercostals
- serratus posterior inferior
- along with some of the accessory muscles including the quadratus lumborum iliocostalis, and longissimus thoracis.

If we included all of the muscles thought to be accessory muscles to forced inhalation and exhalation, we would be listing almost all of the musculature of the trunk. Hence rib dysfunctions can have numerous sources and in turn have numerous consequences.

Joints

The ribs pivot posteriorly on the costovertebral and costotransverse joints (Kapandji 2008; Levangie & Norkin 2011).

The typical costovertebral synovial joints are in ribs 2 to 9. With these ribs the costovertebral joint is composed of a demifacet on a superior vertebral body and a demifacet on the inferior vertebral body and includes the surface of the intervertebral disc (IVD) between them. Within this typical rib joint the radiate ligament has three branches each attaching to each vertebra and the disc. The joint is also divided into two sections or cavities by the intra-articular ligament (interosseous ligament) which travels from the head of the rib to the IVD. These two cavities, however, are in one fibrous capsule.

The costotransverse synovial joint is between the costal tubercle on the rib and the costal facet on the TVP of the vertebra. These joints occur from ribs 1 to 10 on T1 to T10. This joint is reinforced by three strong ligaments: the interosseous (lateral) ligament, costotransverse ligament, and superior costotransverse ligament.

If you draw a line between and through the middle of the costovertebral and the costotransverse joints, then this is the axis around which the rib will elevate (with inhalation) and drop or depress (with exhalation). Each end of the line between the joints is like the end points of a door hinge with the hinge being oriented transversely (rather than horizontally like a door's).

During inhalation, the ribs are lifted and the cartilaginous costochondral joints (at the sternum and ribs) are torsioned. During exhalation, the stored energy in the torsioned cartilage is then used to push the ribs back down into their starting position. This is the principal way that exhalation occurs when it is labelled *passive*. Muscular effort for exhalation is only required and used with forced exhalation when we consciously try to empty the lungs or during exertion.

Figure 13.55 summarizes how ribs have been classically organized.

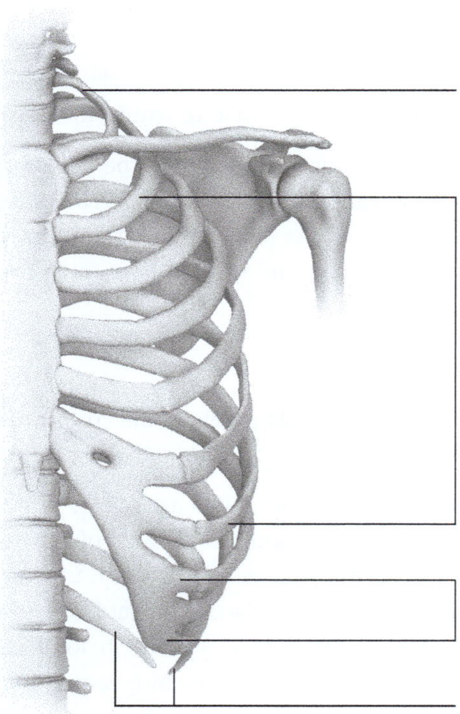

FIGURE 13.55

Organization of the ribs.

First rib

Rib 1 is unique in several ways:

1. It is one of only a few ribs that do not have their costovertebral joint between two vertebrae. (This feature is shared by ribs 10, 11, and 12.) Its joint at the vertebra is to T1 alone.
2. It attaches to the manubrium just below the sternoclavicular joint.
3. It is a flat bone set transversely with the broadest portion facing superior-inferiorly and the thin edges lateral and medial.
4. This broad shelf provides attachment for many muscles: the scalenes and subclavius on top and on its lateral border a finger of the serratus anterior is attached as is a slip of the iliocostalis at its posterior edge.
5. Travelling across its superior surface is the neurovascular bundle to supply the arm and at its anterior area is the attachment for the costoclavicular ligament.

Rib 1 along with rib 2 and the manubrium and the first two thoracic vertebrae are also referred to as the bony borders of the *thoracic inlet* or *outlet*.

First rib dysfunctions are often associated with thoracic outlet syndromes (TOS) and upper respiratory dysfunctions. The basic issues from the first rib's perspective (regardless of consequences) are:

1. The rib can be held superiorly in inhalation. In other words, the rib remains in the position you would find it in if the patient had just inhaled and was holding their breath. The rib is not moving or is hypomobile, and remains lifted while all the other ribs lower in exhalation.
2. The rib can be held inferiorly in exhalation (opposite to number 1). The rib will not lift into inhalation along with the other ribs but rather remains depressed.

The more common of the two is when this rib is being held superiorly and therefore accompanied by shortened and hypertonic or even contractured scalenes.

Palpation of first rib (Figures 13.56–13.58)

Have the patient lying supine; side-bend the head to the side to be tested. Pull the trapezium muscle posteriorly and palate through the soft tissue of the thoracic outlet. Then have the patient breathe in deeply and you should be able to feel the tissue below your fingers (the tissue between your fingers and the rib) rise up and then descend as the patient breathes out.

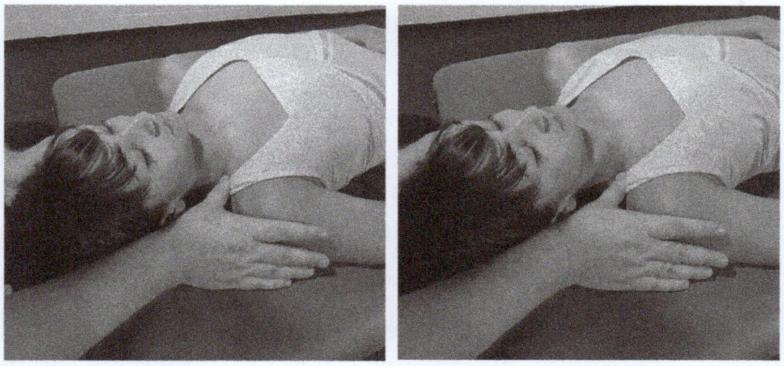

FIGURE 13.56A, B Palpation of first rib

The patient's neck and head are side-bent. Palpate deep (in front of trapezius). Have the patient breathe in and out deeply. Follow the movement of the rib.

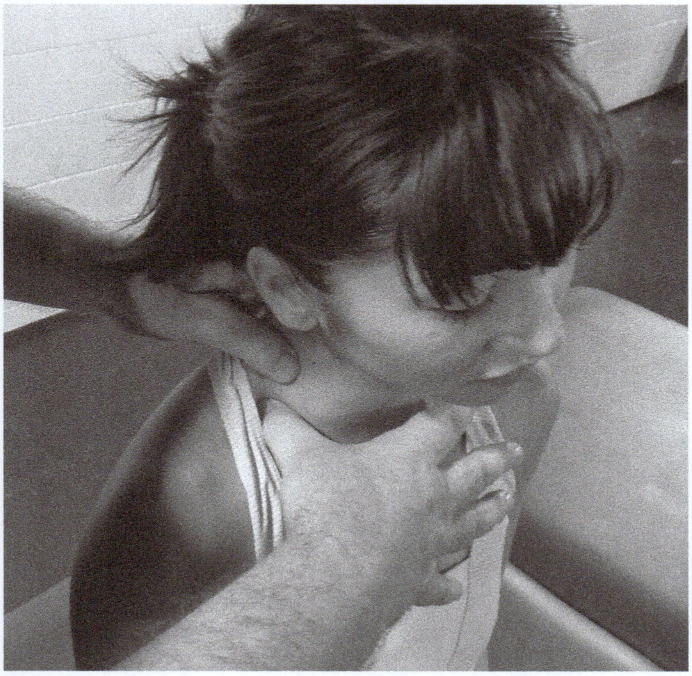

FIGURE 13.58 Palpation of subluxed first rib

Palpate along the first rib to determine whether it is markedly tilted anteriorly.

Palpation of first rib subluxation (Figures 13.57, 13.58)

If you notice that either side (possibly both sides) of the first rib do not display motion during inhalation or exhalation you will have to palpate the first rib heads from the thoracic spine area. If this is the case a first rib may be subluxed superiorly. For this

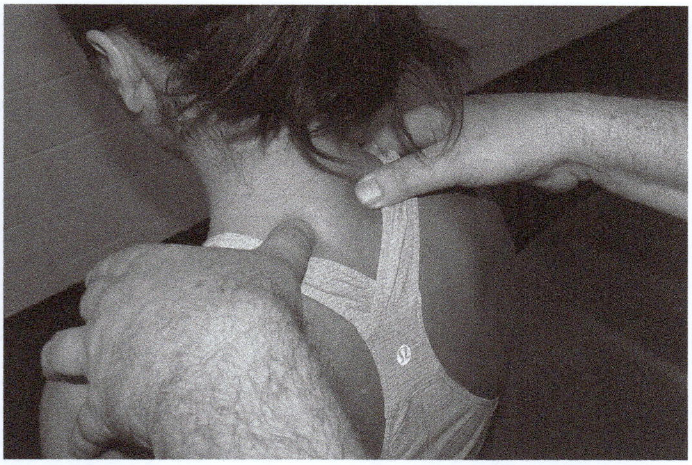

FIGURE 13.57 Palpation of first ribs head

With the patient seated landmark the head of the first ribs bilaterally. Palpate for symmetry of depth.

to have occurred the rib head must have been pulled forward and superiorly around the T1's TVP. This means that the rib has moved substantially and therefore becomes palpable from the back. Landmark and palpate just superior to T1's TVP, and the head of the rib may be felt if the area is not found to be too tender.

Further, if you now palpate through the thoracic outlet the superior posterior portion is distinct if subluxed and the rib will move forward and run clearly inferior. The posterior portion has an unyielding feel (hard end-feel) rather than the normal elastic feel. To properly do this test you must side-bend the head (toward the test side) to loosen the tissues, (especially the scalenes). Next, push trapezius back and palpate obliquely posteriorly feeling for the first rib. Finally, push ribs inferiorly (should feel springiness).

Second rib (Figure 13.59)

The second rib is considered a true rib in that it originates from both T1 and T2's demifacets spanning the intervertebral disc. It too attaches to the manubrium, but also to the sternum. It is often thought of as part of the thoracic outlet bony structures as it also provides a superior surface over which the brachial plexus is taking shape, and the vascular and lymphatics course to the upper limb. It can also be involved in costoclavicular compressions or "crush" scenarios.

Rib 2 motions (elevation and depression) are best felt anteriorly just prior to its articulation with the manubrium-sternum. Place an index finger on each rib 2 which is palpable anteriorly just under the clavicle. Have the patient breathe deeply then normally as you follow the motions.

Box 13.5 describes springing the shoulder girdle to test the upper ribs (Figure 13.60).

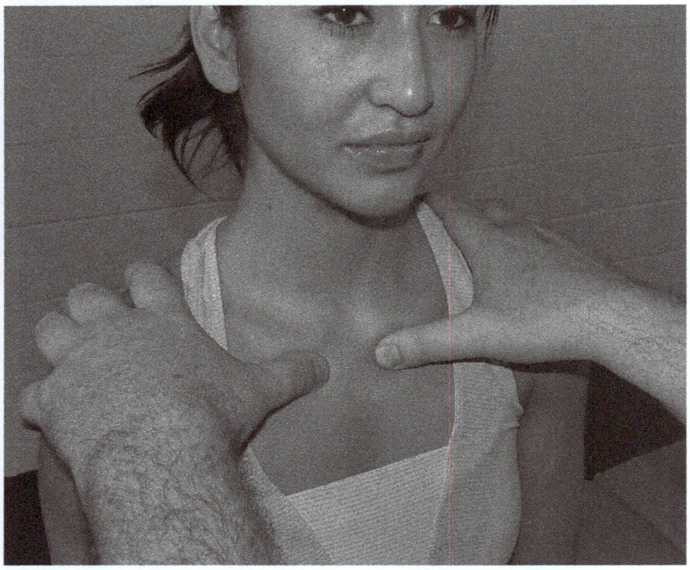

FIGURE 13.59 Palpation of second rib

Landmark the second rib just below the proximal end of the clavicles just lateral to the sternoclavicular joints. Palpate motion as the patient breathes in and out deeply.

The sternomanubrial joint and its palpation (Figure 13.61)

Another joint to consider before we move on is the cartilaginous joint between the manubrium and sternum. As the sternal complex rises on inhalation the manubrium rises superiorly and anteriorly. The sternum will follow superiorly, but the lower end of the sternum will not be allowed to move anteriorly as much due to the lower ribs (Kapandji 2008). Hence, there is a slight hinge motion at the sternomanubrial joint. This motion can be palpated by placing one finger above and one finger below the sternomanubrial joint as the patient breathes. We should feel a springiness if we simultaneously push both the manubrium and the sternum into the chest slightly.

The sternoclavicular joint and its palpation (Figure 13.62)

This motion of the manubrium and the sternum requires that we keep in mind the effect the shoulder girdle will have on the motions of the ribs via the sternoclavicular (SC) joint. The SC joint, being the only bony bridge between the upper limb and the axial skeleton, is therefore not just important to keep in mind for proper clavicular motions during shoulder movements, but for rib motion as well. (It also requires us to keep in mind the possibility of any shoulder dysfunctions as a possible source of rib/respiration problems.)

As the ribcage lifts motion is required at the SC joint. A fixed or restricted SC joint can therefore affect the motion of the ribs

INSIGHTS

Box 13.5 Springing shoulder girdle to test upper ribs

One common palpatory experience that implies that the first few ribs are being held superior or are being held in inhalation is when you push down on the shoulders (Figure 13.60). When sitting at the head of the table with the patient supine and you have a palm of each hand over each of the patient's shoulders (over the AC joint area) you then push first one side inferiorly and then the other. If one side seems stiff or has less "give" when you push then you may want to see if the upper two to four ribs are being held elevated or "inhaled."

Note: This situation is often found when the patient's upper thoracic spine is side-bent. For example, if the spine at T1–5 is side-bent right that implies that on the left the ribs are elevated (convex side of the curve) and so are held in inhalation while the ribs on the right (concave side of the curve) are compressed and tend to be exhaled. Posturally this would appear as a lower right shoulder or conversely an elevated left shoulder. In this example, even though the right ribs are exhaled or compressed the thoracic spine is still willing to side-bend right a little more. It is held side-bent right and is therefore, willing to bend to that side. However, the thoracic spine will resist being side-bent left and so when you apply pressure it resists and feels stiff.

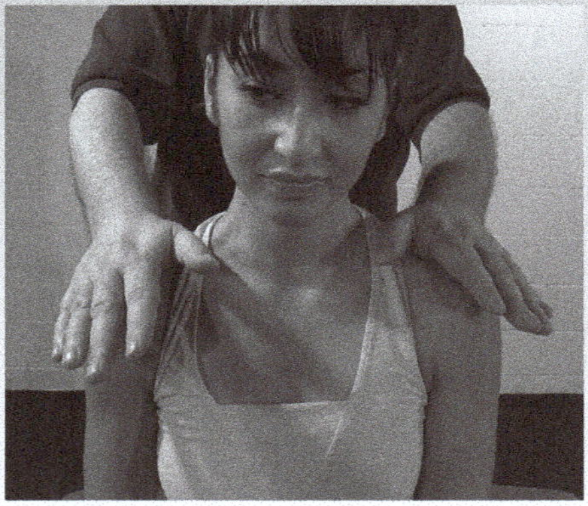

FIGURE 13.60

via the fixating of the manubrium (and hence the sternum and ribcage). This interferes with the elevation of the ribs during inhalation and/or of the descent of the ribs during exhalation. It does so by affecting the amount and quality of motion available to the manubrium (and hence the sternum), and all of this in turn alters the direction of movement (or lines of force/tension) at work in the ribcage (Kapandji 2008; Mitchell 2004).

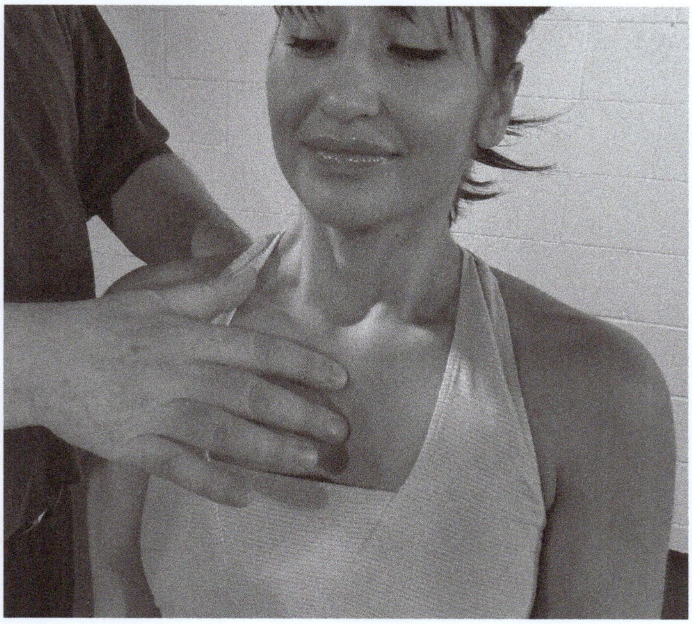

FIGURE 13.61 Palpation of sternomanubrial joint

Landmark and position the finger pad of the index finger on the manubrium with the middle finger on the superior portion of the sternum. Have the patient breathe in and out deeply several times.

With respect to shoulder dysfunctions a quick scan of respiration during the testing/treating could be helpful to gain the information required to help the patient back to full shoulder function. The motion and position of the upper ribs could well affect shoulder motion (through the positioning of the clavicle by the SC joint).

To palpate the SC joint, have the patient supine. Place your index and middle finger of one hand on either side (superior and inferior border) of the proximal end of the clavicle.

Have the patient's arm abducted 90° and grasp their forearm. With the elbow also flexed circumduct the forearm. This internally and externally rotates the shoulder and creates a rolling motion that is transmitted to the clavicle. It induces motion which should be palpable at both the AC and SC joints if everything is moving correctly.

You may try palpating the SC joint during respiration, but usually there is not enough information gleaned (not enough motion generated) to help you decide if the motion of the clavicle is dysfunctional or not. The costovertebral and costotransverse joints are not directly palpable. Palpation of the motion through these joints is made via the rib angles.

General motion of the ribs and a quick scanning of rib motions

The types of movements by groups of ribs (Figures 13.63–13.65) has been organized as such (but the motions overlap):

Rib 1

May elevate or depress

Ribs 2–5

Pump handle motion ribs lift and expand anteriorly

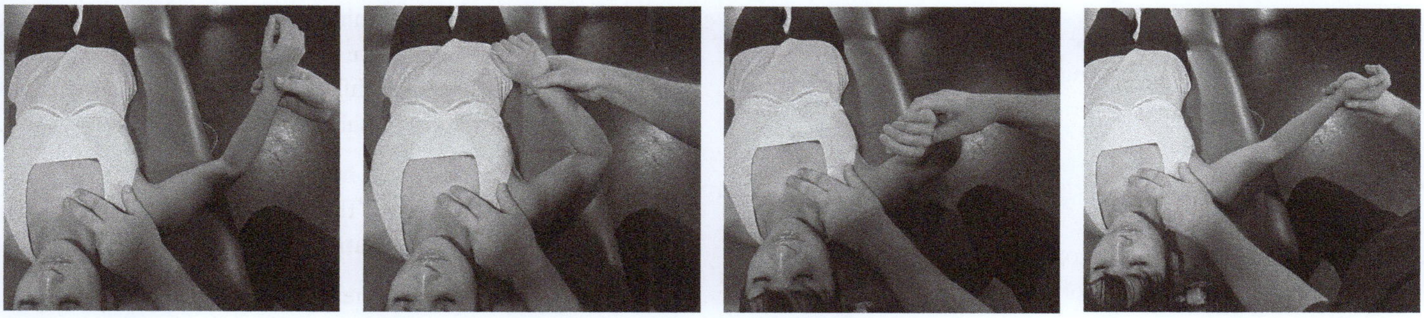

FIGURE 13.62A–D Palpation of sternoclavicular motion

Patient supine. Arm abduct 90°, elbow flexed. Hold the forearm just proximal to the wrist. Palpate over the SC joint. Swing the hand (but not lifting the patient's elbow off the table) in as wide a circle as is permitted by structures. Motion will travel up the arm into the shoulder down through the AC joint to the SC joint. Therefore, you can in turn use this to test motion in the AC joint.

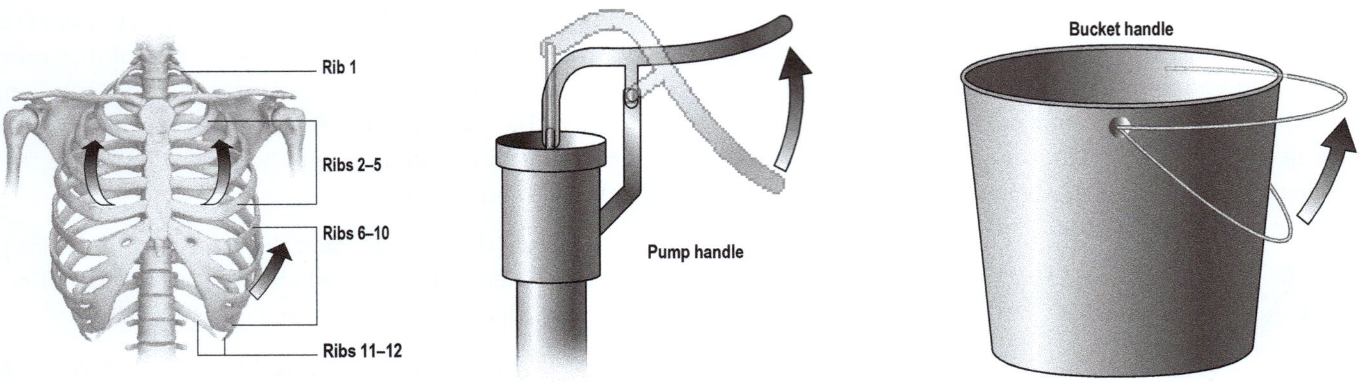

FIGURES 13.63–13.65

Types of movement by groups of ribs.

Ribs 6–10

Bucket handle motion ribs lift and expand laterally

Ribs 11–12

Pincer motion: tips of ribs spread apart or come together in pinching manner.

Possible findings during testing

A sudden sharp pain that comes and goes: If the patient has complained of sharp pains suddenly appearing and then disappearing near the spine or near the sternum ask the patient to take in a very deep breath and hold it for several seconds. If there is a subluxation of any of the rib joints they will become symptomatic when motion to the ribcage is exaggerated by such a deep breath. Often the patient will catch their breath and not be able to continue to inhale. This could also happen on a forced exhalation but clinically it is rare to generate pain from a subluxed rib by exhalation.

Rotation may also provoke pain from a rib subluxation: As the patient (when performing AF-ROM) rotates their ribcage to the right, for example, the right rib needs to roll externally and the left to roll internally.

Palpatory findings

When palpating rib angles, note the quality of motion when pressed, subjective responses of the patient, and also if one or two ribs (angles) seem more anterior or posterior than others. Be sure to compare bilaterally first before jumping to conclusions! Compare to your lateral palpation: where those ribs may have been bulging laterally (i.e., if the rib bulges laterally it will feel deeper at the rib-angle than its neighbors as its anterior to posterior width is less because it is wider at its lateral portion). Check the intercostal spacing. Are they equal bilaterally? Do they seem too close on one side or the other? Is there too large a gap between two on one side?

When palpating the ribs while the patient is breathing note the quality of motion. Is it smooth and even or is there an uneven stuttering type of motion? The latter could imply restrictions to rib motion by hypertonic musculature and/or joint restrictions.

Does one side (or set of ribs) expand more than the other during deep inhalation? Does one side descend more than the other during forced exhalation? Either of these situations implies that one or several ribs are being held inhaled (will rise fully but do not descend fully) or are exhaled (will descend well but will not lift/rise fully). Restrictions can be spread over several ribs or only in one. However, with only one rib dysfunctional it will nonetheless impact on several. Two or three ribs above or below (depending on the dysfunction) will also show restricted motion, but the effect can fade as you move into farther ribs because of tissue stretch.

Example: Rib 7 on the left is held in exhalation. It is descended (fully), but will not rise up on inhalation. Due to the soft tissue that interconnects ribs, the ribs above (5 and 6) will also be held back by rib 7 and are not able to inhale fully. Therefore, a rib held in exhalation will restrict movement (exhalation) to the adjacent ribs above it.

Conversely, if rib 3 is held inhaled it will restrict ribs 4 and 5 from exhaling fully as well. Therefore, a rib held in inhalation will restrict movement (inhalation) to the adjacent ribs below it.

The implications for treatment are:

- If ribs are held in exhalation, begin specific treatment to the lowest rib of the group as releasing it may automatically release those above it.
- If the ribs are held in inhalation, begin specific treatment to the highest rib in the group as releasing it may automatically release those below it.

Palpation of rib motions (Figure 13.66–13.72)

Palpation of rib motions during respiration is often done seated or supine. We need to divide the ribcage into three sections, plus the first rib. After palpating the first rib palpate the pump handle motion of the next three ribs available (ribs 2 to 4). This motion is compared to a pump handle as the motion is seen as primarily happening in an up-and-down motion in the sagittal plane.

Next, palpate the lateral excursion happening between ribs 5 to 10 which is referred to as a bucket handle type of motion. Remember that ribs 3 to 7 will have some combination of these two actions.

The third section is the false ribs 11 and 12. Here motion is usually described as a pincer or caliper type of motion. This motion needs to be palpated seated (best) or in prone.

For a full discussion of ribs motion and their palpation see Mitchell (2004).

Box 13.6 describes a method of testing ribs 7 to 10.

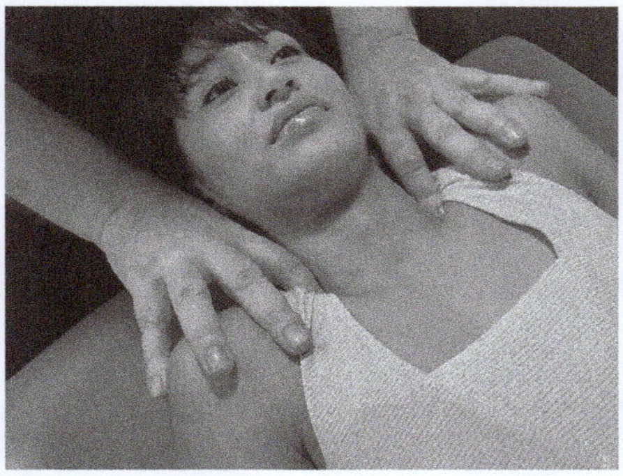

FIGURE 13.66 Palpating elevation first rib

Draw the supine patient's shoulders superiorly (toward you) to loosen tissues. Palpate first rib motion bilaterally as you have the patient breathe deeply.

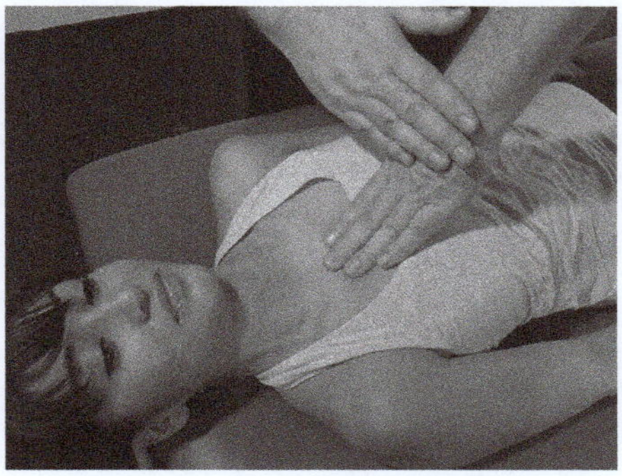

FIGURE 13.67 Palpating pump handle motion ribs 2–4

Palpate over the sternum with your finger pads for group motion. Have the patient breathe deeply. You should feel the sternum move superiorly/cephalad and expanding anteriorly. On exhalation the ribs should all descend equally.

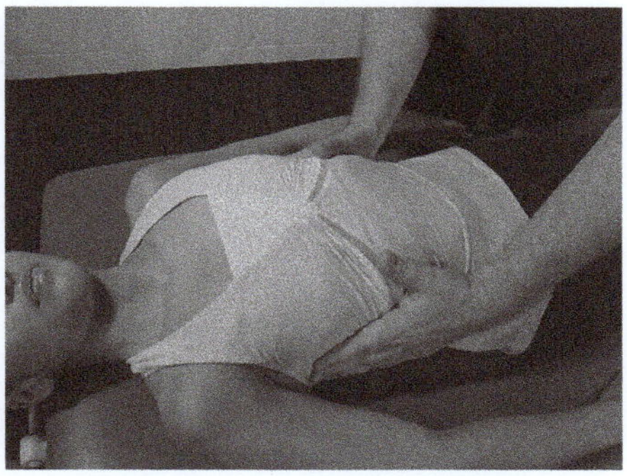

FIGURE 13.68 Palpate bucket handle motions ribs 5–10

Palpate over the lateral area of ribs 5–10. Have the patient breathe deeply. You should feel these ribs move superiorly as they expand laterally. On exhalation the ribs should all descend equally.

Box 13.6 The following action should be pain-free

Gently and slowly push in and out rhythmically on ribs 7 to 10 in an oblique direction (posterior-medially) seven to 10 times (Figure 13.69). Use part of your body-weight to push with relaxed elbows and wrists. There should be a soft springiness felt. If there is any pain, stop right away. This motion is also useful in treatment to test the elasticity of these lower ribs, while it is also useful to loosen the lower ribs and intercostal muscles, if tight.

It is not a bad massage for the internal organs, either, when done very gently and slowly as it helps to move along fluids, nutrients, and gastric products. Especially good for sedentary patients. A variation is to press in slowly then suddenly lift your hands, causing a springing back of the ribs. **Note:** *This is contraindicated for patients with rib fractures, lung disease, enlarged or injured or diseased spleen or pancreas, as well as any liver disease.*

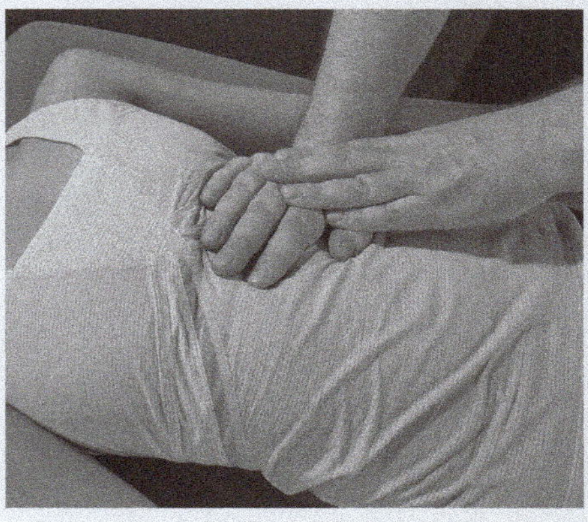

FIGURE 13.69

Prone palpation of rib motion (Figures 13.70–13.72)

When palpating respiration with the patient prone have the patient place the back of their hands on their "glutes" (or if this is not practical then at their waist). This internal rotation of the shoulder helps the scapula to move laterally out of the way for palpation of the rib angles. Motion of the costovertebral and costotransverse joints is not directly palpable. We can, however, palpate at the angle of the ribs to get some idea of how these joints are moving.

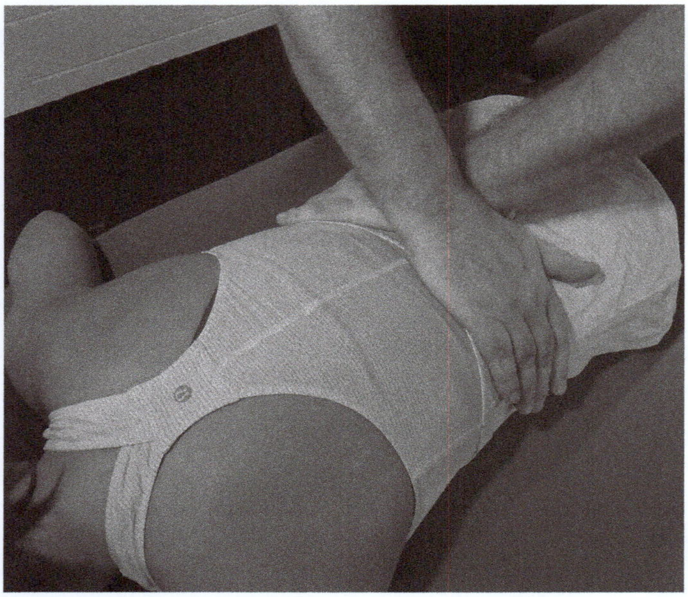

FIGURE 13.70 Palpation of pincer motion ribs 11–12

This is the best position to palpate motion of ribs 11–12. Place your hands over these ribs and you should feel them come posteriorly on inhalation, moving like a pair of calipers or ice tongs.

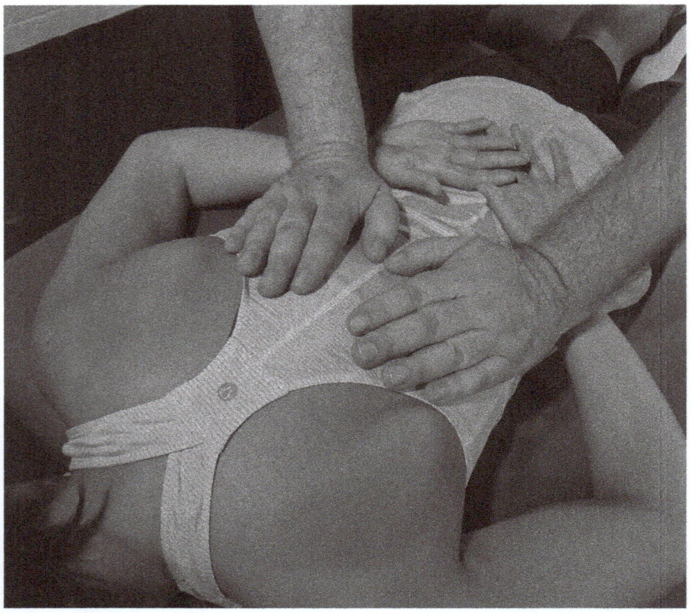

FIGURE 13.71 Palpation of lower ribs

Palpate over ribs 6–10 (approximately). Note the quality and symmetry of motion.

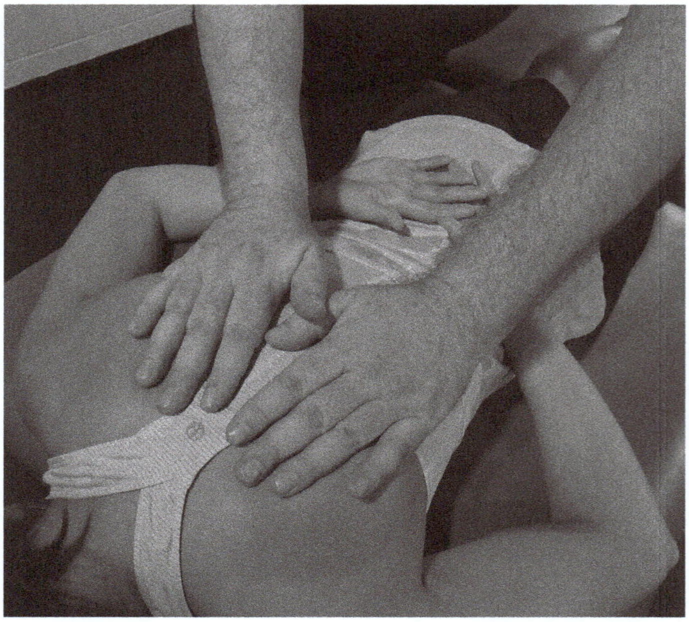

FIGURE 13.72 Palpation of upper ribs

Palpate over ribs 2–5 (approximately). Note the quality and symmetry of motion.

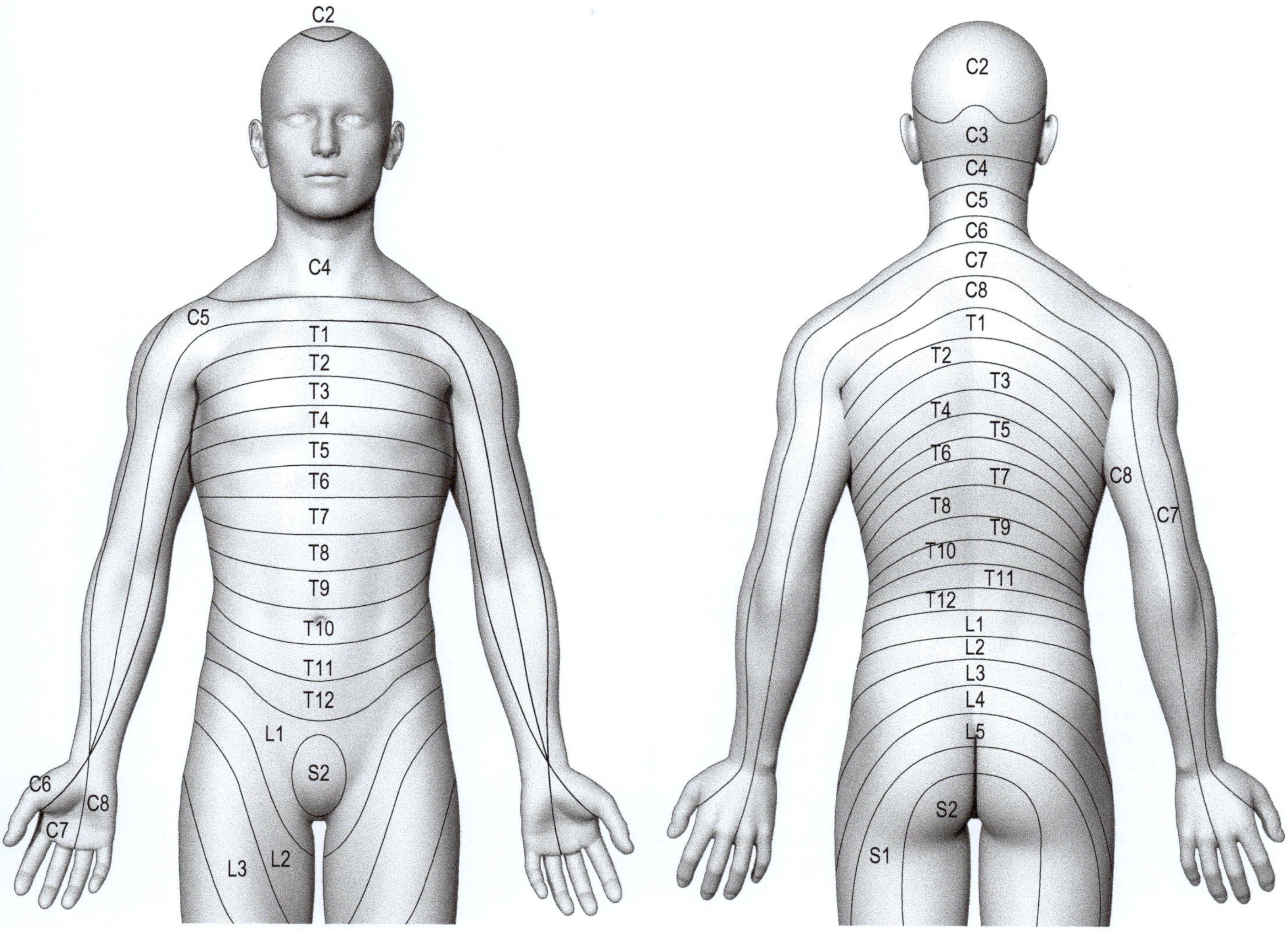

FIGURE 13.73

Dermatome map of the upper body.

CERVICAL SPINE: CHAPTER OVERVIEW

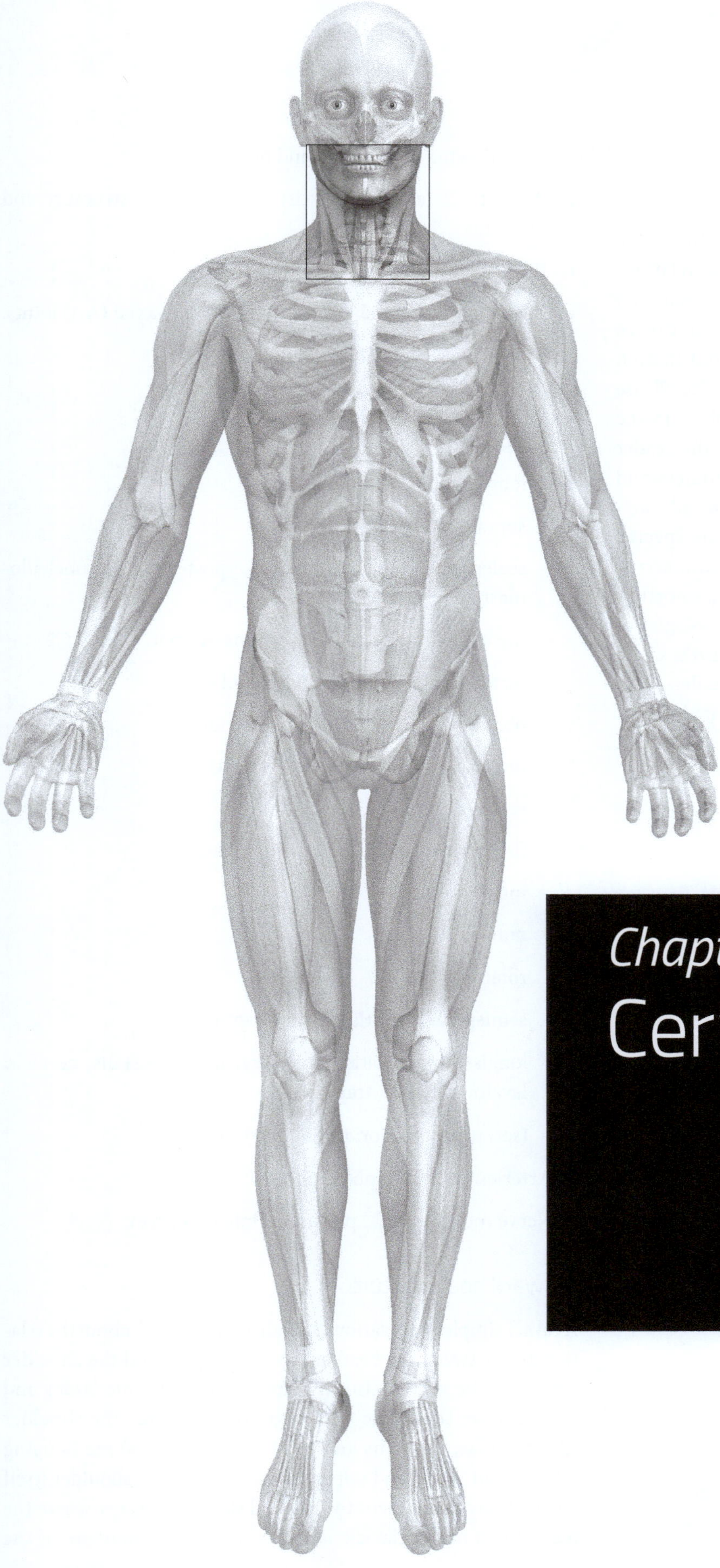

Chapter 14

Cervical spine

Chapter 14

Clinical implications of anatomy and physiology (Figure 14.1)

The following are some anatomical observations that have clinical implications. Understanding the functional relationships (physiology) between structures and tissues (anatomy) will help explain how structures of the cervical spine can be injured, and help us understand how orthopedic and motion tests work to provide the information that they do. Please review the anatomy of the joints and muscles involved in the function of the low back. And, it is suggested that the reader have an anatomy book at hand to more easily understand the information given below. (Either general musculoskeletal or a text that reviews anatomy in detail of this specific area of the body.) The information that has been summarized here has been chosen because of its direct relevance to orthopedic testing and understanding of mechanical pathologies of the cervical spine. (See Agur et al. 2014; Bogduk 2012; Chila 2010; DeStefano 2011; Dutton, 2012; Hertling & Kessler 2006; Kapandji 2008; Levangie & Norkin 2011; Magee 2014; Maitland 2001; Mitchell 2005; Schuenke et al. 2014).

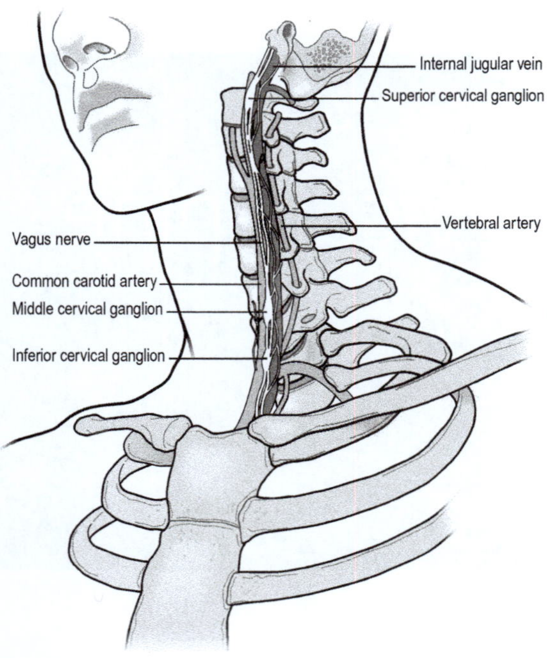

FIGURE 14.1

Location of important veins, arteries and ganglia in the cervical spine region.

The following anatomy should be reviewed:

1. Occiput, C1 (atlas), C2 (axis) – their unique structure and ligaments
   - The occipito-atlanto (OA) joints
   - The atlanto-odontoid joint, and the atlanto-axial (AA) joints.
2. C3 to C7 vertebrae, joints and ligaments.
3. Ligaments.
4. Musculature:
   - longus colli and capitis
   - supra- and infrahyoid
   - scalenes – anterior, medial, posterior; sternocleidomastoid; platysma
   - the intrinsic muscles between the occiput, C1 and C2
   - rectus capitis posterior major and minor
   - oblique capitis superior and inferior
   - rectus capitis lateralis (occiput–C1)
   - rectus capitis anterior
   - the intrinsic muscles between C3 and T1
   - intertransversarii
   - multifidi
   - rotatores
   - semispinalis capitis, spinalis capitis
   - longissimus capitis and cervicis, iliocostalis cervicis; levator scapulae, trapezius
   - (serratus posterior; rhomboids).
5. Arteries, veins, lymphoid tissue.
6. Nerve roots, brachial plexus, peripheral nerves.

Forward head posture

A rather simple observation, though often ignored, about the relationship between the head and cervical spine and the shoulder girdle can be very useful in helping uncover some issues and impairments that these two "regions" can have. The shoulder (the scapulae, the arms and most of the clavicles) are hanging off the head, neck, and upper thoracic spine. The shoulder itself has no bony attachment to the axial skeleton (except where the medial end of the clavicle joins the sternum). Therefore, if the shoulders are held protracted the head will inevitably be drawn forward, much to the detriment of the cervical spine and its tissues and also to the upper trapezius, levator scapulae, rhomboids, to name the most obvious structures and tissues. If the shoulders retract to a more proper alignment then the head will follow suit and resume a more balanced position over the shoulders (when viewed from the side). Kapandji (2008) wrote: "For every inch of Forward Head Posture, it can increase the weight of the head on the spine by an additional 10 pounds." Stress and strain to muscles, joints, ligaments, and neurovascular tissues of the neck and head caused by a forward head posture will affect and impair these structures and their functions.

Suboccipital recti muscles and eye movements (Figure 14.2)

Contraction and motion in the suboccipital muscles can be generated by eye movements alone, because there is a reflex relationship between the muscles controlling the eyes and the suboccipital recti muscles:

> Central connections of the oculo-cervical reflexes ... Ocular muscle proprioceptors send impulses back from the orbit by way of the ophthalmic division of the trigeminal nerve. From the trigeminal ganglion fibers run into the rhombencephalon to the mesencephalic nucleus of the trigeminal nerve. Secondary neuron ramifications run from the trigeminal nucleus into the vestibular nuclei, where third order neurons ramify into the vestibulospinal tracts to synapse with alpha and gamma motor neurons to the occipital recti muscles. (Mitchell 2005; muscle energy technique utilizes this reflex in mobilizing the occipito-atlanto and atlantoaxial joints)

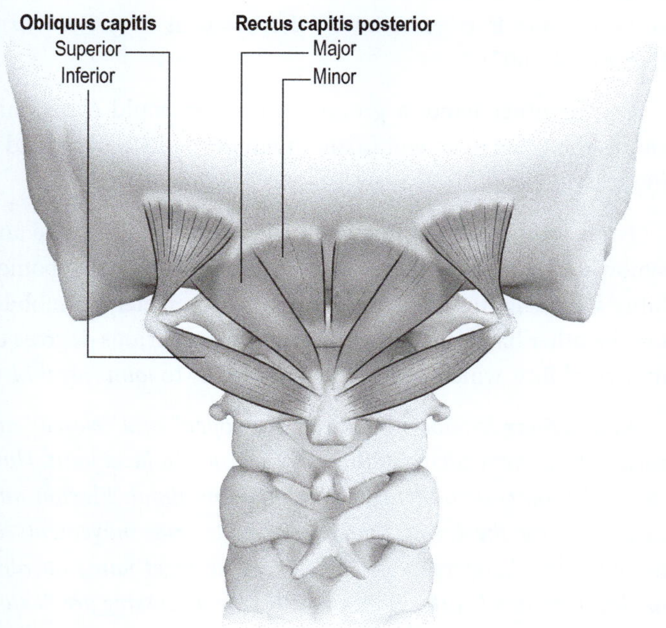

FIGURE 14.2
Suboccipital muscles.

This relationship is palpable: flex your neck forward and place two fingers, from each hand, on each side of the suboccipital area. Relax and let the head hang. Now look up, as if trying to look up into your brain, hold for a count of three, and then look down to your chin. Repeat several times. You will feel the recti muscles tighten when looking up, and relax when looking down (when the longus coli muscle reflexively engages).

Active range of motion for the cervical spine*

Flexion 45–65°

Occipitio-atlanto joint = 5–10°

Atlantoaxial joint = 0–5°

C2–6= 25–35°

C6–T1 = 5–15°

Extension 50–70°

Occipito-atlanto joint = 10–15°

C3–T1 = 40–55°

Side-bending 20–45°

Ocipito-atlanto = 5°

C3–T1 = 20–40°

Rotation 70–85°

Atlantoaxial = 40–45°

C3–T1 = 30–40°

*** NOTE:** The kinematics of cervical range of motion appears to be a hotbed of discussion and dispute. Therefore, what the figures given here in the breakdown of what each portion of the cervical spine contributes are approximations and very speculative. (Compare: Agur et al. 2014; Kapandji, 2008; Levangie & Norkin 2011; Magee 2014; Oatis 2004; Schuenke et al. 2006, 2007; Starkey & Brown 2015; Tillmann 2007).

See the Appendices for charts and tables on muscles (muscle origin, insertion, innervation, action and synergists), joints (actions, ranges, muscles used, tissues stretched and compressed; another table on capsular patterns of restriction, open packed/resting positions and close packed positions) and several charts on neurological testing where any such testing would involve this chapter's region.

Definitions and rules of motion for the cervical spine

A *motion segment* of the spine includes the two vertebrae and the joints between them. We have the cartilaginous joint of the intervertebral disc (IVD) and the two vertebral bodies. And, posteriorly we have a pair of facet joints or zygapophyseal joints (*zygo*, means pair, union or yoke, while *apophyseal*, refers to a natural "swelling" or projection of the spine).

The IVD is a polyaxial joint that allows rotation, forward flexion and extension, and side-bending; as well as shearing, compression, and expansion (Cailliet 1996; Hertling & Kessler 2006; Kapandji 2008; Magee 2014). In the cervical spine, the nucleus pulposus is more anterior within the disc than in the rest of the spine. For more on the IVD, see Chapter 12.

A facet joint is a plane-gliding joint. Motion occurs through two (relatively) flat surfaces sliding on each other. They can gap (open) or compress (close) to accommodate motion in various directions.

Each motion segment has two facet joints posteriorly. They are present from C2 to S1.

The OA joint provides 15° of flexion/extension, which can occur separate from the lower cervical spine. In other words, the OA joint can be flexed while the lower cervicals are extended, and vice versa. There is a minimal amount of side-bending and rotation available here.

The AA joint (joints between C1 and C2) provide approximately 50 percent of the rotation available in the cervical spine. The rest of rotation in the cervical spine comes from several degrees being available from each vertebral motion segment between C2 and C7 (with a small portion coming from the upper thoracics as well, T1–4). Again, it is possible for the AA joint complex to rotate in one direction while the lower cervical vertebrae rotate in the opposite direction. Flexion and extension, along with some side-bending, are also available in the AA joints.

There will be more on this set of joints later in this chapter.

Rules governing side-bending and rotation in the cervical spine

(See Dutton 2012; Hertling & Kessler 2006; Kapandji 2008; Levangie & Norkin 2011; Magee 2014; Mitchell 2005.)

- The OA joint complex *tends* to side-bend and rotate in opposite directions, though the motions available are small.
- The AA joint can move in opposite directions, or the same, when side-bending and rotating.
- The lower cervical spine (C2–T1) motion segments side-bend and rotate in the same direction.

Segmental dysfunction This refers to motion impairment within a specific motion segment. In other words, this refers to a motion impairment between two adjacent vertebrae.

Group dysfunction This is when two or more motion segments (i.e., three or more vertebrae) become collectively restricted in motion.

If the group dysfunction is a restriction in side-bending (which is coupled with rotation) it is called a *rotoscoliosis*, or just *scoliosis*. This can be *structural*, which means that bony changes or deformation of the vertebra's structure hold those involved segments permanently in that pattern. Or, as is the usual case, the scoliosis is *functional*, which means that impaired musculature and/or joint dysfunctions are holding the segments in side-bending and rotation. But if the tension and length of the musculature and joint structures is restored to normal, then the scoliosis will be removed.

Group dysfunctions can also occur that produce a decreased extension curve (lordosis) in the spine; a *hypolordosis*. In severe cases it becomes a cervical kyphosis. When this occurs in the cervical spine it is sometimes referred to as a *reverse curve* (Grob et al. 2007).

On the other hand, a group dysfunction could occur that causes the spine to extend further than normal. This is called a *hyperlordosis*.

Facet joint motion impairments The facet joints, like any synovial joint in the body, can suffer various degrees of hypomobility from slightly restricted motion to completely immobile. On the other hand, they can also suffer from various degrees of hypermobility, which range from *joint laxity* to *joint instability*.

Restrictions to motion *The terms "open" and "closed" are used to help the reader visualize the motion in a facet joint. How much the joints actually open or close is minimal. Flexion and extension are the terms that describe the true movements of these joints. Therefore, when we talk about facet joints opening or closing remember the movements we are discussing are flexion and extension, and all the gliding, rotating, gapping, compressing, etc. that are associated with these movements.*

The joint can be *held closed* either by musculature or other external structures or by intrinsic structures (such as ligamentous or joint capsule fibrosis or adhesions). This fixation of a facet joint means that it is synonymous with the specifically affected joint being held in extension. Saying a facet joint of the cervical spine is in extension means that the joint surfaces are approximated or held closed, regardless of the range of motion the whole cervical spine undergoes. Colloquially we say that the joint is "stuck" closed.

The joint can be *held open* by musculature and also by joint effusion (edema) when inflamed. If held in this position chronically the edema can become fibrous and then it may become difficult to restore mobility. Being held open is synonymous with being held fixed in flexion. Saying a facet joint of the cervical spine is in flexion means that the joint surfaces are held apart (are open) regardless of the range of motion the whole cervical spine undergoes. Colloquially we say that the joint is "stuck" open.

Clinical considerations and more on the OA and AA joints

The cervical spine has been traditionally divided into two sections: the upper and the lower cervical spine or quadrants. The superior portion is made up of the occiput, C1, and C2. These structures and the joints between them are the *upper quadrants*; comprising a left and right quadrant. Though not grammatically correct, this upper cervical portion, as a whole, is often referred to as the *upper quadrant*.

The lower portion of the cervical spine consists of the segments C2–T1 (though, for some schools of thought, the functional cervical spine is thought to extend to T4, which can be felt when the neck is flexed or extended to end-range). This lower portion is often referred to as the *lower quadrant* (with a lower left and lower right quadrant).

It is very important to understand and remember that though the upper and lower quadrants can combine to create significant ranges of motion for the head and neck they can also function *while moving in opposite directions to each other*. For example, the lower cervical spine can be rotated to the left while the upper cervical spine is rotated to the right. Further, the lower cervical spine can be flexed while the upper cervical spine (specifically the OA joint) extends.

The availability of these complementary and contrary motions between these two portions of the cervical spine permits a wide variety of ways that the head can remain balanced. Keeping the head (meaning the vestibular system) level is a necessity for appropriate and balanced movement of the body. The interplay between these two quadrants and the motion segments within each can provide extremely exacting compensations for almost anything that is happening in the trunk and limbs. Further, this cervical complex allows for either quadrant to compensate for the other if one becomes motion impaired.

More on the anatomy of the upper quadrant

The joints between the vertebrae of the upper quadrant are unique in the spine as they contain no intervertebral discs (IVDs). The OA joints are two synovial condylar joints. What is significant clinically about these two joints is that they are not parallel to each other but rather, are closer to each other at their anterior sections than they are at their posterior ends. They are V-shaped in their orientation and provide 15° of flexion and extension for the cervical spine.

The joints between C1 and C2 are called the atlanto-odontoid joint and the atlantoaxial (zygapophyseal) joints (Kapandji 2008). Often, the latter name (atlantoaxial, or AA joint) serves for naming all three joints of this motion segment, called simply the AA joints, collectively. The atlanto-odontoid joint refers to the unique pivot joint that exists between the two vertebrae, made up of the odontoid process and a facet on the posterior surface of the anterior arch of the atlas. The other synovial joints in the AA joint motion segment also help to provide the distinct movements (and hence distinct impairments) between these two vertebrae. These joints can appear as classic facet type joints, as are found in the rest of the spine, if we are only looking at a preserved skeleton (or plastic model). The bony facets appear flat, like those of the spine as a whole. However, in living tissue the cartilaginous surfaces between C1 and C2 are both convex, both rounded, and sitting on each other like two balls, one on top of the other (Figure 14.3).

As mentioned, 50 percent of cervical rotation (45° approximately both left and right) comes from the AA joints. While you would expect to find a great deal of laxity between the two vertebrae (C1 and C2) to allow this much movement, this is not so. The unique convex-convex joint surfaces of the lateral joints of the AA joint complex provides the stability: when in neutral the facet joint surfaces are one on top of the other. As described above, this would appear like two halves of a rubber ball sitting one on top of another (left of Figure 14.3). This holds the two vertebrae

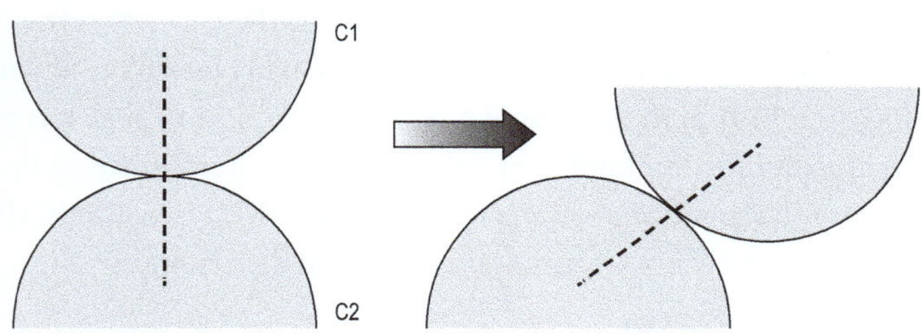

FIGURE 14.3

C1 and C2 in neutral and in rotation.

maximally apart keeping ligamentous attachments (see dotted lines) between the two vertebrae taut. However, when rotation occurs the two surfaces slide down hill on each other (right of Figure 14.3), loosening the ligaments so that more rotation can occur at the pivot joint (atlanto-odontoid joint) (see Hertling & Kessler 2006; Kapandji 2008; Levangie & Norkin 2011; Magee 2014; Mitchell 2005).

You can appreciate that if there is increased muscular tension, especially if shorting or spasming of the suboccipital musculature occurs, this could have consequences for this unique mechanism of the AA joints to become impaired. For one thing, the two convex joint surfaces could be prevented from riding up on each other due to muscular hypertonicity and thus prevented from returning to neutral. This would leave C1 rotated (either right or left) and unable to return to neutral where the rotation to the opposite side would be severely restricted.

Such locking of the AA joints would present as severely restricted rotation. Consequently, the ability to test this joint specifically is crucial for finding the source of loss of rotation. Specifically, how much loss of rotation is coming from the AA joints and how much is due to restrictions (if any) in the lower cervical spine? As rotation from the upper quadrant occurs in a completely different manner than the lower quadrant because of differences in structure, then the ways in which their function becomes impaired differs. This implies that they would most likely need to be treated differently therapeutically. We will provide such a differentiating test later in this chapter.

The lower quadrant

This portion of the cervical spine has the more common joint structure that we associate with the spine as a whole. Each motion segment has an IVD anteriorly and two posterior-lateral facet joints. All of the motions available to the lower cervical spine, such as flexion, extension, side-bending and rotation, involve both the IVD and the facet joints.

A joint specific to the lower quadrant of the cervical spine is the *uncovertebral joint*, also known as "joints of Luschka." If you look carefully at the vertebrae of a cervical spine on a skeleton or in an anatomy textbook you will notice that there is lateral lipping to the superior portion of C3 to C7 which is open anteriorly and posteriorly but cups the intervertebral disc laterally.

To quote Kapandji:

> In the cervical vertebral column movements also occur at two small additional joints – the uncovertebral joints (joints of Luschka). A frontal section … shows the two vertebral plateaus, the disc with its nucleus and annulus, but the disc does not reach the lateral margins of the vertebra. In fact, the superior plateau is raised laterally by two buttresses lying in a sagittal plane. These unciform processes have their cartilage-lined articular surfaces facing medially and superiorly and corresponding to the cartilage-lined semilunar facets of the inferior plateau of the upper vertebra, the latter facets pointing inferiorly and laterally. These small joints are enclosed within a capsule continuous medially with the intervertebral disc. (Kapandji 2008).

During flexion and extension when the body of the upper vertebra slides anteriorly or posteriorly the articular facets of the uncovertebral joints also slide relative to each other. Thus, these uniform ("hook-like') processes guide the vertebral body into this anterior-posterior movement.

It is suggested that as we grow into adolescence this unciform process develops and becomes very supportive to the lateral and posterior portion of the disc. A synovial joint develops between these. How these surfaces engage, especially during flexion and extension is fairly obvious, but lateral flexion (which includes rotation) becomes more complex (Hertling & Kessler 2006; Kapandji 2008).

We can have impairment to just the IVD such as degenerative disc disease (DDD). We can also have degenerative joint disease (DJD) in the facet joints and the uncovertebral joints. When degenerating all these types of joints show a tendency to create osteophytes (bony outgrowth) on the edges of the bony portion of the joint (called *lipping*). Lipping at the facet joints can reduce the size of the neural foramen by growing into the space of the foramen and directly irritate nerve roots as they exit and are rubbed by the rough edges of this bony growth. The osteophytes can also grow onto IVDs (especially along ligaments) and through the uncovertebral joints and eventually meet those growing from above downward causing ankylosing of the spine (e.g., "bamboo spine"). This lipping also occurs in the facet joints.

Presentation of pain in segmental or group dysfunctions

Frequently, a segmental impairment is specifically painful. The patient can often point directly to the acute segments. Less acute pain, pain that has gradual onset, or pain from diverse sources can feel more defuse for the patient. (For this and what follows see: Cailliet 1996; Hammer 2007; Hartley 2000a; Hertling & Kessler 2006; Magee 2014; Mitchell 2001.)

Muscle pain from restrictions to motions such as rotation and side-bending often involve the deep fourth layer muscles which are hypertonic and shortened (if not in outright spasm). These muscles assume a holding and guarding function (*splinting* by muscles) to protect the joint and its supportive tissues and so reduce motion in the joint. This splinting usually includes the larger superficial muscles.

When there is pain during an attempt to move the restricted facet joint: this experience of pain during PR-ROM is known as an *empty end-feel.* This pain can come from the shortened hypertonic muscle(s) contracting and becoming even shorter and therefore, go into a spasm. Of course, the pain can also arise from the joint itself if inflamed or injured which sets off a reflex contraction in the musculature involved in that joint's movement. We can observe this when the patient turns or when we move the patient toward the impaired side and they suddenly pull back. This is a rebound motion done by the patient in order to avoid pain or the increase in pain.

Facet joint pain can be from: compression of irritated or inflamed joint surfaces and structures commonly found in a (facet) joint being held closed; or from the tension placed on inflamed/injured ligaments or the pressure of a swollen joint capsule commonly found in (facet) joints that are being held open or flexed.

Uncovertebral joints can have pain symptoms like any synovial joint and can also suffer from osteoarthritis (DJD). These joints can produce pain during excessive loading or compression of the spine during trauma or postural misalignment. It is clear that degenerative disc disease (DDD), in causing a loss of disc height, will inevitably lead to such overloading and degenerative joint changes in both the uncovertebral and facet joints. It is assumed that these joints can cause local pain and as deep structures they can also refer pain.

Disc pain is sourced in the intervertebral disc (discogenic pain). It remains a controversial topic with respect to finding evidence of it as a source of low back pain (Bogduk 2003; Hertling & Kessler 2006; Levangie & Norkin 2011; Magee 2014). For some theories on this, see Chapter 12.

Nerve root (radicular) pain is felt in the dermatome (refer back to Figure 13.73). In the cervical spine, radicular pain is most common in the shoulder, down the arm and/or into the hand (C4 to T1 nerve root dermatomes). C1 to C3 sensory nerve roots are said to innervate the head and neck. See neurological testing later in this chapter. (For more on nerve pain, see Chapter 4 and Chapter 12.)

Recurring joint pain may be caused by the shortening of fascia (connective tissue components of the muscles, ligaments, and joint capsules) and can become asymptomatic in the sense that the patient does not have a constant experience of pain as they often avoid the motions that produce it. However, the affected joint can be painful on palpation. Further, this situation often has the quality of suddenly flaring up from time to time. This can occur from a sudden re-straining of the tissues and joint (via exertion, etc.) or from a flare-up due to repetitive strain (micro-tearing) or overuse. The latter seems to arise when daily wear and tear at the cellular level of the musculature and/or joint tissues exceeds the ability of the body to heal itself (during rest) and a debt accumulates to the point where the tissues will finally trigger an inflammatory response once the amount of damage reaches a critical mass (Cailliet 1996).

Group dysfunction pain

Group dysfunctions can be initially painful if the onset is sudden, such as in torticollis. The pain is usually due to spasming muscles that are holding the group of segments side-bent and rotated. A patient may report, for example, that they woke up with the pain. They may also report that the neck became locked or stiff upon stopping a certain activity that required the head to stay in one position too long (e.g., computer work). The joints may also become suddenly painful when the surrounding muscles suffer a sudden strain and/or spasm leading to a sudden overloading of the joint tissues of several joints.

Group dysfunctions are also very common postural dysfunctions that are chronic in nature and, with regard to pain, they may often remain asymptomatic for long periods of time. Eventually, if unresolved, they can gradually become painful as the joint tissues start to become inflamed from the constant strain on them (compression or tension). When this occurs on repeated occasions, the patient describes it as a flare-up, which we refer to as an *acute-on-chronic* episode. The patient may say that the pain came on suddenly but, in fact, it may be due to a pre-existing asymptomatic strain or impairment that finally reached a point where the tissues react with an inflammatory response (Hertling & Kessler 2006).

Spinal group impairments (scoliosis or curve in the cervical spine) are often a compensatory response. The curve is adjusting for postural imbalances from above (OA or AA joints) or from below (thoracic curves/scoliosis). The constancy of the curve results in a chronic muscle imbalance with those on one side of the spine (in the concavity) becoming short and those on the other side (of the convexity) becoming long. At first, these lengths may be held solely by the resultant muscle spindle settings appropriate for each length of muscle in their respective groupings. Eventually, the connective tissue will shorten (on the concave side) if it is not stretched/lengthened by normal activity; or it will undergo a plastic change and lengthen if it is not allowed to shorten (the convex side). Shortened muscles tend to become hypertonic and prone to spasm if shortened further, while lengthened muscles tend to weaken (stretch-weakness) and are more easily strained with exertion or trauma (Hertling & Kessler 2006; Janda 1984; Janda & Jull 1987; Magee 2014).

Therefore, with a group dysfunction or impairments, the concave side can be prone to bouts of pain from compressed facet joints and/or shortened muscles spasming. However, the convex side can experience pain due to stretch of the joint capsule and/or from the lengthened musculature becoming fatigued and achy, which results in them exhibiting the signs and symptoms of strain and overuse. ***NOTE:*** The lesson to learn from this is to beware the danger of assuming that when a patient points specifically to one side of their neck that the joints on that side are compressed and the muscles are short and tight. If you do make this assumption but the complaining musculature is long and weak then your treatment (if it includes longitudinal muscle stripping and stretching) may in fact relax them so that the musculature becomes even longer and weaker. If this happens then when the patient returns for their next session they do so with the same (or even a worse) condition.

Segmental pain

Pain from a segmental dysfunction is usually sudden, as the dysfunction occurs. Though they are often immediately painful they may worsen even more over several hours. This worsening pain is often due to the inflammatory process ramping up the swelling and pain. The pain is often initially sharp and bright and often very site-specific. The patient can point to it accurately. Over several days the intensity of pain may stay (or lessen slightly) but it will change in how it is experienced. It may feel deeper to the patient and the edges or border may be enlarged and more vague. Therefore, the patient can become less accurate in pointing to its original source.

See Boxes 14.1 on whiplash grading and 14.2 on migraine for additional information on these disorders.

Comprehensive examination

This testing protocol is usually done when the therapist wants to perform a more detailed postural examination (static and dynamic) of the patient. If several of the tests underlined below are found to be positive then a more thorough examination of the cervical spine needs to be performed. As presented in the rest of this chapter. Pain, asymmetries, and other impairments on-site at the cervical spine area can occur with standing, sit-

Box 14.1 Whiplash associated disorders (WAD)

Grade according to assessment findings:

WAD 0: Patient reports no pain or discomfort. Therapist finds no physical signs of injury.

WAD I: Patient reports neck pain, stiffness or tenderness. However, therapist finds no impairment to ROM etc.

WAD II: Patient reports neck pain, stiffness, or tenderness. Therapist finds one or more of the following: changes in range of motion, restriction in motion, edema, some physical signs of injury (bruising, wound, etc.); palpation finds point tenderness.

WAD III: Patient reports pain, stiffness or tenderness. The therapist may find any number of physical findings (per WAD II) plus therapist finds neurological signs of injury, such as changes to reflexes or muscle weakness.

WAD IV: Fracture or dislocation of the neck, in addition to musculoskeletal findings.

INSIGHTS

Box 14.2 Migraines can be a pain in the neck

Non-pathological (not from high blood pressure, tumors, etc.) migraines, sometimes called "common migraines," can often be traced back to pain originating in the suboccipital muscles, joints of occiput-C1-2-3, and their ligaments. There are important neurological connections that explain how upper cervical pain may lead to headaches and migraines. The following will trace a number of these connections, and show how the symptoms of headaches, pseudo-ear infections, and pseudo-sinus headaches, and the common migraine can be generated in the suboccipital area. This is a brief review, however, and therefore over-generalization may be unavoidable (for much of the anatomy see Schuenke et al. 2007).

Contraction of the suboccipital recti muscles tenses the connective tissue "curtain" between the deepest tissue layers and the spinal cord's dura mater, in the spaces between the occiput-C1 and C1 and C2. Some of the muscle fibers reach right through this curtain of connective tissue and are attached to the dura mater. Hypertonicity of these suboccipital muscles will sustain this tension. Nerves and blood vessels are compressed as they pass through these tense muscle tissues and the curtain created by their connective tissue, as they pass in and out of the brainstem/spinal cord. The occiput and the atlas (C1) are approximated (in extension) because of these short and hypertonic muscles, adding further compressive forces from bony structures onto these nerve fibers and blood vessels. This can cause impaired signaling and facilitation of the affected nerves while reducing blood flow into the posterior brain.

There are sensory and motor connections running from the upper cervical joints, the recti muscles and tissues overlaying them, that enter into the trigeminal nerve's nuclei in the brainstem. This area is therefore referred to as the "trigemino-cervical complex." This route is also one of the access points for the sympathetic system entering into the cranium (via the superior cervical ganglion). Nerve impulses from upper cervical pain sensations, impulses from the sympathetic nervous system, along with proprioceptive information, run along with the trigeminal nuclei and travel with the input from the trigeminal nerve up into the higher centers of the brain to be processed, and a misinterpretation of cervical sensations (pain) as trigeminal sourced pain occurs (Puledda et al. 2017), thereby generating cervicogenic headaches and migraines.

The trigeminal nerve breaks into three branches. The lowest branch, the mandibular division (CN V-3), travels to the muscles of mastication: masseter, temporalis, and pterygoids. Facilitation from suboccipital sensory nerves and from the sympathetic chain can cause these muscles to become hypertonic, or even spasm. This spasming, especially in the case of the temporalis muscle, can present as one-sided head pain. It is well-known that jaw (TMJ) pain can refer into the ear. The pathway for this referral may be the branch of V-3 innervating the tensor tympani muscle that controls the tension on the eardrum. The greater the tension on the eardrum, the greater the volume we get from sound. If this muscle is over-activated, it will tighten to the degree that sounds become more intense. Further, if this tension is very high it can be interpreted as (feel like) an ear infection or as a "plugged ear." This referral can in turn affect the vestibular sense, causing dizziness (even vertigo) and nausea. V-3 exits the mandible via the mental foramen, being the sensory nerve for the skin over the mandible. It seems to be very rare for the higher centers of the brain to misinterpret upper cervical pain sensation as coming from this branch. V2 and V3 are much more prone to this.

The maxillary division of the trigeminal nerve (CN V-2) is the sensory nerve for the upper jaw (and teeth), maxillary sinuses, and the interorbital area. Over-stimulation of the interorbital sensory nerves can give rise to feeling pain behind the eye. V-2 exits the skull through the infraorbital foramen, being the sensory nerve for the area around the cheekbones.

The ophthalmic branch (CN V-1) travels to the eye, the sinuses, and the forehead: with respect to the eye, one portion of V-1 innervates the ciliary ganglia. The sensory part of this ganglia receives pain signals from the surface of the cornea. The motor part of the ganglia controls how the pupil opens (dilates) and closes and corneal reflexes. If this motor signal is not as it should be (too much stimulus entering the ciliary ganglia) then the pupil does not respond to light correctly, staying dilated. This is why migraine and other headache sufferers can be so sensitive to light. They find bright or flashing light to be painful, and often experience the eye itself as painful. Further, ciliary muscle fiber in the eye shapes the lens of the cornea and again, if inappropriate signaling is involved, the lens may be distorted, resulting in optical distortions such as wavy lines, spots, etc., in the periphery of vision and difficulty focusing the eye when reading, etc., elements of the classic auras experienced by migraine sufferers.

ting, or motion from above or below and therefore demand further investigation. For more detailed information and pictures see Chapter 10.

Observation and landmarking during motion gives us the most clues about which part of the spine has the greatest impairment.

Standing postural views: front, side, side and back:

1. Looking for relationships with a gravity line. With a plumb line check vertical landmarks, observe horizontal landmarks (again, see introductory remarks for spinal assessment for details). Note asymmetries and tissue texture changes.

Sitting behind the patient, note any asymmetries and any restrictions to range of motion:

1. Landmark levels of arches of the feet, ischial tuberosities, trochanters, PSISs, iliac crest heights, (creases of) waist, inferior and superior angles of scapulae, mastoid processes.
2. Return to PSISs. While landmarking PSISs, have the patient bring the chin to the chest, then slowly roll down to lumbar

flexion while noting movement of the PSISs (standing flexion test). Then check the spine for flat spots, excessive curve, bulking of the erector spinae, lateral curves, and the like. Then, have the patient return to standing straight. Ask the patient to look up to the ceiling (while you leave your hands on the patient's hips for their stability) and have the patient extend their back while you observe changes to the curves of the spine (lordosis-kyphosis).

3. Have the patient bring the ear to the shoulder; then have them slide the hand down the side of the leg to the knee, observing how the spine curves during side-bending (from above). Check both sides.
4. Have the patient flex one knee while the other remains locked. Note lumbar side-bending (from below). Check both sides.
5. Hold the patient's hip stable. Have the patient bring their chin over a shoulder and note head and cervical rotation. Then have them bring that shoulder back toward you, observing upper thoracic rotation. Also note the difference in the amount of resistance required at the hips to resist lower trunk rotation (ease versus effort).
6. Challenge sagittal plane (anterior-posterior) stability (via the manubrium and T2).
7. Challenge coronal plane (side-bending) motion, either by pressure on the acromions or an inferiorly directed tug on the wrists.

Have the patient sitting:

1. Re-check iliac crest heights, PSISs, shoulder/scapulae landmarks, tissue bulk, etc. Observe all changes of orientation to landmarks, tissue changes, etc., during the following motion.
2. Seated flexion test. While landmarking PSISs, have the patient flex forward. Check for asymmetry of tissue bulk on either side of the spine.
3. Side-bending: with the elbow at 90°, the patient brings the ear to the shoulder, then lowers it toward the table.
4. Rotation: turn the chin toward the shoulder and, at end-range, push the shoulder back. Challenge to side-bending: push down alternately on each shoulder cap.
5. Patient supine (after traction of legs or other corrections to patient's orientation on table).
6. Note medial malleoli levels.
7. Check the ASISs
   - level (innominate rotation)
   - heights from table (pelvic rotation)
   - distance from mid-line (inflare/outflare).
8. Check rotations (fascial exam). Compare the height from the table of the hips (ASISs, as above), lower ribcage, upper ribs, anterior shoulders, L and R occiput, i.e., height from the table compared to the norm and compared one to the other bilaterally, and then compare directions of rotation from one set of landmarks to the next.
9. Push the following side to side comparing ease/bind, (testing side-bending): at waist (lumbars), mid-ribs (thoracic) and neck (cervicals).

When, or if, specific testing has the patient prone check the following:

1. Levels of the plantar surface of the heels, ischial tuberosities, PSISs (and height from table); and the lateral curves in the spine, tissue bulk of the erector spinae, and scapulae orientation.

The protocol for testing the cervical spine can be extensive or simple. See p. 413 for further comments and an example of the complete protocol.

Case history (specific questions)

- Ask the patient if they have experienced any headaches: tension, cluster, migraines, or sinus. Ask them for the source of the diagnosis.
- Ask them if they are prone to headaches. What type(s)? Frequency? Duration? Intensity? Do they know of any triggers? Allergies?
- Ask about head injuries. Whiplash (MVA)? Falls or other traumas? History, number and severity? Treatments/interventions? Jaw injuries or temporomandibular joint diagnosis? Amount and type of dental work done?
- Blood pressure issues? Blood disorders?
- Diabetes? Hypo/hyperglycemic? Digestive issues/conditions?
- Vision problems? Hearing or balance issues?
- Ask about neurological issues/conditions in head or neck, if warranted by their intake form.
- Any issues in, impairments to the shoulders or arms and hands?

Note any obvious deformities and consider their implications. Is the deformity a contributing factor to the patient's chief complaint?

Observations

See the postural assessment material in Chapter 3 for more detail.

Standing postural exam. Note that it is important to have the patient standing in a natural pose. To help with this have the patient look up slightly (i.e., you do *not* want them looking at their feet) and take a couple of steps while staying in place. Ask the patient to try and not correct their feet positions, head positions, etc. You are trying to have them stand as they naturally do or as near to it as is possible given they are in a clinical setting.

NOTE: Much of this standing postural information is needed to compare with supine and prone examinations so that we are not misled by what we see (or will not see) when the patient is on the table.

- Observe the general orientation of the upper body – especially rotations and side-bending of the shoulders and spine, with a particular focus on the cervical spine and head.
- Observe the general orientation of the hips, thighs, knees, tibias, ankles, and feet while noting if the hips are shifted right or left over a leg. Note proportions (tissue bulk) and orientation of the thigh and lower leg (rotations throughout the course of the limb down to the feet, varus or valgus of knees or ankles, arches of the feet, etc.).

During observation, be specific with the following:

- Check iliac crest and greater trochanter heights.
- Record ASIS and PSIS heights from the anterior, posterior, and lateral views. Compare the heights of the ischial tuberosities.
- Note pelvic obliquity. This is a change in the height of one hip compared to the other, usually due to a unilateral anterior or posterior rotation of the innominate.
- Note whether the pelvis appears rotated around a vertical axis. In other words, does one ASIS (hip pointer) appear more anterior than the other (in the coronal plane), whether the ASISs are level with each other or not.
- Is the head rotated left, or right? Tilted?
- Note whether one shoulder is higher than the other (landmarking the AC joints). Do the same for the scapulae (landmarking with the inferior angle).
- Is one shoulder more forward than the other? If so, it is often the lower shoulder as well, and is often closer to the mid-line than the other shoulder.
- Is the upper thoracic cage rotated? If so, you will often notice the lower and more forward shoulder is rotated to the other side.
- The patient is said to be compensating when the rotations at various levels are alternating. The patient is said to be uncompensating when the rotations are (usually) to the same side.
- Observe if the patient has shifted their pelvis to one side over a leg, which then usually becomes the principal weight-bearing leg.
- Note any lateral curves in the spine (scoliosis).
- Note whether the patient has a hyperlordosis or a hypolordosis of the lumbar spine or of the cervical spine. Observe whether any part of the spine seems rotated and/or side-bent.
- Note whether the thoracic spine is hypokyphotic or hyperkyphotic.
- Note whether the cervical spine is hypolordotic (reversed curve) or hyperlordotic.
- Is there a forward head posture?
- Is there a protracted or retracted chin?
- Is there notable asymmetry to the look and shape of the ribs?
- Note the shape and orientation of the thoracic cage. Does the ribcage look inflated or inhaled (as if the patient is holding their breath in), or does it look exhaled (as if the patient had completely breathed out and is holding that position)? Is there any abnormal shape to the ribcage?

From your observations consider if you have found any possible causes or suspicions for the patient's chief complaint(s) and secondarily, if you have found any postural or other structural faults that may *predispose* the patient to further impairments (that are not yet present or experienced). Some of these questions can be answered by deciding which muscles may be short and tight or long and weak. You may also discover which joints are under extra tensile or compressive stress and whether the neurovascular flow to the upper extremities (or anywhere else) is possibly being compressed.

The upper cross (X) syndrome (Janda & Jull 1987)

Figure 14.4 can provide clues as to which tissues may be short and which may be long, which muscles may be short and tight and which are long and weak; see Figure 14.5 for examples.

Posturally challenging the chief complaint (Figure 14.6)

As a final step of observation and inspection, look at how the patient naturally stands and correct their posture with gentle

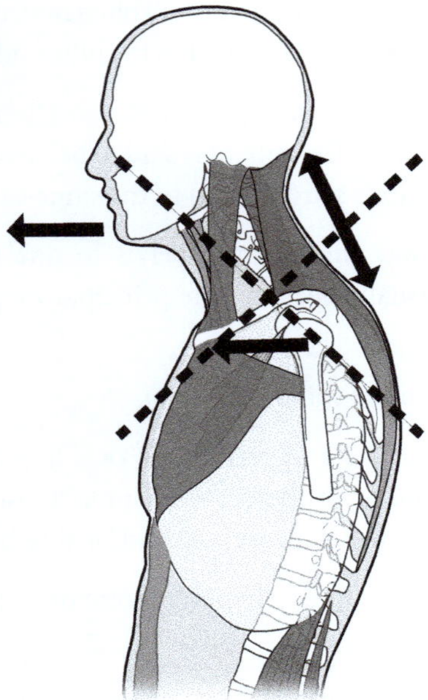

FIGURE 14.4 **The upper cross syndrome**

The chin moves forward into protrusion; the shoulder rolls forward or is protracted. The occiput is extended so the upper cervical vertebrae are held in extension while the lowest cervical and upper thoracic are held flexed. Thoracic kyphosis exaggerates and the musculature and posterior ligaments are under stretch.

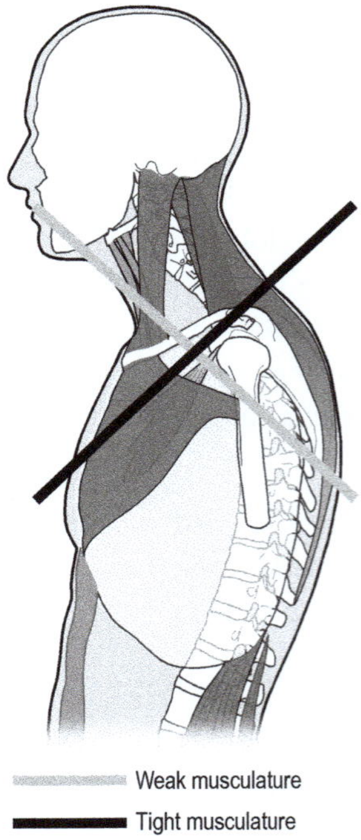

FIGURE 14.5

Weak: deep flexors of the neck, rhomboids, infraspinatus and teres minor, middle and lower trapezium.

Tight: suboccipitals, upper trapezium, and levator scapulae, SCM and scalenes, teres major and latissimus dorsi, pectoralis major and minor, serratus anterior.

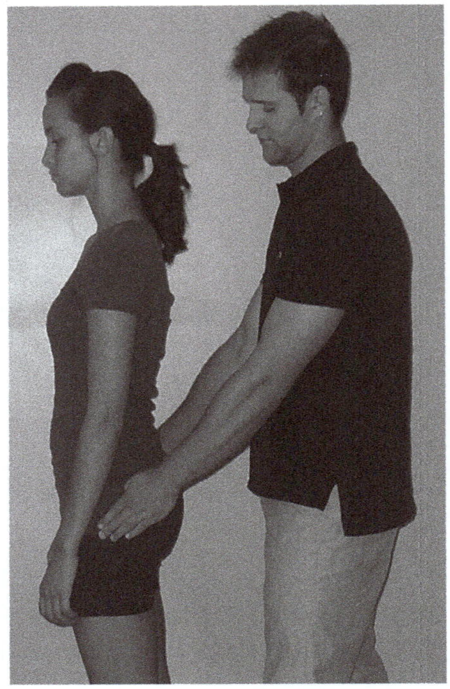

FIGURE 14.6

Exploring how the chief complaint fits into the whole.

movements. For example, push the hips back, unlock hyperextended knees, re-position a forward head over the shoulders and the like. Note what changes occur above and below. Ask the patient to sustain this corrected position (if possible). As they do so, a growing tension or discomfort/pain they experience from sustaining this corrected posture may point to injured, shortened, weakened, or stressed tissues or structures that need to be included in your assessment and treatment. This will help reveal problems that have a global effect (predisposing them to impairments) as well as possibly being intimately connected to the specific impairment that makes up their chief complaint.

Light inspection palpation

Assess tissue texture changes to the skin and connective tissue of the upper back and neck. Also include a brief examination from neck to shoulder, down the arm and hands. Check for heat or coolness over joints and the musculature The appearance and feel of tissue texture changes can be covering an underlying joint impairment. On the other hand, it can also be radiating from a specific nerve root to its dermatome via the sympathetic system. Symptoms include dryness, excessive moisture, trophic changes, goosebumps, and the like. The sympathetic ganglion controlling autonomics for the head are T1–4 and for the arms and hands, T5–7.

Use *light* palpation at this time as techniques such as skin rolling may cause pain and interfere with testing results. Many of the palpable skin changes come from altered neurovascular perfusion to the tissue and a common reason for this is an altered sympathetic response to impairments in the joints and tissues associated with that area.

Rule outs

Ruling out the shoulder (Figures 14.7, 14.8)

To rule out the shoulder joint as the source of neck pain, we need do only two active free movements: abduction and forward flexion, and add over-pressure (O-P) to both if the AF is pain-free (Hartley 2000a). If there is a dysfunction in the glenohumeral, acromial, or scapulothoracic joints these actions with O-P place enough stress on the structures and tissues to elicit a sufficient positive response which is pain and/or reproduction of the patient's chief complaint. These actions can give us enough information to tell us if we need a more thorough testing of these areas.

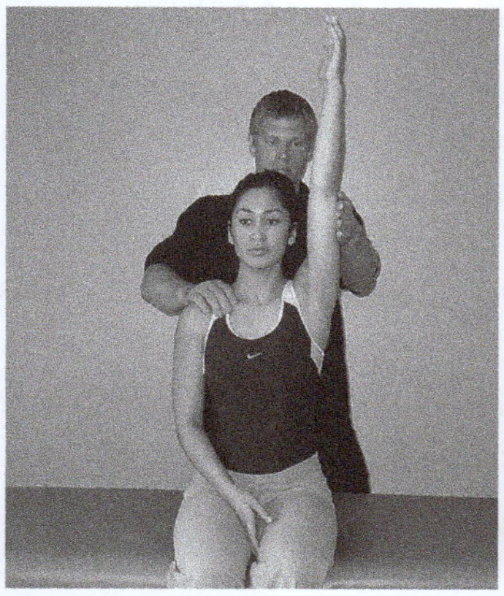

FIGURE 14.7 1. Rule out with AF abduction, then O-P

Have the patient abduct the arm; if this is pain-free apply over-pressure.

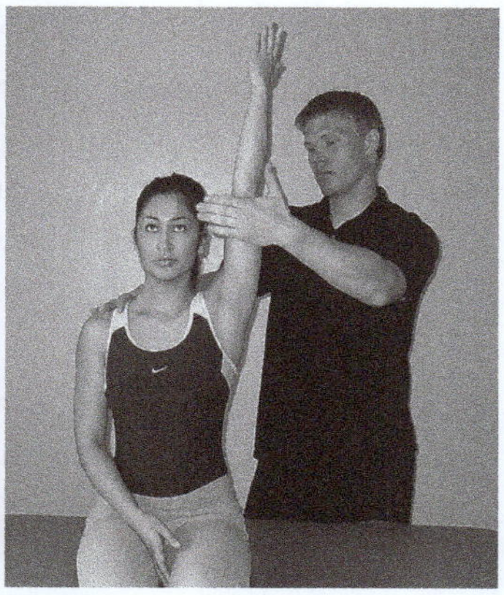

FIGURE 14.8 2. Rule out with forward flexion, then O-P

Have the patient fully forward flex the arm; if pain-free apply over-pressure.

Since there is such a close connection between the functioning of the head, neck, and shoulders the rule outs suggested may aggravate the patient's chief complaint in the cervical spine, especially if the musculature that runs between the scapula and the head and neck is involved. However, one advantage of doing these rule outs and getting a positive response is that we would now know that we need to investigate more than just the cervical spine. We may need to investigate the *occiput-cervical spine-shoulder girdle complex.*

Temporomandibular joint (Figures 14.9–14.12)

To rule out the temporomandibular joint (TMJ) have the patient do the following actions. The therapist should be observing for deviations, etc., as the jaw opens or closes; palpating the TMJ and other related tissues while asking about pain, etc.

It helps the patient when doing protrusion and retrusion (Figure 14.12) if they place the web space of thumb and index

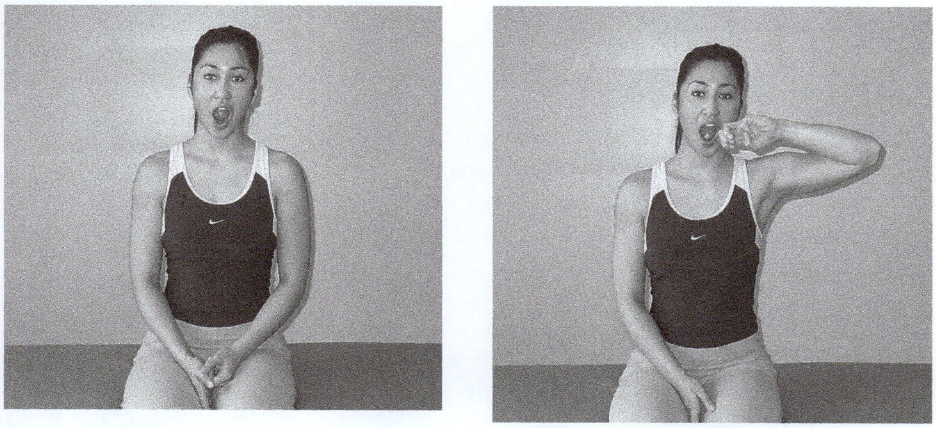

FIGURE 14.9A, B 1. Active mandible depression

Observe if patient can open jaw wide enough to equal three of their finger widths. Palpate TMJ joint as patient performs this action. At end-range, apply a slight,gentle O-P via patient's chin using the web space between your thumb and index finger.

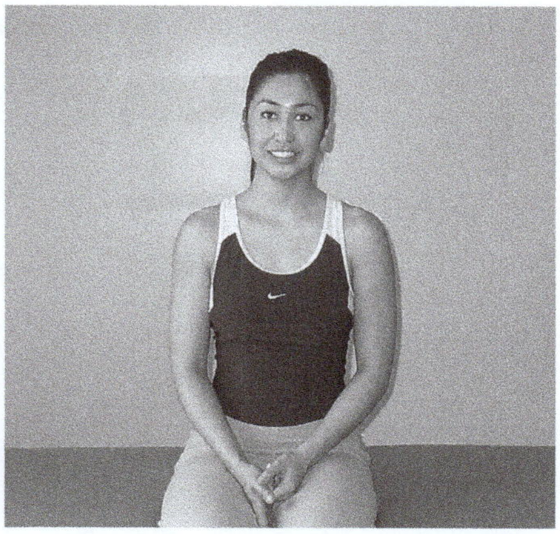

FIGURE 14.10 2. Active mandible elevation

The patient brings the teeth together gently. For O-P, the patient clenches the teeth. This reveals not only joint problems but also shows muscular problems. As the patient holds the clench, you should palpate the masseter and temporalis muscles and TMJs.

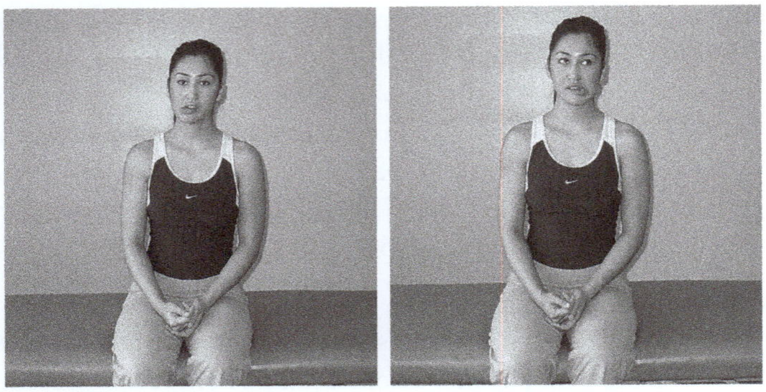

FIGURE 14.11A, B **3. Active lateral excursions, left and right**

Have the patient move the mandible left; apply gentle O-P if pain-free. Move the mandible right and then O-P if pain-free.

finger on their chin and feel the jaw while they are protruding and retracting. Their hand is there for sensory feedback purposes only. The patient is not to push the jaw backward or grasp the mandible and pull it forward. O-P is applied by the therapist only if the action has been pain-free.

The vertebral artery test (Figures 14.13–14.16)

This is to test for occlusion/compression of the vertebral artery. It should always be done if the patient has reported symptoms of dizziness or light-headedness during their case history taking for any cervical dysfunction. First, review the steps below carefully before performing the test, especially noting the positive signs for occlusion.

- With the patient supine, reach under the cervical spine and place your fingertips in the laminar groove on either side of the

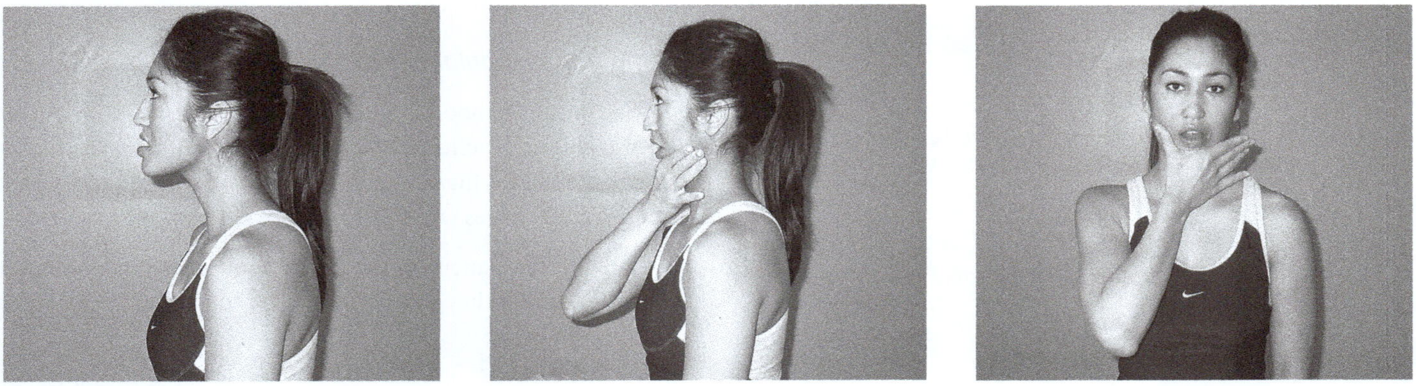

FIGURE 14.12A–C **4. Active protrusion and retrusion (retraction)**

(A) After the patient protrudes the chin, place your finger-pads along the line of the jaw and traction it forward gently and slightly inferiorly (not shown). (B) After the patient retracts their jaw, ask about pain. If there is none, then for O-P for retraction replace the patient's hand with yours (over the chin), or place your hand over theirs. Apply slight O-P.

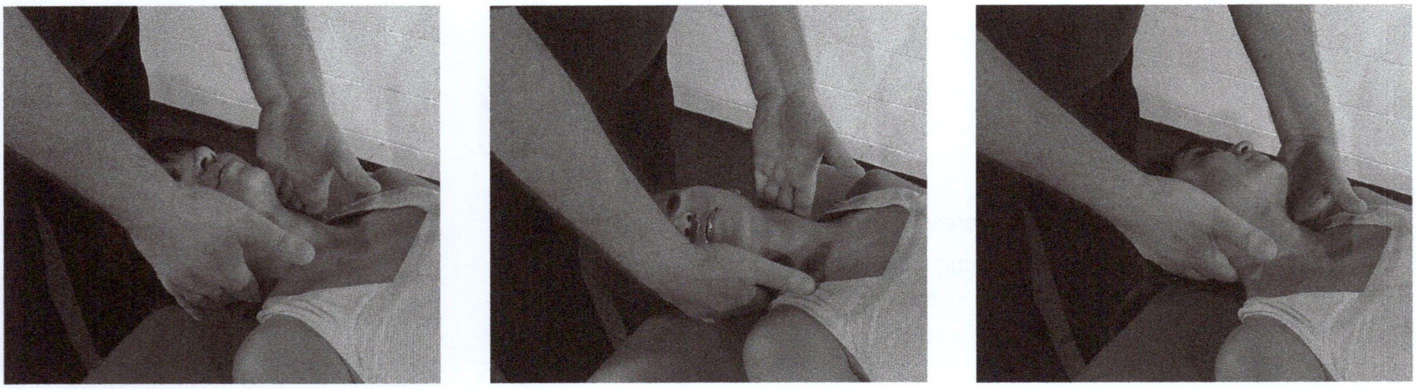

FIGURE 14.13A–C **Vertebral artery test**

The supine patient's neck is passively extended by lifting C3. Look for symptoms. If none, then rotate to one side while observing. Repeat rotation to the other side (only if the first side was negative) and make observations.

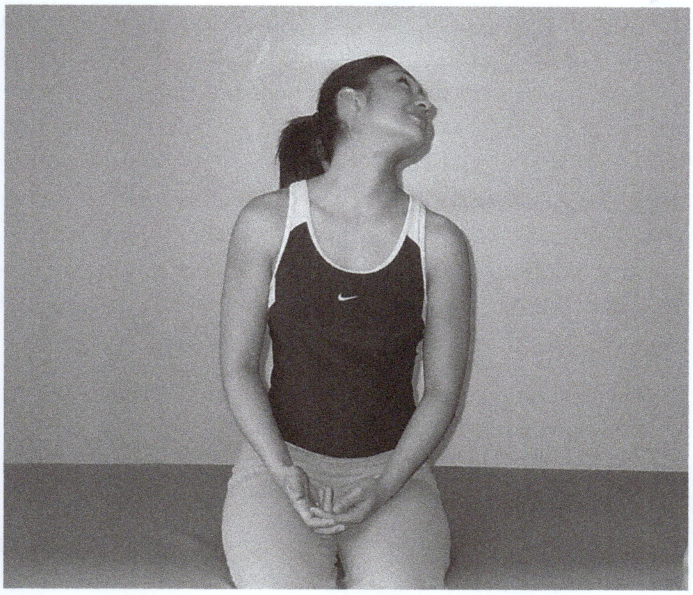

FIGURE 14.14 Alternative vertebral artery test

1. Have the patient seated for safety. Stand close to the patient or even have a hand on their back so they feel secure during actions and you are able to quickly support them if need be. Ask the patient to look back and up over their shoulder moving only their head and neck. Watch for symptoms while standing just beside or behind the patient. Repeat on the other side if the first side is negative.

mid-portion of their C-spine. Tell the patient to lift their chin as high up as they can (or point their chin up toward the ceiling). You can assist while they do this by lifting the spine up anteriorly, increasing the lordosis and thus taking the spine into extension.

- Now, side-bend the head and rotate it to one side holding for at least 30 seconds. Then side-bend the head and rotate it to the other side.
- Tell the patient to keep their eyes open and keep your attention on their eyes.
- Hold for 30 seconds on each side or until the test is positive.

The clearest positive for this test is if *nystagmus* (dancing eyes/rapid twitching of the eyeball) is noticed. The eyeball itself fasciculates. Blinking is not a positive. However, the test is also positive if there is any re-creation or exaggeration of the patient's symptoms of dizziness, ringing in the ears, or changes to eyesight (going black, fogging out or going white, tunnel vision, etc.). Slurring of speech is also positive and because of this you should continue throughout the test to ask about symptoms (or any case history sort of question) while doing the test and note any changes to the patient's speech, asking the patient to verbally respond if they do not.

If you get a positive test, then refer the patient to their physician. If symptoms are present in everyday activity for the patient, then refer them immediately to a hospital emergency room.

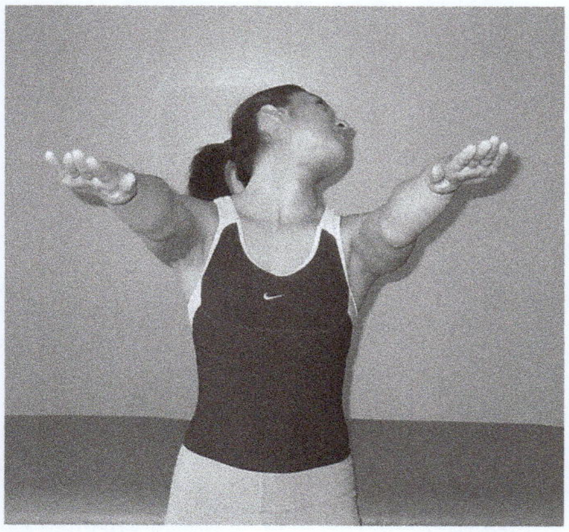

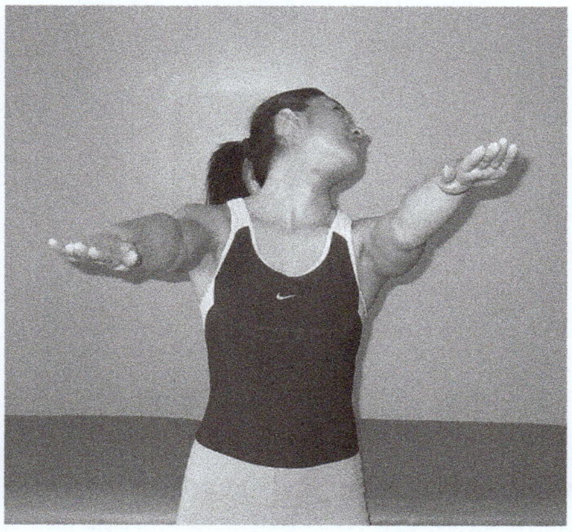

FIGURE 14.15A, B Alternative vertebral artery test

2. Have the patient place the head as in test 1. Have them hold their arms out straight. While watching for symptoms you can also note if one arm begins to droop. This is positive sign. Repeat on the opposite side if the first side is negative.

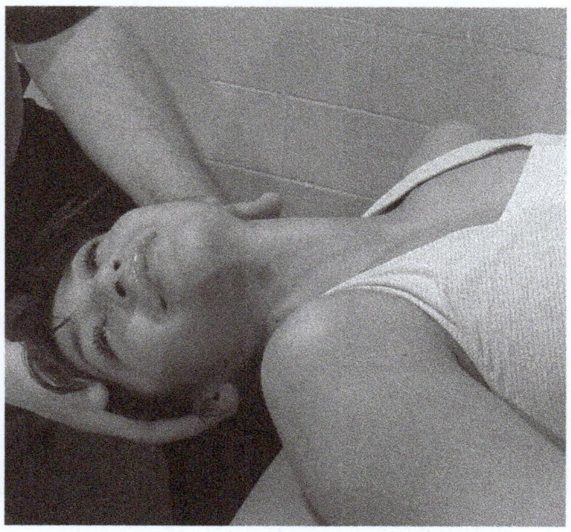

FIGURE 14.16 Classic vertebral artery test

The supine patient's head and neck are off the table. With their eyes kept open, take their head and neck into extension, side-bending and rotation to one side. Observe. Repeat to the opposite side (if negative).

Classic vertebral artery test (Figure 14.16)

The classic version is to have the patient's head off the table. Many patients can be uncomfortable or unable to relax even though you are providing firm yet comfortable support for their head. However, one advantage of this position is that the weight of the patient's head can be used to slightly traction the C-spine which adds a further provocation to the test. Some may say that this is an unnecessary step and possibly also not safe as it could be too provoking for fragile blood vessel tissues. Therefore, *use this original version with caution* (if you use it all).

Range of motion testing (ROM)

Active free range of motion (AF-ROM) (Figures 14.17–14.27)

When testing a patient's AF-ROM it may be best to have them seated for their security and comfort as cervical injuries and dysfunctions can often have dizziness and lack of balance as a consequence.

Have the patient do the following actions and see if they reach the usual normal degrees of movement. Remember that 20° loss of range in general in all planes of motion is not abnormal for the elderly due to the natural shrinkage of the intervertebral discs that leads to the facet joints to engage sooner than when they were younger. Note any pain or limitation of their range. Always note how much movement occurs in the upper thoracic spine. A small amount is expected but note if they try to use motion through the thoracic spine to compensate for loss in the cervical spine.

The contributions to flexion by the upper cervical and lower cervical spine are examined in Box 14.3.

Cervical flexion

Range is considered normal if the patient can get their chin to within one or two finger widths of their chest with their mouth closed. Have the patient first tuck their chin in, or nod their head forward as 10° of flexion can come from the OA joint (O–C1) alone. As the upper cervical motion can be in the opposite direc-

INSIGHTS

Box 14.3 Contribution to flexion by the upper cervical and lower cervical spine

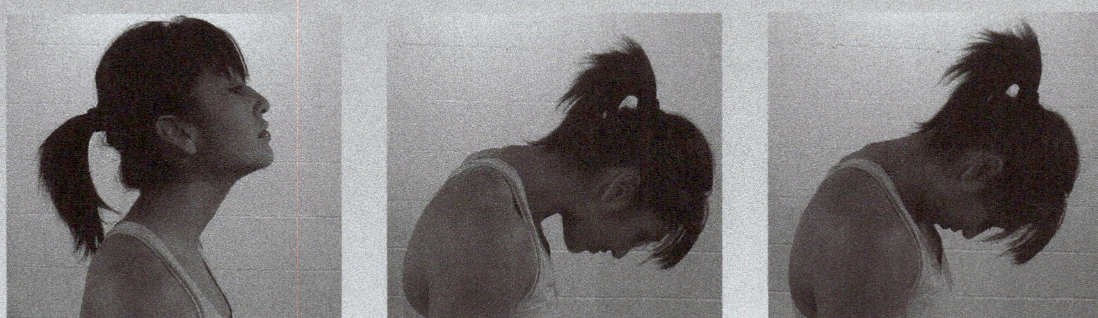

FIGURE 14.17A–C

Flexion with restricted upper cervical spine motion.

Many patients with loss of range in flexion may have restricted their upper cervical spine motion to avoid stretch or pain in the suboccipital area (see the first two photos in Figure 14.17). They do this by jutting the chin forward to avoid flexing the upper cervical vertebrae. You can perform the experiment to see this for yourself. Jut your chin forward (extending the upper cervical spine). Hold this position and now flex the rest of the neck forward. You will find that you can bring the chin quite close to the chest. Now, return to neutral and first tuck the chin in and, only then, bring the chin to chest. You may go further, or you may go less and may now notice tension in the posterior suboccipital muscles that you may not have noticed before (final picture shows flexion after chin tuck). In other words, the lower cervical spine can flex while the upper cervical spine is extended, and vice versa. They can rotate to opposite sides, side-bend to opposite sides.

tion to the lower cervical spine we need to ensure that the upper cervical spine is also in motion along with the lower cervical spine when we are doing our testing.

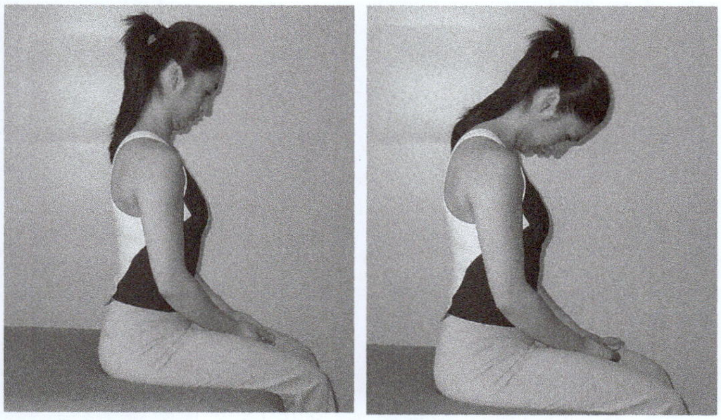

FIGURE 14.18A, B **Cervical flexion 50–65°**

Have the patient tuck in the chin. This flexes the upper cervicals. Then have the patient bring the chin to the chest. This flexes the lower cervicals. The patient should be able to get the chin within two (of their) finger widths of their chest. Also, note if the patient slumps forward with the upper thoracic spine in an attempt to get more range.

Box 14.4 contains further information about observing OA impairment.

Side-bending/lateral flexion

In side-bending there is usually some rotation to the same side because in the lower cervical spine rotation and side-bending are usually coupled to the same side. However, the patient can keep the head straight forward in side-bending by using the AA joint to rotate slightly in the opposite direction and hide the rotation that is happening in the lower cervical spine.

Side-bending/lateral flexion 20–45°

Ask the patient to bring their ear on one side to that shoulder, and then repeat on the opposite side.

If when side-bending to one side there seems to be excessive rotation of the head and the patient cannot compensate for the rotation and look straight forward when asked to without losing range of motion, then this implies impairment. In this case, the patient is using rotation in the AA joint to have the chin move lower to the shoulder to compensate for loss of side-bending. *Leading with the chin*, you could say. Whether the restriction or impairment is from joint or muscle, or both, we cannot yet tell.

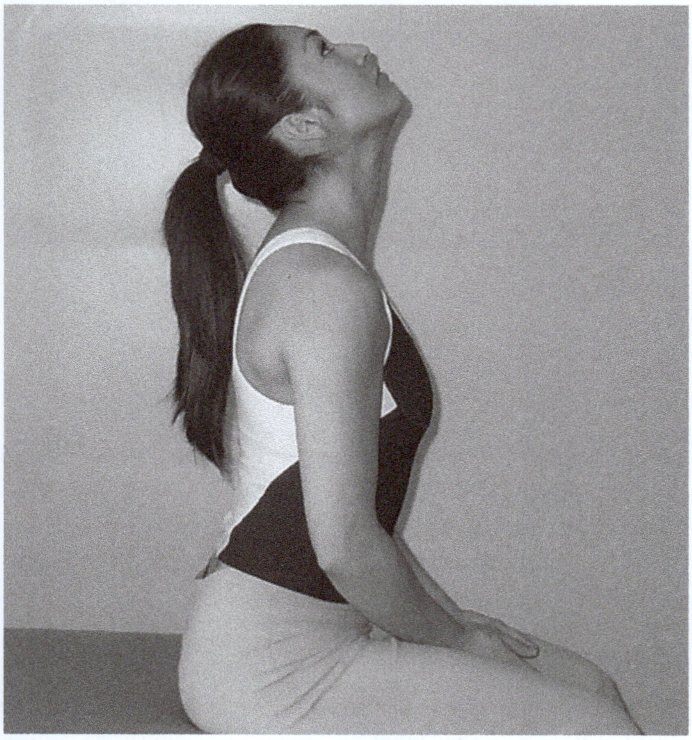

FIGURE 14.19 **Cervical extension 50–70°**

Ask the patient to first look up to the ceiling to ensure that the upper cervical spine is in motion. Then, have the patient extend their head as far as possible. Normal range is when the forehead is level or horizontal. Make sure the patient is not leaning back from the low back or hips to increase the appearance of their range. The first 10–15° can come from the OA joint. Make sure that when the patient extends their neck and that their mouth is closed (due to tight or short hyoid muscles the patient may open their mouth to get more range). If the patient seems limited in extension, ask them to then open their mouth to see if more range is available. If so, the hyoids may well be involved in the loss of extension.

Extension may induce spasming of the suboccipital musculature and/or other larger posterior cervical muscles and therefore extension can increase the intensity of a patient's headache or migraine. Note if the patient is extending either the thoracic or the lumbar spine in order to achieve the appearance of normal cervical spine extension.

INSIGHTS

Box 14.4 Observing OA impairment

You may notice in AF-ROM (or in PR-ROM for that matter) that when the patient flexes or extends the cervical spine, the chin may deviate to one side. This could be a clue that: (1) one or other of the OA joints is dysfunctioning (hypomobile); or (2) some facet joint(s) in the lower cervical spine are being held (stuck) open/flexed or closed/extended. Any of these unilateral restrictions will cause the cervical spine to rotate, making the chin go off to one side. The side stuck or fixed in place is acting as a pivot point around which the structures above will rotate.

The deviation may be due to an OA joint, AA joint or lower cervical joint impairment and the musculature involved. The only sure way to figure out where the loss or restriction is requires very specific testing of the joints of both the upper and lower quadrants. The motion palpation testing presented later in this chapter will help you locate any specific OA joint, AA joint, or any facet joint impairment. These deviations are most apparent when observing a supine patient from the head of the table (Figures 14.20–14.22).

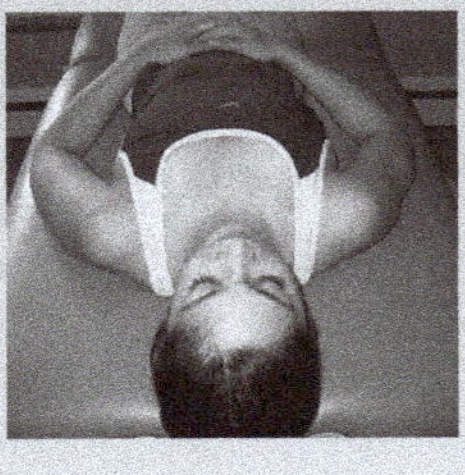

FIGURE 14.20
Normal symmetry of cervical spine in neutral.

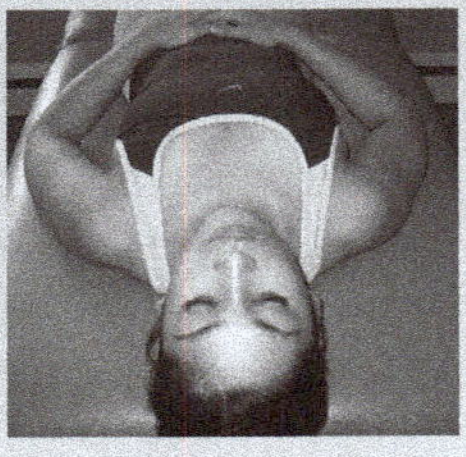

FIGURE 14.21
Normal symmetrical extension of cervical spine.

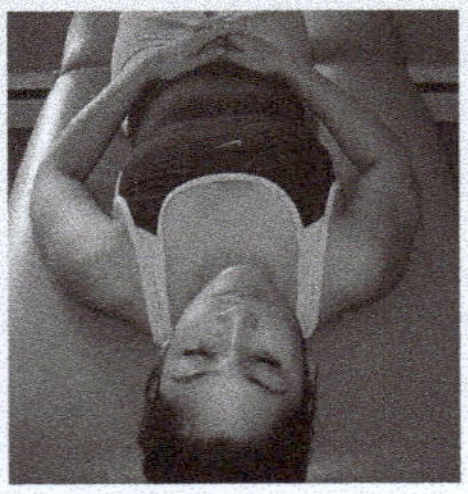

FIGURE 14.22
Asymmetrical extension, seen by deviation of chin to right. Facet(s) on right will not extend/close.

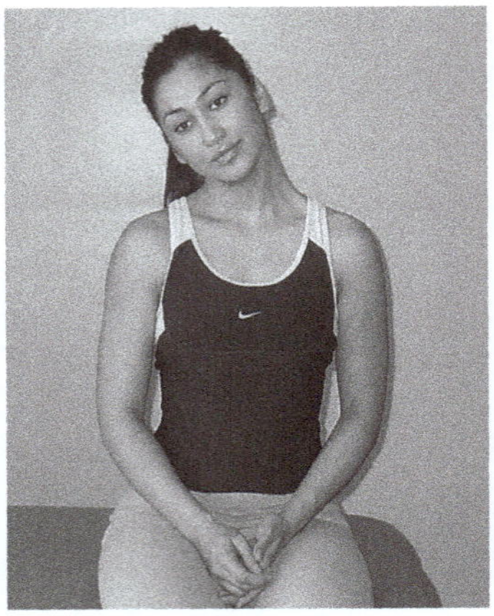

FIGURE 14.23
Side-bending right.

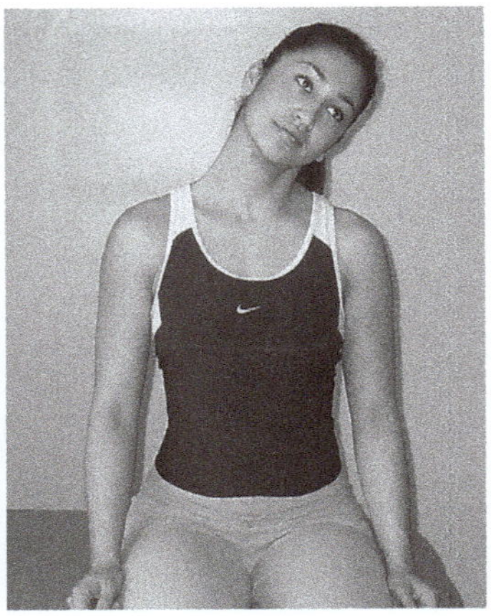

FIGURE 14.24
Side-bending left.

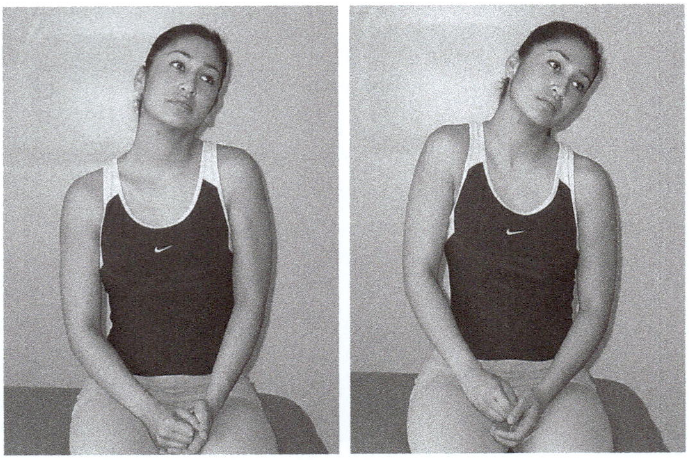

FIGURE 14.25A, B Patient compensating for loss of range
The patient may try to compensate by raising their shoulder to their ear, or by side-bending through the thoracic spine, which will cause the contralateral shoulder to rise.

Rotation 70–85°

Approximately 50 percent of cervical rotation is considered to be from the AA joint. Rotation always includes some side-bending of the cervical vertebrae. Hence, the chin may dip slightly toward their shoulder as they approach end-range. This is normal if done equally to both sides.

Motion palpation testing of the upper cervical spine

The purpose of motion palpation of the spine is not just to locate areas of pain or impairment but, more importantly, to help us

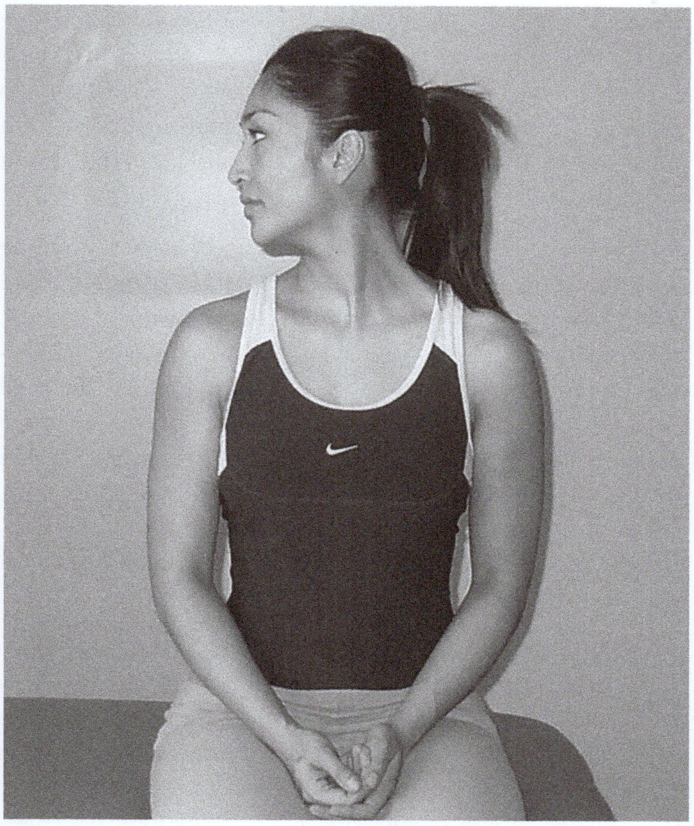

FIGURE 14.26 Rotation right

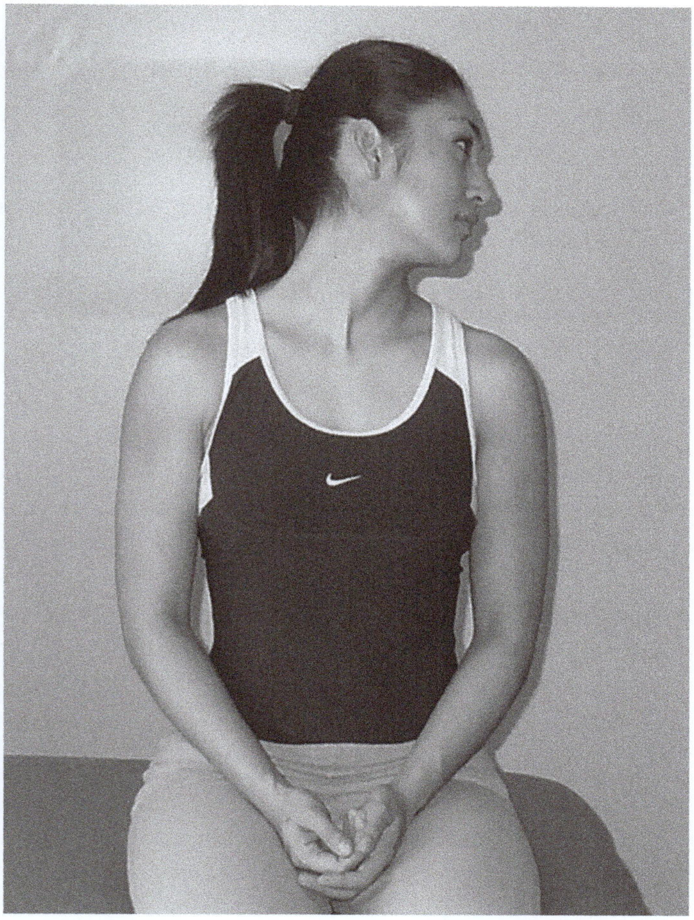

FIGURE 14.27 Rotation left

Record the amount of rotation to either side. ***NOTE:*** The patient shown has to use more side-bending when rotating left in order to achieve the same rotation they have to the right.

understand exactly what the problem or restriction of motion is due to. Is the facet joint impairment due to the facet joint being held closed? Or is it due to a joint being held open? Is it impairment at just one segment, several separate segments, or is it impairment of a group of vertebrae – a scoliosis? This form of testing is done by observation and motion palpation (Chila 2010; DeStefano 2011; Mitchell 2005).

Classical orthopedic testing of the cervical spine may at times help to locate where joint dysfunctions are but they do not help us to understand the nature of the impairment as motion palpation can.

This portion of the chapter is intended to be a mixture of lecture and practice experiments. It requires you to take the time to absorb the information slowly. You should only proceed as each paragraph is understood and to proceed only as each practice or palpatory exercise has been done. I assure you that the knowledge you will gain, both factual and as experiential, will be of great benefit to you as a therapist and to your patients' well-being.

Palpating the cervical spine while it is moved either actively or passively through various ranges and actions affords much more information about how the spine is functioning mechanically than can be gained by just observing active free range of motion. In its most simple form, motion palpation of the cervical spine is the art of looking for asymmetry of motion as the cervical spine is passively moved through its anatomical ranges while your fingertips palpate structures and tissues of the cervical spine at various levels. It is more than just holding the head and performing passive relaxed motion to the spine. Motion testing helps us to see both how the individual structures of the spine are working separately and how they are working together as a whole.

We are looking for:

- symmetry/asymmetry in vertebral alignment – both static and in motion
- restriction of motion, or even hypermobility
- tenderness or any reproduction of the patient's complaints or impairments.

We can look at the spine standing, seated, or prone.

Motion palpation and testing of occipitoatlantal (OA) joints

This motion testing of the OA joints, along with the AA joint and facet joints that follow, are presented here ahead of classic orthopedic testing (PR-ROM, AR-ROM, and the special tests). The primary reason for this is because typical orthopedic tests including PR-ROM with over-pressure (O-P) can be highly provoking when neck pain is part of the chief complaint. This experience of pain by the patient usually results in muscle guarding that will skew the results of any passive motion tests as presented here.

There are three levels of testing for the OA joints explained. They are presented in order of increasing precision, which is matched by the increasing subtleness in palpation required. As competency is attained for each, the reader can move on to the next. When all are mastered, choose the one that you find most useful, though the third method is considered best by most manual practitioners (Chila 2010; DeStefano 2011; Mitchell 2005).

When beginning to learn how to test this portion of the upper quadrant of the cervical spine, it is helpful to start with the first of the following three tests and then proceed to each more precise test. This certainly requires taking more time initially. However, you will quickly develop your palpation skills and learn to feel and recognize the amount of normal and abnormal play within and around the joints. With practice you will learn to quickly yet efficiently test this crucial area of the spine. The result of this practice is the development of acute and accurate palpatory skills which ultimately save you time assessing and treating musculoskeletal impairments.

The positive sign for motion testing is principally asymmetry of motion, the degree of restriction and/or pain. Philip Greenman D.O. (following many others, such as Mitchell 2005) summarizes how impairments/somatic dysfunctions are found and analyzed by the acronym: ARTs. This stands for *Asymmetry*, *Restriction of motion*, and *Tissue texture changes*, all of which are objective findings. An "*s*" is added to take into account the subjective finding of sensitivity or pain experienced by the patient (DeStefano 2011). Therefore, we will be focusing in this section on asymmetry and restricted range of motion as well as the patient's experience of pain as the principal clues to an impaired structure. Tissue texture changes associated with impairments or somatic dysfunctions are discussed in Part I of this book.

Postural cues such as a forward carriage of the head (leading with the chin) imply that the OA joints are in extension in order to compensate for a forward flexion of the upper thoracic spine. The protraction of the shoulders leads to the upper thoracic spine becoming more flexed (hyperkyphotic). The head would be bent toward the ground if the cervical spine did not compensate by extending. This constitutes the hyperlordosis of the cervical spine seen with the forward head positioning. We need to test it to see if the chronicity of this postural positioning has affected the motion in these joints and if so, to what degree.

Patients presenting with occipital and upper cervical headaches (with or without the referral to behind the eyes) require us to see if the suboccipital muscles are in spasm and/or have active trigger points (TrP). Feelings of dizziness or nausea can come from a dysfunctional OA joint due to the high number of facilitated proprioceptors embedded in the joint structures and musculotendinous units involved in these muscles and joints. Further, the vertebral artery may be partially occluded if the occiput is held in excessive extension and cause similar symptoms.

We also need to be able to differentiate between the upper and the lower cervical spine as the sources for losses in flexion and extension (along with some side-bending). As the upper cervical spine's anatomy/structure differs from the lower cervical spine so too do they differ in function. Therefore, we need to know how much loss is coming from either quadrant as our approach to treatment may also differ between these two quadrants.

These are just a few of the obvious reasons to focus on testing the motion in the OA joints.

First method of testing OA joints (Figures 14.28–14.30)

We can explore the nodding motion (flexion/extension) of the OA joint by translating the joint in the sagittal plane, in other words, in an anterior-posterior direction. This is a classic joint mobilization maneuver used to test the OA joints (and with gentle repetition can be used to treat the restriction).

With the patient supine (Figure 14.28) gently cup the head in your palms. Apply a *little* traction *to only slightly gap* the cervical

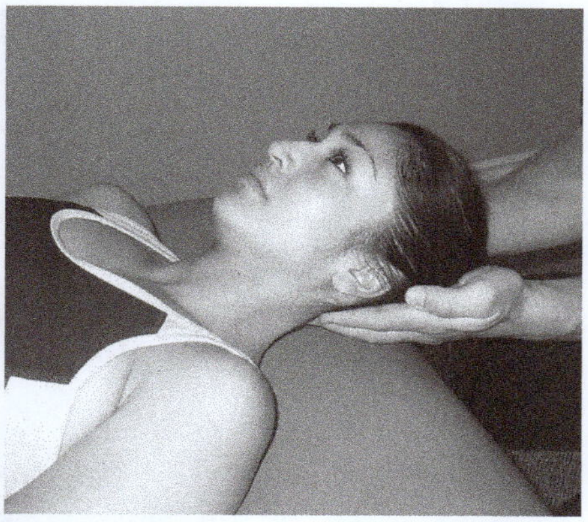

FIGURE 14.28 First OA test positioning
Hold the occiput in the palm of your hands. Traction slightly.

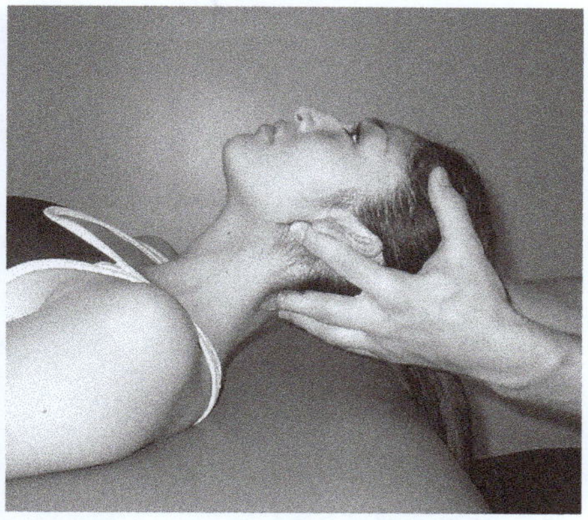

FIGURE 14.29 OA joint extension
Lift the occiput up as you palpate for ease and symmetry of movement.

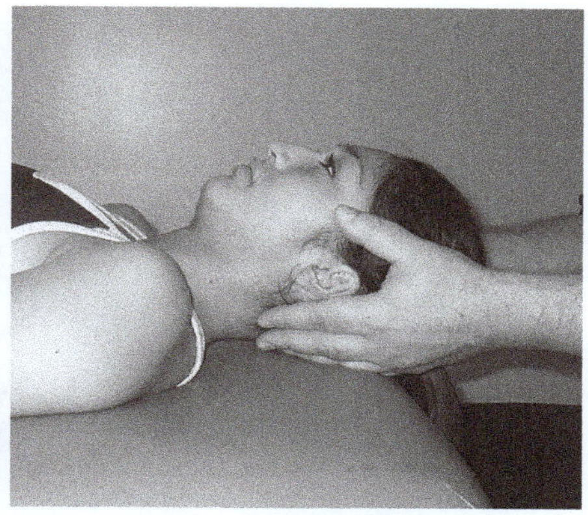

FIGURE 14.30 OA joint flexion
Use the cheekbones to tuck the chin in.

joints. Taking up all the slack in the joint structures will restrict their motion and distort the results of testing. Be sure you are holding the head only and not any cervical vertebrae!

Then lift the head toward the ceiling (Figure 14.29), while keeping it parallel to the table. ***NOTE:*** The movement has been exaggerated for clarification purposes. Lifting the head (while keeping the chin level with the forehead) will take the OA joints into extension. To feel this movement, you may initially have to lift the head quite far (as shown). Eventually, as you gain palpatory experience and precision, you will only minimally "bob" the head up and down.

Lower the head back to neutral. To bring the cervical spine, and especially the OA joint, into flexion tuck the patient's chin in (Figure 14.30); in other words, nod the head forward. Note the positioning of the therapist's thumbs on the superior border of the cheek bone (zygomatic arch). Using the cheek bone the therapist can apply a gentle pressure inferiorly and posteriorly to further increase the flexion motion of the OA joint. This also encourages the patient to let flexion happen (if it is available). If you feel the patient is holding and preventing movement, ask them to let their chin tuck in or drop. ***NOTE:*** *The therapist has not flexed the lower cervical spine.* The point is to feel the occiput "rock" into flexion on C1, the atlas.

A positive sign for restriction is palpating less motion on one side. If severe the head will rotate away from the restricted side when you elevate the occiput and conversely the head may roll toward the restricted side when you bring the OA joint into flexion.

Try to practice with as many different people as you can. Eventually you will be able to do a gentle anterior-posterior wobble or wave-like motion. The latter action can be a good way to get the musculature and the joints of the OA to relax and let go.

Second method of testing OA joints (Figures 14.31, 14.32)

Start as in the first method of testing: with the patient supine gently cup the head in your palms. Apply a little traction *to only slightly gap* the cervical joints. Be sure you are holding the head only and not any cervical vertebrae. While cupping the head traction slightly and rotate it approximately 30° to one side (rotated left is demonstrated in the Figure 14.31). As an example this rotation to the left will orient the left OA so that the joint is now perpendicular to the table (see Figure 14.32). Now, if you lift the head a quarter of an inch or so straight up then the left condyle of the occiput can glide through the length of the right joint surface on the superior aspect of the atlas, C1. Now draw the head back to neutral and then a little further.

Again, you will want to practice this until you can do the sliding movement within the natural play available in the joint (about an eighth of an inch). This motion should be felt as a very small sliding movement up and down, a gentle oscillation motion. Do both sides and compare.

The orientation of the OA joints are is an inverted V-shape or wedge shape with the anterior (toward the face) joint surfaces closer together while the posterior surfaces are farther apart. In Figure 14.32 when the head is rotated 30° the left the OA joint is perpendicular. Lifting the head will cause the left occipital condyle (joint surface) to slide anteriorly. Meanwhile the right side can only move slightly in rotation and side-bending and thus acts more as a pivot point or axis for the motion.

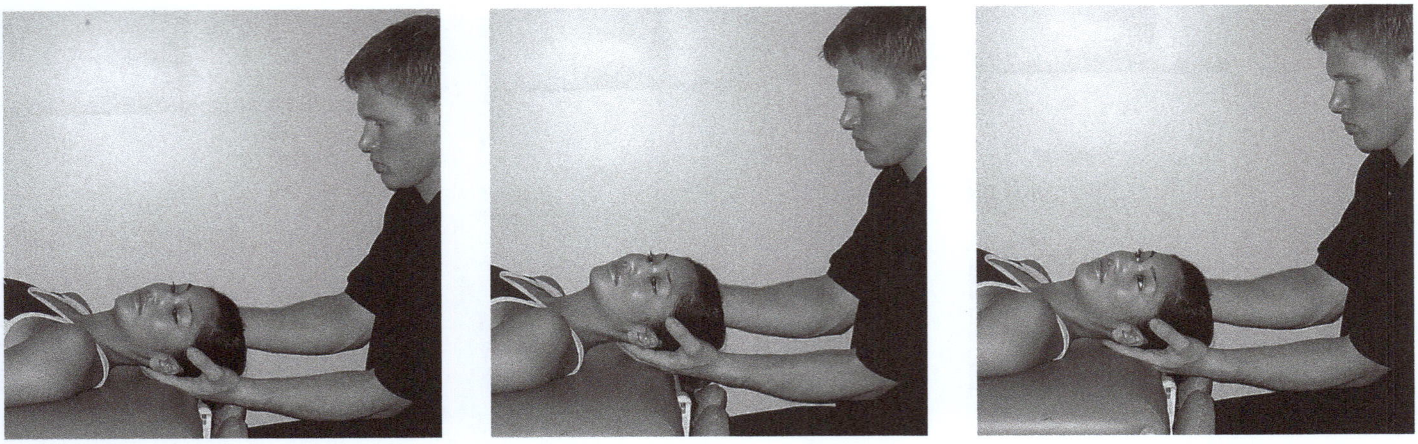

FIGURE 14.31A–C Glide of perpendicular OA joint surface

Turn the head 20–30° (e.g., left). Lift head straight up to barrier (extension); bring head down letting chin tuck/drop slightly (flexion). The dysfunctional side will show a marked reduction in motion. The lift is very slight (you may notice the amount more clearly by the therapist's fingers, how they are sunk into the table in the first image, less so in the second, then back into the table).

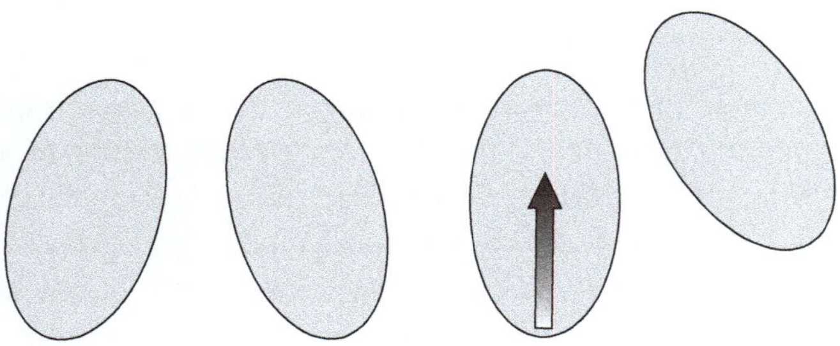

FIGURE 14.32

(left) Normal orientation of OA joints. (right) Head rotated 30° left making left OA joint surfaces perpendicular.

With time, you can not only feel restrictions when they occur in either left or right joints but you will also be able to tell if the joint is restricted in flexion or extension. The secret is in realizing that when a joint is held in flexion or in extension it is still willing to move slightly in that direction but is unwilling to move in the other. For example, if the left OA joint is held in flexion then you will still be able to glide or draw the joint down at least a little (as it would when nodding forward into flexion). However, it will not want to glide or move superiorly/forward. (This is to say that when the joint is being held fixed in flexion it is willing to flex a bit more but it cannot move into extension and when the joint is held in extension it may allow more extension but it cannot move into flexion.)

When held in flexion you can feel the musculature "grab" ("bind") when you try to lift the head (try to move the OA joint into extension) as it resists this motion. However, as you move into flexion (when you let the chin "tuck" or drop to flex the OA joint) the tissue gives a little; there is a sense of "ease" to the movement. Developing this palpatory sense of *ease* and *bind* is very important for manual therapists. This is an excellent exercise to develop such a sense.

Third method of palpating motion in OA joints (Figures 14.33–14.38)

This method requires good palpation skills and an acquired awareness of how normal and impaired motion in these joints feel. It includes a variation of a second test. You begin as you have in all of the previous methods of testing or palpating motion by first holding the patient's head gently in your hands and applying slight traction.

The next step in the test requires practice to acquire the dexterity of the hand to do the action and with a good palpatory/proprioceptive sense or feel. This comes with practice so you can still proceed to the next steps even if you are not sure or are yet unable at first to feel the small movement that you are being asked to feel.

This time you support the C1 vertebra with your finger pads (Figure 14.34) and then let your thenar eminences or the palms of your hands "drop" or "give way" just slightly (about two or three millimeters, or about an 1/8 of an inch) and so let the

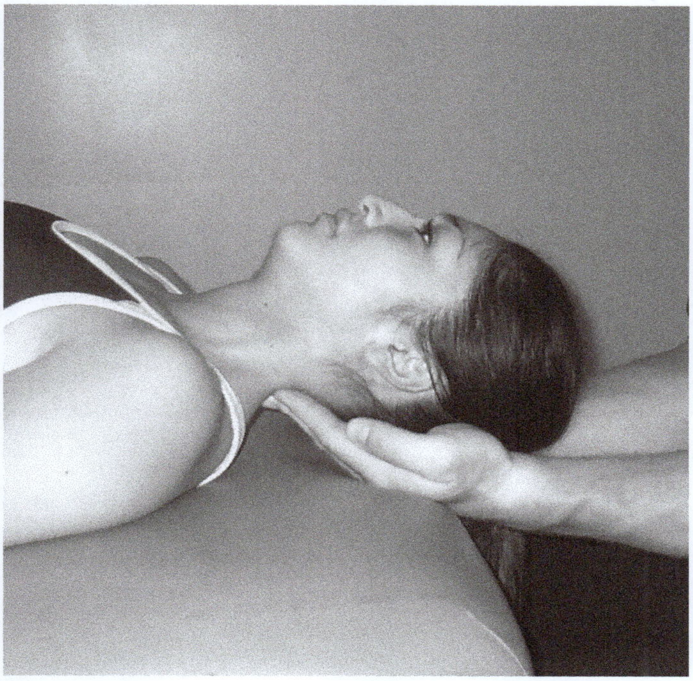

FIGURE 14.33 1. Positioning for testing OA joints

Cup the occiput with the palms of both hands. Finger pads support C1.

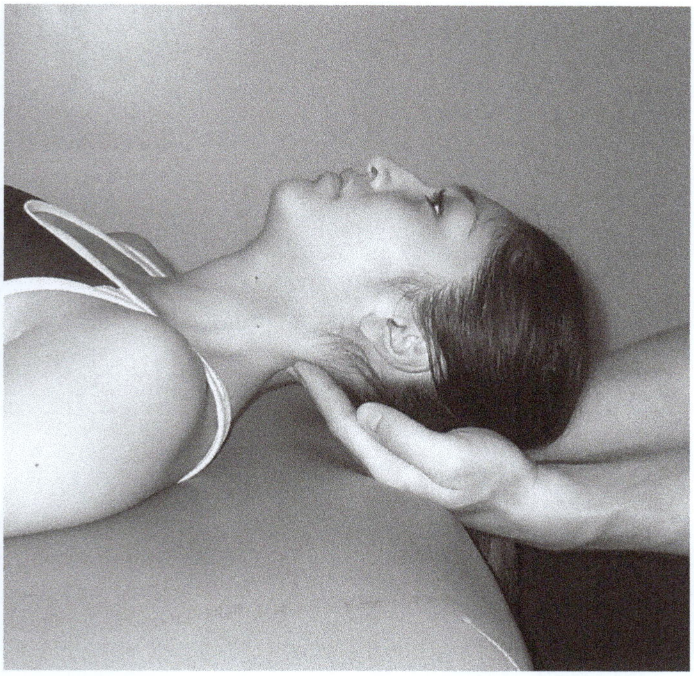

FIGURE 14.34 2. Posterior glide of occipital condyles on Cl: testing flexion

Hold C1 in place while you let the palms of your hands drop slightly. You want to feel the occiput slide down into your palms while C1 remains where it was. If you hold this position and wait for the OA joints to slowly release (when they are restricted) this is what is usually referred to as a suboccipital release. (In this way, you do not push C1 superiorly/forward but rather you let the occiput (head) slide inferiorly if it is willing to. A much less aggressive approach.)

occipital condyles slide posteriorly (which lets the occiput slide posteriorly on the atlas). This allows the occipital condyles to slide to the posterior edge of the OA joint surfaces of C1. Note any restriction to movement, bilaterally or unilaterally. You are testing OA joint flexion.

For a gentle treatment for extension lesions of the OA joints hold the position in Figure 14.34 for 30 seconds to 2 minutes while the patient breathes. Breathing in assists flexion of cervical spine so after the patient takes in a deep but relaxed breath have them pause for a count of three before breathing out. You can have the patient further assist by looking down toward their toes with every "breathe in and hold" (causing gentle activation of the suboccipital flexors of the head) and then have them look up to their eyebrows on the out-breath. You have then used both breath and the ocular-suboccipital muscle reflex to assist in the release. Extension lesions are very common, especially with patients with a forward head posture.

OA joint diagonal glides to test extension

Now, remove any contact with the cervical spine and again hold only the head. You now test each OA joint separately by lifting the head about a quarter of an inch in a diagonal direction (see Figures 14.35–14.37). For example, lift your right hand in the direction toward the patient's left eye. This induces a small movement along an approximately 30° angle. You are attempting to glide the occiput's right condyle along the length of the right joint surface on C1's superior surface. Return to neutral. Now lift your left hand toward the right eye. (The movements in Figures 14.36–14.38 are slightly exaggerated for clarity; the movements described can be seen by observing the position of the chin in relation to the mid-line, the suprasternal notch.)

You may wish to shift back and forth from one hand to the other as the joints are often hypomobile at first (i.e., "stiff" or "tense") but will often loosen up with just a few glides back and forth. You will then be able to get a more accurate appraisal of any impairment to motion at that specific joint.

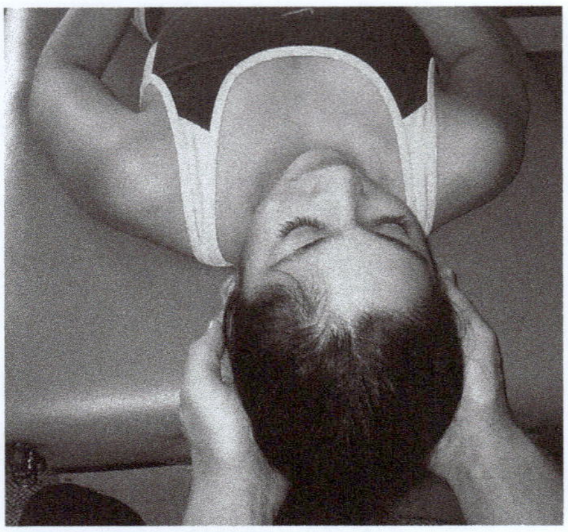

FIGURE 14.35 Diagonal glide through the OA joints: testing extension

Cup the occiput in the palms. The finger pads are not in contact with C1 or any part of the cervical spine. The head is in neutral. Traction the head slightly to disengage the OA joints.

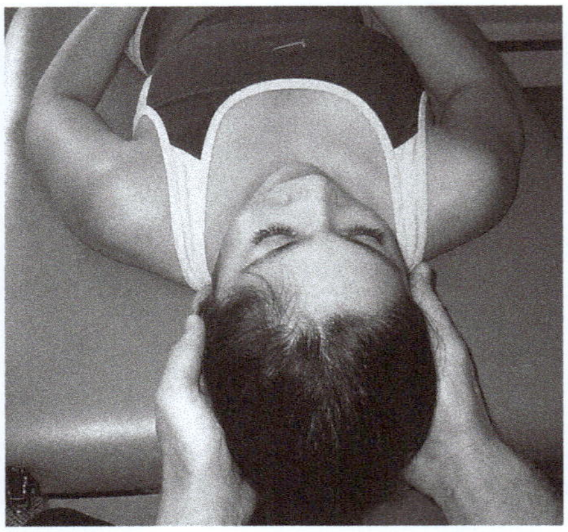

FIGURE 14.36

Move the head diagonally with the left hand toward the right eye. End-range is reached when the cervical spine begins to move.

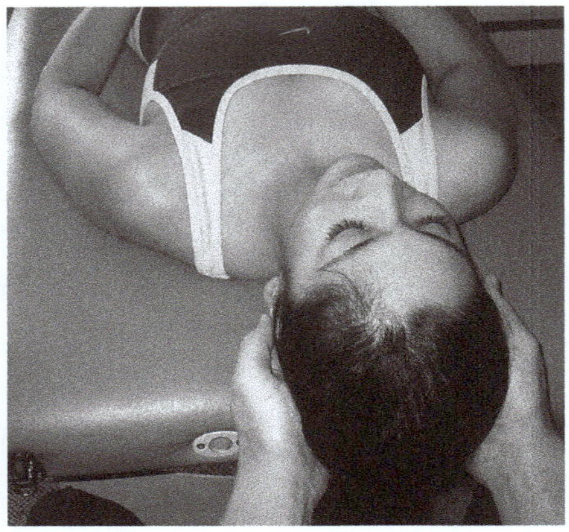

FIGURE 14.37

Move the head diagonally with the right hand toward the left eye. End-range is reached when the cervical spine begins to move.

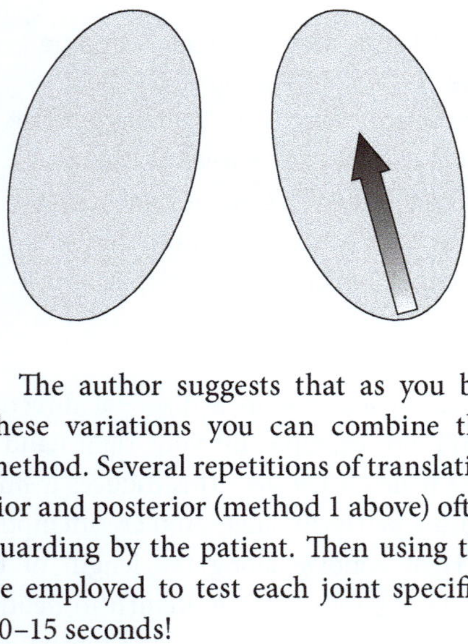

FIGURE 14.38

Lifting the occiput through its right OA joint.

The author suggests that as you become proficient with these variations you can combine the first and the third method. Several repetitions of translation (or *oscillation*) anterior and posterior (method 1 above) often releases holding and guarding by the patient. Then using the third technique can be employed to test each joint specifically. All of this takes 10–15 seconds!

Summary of preferred testing protocol for OA joints

1. Testing extension/flexion by anterior-posterior oscillation. To relax musculature and palpate for any sense of restriction.
2. Posterior glide to OA joints. More specific palpation of OA joints ability to flex.
3. Testing each joint by lifting in diagonal (left hand toward right eye tests left OA joint and vice versa).

Motion palpation and testing of the atlantoaxial (AA) joints (Figures 14.39–14.42)

When we have observed a loss of cervical rotation during AF-ROM we then need to differentially test for loss of range coming from the upper cervical versus the lower cervical spine. To do this we first note the range of motion when doing AF-ROM rotation of the cervical spine, recording the patient's approximate ranges in rotating left and right. We then do the following test to see how much loss of motion may be due to, if at all, the AA joint. (Remember the AA joint is responsible for approximately half of normal rotation of the cervical spine; 40–45° of rotation in each direction from neutral.)

Compare loss, if any, with what is seen in PR-ROM (which is described below) and then calculate how much of the loss is from the AA joint and how much is from the lower cervical spine. (Examples of such calculations follow after the descriptions of testing.)

To test the AA joint (between C1 and C2) we again start with the patient's head cupped in your hands.

Note the approximate degrees of motion available to each side and compare with ranges seen in AF-ROM and PR-ROM. You can then calculate the percentage (or approximate degrees) of motion lost from the AA joint in comparison to the lower cervical spine.

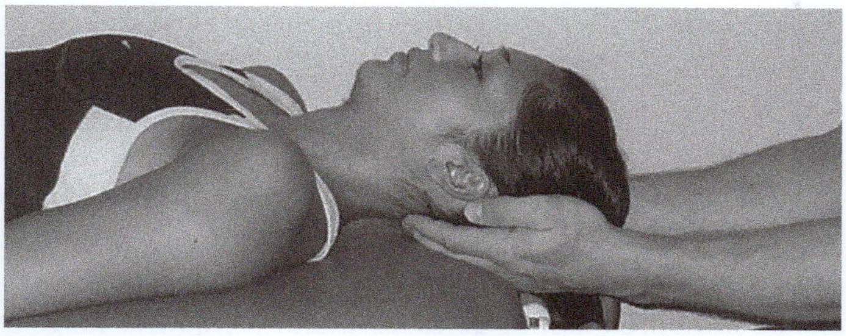

FIGURE 14.39 1. AA joint test starting position

Cup the head in the palms of your hands.

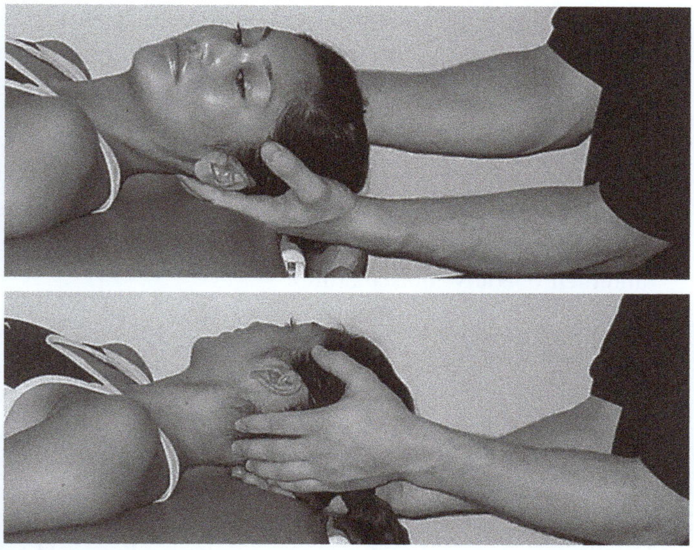

FIGURE 14.40A, B 2. Perform PR-ROM testing

Passively rotate the head and cervical spine to left and right. Note total ranges. *Do not apply O-P.* Return the head and neck to neutral. Now take the cervical spine into flexion by first tucking the chin in (which also takes up the slack in the OA joint). Then move into the total full flexion available to the cervical spine. Full flexion takes up the slack within the facet joints of the lower cervical spine which will help restrict movement coming from them during this test. The therapist stands up when forward flexing the cervical spine. This allows the therapist to easily and securely hold the weight of the patient's head and it prevents excessive extension of the wrists as can occur should one remained seated.

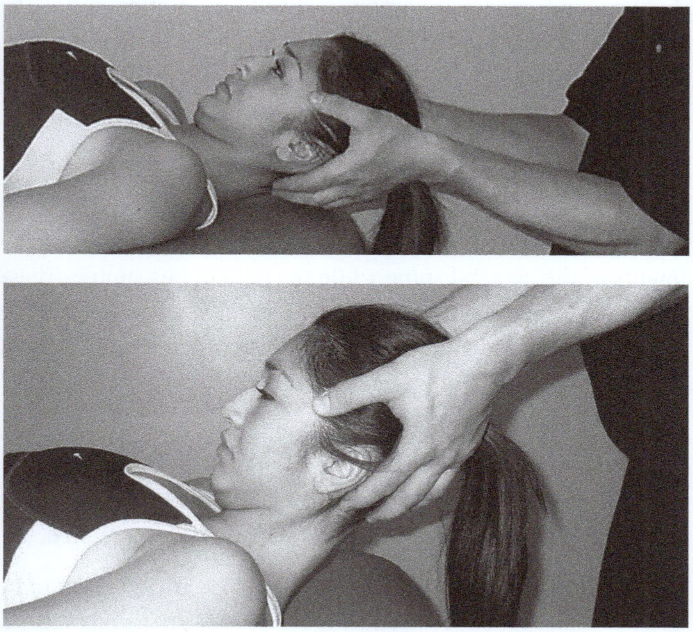

FIGURE 14.41 3. Positioning for AA joint testing

Starting from neutral: tuck the chin in, flexing the OA joint, and continue flexing the cervical spine until end-range. This locks all the joints except the AA joint. Ask the patient if they are in any discomfort. If not, then proceed.

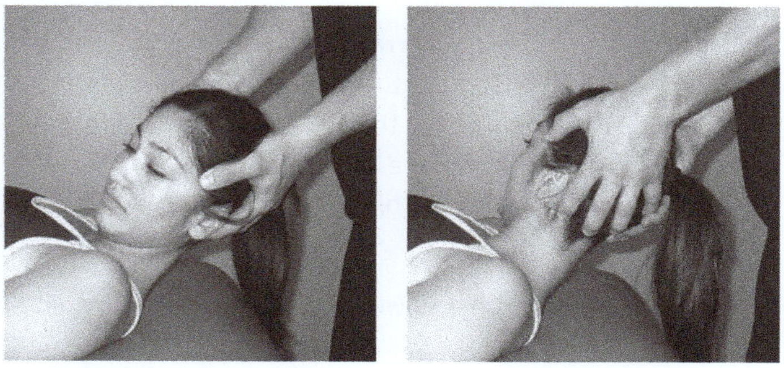

FIGURE 14.42 4. Testing ROM of AA joint

Rotate the head to the left. Note the range. Rotate the head to the right. Note the range. Compare results. Should achieve roughly 45° in either direction.

Calculating ROM loss in AA joint, compared to lower cervical joints

1. If during AA joint testing *we get less rotation* than normal (on either side, or both) then the AA joint is probably involved in the patient's loss of rotation.
2. *If this loss equals the total loss* seen in PR ROM testing, then the AA joint is fully responsible for the loss and it is the area to work on.

3. *If it is only part of the loss* as seen in PR-ROM tests, then both the upper and lower cervical quadrants are contributing to loss of rotation. (We will discuss specific testing for each level of the lower cervical spine shortly).
4. *If the AA appears normal* but PR-ROM of the whole cervical spine had shown loss of rotation, then that loss should be coming from the lower quadrant (the patient's facet joints and their operative musculature).

In the images above it is noted that the patient had difficulty rotating the whole cervical spine to the left during PR-ROM testing of the whole cervical spine. Yet AA rotation to the left appears normal. Therefore, we would suspect that the lower cervical spine is responsible for the loss of range of motion.

NOTE: We observed some impaired motion to left rotation with this patient during AF-ROM testing – see above – but could not then yet say where the impairment might be. Now we know it is from the lower cervical spine. We will be able to pinpoint the impaired segment(s) and understand the nature of the impairment – (which side will not open/flex or close/extend) – if we test via *Motion palpation of the lower cervical spine.* That testing can be found at the end of the chapter (p. 404). The author thought it best at this point to continue at present with the more traditional orthopedic testing so as to sustain the flow of range of motion testing. However, in his own practice the author would perform the motion testing of the lower cervical region right before PR-ROM, especially if over-pressures are to be used in PR-ROM. O-P may cause discomfort or pain and so produce holding and guarding compromising these motion tests. The same holds true for AR-ROM and many of the orthopedic special tests as they seek to provoke pain as their positive sign.

Box 14.5 looks at a rotated C1 impairment.

Box 14.5 Rotated C1 impairment

Sometimes the rotated C1 can be a very distinct presentation with a high degree of loss of rotation between C1 and C2 to one side.

As mentioned in the anatomy section, the facets between C1 and C2 are both convex (in the living body) – like two halves of a rubber ball with their curved surfaces touching and one balancing on the other. As rotation occurs (let us say to the right) both convex surfaces of C1 slide down on the convex surfaces of C2. This slackens the ligaments and the musculature between the two vertebrae which then permits the usually high degree of rotation that is possible between them.

If, while the AA (C1–2) stays rotated to the right, the suboccipital and/or other musculature attached to the occiput and C1 go into spasm, then, as the patient attempts to rotate back to normal (or turn to the left), the taut musculature will not let the convex surfaces of C1 "ride up" or "go up hill" on the convex surfaces of C2.

The patient may present with the head slightly rotated right (though the lower cervical spine may compensate and rotate left to have the patient able to face forward), and turn to the right at the AA joint but seem unable to turn left much, if at all, at that joint. The patient (or other therapists) will often describe this as the neck being locked on one side. This is also often described by other health care practitioners (usually chiropractors) as a rotated C1 diagnosis.

Passive relaxed range of motion (PR-ROM)

The therapist should do passive relaxed range of motion movements of the cervical spine while the patient lies supine. These movements *may* be done with the patient's head off the table supported securely in the therapist's hands. However, a patient is often unwilling to relax and therefore this approach can defeat the purpose of passive testing.

Much can be learned by moving the C-spine passively through the whole range of motion. That is why carrying out passive movement in the C-spine is strongly recommended.

The range of motion which is seen during PR-ROM is can be greater than the range seen during AF-ROM, when done supine. This is because the patient can more fully disengage (relax) muscles that were being used to hold the head erect when they were seated doing AF-ROM. The normal end-feel here is tissue stretch with the possible exception of flexion on occasion being a bony block if the chin hits the sternum.

As always, when end-range has been reached and only if there is no pain apply slight O-P to determine the joint's end-feel*; but never apply O-P to extension!*

Remember that the capsular pattern of restriction for the C-spine is first and foremost loss in side-flexion and rotation, then some loss of extension while flexion may remain free and full (Hertling & Kessler 2006).

When performing PR-ROM With O-P

Do not have your hands over the mandible, the TMJ, or the ears when holding and moving the patient's head.

Make sure that both shoulders are in neutral or what is neutral for the patient (as seen in AF-ROM, etc.). Place your hands over each shoulder cap and gently push both shoulders inferiorly once or twice then push one at a time two or three times each. Ask the patient to take in a deep breath while they look straight up at the ceiling and fully breathe out and relax. This should help to place the patient's shoulders in a relaxed neutral position.

Also, make sure you return the patient's head and neck to neutral and always ask if returning to neutral in itself causes any pain or symptoms, or how it affects any pain or symptoms they may have experienced in moving to and/or when reaching end-range, with or without O-P.

PR-ROM cervical flexion (Figures 14.43–14.47)

Now, take the patient to the end of range of forward flexion. End-range is reached when all the slack has been taken up, when further movement would start to lift the patient's upper back off the table. Note, however, that some flexion of the first two thoracic vertebrae will often occur in order to generate enough tension to fully flex all the lower cervical spine's vertebrae. This is acceptable and one of many reasons that some professionals (especially osteopaths) consider the first two or three thoracic vertebrae as part of the cervical spine complex (Chila 2010).

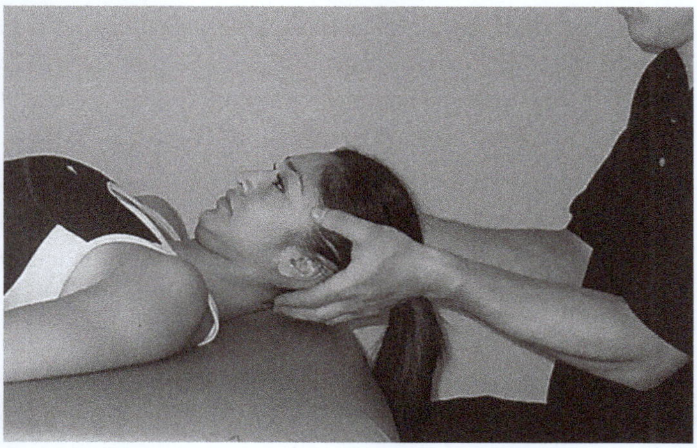

FIGURE 14.43 PR-ROM cervical flexion

Flex the upper cervical spine by tucking in the chin for the patient. Ask the patient if there is any pain or symptoms and if there is not proceed to apply firm but gentle O-P. Ask if there is now pain or return of symptoms especially if they are reproductions of their chief complaint they presented to your clinic with. Return to neutral and again ask if the return provoked any pain or symptoms.

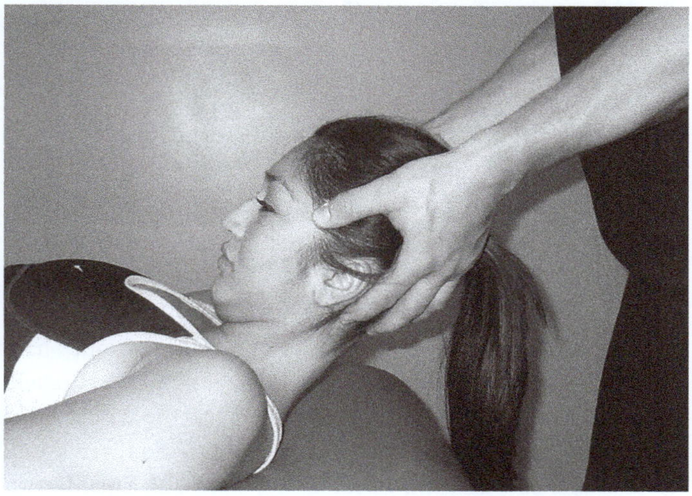

FIGURE 14.44

Full flexion with O-P. Take the patient to the end of range in flexion. Make sure the scapulae do not lift off the table. Ask if there is any pain or symptoms and if not proceed to apply firm but gentle O-P. Ask if there is now pain or return of symptoms. Return to neutral and repeat the questions. Achieving full flexion is made easier if the therapist stands.

PR-ROM cervical side-bending (aka lateral flexion)

To test side-bending bend the head toward the shoulder taking up the slack until the contralateral shoulder begins to lift or follow the head. This lifting means the thoracic spine is now side-bending. As soon as that shoulder begins to move, end-range for the cervical spine has been reached. Before applying O-P (after asking about pain, etc.) you need to stabilize the contralateral shoulder.

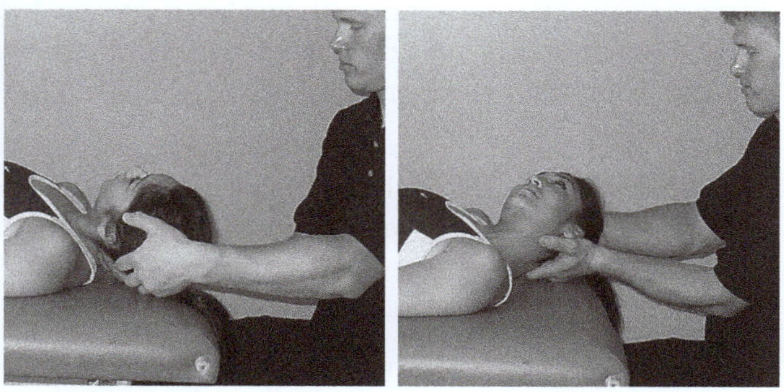

FIGURE 14.45A, B PR-ROM cervical side-bending

Side-bend until discomfort or when the contralateral shoulder begins to move. Ask about pain or other symptoms.

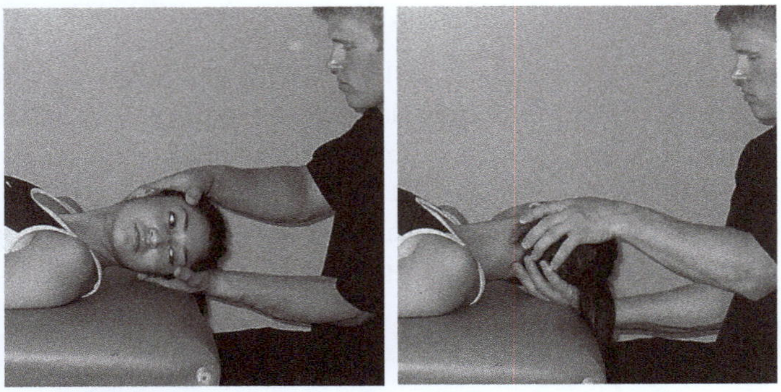

FIGURES 14.46, 14.47 Rotation with O-P

O-P shown. Rotate the head to one side. Try not to flex the neck. Ask the patient about dizziness or changes to vision (re: vertebral artery compression). Ask about pain and symptoms. If all negative then apply a small O-P cautiously. Test the other side, asking all the questions again before applying O-P.

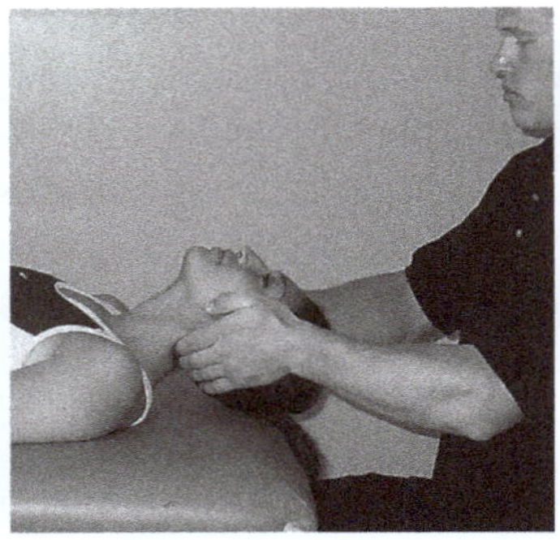

FIGURE 14.48 Extension of cervical spine: no O-P

Using the finger pads, lift the cervicals by C3–5 up toward the ceiling.

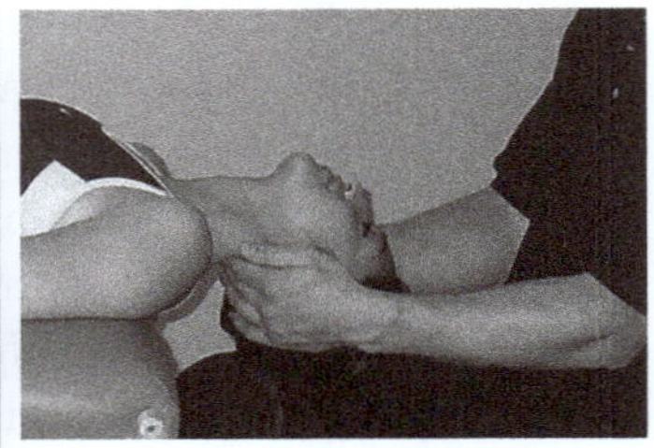

FIGURE 14.49 Extending cervical spine off table: no O-P

Use with caution. Ensure the weight of the patient's head is negated by your support so that no excessive tractioning occurs.

Side-bending with O-P To stabilize, take one hand (i.e., when side-bending right, take the right hand; when side-bending left, take the left hand) and block the contralateral shoulder so that it cannot move. Only when so stabilized should O-P be applied – and still with caution. Start with a gentle pressure and slowly increase. Repeat all questioning about pain, etc.

PR-ROM extension of the cervical spine (Figures 14.48, 14.49)

Following the principle of not causing the patient to move about too much (i.e., switch positions too many times), testing extension of the cervical spine does not necessarily require you to take the patient's head off the table. You can place your finger pads in the laminar groove on both sides of the cervical spine and lift toward the ceiling. Some therapists find it useful to stand up as this helps them to position their hands properly without too much ulnar deviation of the wrists.

Many therapists will test extension of the cervical spine by taking the head and neck off the table. However, most patients feel insecure and apprehensive in this position, which usually leads to them engaging their cervical musculature. This holding and guarding will make the test results inaccurate.

Further, the weight of the head if not negated by the therapist's support will traction the neck. If the patient has suffered a whiplash or similar injury where there has been ligamentous damage or stretching (making the vertebrae unstable) this position may stress such tissues and re-injure them. Therefore, never use this position for patients with new or recent neck injury.

Because the vertebral and carotid arteries could undergo excessive stretch never use this positioning on a patient suffering from any *arteriosclerosis obliterans* or friable vascular tissue, etc.

Active resisted range of motion (AR-ROM)

AR-ROM testing can be done seated or supine. The choice can be made for you by simply continuing with the patient in the position they are in from their last testing, if that was done in seated or supine. The most important thing to remember is to properly stabilize the patient to prevent unnecessary movement and to protect the patient from injury.

When testing the cervical spine isometrically it is best to have the patient initiate movement in order to protect them from you overpowering them too easily and moving the spine. Also, many muscles in the neck could be easily strained or other structures injured if the patient is overpowered.

Remember to tell the patient to push gently at first and only then to slowly increase the strength used until they are using full strength. Remind the patient that you then want them to try and hold at full strength as you count back down from five to zero. After you reach zero the patient should then slowly ease off. Emphasize to the patient that they should under no circumstances quickly engage the muscles and try to go right to full strength. Nor should they relax or let go suddenly. Instruct them to tell you the moment they feel that either pain or a feeling of weakness is going to stop them from pushing by saying either "I can't hold!" or "I have to stop!" This requires you to stay very focused and ready to change your resistance quickly if need be.

Seated AR-ROM (Figures 14.50–14.53)

To test flexion of the cervical spine stabilize the upper back with one hand and have the other against the patient's forehead to resist movement. When testing seated it is best for safety reasons to have the head in slight flexion (nodding forward) to avoid excessive strain to the musculature involved.

NOTE: When testing forward flexion the patient's chin may thrust forward and this response implies that the forward flexors of the neck are weak (Kendall et al. 2005).

The therapist should test both sides for side-bending and then move on and do rotation to each side. However, if the therapist thinks it is appropriate they may choose to test side-bending

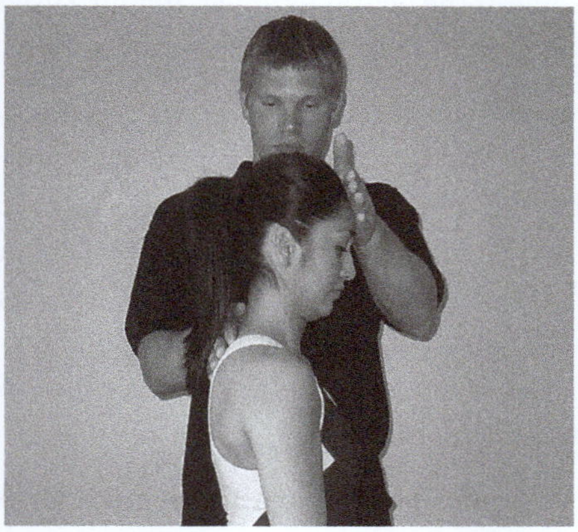

FIGURE 14.50 AR-ROM cervical flexion

Stabilize the patient at the upper thoracics and lowest cervicals. With the patient's neck in slight flexion place the palm of your hand on their forehead. Ask the patient to push gently then slowly increase to full strength. Ask about pain or weakness.

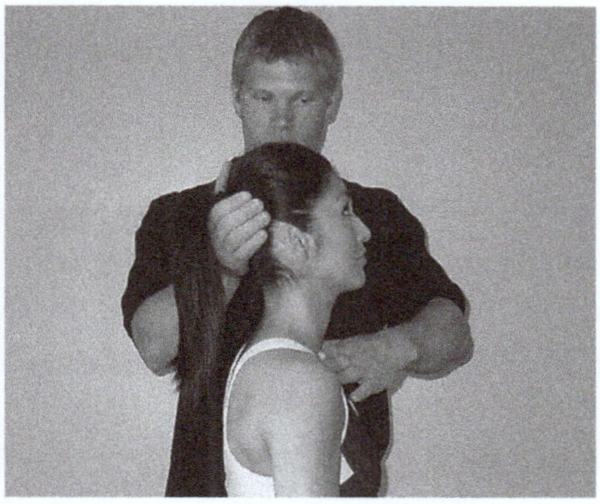

FIGURE 14.51 AR-ROM cervical extension

For resisted extension support the patient's slightly extended head by cupping the occiput. With the finger pads of the other hand support the clavicle. Ask the patient to look up and gently take the chin toward the ceiling. Have them continue, with increasing effort.

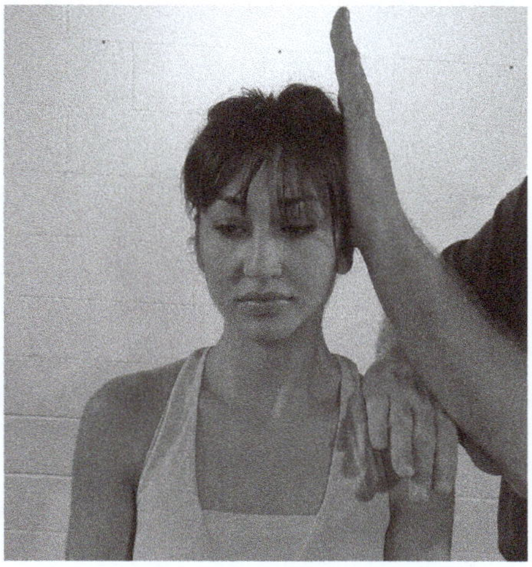

FIGURE 14.52 AR-ROM cervical side-bending

Stand to the side of the patient and stabilize their shoulder with one hand and resist with the palm of other hand above the ear. Compare sides.

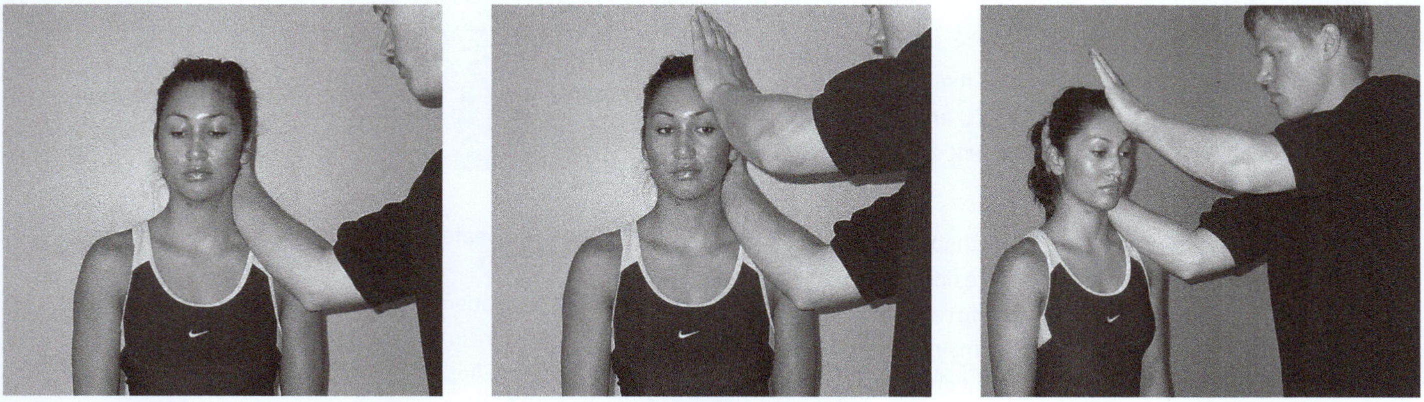

FIGURE 14.53A–C AR-ROM cervical rotation

Stand to one side but slightly in front of the patient. Block the shoulder with your forearm (and cup that hand over the back of their head) and resist at the lateral portion of the forehead (*not* over cheekbone or ear!). The patient's head may be slightly rotated away. Have the patient at first gently try to rotate their head toward you, with increasing effort. Compare sides.

and then rotation on one side and then move over to the other side. The latter approach does save time and often appears to the patient as being more organized.

INSIGHTS

Box 14.6 Shortfalls of some orthopedic testing of the cervical spine

It must be noted that though some of the following orthopedic tests may find, or imply, facet joint dysfunction they do not always tell us exactly where the impaired joint is, due to pain referral. The patient may point to where they feel pain but often that is not where the pain has its source. Nor do these tests tell us if the joint is fixed closed or open (held flexed or extended). Therefore, we do not know what the mechanical impairment is. Further, some of these tests simultaneously stress different types of tissues.

The orthopedic tests on the following pages of this chapter should always be done after motion palpation testing if you intend to use the latter. Remember that provoking pain and the muscle guarding/splinting that can come with that can compromise any motion palpation test.

Many orthopedic tests produce pain and compromise further testing. This is probably one of the principal causes of health professionals taking an educated guess about what is wrong and going right to the most likely special test. They may worry that doing range of motion testing or other screening tests (to rule out other issues) will cause enough discomfort that they will skip all of that the results of further specific testing may become unclear.

Still, some of the orthopedic joint tests may be useful even if the patient's tissues are hypertonic (HT) and will not permit motion testing (use your clinical judgment as to whether any testing is possible that day).

Regardless of your opinion about orthopedic testing you need to understand how these tests are done and what they are meant to tell the therapist so that you can understand the testing other health care professions may have performed. A knowledge of these tests improves our ability to communicate with other therapists or medical specialists.

As with the lumbar spine, many of the special orthopedic tests for the cervical spine are investigating neurological issues rather than mechanical. These can be the most import tests to know and have facility in performing.

Box 14.6 examines shortfalls of some orthopedic testing of the cervical spine.

Special tests

Compression test (Figures 14.54, 14.55)

Originally used to test if the nerve root is being pinched or compressed as it exits the spine at the neural foramen. It is also used to test for acute arthritic facet joints.

A positive test for nerve root compression is the reproduction of neurological symptoms down into the patient's upper extremity following that nerve root's dermatome pattern (refer back to Figure 13.73, p. 351). The compression may be from a herniated disc (though not as common in the cervical spine as in the lumbar area) or the consequence of degenerative disc disease or arthritic (osteophytes) formations causing the nerve to be compressed in the neural foramen.

A positive test for an acute facet joint is the reproduction of local pain around the affected facet joint and/or interscapular area. The test appears to be good (sensitive) for getting a positive result when there are arthritic changes in the facet joints but also gets a lot of false positives if used specifically as a test for arthritis, i.e., other sources of pain are just as possible (Starkey & Brown 2015).

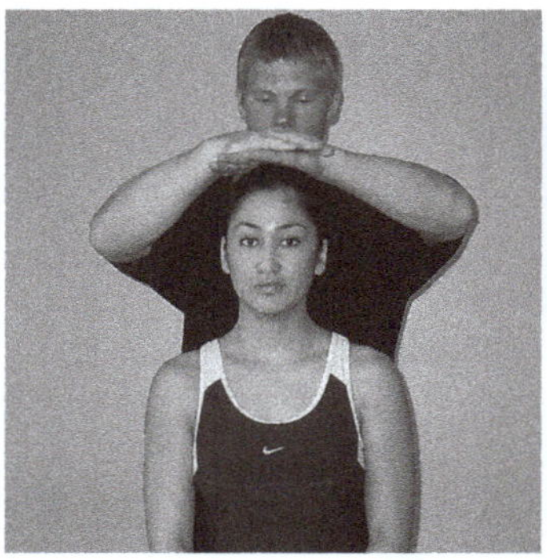

FIGURE 14.54 Seated compression test

Make sure the patient's head and neck are in normal neutral position. Apply pressure inferiorly, directed down spine, increasing from light to heavy slowly, constantly asking about pain or return of signs and symptoms.

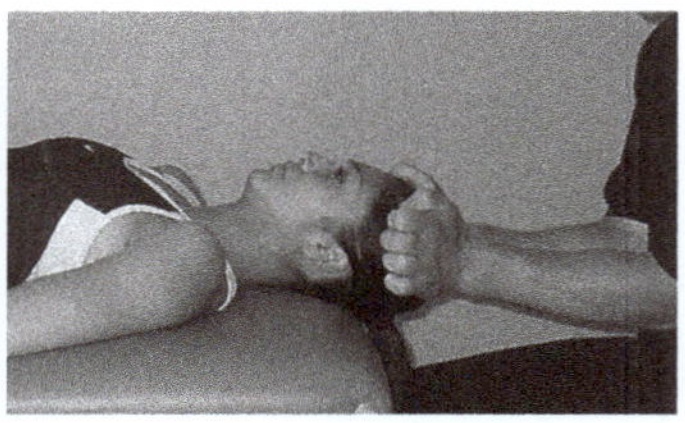

FIGURE 14.55 Supine compression test

Apply a pound or two of pressure first; ask about any pain or return of/or increase in symptoms or discomfort. If none then proceed with applying more pressure. As above, the head should not move about or wobble. All of the pressure is coming from the palm of the hand (*the fingers are shown here curled so they do not block the view*).

Have the patient supine or seated sitting up straight. Further, place patient's neck in anatomical neutral if possible, not necessarily in their neutral (i.e., avoid pressure on a hyperlordotic curves). Place one hand on the top of the head and the other on top of that hand. Let your hands mold so they cup the top of head in order to stabilize the head and neck in neutral as you compress. First, just let the weight of your hands and arms apply the compressive force. Imagine that your force is directed straight down through the whole spine (called axial pressure). Ask if there is any pain or return/increase in symptoms. If there is stop here; you have your positive sign. If the patient reports no pain, then press straight down through the cervical spine, using a slowly increasing pressure. If no pain or symptoms show themselves then slowly release the pressure. The head should not move about or wobble during the test.

If the patient is supine move the patient's head and neck into neutral. Make sure that the lordosis of the cervical spine is not exaggerated and the head is not extended. Cup the head as above (your elbows should be out to the side).

Decompression test (traction/distraction test) (Figures 14.56, 14.57)

This test should always follow the compression test. If tractioning the cervical spine results in a decrease of the patient's symptoms then the test is positive. Record as "+ decomp." under cervical tests. No change in the patient's symptoms is a negative. However, if symptoms worsen then you can record this positive as "+ S/S traction" (positive sign for an increase in signs and symptoms during traction).

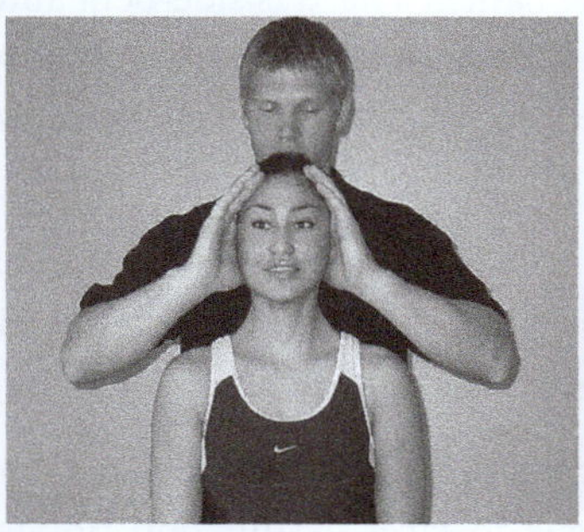

FIGURE 14.56 Seated decompression test

Have your thumbs under the occiput with your thenar eminence on the mastoid process. Traction gently straight up.

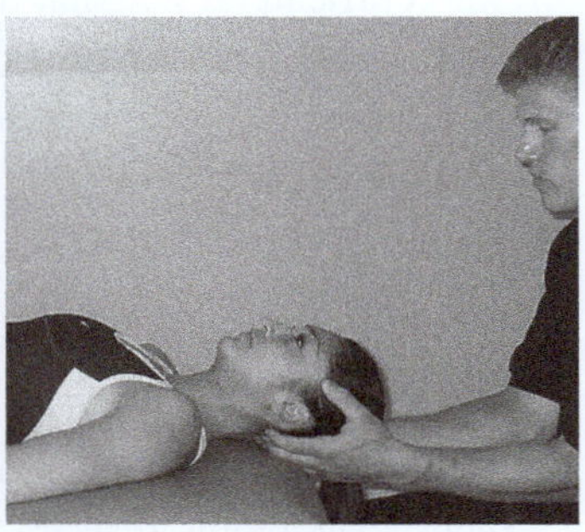

FIGURE 14.57 Supine decompression test

Place the finger pads at the base of the skull. Lean back (rather than pull) to generate traction.

If the compression test was done with the patient seated then keep them in that position to do the decompression test. Bring your hands down to the side of the head. Have the fingertips pointing straight up to the ceiling. Gently but firmly grasp (cup) the base of the skull on either side with the thenar eminences. The hypothenar eminences should rest on the posterior border of the mastoid processes on either side. Place the finger pads on the head but leave the palms of the hand off the head so as to avoid putting pressure on the ears. Ask the patient if your grip is comfortable and then lift the head straight up. Hold the traction for 5–10 seconds, asking the patient to tell you if they feel more pain or less (feel any symptom of their chief complaint increasing or decreasing).

If you are doing the test while the patient is supine cup the subocciptial area with your finger pads (do not poke), place the thumbs at the temples (the hollow created by the sphenoid bone). Ask the patient if the grip is comfortable and if so proceed with decompressing the cervical spine by traction.

If no change occurs in symptoms with traction have the patient move their shoulder by abducting or flexing their upper arm to 90–100° and then bring it back down and relax the hold completely. This repositioning may help shift compressive tension on the neck and aid in decompressing the cervical spine and bringing relief of symptoms as you then re-do the test.

Spurling's test and the cervical lower quadrant test

Spurling's test is more specific to nerve root involvement because it is more provoking than the straightforward compression test. However, this test should be done in two steps. The first step is to perform the lower quadrant test. This test is moderately provoking. Only if this is negative do we proceed to adding compression to perform Spurling's test.

The position for both of these tests is identical to the position the patient is placed in for the vertebral artery test (see Rule outs). The possibility of occlusion to the vertebral artery is another reason to do the test in two steps.

What follows is this author's procedure to safely apply the test. First is a quick summary and then more detail follows on how to do the testing. In fact, five tests are being done here. What is meant by this is that there are five results possible and we would record each as a distinct result. Thus, the result of the testing that follows determines what we name the test.

The first three tests are done simultaneously by placing the patient's neck into the test position. This position is having the cervical spine side-bent, rotated and extended, without yet applying O-P.

This position tests three different tissues and if positive implies an acute stage impairment.

1. If the patient reports dizziness, nystagmus, etc., we have a positive vertebral artery test.
2. Testing of nerve roots has occurred when there is a positive dermatomal referral of pain, numbness, or tingling in the upper limb.
3. A report of local pain at the site of a facet joint and/or intrinsic muscles of the spine tells us that we have a positive lower quadrant test for facet joint impairment (Hartley 2000a).

If this positioning results in a positive sign for any of the above tissues/structures do not proceed to the following. Only if the testing has been negative would you proceed.

The next tests occur when compression is added to this testing position and can imply a more chronic or at least sub-acute scenario. In other words, the addition of compression is what makes this a highly provocative test.

- Testing of nerve roots (Spurling's test completed) with nerve root compression symptoms.
- Testing of facet joint structures (lower quadrant test with compression or with O-P) when there is pain (usually local) but no neurological symptoms.

Lower quadrant test (Figure 14.58)

The patient is supine or seated. Ask the patient to keep their eyes open. First extend then rotate and side-bend their head to one side. This is referred to as positioning without O-P. Extending, rotating and side-bending to one side will close and slightly compress the facet joints of the lower cervical spine.

This will shorten musculature which if impaired can spasm. This usually provokes localized pain.

This positioning to one side also closes the neural foramens on that side of the cervical spine as small as is possible. This narrowing of the foramen can compress an inflamed swollen nerve root or have osteophytes around the foramen press onto the nerve as it exits the foramen. You get neurological results usually in the upper limb on that side. The extension with rotation and side-bending also closes the space between the occipital bone and C1 making it a site for possibly compressing and occluding the vertebral artery as it makes its way to the foramen magnum between these two bones.

Further, the rotation of the vertebrae puts tension and stretch on the vertebral artery as it travels through the artery's foramen

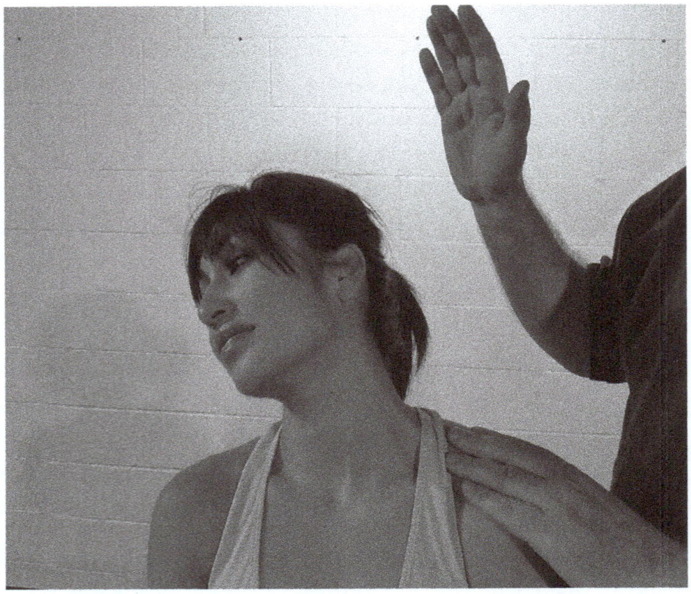

FIGURE 14.58 Lower quadrant test

The cervical spine is extended, rotated, and side-bent to one side, either seated or supine. Watch the eyes for nystagmus and ask about any vision changes, dizziness, or slurred speech, all of which can be signs of vertebral artery occlusion. Ask about pain that is local or referred into the head or the extremity on the side rotated to.

in each cervical vertebra's TVP. This is done as each successive vertebra rotates on the one below, opening the TVPs like a fan or a flight of stairs. The vertebral artery is under maximal stretch on the contralateral side that the patient's head is side-bent and rotated to, which narrows the diameter of the artery. The artery is more likely to be compressed on the same side the head is side-bent and rotated to.

If the patient has any pain and/or you observe any signs of vertebral artery occlusion then you must stop the test and return the patient's head and neck to neutral.

- Pain usually means an acute condition is present. If the patient reports symptoms that are due to facet dysfunction (joints and supportive tissues) it is recorded as + C-SP quad R. This means that positioning alone caused the lower quadrant of the cervical spine on the right to be symptomatic for facet joint lesions.
- If the positive is a reproduction of their neurological symptoms you record it as + Spurling's R w/O-P. This means that the test was positive without applying compression (O-P) when done to the right cervical spine.

As the symptoms recurred prior to compression you know that the neural tissues or the joint structures are quite inflamed and swollen and to then apply compression would only add injury to insult, or even assault to the injured.

- If acute provide the appropriate therapy and refer the patient to their physician. Any reports from scans (X-rays, ultrasounds, etc.) would be of benefit to you.
- If you have symptoms of vertebral artery occlusion you have a + vertebral artery test (+VAT) and should refer out for immediate medical attention.

Spurling's test (Figure 14.59)

If after doing the lower quadrant portion of this testing the patient reports no symptoms and there are no signs of vertebral artery occlusion then proceed to do Spurling's test.

A compressive force is directed down the cervical spine. Make sure that the vector of pressure is directed straight down into the spine and that you are especially *not* increasing the extension and at most only minimally increasing the side-bending or rotation. The purpose here is: (1) to compress the discs to make them bulge and see if they compress a nerve root or ligament; (2) further narrow the neural foramen to see if compression happens there; and (3) to approximate the facet joints and by compression apply a maximum load through the articular structures.

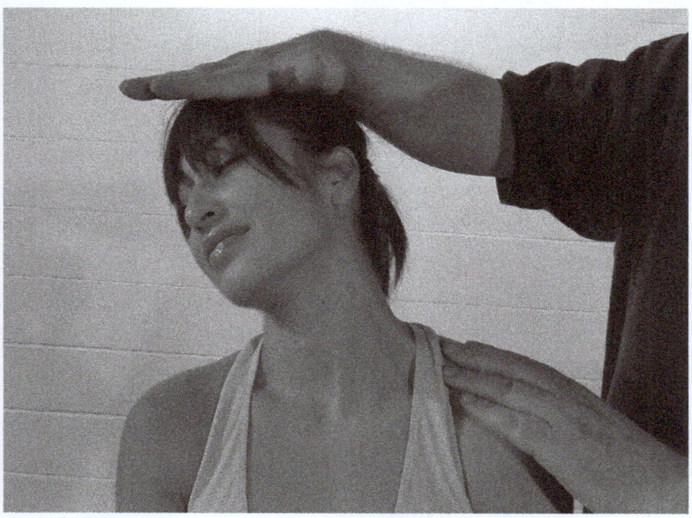

FIGURE 14.59 Spurling's test

Press straight down on the most superior portion of the head (as in this position). Begin gently, slowly increasing pressure. Avoid increasing the extension, side-bending and rotation.

Ask the patient to report any pain or symptoms immediately. Further, be sure to slowly increase the pressure and stop when positive. If no positive sign occurs then slowly release the pressure.

A positive result that has local pain implies that there is facet joint and supportive tissue injury (including intrinsic deep muscles). *This has been a lower quadrant test with O-P.* Soft tissue pain in surrounding areas may be referred pain or the result of complaints from accessory or compensatory tissues. A common area for soft tissue referral for the cervical spine is into the interscapular-vertebral area of the upper thoracic spine (Bogduk 2003).

If you get positive facet joint results to this testing then you may record them as follows: "+ R C3-4 quad w.O/P." In long hand this means: *A positive test found on the right for facet symptoms at C3–4 using the lower quadrant test with over-pressure.* However, if you reproduce the patient's neurological signs and symptoms in the upper limb when doing this test that constitutes a positive Spurling's test. Though this test can be negative (false negative) while there is in fact a compression of a nerve root in a neural foramen when positive for nerve root impingement at the foramen it is often right (Starkey & Brown 2015). Which nerve root is affected is known by the patient reporting symptoms occurring in a recognizable dermatomal pattern (see neurological testing later in the chapter and refer back to Figure 13.73). Use "+ R Spurling's" to record reproduction of various neurological impairments as that is what that test was designed to find. Add to your notation as to what nerve root(s) appear to be affected.

Box 14.7 examines at the impact of extended, rotated, and side-bent positions on the arteries, veins, and nerves.

Valsalva's test (Figure 14.60)

By increasing the intrathecal pressure in the spinal cord the positive sign of pain will be elicited if there is a space occupying lesion such as a tumor, herniated disc, or osteophytes that then increase their compression on a nerve root. Where the symptoms recur and to what dermatome they may refer will tell you at what level of the spine the lesion is. Refer to the primary physician and treat appropriately.

If there is local pain in the spine with or without referral ***this is a red flag:*** refer the patient out to seek imaging testing (X-rays, etc.). However, some local pain can be generated from this test if the disc bulges onto a ligament.

Have the patient, seated or supine, take a deep breath and pretend they are trying to blow up a balloon but cannot let the

INSIGHTS

Box 14.7 Impact of extended, rotated, and side-bent position on arteries, veins, and nerves

- Stretching (on the one side) will reduce the diameter of the artery, and if there is plaque build-up then blood flow can be significantly decreased. Excessive stretching could also cause some of the plaque to break off from the wall and induce a stroke. The carotid artery on this side is also stretched, which can also reduce blood flow through it.
- The compression (on the other side) occurs as the TVPs approximate and rotate, creating a significant bend between each motion segment. Unlike the side that is stretched, where there is some advantage to having space for the artery to spread the bending over a greater distance and so decrease the likelihood of a sharp severe bend, this is not so for the shortened compressed side. The superior TVP in each motion segment presses (shears) into the anterior portion of the artery coming from below, while the inferior TVP presses into the posterior portion of the artery leaving it.
- The jugular vein, as it exits the skull, can also become compressed between the occiput-temporal bone and the lateral mass of C1. Slower drainage of blood to the skull means slower arterial flow in as well.
- The vagal nerve (CN X) and the glossopharyngeal nerve (CN IX) also exit through the jugular foramen. They too can be subject to compression when the head is rotated, side-bent, and extended to that side. Note that the patient's case history may include gastrointestinal impairments due to vagal impairment. Though by no means a main reason for irritable bowel syndrome, many patients with chronic suboccipitally generated headaches and neck injuries will report irritable bowel symptoms.
- Note that in a whiplash injury (especially from behind, or the side) all of these structures can be injured from compression or stretch. Other nerves can also become compressed between the occiput and the atlas, for example: sympathetic nerves from the superior ganglion, the accessory nerve (CN XI), occipital nerves, as well as the C1 nerve itself.

air out; or hold the breath in while bearing down as if having a bowel movement. ***CAUTION:*** After performing this test patients can become dizzy.

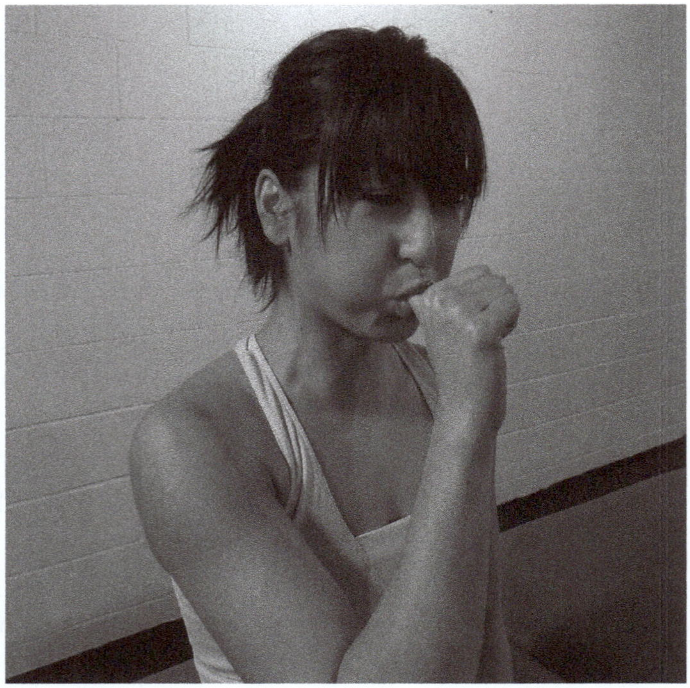

FIGURE 14.60 Valsalva's test

Ask the patient to take a deep breath, place the tip of the thumb in the mouth, and pretend they are blowing up a balloon, but let no air escape.

Swallowing test (Figure 14.61)

This test is positive if the patient has the sensation of a lump in the throat when swallowing. This is caused by a space-occupying lesion in the cervical spine that protrudes into the anterior longitudinal ligament and in turn, protrudes into the esophagus. The lesion could be an anteriorly herniated disc, a hematoma (from a whiplash, for example), or a tumor, to mention the most obvious possibilities. A positive result requires a referral back to the patient's primary physician. If the patient has trouble swallowing (for example, from a dry throat) have them sip some water and swallow that.

Tinel's sign at the neck (door bell test) (Figure 14.62)

This test shows if the nerve roots as they exit out of the intervertebral foramen are inflamed.

The therapist applies pressure with the pad of their index finger over the cervical nerve root as it exits the neural foramen ("*presses the door-bell button*"). The pressure is applied to the patient's slightly laterally flexed and rotated neck just behind the sternocleidomastoid muscle (SCM) which will be over the

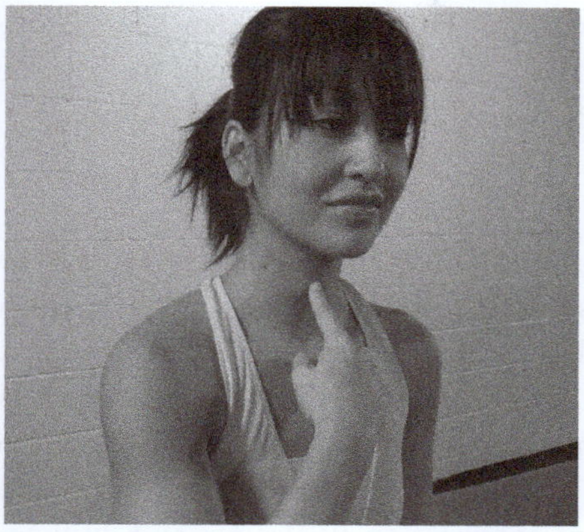

FIGURE 14.61 Swallowing test

Have the patient swallow and report if they feel a lump in the throat or have difficulty swallowing. If so, refer out.

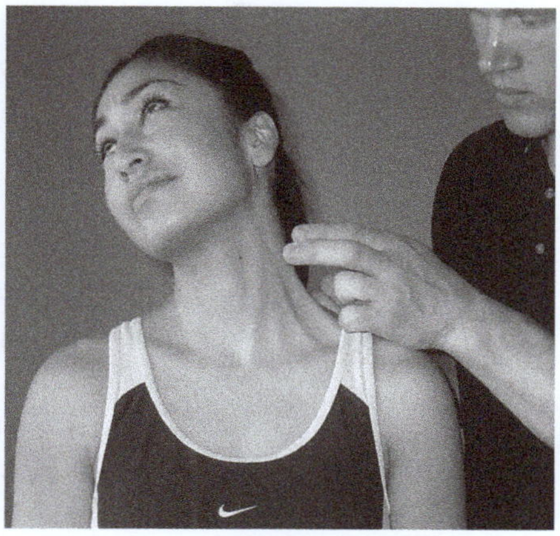

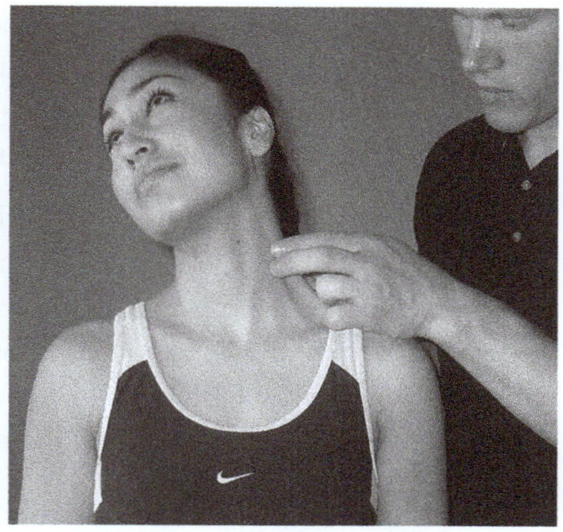

FIGURE 14.62A, B Tinel's sign at the neck

The patient side-bends and rotates to one side. The therapist lightly presses (momentarily) or "taps" over the tips of TVPs behind the SCM.

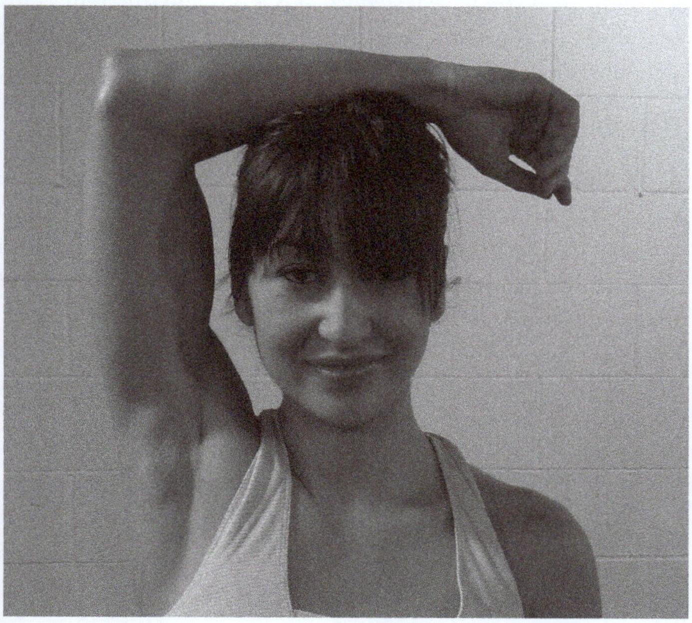

FIGURE 14.63 Test for Bakody's sign

The patient places their forearm on top of their head. Reduction of symptoms is positive.

nerve roots as they exit the spine. The patient may be seated or supine. The positive sign is reproduction of the patient's neurological symptoms in the upper limb ("*and the door-bell rings*"). This test is often unproductive or inconsistent in its results. Local pain where pressure was applied is not positive for nerve root pathology.

Bakody's sign

Another way to check if a nerve root is involved in shoulder or arm pain is for the patient to place the affected side's forearm on top of their head. If this brings clear relief it is a positive Bakody's sign. The test works by lifting the clavicle and shortening the distance the nerve needs to travel to the brachial plexus and upper arm. This action reduces the pull on the nerve roots and it may possibly reduce symptoms of neural compression.

However, it may also be reducing symptoms originating not from the cervical spine per se but from other soft tissue and joints such as entrapment between the clavicle and the first two ribs. Nonetheless, when it does reduce symptoms it has traditionally been said that it indicates that the nerve root lesion exists at the C5 or C6 region. At best this is a "screening test" that when positive suggests a need for further detailed testing.

Introduction to specific neurological testing

If the patient tests positive for any neurological test refer them to their physician. It would be wise for you to write a note that they can take with them explaining what testing was positive during the neurological assessment and at what levels so that their physician knows what testing to do to try and repeat your results.

Dermatome testing

Initially the therapist may wish to do some quick testing for sensory nerve enervation dysfunctions relating to sensory nerve roots. This can be done with the patient seated or standing. Test bilaterally at the same time by brushing over both arms and hands simultaneously. Inform and show the patient what you are going to do. By brushing we mean to lightly drag over the patient's skin using your relaxed fingers. Repeat over each dermatome several times (refer back to Figure 13.73).

Ask the patient if they notice any difference side to side and if there is any change in the quality of sensation on either arm in any specific area. Often a delayed response or uncertainty on the patient's part can be considered a possible positive sign (of a mild problem). If you wish you can repeat this with deep touch, hot and then cold, two-point discrimination and vibration.

If the patient reports any changes or absence of sensation note which dermatome area those changes are in. You can then brush each specific dermatomal area (always bilaterally) several times and ask each time if the patient notices any difference one side to the other or to the prior area tested. Even if you feel that you have already identified the dermatome through case history questioning then perform the testing in several of the dermatomes above and below and never test just the one you suspect. Remember that if the patient has not seen their primary physician regarding any positive results then they need to be encouraged to do so. If you do not find any positive results but the patient's symptoms seem to be neurological and you find no other cause (like trigger point referral zones) then also refer them back to their primary health care provider.

The areas to brush listed below correspond to the generally undisputed areas of the various dermatome maps developed over the last 100 years or so. Further, dermatomes overlap to some degree in everyone. Therefore, it is suggested you test the central areas of each dermatome.

Red flag

If two or more dermatomes are affected the patient may be suffering from stenosis of the spinal canal; in other words a compression within the spinal canal. A stenosis can also cause bilateral loss. *This is a red flag* and the patient should be advised to see a physician promptly. However, having a positive may also point to a peripheral nerve lesion. Remember that peripheral nerves also suffer from compression syndromes and dysfunction. Compare your dermatome findings especially if the results are not clear with a map of peripheral nerve sensory innervation. (See peripheral nerve testing on the pages following dermatome testing.)

NOTATION: To record your findings of brushing write them as C3 Derm +. If you have tested various levels and different kinds of sensations note them accordingly, e.g., C3 Derm + light touch and vibration.

Dermatomes

Table 14.1 is a dermatome chart. Compare this chart with the peripheral nerve chart presented later in this section. Comparing your findings with these charts and maps will help to differentiate between nerve root dermatomes and peripheral nerve cutaneous enervation.

TABLE 14.1
Sensory areas of the dermatomes

Dermatome	Sensory area
C1 and C2	C1 Back of the head, or behind the ears
C3	Above the clavicle
C4	Below the clavicle
C5	Lateral shoulder and arm down into the lateral elbow
C6	Whole thumb, and up into the lateral wrist
C7	Both dorsal and ventral surfaces of the middle finger
C8	Ulnar border of little finger and wrist and distal forearm
T1	Medial forearm up to the elbow

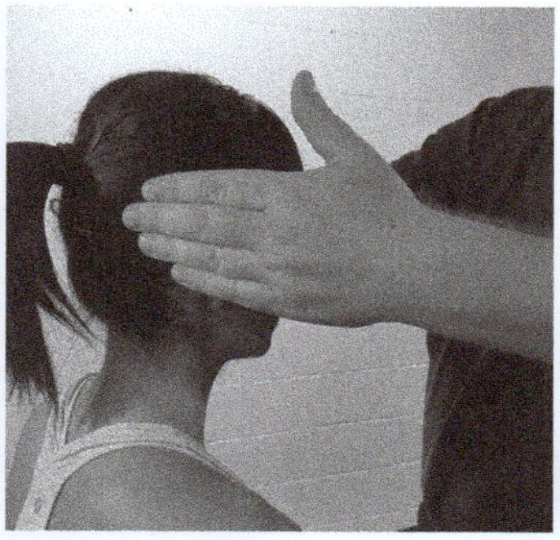

FIGURE 14.64 C1 and C2 dermatome test

The therapist brushes the back of the patient's head or behind the ears.

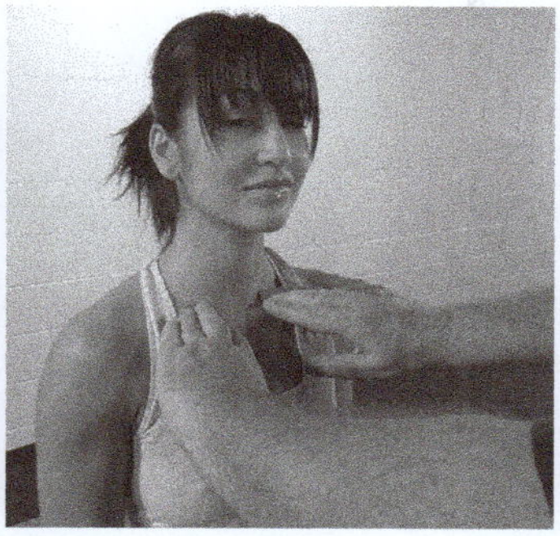

FIGURE 14.65 C3 dermatome test

Brush above and along the length of the clavicle.

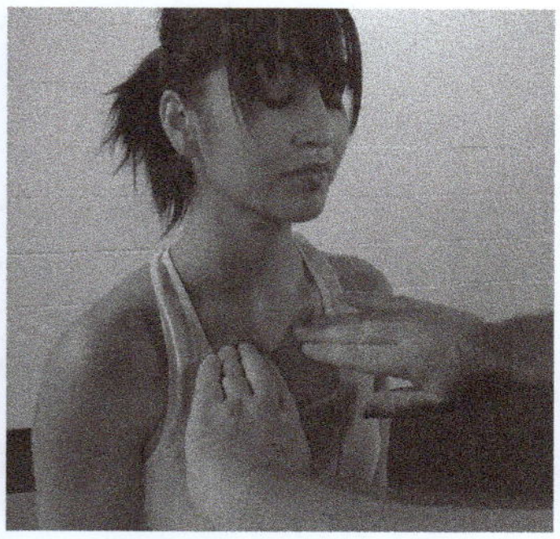

FIGURE 14.66 C4 dermatome test

Brush below and under the clavicle along its entire length.

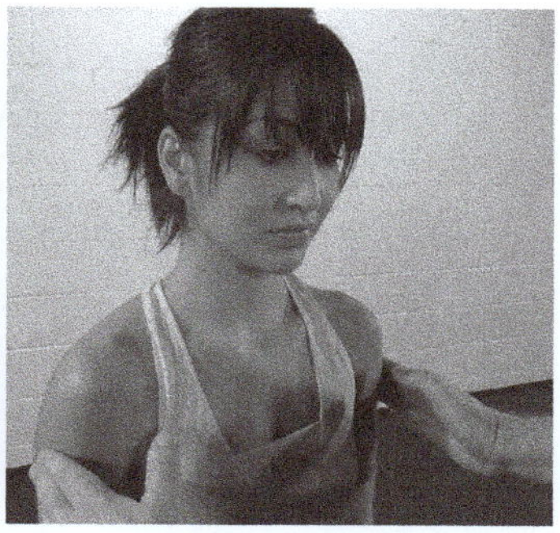

FIGURE 14.67 C5 dermatome test

Brush the lateral portion of the deltoid, down toward (but not to) the elbow.

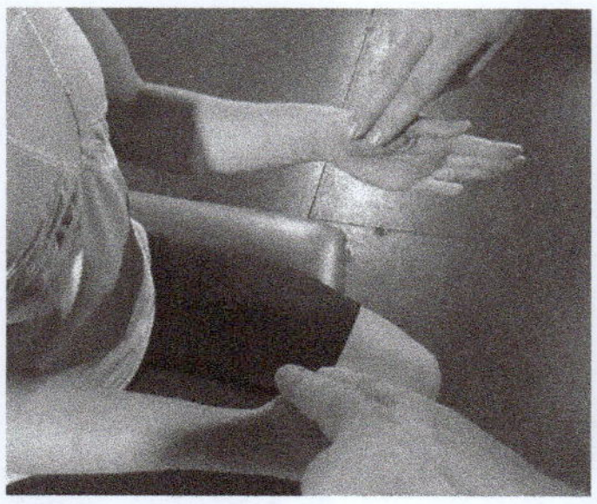

FIGURE 14.68 C6 dermatome test

Brush from the base of the thumb, along its lateral side down to the tip of the thumb.

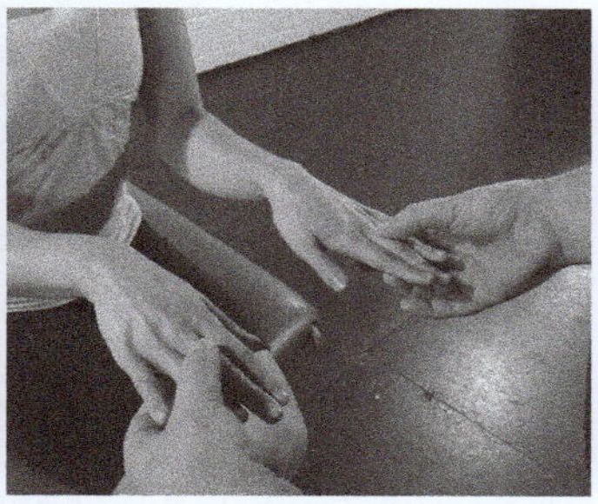

FIGURE 14.69 C7 dermatome test

Brush the middle finger's dorsal and ventral sides from the MCP to the fingertip.

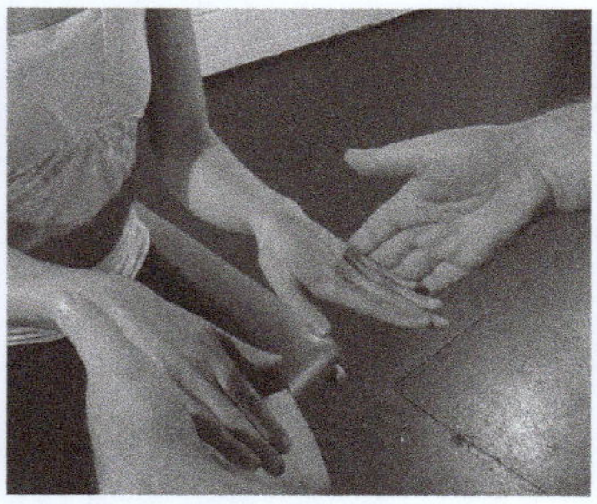

FIGURE 14.70 C8 dermatome test

Brush the ulnar border of the little finger from the wrist to the fingertip.

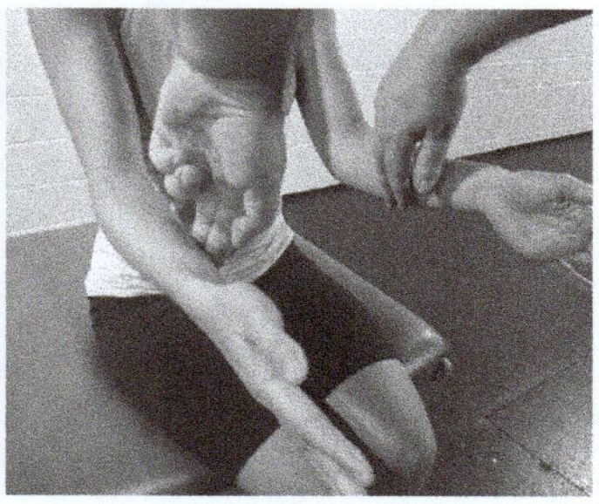

FIGURE 14.71 T1 dermatome test

Brush the proximal ulnar border of the forearm up to the medial elbow.

Dermatome tests (Figures 14.64–14.71)

This testing can be done very quickly.

Sensory testing of the face (Figures 14.72–14.74)

The face is enervated by the three divisions of the trigeminal nerve (CN V). See the peripheral nerve map in Figure 14.75.

Peripheral nerve testing

For suspected peripheral nerve impairments see Table 14.2 and Figure 14.75. For other means of testing these nerves see Chapters 15, 17.

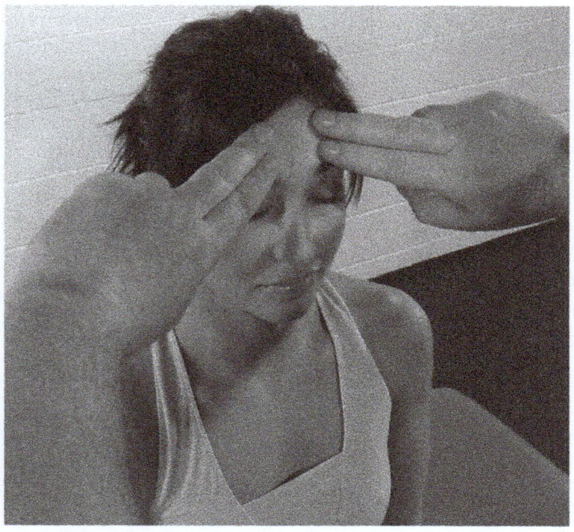

FIGURE 14.72 Testing CN V1 – opthalmic nerve

Brush over the eyebrows.

Table 14.2
Sensory areas of peripheral sensory nerves

Peripheral sensory nerve	Sensory area
Axillary (C5–6)	Lateral arm and deltoid area on upper arm – but distinctive is total loss of circular area mid-lateral deltoid – down to elbow and over to medial forearm
Musculocutaneous (C5–6)	Lateral forearm
Radial (C6–T1)	Dorsal surface of lateral hand and onto thumb; and also dorsal surface index, middle finger and lateral portion of the 4th finger, all up to DIP joint but not including surface of the distal phalanges
Median (C6–7)	Tips of index, middle and medial side of 4th digit, and ventral surface of those fingers and the palm of the hand
Ulnar (C8–T1)	Dorsal and ventral surfaces of little finger and lateral half of the 4th digit

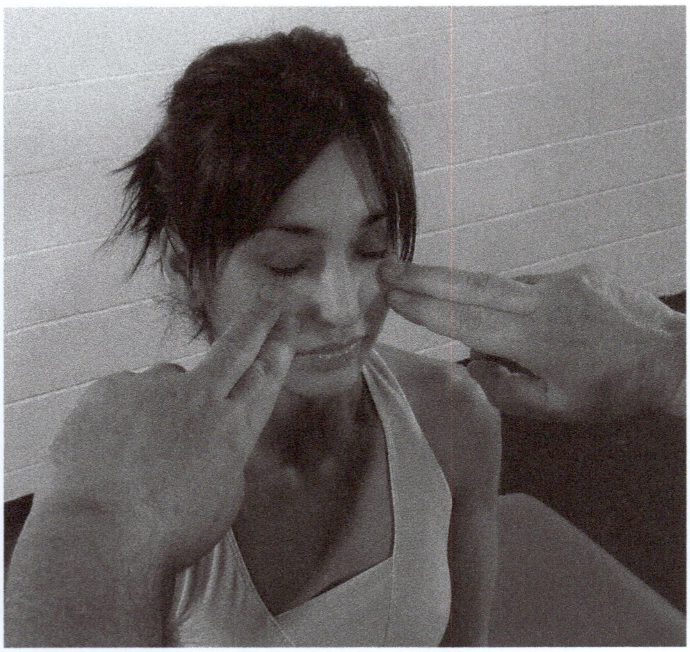

FIGURE 14.73 Testing CN V2 – maxillary nerve
Brush from under the eyes over the cheek bones.

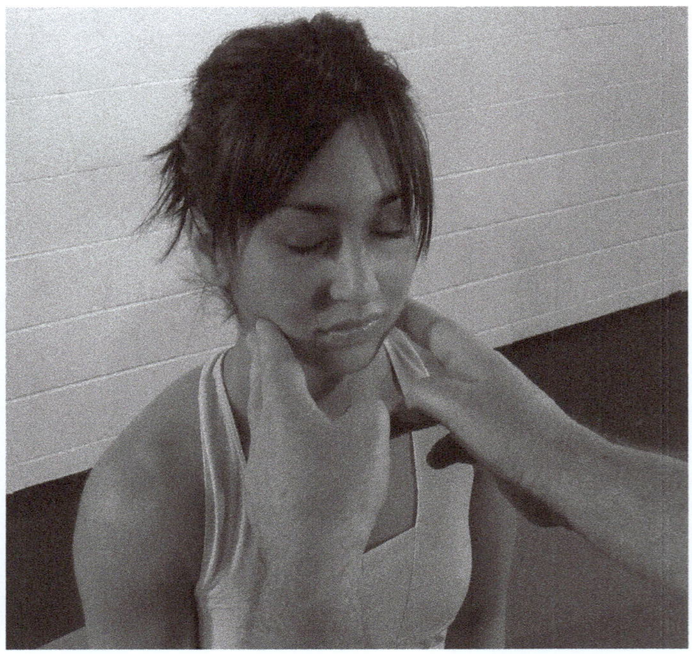

FIGURE 14.74 Testing CN V3 – mandibular nerve
Brush along the mandible, from its angle toward the chin.

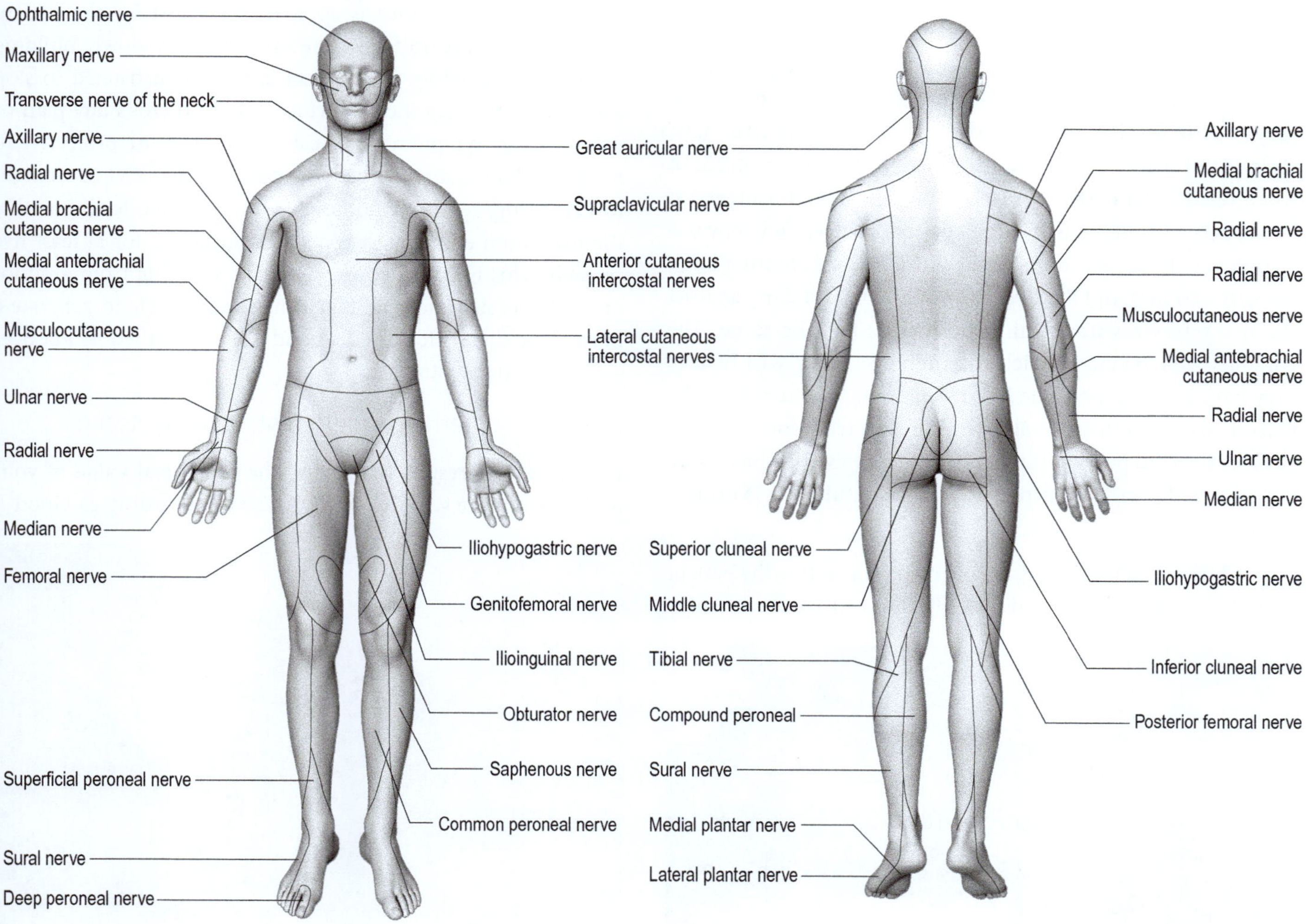

FIGURE 14.75

Peripheral nerve map.

Myotome testing for the cervical spine (Figures 14.76–14.83)

Patients must use their full strength in neurological tests or when doing any strength testing for that matter because they may inadvertently mislead the therapist about the true strength of a muscle. If you ask for only half their strength when testing the patient will often only be able to gauge that by the resistance they feel being applied. Hence, they may use 50 percent of their strength on the uninjured side of their body being tested first and 70 percent on the other; pushing against the therapist's resistance until both sides feel the same. The patient is not trying to trick the therapist. They will believe they have applied the same force because it felt the same. The reason given for using half-strength has traditionally been cited as a way to prevent further injury. However, if the testing is performed correctly (progressively) then this rule is unnecessary.

Just like AR-ROM testing, during myotome testing the patient should be instructed to begin their effort or resistance with minimal effort and take a good five seconds to build up to maximum strength. If the therapist is applying the effort for the patient to resist they need to follow the same rules by slowly building up to maximal effort. The patient is further instructed to stop and slowly decrease their effort as soon as there is any pain or recurrence of symptoms. This can in fact be more protective to re-injury than giving the patient some specific level of strength to use during testing. Another rule of myotome testing is that the maximum effort by the patient is sustained for at least five seconds. This is done because a muscle suffering from a minor or moderate neurological deficit may still be able to generate a normal maximal effort for a second or two but then will noticeably begin to lose strength.

Scale for isometric strength testing of myotomes

Record testing results by placing the numerical value of your finding over 5, e.g., 4/5 R Myo C5, or by recording as Good R

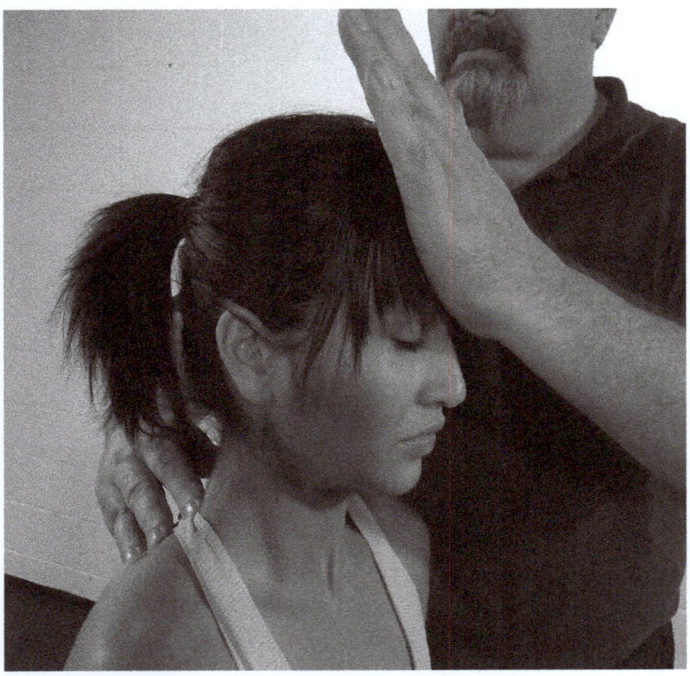

FIGURE 14.76 Testing C3 myotome

Forward head nodding (from OA joint, rather than neck flexion). Resist movement at the forehead. Ask the patient to tuck the chin in rather than just telling them to push the forehead into your hand.

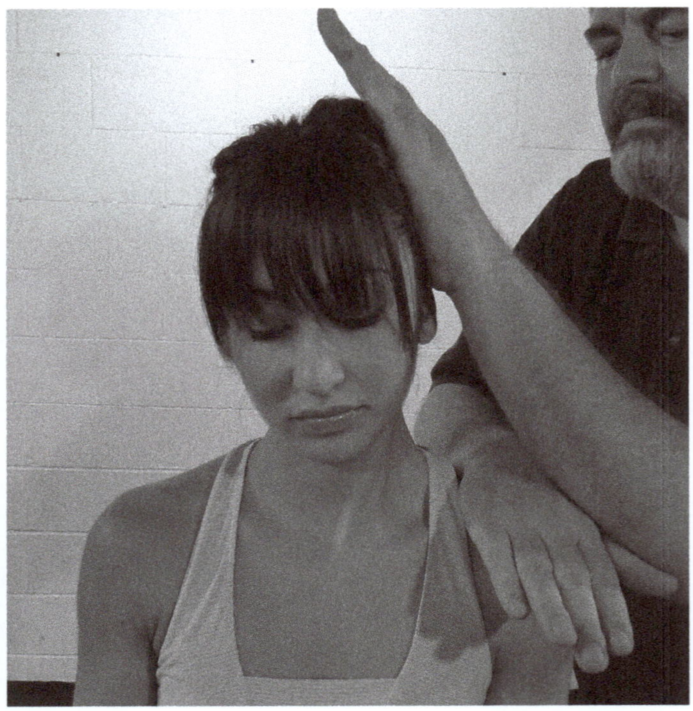

FIGURE 14.77 Testing C1 and 2 myotome

Side-bending. Resist the patient at the side of the head and the ipsilateral shoulder using crossed forearms. The therapist can bring the forearm down on top of their hand for better leverage for both resisting side-bending and lifting of the shoulder. Ask the patient to bring the ear down to the shoulder but try not to bring the shoulder up to the ear.

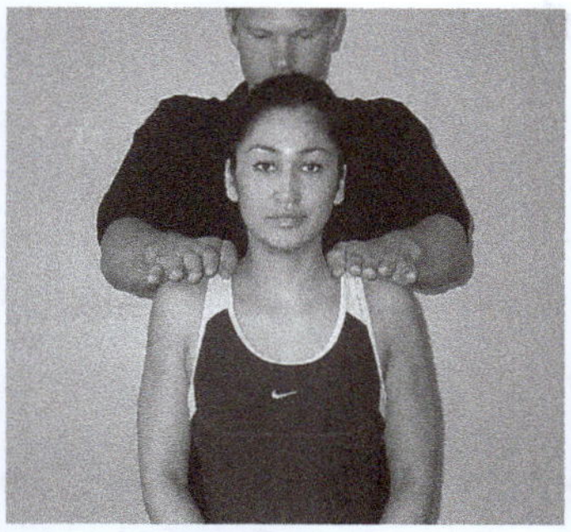

FIGURE 14.78 Testing C4 myotome

Resist shoulder elevation bilaterally. It is best if the patient lifts the shoulders first then the therapist pushes the shoulders down while the patient resists.

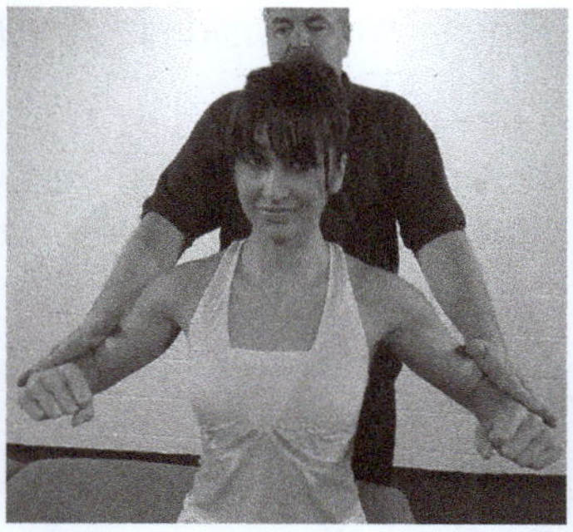

FIGURE 14.79 Testing C5 myotome

Shoulder abduction. Have the patient hold the upper arms at 45° then apply resistance to engage the deltoid muscle (this also tests the axillary nerve).

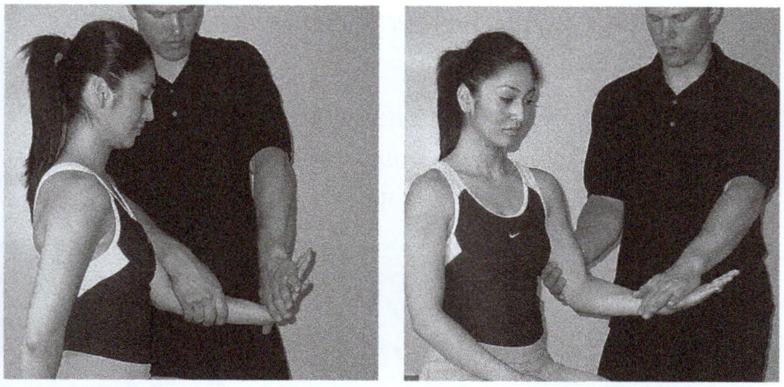

FIGURE 14.80A, B Testing C6 myotome

Wrist extension is fairly specific, while testing elbow flexion draws on C5 and C6. Resisting elbow flexion also tests the musculocutaneous peripheral nerve.

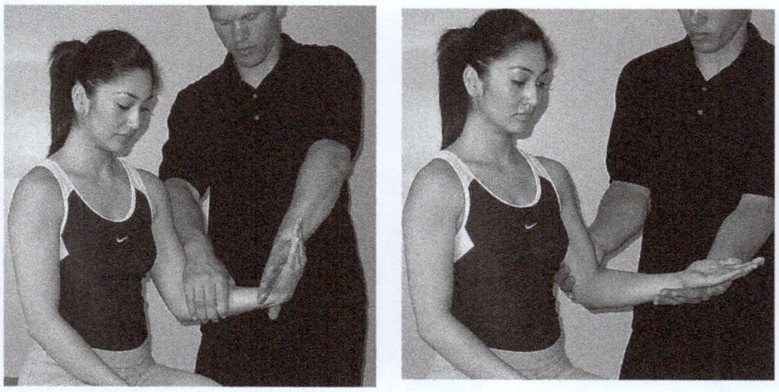

FIGURE 14.81A, B Testing C7 myotome

Wrist flexion is more specific; some test elbow extension. Both tests will challenge radial nerve.

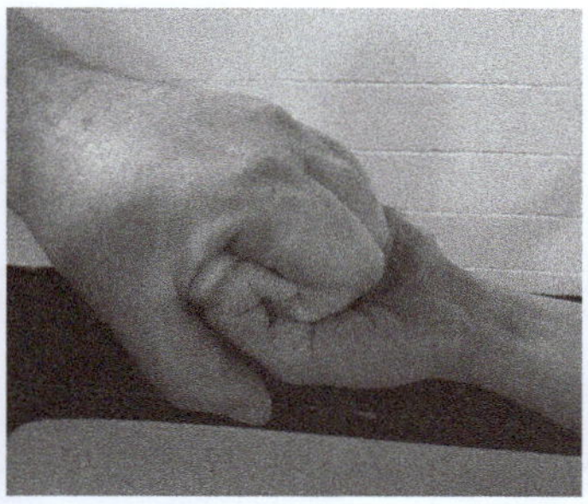

FIGURE 14.82 Testing C8 myotome

Finger flexors. Have the patient grasp your fingers and tell them to not let you open their hand.

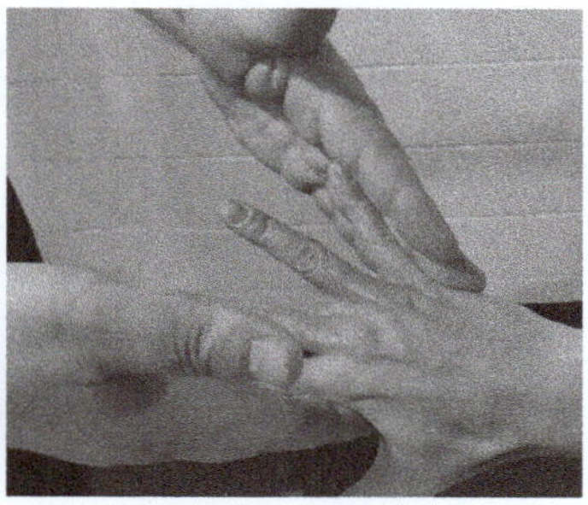

FIGURE 14.83 Testing T1 myotome

Abduction of fingers. Abduction of the little finger on its own is sometimes used to test the ulnar nerve.

Myo C5. Kendall et al. (2005) suggest that a negative (-) or positive sign (+) can be added to the number or term applied to the finding in order to fine tune them to the variety of functionality observed in clinical settings.

5 = Normal: full strength available with strong resistance applied.

4 = Good: can resist with only slight resistance applied.

3 = Fair: can only resist the affect of gravity alone.

2 = Poor: cannot resist gravity but can move the limb in the horizontal plane.

1 = Trace: no movement, only "flickering" of muscle present.

0 = Zero: no trace, no flickering, flaccid.

Do the following resisted testing either having the therapist resist the patient's movement or better still, have the patient hold their position while the therapist applies force. The actions resisted below to test the myotomes have been chosen for their specificity, and for the ease of comparing bilaterally.

Testing motor function of peripheral nerves (Figures 14.84–14.95)

NOTE: Axillary, musculocutaneous and radial nerve tests are very similar to myotome testing, while the ulnar and median nerve motor tests can be more specific (Waxman 2000).

Upper limb tension testing (ULTT)

This is also referred to as brachial plexus tension testing. It is a series of provocative tests of the peripheral nerves done by stretching (placing tension on) a specific peripheral nerve when possible. This is done through positioning the various joints and

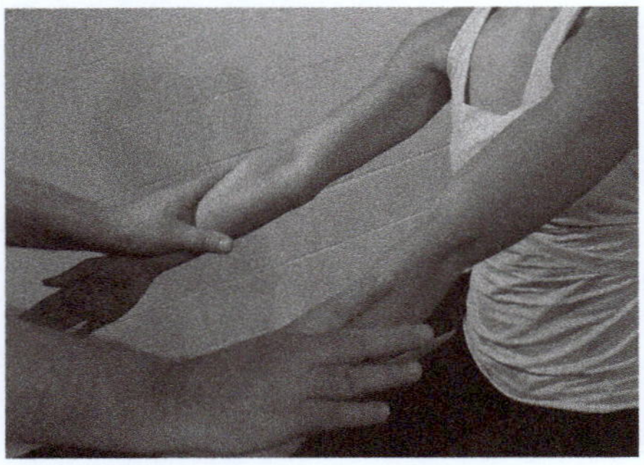

FIGURE 14.84 Axillary nerve test

Have the patient forward flex their extended arms and tell them to hold position while you place your hands on their forearms and try to push their arms down. The purpose here is to test the (anterior) deltoid muscle.

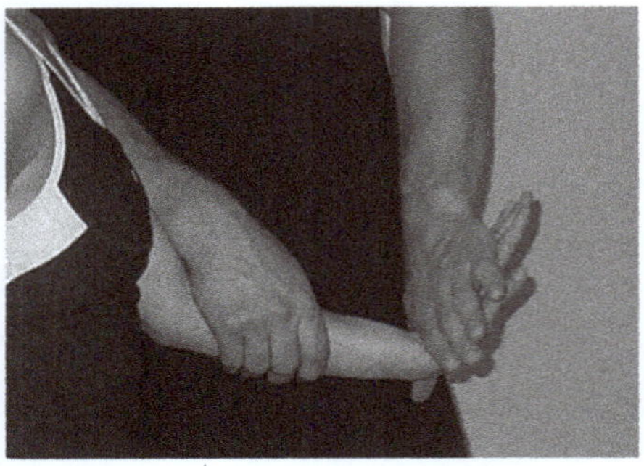

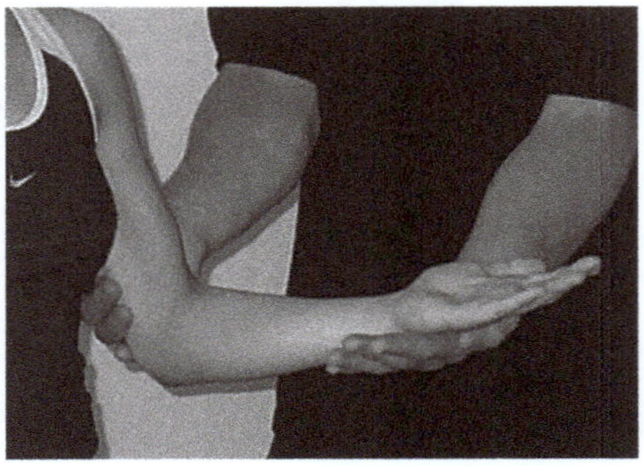

FIGURES 14.85, 14.86 Radial nerve test

The radial nerve innervates most extensor muscles; hence, we can test the lower portion by testing the extensors of the wrist or the upper portion by testing triceps.

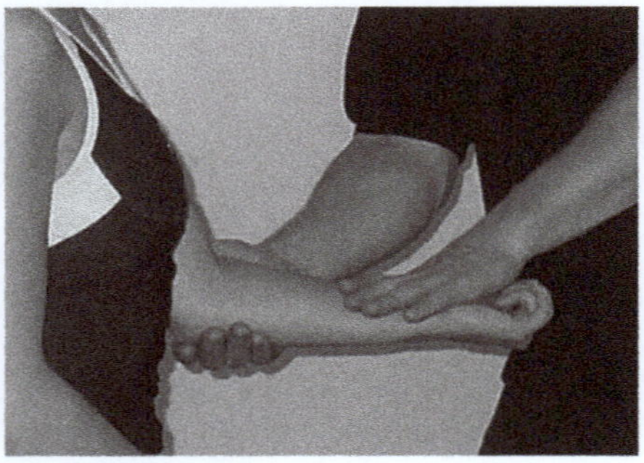

FIGURE 14.87 Musculocutaneous nerve test

Biceps brachii is tested. Though this muscle is often used to test the C6 myotome it is not that specific to a single nerve root and thus, more accurate to musculocutaneous nerve.

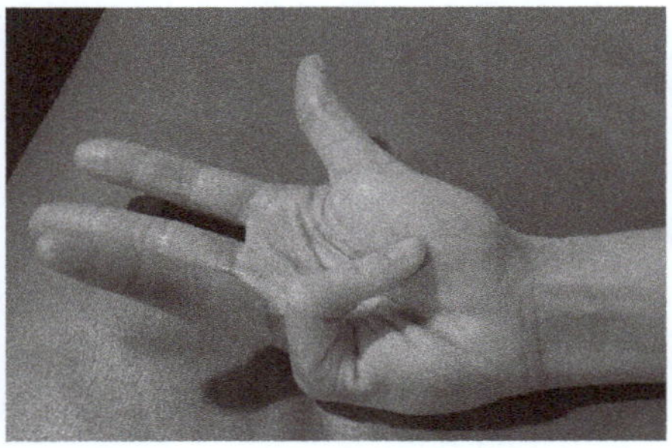

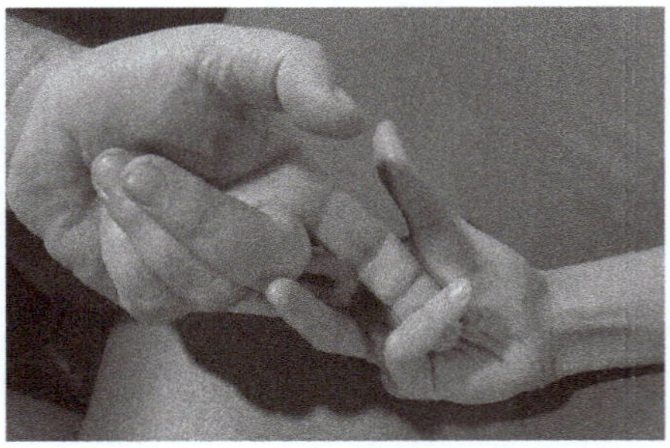

FIGURE 14.88A, B Ulnar nerve motor test

To be very specific to the ulnar nerve and not use the thumb (which can be synergistically making use of the median nerve) have the patient supinate the arm. Demonstrate and ask them to move the little finger until its tip touches the base of the thumb. First, see if the patient can complete this maneuver. If they cannot, yet there is no pain, the ulnar nerve may be severely impaired. To ensure they are not prevented from doing the maneuver by fascial or other restrictions see if you can complete the movement passively for them. Second, if the patient completes the maneuver then hook your index finger under their little finger and slowly and gently increase your effort to lift the little finger away from the palm of the hand as the patient resists.

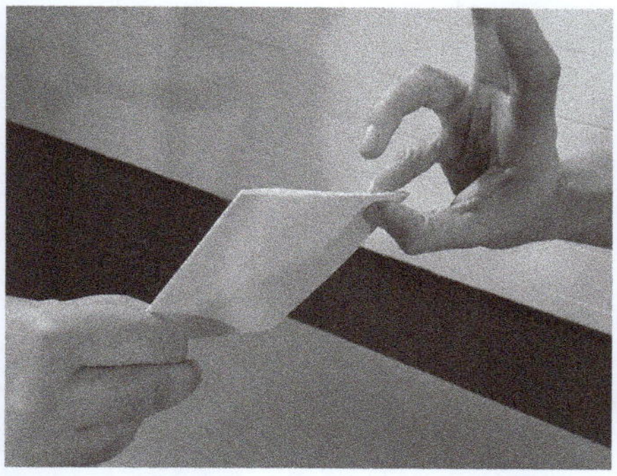

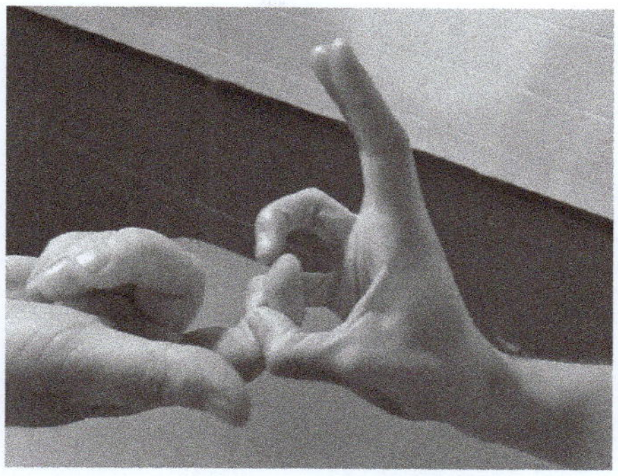

FIGURES 14.89 and 14.90 Fromet's sign and alternate Fromet's sign

A common test for the ulnar nerve. The patient places the tips of little finger and thumb together in opposition. Ask the patient to hold a piece of paper between the digits and not let you pull it out. Alternatively, you can also just hook your index finger into a circle made by the patient's thumb and little finger and try to pull the tips apart by pulling your finger through them while the patient tries to prevent you from doing this. If at first it appears that there is weakness (a positive sign) then repeat two or three times to confirm and ensure the patient is trying hard to resist you.

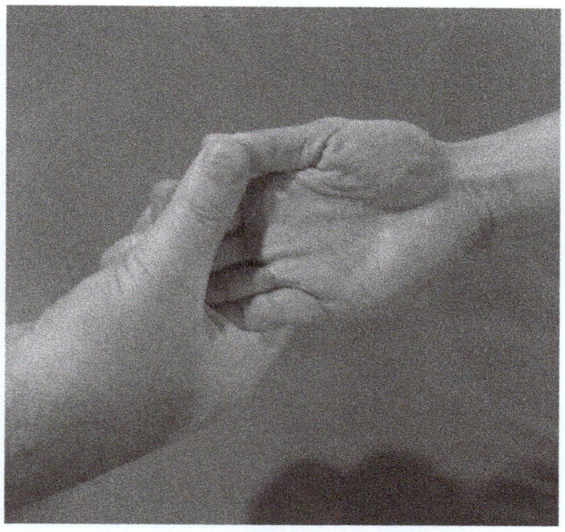

FIGURE 14.91 Median nerve motor test

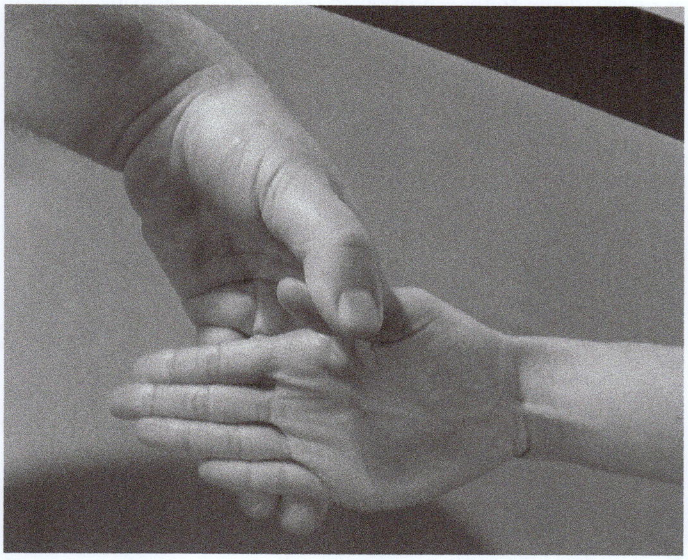

FIGURE 14.92 Alternate median nerve motor test

To test the median nerve resist the patient's attempt to flex their extended thumb across the palm of the hand. You resist at the distal phalange. Alternatively, you can have the patient abduct their thumb and tell them to hold the position as you attempt to push the thumb toward the lateral border of the palm.

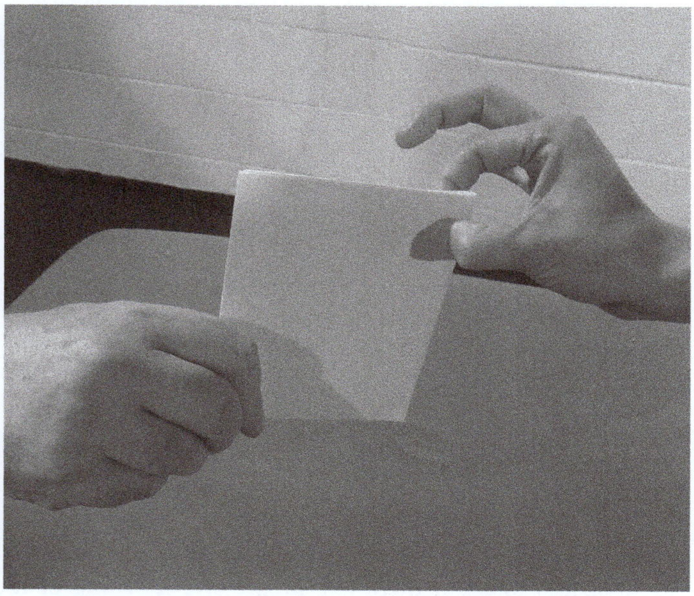

FIGURE 14.93 Alternate median nerve test 2

The patient pinches the thumb and index finger as in making an okay gesture. Then have the patient do this with a piece of paper pinched between the tips of the fingers. The therapist tries to pull the paper out from the pinch. Positive sign is the patient unable to hold.

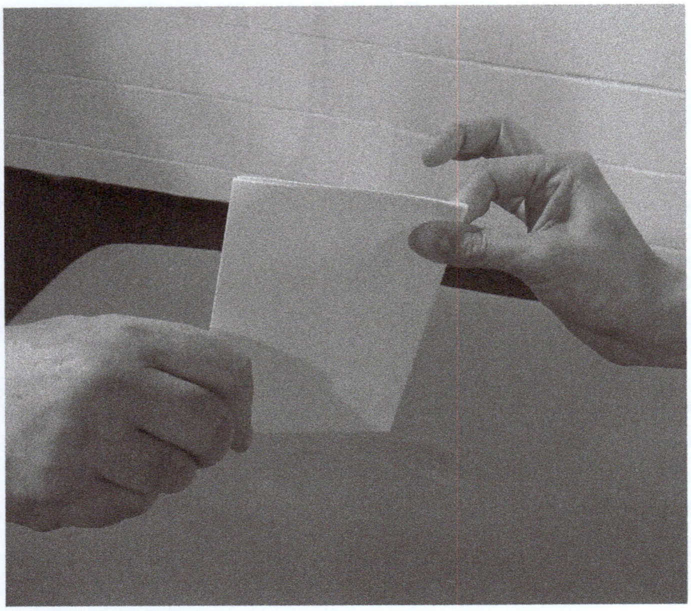

FIGURE 14.94 Alternate 2: positive sign

The test is positive for median nerve root dysfunction even if the patient can hold the paper but does so only if the finger and thumb extend and cannot hold tip-to-tip. Digits collapse and the paper is held by the finger pads. If this happens, repeat the test and ask the patient to try to sustain tip-to-tip pinching only. If the patient is unable to do so and involuntarily reverts to a pad-to-pad grip this is considered a positive sign.

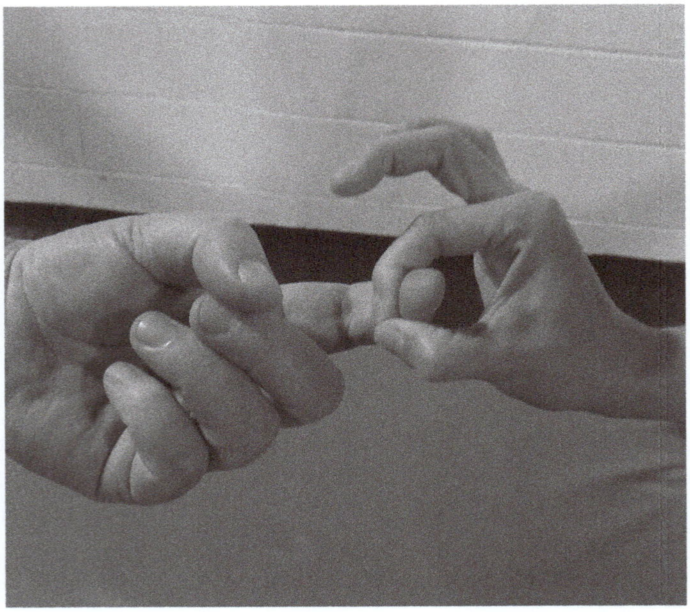

FIGURE 14.95 Alternate median nerve test 3

Alternatively, to test the median nerve you can also just hook your index finger into a circle made by the patient's thumb and index finger. Now try to pull the tips apart by pulling your finger through them while the patient tries to prevent you from doing this. If at first it appears that there is weakness (a positive sign) repeat two or three times more to confirm and to make sure patient is trying hard to resist you.

sections of the upper extremity/limb (i.e., the shoulder, arm, forearm, wrist and fingers) in specific patterns or positions.

Instructions for upper limb tension testing (ULTT) for peripheral nerves are shown in Chapter 15.

Deep tendon reflexes (DTR) (Figures 14.96–14.98)

Rather than the classic one strike or two with a reflex hammer it is wise to test each DTR on each side of the body with seven to 10 strikes to see if there is a progressive lessening of the response. This decreasing response is a positive sign.

The obvious positive sign for DTRs is a difference bilaterally. You can have a decreased or absent reflex on one side as a positive sign or you could have a hyper-reflexive response on one side as a positive sign. If you get little or no response from both sides that is what is normal for that person and in no way is it a positive sign. Lack of response is due to the fact that we are using a stretch reflex to test innervation. If the muscle is long or low in tone the response could be minimal or absent.

Reflex grading scale

0 = No response. Pathological if unilateral; if bilateral the test is considered negative.

1 = Hyporeflexive, trace of movement. Pathology may be present if response is unilateral; if bilateral it may be due to hypotonicity or deconditioning.

2 = Normal response.

3 = Brisk or greater than normal response. May be pathological if unilateral; if bilateral it may be due to hypertonicity of the musculature involved in the reflex.

4 = Non-sustained clonus or a repetitive contraction-relaxation (vibratory) movement in the muscle for a short period of time; or hyper-reflexia, a gross exaggeration of movement.

5 = Sustained clonus or a prolonged contraction-relaxation of the muscle involved; or hyper-reflexia that seems to spread to other muscles nearby.

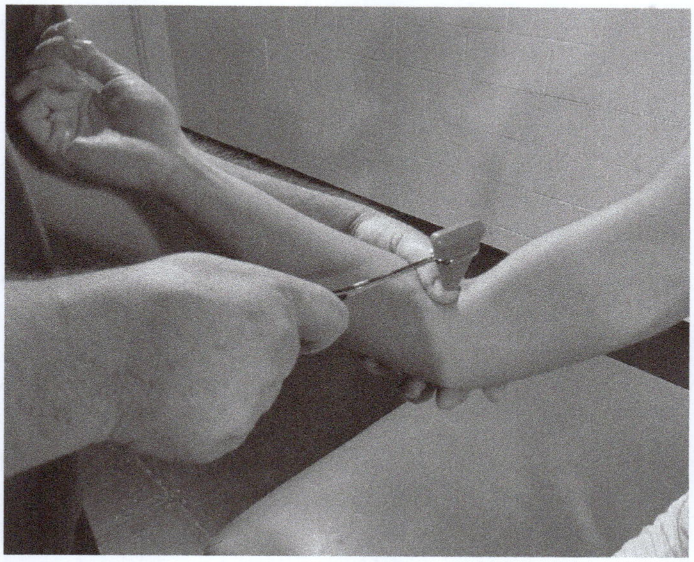

FIGURE 14.96 C5–6 DTR (at biceps tendon)

Place the patient's forearm over your forearm and ask them to relax. Place your thumb over the biceps tendon at the elbow and hit your own thumb. You may not see a response of reflex but rather just feel the tendon go tense and firm.

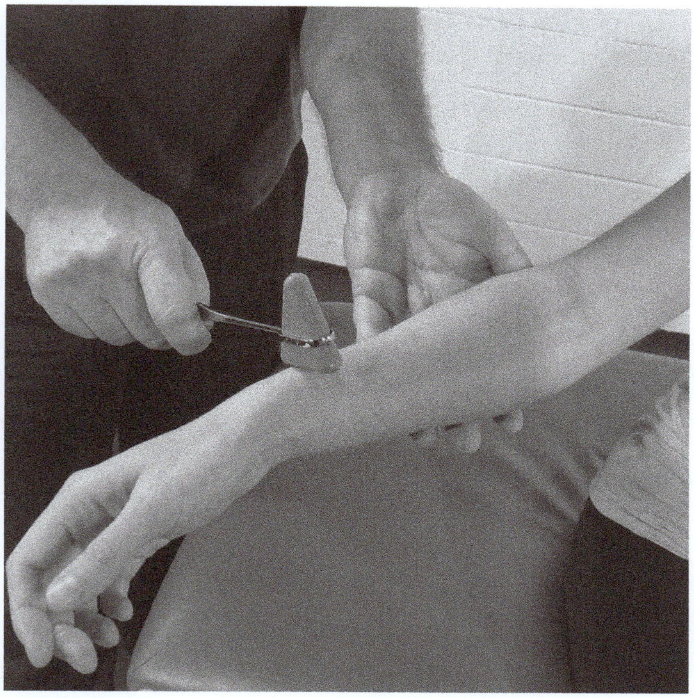

FIGURE 14.97 C5–6 DTR (over brachioradialis)

Hard to find and even harder to get a reliable response. Some health care professionals will lay their fingers over the site of the tendon and then strike their middle finger (at the middle phalange) to aid in getting a response. It is thought that this spreads the tap of the hammer over a wider area and there is an increased chance of hitting the appropriate site. Note that a positive sign of this test is observing flicking of the wrist (radial deviation), which occurs because of a slight but quick flexion of the elbow (i.e., the muscles quick active flexion of the forearm and then its sudden drop due to gravity).

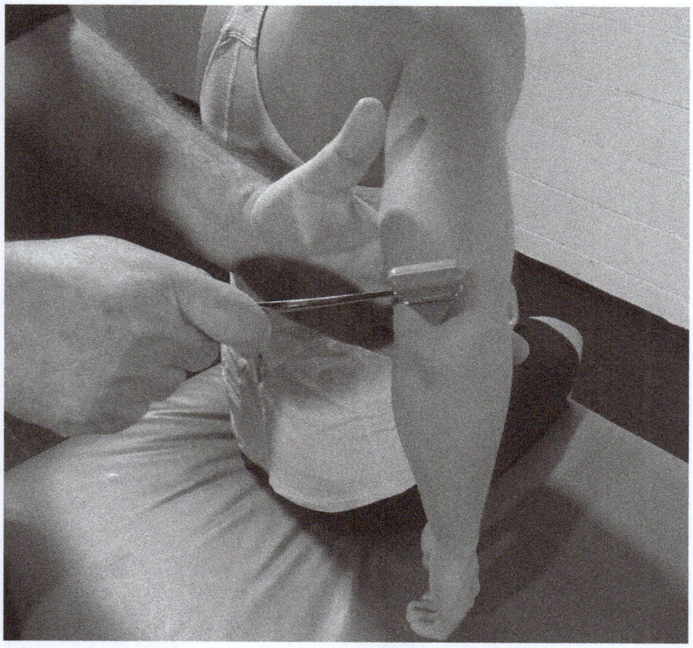

FIGURE 14.98 C7 DTR (triceps tendon in olecranon fossa)

The trick here is to get the patient to relax the arm enough to let you get a reflex.

To record your findings place the numerical equivalent over 5. Examples: 3/5 DTR R C6 equals a finding of number 3 grading on the right for the biceps tendon DTR; 0/5 DTR R C7 equals number 0 grade for the right triceps tendon reflex. These notations imply that the contralateral side is normal.

Responses 0 and 1 can be normal if bilateral (though a few do regard 0 as abnormal). They are usually only considered positive if seen unilaterally. 3 can be normal if bilateral. It may be abnormal if seen unilaterally if there is no reason for that side's muscle to be hypertonic (e.g., due to strain or overuse). 4 and 5 are considered positive. If bilateral there may be a systemic pathology or the presence of an upper motor neuron lesion (UMNL), i.e., a lesion in the central nervous system.

Pathological nerve impairment testing: upper motor neuron testing (Figures 14.99, 14.100)

Babinski's is the classic test for upper motor neuron dysfunction or pathology which means there is a lesion in the brain and/or in a neuron as it extends down into the spinal cord (specifically, the corticospinal tract). The sole of the foot is stroked with a fingernail or the pointed end of a reflex hammer. Start at the lateral side of the heel and run up the lateral side of the sole of the foot and across the metatarsal heads toward the big toe. A positive sign is that the big toe extends upward toward the head and the other toes splay (abduct). A negative sign (or normal response) is that the toes flex. This negative sign is only seen in those over two years of age. Babinski's sign is normal in newborns and disappears once the child learns to walk. After that it is a pathological reflex when present.

Spastic paralysis versus flaccid paralysis

Upper motor neuron lesions (UMNL) also present differently symptomatically. Initially, there is weakness or a loss of tone in the affected muscles (hypotonia) but the muscles will soon (in two or three weeks) develop resistance to passive movement (known as spastic paralysis) where the tissues will resist sudden passive movement of the applicable joint. This stage is accompanied by hyper-reflexia of DTR. This progression is highly distinctive for an UMNL.

In contrast a lower motor neuron lesion (LMNL) presents as weakness or even paralysis known as flaccid paralysis. This is accompanied by loss of DTR. The muscle often presents with distinctive tremors or fasciculation for two or three weeks after paralysis which then disappears. ***NOTE:*** If fasciculation begins again several weeks later this can imply that the nerve is regenerating.

There are a number of tests for UMNL but Babinski's test remains the most common and works well in providing a clear positive or negative sign.

Trigger point referral symptoms

Although there are many steps in doing a thorough neurological examination and this may not seem the time to mention any further complication of the issue we would be remiss if we did not mention at least one of the most common mimics of neurological symptoms: trigger point (TrP) referral.

TrP referral is not limited to pain. TrP referral can also manifest as weakness, tingling, or burning (i.e., paresthesia) as possible symptoms experienced by patients suffering from TrPs. By using charts that map TrPs and their common referral zones you can test (using appropriate palpation techniques) for the TrP that could be causing a referral into the area of the body that

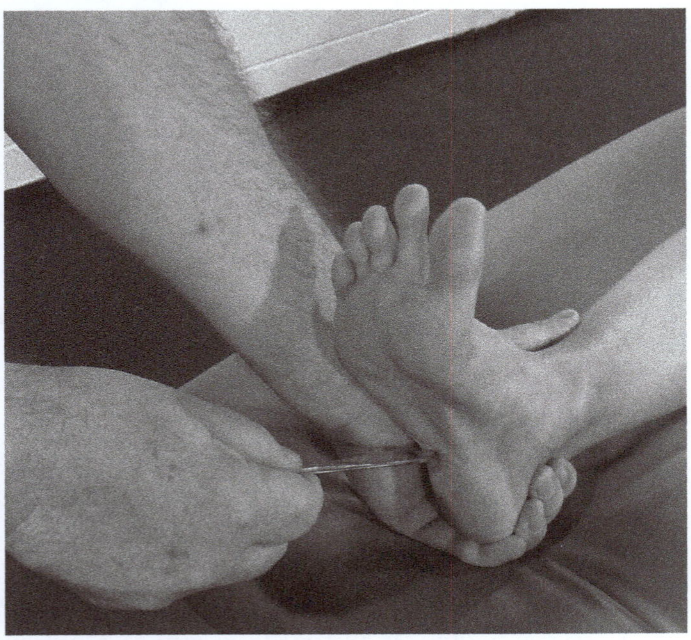

FIGURE 14.99

Babinski's sign or reflex (positive).

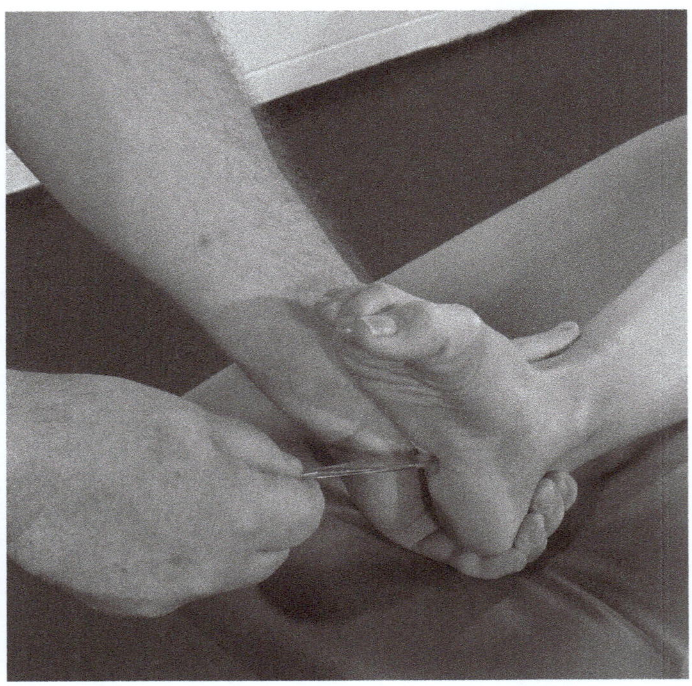

FIGURE 14.100

Babinski's sign or reflex (negative).

the patient describes they are experiencing their symptoms in. For a definition, signs of, and palpation techniques for TrPs see Chapter 4 (Travell et al. 1999).

Temporomandibular joint (TMJ) testing: an introduction

Review the anatomy and movements of the temporomandibular joint. Note how the masseter and the medial pterygoid create a sling to hold the mandible. This sling of muscles, ligaments and joint capsule is what holds the joint together. These muscles, along with the temporalis, work in concert to help close the jaw. See Box 14.8 for more on how these muscles function. When reviewing the anatomy of the TMJ pay close attention to the meniscal pad between the joint surfaces and the role it plays as the mandible slides forward when the jaw opens, and retracts as the jaw closes. Disruption of this disc's placement or degeneration through impairment to joint motion and function are the most common reasons for chronic TMJ problems. However, in turn, the most common source of this wear and tear on the disc is muscle imbalance or spasming.

Another principal cause of TMJ impairments is stretching or lesioning of the ligaments that guide movements in the joint and the displacement of the meniscus. Spasming of the pterygoid muscles can restrict motion by disrupting the unique biomechanics of this joint. Plus bruxism (grinding of the teeth) uses the lateral and medial pterygoids to grind back and forth, and side to side while the masseter and temporalis muscles hold the jaw closed.

Recent studies indicate that 30 percent or more of the superior lateral pterygoid muscle attaches to the meniscal pad (Okeson 1996). The rest of the superior pterygoid and all of the inferior lateral pterygoid attach to the neck of the condyle of the mandible. When the jaw opens and the lateral pterygoids draw the condyle (mandible) forward the fibers of the superior lateral pterygoid that attach to the meniscal pad help to draw the pad forward in concert with the condyle of the mandible. Thus, the pad stays between the condyle and the joint surface above on the temporal bone.

The lateral pterygoid works with the digastric muscle to open the mouth while the temporalis and masseter close the mouth. Acting together in bruxism puts all of these muscles at odds with each other and the hypertonicity created by bruxism further upsets the muscle balance required for a properly functioning jaw. Bruxism also needs the head to be stable and fixed which is why posterior cervical muscles are also usually involved and become hypertonic.

The masseter is the strongest muscle closing the jaw. It can refer pain into the side of the head but also note that it commonly refers into the ear. Many patients will arrive at your clinic complaining about ear infections (or just plugged ears) that their physicians cannot find any evidence of. Work the masseter and the pain in the ear disappears or becomes unplugged. The temporalis helps to both close and retract the jaw. It is notorious for creating headaches on its side of the head. The tendon itself can be particularly tender as it passes classic pain in the temple area.

Note that the temporalis is also susceptible to being set off as a satellite trigger point by an active trigger point in the upper trapezius muscle (Travell et al. 1999). Note also that as a person feels referred pain into the temporalis they will often tighten that temporalis which, in turn, now unbalances the tension in the musculature of the TMJ. This can lead to impairment of the TMJ.

Imbalance in the lateral pterygoids is one of the principal causes in TMJ dysfunction. This occurs because a spasming (or very hypertonic) pterygoid can lock the joint on that side in a forward (protruded) position even when the mouth is closed and the mandible should be retracted. Those superior lateral pterygoid fibers attached to the meniscal pad/disc will keep pulling this pad forward, resisting its retraction. This fixation in a forward position on one side will cause the ligaments that should be guiding and assisting in pulling and retracting the meniscus and mandible back into place to become stretched. Further, the temporalis will be trying to retract the mandible on that side, setting in motion a chronic strain on this muscle. If this imbalance continues for some time irreparable impairment to the ligaments and the meniscus will occur and adversely affect that temporomandibular joint's ability to function correctly.

INSIGHTS

Box 14.8 Chewing: more than just opening and closing the jaw (Kapandji 2008; Levangie & Norkin 2011)

The action of chewing food is not as simple as opening and closing the jaw. Grinding of food requires translatory (side-to-side and front-to-back) motions as well.

The action of chewing is one of the principal reasons that the jaw protracts on opening and retracts on closing. This is the anterior-posterior translation of the mandible (on the stable maxilla). This action assists in the bolus (the bite of food being masticated/chewed) being drawn into the mouth and onto the tongue, which carries the bolus back near the molars.

The jaw is drawn forward, or protruded, by both lateral pterygoids while the digastric muscle opens the mouth. In closing the mouth, the anterior and superior portion of the temporalis helps to pull the mandible up, assisting the masseter, while the inferior and posterior portion of the temporalis also draws the mandible back (retracts it). All of this combines to create an elliptical rotary motion in the sagittal plane: an opening and translating forward and then closing and translating posteriorly.

The mandible also translates from side to side. For example, while the right masseter and temporalis is contracting fully on the right, the left medial pterygoid contracts and so pulls the mandible off to the left, i.e., translates it left. Yes, there is some contraction in the left masseter and temporalis, but very much less than on the right side. Again, opening and closing in conjunction with translation left results in an overall elliptical and rotary motion but in a mix of the transverse and coronal planes. The jaw will usually repeat this action on one side three times (on average). Then, there is a reflex alteration to the opposite side. Now, the left masseter and temporalis maximally contract in combination, with the right medial pterygoid translating the mandible right. Again, this pattern happens three times.

The jaw will continue in this alternating pattern until the person swallows. It all starts over with the next bite. Also, the tongue will move the bolus from one side to the other side as the jaw alternates this lateral translatory action.

The buccinator muscle (in the cheek) will relax when the bolus is initially coming to that side, creating a pouch in which the food sits. This buccinator begins to tighten, pushing some of the bolus under the molars while the maximally contracting temporalis and masseter grind down onto this portion of the bolus. Meanwhile the contralateral medial pterygoid pulls the mandible toward it. This adds a translatory grinding motion to the mandible's molars, away from the side grinding the food. This translatory motion will assist in moving that ground food (a portion of the bolus) onto the tongue as the jaw closes.

The buccinator continues to tighten in order to help shove more of the bolus between the molars (as the jaw opens for another chew). As the buccinator continues to shorten and the tissues of the cheek press the food toward the molars it is also assisting in moving the food onto the tongue. Thus, it prevents the already ground food from coming back to that side. This growing tension in the buccinator in turn tightens the tissues of the cheek so that it does not itself get drawn under those molars as the food shifts over. In other words, the buccinator keeps the food moving over to get ground between the molars while it prevents us from biting the inside of our cheek as we eat (most of the time, anyway).

One dramatic example of all of this going awry is when someone has a stroke and one side of the face is paralyzed. The buccinator (and other musculature) does not function correctly, and the person will consistently bite the inside of their cheek and tongue on that side.

Assessing the TMJ (Figures 14.101–14.106)

Assessing the TMJ can be extensive and detailed. However, we are going to present only a brief testing protocol here. If impairments are found the therapist needs to use their clinical judgment as to whether they have sufficient training to treat. Massage therapists can receive specific training in assessment and treatment of TMJ impairments, usually as graduates.

If you believe your training to date on this specific topic is insufficient then refer out. If treating you should advise the patient to inform other health practitioners that they may have TMJ issues. Within the medical community TMJ requires a diagnosis and for most jurisdictions massage therapists are not considered as a diagnosing profession (by legislation). Therefore, be clear with the patient that though this is your assessment they should receive a diagnosis from a physician, dentist, or (where applicable) a physiotherapist.

When assessing the TMJ a therapist should place two fingers (index and middle) directly in front of the ear just below the cheekbone. This placement will put your finger pads over the joints. Palpate for crepitus, sudden movements (jumping, popping, clunking, or grinding). While observing motions of the jaw note if the mandible moves off to one side or appears restricted in its motion. One of the most important impairments to notice is when and where the first restriction of movement is.

A pause (just prior to a click, or jumping motion) on one side when the jaw is opening tells us which side is principally restricted. The patient may present with pain on either or both sides, however. The restricted side may be painful because of the spasming muscles involved or damage to the TMJ on that side. Yet, the other side may be painful because it has been used the most; doing the most work when chewing, for example.

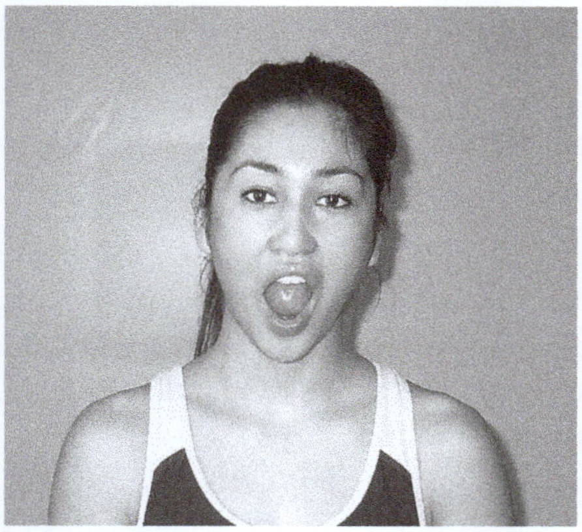

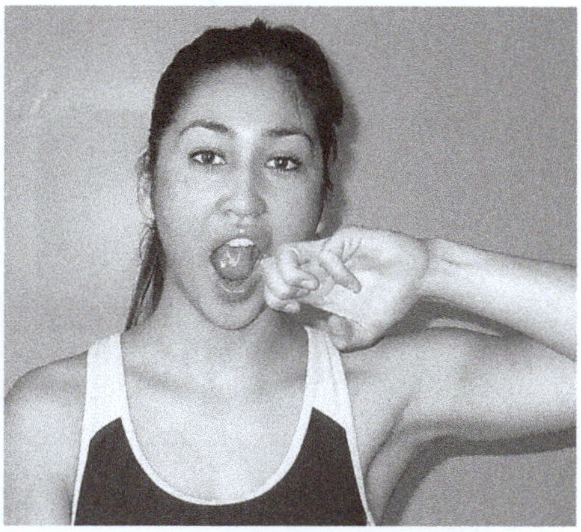

FIGURE 14.101 Active TMJ depression

Observing and palpating the motion of the jaw. See if the patient can open the jaw enough to equal three of their finger widths.

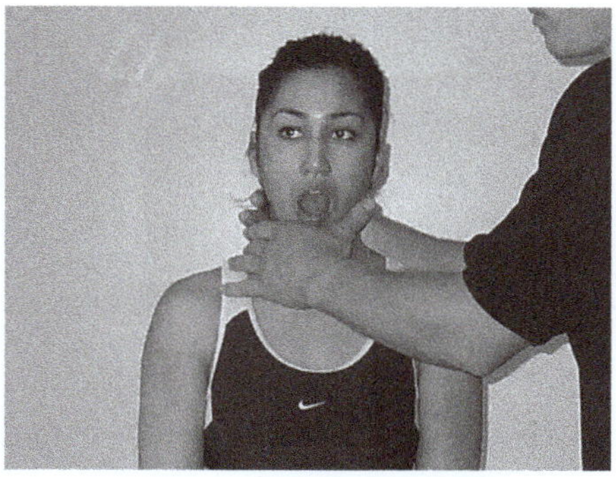

FIGURE 14.102 TMJ depression with O-P

If there is no pain from AF-ROM hold the mandible with the web space of the hand. Press down gently for O-P.

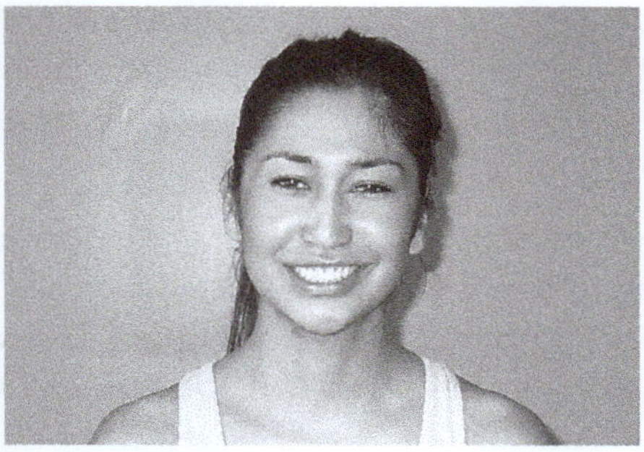

FIGURE 14.103 Active elevation (closing mouth)

Have the patient close the mouth and then clench the teeth for O-P. Clenching clearly reveals not only joint problems but also displays muscular problems.

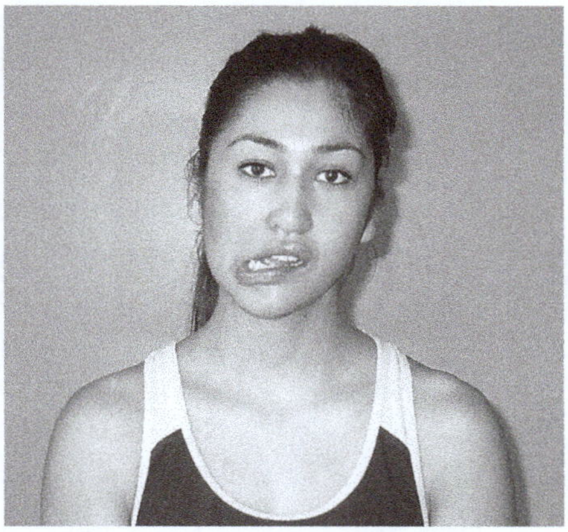

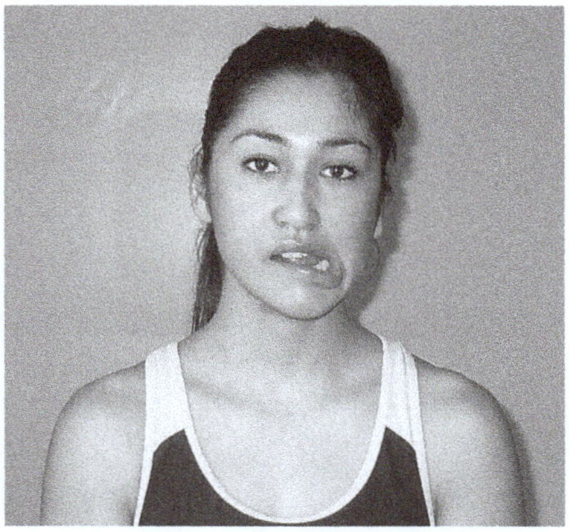

FIGURES 14.104, 14.105 Active lateral excursions right and left

Have the patient shift the mandible right and then left.

If there is impairment at the TMJ, sometimes the mandible may shift with one smooth arc but usually it does so suddenly. It may jump or shift with or without crepitus. The jaw can shift to one side then back to the center, or over to the other side. Or it may shift or jump over to one side several times as it depresses. To test the TMJ have the patient do the following actions slowly; if they are pain-free then gentle O-P may be used with caution. Though not shown here the therapist should palpate lightly over the TMJ, which is just in front of the ear lobe. ***NOTE:*** The O-P applied is *not meant to move* the jaw further in any direction as much as it is to slightly increase the tension within the involved tissues.

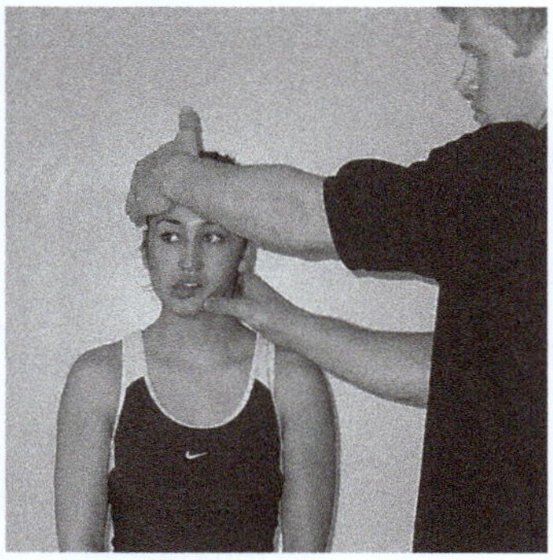

FIGURE 14.106 Excursion with O-P

When the patient reaches the end-range of excursion without pain, have them relax. Gently apply PR-ROM back to end-range and add very gentle O-P.

Box 14.9 Treatment tips

The therapist can use excursion to perform a post-isometric stretch (PIR) to the lateral pterygoid. For the mandible to go to the left, for example, the right lateral pterygoid has to relax and stretch.

- Have the patient go to end-range excursion to the left (AF-ROM). The therapist stabilizes the mandible on the right side and asks the patient to relax, while not letting the mandible move back to the right.
- While resisting on the right side instruct the patient to gently try to bring the mandible back to neutral (i.e., move it to the right). Do not let the mandible move. Less pressure is needed to resist than you might think.
- After 3–5 seconds ask the patient to stop trying and relax. Only after you feel the muscles relax, gently take the mandible more to the left, stretching the right pterygoid. Repeat two or three times. Make sure the patient understands that they are to tell you if any pain arises, and, if it does, stop the stretching.

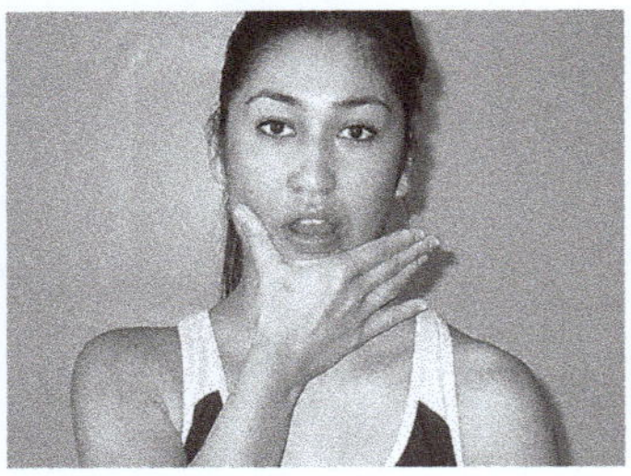

FIGURE 14.107 1. Sensory feedback

Have the patient place the hand around the chin.

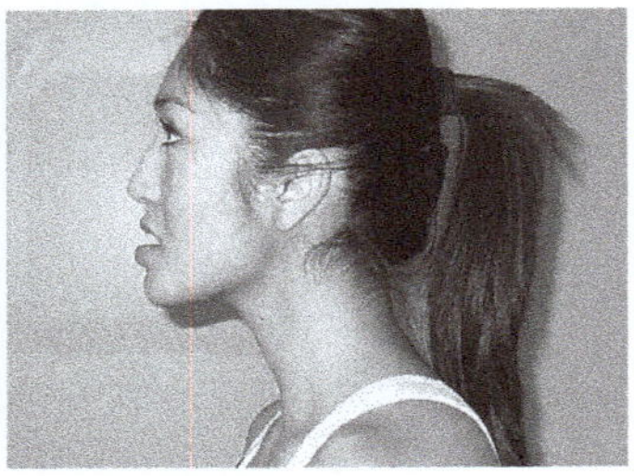

FIGURE 14.108 2. Active protrusion

The patient protrudes the jaw.

Box 14.9 lists some treatment tips for stretching the lateral pterygoid.

Active protrusion and retrusion (retraction) (Figures 14.107–14.111)

It often helps the patient if they place the web space of the thumb and index finger on the chin and "feel" the jaw while they are protruding and retracting. Note: The patient is not to push the jaw backward or try to grasp the mandible and pull it forward. The hand is there for sensory feedback purposes.

PR-ROM and joint mobilization for TMJ (Figures 14.112–14.115)

Therapists need to have good palpatory skills to be able to sense tension in the joint and musculature. It is very important to have a signal for the patient to let you know about pain, apprehension, or for that matter, to just stop the testing (withdrawal of consent). The best is to have the supine patient place one hand on their abdomen and when they wish to signal you they simply lift their hand off by extending at the wrist or lifting the hand and forearm as a whole up off their body.

Also, the patient needs to relax the jaw as best they can so that you can move it passively. This very hard for patients to do even for those who have no TMJ impairments. You will find that when you change to the next PR-ROM the patient will have to be reminded to let go and let you move the jaw. Be prepared to keep asking the patient to let go and try not to get frustrated at having to continually ask this of them. Ask the patient to separate the teeth slightly.

Use a light touch and do not force any movement. Broad contact is best. Therefore, do not just use the finger pads but as much of the dorsal side of the finger surface as possible. Mostly, the index and middle fingers are in contact with the mandible. Palpate for crepitus, jumps, shifts, clicks, etc. Some therapists use the palm of their hands but be careful not to over-compress into the mandible.

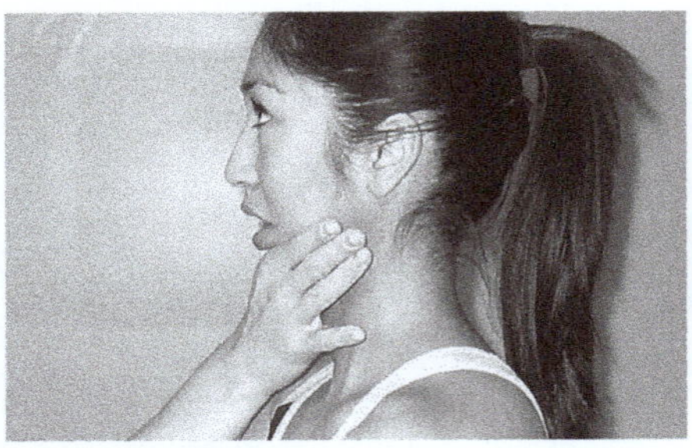

FIGURE 14.109 3. Active retrusion

The patient retracts the jaw.

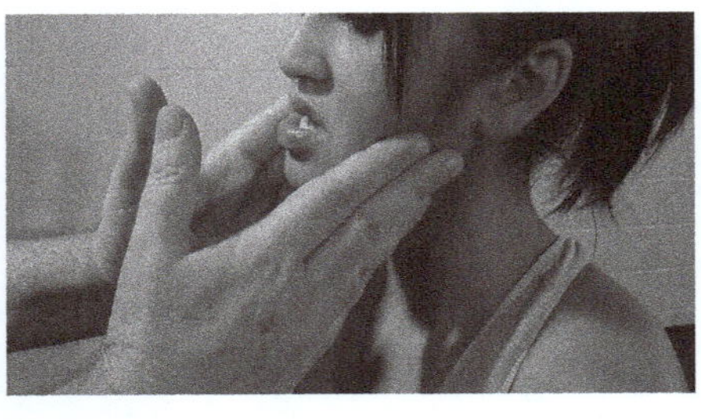

FIGURE 14.110 O-P protrusion

Place the fingers of both hands along the sides of the mandible and draw forward.

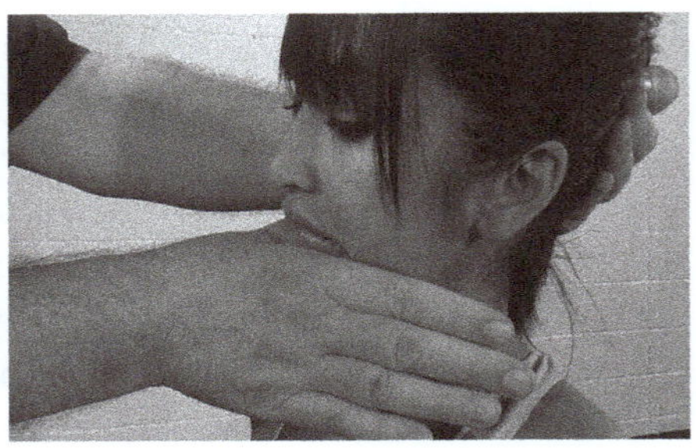

FIGURE 14.111 O-P retraction

Gently apply O-P to the retracted jaw.

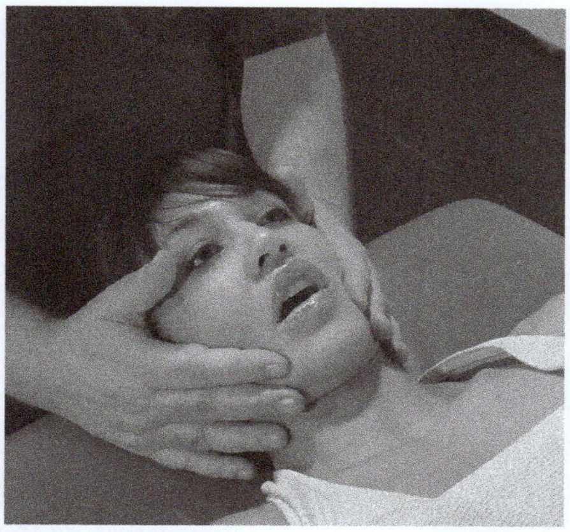

FIGURE 14.112 PR-ROM TMJ depression

With your finger pads near the chin, gently draw the mandible forward and down taking the jaw into depression. If pain-free, apply gentle O-P.

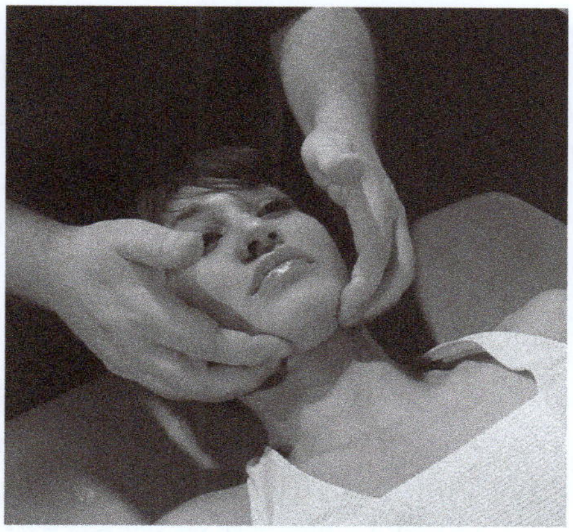

FIGURE 14.113 PR-ROM TMJ elevation

Rotate the fingers so the lowest is on the posterolateral edge of the mandible. Draw up gently. If pain-free, use very mild O-P.

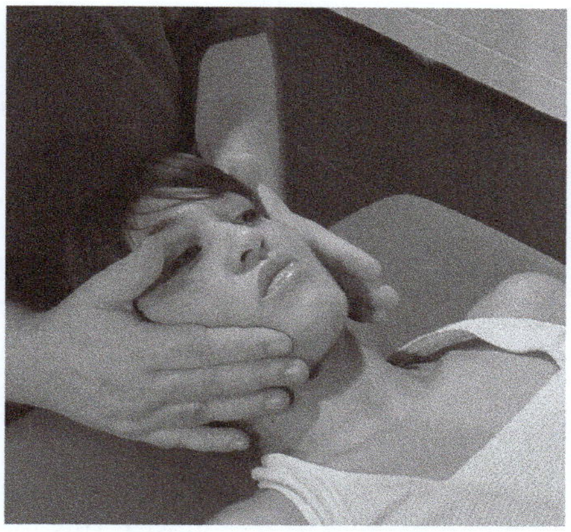

FIGURE 14.114 PR-ROM TMJ excursions

With the finger pads near the chin apply pressure to one side in order to slide the mandible in that direction. Then gently apply O-P if appropriate. Repeat to other side.

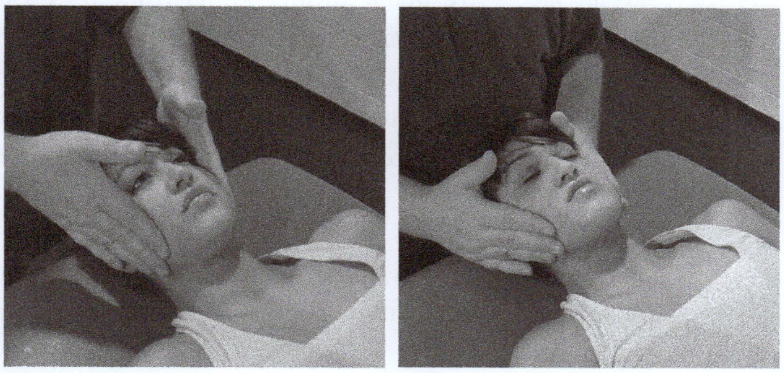

FIGURE 14.115A, B PR-ROM TMJ protraction

Slide (without pressure) finger pads back to the angle of the jaw as you turn your hands vertically (45°). Re-apply contact for movement. With a scooping motion, push down gently (tractioning the joint inferiorly) while moving the mandible forward into protrusion. The fingers may glide a little on the skin as you press into protrusion. Apply gentle O-P.

The patient is supine for all of the PR-ROM testing. In all movements, even with elevation, always begin with gently drawing the mandible inferiorly, i.e., very slightly tractioning the TMJ inferiorly. This disengages the joint and helps relax the musculature.

Box 14.10 looks at the TMJ and cranial osteopathy.

Box 14.10 TMJ and cranial osteopathy

PR-ROM protraction, if sustained, will decompress the TMJs (temporomandibular joints). It will also apply a gentle stretch to the temporalis, masseter, and medial pterygoid muscles.

Within cranial osteopathic manipulation, the connection between the TMJ and the sphenoid is considered quite important. One of the most important connections is that the lateral pterygoids attach onto the sphenoid bone. It is believed that TMJ impairments will impair the cranial motions of the sphenoid, which is considered the most important cranial bone. The sphenoid is considered the principal axis for all movements of the cranial bowl as it contacts all of the bones that make up the cranium.

The bulk of the medial pterygoid also attaches to the sphenoid (and some on the maxilla). The masseter attaches onto the zygomatic arch, consisting of the zygomatic temporal bone. The temporalis also attaches to the temporal fossa on the temporal bone. The suprahyoid also attaches to the temporal bone via the mastoid process. Therefore, treatment of TMJ impairments is considered an important component of cranial osteopathic manual practice (Upledger & Vredevoogd 1992).

Motion palpation of the lower cervical spine

We will now resume instruction in motion palpation and focus on facet joint lesions in the lower cervical spine (C2–T1).

The purpose of motion palpation of the spine is not just to locate areas of pain or impairment but more importantly to help us understand exactly what the problem or restriction of motion is due to. Is the facet joint impairment due to the facet joint being held closed/extended? On the other hand, is it due to a joint being held open/flexed? Is it impairment at just one segment, several separate segments, or is it impairment of a group of vertebrae, a scoliosis? This form of testing is done by observation and motion palpation (Chila 2010; DeStefano 2011; Mitchell 2005).

Classic orthopedic testing of the cervical spine may at times help to locate where joint dysfunctions are but they do not help us to understand the nature of the impairment, as motion palpation can.

This portion of the chapter is intended to be a mixture of lecture and practice experiments that require you to take the time to absorb the information slowly. You should only proceed as each paragraph is understood and only as each practice or palpatory exercise has been done. I assure you that the knowledge you will gain, both factual and experiential, will be of great benefit to you as a therapist and to your patients' well-being.

Palpating the cervical spine while it is moved either actively or passively through various ranges and actions affords much more information about how the spine is functioning mechanically than by just observing active free range of motions. In its most simple form, motion palpation of the cervical spine is the art of looking for asymmetry of motion as the cervical spine is passively moved through its anatomical ranges while your fingertips palpate structures and tissues of the cervical spine at various levels. It is more than just holding the head and performing passive relaxed motion to the spine. Motion testing helps us to see both how the individual structures of the spine are working separately and how they are working together as a whole. We are looking for:

- symmetry/asymmetry in vertebral alignment, both static and in motion
- restriction of motion, or even hypermobility
- tenderness or any reproduction of the patient's complaints or impairments.

In the lower cervical spine we do this by noting whether the TVPs appear to be more prominent on one side of the spine than the other. If a group of vertebrae is rotated to one side, the TVPs moving posteriorly lift the tissue above them, giving the appearance of more bulk to the tissue on that side of the spine.

We may note a group of TVPs on one side and should see some side-bending (scoliosis) toward the opposite side of the prominent TVPs, or we may note a single prominent TVP.

We can look at the spine standing, seated or prone.

It is certainly true that impairments to movement in the lower cervical spine can be seen and palpated during AF-ROM. However, the nature of such lesions is often unclear unless the therapist has first gained experience in accurately assessing the types of impairments that can occur. Therefore, though the following method of assessing the lower cervical spine may take some time to master, it is the most reliable testing for this area of the cervical spine. With time, the therapist can refine and simplify their testing. ***NOTE:*** Overall, you can assume that the term cervical spine used in the section below refers to the lower cervical spine.

Joint mobilizations (Figures 14.116–14.118)

As the cervical facets are plane-gliding joints (roughly on a 35–45° angle with the anterior portion higher) they are able to slide (glide) side to side or as it is sometimes put, they have the ability to *translate*. This lateral glide along with rotation is required for side-bending to occur. They also have the ability to:

- glide anterior-superiorly (as in flexion, opening of the joints)
- glide posterior-inferiorly (as in extension or closing the joint when its surfaces are approximating and taking on more mechanical stress)
- rotate on each other, each moving in different directions.

When all of these movements are combined they provide great ROM to the cervical spine.

As with almost all joints of the body, movement in one direction *within the joint* is going to limit the motion available in other directions. Joint capsule (shapes), ligaments, and muscles are all involved in guiding joint motion. When combinations (or types) of motion in different directions happen *within* a joint these tissues also come into play to reduce any secondary or tertiary motions taking place, and will even take back, or retract, some of the initial motion. Therefore, only movement done in one specific single direction or anatomical plane of motion can have its greatest range available.

Investigation by joint mobilizations for the play (free motion) available within a joint is done by inducing glide *in a specific direction* through the joint. We test glide by using or performing a *translatory* motion through each motion segment (i.e., between two adjacent vertebrae) after we have disengaged the joint (applied a slight traction to gap the joint surfaces slightly). This slight gapping is meant to counteract any compressive forces between the joint surfaces that may limit motion. Further gapping which is also known as *distraction* or disengagement, tends to reflexively relax the musculature somewhat. We can translate through the facet joints because the intervertebral discs between C2 and T1 as polyaxial joints allow this movement by being able to accept a small amount of shearing motion.

When doing lateral translation we start at the T1–C7 level. Have the fingers at the level of C7's TVPs but in the lamina groove on either side. The ends of the TVPs are generally too sensitive an area to hold. On the other hand, pushing on the spinous processes can also feel tender or painful to the patient, but more than that, you will more likely induce rotation than translation.

Positioning for lateral glide

To begin palpating lateral glide of the lower spine start with the heels of the hands supporting the occiput and the fingertips in the lamina groove at C7. Translate (slide) the head and the whole cervical spine down to C7 from side to side, as if it is one fixed structure. Holding all of the cervical segments fixed and moving over T1 places the movement specifically between C7 and T1's facet joints. We translate left and right noting any restriction or asymmetry in motion.

The motion available is not only palpable but is usually also visible. We can measure it by eye by looking at the amount of movement the chin undergoes as it moves left and right during our translating of the patient's cervical spine. The mid-line used to measure from is provided by the sternum or more precisely the sternal notch. Motion side to side should appear symmetrical.

A line running between the patient's eyes through the nose and the chin should be seen to move perpendicular, shifting slightly to the left and to the right of the sternal notch.

Restrictions are seen when the chin moves less to one side than the other, producing asymmetry of motion. Restrictions are felt by the palpating hands, often as if the vertebra is tethered (as with a rope) and when it tries to go in one direction it stops short. It has a firm end-range feel. Make sure that you are moving the whole head laterally and are not actually side-bending the head. In other words, make sure that the head remains perpendicular. Think of the head as always remaining at 90° to a straight line running from one shoulder to the other. Further, when supporting the head you are negating gravity, there is just enough support (lift) so that the head *floats*.

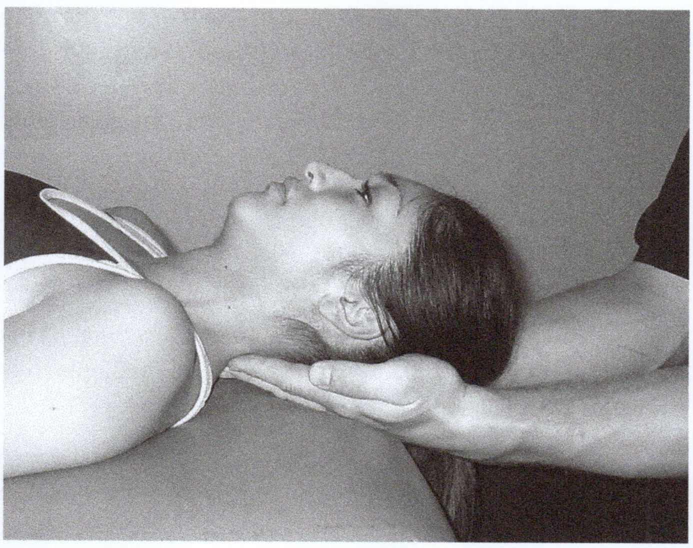

FIGURE 14.116 Starting position for lateral glide

The head is supported by the therapist's thenar eminences with the fingers supporting and palpating within the lamina groove.

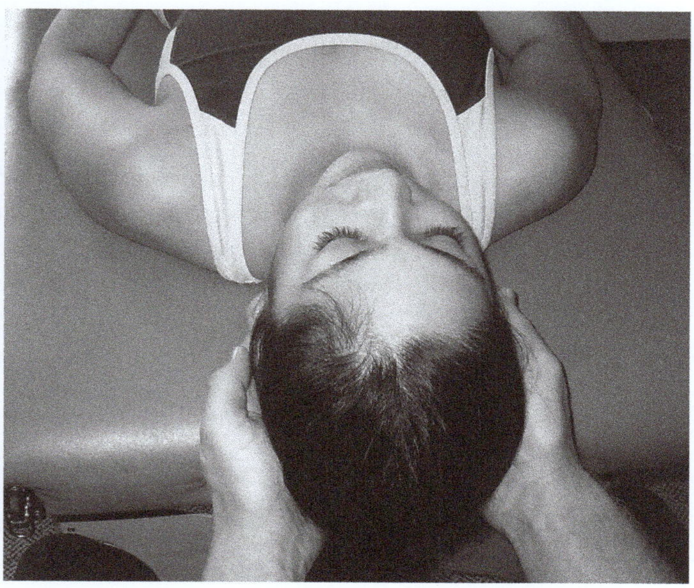

FIGURE 14.117 Cervical spine neutral

Holding the spine in neutral.

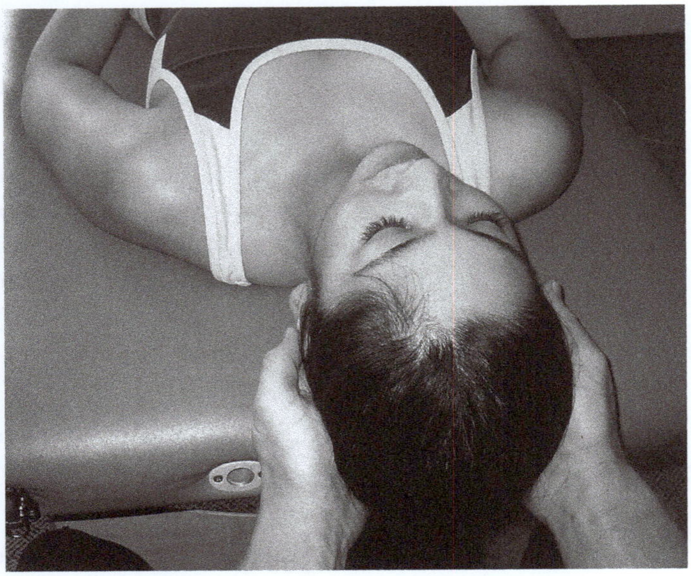

FIGURE 14.118A Lateral translation right

Translate the lower cervical spine to the right, which tests side-bending left.

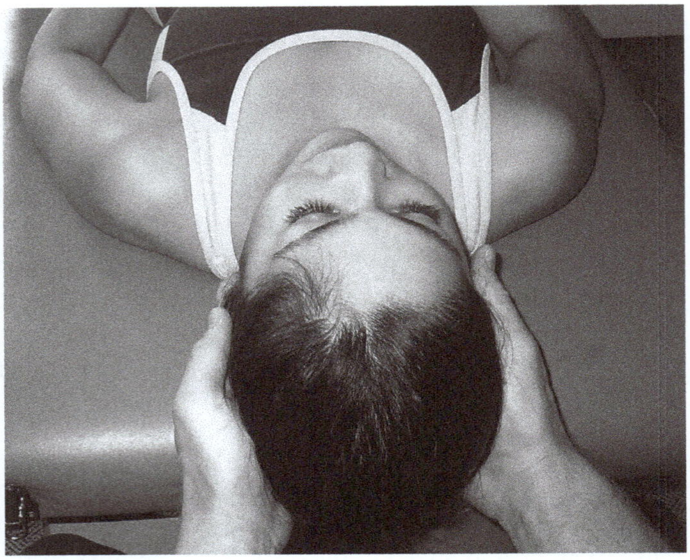

FIGURE 14.118B Lateral translation left

Final step in testing of motion segment, translate left, testing side-bending right.

Now, move up one level with the fingertips in the lamina groove adjacent the TVPs of C 6. Translate through the facet joints of C6 and C7. Continue to work your way all the way up testing all the segmental levels up to C2–3.

We may find restriction at only one level or at several levels. Up until this point we have tested for restrictions in neutral. If any restrictions are found then we will next test the lower cervical spine held in flexion and in extension.

The positive sign in motion testing is the observation of asymmetry of motion as is noted by the motion of the chin *and* by the palpation of ease of motion or a sense of bind, a sense that motion is blocked. Hence, for the lower cervical spine we will be looking for motion asymmetry at each segmental level as we translate each level from one side to the other. However, it is possible that the patient could experience pain during such passive motion testing but that is not a positive sign for impaired motion in a motion segment. Asymmetry of movement side to side is the key positive sign in any motion palpation. In fact, if the patient experiences pain during translatory motion it would be wise to stop this form of motion testing. You may be using too much force for what should be a very gentle movement. Some reasons for the patient to experience pain when you have your fingers in the lamina groove is that the joint capsule is inflamed and swollen or muscular tissue under your fingers is inflamed and sensitized.

If the patient is willing and able then use other special tests (discussed earlier in this chapter) to investigate further. However, when the technique is done properly as a gentle form of testing, then any occurrence of pain speaks to an acute situation. Moreover, in the worst case scenario, pain may indicate an unstable segment (for example, ligamentous and/or joint capsule tearing). This may be extremely painful and is often accompanied by muscle spasming (which will prevent any translatory motions). If there are multidermatomal neurological symptoms and possibly autonomic signs refer out as a possible emergency.

What type of restrictions are we finding by this lateral glide?

We use lateral glides or translations to test not just for glide but also for the ability of the facet joints at one level (or motion segment) to flex and extend.

For the vertebrae (of the lower cervical spine) to side-bend to one side (for example, to the left) the upper vertebra of a motion segment slides/glides away slightly from the side to which it bends (i.e., *slides right and tilts left*). As the superior vertebra slides slightly to the right, the left side of the disc can slightly compress, which pushes the nucleus pulposus (which cannot be compressed) toward the right. This shift increases the height in the right side of the disc. Thus, the top vertebra in the motion segment tilts to the left. Therefore, side-bending of the cervical spine requires the facet joints to be able to flex (open) extend (close) *and* for one vertebra to laterally glide/translate over another (Kapandji 2008). This is called *coupled motion*. In other words, side-bending in the cervical spine is a coordinated set of movements in several planes of motion. In fact, some rotation must happen as well within motion segments. Consequently, rotation is also tested to some degree. (This is discussed more below.)

It is suggested that before you proceed you look at Box 14.11.

The ability of the vertebrae *to translate* to the right is an *intrinsic joint motion within the motion segment* that is required for the facet joints of the vertebrae to be able to side-bend to the left. And further, for side-bending left to occur the right facet must open and the left must close. Therefore, when we are investigating or testing the lower cervical spine and we find a restriction in one direction what we are feeling is result of either:

- one side of a motion segment's facet joint being held open (flexed) and it will not close, or
- the other side being held closed (extended) and so will not open.

Side-bending and rotation are coupled motions in the spine and they usually occur to the same side in the lower cervical spine (Cook 2007; Hertling & Kessler 2006; Kapandji 2008; Mitchell 2005) and a finding of loss of side-bending implies a loss of rotation. As side-bending requires facets to open (flex) and close (extend) we are also testing flexion and extension abilities. Thus, *lateral translation testing of the lower cervical spine tests all the motions available to the facet joints*. However, when translating in neutral we cannot yet tell which motion is being restricted. We only know that there is a restriction to motion at that level. We need to now repeat these lateral translations with the lower cervical spine held slightly flexed, and then slightly extended, in order to be able to tell which facet joint (of the two) is restricted in opening or in closing in any motion segment (which is two vertebrae and the joints between these two).

Box 14.11 A motion palpation experiment

Before proceeding, I encourage you to do the following motion palpation experiment. Note that when you side-bend your head to the left, your chin tends to go off to the right, and when you side-bend right, your chin goes off to the left. Now, place the index finger of each hand on the side of your neck. Imagine that your left index finger is pushing to the right when you side-bend left (and your chin goes right). When you side-bend right (chin left), it is as if you were pushing (translating) the spine to the left. Keep this simple observation in mind as you read on.

INSIGHTS

Box 14.12 Further comments on translation movements

When first learning to do side-to-side translations, it is best to translate to either side as far as is possible in a pain-free manner until reaching end-range. At the lowest level (C7–T1), there should be only a slight side-to-side movement, equal to each side. T1 and below restrict the mobility of these lower segments because of the connection they have to the ribs. We are, however, moving the thoracic segments slightly.

As the therapist moves up the cervical spine, testing segment by segment, the movement to either side will become greater. The reason for this is that there are now a number of the lower cervicals moving below the segment you are holding. We start at the lowest level of the cervical spine precisely because the segmental levels below that will move when testing a specific motion segment, and we are not testing these thoracic segments here. Once the lowest segment of the cervical spine has been tested and results noted, then we proceed on up the spine. Nevertheless, try not to move with so much force that motion travels excessively down into the thoracic spine.

With practice, the therapist will be able to see and feel restrictions with quite small movements in translation. Eventually a very short translation within the play of the joints is available and this will become clearly palpable without grossly moving the joints below that segment. At this level of expertise the motion of the chin (and head) is almost imperceptible to any third person watching the testing. By this time your testing will in fact increase in accuracy as you avoid involving other tissues in a motion that should be as specific as possible to just the joints at the level of the spine you are testing.

Further comments on translation movements can be found in Box 14.12.

Discovering which side is impaired

Now that we understand how side-bending and translation left and right are related and that translation requires flexion and extension for it to occur we need to go a step further. With the testing done in neutral (spine neither flexed nor extended), we are able to tell that we have restriction to lateral translation to the left, for example, thus side side-bending is restricted to the right. However, what we do not know is which facet

TABLE 14.3
Summary of findings while testing in neutral

Position of spine:	Direction of translation	Side-bending to the:	If restricted, lesion is:	Side of lesion
Neutral	To the right	Left	Unknown	Unknown
Neutral	To the left	Right	Unknown	Unknown

has the problem, the left or the right. Right side-bending, for example, is restricted by either the left facet not opening (fixed in extension) or the right facet not closing (fixed in flexion). How do we sort this out? How do we discover which side is impaired?

Table 14.3 presents a summary of findings while testing in neutral.

Restrictions seen while translating in flexion: searching for extension lesions (Figure 14.119)

When we test using translation while holding the cervical spine in flexion, we will be looking to see if a facet will not close or extend. We flex the neck a little more than half-way toward full flexion and we then translate left and right. We do not fully flex the neck, otherwise we would not have enough slack left in the joint capsule to be able to move laterally (due to the stretched joint capsules restricting movement). Therefore, with the neck in some flexion but not full flexion we can still get the vertebrae to translate.

Both facets are slightly opened/flexed at the level we are testing. What is going to be most restrictive to lateral motion (side-bending) in this situation is if a facet will not close or extend. In fact, the restricting facet that is closed/extended will often exaggerate the asymmetry that was seen testing in neutral when we translated side to side. The positive sign of an impairment of a facet to extend or to close is increased asymmetry in lateral translation when the spine is held in flexion. Therefore, we will see that the chin moves less in one direction and we feel a firm *bind* or block to further movement laterally at that level.

If, for example, translation is done while the neck is flexed and we find even greater restriction when we try to translate left then the dysfunction is on the left side: C6–7's facet on the left is fixed closed (is in extension). It will not open/flex to allow side-bending to the right.

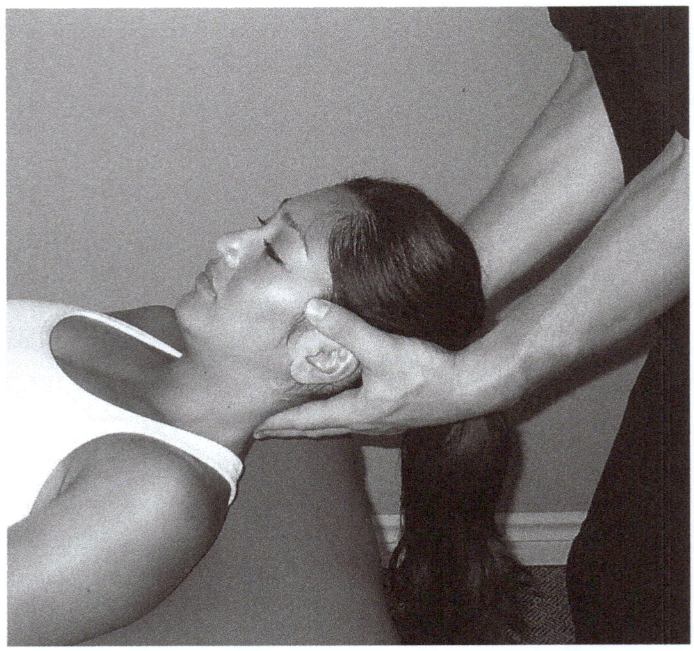

FIGURE 14.119 Testing in flexion
Hold the head with the finger pads on C7. The cervical spine is slightly flexed. Translate left and right.

Conclusions

We can conclude that, as a rule, when we find a restriction in translating while holding the cervical spine in flexion, such restriction:

1. reveals extension lesions (facets held closed/extended), and
2. the dysfunction is on the same side as the side the segment is being translated toward.

Findings for impaired flexion are summarized in Table 14.4.

TABLE 14.4
Summary of findings for impaired flexion

Position of spine:	Direction of translation	Side-bending to the:	If restricted, facet is:	Side of lesion
Flexed	Left	Right	Extended	On the left
Flexed	Right	Left	Extended	On the right

INSIGHTS

Box 14.13 Don't make assumptions

While some restriction may have been noticed when translation was done in neutral, a "negative sign" (no restriction seen) may happen when then translating in flexion or in extension (in one or the other).

For example: if a facet that was held flexed or open was the cause of restriction seen in neutral, that restriction will decrease or even disappear when translation is done in flexion – we may see more symmetry, not less! Remember, we will find extension lesions when testing in flexion. Also, if a left facet is stuck open (is flexed) then when translating right while the spine is in flexion we may find some slight restriction in that direction because the left side will not close. However, we do not necessarily get a clear enough lack of motion to know for sure what the restriction is. After all, the facets remain open to some degree as we translate while holding the spine in flexion. However, when we translate in extension then the nature of the restriction will be more clear.

Of course, it may be true that while doing the testing above with the neck in flexion one side of a segment may be stuck flexed. But that will not show (or impact on the test) when testing the neck in flexion. Testing in flexion only reveals problems if a facet stays extended.

Box 14.13 warns against making assumptions.

Restrictions seen while translating in extension: searching for flexion lesions (Figure 14.120)

Let use an example where we have a restriction when translating left while testing in neutral.

However, let us say that while testing in flexion the translation left becomes less affected than it was than when done in neutral and so movement left and right appears more symmetrical.

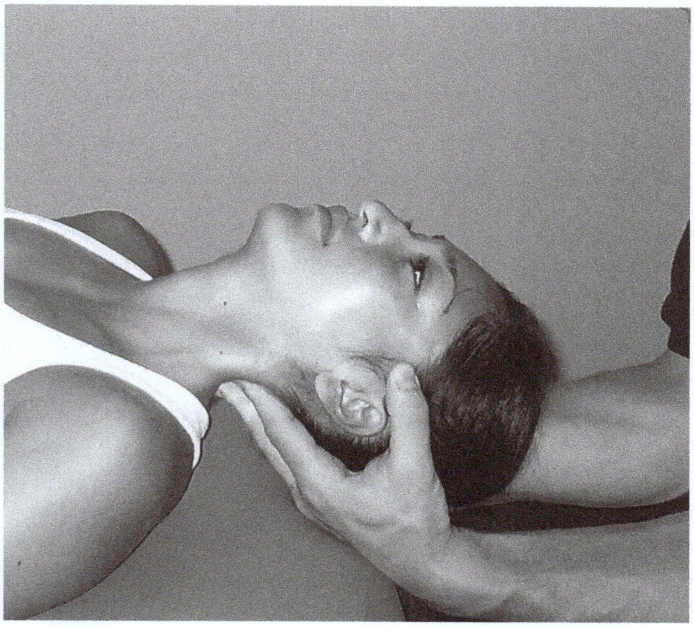

FIGURE 14.120 Testing lateral translations in extension
Lift the patient's neck into hyperextension. This is safer for the patient and easier for them to relax than having their head off the table. Stabilize with finger pads the superior vertebra of a motion segment. Translate left and right looking for symmetry.

We get a negative finding when testing in flexion. This implies that the left facet will open.

Therefore, we will then proceed to test lateral translation while the neck is in extension.

When translating in extension we are investigating whether the facets will, or will not go into extension (close or not close). If it will not extend it must be that a facet joint is being held in flexion.

EXAMPLE: When translating at the C6–7 level while the neck is extended a limitation in translation is found when going to the

TABLE 14.5
Summary of findings for impaired extension

Position of spine:	Direction of translation	Side-bending to the:	If restricted, facet is:	Side of lesion
Extended	To the left	Right	Flexed	On the right
Extended	To the right	Left	Flexed	On the left

When the cervical spine is tested while in extension, the flexion impairment is on the opposite side to the side the segment is being translated toward.

left (while free when going to the right). We may now even see *more asymmetry* than was seen in neutral translation.

Remember that translation to the left requires the facet on the right to close (as the segment is side-bending right).

Therefore, the dysfunction is due to a facet that will not close: the facet on the right side of that spinal motion segment is being held flexed/open (and will not extend or close).

We can conclude that when we find a restriction during translation of the cervical spine that is in extension there are flexion lesions present (facets that are held open/flexed) and the dysfunction is on the opposite side to that which the motion segment is being translated toward.

Table 14.5 summarizes findings for impaired extension, Box 14.14 describes another way of expressing the rules for flexion/extension lesions during translations, and Box 14.15 summarizes what we may have observed in cervical AF-ROM.

Group dysfunctions

Assessing a rotoscoliosis These are group dysfunctions where three or more vertebrae are all held side-bent and, hence, rotated to one side or the other.

We will assess as above. However, we will find two or more motion segments in a row showing the same impairment. Two successive motion segments (three or more vertebrae) are more side-bent and rotated to the right or to the left. Through our testing we will be able to clarify if they are successive flexion lesions or impairments or successive extension lesions.

- Based on what we have discussed so far we can say that if they are flexion lesions (fixed open) then the vertebrae affected bend and rotate away from that lesioned side.
- Alternatively, if they are extension lesions then the vertebrae are bent and rotated toward the side with the lesions.

Box 14.14 Another way of expressing the rules for flexion/extension lesions during translations

When the cervical spine side-bends, the facet(s) on the side it side-bends toward must close. The facet joint(s) on the side opposite the side to which it is bending must open.

Therefore, when translating in flexion, the side that will not open will most restrict side-bending:

- on the same side as the one to which translation is directed, or
- on the opposite side to the one to which the cervical spine at that level is trying to side-bend.

The facet joint that will not open is, therefore, said to be extended.

When translating in extension, the side that will not close will most restrict side-bending:

- on the opposite side to the one to which translation is directed, or
- on the same side as the one to which the cervical spine at that level is trying to side-bend.

Notation and examples

Having found impairments, we now need to name them. To imagine the following, note that we are talking about the cervical spine being in neutral (except for the lesion), and remember that impairments or lesions are named for the superior vertebrae in a vertebral motion segment. Labeling an impairment C4 means we are talking about the positioning of C4 sitting on top of the relatively neutral C5. That being said:

When we find C4 held flexed (open) on the right, it implies that it will be side-bent and rotated to the left. It can be written out as FRSl which expands to mean Flexed (on the right) while Side-bent and Rotated Left.

Let us say we found the opposite:

When we find C4 held extended (closed) on the right, it implies that it will be side-bent and rotated to the right. This can be written out as ERSr which expands to mean Extended, Side-bent, and Rotated Right.

The following is meant to be used for the purpose of review:

ERSr

Saying that the right facet is extended, equals saying it is being held closed.

- It will not open/flex on the right.

Saying that the right facet is extended, equals saying the vertebra is side-bent right.

- It will not side-bend to the left.

Saying that the right facet is extended, equals saying the vertebra is rotated right.

- It will not rotate to the left.

FRSr

Saying that the left facet is flexed, equals saying it is being held open.

- It will not close/extend on the left.

Saying that the left facet is flexed, equals saying the vertebra is side-bent right.

- It will not side-bend to the left.

Saying that the left facet is flexed, equals saying the vertebra is rotated right.

- It will not rotate to the left.

Summary of testing the cervical spine by translations

Let us summarize what we have said about motion palpation of the lower cervical spine.

1. We first test in neutral starting at the lowest motion segment (C7–T1) and move up from there laterally translating left to right.
2. When we translate the spine laterally we are testing side-bending and rotation (as they are coupled actions) occurring to the same side. Side-bending also requires one side of the vertebra to open/flex as the other side closes/extends. Therefore, when translating laterally in the cervical spine, we are also testing the facet joint's ability to flex and extend.

INSIGHTS

Box 14.15 What we may have observed in cervical AF-ROM

If the patient has a C4 FRS_L, then certain ranges of motion will appear normal in AF-ROM.

The patient may be able to:

- forward flex normally
- rotate left normally
- side-bend left normally.

However, we would find that the patient may not have good range, i.e., they may show some restriction when they:

- extend
- rotate right
- side-bend right.

If they experienced pain in a localized area, they may well point to the C4–5 facet joint area on the right side of their neck, as that is the side of the impaired or lesioned joint.

Conversely, *if the patient has a C4 ERS-R*, then certain ranges of motion will appear normal in AF-ROM. The patient may be able to:

- extend normally
- rotate right normally
- side-bend right normally.

However, we would find that the patient may not have good range when they:

- forward flex
- rotate left
- side-bend left.

If they experienced pain in a localized area, they may well point to the C4–5 facet joint area on the right side of their neck, as that is the side of the impaired or lesioned joint

NOTE: In these two examples of different lesions, with restrictions in AF in *opposite* directions, nonetheless, their impairment or lesion (and possibly their pain) are found or felt on the *same* side of the C4–5 segment – on the right side!

3. When we test lateral translation with the head held in flexion we are testing for extension lesions. Finding restrictions in

motion while translating in flexion means that a facet will not open/flex: that facet has an impaired ability to flex. Therefore, that facet is stuck in extension. In addition, that *restriction is on the same side to the one we are translating.*

- ***EXAMPLE:*** Restriction in translating left during forward flexion implies that the left facet is being held closed/extended. It is not being allowed to open or flex.
- An extension lesion is like a gate that will not let the vertebra move toward it when translating toward that side. It only allows translation away from itself but not toward itself.

4. When we test lateral translation with the head held in extension we are testing for flexion lesions. Finding restrictions in motion while translating in extension means that a facet will not close/extend – that it has an impaired ability to extend. Also, that *restriction is on the opposite side to the side we are translating toward.*
   - A flexion lesion is as if the vertebrae is tied by a rope to a post: it may move in one direction but only as far as neutral in the other direction and no further. It has reached the end of its rope. It will only allow movement toward the side which will extend (as this slackens the rope, so to speak) while the other side opens/flexes but cannot move toward the side that can only flex.
5. We name the lesion (impaired motion segment) for what it is willing to do and not for what it will not do. We are naming it for the position it is in. When a facet is held extended (cannot flex), it is called an extension lesion. When a facet is held flexed (cannot extend), it is a flexion lesion.

Other impairments and red flags

Some of the following assessments could be found at this point in our testing.

Simultaneous lesions These are said to occur when one facet is held extended and the other in flexion. This is most likely to be found in a motion segment that has been held side-bent and rotated for some time, leaving both facet joints *fibrosed.* In this case you will find a positive when translating in neutral, in flexion and in extension. Neither facet has mobility.

Bilateral lesions Is it possible for a motion segment to be bilaterally fixed or held in either flexion or extension? Yes, it is. We would find symmetrical restriction in both directions of lateral translation through that motion segment when done either in flexion or in extension, *but not in both.*

With bilateral flexion impairment to a motion segment we would find symmetrical restriction when translating in extension. They would clearly appear "locked." While the lateral translations in flexion may not appear to have quite the expected or normal range, nonetheless, those translations would have some movement.

With a bilaterally extended impairment to a motion segment, we would find symmetrical restriction when translating in forward flexion.

Some further points:

- We can often find bilateral restrictions in one segment or in several, such as in a hyperlordosis of the cervical spine or in a flat (reversed curve) cervical spine. Movement in the segments directly above and below those with impaired motion can be full or even hypermobile. The latter hypermobility often occurs as compensation by the spine above and below the hypomobile segment as an attempt to retain overall range of motion with respect to the cervical spine as a whole.
- ***NOTATION:*** We need only record a single segment's bilateral impairment as, for example, C5 Extended. We can record a group dysfunction as C3–6 Extended, or simply a C3–6 hyperlordosis.

Complete immobilization to a motion segment If you find restriction in a motion segment that appears in neutral, flexion, and extension, then you may have a motion segment that has ankylosed; all the intervertebral joints have calcified. ***This is a red flag***, and a possible contraindication to treatment. This segment needs to be imaged (X-ray, etc.) before any attempt is made to increase motion above or below.

If the whole cervical spine showed decreased range of motion at every segmental level then we need to look more globally for the reasons for that. Extensive degenerative disc disease (DDD), or extensive degenerative joint disease (DJD), large fascial disturbances/diseases, whiplash, aging, etc. Imaging should be done, if none has yet been done.

We need to keep in mind that a vertebral motion segment could suffer from DDD and as a result the vertebral bodies are much closer together. Consequently, the motion between them can have:

- bony blocks (bony portions of each vertebra coming into contact with each other and restricting motion)
- muscle spasming around that motion segment to prevent instability (hypermobility) at that level.

If the patient has recurring symptoms that last for only a few hours or a day and then return as even more intense or acute, refer the patient out.

Be careful not to remove the splinting of an unstable segment. Restoration of normal motion appropriate to the tissue's health is the goal, but instability in a joint creates its own unique environment and appropriate compensations need to be found. Therefore, do not try to get maximum quick results. Massage techniques are like medications. Do not over-medicate and overdose the patient!

The order of the protocol for the cervical spine can depend on the purpose of the assessment and on what pre-existing pathologies patients come with, such as carotid artery partial occlusions, concussions, motor vehicle accidents (MVAs), etc. What is presented below encompasses the complete testing presented in this chapter. However, many elements may be omitted or tested at a later time, depending on the chief complaint the patient arrives with.

Box 14.16 Protocol for assessing the cervical spine

Case history

Observations (may include a comprehensive postural examination)

Light inspection palpation

Rule outs

Shoulder

Temporomandibular joint (TMJ)

Vertebral artery tests

Active free range of motion (AF-ROM)

Motion palpation testing of the occipito-atlantal (OA)

Motion palpation testing of the atlanto-axial (AA)

(Preferred placement of Motion palpation of the lower cervical spine)

Passive relaxed range of motion

Active resisted range of motion

Special tests

Compression test

Decompression test

Quadrant testing

Lower quadrant test

Spurling's test

Valsalva's test

Swallowing test

Tinel's sign at the neck

Bakody's sign

Neurological testing

- Dermatome testing
- Sensory testing of the face
- Peripheral nerve testing
- Myotome testing
- Motor testing of peripheral nerves
- Upper limb tension testing (ULTT – see Chapter 15)
- Deep tendon reflex (DTR) testing
- Pathological nerve impairment testing

Temporal mandibular joint testing

- Active-free range of motion testing
- Passive relaxed range of motion and joint mobilization for TMJ
- Motion palpation of lower cervical spine
- Joint mobilizations

THORACIC OUTLET: CHAPTER OVERVIEW

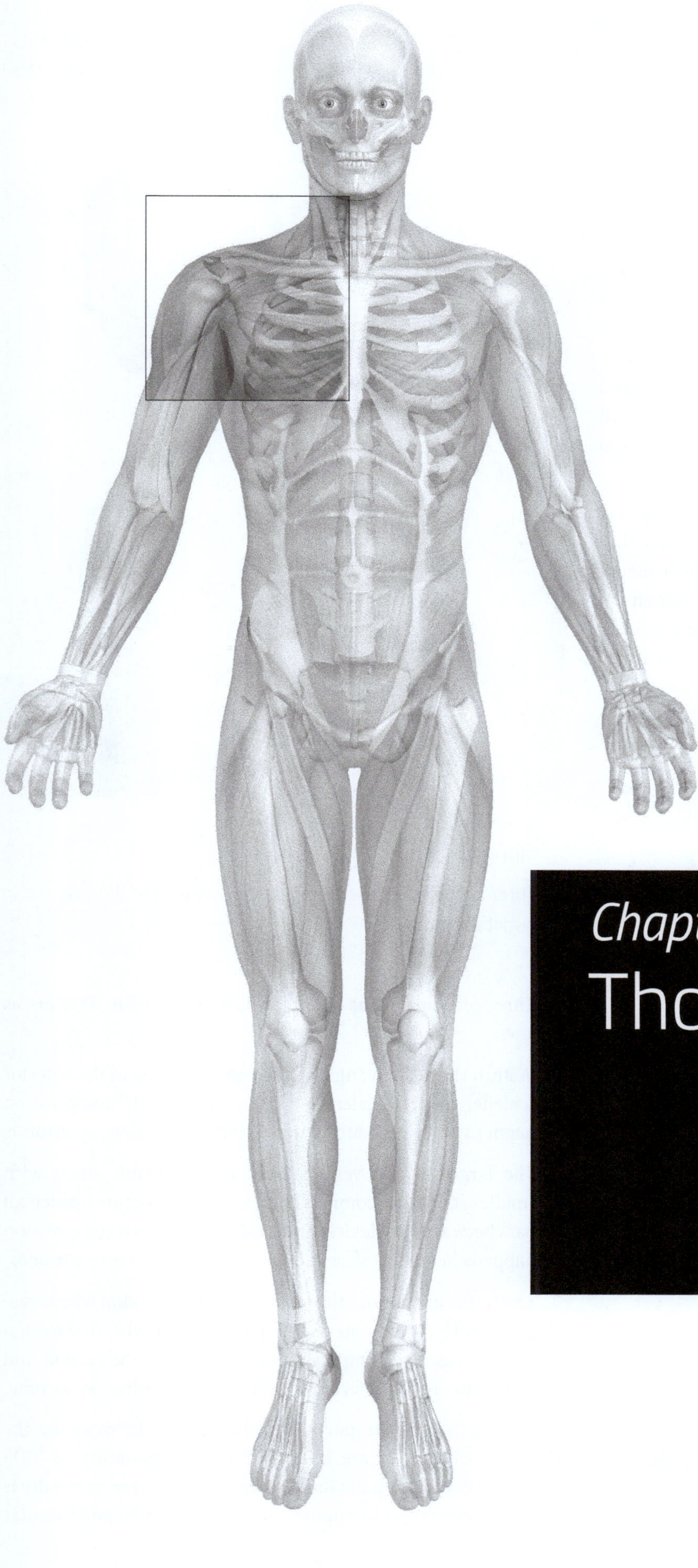

Chapter 15

Thoracic outlet

Chapter 15

Clinical implications of anatomy and physiology

Thoracic outlet syndromes (TOS) (Figures 15.1, 15.2)

Though the area we are speaking of is referred to anatomically as the thoracic inlet, we will use the word "outlet," as it remains the principal term used by most health professionals and the acronym TOS is extremely common. ***NOTE:*** The term thoracic outlet is actually used anatomically to refer to the area around the bottom of the ribcage and the diaphragm through which structures pass. The term thoracic inlet is the correct anatomical name for the superior aperture.

TOS refers to a number of impingement syndromes that involve the vascular structures that exit from the superior thoracic aperture and also the brachial plexus. However, their sites of compression are not only at the aperture, but also at the sites mentioned below (Agur et al. 2014; Dutton 2012; Hertling & Kessler 2006; Magee 2014; Schuenke et al. 2014; Travell et al. 1999).

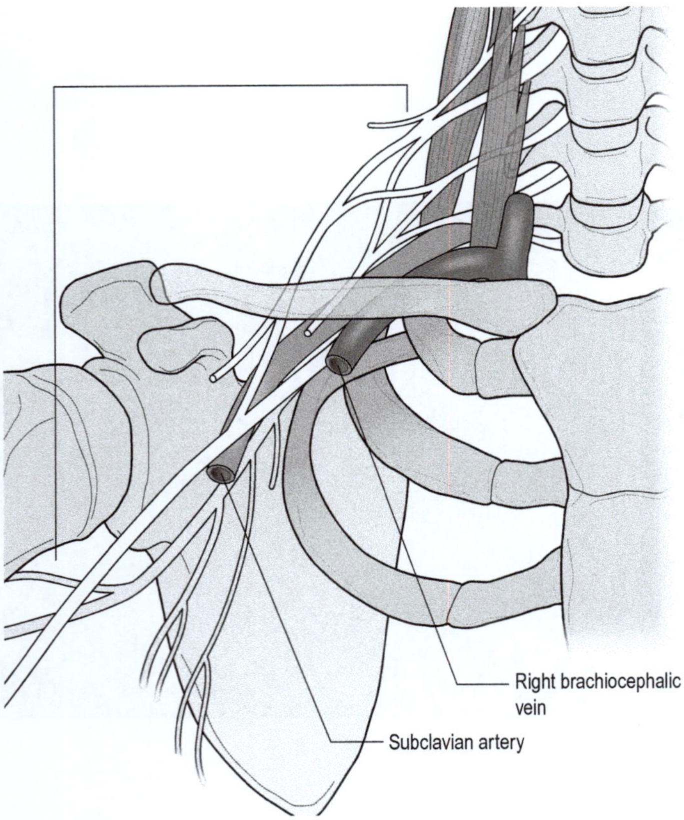

FIGURE 15.1

Some of the vascular structures that exit from the superior thoracic aperture and also the brachial plexus.

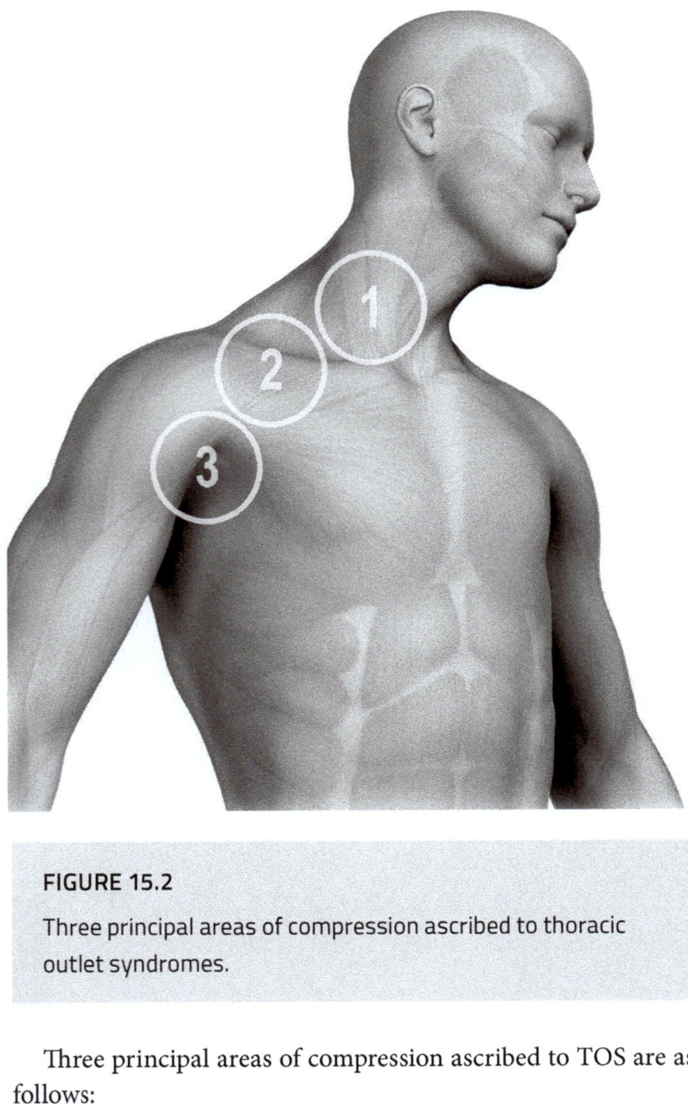

FIGURE 15.2

Three principal areas of compression ascribed to thoracic outlet syndromes.

Three principal areas of compression ascribed to TOS are as follows:

1. Within the bottom angle of a triangle made up of the anterior scalene, medial scalene and the first rib. If compression happens here, it is referred to as an anterior scalene syndrome.
2. The larger artery, vein, and lymphatic trunk along with smaller (but more complex) neurological structures which all pass between the clavicle and the first rib. When compression happens here it is referred to as a costoclavicular syndrome.
3. Lastly, the area under the pectoralis minor tendon where vascular and lymphatic structures pass and can, when the tendon spasms, become compressed between it and the second and third ribs. This is referred to as a pectoralis minor syndrome.

One of the most important distinctions to be made by the therapist when they are investigating the possibility of TOS being involved in specific impairments in the upper extremity is between neurological symptoms (neurogenic TOS) and vascular symptoms (vascular TOS). The assumption of neurological impingement is made far too often to explain both the sensations felt by the patient in the upper limb and the results of TOS testing as found by the therapist.

A presenting complaint of tingling pain and/or weakness by the patient can be the result of a neurological and/or vascular deficit to the arm, forearm, or hand. Vascular insufficiency itself can be a source of any, or all, of these symptoms. Reduction of arterial supply or venous return may well in fact be the most common source of impairments uncovered by TOS testing.

Further, because of the size of the vascular structures as compared to the neurological structures, the artery is more at risk as it passes through the three areas involved in TOS. The classic signs of arterial insufficiency are:

- general symptoms, such as paleness of the limb
- a generalized non-specific tingling or paresthesia
- a feeling of general weakness in the limb or a proneness to fatigue in the musculature of the limb; and/or
- a sense of heaviness to the limb.

We will consider how the vascular and lymphatic structures are affected when we discuss the specific syndromes. Variations in possible nerve impingement impairments will also be addressed with the syndromes that they are most associated with.

Anterior scalene syndrome

If you look carefully at the anatomy of the pectoral girdle, it becomes obvious why arterial supply is most at risk in anterior scalene TOS. The artery lies at the most anterior-inferior end of the scalene-first rib triangle, which is the premier site for compression in anterior scalene TOS. The arterial supply to the upper limb, the subclavius artery, passes within the triangle created by the two scalene muscles and the first rib precisely at the most vulnerable position, lying at the inferior-anterior angle created by the anterior scalene and the first rib.

With respect to compression of venous return at the scalene area, note that the subclavian vein lies outside the scalene-first rib triangle. It does pass over the first rib, but just in front of the attachment of the anterior scalene. Its greatest risk of compression here is between the first rib and the clavicle (and/or the subclavius muscle) lying just above it. Compression can be due either to the rib being elevated by a spasming scalene muscle or the clavicle being pulled down by a shortened spasming pectoralis major or subclavius muscle. Hence, compression of the vein here is a costoclavicular syndrome. Note that arteries have a significant smooth muscle component in their walls while veins do not, making venous structures more likely to be compressed in general.

The neurological symptoms that would most likely show up in an anterior scalene syndrome relate to the peripheral nerves composed of C7, C8, and T1 nerve roots. This is because those nerve roots could be compressed in this syndrome just prior to their intermingling in the brachial plexus, becoming the peripheral nerves of the upper extremity.

Therefore, one of the most common peripheral nerves affected is the ulnar nerve, along with some fibers of the median nerve. Tingling from a neurological impingement during TOS is most often felt in the fourth and fifth digits and the ulnar border of the hand (and possibly into the forearm). Weakness, if it occurs, is most often found in the intrinsic muscles of the hand. That is why clumsiness is often mentioned by the patient, or a tendency to drop things. It can also explain a tendency for the hand specifically to feel achy or to fatigue quickly (Hartley 2000a; Hertling & Kessler 2006; Magee 2014; Travell et al. 1999).

The costoclavicular syndrome

The second general site of compression of the neurovascular bundle is between the clavicle and the second rib. The arterial supply by the subclavius artery is one of the largest components of that neurovascular bundle, which is composed also of the trunks and branches of the brachial plexus, the brachiocephalic/subclavius vein, and the subclavius lymphatic trunk.

The classic signs of occlusion of venous return are a dark color to the limb affected and a swollen engorged look. The most distinct sign of venous congestion is that the veins on the back of the hand stand out. (However, take note that the veins can be more prominent just post-work/exercise, and also if the patient has been in a warm environment.) Impaired venous return will also reduce the flow of blood through the tissue and muscles of the limb, thus reducing oxygen exchange. This results in reduced strength or endurance during activity. Because of the engorgement of blood in the arm and hand there can be a complaint of a feeling of heaviness to the limb. A wrist and hand which is of a normal color but has a swollen, engorged look can occur if the lymphatic trunk is compressed.

The arterial symptoms parallel those described above. The neurological signs can be more equally divided between the ulnar and median nerves; and in extreme impingement the radial nerve may also be involved. These nerves are not as yet differentiated at the site of compression at what are the brachial nerve trunks that contain the nerves as they start organizing themselves into the peripheral nerves of the upper extremity.

Pectoralis minor syndrome

The third site that TOS testing investigates is under the pectoralis minor tendon and between it and the ribcage. The brachial plexus has just about finished its "weaving" of the trunks into the peripheral nerves of the arm at this point. Also, the nerves generally surround the vascular-lymphatic vessels as they pass through this aperture. Hence, at this site of compression the nerves can be as commonly affected by compression as the vascular structures. Compression here generally happens when a person is engaged in an activity that requires their arm to be held above their shoulder.

Other structures that can be involved One needs also to take into account fascial restrictions in the coracoclavicular fascia, which provides a pathway and protection to the neurovascular bundle as it travels from the cervical region into the arm. Due to injury or inflammation of this pathway, the neurovascular bundle can become adhered to the fascia rather than being able to slide freely within the sheath as it adjusts for cervical and arm motions.

Though the coracoclavicular fascia and the neurovascular bundle will both have to adjust to changes in the limb and spine, the neurovascular bundle needs to be able to slide and move freely within its fascial sheath. If there are adherences between these tissues, whenever the fascia is moved so is the neurovascular bundle, and in the same way. This results at times in the stretching or compression of the bundle.

Clinical experience in many medical professions has encountered what is referred to as a *double crush*. This means that more than one site is implicated in compressing the neurovascular bundle.

This makes good anatomical sense: if we have a compression occurring at the anterior scalene site, those hypertonic/spasming scalenes are also lifting the upper two ribs and dramatically narrowing the costoclavicular space (Hartley 2000a; Hertling & Kessler 2006; Magee 2014).

Or, we can have a double crush at the pectoral minor area and costoclavicular. When hypertonicity and shortness occurs in pectoralis minor the pectoralis major is usually short as well. Therefore the pectoralis major pulls the clavicle down onto the upper ribs (costoclavicular compression) while the pectoralis minor further compresses the neurovascular bundle, especially if the arms are held up over the head.

If the person is also looking overhead while working overhead we could get a triple crush! For example, with restrictions/compressions at either of the other two sites (pectoralis minor and clavicle) by the patient working with their arms over their head and looking up, the anterior scalene is put on stretch. This lifts the first rib (worsening the costoclavicular compression) and with the anterior scalene, compresses the nerve roots and artery at this site.

Because of the possibility of the double crush (or multi-crush) scenario we should not be surprised to find more than one of the classic tests positive. And remember, just because we do find TOS does not mean that nerve or vascular compressions are not also taking place at the nerve root or somewhere else down the course of the nerves as they travel through the limb. A positive test only speaks to us about the specific tissues involved in that test. A positive test tells us nothing about other structures and tissues that can be involved somewhere else along the course of the neurovascular bundle. Therefore, a therapist could get an incomplete assessment if they stop their TOS testing when they find their first positive test.

Case history (specific questions)

If the patient complaint centers around the upper limb the therapist needs to ask:

- What sensations are you feeling in the arm or hand?
- Does the whole hand have these symptoms, or only particular fingers or portion of the hand?
- Are these constant? Do they vary over time?
- What activities seem to bring on or aggravate these symptoms? What activities seem to help?
- Times of day when worse or better?
- Any changes to the color of the affected arm? Pale, bluish?
- Does the limb (or part of it) feel cold compared to the other?
- Does the arm or hand look swollen at times, less so at other times?
- Do you experience any weakness with that arm/hand?
- Do you find yourself dropping things, or losing your hold on things?

Observations prior to specific TOS testing

Postural observations that should be made:

1. Orientation of head and cervical spine.
2. Orientation of the shoulders and clavicle.
3. Orientation of the thoracic spine and ribs.
4. Orientation of the lumbar spine.

Some of the specific things to check out during these observations:

- The position of the head observed from the side, front and back.
- The quality of the lordosis of the cervical spine; excessive lordosis, or a reversed curve where the lordosis has disappeared (for more details, see observations in the cervical section).
- The orientation of the shoulder (clavicle, scapulae, and positioning of the glenohumeral joint).
- How the affected arm is carried (is it internally rotated, for example?).
- General tissue health in the affected upper limb (edema, hyper- or hypotonic musculature, condition of the skin, blood flow, venous drainage, etc., as compared to the other limb).
- Specific observation of the hand and forearm being pale with relative coolness to the tissue, suggesting an arterial compression. A darker shade to the affected arm and hand can suggest venous return restrictions. (Usually the veins are engorged on the dorsum of the hand. Compare both hands carefully, however, as recent physical exertion or being in a hot environment can cause this in both hands. The unilateral observation is merely suggestive here.) The hand can also be cool with restricted venous return as it prevents proper perfusion of the tissues. Edema on the affected side (with no history of recent trauma) may indicate compression or occlusion of the lymphatics. A referral back to the patient's physician is warranted if they have not already discussed this with their MD.
- Quality of the lumbar lordosis. Excessive lordosis, or the lack of a lordotic curve in the low back, can be the start of compensatory changes that cause postural faults up in the shoulder girdle and upper thoracic and cervical spine. Note: Any curve of the spine (anterior-posterior, lordosis-kyphosis), when exaggerated or lost, will eventually produce similar changes in the other curves.
- And finally, observe the condition of the pelvis and lower limbs and look at how they might be participating in the patient's complaints and impairments. For example, a lower limb and/or pelvic dysfunction can cause the sacral base to be unlevel, which affects the spinal curves and in turn, cervical and shoulder orientation, both of which have a huge impact on classic TOS.

Rule outs

NOTE: The following is a brief summary of the possible other sources of neurological symptoms in the upper limb. It is assumed that the therapist has done such testing (which has been described in the appropriate chapter), and what is listed here is meant to act as an inventory that can be used to make sure that all avenues of testing have been explored when testing for compression syndromes in the upper limb. A summary of the rule outs of the cervical spine is provided below. Also provided is a list of the rule outs of the shoulder, elbow, and wrist joints that can be of help in making sure that they are not a source of the patient's complaint.

First, here is a list of tests for nerve root sources for the patient's symptoms outside of TOS that need to be ruled out. See the appropriate pages in Chapter 14 for details on the following:

Cervical spine quick rule out

1. AF-ROM: flexion, side-bending, rotation and if pain-free, apply over-pressure (O-P). Lastly, extension, with no O-P.
2. Compression and distraction: only if negative, proceed to the following.
3. Lower quadrant test (side-bending, rotation, and extension, all to the same side. Always watch for the signs of vertebral artery occlusion!). If pain-free, apply O-P (Spurling's test).

Shoulder girdle, elbow, and wrist

These tests are composed of AF motions and if pain-free, then O-P can be applied after you take hold of the limb and ask the patient to relax. The following tests take only a few moments to do. The shoulder motions should be done last, if at all, because the rule outs for the shoulder contain movement that could aggravate TOS compression at the three sites discussed above, since they will move the clavicle, stretch the pectoralis minor, put tension through the brachial fascia, etc.

Elbow

- AF ROM of flexion, if pain-free, apply O-P.
- AF ROM of extension, if pain-free, apply O-P.

Wrist

- AF ROM of flexion, if pain-free, apply O-P.
- AF ROM of extension, if pain-free, apply O-P.

Shoulder girdle

- AF-ROM of abduction, if pain-free, apply O-P.
- AF-ROM of full forward flexion of the shoulder, if pain-free, apply O-P.

These movements provide sufficient stress of joints and ligaments to rule them out. Usually they will also provoke neurological symptoms (often distal to the site) if an impingement is occurring near or at the relevant joint. (See the appropriate chapters for these joints for peripheral nerve impingements.)

Thoracic outlet tests

IMPORTANT: You will note that all of the three TOS tests use the loss of pulse as a positive sign. Remember, however, that the loss of pulse only means that the blood flow is restricted. The test is positive only if it reproduces the patient's signs and symptoms. Further, it does not necessarily mean there is compression of nerve structures. Clear neurological symptoms must be reproduced from the test in order to claim that the patient's neurological symptoms are due to a thoracic outlet compression syndrome. Therefore, you need to be clear about noting your results: vascular compression and/or neurological compression. Neurological compression syndromes felt in the hand tend to address *specific parts* of the hand and fingers (*see neurological testing in Chapter 14 for details*). Blood flow compression usually results in numbness and/or tingling in the *whole* hand.

Adson's maneuver or anterior scalene syndrome test (ASST) (Figures 15.3, 15.4)

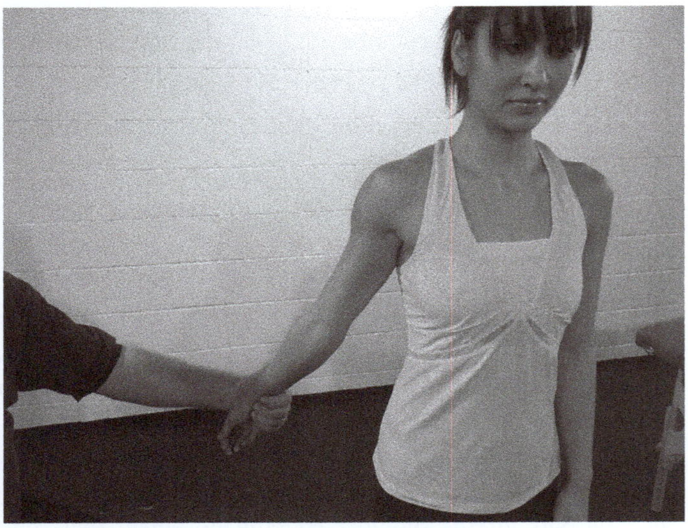

FIGURE 15.3 1. Adson's test preparation

Stand at the side, slightly behind the patient. Find the radial pulse of the arm that is extended and slightly abducted. Once the pulse is found, apply a slight traction to the arm (by making your hand heavy).

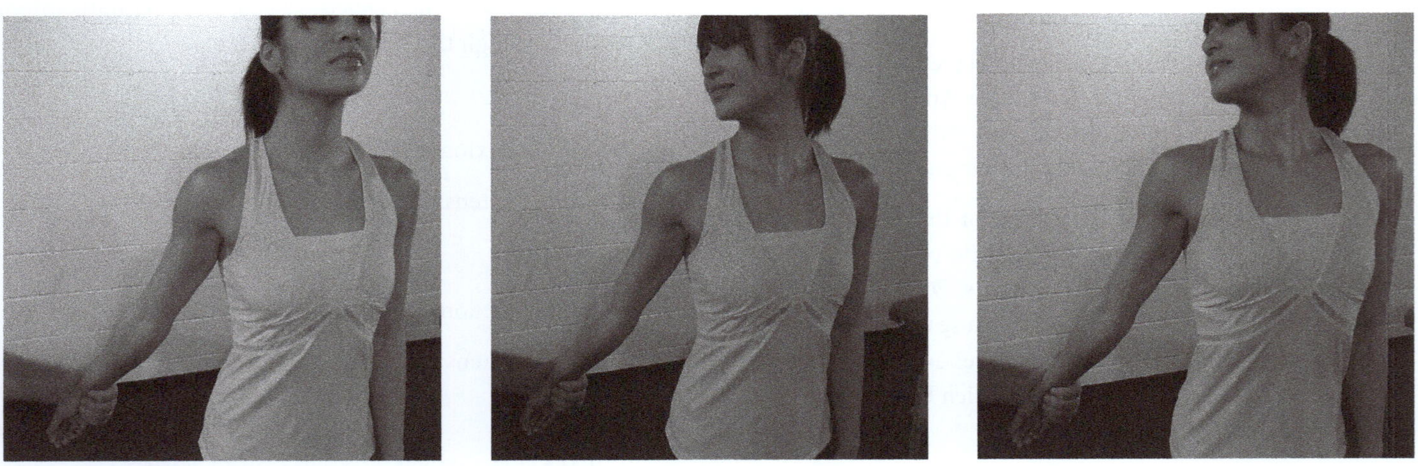

FIGURE 15.4A–C 2. Adson's test

(A) Have the patient hold the chin up (or slightly extend the cervical spine). (B) Have the patient turn their head (to face you), and (C) take in a deep breath and try to hold for 30 seconds, if possible. The test is positive if the pulse disappears and symptoms return.

Box 15.1 describes variations on Adson's test.

Box 15.1 Travell's variation of Adson's

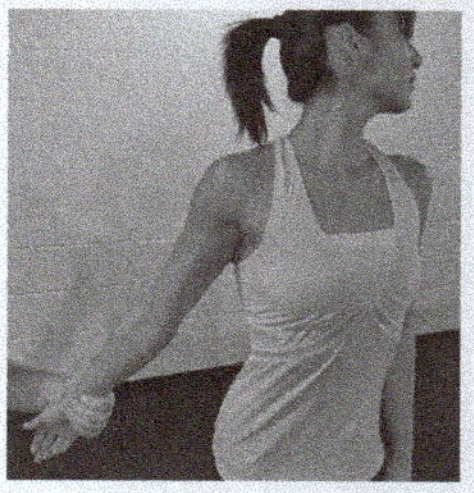

FIGURES 15.5

Travell's variation on Adson's test.

Dr Janet Travell suggests that having the patient turning away from (instead of toward) the therapist will put a stretch on the muscle, and further tension on the muscle will happen when the patient then contracts it by taking a deep breath. Travell postulates that this will increase the compression on the neurovascular bundle as it passes through the scalene–first rib aperture. Other than that, the test procedure is the same (Travell et al. 1999).

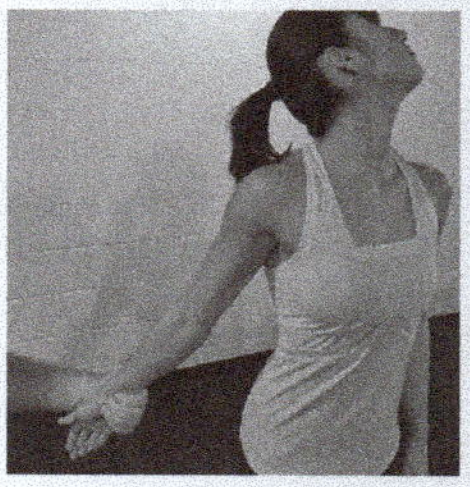

FIGURES 15.6

The Halstead maneuver.

Halstead maneuver

Another variation is called the Halstead maneuver, where the therapist is positioned the same as for Adson's, but the patient looks up, extending the head. This is to stretch the scalenes. This may be positive for anterior scalene syndrome. However, in lifting the first and second rib, it could be positive for a costoclavicular syndrome. In other words, it could reproduce a *double crush*.

Costoclavicular syndrome test (military position test) (Figures 15.7–15.9)

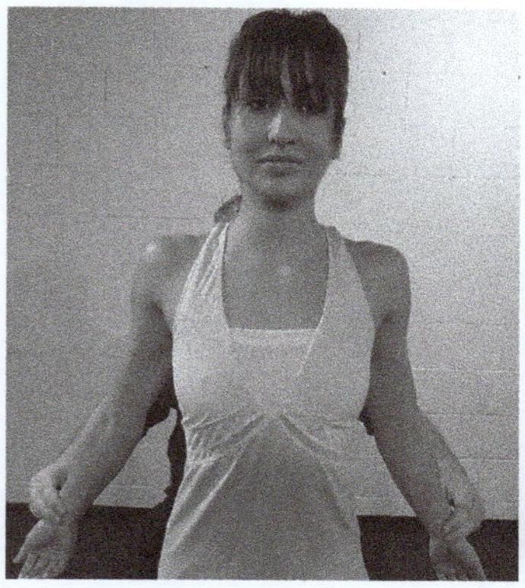

FIGURE 15.7 1. Costoclavicular test positioning

With the patient seated or standing, take both of the patient's arms back into extension and slightly abducted. Find the radial pulse on both wrists.

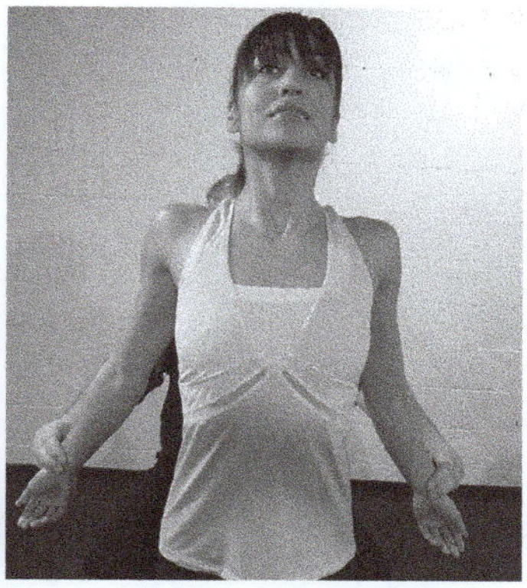

FIGURE 15.8 2. Costoclavicular test positioning

Have the patient strike a military-like posture. That is, have them depress their shoulders, pull their shoulder blades together, stick out their chest, and hold their chin up (extending cervical spine).

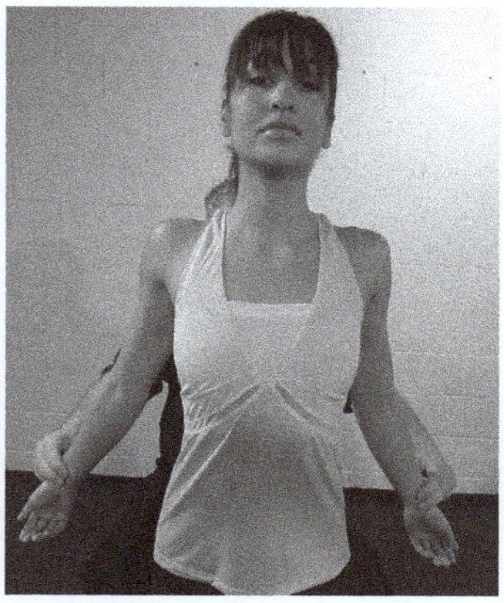

FIGURE 15.9 3. Costoclavicular test

Have the patient take a deep breath to raise the ribcage and have them try to hold their breath for as long as 30 seconds. Again, a positive sign is loss of pulse and/or a return of their symptoms on the affected side.

Wright's hyper-abduction test (pectoralis minor syndrome test) (Figures 15.10, 15.11)

NOTE: This test would be contraindicated if the patient has suffered an anterior dislocation of the shoulder. You may wish to do a dry run with the patient first so that they understand the passive movements that are going to occur during testing after they hold their breath.

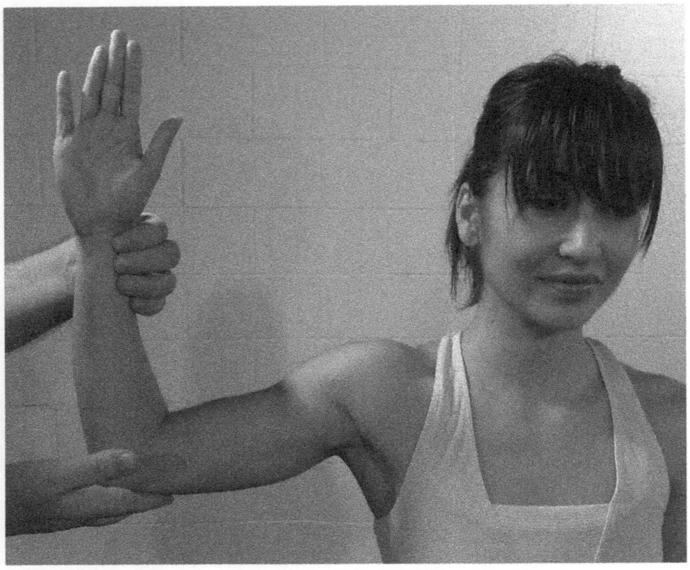

FIGURE 15.10 Pectoralis minor syndrome test 1

Have the seated patient's affected arm slightly abducted with the elbow flexed and the hand pointing straight up, level with the head. Palpate for the radial pulse. Once found, have the patient take a deep breath and to try to hold the breath for 30 seconds.

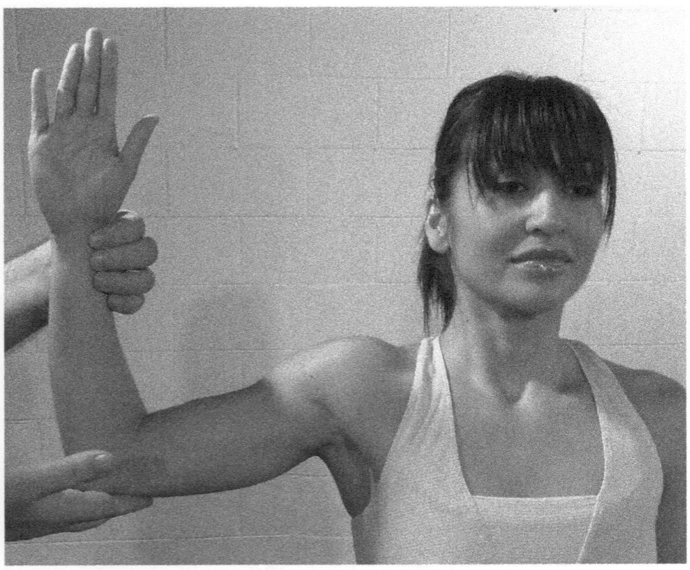

FIGURE 15.11 Pectoralis minor syndrome test 2

Passively abduct the patient's arm to 90°, with the elbow flexed at 90°. The shoulder should be externally rotated. The patient looks upward while breathing in deeply. Positive sign is a loss of pulse and/or a return of symptoms.

Some suggest that the patient then look up to the ceiling. Looking up adds to the test being more likely to imitate the actions of someone using their arms over their head. However, to do this would increase tension on the anterior scalene, which in turn could also be causing compression under the clavicle or at the anterior scalene and first rib. Therefore, if the test with the head in neutral is negative, repeat it with the patient looking up.

Cervical rib

TOS can also be caused by a cervical rib, which is a lengthened transverse process (TVP), if the rib is large enough to extend into the area between the medial and anterior scalenes. This may be revealed by palpation but would require an X-ray to confirm. It may play a role in all of the tests shown but Adson's test is thought to be the most effective in catching it.

It sometimes causes pain (via soft tissue compression) when the patient rotates to the affected side.

There are other anatomical abnormalities that can be causative, such as an unusual shape to the clavicle. Other causes of TOS include: trauma to the any of the structures mentioned above that make up the common areas of compression (e.g., a bony callus around the site of a clavicle fracture); and vascular pathologies, both local and systemic.

Upper limb tension tests (ULTT)

These tests are done to assess for brachial plexus and upper limb peripheral nerve compression syndromes. They may be useful in locating multiple crush sites where compressions at several sites along the nerve's path are occurring. Hence they are good tests to perform if you have a positive TOS test and wish to specifically explore if there may be more than one site of compression from nerve root to fingers. Also, they can be of help in exploring specific peripheral nerve pathways. Lastly, they are important to do if neurological testing of the cervical spine, TOS testing, and/or peripheral nerve compression tests have all shown to be negative or unclear, and yet the patient's complaint seems to have a neurological component. (See Cleland & Koppenhaver 2011; Hertling & Kessler 2006; Magee 2014; Schuenke et al. 2014. The best accessible source of information and instruction for this type of testing and treatment options for massage therapists is the DVD *Nerve Mobilization for the Neck, Arm and Hand with Doug Alexander*, from Real Bodyworks Presents.)

Box 15.2 examines some of the pros and cons of ULTT.

The ULTT for specific nerves are most revealing if the various steps are done in a specific order: the order systematically

Box 15.2 Pros and cons of ULTT

There is an argument that can be made for claiming that upper limb tension tests (ULTT) should be the first form of testing when investigating neurological TOS impairments or any neurological impairment of the upper limb. By design, the progressive steps of increasing tension on the nerves can reveal impairment or obstruction of nerve flow all the way from the nerve roots to the fingers. This is especially true if the therapist is well versed in this form of testing and clearly understands what constitutes a positive sign.

The positive sign is *reproduction of the patient's neurological signs and symptoms*. Further, *always* test the unaffected side first to see if this testing will produce seemingly positive signs, and so may well produce false positives in that specific patient.

The symptoms we are testing for, and trying to provoke, include burning, tingling, and paresthesias that the patient has experienced prior to the testing. Simply getting sensations of pain, burning, tingling, aching, or intense stretch during these tests is not necessarily a positive sign. Stretching of connective tissue, vascular structures, or tissues containing myofascial trigger points can create some or all of these sensations and can be mistaken as neurological symptoms. Remember that myofascial trigger points or connective tissue adhesions can produce these, as can autonomic or visceral (including vascular) referral. This form of testing therefore, can produce a high number of false positives (Starkey & Brown 2015).

provides tension (provocation) on the nerve beginning at the brachial plexus and then step by step down into the limb. The therapist can trace the sites of compression as symptoms occur and are further provoked at various stages of the testing procedure as the nerve is stretched.

Critical issues

First and foremost, the following rule should be strictly followed: whenever neural and/or vascular symptoms arise during the several steps that need to be done for each ULTT, the therapist needs to release the tension and ask the patient if the symptoms have now subsided. If the provoked symptoms do not subside immediately, or within a second or two of the tension being released, then all the testing should be stopped immediately. In other words, all of the stretching steps need to be released, not just the last step done prior to provoking the symptoms.

The continuation of symptoms indicates that the nerve (or other tissue) is not just sensitized by the test but is being injured. At each stage of the test, ask the patient about their symptoms and have them tell you where they are feeling them.

The following require good clinical judgment and of course the consent of the patient. You must feel confident that no tissue's health is being compromised.

- If mild or faint symptoms (sensitization) disappear quickly with the release of tension, then the tension is again placed on the nerve and the next portion of the nerve is stretched. If that now also causes a further provocation (increase in symptoms), then you again have found another area of compression. If no further increase occurs, then proceed with each of the further movements of the test, checking in with the patient constantly.
- Remember, as mentioned above, each time the nerve is sensitized by a movement (stretch), the therapist is to remove the stretch (back off). Ask the patient if this diminishes the symptom. If it does not, then the test is ended.
- It is common to find a multi-crush scenario where a specific site is more provocative than any other site found. This means that the sites can be prioritized. The most provoked or sensitized site is considered the principal compression and the others are secondary, or even tertiary.

General ULTT (Figures 15.12–15.15)

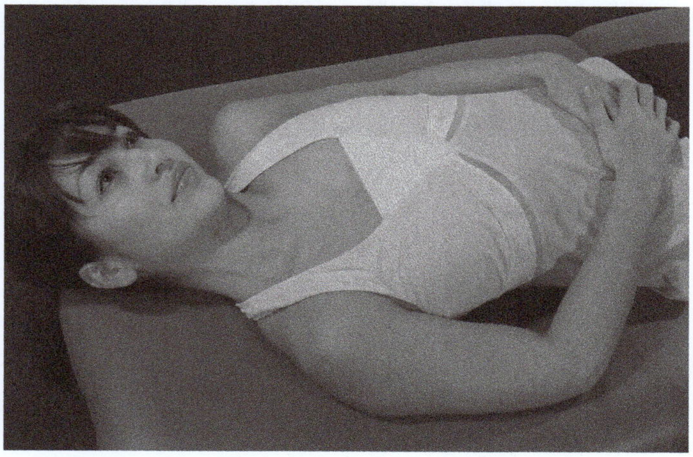

FIGURE 15.12 1. General ULTT

Side-bend thehead away from the side to be tested. The nose should stay pointed to the ceiling, i.e.,the patient's head is not rolled/rotated one way or the other.

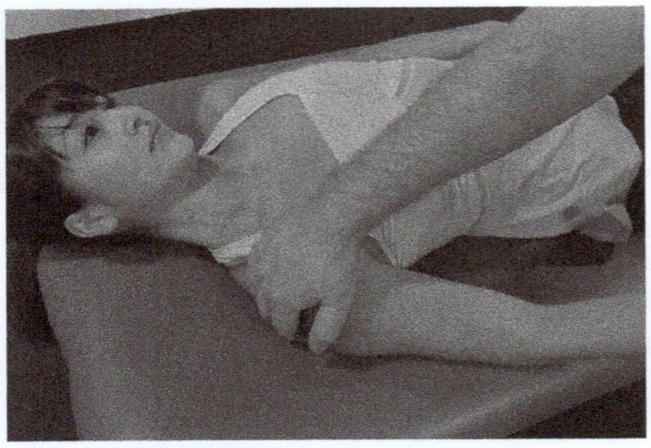

FIGURE 15.13 2. General ULTT

Cup the patient's shoulder and depress it.

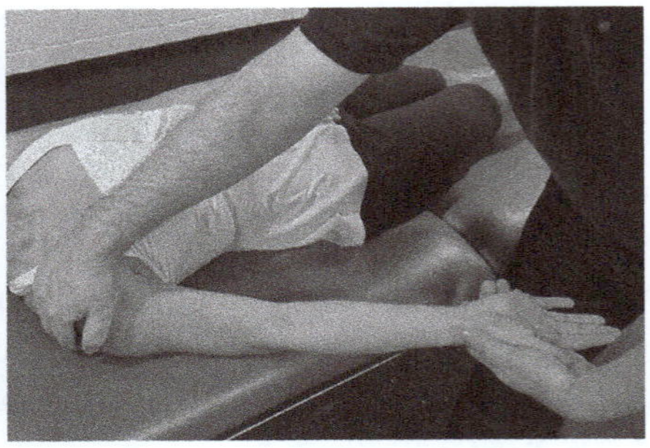

FIGURE 15.14 3. General ULTT

Abduct the patient's arm 20°, externally rotating the humerus and supinated forearm.

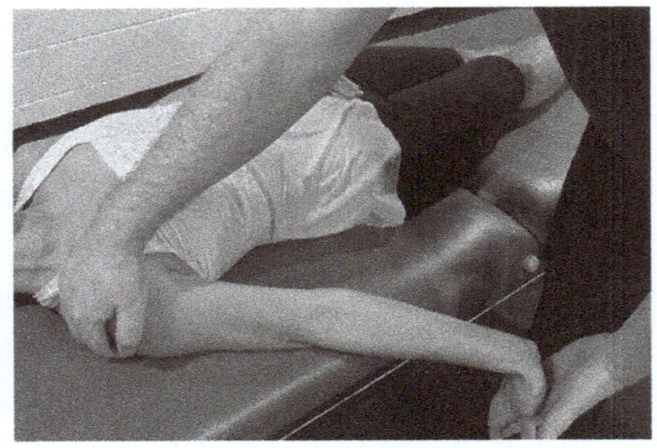

FIGURE 15.15 4. General ULTT

Extend the wrist and fingers. General test complete.

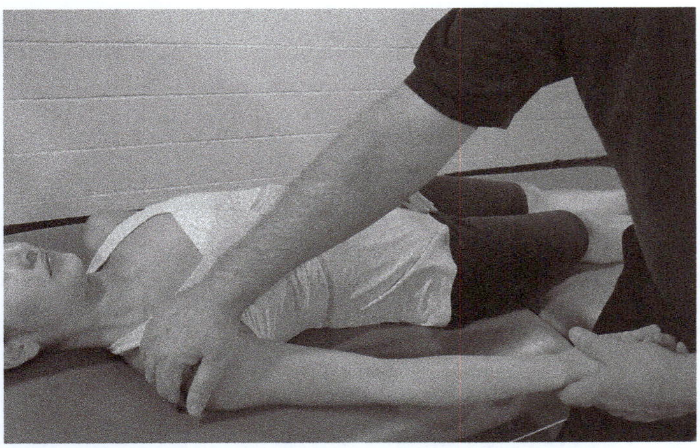

FIGURE 15.16 1. Median nerve bias ULTT

With the patient's head in neutral, cup the shoulder and depress slightly. If symptoms occur at this point, they may imply nerve root or brachial plexus compression. Do not push the shoulder into the table.

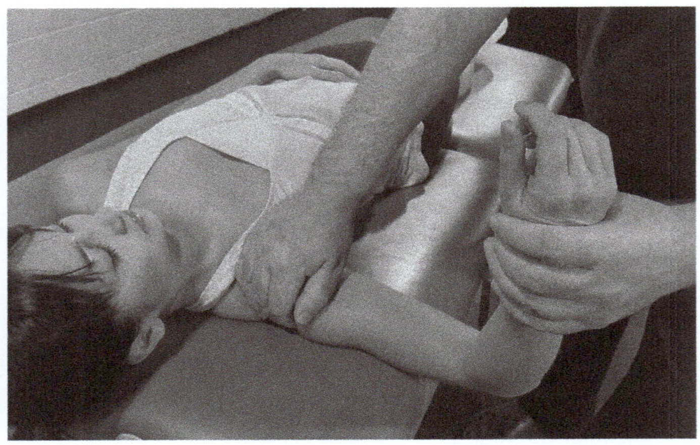

FIGURE 15.17 2. Median nerve bias ULTT

Grasp the wrist and bend the elbow about 90°. Lift the upper arm an inch or two off the table by taking the wrist toward the ceiling. Should be a comfortable (resting) position for shoulder. Abduct the shoulder to about 110°.

For median, axillary and musculocutaneous nerves. Remember that asking about the presence or increase in symptoms is to be done after completing each step.

The following are specific ULTTs for the median, radial, and ulnar nerves. Hence, the use of the term "bias," meaning that though tension will be put on some sections of all the peripheral nerves, some steps in the test may actually release tension on sections of some nerves. Therefore, the specific steps for each of the following tests are designed to place the most tension on all sections of one specific peripheral nerve.

Median nerve bias ULTT (Figures 15.16–15.21)

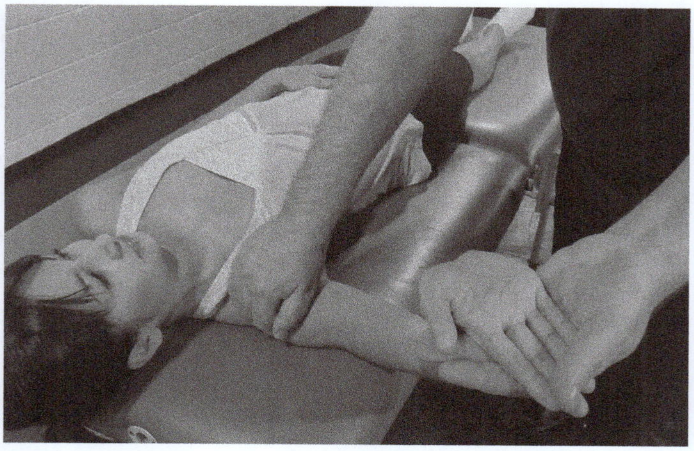

FIGURE 15.18 3. Median nerve bias ULTT

Turn the palm and forearm so they now face the patient (i.e., supination of the forearm); extend the wrist and fingers. Adds stretch through wrist and also increases tension from the elbow to the wrist, especially the anterior interosseous portion of the median nerve.

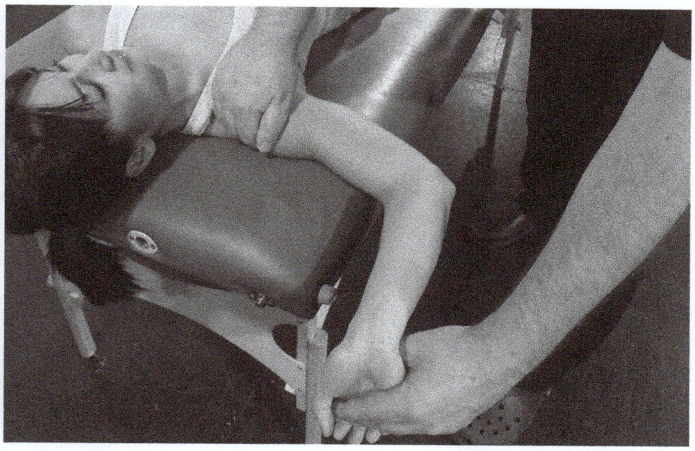

FIGURE 15.19 4. Median nerve bias ULTT

Externally rotate the humerus, leaving the hand/forearm parallel with the table. This hyper-abducts the shoulder. This increases compressive forces at the pectoralis minor area. ***NOTE:*** Contraindicated for a previously dislocated shoulder.

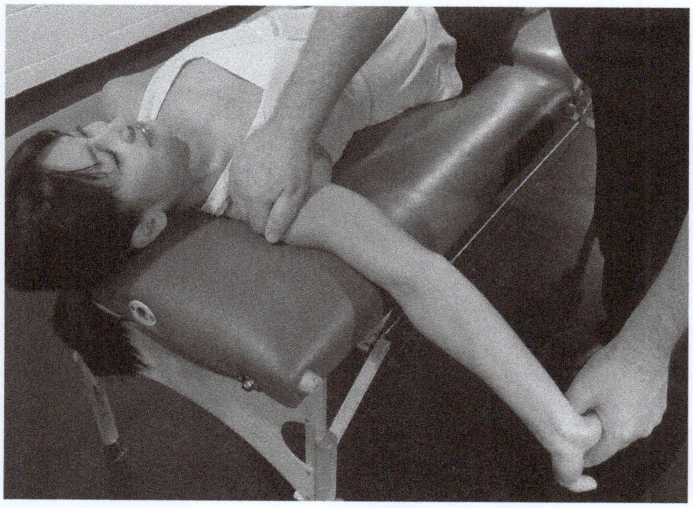

FIGURE 15.20 5. Median nerve bias ULTT

Now, extend the elbow (which is said to stretch the nerve from shoulder to fingertips).

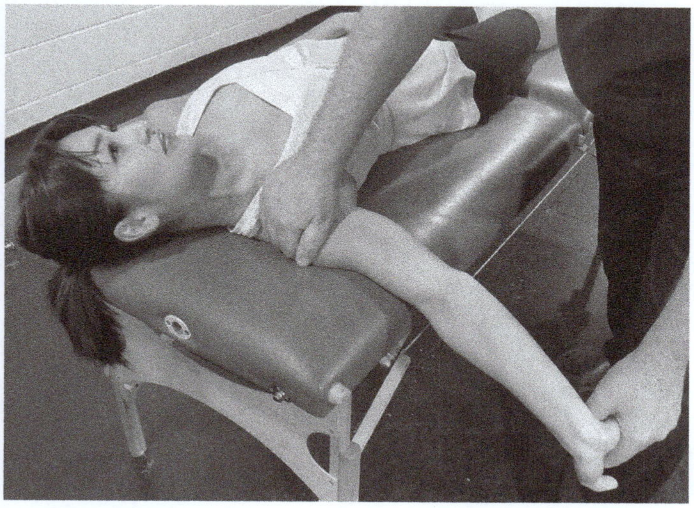

FIGURE 15.21 6. Median nerve bias ULTT.

The patient bends (not rolls) the head away from the arm being tested. The nose is pointed toward the ceiling as they side-bend away at the neck. This increases stretch all the way down the nerve, but can specifically increase tension from the neural foramen, through scalenes, costoclavicular, and to pectoralis minor apertures.

Radial nerve bias ULTT (Figures 15.22–15.25)

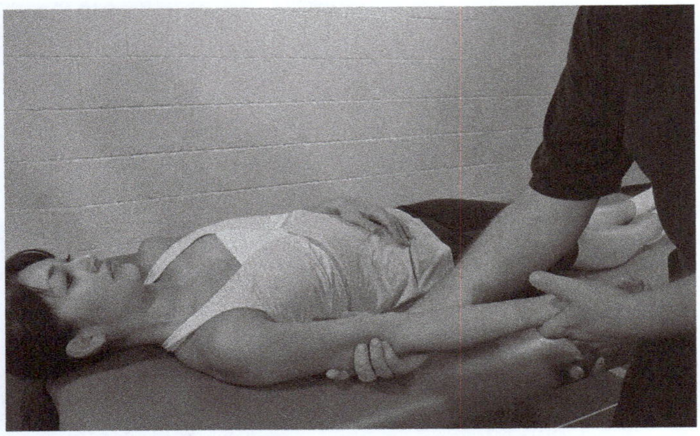

FIGURE 15.22 1. Radial nerve bias ULTT

Abduct the patient's arm about 15–20° and grasping just proximal to the elbow, pull the shoulder interiorly, depressing the shoulder (tractions brachial plexus). The therapist uses the hand closest to the patient.

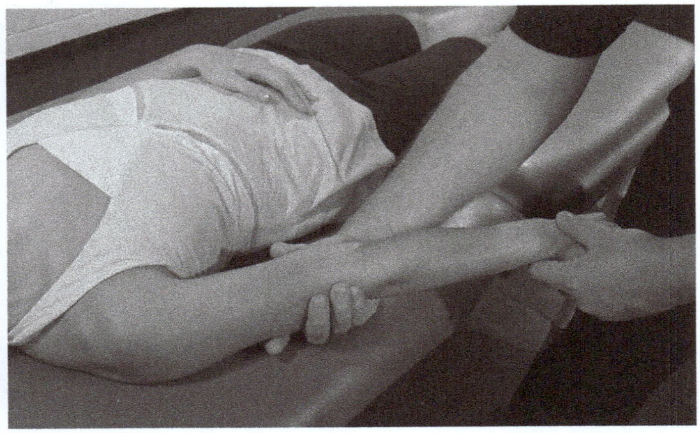

FIGURE 15.23 2. Radial nerve bias ULTT

With the other hand pronate the forearm and internally rotate the humerus. Keep the elbow extended. Increases tension on the radial nerve as it courses around the humerus and runs across the elbow, down into the hand.

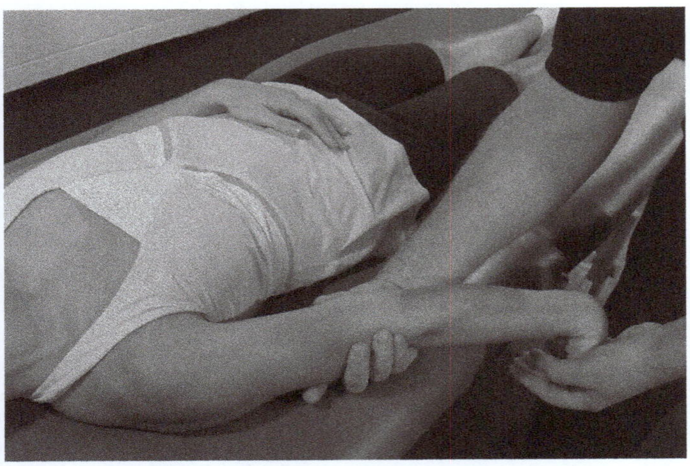

FIGURE 15.24 3. Radial nerve bias ULTT

Flex the patient's fingers and wrist, with ulnar deviation of the wrist. This increases the stretch of the radial nerve, especially over the wrist.

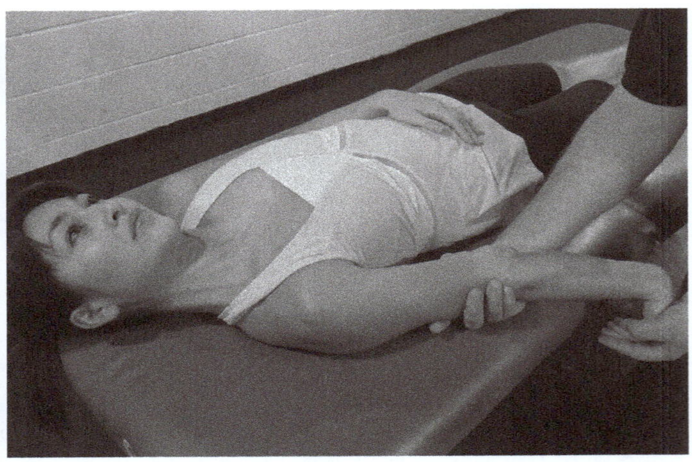

FIGURE 15.25 4. Radial nerve bias ULTT

The patient bends (not rolls) the head away from the arm being tested. The nose is pointed toward the ceiling as they side-bend away at the neck. This increases the stretch all the way down the nerve but can specifically increase tension from the neural foramen, through the scalenes, costoclavicular, and to pectoralis minor apertures.

Ulnar nerve bias ULTT (Figures 15.26–15.30)

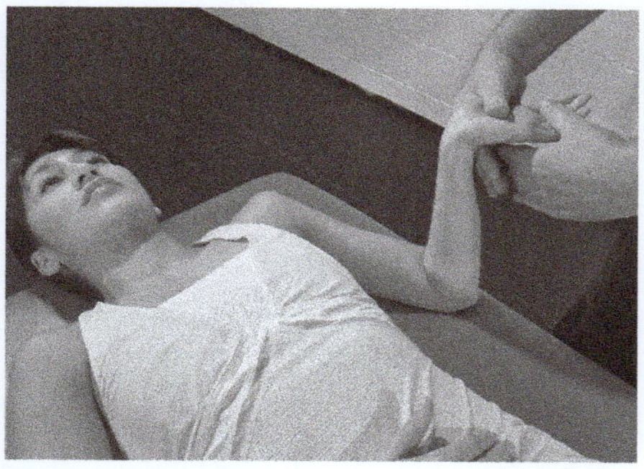

FIGURE 15.26 1. Ulnar nerve bias ULTT

With the patient's elbow flexed and the palm up, extend the fingers and wrist. This stretches the ulnar nerve over the wrist and through the tunnel of Guyon that is between the hook of the hamate and the pisiform.

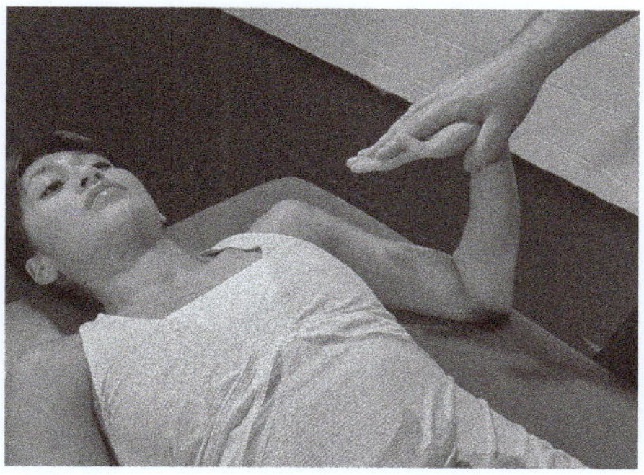

FIGURE 15.27 2. Ulnar nerve bias ULTT

Pronate the forearm by turning the patient's hand so that the fingers point to their shoulder. This further stretches the ulnar nerve from elbow to wrist.

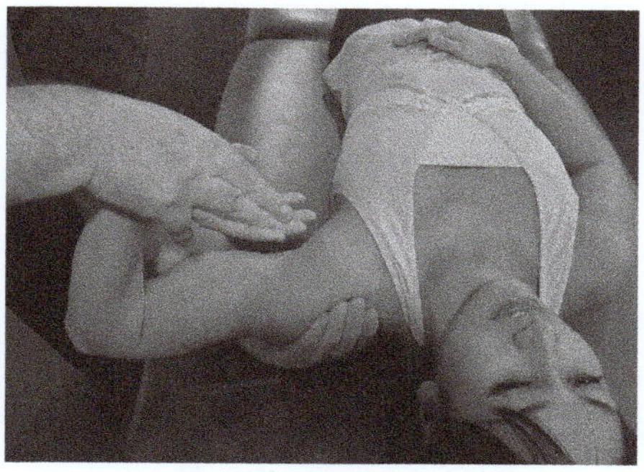

FIGURE 15.28 3. Ulnar nerve bias ULTT

Abduct the patient's shoulder until tension is felt. At this point the patient's palm is facing their ear. This maximizes stretch of the ulnar nerve around the elbow.

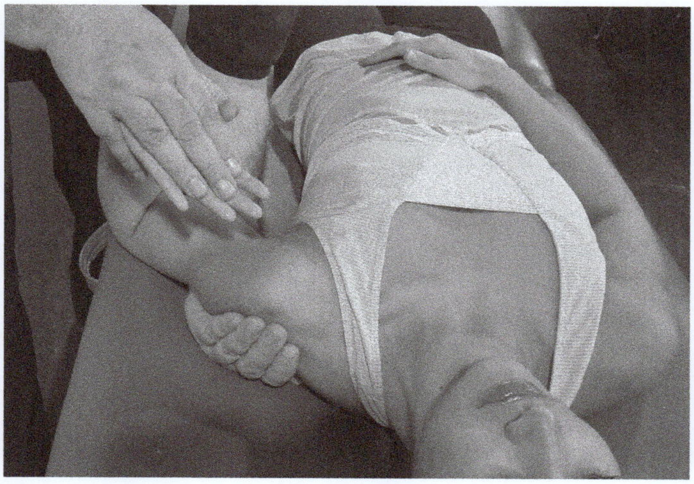

FIGURE 15.29 4. Ulnar nerve bias ULTT

While holding the wrist in extension, use the other hand to slide under the patient's scapula and cup the shoulder, which you draw inferiorly. You may have to then take that hand away, letting the weight of the body hold the shoulder in place; especially if you need to push the elbow down in case it has lifted up off the table. This increases stretch through the brachial plexus area.

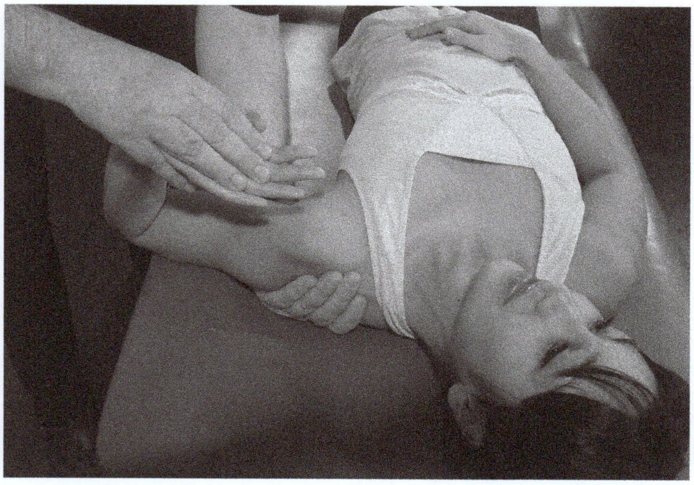

FIGURE 15.30 5. Ulnar nerve bias ULTT

The patient bends (not rolls) the head away from the arm being tested. The nose is pointed toward the ceiling as they side-bend away at the neck. This increases stretch all the way down the nerve but can specifically increase tension from the neural foramen, through scalenes, costoclavicular, and to pectoralis minor apertures.

SHOULDER: CHAPTER OVERVIEW

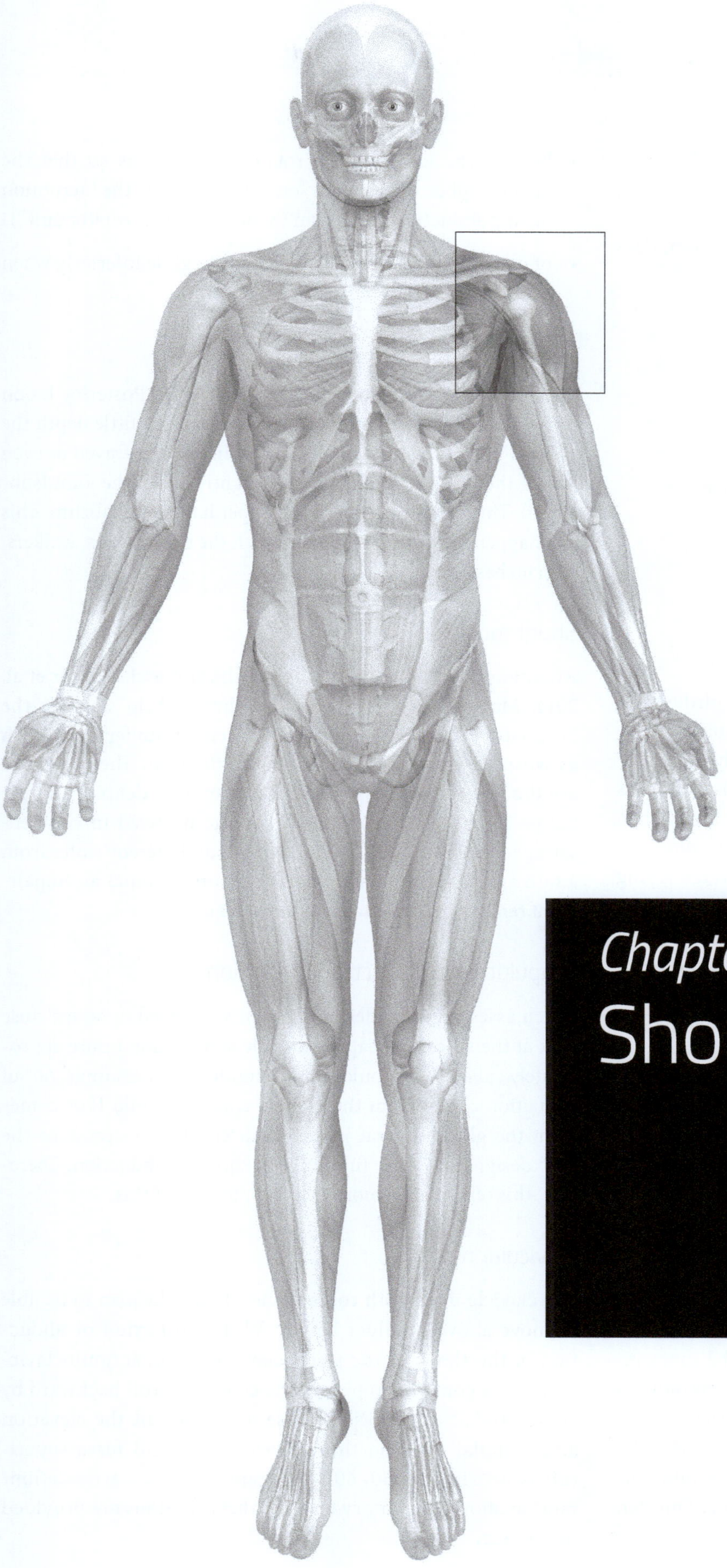

Chapter 16
Shoulder

Clinical implications of anatomy and physiology

The shoulder, or more accurately *the shoulder girdle*, comprises the following:

- humerus
- scapula
- clavicle
- sternum (manubrium).

Between these structures we have the following joints:

- glenohumeral joint (GH)
- scapulothoracic articulation
- acromioclavicular joint (AC)
- sternoclavicular joint (SC).

The great mobility and complexity of the shoulder girdle gives great mobility to the arm at the expense of the stability of the joint and soft tissues (Hertling & Kessler 2006). The interrelationship between these structures and their soft tissue means that we often encounter more than one lesion at a time when dealing with a shoulder injury. Further, numerous complications will inevitably arise from tissues and structures trying to compensate for the original impairment. At times this complexity also makes it difficult to access and pinpoint exactly what tissues are injured and to what degree (sometimes even to know which came first). In chronic or insidious onset situations sorting out primary impairments from their compensations or consequences often can become difficult and confusing (Levangie & Norkin 2011; Magee 2014).

The glenohumeral joint

This is a multiaxial ball-and-socket synovial joint, and it is highly mobile. This extensive range of motion is due to lack of depth in the socket along with laxity of the ligament and joint capsule. This speaks to the joint's lack of stability.

Some stability is achieved by the rotator cuff. The rotator cuff musculature is so called because the tendons of the supraspinatus, infraspinatus, teres minor, and the subscapularis muscles unite around the head of the humerus looking like the cuff of a shirt. This "cuff" of tendons not only helps to stabilize the glenohumeral joint but also helps to guide and move the humerus through several movements required for basic ranges of motion available in the shoulder. For example:

- helping the joint capsule rotate the humerus so that the greater tuberosity moves out from under the acromion during abduction of the arm (hence the term "rotator cuff")
- or assisting the head of the humerus to glide inferiorly when the arm moves above shoulder height.

SLAP lesion

This stands for Superior Labrum Anterior to Posterior lesion or tear. The cartilaginous labrum provides what little depth the glenoid side of the joint possesses. It can become frayed or even torn if the humeral head is forced slightly out of the joint (subluxed). This usually occurs to the upper half of the labrum. This can happen in sports injuries and with the use of canes, walkers, or crutches.

Shunt muscles

Attention should also be paid to the shunt muscles (Agur et al. 2014; Magee 2014). These muscles further help stabilize the humerus in the glenohumeral joint when it is under strain such as when carrying something in/with the arm. These muscles are the coracobrachialis, long head of triceps, deltoid, and the biceps brachii. They commonly become involved in compensating for impaired rotator cuff muscles and thereby suffer from strain and tendonosis the longer (or more chronic) an impairment remains in the rotator cuff complex.

Scapulothoracic articulation/motion

When assessing shoulder impairments, we need to take a close look at the so-called scapulothoracic articulation (more appropriately called the scapulothoracic motion). For example, 60° of abduction comes from the scapula rotating, while 120° comes from the glenohumeral joint, which continue to produce the 180° designated as the full range of shoulder abduction. Therefore, this text offers a more thorough testing of this.

Clavicular motion

The clavicle must both roll and elevate for the arm to be able to move above shoulder height. With full flexion or abduction of the shoulder the sternoclavicular and acromioclavicular joints combine to permit the clavicle to roll backward by about 30–50°. In addition, these joints permit the elevation and scapular rotation that moves the glenoid fossa superiorly approximately 30–60° (see scapulothoracic articulation/motion above). Palpatory tests for these motions are provided in the text.

Thoracic and cervical spine

It is important to observe how these structures participate or react to shoulder girdle movements.

For example, in forward flexion of the shoulder the thoracic spine needs to extend and side-bend slightly away to complete the range of motion. However, excessive motion of the spine can hide impairments of the shoulder. Experience is the best and only way to judge when this is occurring.

Palpation

The following landmarks are important for testing purposes. You should review their anatomy:

- manubrium
- sternoclavicular joint
- clavicle
- acromioclavicular joint
- scapula
- medial and lateral borders, superior, and inferior angles spine of the scapula and the "root of the spine of the scapula," acromion, coracoid process
- humerus; greater and lesser tubercles and also the bicipital groove
- cervical and thoracic spine (spinous processes), and the first six to eight ribs.

Active range of motion of the shoulder

Forward flexion = 160–180°

Extension = 50–60°

Abduction = 160–180°

Adduction = 50–75°

Internal rotation = 60–100°

External rotation = 75–90°

See the Appendices for charts and tables on muscles (muscle origin, insertion, innervation, action, and synergists) joints (actions, ranges, muscles used, tissues stretched and compressed; another table on capsular patterns of restriction open packed/resting positions and close packed positions), and several charts on neurological testing where any such testing would involve this chapter's region.

The protocol (Box 16.1) begins with the case history.

Box 16.1 Protocol

Case history (specific questions)

Observations

Rule outs

Active free range of motion (AF-ROM)

Passive relaxed range of motion (PR-ROM)

Motion testing of the scapula and glenohumeral joint

Active resisted range of motion (AR-ROM)

Special tests

Case history (specific questions)

The following questions should be included in the interview with the patient if these concerns do not come up on presentation:

- Have you previously or just recently been diagnosed with any liver or gall bladder problems? Have you ever injured your diaphragm muscle? (These can refer to the shoulder area.)
- Have you any respiratory problems, asthma, etc.? Chronic bronchitis? Pneumonia?
- Have you ever broken any ribs? ... collar bone? ... or bones in your arm?
- Have you ever dislocated or separated your shoulder?
- Any weakness, numbness or unusual sensations in the arm/hand? Constant? Occasional?

Observations

Regional assessment within the context of the whole

As with every area of the body being investigated by orthopedic testing (specific view), remember to always look at that joint or tissue within the context of the surrounding joints and structures (regional view). What is the interplay of impaired tissues or structures with the rest of the tissues in that region? In turn take into consideration the global view – how are that joint and region affecting the whole body? How is the whole affecting or influencing the region and the specific site(s) of impairment(s)?

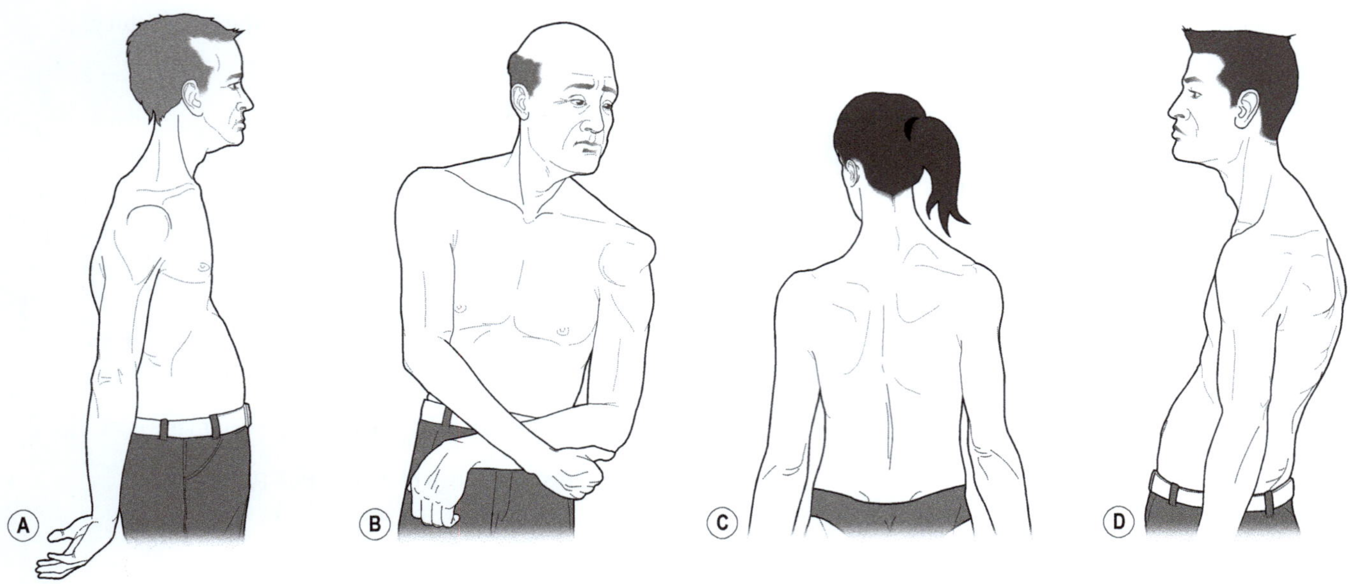

FIGURE 16.1

Left to right: Erb's palsy (paralysis of C5 and C6); dislocation of the humerus; Sprengel's deformity (partially undescended scapula); Scheuermann's disease (significant thoracic kyphosis).

Just as with treatment, the approach to assessment also moves from general-to-specific-to-general.

Not all the preconditions for an impairment exist on-site or in the surrounding region; they can come from the totality of the body the person and their environment.

REMEMBER: Observation begins the moment a patient enters the clinic. Perform a postural scan from each side and from the front and back. Deformities are visible signs of impairment that result from either severe genetic or long-standing conditions. These deformities will have caused clear compensatory changes to the structures in support of those areas.

Note obvious deformities (Figure 16.1) and consider their implications. Is the deformity a contributing factor to the patient's chief complaint?

Observations and inspection

In the lower body look for asymmetries such as in the position and structure of the feet, tibial rotations, varus/valgus, or flexed/extended knees, lateral shifts of the hip, or hip rotations. Check your landmarks for discrepancies side-to-side in height or positioning (e.g., ASISs, PSISs, iliac crests, greater trochanters, ischial tuberosities, posterior crease of the knee, arches of the feet, and orientation of the patellae).

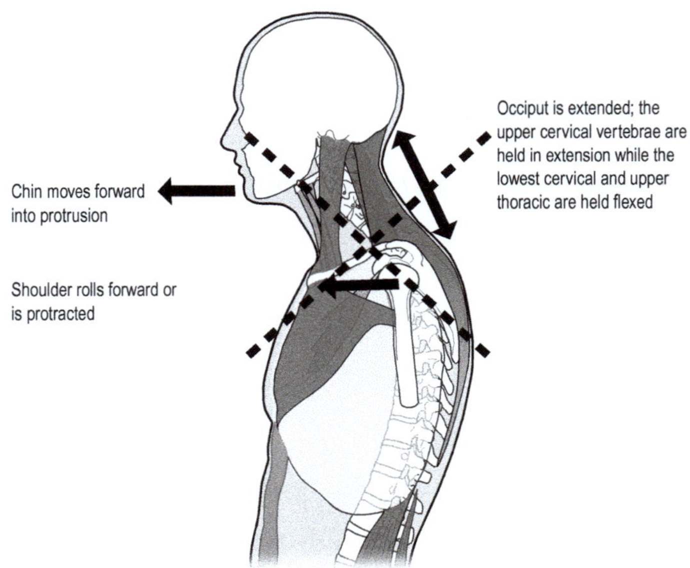

FIGURE 16.2

This diagram can provide insight as to which tissues may be short and which may be long, which muscles may be short and tight, and which are long and weak.

Perform a slightly more thorough scan of the upper body: besides checking for asymmetries of landmarks (such as creases of the waist, inferior, and superior angles of the scapula, acromions, etc.) note from both posterior and lateral views the curves of the spine, head position, and position of the shoulder girdle. These observations can be done separately as a postural examination or these static views can be observed while doing range of motion testing just prior to asking the patient to perform various movements. For an example of what could be observed in a lateral view see Figure 16.2.

The upper cross (X) syndrome (Figure 16.3)

(See Janda & Jull 1987; Janda 1984; Hertling & Kessler, 2006)

Posturally challenging the chief complaint: exploring how the chief complaint fits into the whole (Figure 16.4)

As a final step of observation and inspection look at how the patient naturally stands and correct their posture with gentle movements if possible (e.g., push the hips back, unlock hyper-extended knees, re-position a forward head over the shoulders). Note changes that occur above and below. If the patient can sustain this corrected position then tension or pain that they now experience may point to injured, contractured, weakened, or

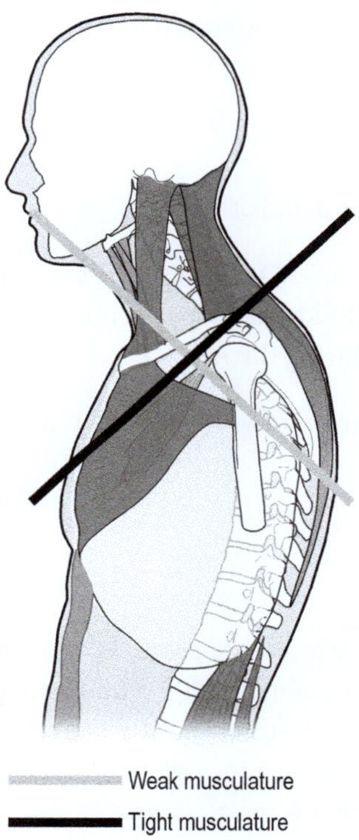

FIGURE 16.3 The upper cross syndrome

Weak

Deep flexors of the neck

Rhomboids, infraspinatus and teres minor, middle and lower trapezium

Tight

Suboccipitals

Upper trapezium and levator scapulae

SCM and scalenes

Teres major and latissimus dorsi

Pectoralis major and minor

Serratus anterior

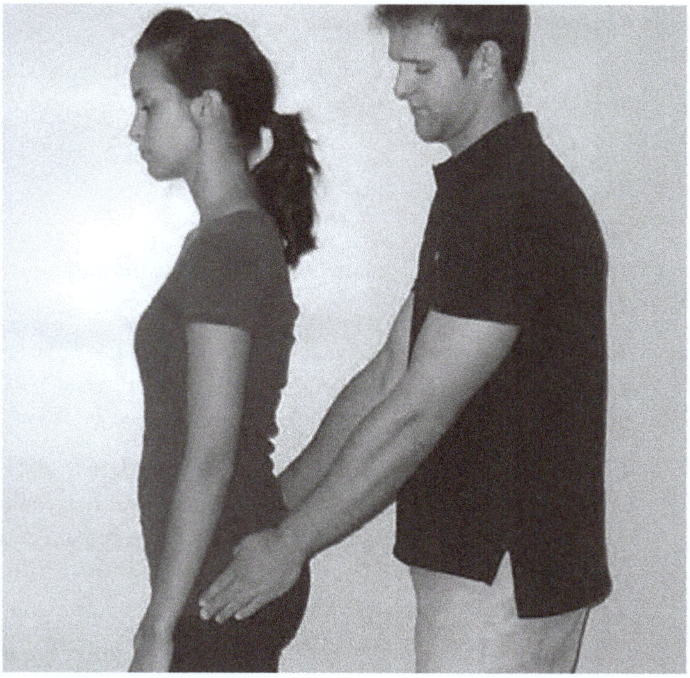

FIGURE 16.4

Observe how the patient naturally stands and correct their posture with gentle movements if possible.

stressed tissues or structures that need to be included in your assessment and treatment. This will help reveal problems that both have a global effect and are intimately connected to specific impairments.

Take note of postural issues especially in the thoracic and cervical spine and their effect on the orientation of the shoulder girdle. For example, protracted shoulders that may accompany a hyperkyphosis will tilt the glenoid fossa downward, which can put more strain on the joint capsule as well as the rotator cuff musculature as they work to stabilize the glenohumeral joint.

Rule outs

The following joints need to be ruled out before testing the shoulder girdle to ensure that their structures are not referring symptoms into the shoulder (Box 16.2).

Cervical spine

(See Chapter 14 for details of these movements.)

This is done by AF-ROM – flexion, rotation, and side bending – followed by over-pressure (O-P) if there was no pain reported with these movements. Finish with extension; do not apply O-P as this could be harmful to anterior and posterior structures.

If neurological signs and symptoms have been noted during the case history taking or when doing the above rule outs a cervical assessment should be carried out. The focus of such testing would be to perform the following neurological tests: Valsalva's test, deep tendon reflexes (DTR), myotomes, dermatomes, a compression and a decompression test, then Kemp's/Spurling's test bilaterally. In turn thoracic outlet syndromes may need to be considered.

The elbow joint

(See Chapter 17 for details.)

This is done by AF-ROM – flexion, extension, pronation, and supination, each followed by performing over-pressures if no pain is reported during the AF-ROM.

Box 16.3 examines why we need to test both sides simultaneously.

Box 16.2 Ruling out the joints above and below the patient's chief complaint

Once you have decided which joint or region of the body you are going to investigate for the source of the patient's chief complaint, you must first rule out the joint above and below.

It is imperative to determine whether the joints/areas above and below the primary joint or region could be referring to the impaired joint or tissue. If a specific rule out test does not reproduce the patient's chief complaint, then that joint is said to be ruled out and not in need of immediate further testing.

REMEMBER: The patient may experience pain or other symptoms or impairments with the rule out testing but if they do not provoke or reproduce the chief complaint then they are set aside and may be returned to at another time.

These quick tests stress the principal tissues involved in each of the joints to be ruled out. They primarily focus on the non-contractile elements. Therefore, you begin by having the patient do specific AF-ROM tests of each joint. When the end-range of each AF motion is reached, ask if the patient is experiencing any pain (even if other than their chief complaint).

If no pain or impairment is present, grasp and support the limbs or structures and tell the patient to relax and let you now move it. You will now apply over-pressure (O-P) as if/when performing passive relaxed range of motion (PR-ROM) testing. It is O-P that stresses the inert or non-contractile tissues of that joint. Having applied the O-P, again ask the patient if they feel any pain or impairment with the O-P.

If no pain is experienced, proceed to the next AF ROM and continue as above. However, if they do experience any pain, etc., then further clarify by asking if the pain is the same as the pain they came to see you about, or something different. If you get a positive reproduction of their chief complaint when doing a rule out, that joint needs to be included in your protocol of testing and considered ruled in. A chief complaint may include more than one joint.

If you get pain with or without other impairments, but these are not part of the patient's chief complaint, then record these but return to your testing of the area indicated by the patient's complaint. These extra findings can be further investigated at a later time. If neither joint reproduces the patient's chief complaint during either the AF-ROM or the PR-ROM with O-P portion of these rule outs, then proceed onward to do the regular AF-ROM testing of the joint or structures that are the focus of the day's testing.

Box 16.3 Why we test both sides simultaneously

With reference to the spine, we need to keep an eye on the thoracic spine and the upper ribcage during AF-ROM. We have to learn by experience to recognize when the patient is compensating for an action by replacing it with excessive movement of nearby joints.

Yet we also need to recognize when we have motion in these nearby joints that would be considered normal occurrences, as they are meant to participate to some degree during the motion of the upper limb.

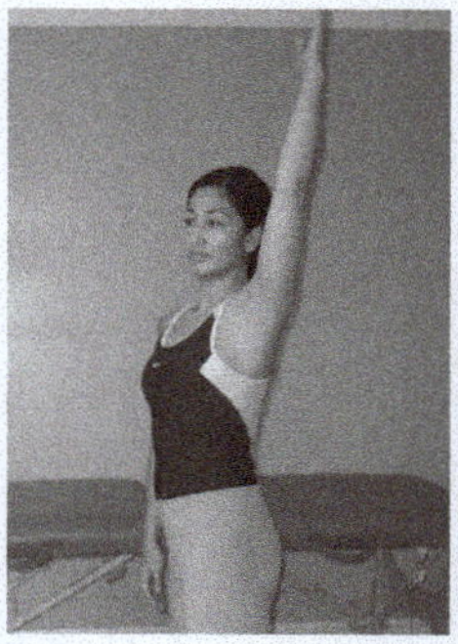

FIGURE 16.5

For example, if you have a patient do forward flexion at the shoulder unilaterally (Figure 16.5), you may see that a lot of the flexion near end-range is actually achieved through rotation and extension in the thoracic spine. Another example is the involvement of the thoracic spine and ribcage in abduction (especially when done unilaterally).

We would see side-bending and rotation of the vertebrae along with opening of the ribs on the ipsilateral side of movement and closure on the contralateral side. It can become hard to judge when such movement is excessive.

Therefore, it is best when testing the shoulder in AF-ROM to have the patient perform flexion, extension and abduction along with internal and external rotations simultaneously with both arms to minimize compensatory motions.

When the patient moves simultaneously we still need to watch carefully. For example, to reach the end-range of forward flexion (sometimes called hyperflexion), the thoracic spine's kyphotic curve has to flatten and the ribcage has to take on the position of inhalation. These can be acceptable motions to occur. However, if we see the thoracic spine reversing its curve, and/or that the motion also moves down into extending the lumbar spine, then we would consider that excessive and compensatory.

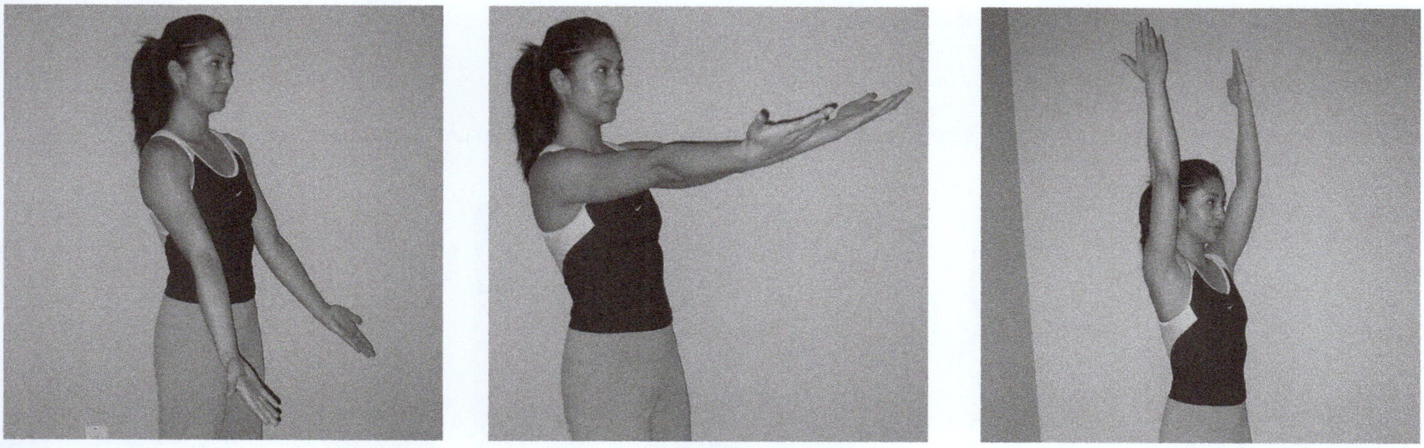

FIGURE 16.6A–C Forward flexion 160–180°

If the shoulder impairment is not acute and ROM is not painful for the patient the therapist may wish to check the movement of the clavicles during forward flexion.

Range of motion testing (ROM)

Active free range of motion (AF-ROM) (Figures 16.6–16.16)

The therapist may wish to demonstrate each motion they are asking the patient to perform and then have the patient follow along.

Take note of whether there is a *painful arc*. The beginning phase of abduction is pain-free, mid-phase painful, and end-phase of motion is pain-free again. This often implies an impingement or compression of tissue between greater tubercle of the humerus and underside of the acromion process. While abducting, the greater tubercle at the head of the humerus may

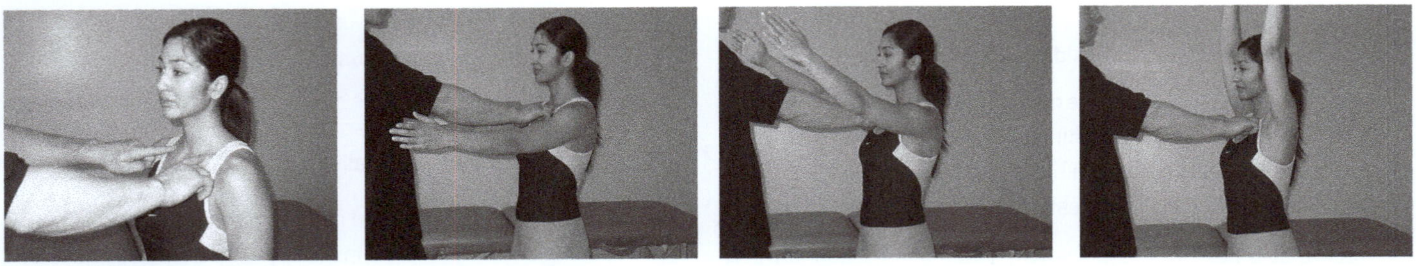

FIGURE 16.7–16.10 Checking clavicular motion

Repeat forward flexion while checking rotation of the clavicles at the same time. Find and palpate mid-point along the length of the clavicle as the patient again performs forward flexion of the shoulder. You should feel the clavicles roll back and sink into the tissue. Again, if pain prevents both done simultaneously then have the patient perform one at a time.

FIGURE 16.11A, B Extension 50–60°

The patient extends both arms with the elbows bent. This allows for more accurate evaluation of joint extension.

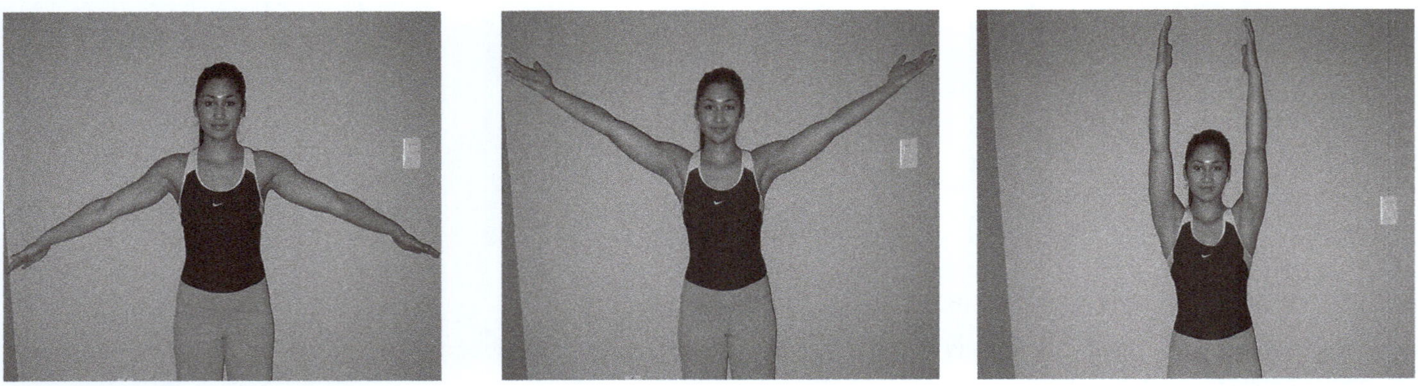

FIGURE 16.12A, B, 16.13 Abduction 160–180°

Have the patient standing with their arms at their sides. First have the patient abduct both arms up as high as they can. If the patient cannot get full range because of pain in the impaired shoulder, then have them abduct the unimpaired side first, then follow with the impaired side. Note the start of any compensatory movements (like side-bending of the trunk). This start of the compensatory movement marks the end of range for abduction.

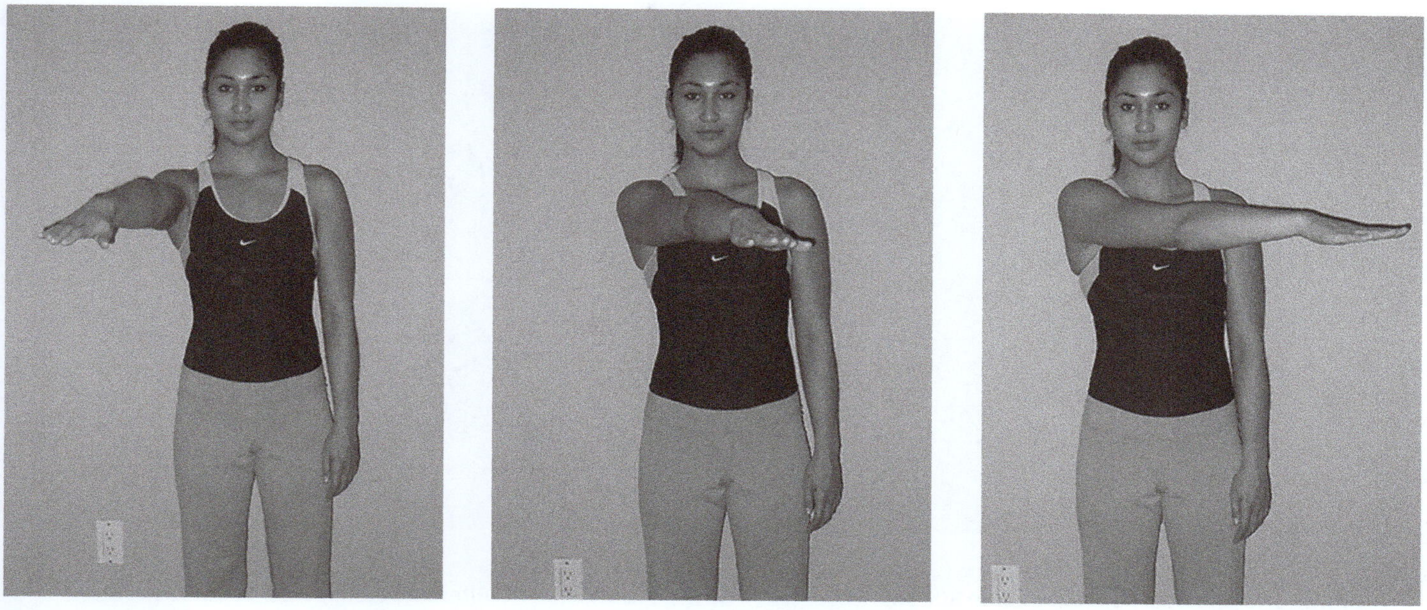

FIGURE 16.14A–C **Abduction (cross adduction) 50–75°**

This is "cross-adduction" where the patient should forward flex the arm up to 90° first and then bring it across the front of the body.

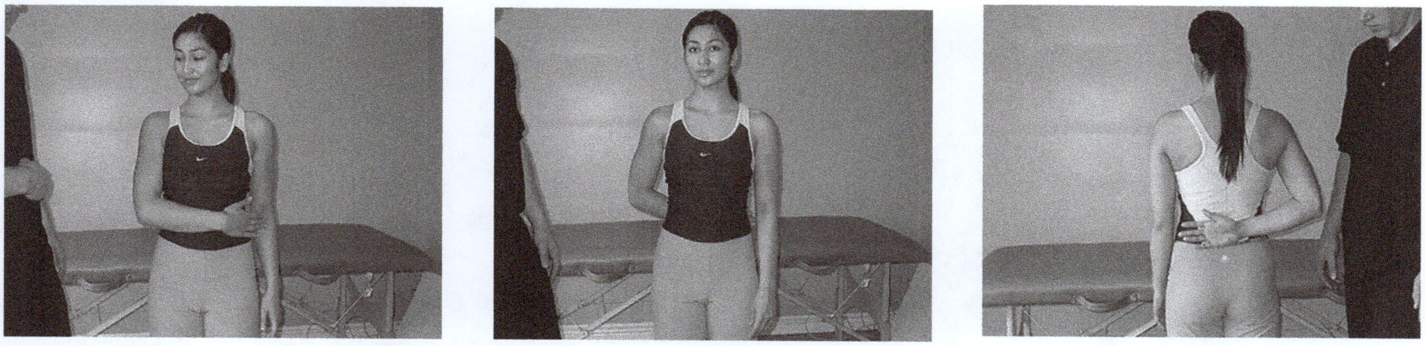

FIGURE 16.15A–C **Internal (medial) rotation 60–100°**

Have the patient bring the arm to the abdomen. If pain-free, take the hand behind the back. The ability to place their hand behind the back gives valuable information about patient's functional abilities with respect to activities of daily life (ADL). This helps up to understand the patient's limitations of daily activities.

not rotate away from under the acromion, pinching a (swollen) bursa or supraspinatus tendon. A test to confirm impingement is described later under special testing.

Alternate testing for rotations (Figure 16.17A, B)

Internal rotation is sometimes done standing as shown in Figure 16.17. This gives the therapist information about the internal rotation available; however, it does not provide an accurate picture of the patient's limitations of daily activities, i.e., loss of ability to dress.

Scapulothoracic articulation (Figures 16.18–16.21)

There are four AF-ROMs of the scapula to investigate: elevation, depression, protraction, and retraction.

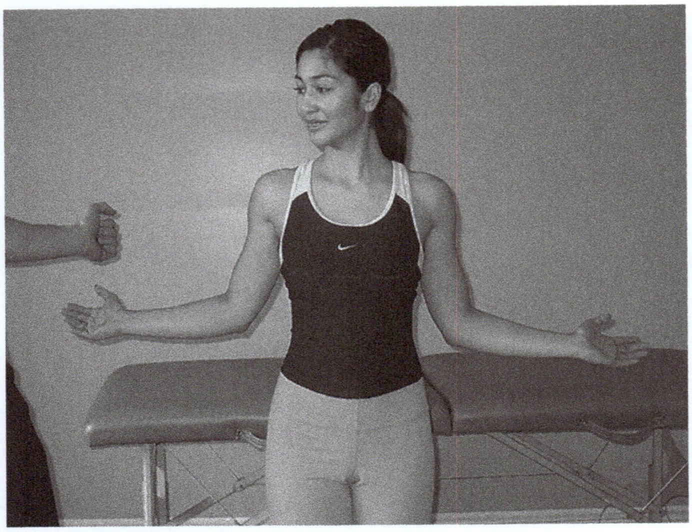

FIGURE 16.16 External (lateral) rotation 80–90°

With elbows bent at 90° and at their sides have the patient turn their arms externally.

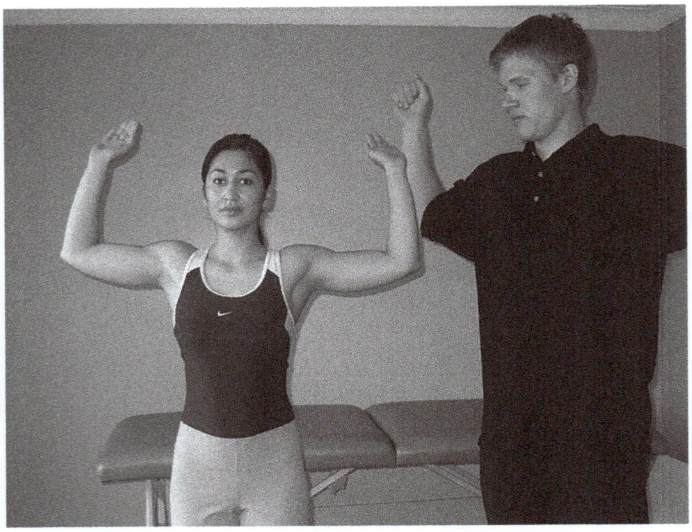

FIGURE 16.17A Alternate testing internal rotation

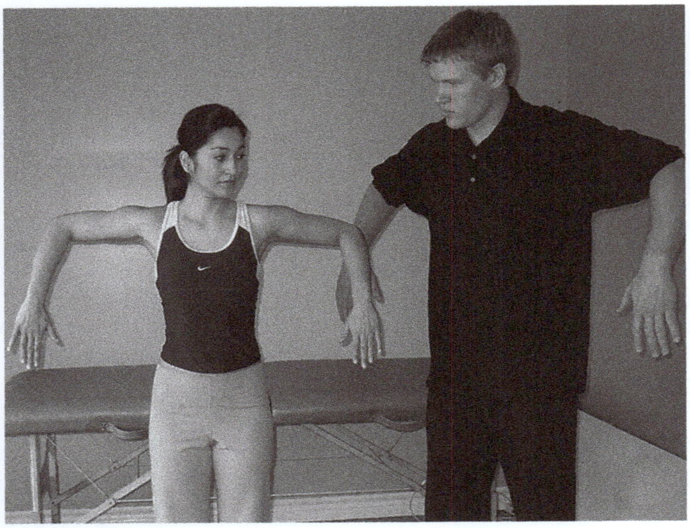

FIGURE 16.17B Alternate testing external rotation 75–90°

Externally rotate the shoulders with elbows flexed to 90°.

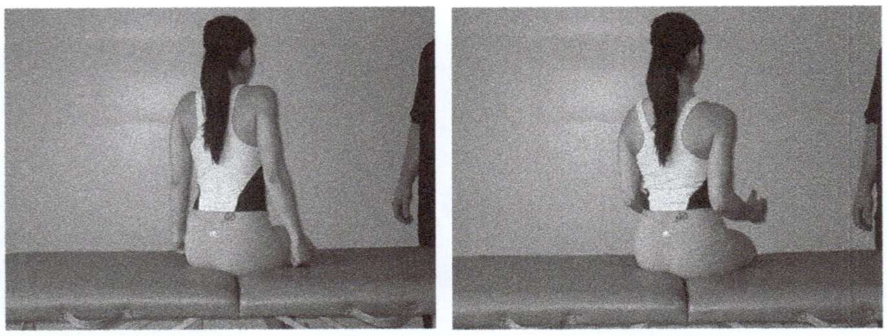

FIGURE 16.18A, B Elevation of shoulder girdle

Have the patient shrug their shoulders and hold. Excessive lateral rotation during this movement indicates the superior angle of the scapulae is fixed or adhered to surrounding tissue. Elevation may be performed with the arms either straight or flexed. If straight, then make sure the patient does not push down on the table to assist in elevating the shoulders.

Apley's scratch test (Figure 16.22A, B)

Once AF-ROM is completed the therapist may have the patient to do Apley's scratch test. This involves a combination of motions through two or more anatomical planes of motion. This tests for functional impairments that can impact on activities of daily living. If you use Apley's scratch test as a quick test and skip some of the tests outlined and you find a restriction or impairment then you need to go back and do the testing in

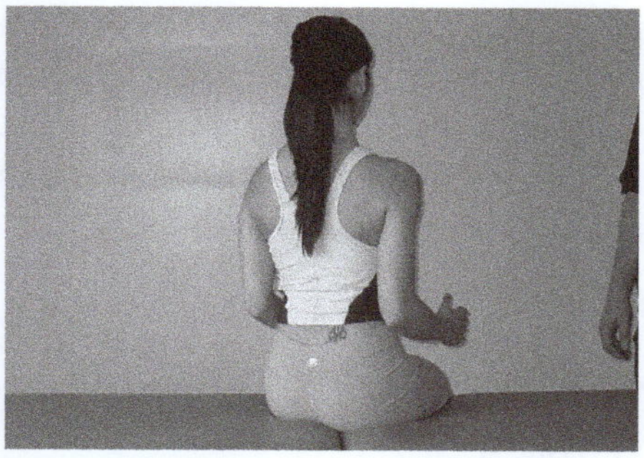

FIGURE 16.19 Depression

Have the patient bring the shoulders down not back as in assuming a military stance. You may ask them to reach straight down toward the ground. Make sure the inferior angle of the scapula moves slightly lower.

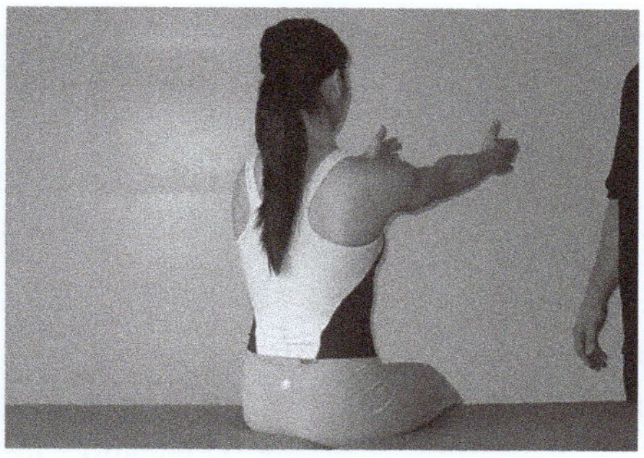

FIGURE 16.20 Protraction

Have the patient roll the shoulders forward or ask the patient to reach forward to touch something just beyond their grasp. The scapula should slide laterally increasing the space between the spinous processes of the vertebral column and the medial border of the scapula.

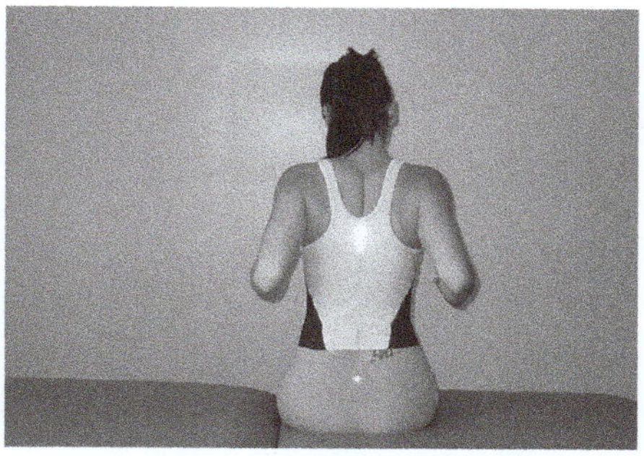

FIGURE 16.21 Retraction

Tell the patient to try to bring the shoulder blades together thereby decreasing the distance between the medial border of the scapula and spinous processes.

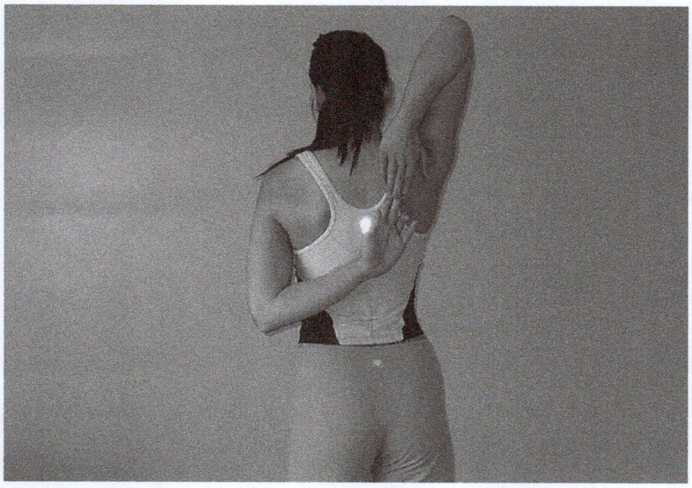

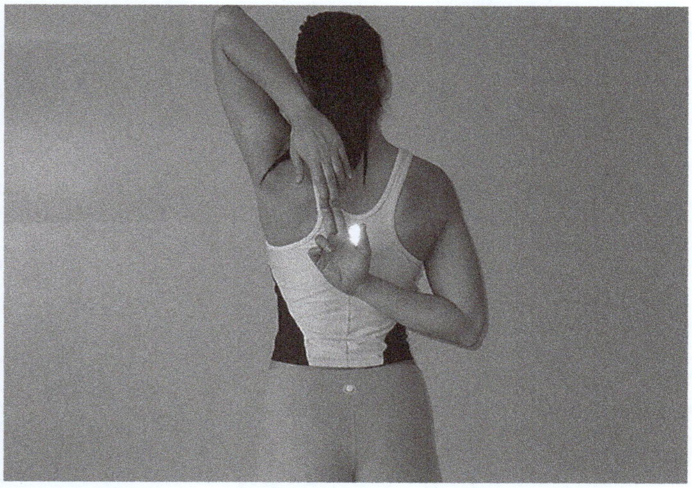

FIGURE 16.22A, B Apley's scratch test

The upper arm is slightly forward flexed, abducted, and externally rotated while the lower arm is adducted, extended, and internally rotated.

single anatomical ranges. Further, if pain has been provoked with this testing any AF-ROM testing may be compromised as the pain may now make the patient more hesitant to complete a motion they might otherwise have available.

There is usually a difference seen when the patient switches arms due to "handedness"; for example, a right-handed person tends to have more mobility in their right shoulder due to it being moved more during the day and into the end-ranges of motion, both of which help keep the tissues soft and pliable or even stretched. However, the left arm/shoulder is often tasked with holding and stabilizing things, usually in mid-range. Therefore, the left shoulder may not be used as much as the right and usually moves through the day in a manner that avoids going anywhere near end-range. Because of this tissues on the left shoulder are often shortened and usually stronger in mid-range.

Left-handed people are more symmetrical because they are forced to use their right hand since they live in a right-handed world. The dominant side, or motor side of the body, often has greater range flexibility and dexterity but it can be weaker. If the person exercises in a way that impacts both sides of the body equally they may not clearly display a dominant side.

Passive relaxed range of motion (PR-ROM) (Figures 16.23–16.34)

When over-pressure is applied do not change the basic orientation of the joint and try not to engage or move other surrounding tissues or structures any more than is necessary.

Begin testing with the patient seated on a stool so that you can have a high enough position to move their arm freely and confidently. Take note of any crepitus as you move the joint. When end-range has been reached (and only if there is no pain) apply slight over-pressure to determine the joint's end-feel.

End-feels are as follows:

- forward flexion – normally tissue stretch
- extension – normally tissue stretch
- internal rotation – normally tissue stretch
- external rotation – normally tissue stretch
- abduction – normally bone-to-bone or tissue stretch
- cross-adduction – normally tissue approximation.

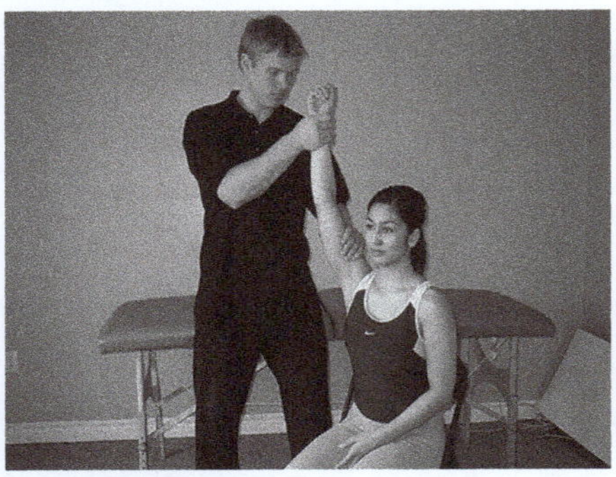

FIGURE 16.23 Forward flexion

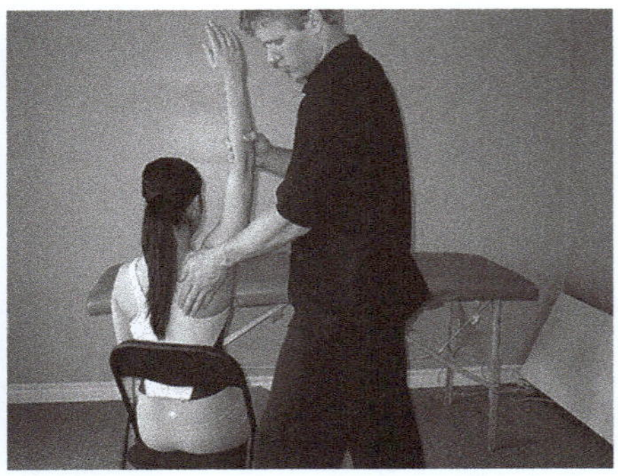

FIGURE 16.24 Forward flexion with O-P

Stabilize scapula. Take the shoulder into hyperflexion. End-feel is normally tissue stretch.

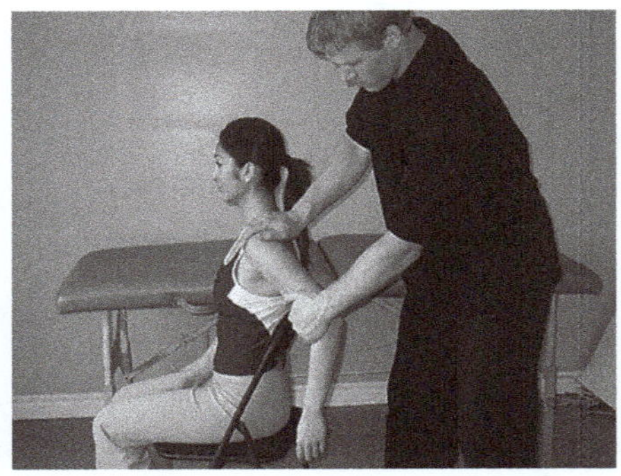

FIGURE 16.25 Extension

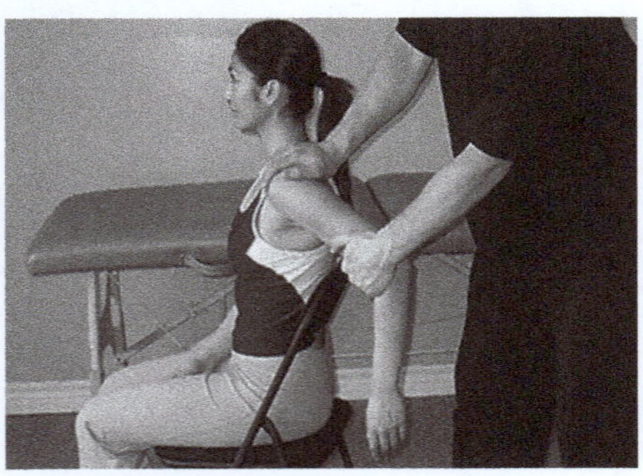

FIGURE 16.26 Extension with O-P

Stabilize the scapula and continue movement while applying O-P. End-feel is normally tissue stretch.

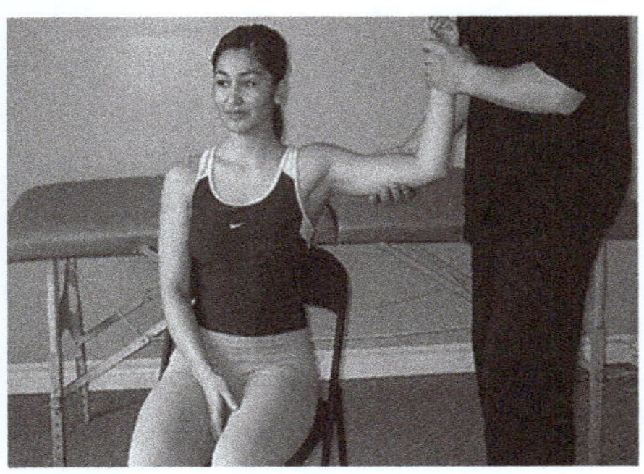

FIGURE 16.27 External rotation

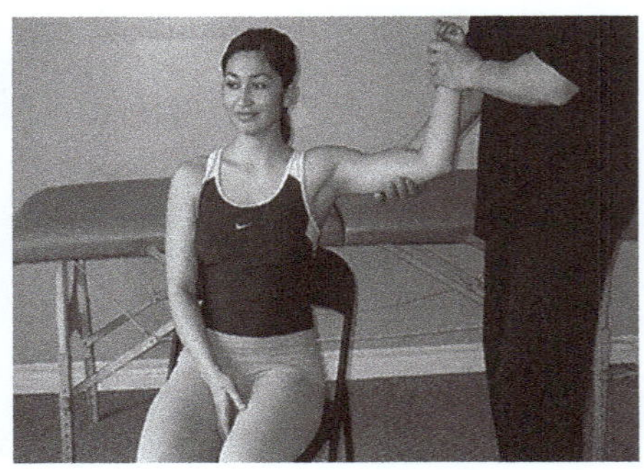

FIGURE 16.28 External rotation with O-P

Stabilize the arm and continue movement while applying O-P. End-feel is normally tissue stretch.

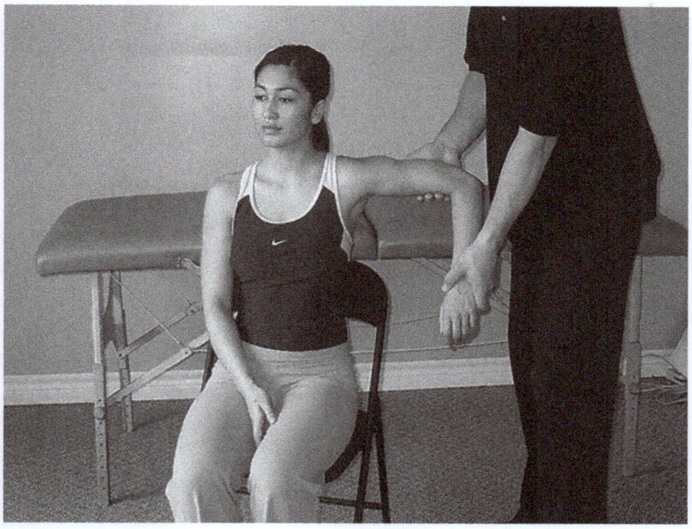

FIGURE 16.29 Internal rotation

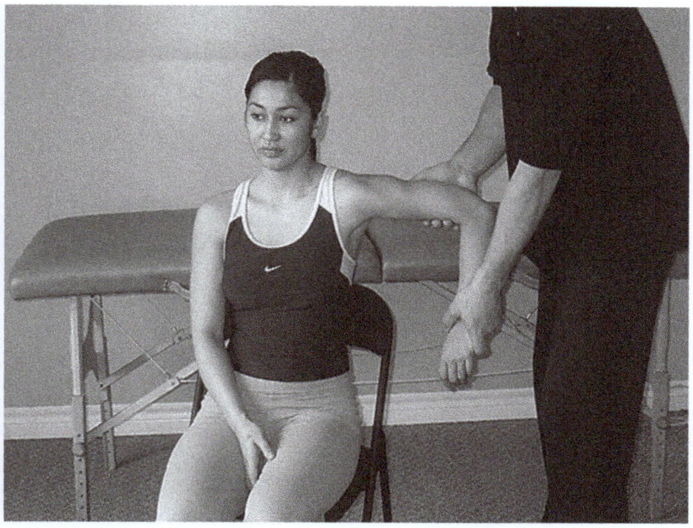

FIGURE 16.30 Internal rotation with O-P

Stabilize the arm and continue movement while applying O-P. End-feel is normally tissue stretch.

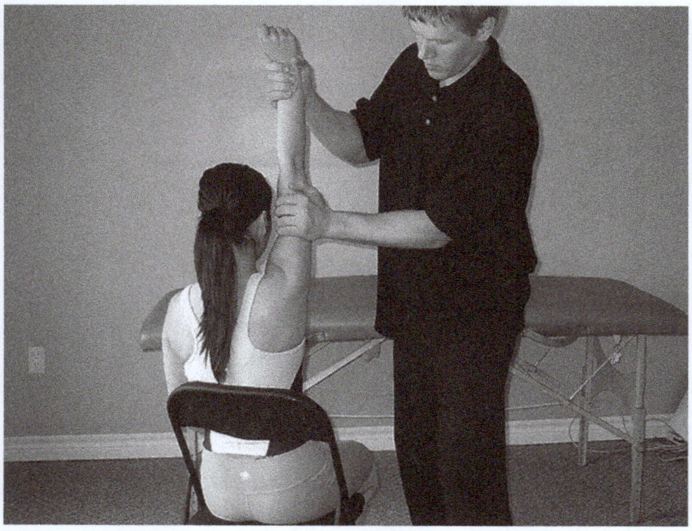

FIGURE 16.31 Abduction

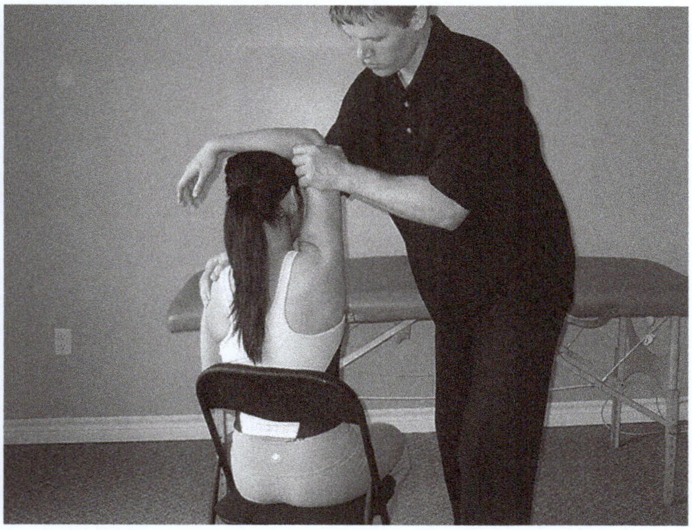

FIGURE 16.32 Abduction with O-P

Stabilize the opposite shoulder while applying O-P. End-feel is normally bone-to-bone or tissue stretch.

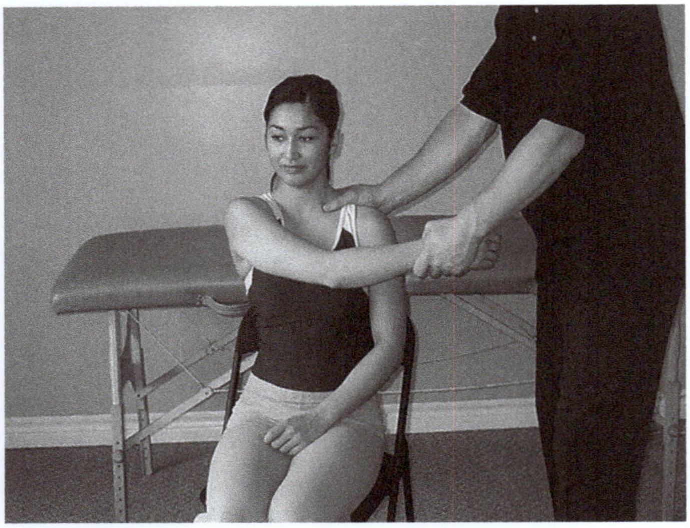

FIGURE 16.33 Cross-abduction

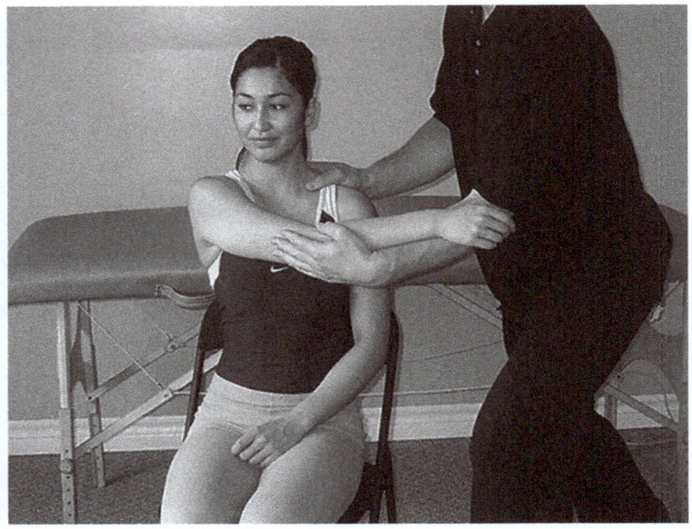

FIGURE 16.34 Cross-abduction with O-P

Stabilize the opposite shoulder while applying O-P. End-feel is normally tissue approximation.

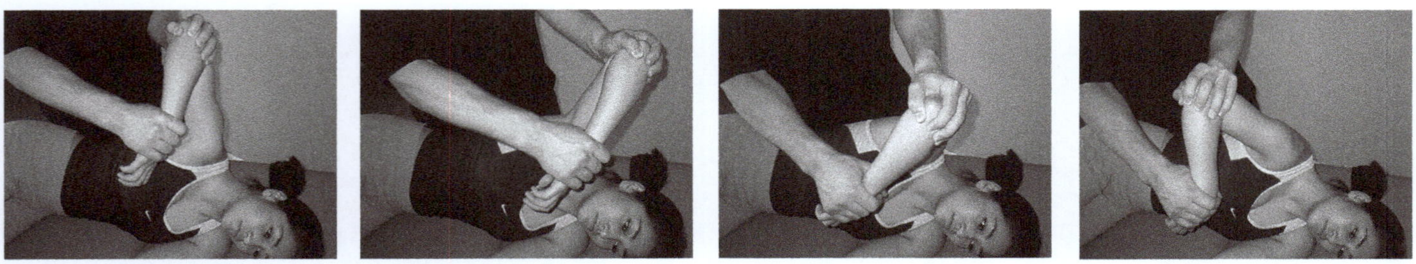

FIGURE 16.35A–D Scouring test for shoulder

Apply pressure through the flexed elbow down into the joint. Slowly circumduct two or three times clockwise and then repeat counter-clockwise.

Circumduction with over-pressure (Figure 16.35A–D)

Apply circumduction with over-pressure to test the glenohumeral joint surfaces. This is sometimes regarded as a special test known as the scouring test.

Positive (+) sign of dysfunction is a feeling of roughness, bumps, or jumps felt by the therapist and/or pain felt by the patient within the joint. Further investigation is required.

Assessing the acromioclavicular and sternoclavicular joints (Figures 16.36A, B, 16.37A, B)

This is the time to test the acromioclavicular (AC) and sternoclavicular (SC) joints, unless impairments found so far would indicate that such testing is compromised. It is best to test these joints now so you can begin to make sense of any impairments seen up to this point. Also, the therapist needs to know if these joints have impaired function so that testing of specific structures does not produce confusing results by these joints causing false positives.

The first test suggested below for AC joint dysfunction will also place sufficient stress through the SC joint to reveal any dysfunction there. The testing is done by placing a shear force through the AC joint and a compressive force through the SC joint.

Alternative shear test

This test can be done if the patient cannot tolerate the position of cross-adduction needed in the first test. It also stresses the AC joint (and only slightly stresses the SC joint) but does so with less involvement of other tissues and other component joints of the shoulder. It is often listed as a special test.

Joint play inspection of the glenohumeral joint

Note excess motion or a complete lack of motion (or "give"). Have the patient tell you immediately about discomfort pain or any altered sensation *during and after* each application of mobilization.

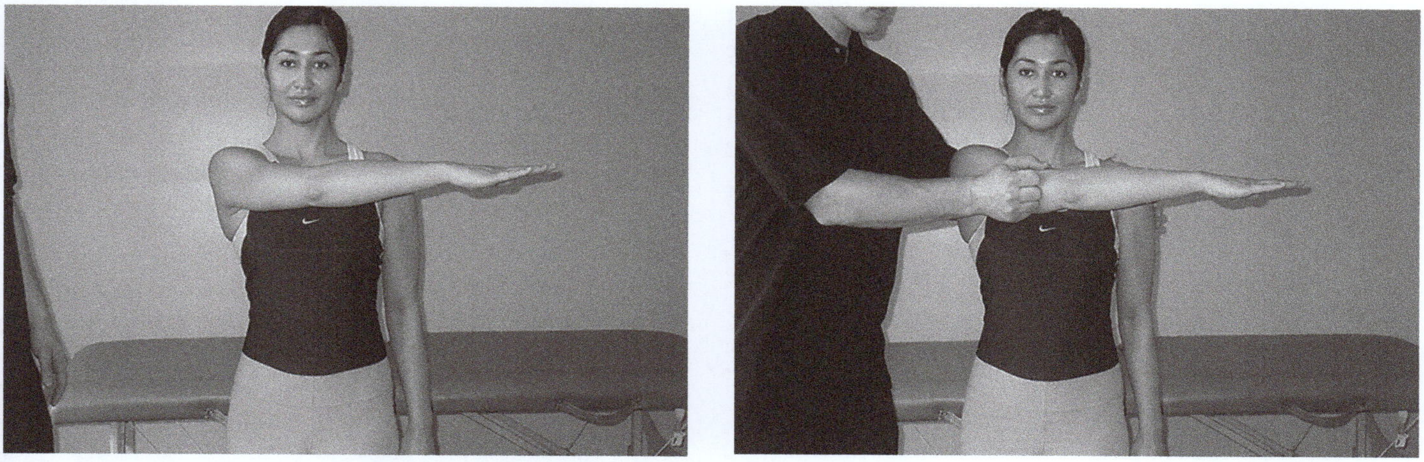

FIGURE 16.36A, B Assessing AC and SC joints

Have the patient standing or seated on a low stool. Have the patient cross-adduct arm (at 90° of flexion) and if pain-free apply O-P. Ask the patient to report pain and point to where it is. Positive test is pain in the joint and/or abnormal movement of the clavicle.

NOTE: The therapist stabilizes the patient through the contralateral shoulder in this position.

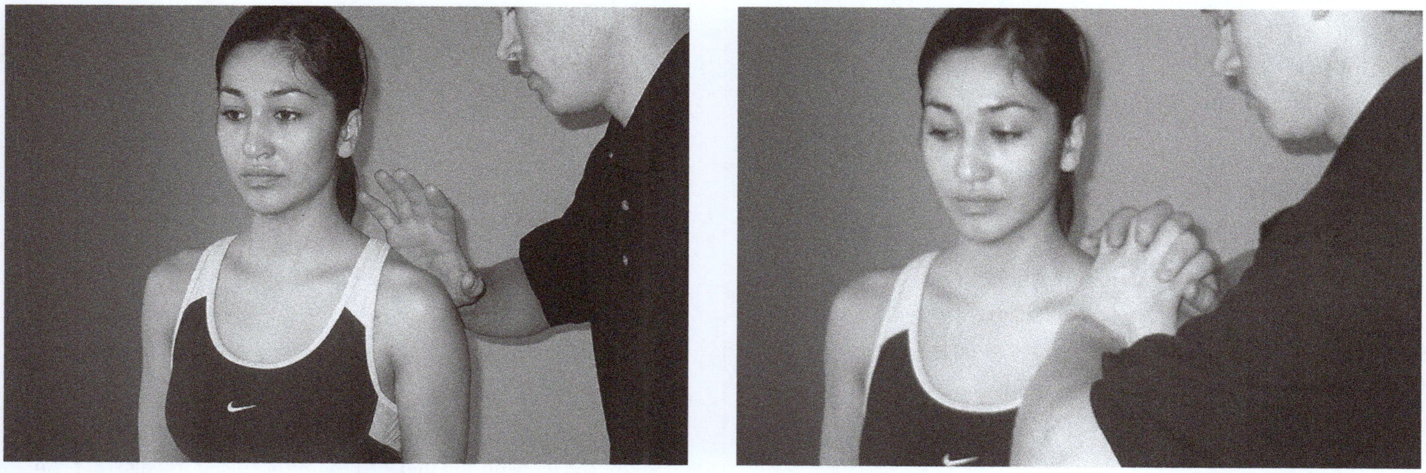

FIGURE 16.37A, B Assessing AC joint

With the patient seated, the therapist puts the base of the hand (pisiform to base of thumb) along the spine of the scapula. The therapist next places the base of the other hand along the middle-to-lateral portion of the clavicle. Interlace the fingers. Apply a squeeze to put a shear force through the AC joint. To place more stress on the SC joint move the anterior hand on the clavicle more medially. The positive sign is pain, hypermobility (laxity), and hypomobility (stiffness). The negative sign (normal) is a firm springiness.

In most joints mobilization tests of the accessory motions available are in general going to be stressing ligaments and joint capsules. Because of the laxity of the ligaments in the shoulder (to allow for the large ranges of motion) the four rotator cuff muscles and the "shunt muscles" can often take the brunt of the force of shearing/gliding motions involved in joint mobilization techniques. (For more on the rotator cuff and shunt muscles see the anatomy and physiology review at the beginning of this chapter.)

Therefore, especially when testing the glenohumeral joint with mobilizations, the therapist needs to keep in mind that the restrictions found in joint mobilizations (or assessing joint play) need not necessarily come from intrinsic structures of the joint (joint capsules or ligaments) but may also be caused by hypertonus in muscle(s) that prevent movement in either general or accessory joint motions under assessment.

(For more details and instruction see Part I, Chapter 3. See the following for even more information and optional positioning of patient or limb and variations or additional tests: Edmond 2006; Hertling & Kessler 2006; Kaltenborn 2006; Kisner & Colby 2012; Magee 2014; Starkey & Brown 2015.)

Box 16.4 Follow rules of joint mobilization techniques

This form of passive testing is specific to glide, one of the accessory movements within the shoulder that contributes to the voluntary motions observed during ROM testing, or any joint movement. For example, when the shoulder abducts at the glenohumeral (GH) joint, the humerus must roll superiorly and also glide inferiorly on the joint surface of the glenoid fossa.

Follow the rules that you have learned for joint mobilization techniques to ensure both the safety of the patient and clear results of testing (see Chapter 3, pp. 43-46).

NOTE: The information that follows does not constitute complete instruction in joint mobilization techniques. The purpose is to remind those trained in the use of joint mobilization which movements or glides need to be tested when specific anatomical motions are seen to be restricted in the patient during ROM testing. Having found restrictions, the appropriate use of the testing technique can transform it into a treatment technique.

The author strongly encourages all students of massage to get appropriate training in joint mobilization techniques in order to increase the effectiveness of their assessment and treatment skills.

Always try to use body-weight (rather than pulling or pushing from the shoulders) to move the limb. Remember the orientation of the glenoid fossa; it faces laterally and slightly anteriorly and superiorly. Ask about pain or any other symptoms and take note of both the quality and quantity of motion available in the joint.

Box 16.4 has some suggestions for learning joint mobilization techniques.

Positive signs of joint play testing (Figure 16.38–16.42)

Pain and/or restriction in, or loss of, joint play are all signs of joint dysfunction. If loss of abduction is seen during ROM testing the inferior glide of the GH joint, then the inferior glide of the AC and SC joints, the lateral glide of the AC, and compression of the SC joints should also be tested.

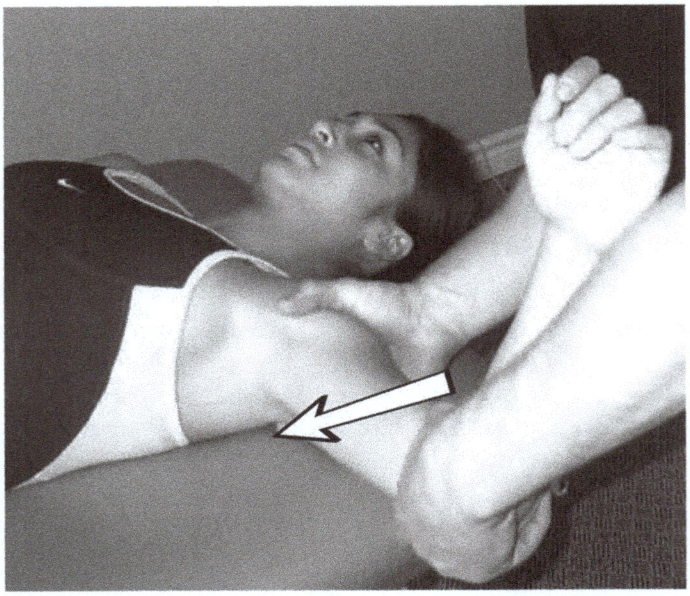

FIGURE 16.38 Inferior glide of GH joint

Abduct the patient's arm 90°. The therapist stands above and to side of the test shoulder. With the hand closest to the joint encircle the superior portion of the head of the humerus close to the GH joint line. Stabilize the arm at the elbow to keep the humerus level during glide. Remember to slightly distract the joint first then press slowly but firmly in an inferior direction. The positive sign for joint capsule restriction for inferior glide is pain or loss of joint play (no slack available in an inferior direction). This positive sign means joint capsule restriction or adhesions are contributing to a loss of abduction in shoulder.

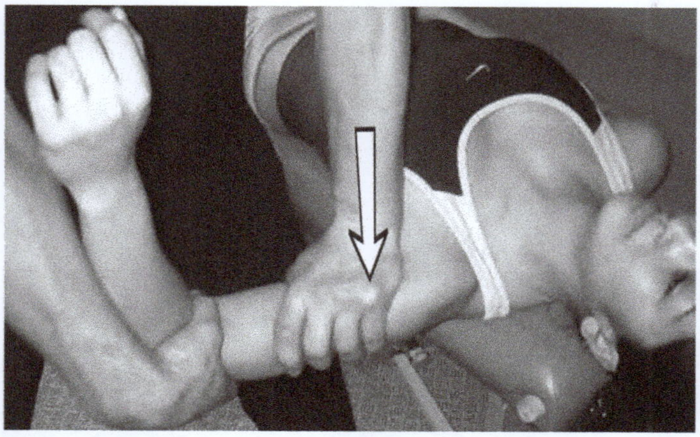

FIGURE 16.39 Posterior glide of GH joint

Have the patient supine with the arm abducted to 90°. Have the scapula on the table but have the head of the humerus (up to and including the joint line) off the table. Stabilize at the elbow to keep the humerus level during glide "gap" or distract the joint and apply a firm posterior pressure through the head of the humerus, taking the whole arm with it. When loss of flexion or internal rotation is seen during ROM testing check for restriction in posterior glide of the GH joint.

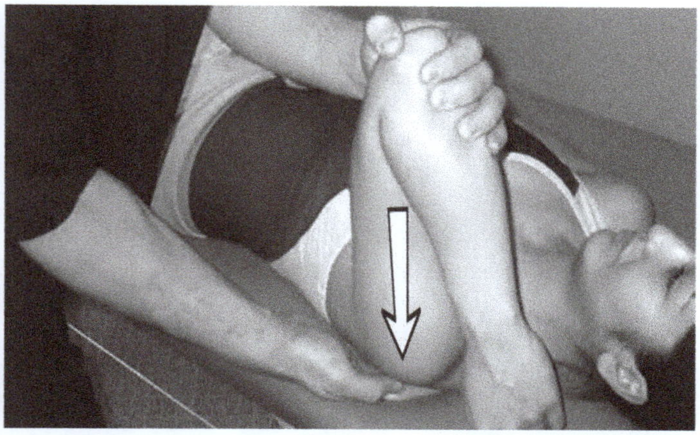

FIGURE 16.40 Alternative posterior glide of GH joint

This version is more specific for internal rotation. The inferior hand is stabilizing the scapula (with the assistance of the table). The other hand encircles the flexed elbow and applies a downward pressure. Movement of the head of the humerus will be also be felt in the palm of the therapist's stabilizing hand. This is a good position to test (or treat and stretch) the posterior fibers of the joint capsule.

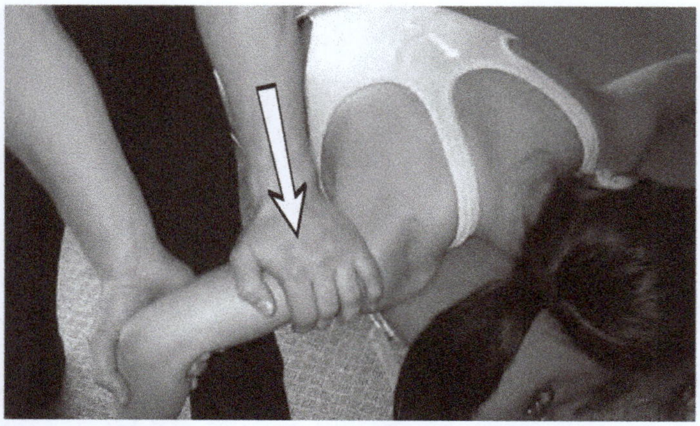

FIGURE 16.41 Anterior glide of GH joint

For loss of extension and/or external rotation seen during ROM testing check anterior glide and acromioclavicular superior glide. Position the patient prone on the table with the arm and GH joint line off table. Anterior movement of the scapula is blocked. Stabilize the arm at the elbow to keep the humerus level during glide. Distract the joint. Use firm pressure as usual. This position blocks anterior motion in the chest keeping glide or translatory motion cleanly through the joint.

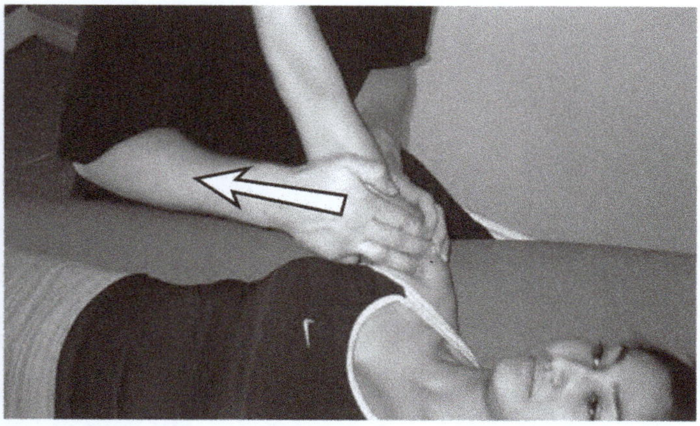

FIGURE 16.42 Dynamic testing of inferior glide

(and treatment technique to increase glide). Encircle the head of the humerus with the fingers and ask the patient to press their straightened arm down onto the therapist's shoulder. You should feel the humeral head move inferiorly as the muscles engage. If movement is limited then the therapist can repeat while adding pressure in an inferior direction to help the muscles inferiorly glide the head of the humerus.

Joint play inspection of the clavicle and associated joints (Figures 16.43–16.49)

Glides for the SC joint

The following glides are designed to test the motions available to the SC joint.

Glides for the AC joint

The following glides are designed to test the motions available to the AC joint.

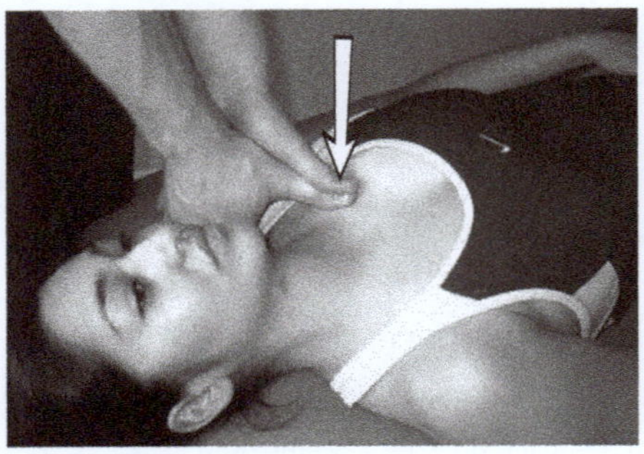

FIGURE 16.43 Posterior glide of clavicle through SC joint

Place the thumb on the clavicle, just before the joint with the manubrium. Press downward into the table.

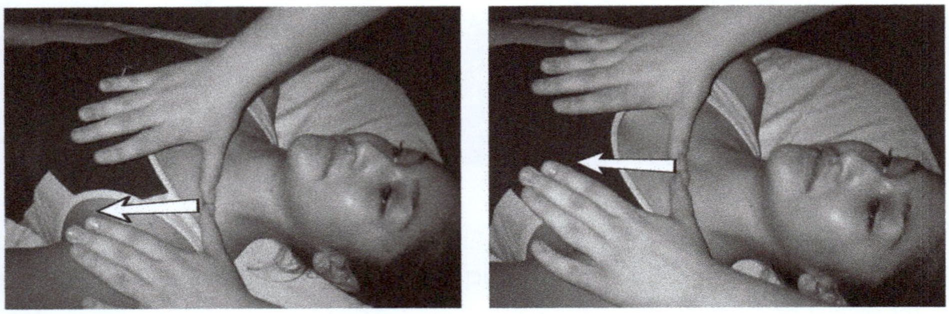

FIGURE 16.44A, B Inferior glide of AC and SC joints

Place the thumbs on the superior lateral surface of the clavicle and move inferiorly appropriately. To stress the SC joint more move the thumbs over to the medial and superior surface of the clavicle.

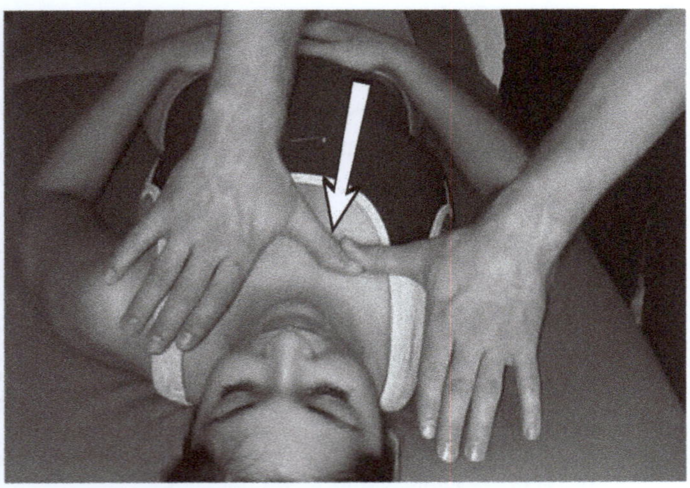

FIGURE 16.45 Superior glide of AC joint and SC joint

To generate superior glide of the AC joint (and SC joint) place the thumbs on the inferior surface of the clavicle. Shifting the thumbs more laterally will add more pressure through the AC joint, while moving the thumbs to a more medial portion on the clavicle will put a more specific motion through the SC joint.

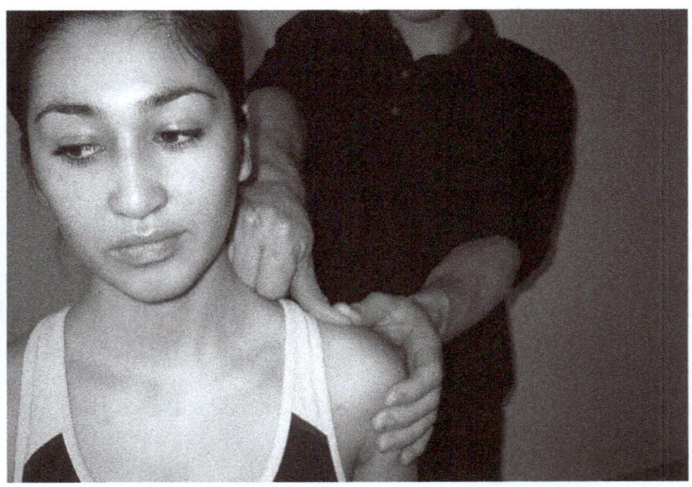

FIGURE 16.46 Anterior glide of AC joint

Seated position. Press anteriorly on the lateral end of the clavicle.

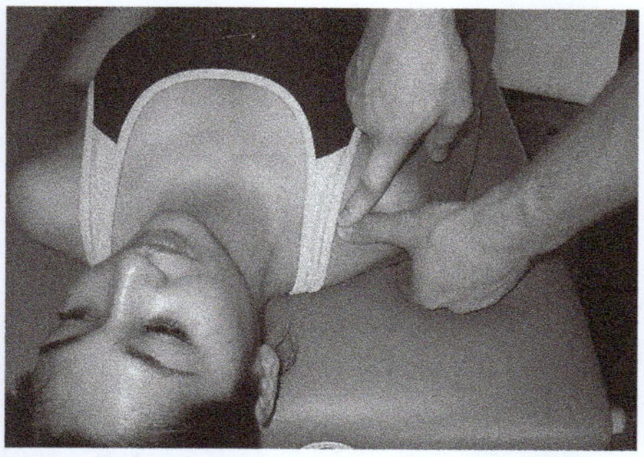

FIGURE 16.47 Posterior glide of AC joint

Press posteriorly on the lateral end of the clavicle.

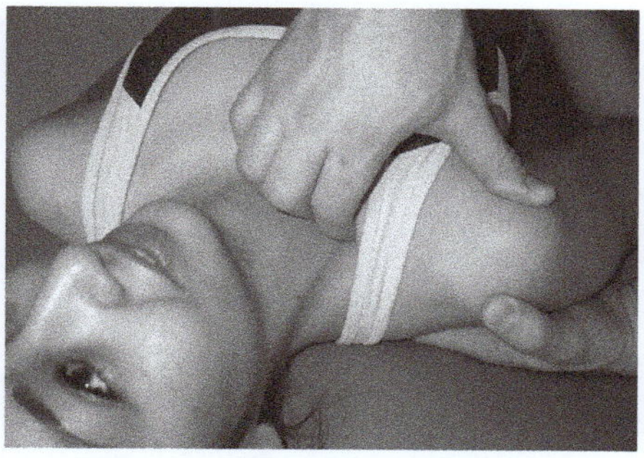

FIGURE 16.48 Inferior/anterior glide of both AC and SC joints

Slip the fingers under the clavicle; pull anteriorly and inferiorly. You may need to side-bend head toward the side being tested to slacken the musculature above the clavicle so that you can grasp it.

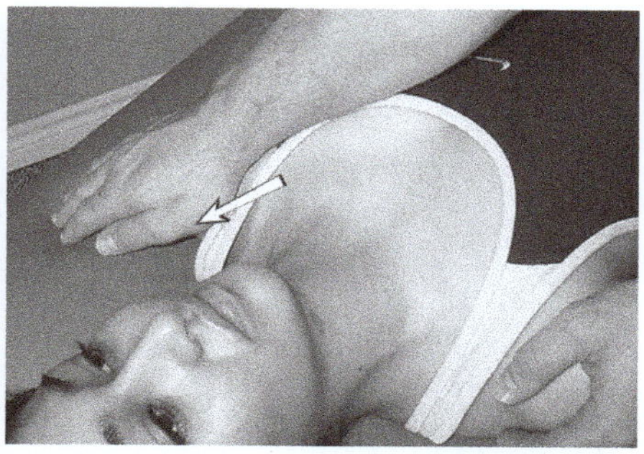

FIGURE 16.49 Lateral glide of AC joint and distraction of SC joint

Lightly grasp the shoulder not being tested to stabilize. Place the palm of the other hand over the lateral third of the clavicle being tested. Push along the shaft of the clavicle as if trying to push it diagonally off the acromion.

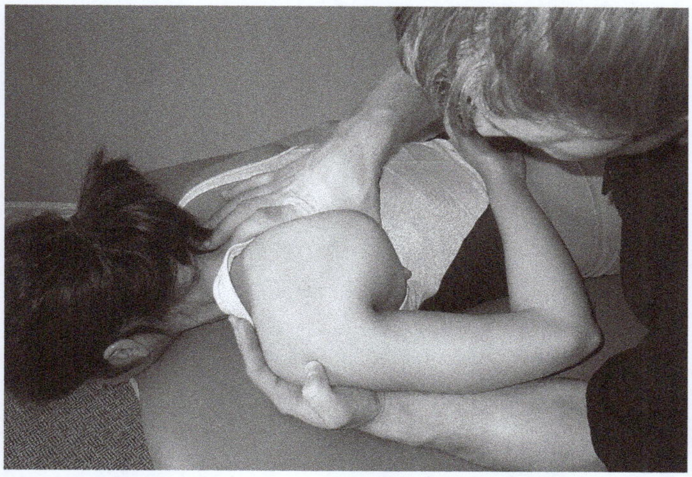

FIGURE 16.50 Lifting scapula off wall of trunk

The patient has their hand behind their back. Slip your fingers under the medial and inferior border of the scapula. Cup the anterior shoulder and lift off the trunk.

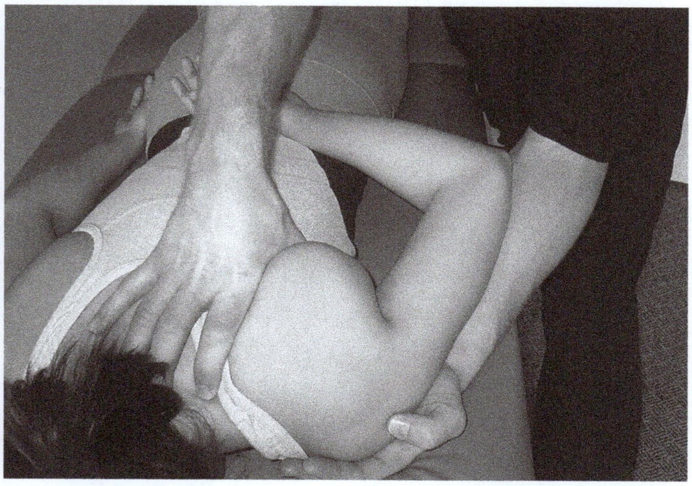

FIGURE 16.51 Inferior glide of scapula

Slip the fingers under the medial and inferior border. Cup the anterior shoulder. Lift and push the scapula inferiorly.

Joint mobilizations of the scapula (Figures 16.50–16.55)

Motion testing of the scapula and glenohumeral joint (Figures 16.56–16.62)

This motion testing is designed to clarify the relationship between scapulothoracic motion and the glenohumeral joint in shoulder dysfunctions. If it has been noted that there is a dysfunction with abduction or flexion then these tests need to be done in order to see how much loss of ROM is due to loss from the glenohumeral joint specifically and how much is from the scapula's own impairments. Note that these are not meant as provocation tests but are more in line with motion testing.

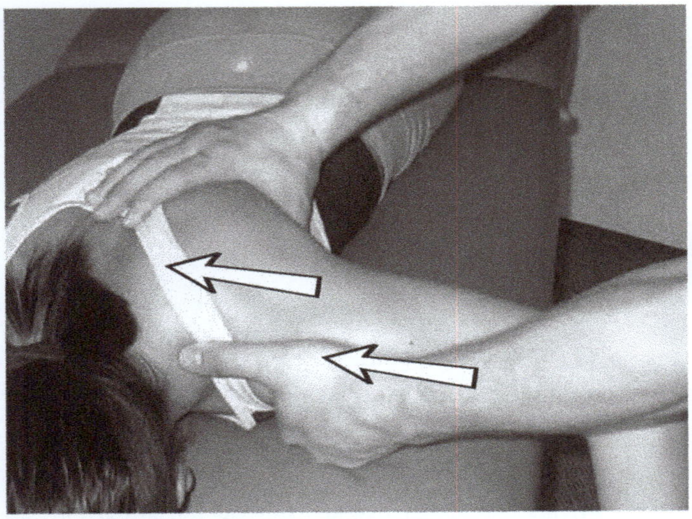

FIGURE 16.52 Medial glide of scapula

With the hands move the scapula as a whole medially.

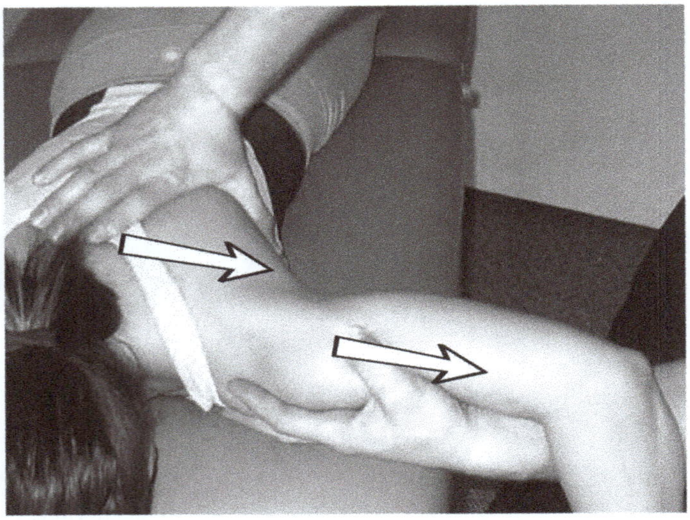

FIGURE 16.53 Lateral glide of scapula

With the hands pull the scapula and arm laterally.

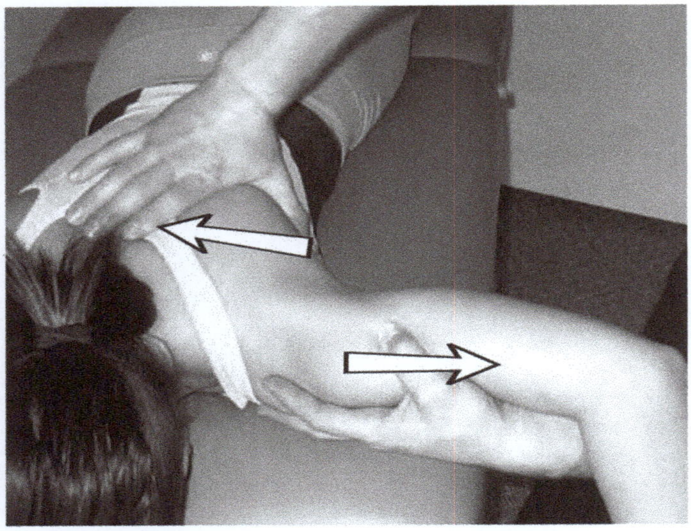

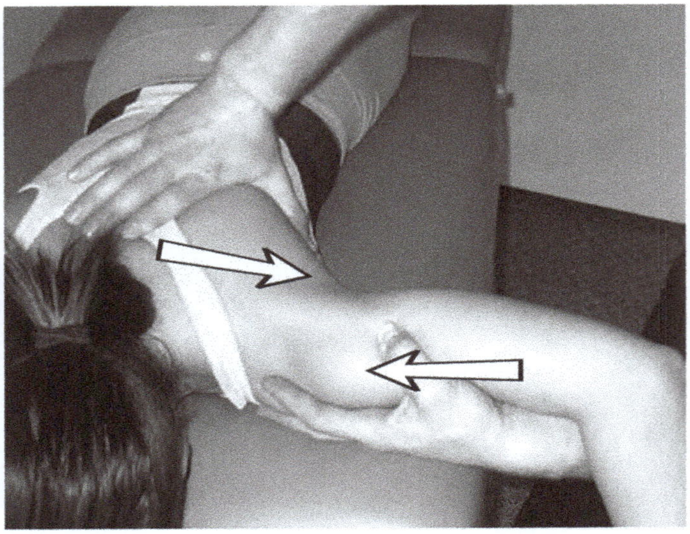

FIGURES 16.54, 16.55 Rotation of scapula

To assess rotation of the scapula, engage tissue as shown above. Step 1: Have the inferior and superior hands go in opposite directions. Step 2: Reverse directions. This will check both the lateral and the medial rotation of the scapula.

Motion test 1

This test is designed to investigate if the rotator cuff musculature is engaging appropriately during AF-ROM. A positive sign is that the scapula (and hence the musculature) engages too early or too late on abduction of the scapula.

Motion test 2

This test is used to investigate if the rotator cuff musculature is engaging appropriately during passive relaxed motion. This can help clarify tissues involved in active free motion dysfunctions. Positive signs include: (1) noting that the scapula is moving

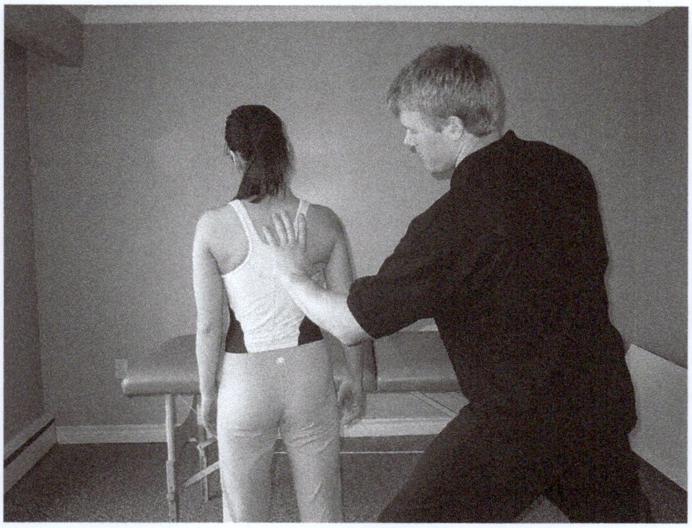

FIGURE 16.56 Motion test 1

While standing behind the patient's shoulder cradle the inferior angle of the scapula between your thumb and your index finger. With the other hand lightly hold the patient's upper arm and have the patient slowly begin to abduct it.

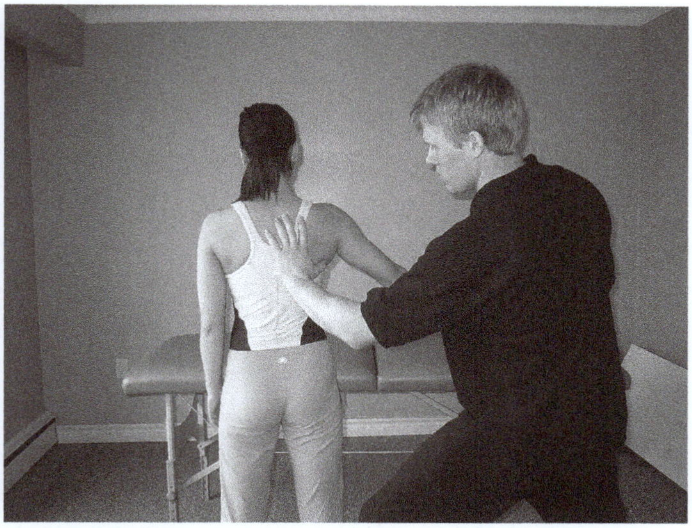

FIGURE 16.57 Motion test 1

Note when the scapula starts to move as the patient lifts the arm. If it moves before 15° there is a restriction.

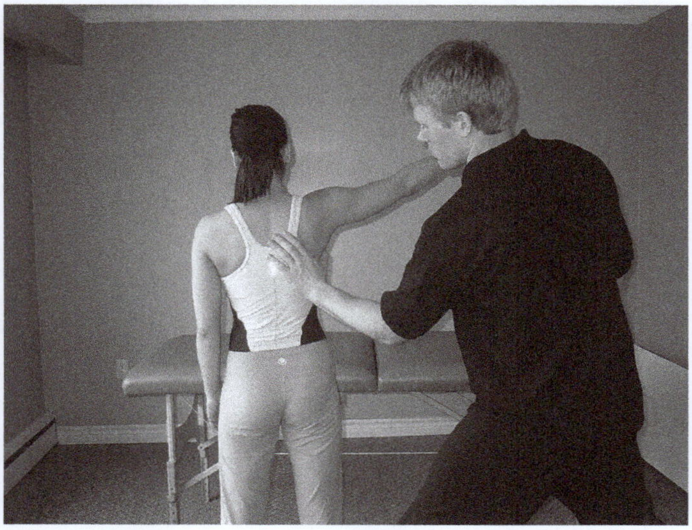

FIGURE 16.58 Motion test 1

NOTE: If there is no movement of the scapula until some time past 30° of abduction then rotator cuff muscles should be investigated as this indicates that muscles are inhibited, weakened, or injured.

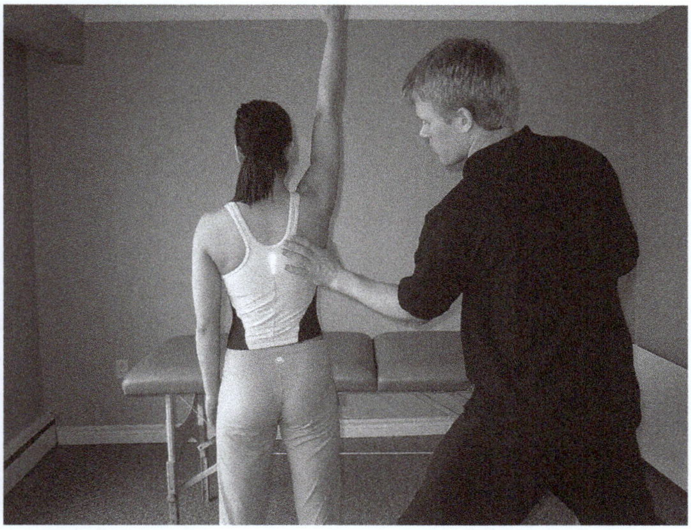

FIGURE 16.59 Motion test 1

The patient continues to lift the arm.

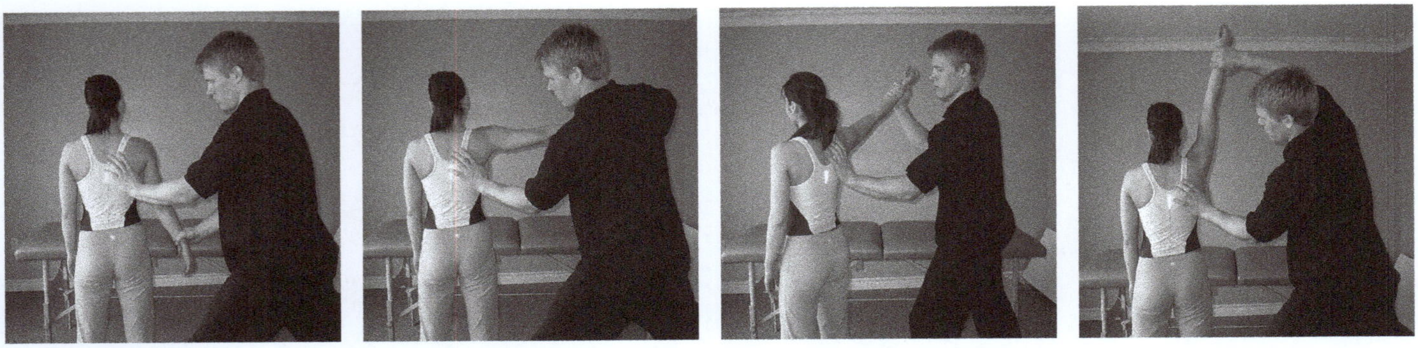

FIGURE 16.60A–D Performing motion test 2.

While standing behind the patient grasp the inferior angle of the scapula between your thumb and index finger. With the other hand grasp the forearm and ask the patient to relax and slowly abduct. Note when the scapula begins to move. As the test proceeds, externally rotate the arm to allow the greater tubercle of the humerus to rotate out from under acromion.

too soon. If motion begins significantly before 80° it is because of taut tissue. This may be due to either the rotator cuff musculature engaging too soon when it should remain relatively quiet or because of restrictions in the joint capsule; (2) if the scapula does not move until after 100°, and you do not feel the muscles engage until then, the scapula is only moving because of tissue stretch. Note: This test for scapulothoracic motion is a PR-ROM.

Note that the scapula moving before 80° may imply capsular restriction. If muscles spasm as tissues are stretched it could indicate injury to individual muscles or muscle groups. Differential muscle testing (see Special tests) will help locate and evaluate muscles and clarify how many are involved. Palpation can help determine this; with the hand positioned as shown in Figure 16.61 muscle engagement or fasciculation can usually be felt.

If there is a sense of early muscle engagement (or to just more accurately test for this) the therapist can repeat the motions with their fingers spread. Leave the thumb where it is (for the teres muscles) with the index and middle finger over the infraspinatus muscle and the last two digits over the rhomboid and middle-lower trapezius area.

NOTE: The fiber direction of the infraspinatus and the teres muscles are almost identical. These are often seen impaired together.

Motion test 3: isolating glenohumeral joint motion

Motion test 3 tests the movement within the glenohumeral joint itself. Positive signs: if the joint does not reach approximately 120° then it is hypomobile. If the joint exceeds 120° then it is hypermobile.

NOTE: If you reach 120° you can be confident that any loss of range of motion that may have been observed during the AF-ROM of abduction is not coming from the glenohumeral joint. This indicates that the restriction of movement is coming from the tissues in which the scapula is contained. Palpation and differential muscle testing will be performed to identify which tissues may be involved.

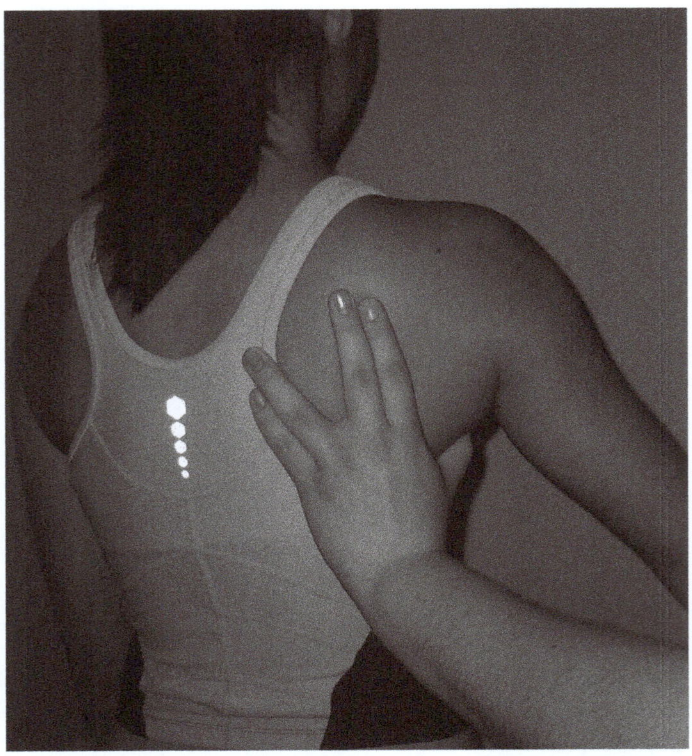

FIGURE 16.61

Hand position for palpation of muscle engagement.

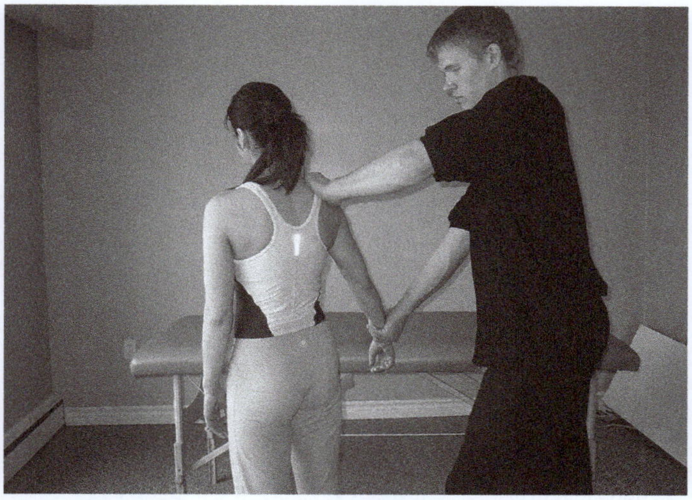

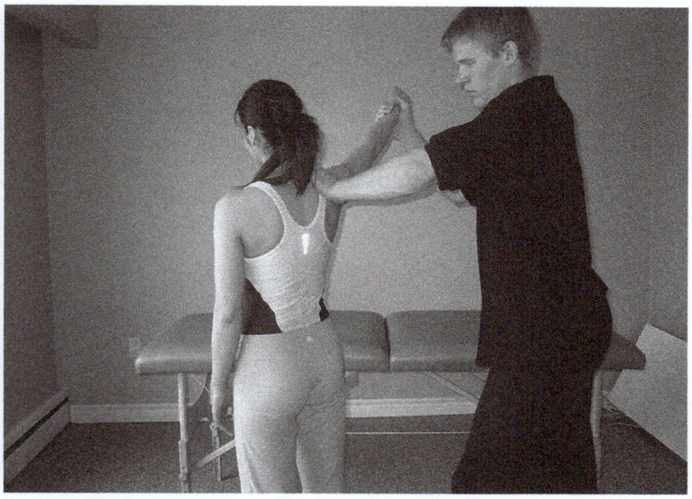

FIGURE 16.62A, B Motion test 3

Stand behind the shoulder being tested. Place one hand on top of the acromion. With your other hand grasp the forearm and ask the patient to relax, allowing you to move the arm slowly into abduction. As you passively abduct the humerus prevent the scapula from lifting with the other hand by applying gentle but firm pressure downward.

Active resisted range of motion testing (AR-ROM)

See Part I, Chapter 3 for a discussion of active resisted testing and what we learn from such testing including a grading scale 0 to 5. (See Kendall et al. 2005 for a truly comprehensive exploration and instruction in muscle testing; see and compare: Dutton 2012; Hartley 2000a; Hertling & Kessler 2006; Magee 2014; Petty 2011.)

CLINICAL NOTE: Have the patient begin the following isometric testing using only a portion of their strength and then over a count of five build up until maximum exertion is reached. If the therapist is concerned that a patient may overpower them then they should tell the patient to resist the pressure that they apply but only with an equal counter-pressure. Then have the patient match the increasing pressure being applied by the therapist over a count of five. The patient is supposed to immediately report if pain is felt and the isometric testing should stop to prevent further injury to tissue or structures.

The patient needs to reach full exertion if that is possible, to see if: (1) there is full strength with only minor pain which indicates a mild strain to the tissues; (2) if weakness is encountered without any pain, which is a neurological **red flag**. This requires a referral back to the primary physician. Weakness with pain implies a severe strain. Hence if the patient is told to use only part of their strength then both (1) and (2) could be missed.

AR-ROM of glenohumeral joint (Figures 16.63–16.68)

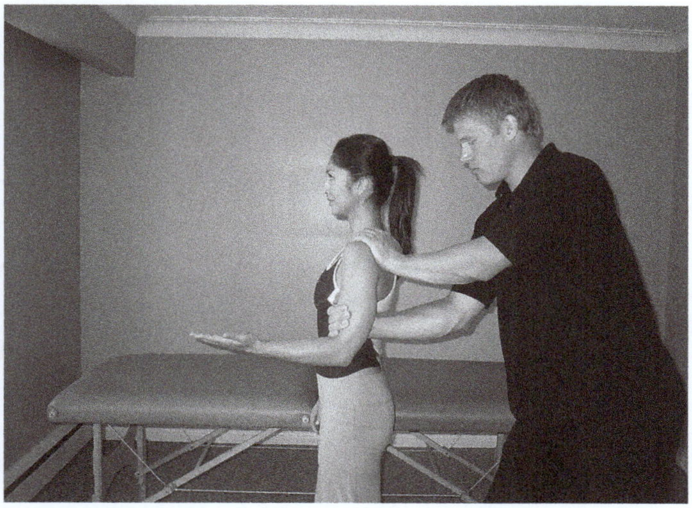

FIGURE 16.63 AR-ROM flexion

Stand behind the patient, centered behind the arm being tested. Place one hand on the patient's scapula to stabilize it. Reach forward and grasp the arm just above the elbow. Resist forward flexion. You are primarily testing the anterior deltoid, coracobrachialis, biceps brachii, and pectoralis major.

REMEMBER: If the patient experiences pain and/or weakness you will have to test these muscles individually later.

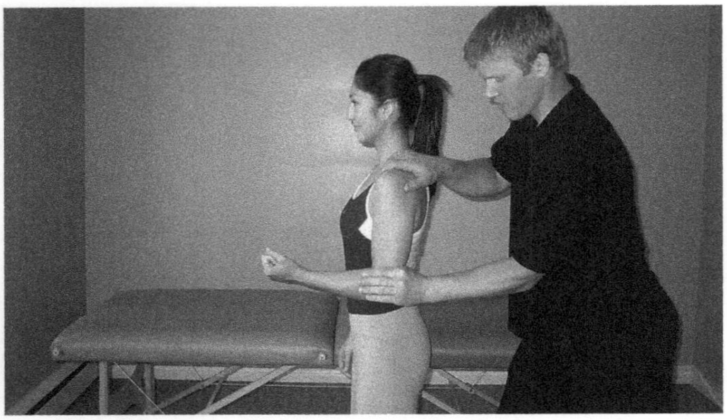

FIGURE 16.64 AR-ROM extension

Place your resisting hand just above the patient's elbow. You should be standing far enough back from the patient to have your resisting arm extended but your elbow still slightly flexed. This provides a mechanical advantage and prevents you from being pushed back and/or losing balance. Have the patient extend their arm while you resist. You are primarily testing latissimus dorsi, posterior deltoid, and teres major. ***REMEMBER:*** If the patient experiences pain and/or weakness you will have to test these muscles individually later.

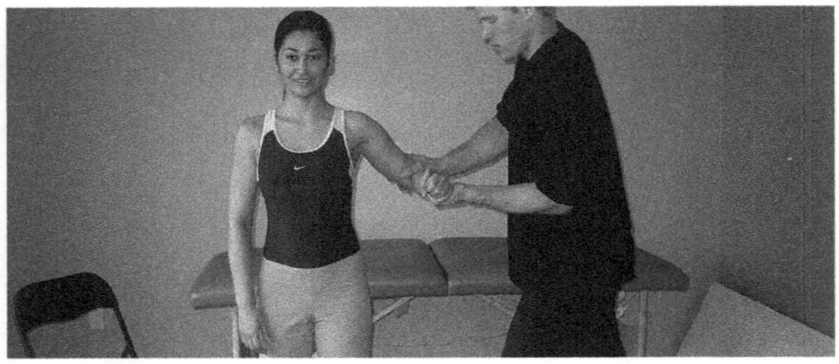

FIGURE 16.65 AR-ROM abduction

Have the patient abduct the arm at least 45° with the elbow flexed to 90°. While at the patient's side place the resisting hand just proximal to the elbow. Resist the patient's abduction. If the patient shrugs the shoulder while trying to abduct the arm re-do the test with a stabilizing hand on top of the shoulder (to prevent shrugging). You are testing primarily middle fibers of deltoid and supraspinatus. If the patient experiences pain and/or weakness you will have to test these muscles individually later. Pain localized to the insertion point of supraspinatus may indicate tendonitis. Pain felt deep in the shoulder after the patient releases pressure of resistance (rebound pain) may indicate bursitis.

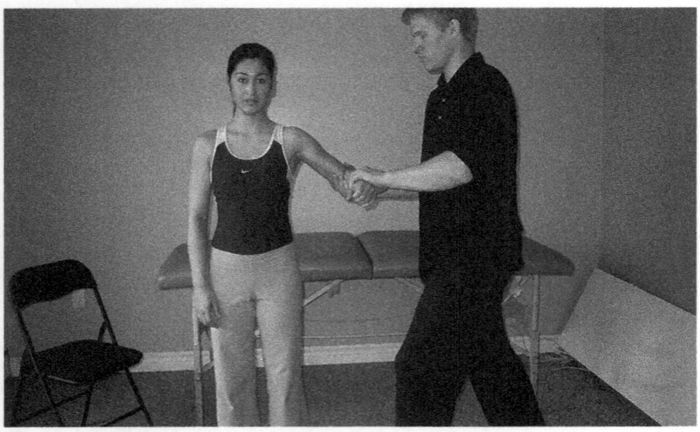

FIGURE 16.66 AR-ROM adduction

While still standing at the patient's side have the patient's arm abducted 25–45°. Cup the hand around the upper arm just above the elbow (you may also choose to stabilize their shoulder with your other hand), resist the patient's adduction. You are primarily testing pectoralis major, teres major, and latissimus dorsi. If the patient experiences pain and/or weakness you will have to test these muscles individually later.

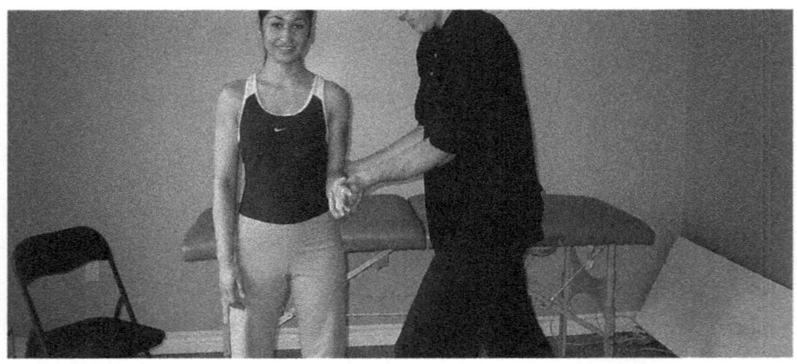

FIGURE 16.67 AR-ROM external rotation

Have the patient hold the arm at the side. Flex the elbow to 90° so the forearm is pointed straight ahead. Stabilize the upper arm just above the elbow, making sure the arm stays against the body throughout the test. Place your resisting hand just above the wrist. Have the patient attempt to externally rotate their shoulder. Primarily testing infraspinatus and teres minor. You can repeat this test with the arm now abducted to 90° in order to bring accessory muscles of external rotation into play. If the patient experiences pain and/or weakness you must test these muscles individually later.

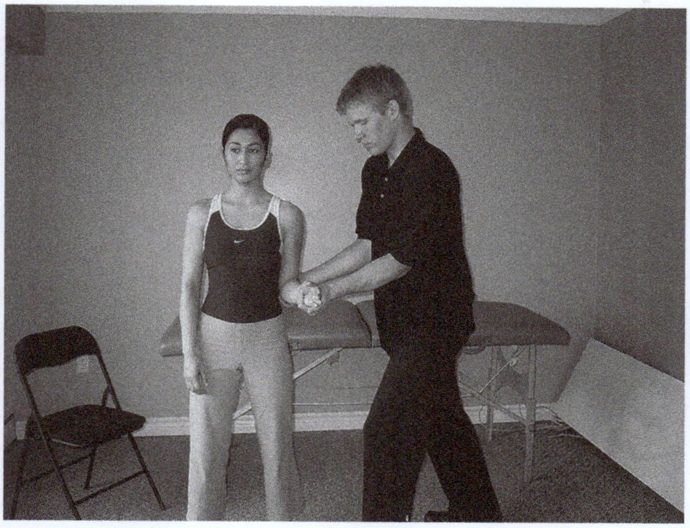

FIGURE 16.68 AR-ROM internal rotation

Cup the wrist proximally with your resisting hand. Stabilize at the elbow as the patient attempts to internally rotate their shoulder. Primarily testing the subscapularis, pectoralis major, latissimus dorsi, and teres major. If the patient experiences pain and/or weakness you must test these muscles individually later.

Resisted scapular motions (Figures 16.69, 16.70)

Special tests

Differential muscle testing

The therapist uses differential muscle testing on those muscles that have been possibly implicated as impaired during AF-ROM or AR-ROM testing or in which the patient's description of pain and/or dysfunction implicates the muscle (see Kendall et al. 2005). The musculature around the shoulder girdle is manifold and synergistic in many ways in varying combinations. Further a detailed testing of the musculature is highly beneficial when the chronicity of an injury persists and/or the injury is unclear. While functional impairment may be obvious, specific musculature and joint impairments may be difficult to assess if no differential muscle testing is done.

Where are we in our protocol?

In AR-ROM we have only tested muscle groups. It is necessary to grade the acuity of impairment of the muscles within groups. It is important to investigate whether there is one muscle within a group that is more impaired than the others. Remember we are trying to recreate or elicit the patient's chief pain/complaint while taking note of other pain created that may be secondary or compensatory.

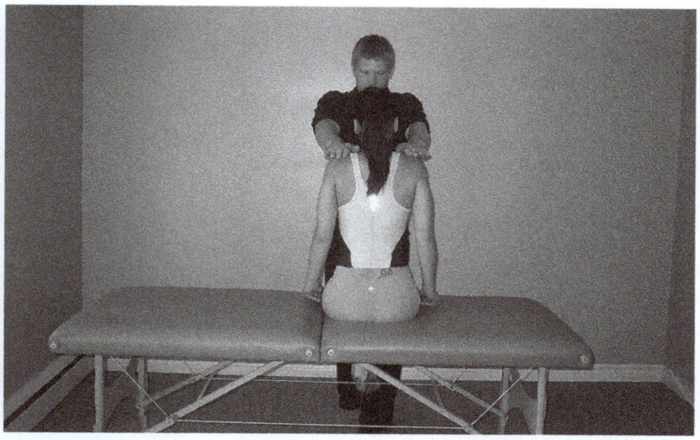

FIGURE 16.69 AR-ROM elevation (shoulder shrug)

The patient elevates the shoulders then the therapist presses downward. Any patient should be able to resist downward pressure. Primarily testing the upper trapezius and levator scapula.

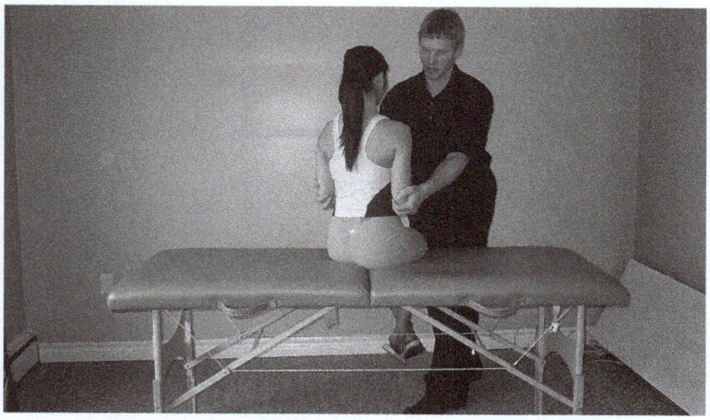

FIGURE 16.70 AR-ROM depression

The patient draws the scapulae toward the ground. Then the therapist attempts to elevate the patient's shoulders by grasping under the patient's flexed elbow and lifting superiorly. Principally testing serratus anterior, lower trapezius, latissimus dorsi.

Testing scapular muscles (Figures 16.71–16.78)

The three muscles in Figures 16.71–16.73 can be differentiated by stressing each in the way that uses their fiber direction.

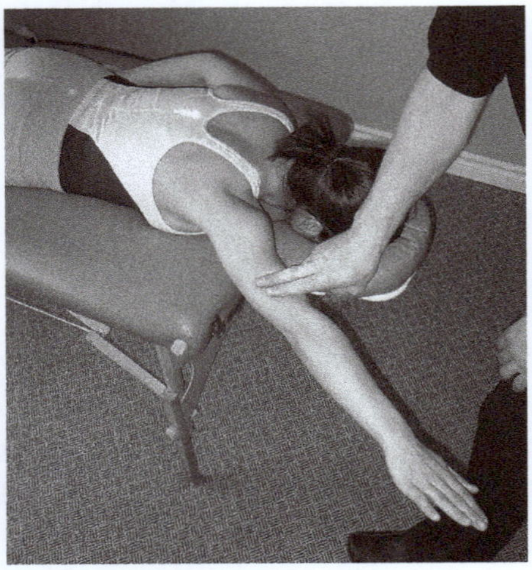

FIGURE 16.71
Lower trapezius.

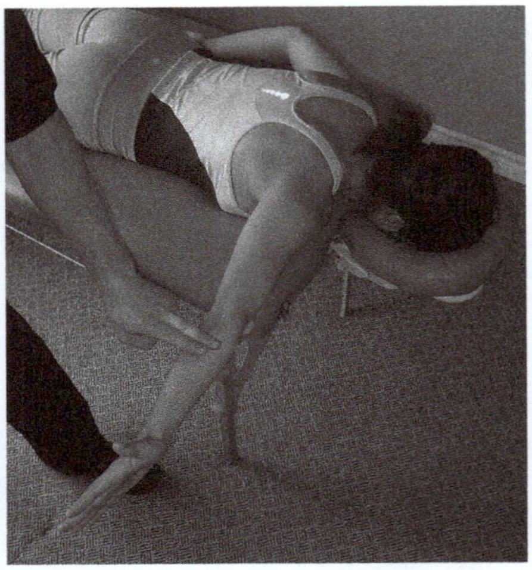

FIGURE 16.72
Middle trapezius.

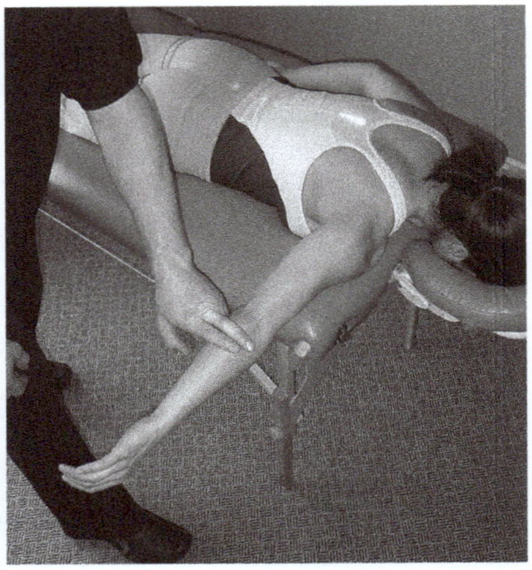

FIGURE 16.73
Rhomboids.

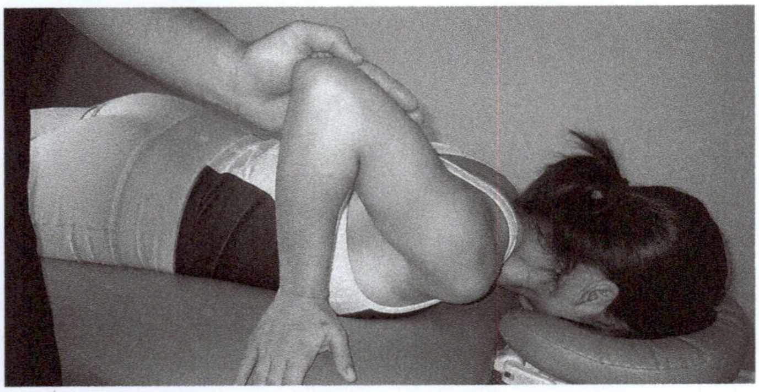

FIGURE 16.74 Rhomboids test

Fully extend the elbow and have the patient pull the arm tight to the body in adduction. Then ask the patient to lift the hand off the table as far as possible. The therapist cups the elbow and pushes out (abduction) and up (superior), attempting to protract the scapula and swing inferior angle laterally.

Have the patient lying prone and use the arm as a lever to stress tissues.

- For lower trapezius: have the patient's arm abducted about 150° and then extend the arm slightly. Place pressure downward in the area above the elbow so that you do not easily overpower the patient and therefore not have sufficient resistance for adequate bilateral comparison.
- For middle trapezius: have the patient's arm abducted to 90° and again in slight extension. ***NOTE:*** The patient's thumb is

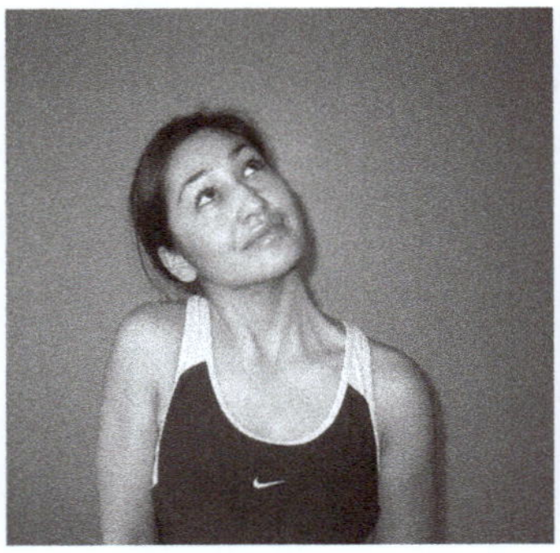

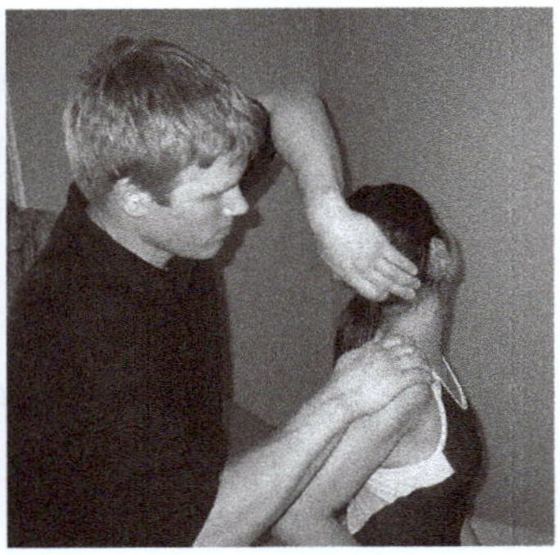

FIGURE 16.75A, B Upper trapezius versus levator scapula

Have the seated patient lift the shoulder up on the side to be tested, then have the patient look up and turn the head away from the side being tested. This shortens both muscles but levator scapulae is now too short to do more work (it is rendered "insufficient"). However, upper trapezius can still function. The therapist places one hand on the shoulder, the other at the posterior-lateral surface of the skull, then tries to push them apart as the patient tries to hold the position. If upper trapezius is of normal strength the patient can resist easily and no movement will occur. If there is no return of symptoms (e.g., pain) with this positioning, then one can surmise that the levator scapulae is the chief complainant. If it recreates the patient's pain then the upper trapezius is involved, with the levator possibly involved as well.

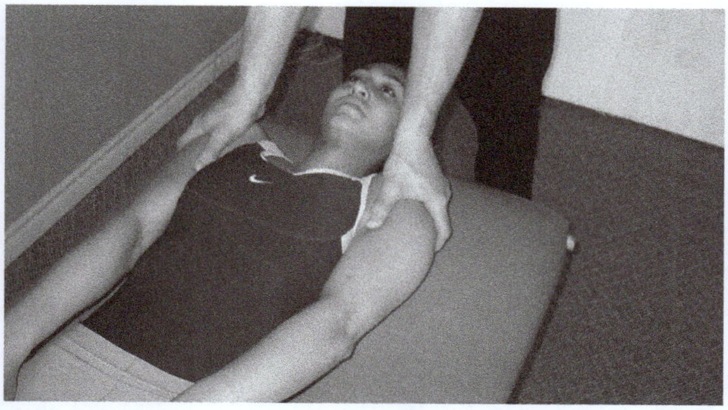

FIGURE 16.76 Pectoralis minor supine test

Have the patient roll the shoulders forward off the table. The patient then tries to push both shoulders back down to the table. Any patient should be able to resist this.

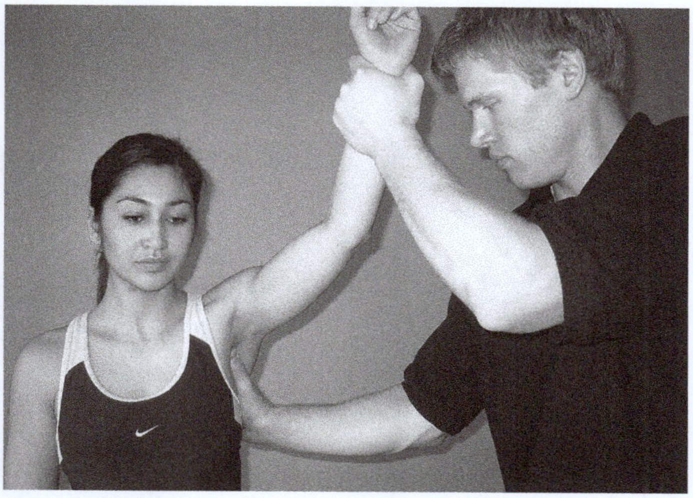

FIGURE 16.78 Serratus anterior

This muscle stabilizes the scapula as the arm performs various movements particularly when the flexors or abductors of the arm are under load. The patient has the arm forward flexed to 120°. The therapist places the thumb and hypothenar eminence of one hand against the anterior-lateral border of the scapula. With the other hand grasp the patient's forearm and try to pull the arm down as the patient resists. To fully test serratus anterior simultaneously push posteriorly on the anterior-lateral surface of the scapula trying to cause the scapula to "wing" posteriorly. This puts a maximum load onto the serratus anterior muscle.

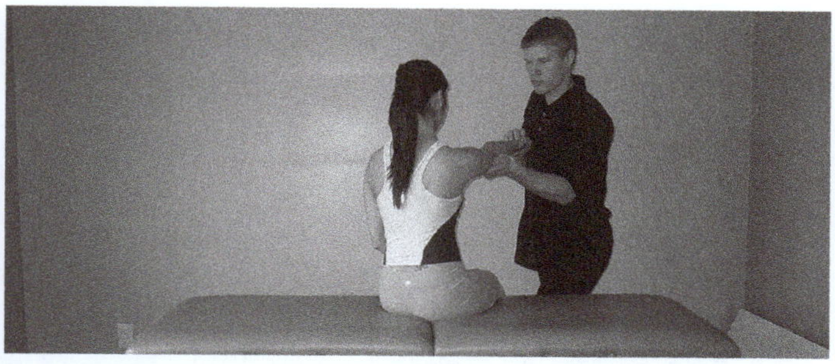

FIGURE 16.77 Pectoralis minor seated test

Have the patient reach forward as far as possible with a straight arm or pretending to punch something just out of range. This protracts the shoulder. The therapist tries to push the arm back to attempt to retract the shoulder. The test will be a false positive if the scapula lifts off the thorax or "wings."

NOTE: Anterior serratus is also involved in this test. If there is a positive result (pain or weakness) further differentiation is required. See serratus anterior test described next. The patient pointing to a specific area of pain can help distinguish between the muscles.

pointing up. It is wise to stabilize the opposite scapula so the patient does not roll on the table.

- Figure 16.73 shows the commonly used rhomboids test position. Positioned as for middle trapezius test but with thumb down. Note: This is not the author's preferred positioning; that is shown in Figure 16.74.

Rotator cuff muscles (Figure 16.79–16.81)

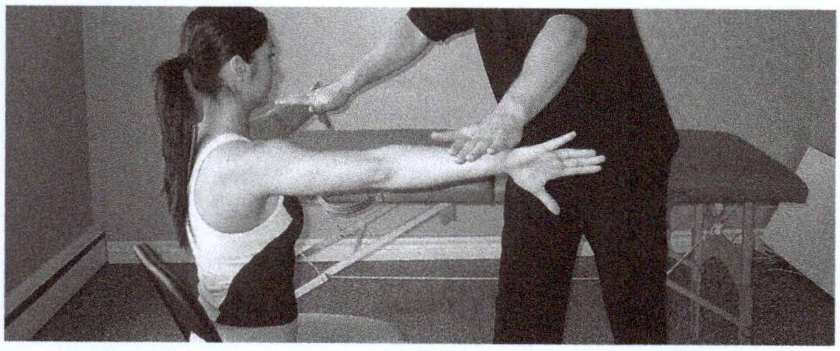

FIGURE 16.79 Empty can test (supraspinatus test)

The patient abducts the arms to 90° and brings them 30° forward. The patient pronates the forearms (as if emptying a can) and then resists downward pressure. This stresses supraspinatus more than deltoids thus making it specific to supraspinatus.

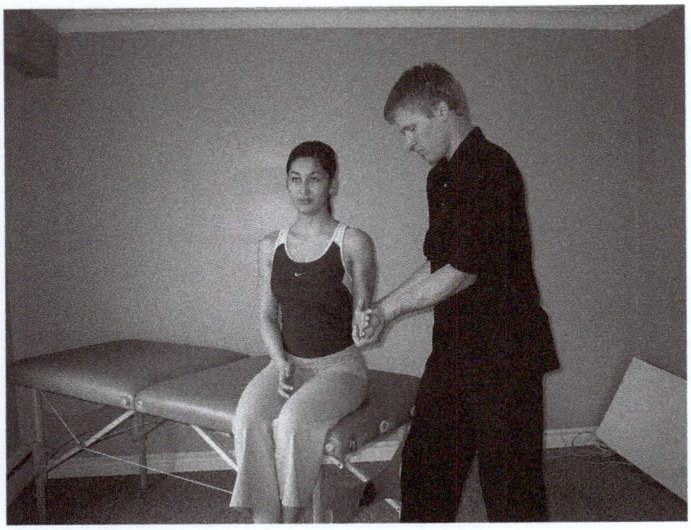

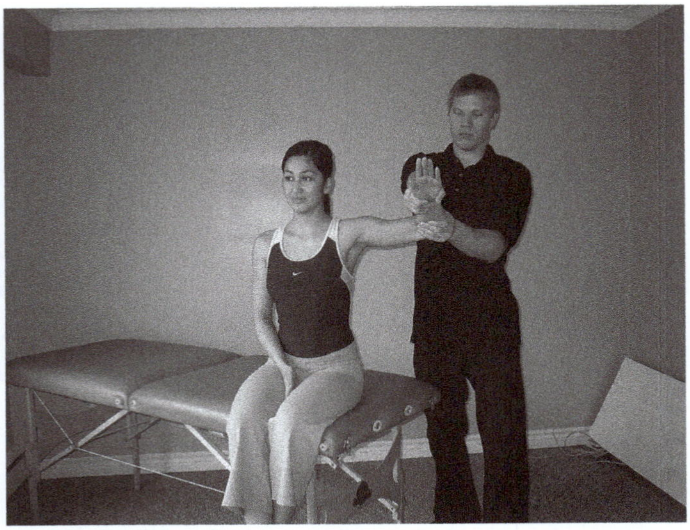

FIGURES 16.80, 16.81 1. Infraspinatus and teres minor, and 2. teres minor specific

Stabilize the patient's lateral elbow and wrist. Resist the patient's external rotation. If a positive sign of pain and/or weakness is noted then differentiate with the teres minor specific test. As positioned in the specific test the teres minor must work harder and it will therefore complain more if injured.

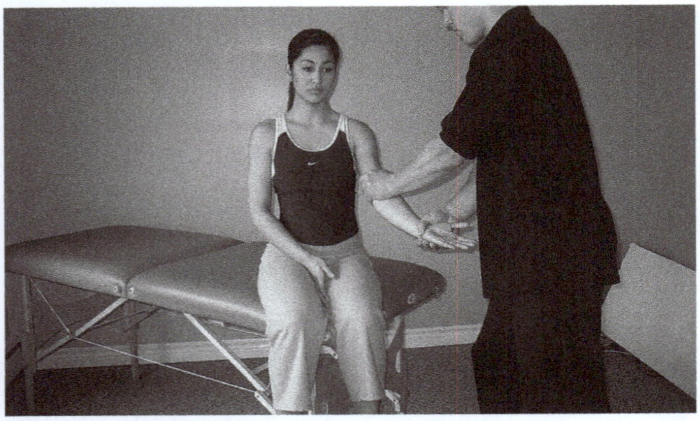

FIGURE 16.82 1. Anterior deltoid, biceps brachii and coracobrachialis

Use resisted forward flexion at 30° of shoulder flexion to provide a base line for group action of these three muscles. Forward flexion helps neutralize the pectoris major (a strong synergist). Have the elbow somewhat extended to enable the biceps brachii to generate enough tension to provoke symptoms.

Glenohumeral muscles (Figures 16.82–16.85)

The first four tests are performed in a specific order to progressively uncover the degree of impairment for each.

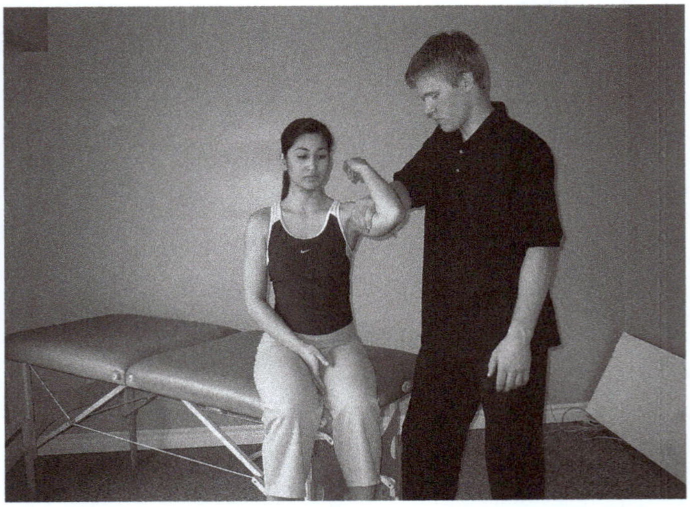

FIGURE 16.83 2. Anterior deltoid and coracobrachialis

To make the biceps brachii insufficient (too short to generate enough tension to provoke response) flex the shoulder to 90° and nearly fully flex the elbow. The patient resists downward pressure on the arm. Here only anterior deltoid and coricobrachialis work in a manner that creates enough tension for them to be symptomatic. ***NOTE:*** If pain was felt in test 1 but not here then the biceps is implicated.

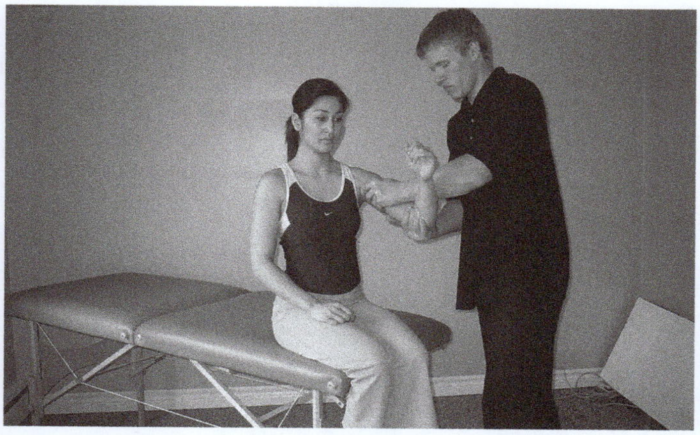

FIGURE 16.84 3. Coracobrachialis

If symptoms of impairment persist perform the following: to make coricobrachialis work hardest change the vector (direction) of downward pressure applying force down and away from the body. If this recreates impairment then coracobrachialis is indicated. If it does not make any difference then the deltoid may well be the principal structure involved. Confirm this with the next test.

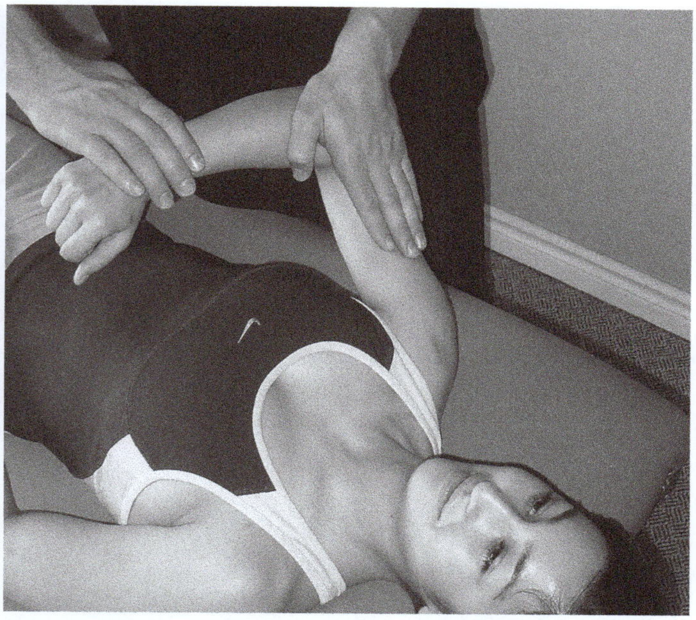

FIGURE 16.85 4. Anterior deltoid

This position with resistance stresses the anterior deltoid most specifically. (*Shown supine but can be done seated.*)

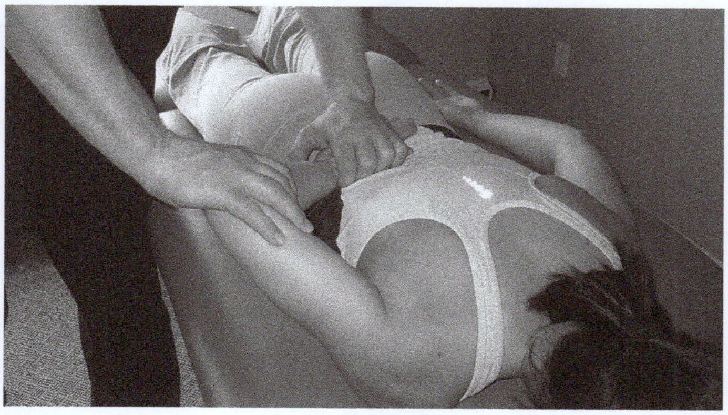

FIGURE 16.86 1. Teres major

Positioning isolates this muscle. The patient is prone with their hand behind their back. Lift the elbow (arm in this much extension and internal rotation makes latissimus dorsi insufficient) and have the patient resist your effort to bring their arm down and out. Compare results with test 2.

Teres major versus latissimus dorsi (Figures 16.86, 16.87)

These two tests help differentiate between these two muscles.

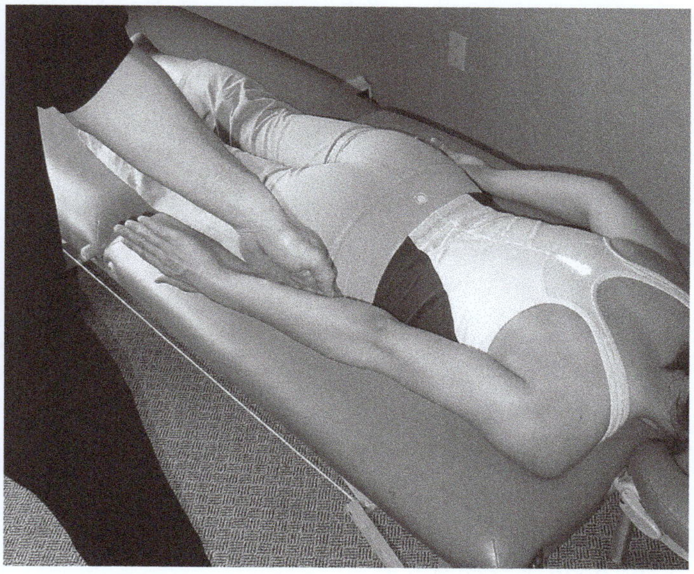

FIGURE 16.87 2. Latissimus dorsi

The patient is prone with the arm at the side. Lift the arm off the table. Have the patient resist your effort to push the arm down and out. ***NOTE:*** The therapist's pressure should be at the elbow so as not to easily overpower the patient's effort.

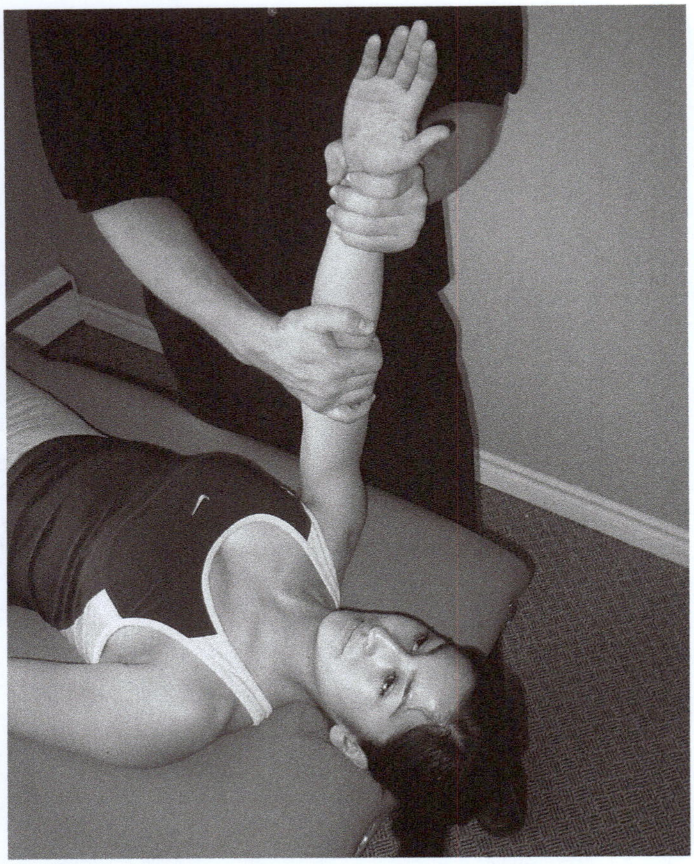

FIGURE 16.88 1. Clavicular division

Have the patient lying supine with the elbow extended and the shoulder flexed to 90° with the hand facing straight across the chest, aimed at the contralateral clavicle. This helps the patient focus on the action the therapist wants to resist. Ask the patient to try to cross-adduct the arm.

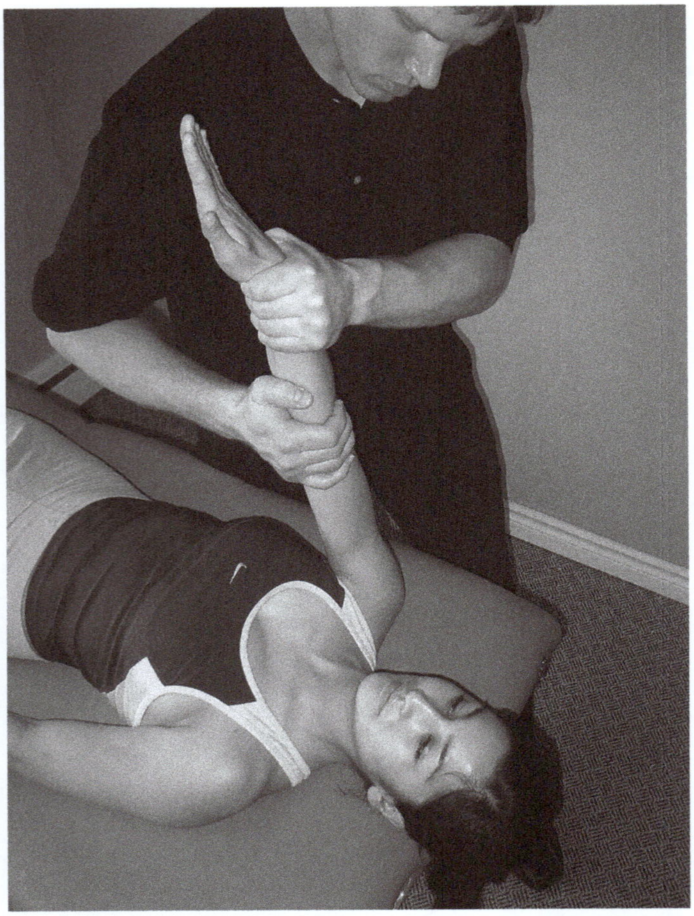

FIGURE 16.89 2. Sternal division (diagonal fibers)

Have the patient in the same position but with the hand facing the opposite hip. Ask the patient to try and take the straight arm toward that hip.

Pectoralis major clavicular versus sternal division (Figures 16.88, 16.89)

These tests show how to differentiate between two portions of the pectoralis major, which having different lines of pull can be impaired to different degrees.

Long head of triceps (Figure 16.90)

This muscle is often overlooked when investigating shoulder impairments since the triceps as a whole is only brought to mind when thinking of elbow impairments. The long head of the triceps helps to adduct the arm as it crosses the shoulder joint. It also helps to stabilize the GH joint. Further, because of its attachment on the infraglenoid tubercle which, when injured, can cause pain in an area nearby (under) the infraspinatus and teres minor attachments on the humerus. This can be mistaken as an injury to those rotator cuff muscles.

Yergason's test (transverse ligament integrity test) (Figures 16.91–16.94)

This tests the stability of the long head tendon of biceps brachii in the bicipital groove of the humerus; it tests whether the transverse humeral ligament that holds the tendon in the groove is intact. Biceps tendonitis can also be revealed by pain in the tendon. If the ligament is ruptured then the positive sign will be when the tendon slips out of the groove and causes pain (usually with a snap).

The test is more effective if you allow some movement in all three actions rather than doing the test purely isometrically.

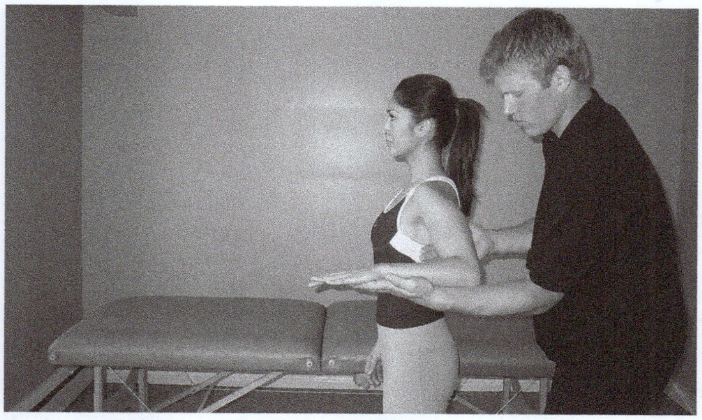

FIGURE 16.90 Long head of triceps

Position the patient as when testing extension but have the arm abducted about 45°. Have the patient try to extend the elbow while simultaneously trying to adduct the arm. Pain may be felt in the posterior arm and/or over the area at the attachment site on the scapula (often diffused over the lateral scapula).

The therapist applies enough resistance so the biceps muscle fully engages but not so much that movement is prevented. Use just enough resistance to slow the movement. Without movement, the tendon may not move out of the groove and the test would not show a positive sign (ruptured transverse ligament).

Speed's test (long head of biceps tendonitis test) (Figures 16.95–16.98)

The tests below are for tendinopathy of the long head tendon of the biceps brachii. The classic test (Figure 16.95) is done isometrically, while the alternative test shown (Figures 16.96-16.98) allows movement under load. Again, the author prefers the alternative version of this test.

Supraspinatus tendonitis tests (Figures 16.99, 16.100)

These two tests focus on the integrity of the rotator cuff musculature, especially the supraspinatus tendon. The drop arm test is more general in nature while the empty can test places more stress on the supraspinatus specifically. The drop arm test works because even though the lateral deltoid is not injured it will reflexively be weakened (like using a dimmer switch) so that strain is not permitted to be placed on the supraspinatus tendon.

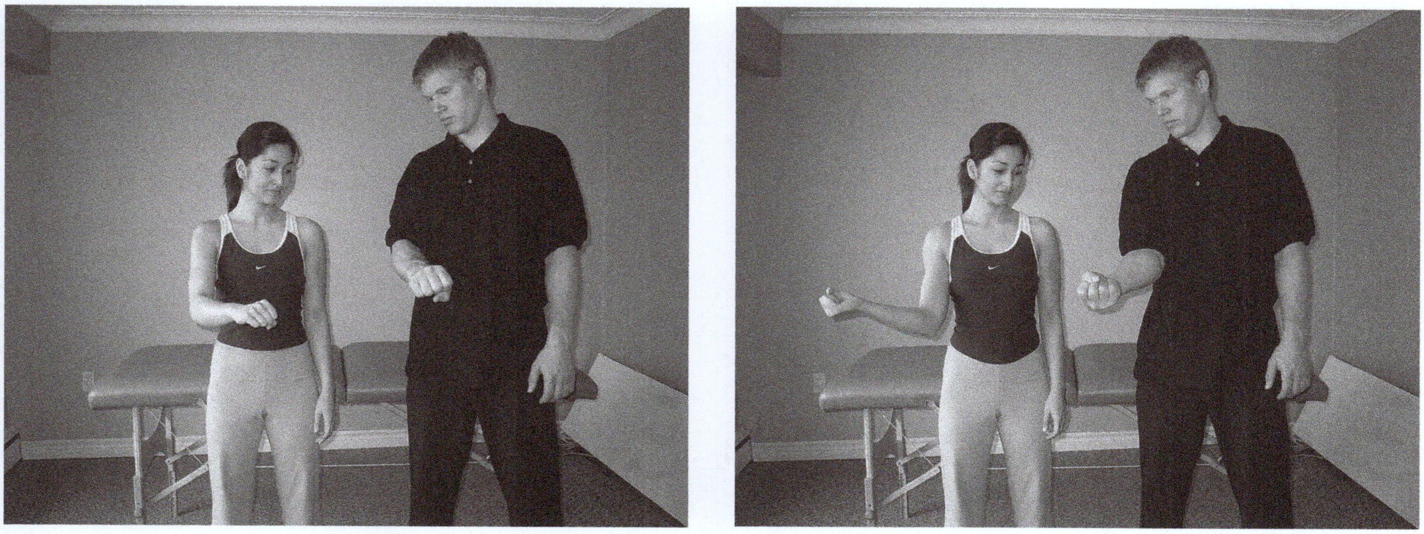

FIGURE 16.91A, B Demonstrating Yergason's test to patient

Demonstrate what you want the patient to do. It can be explained by telling the patient to imitate the action of taking a lid off a pot. Have the patient high-sitting with the elbow flexed to 90° and the forearm pronated (palm facing down). The therapist grasps the forearm just above the wrist. Apply resistance as you have the patient try to supinate the forearm, flex the elbow, externally rotate the arm. Be mindful of keeping the shoulder abduction to a minimum. The therapist must palpate over the area where the biceps brachii long head muscle's tendon lies in the bicipital groove to feel if the tendon lifts out. Positive sign: palpation of movement of the tendon out of the groove. The patient may or may not feel pain depending on how inflamed or irritated tissue is.

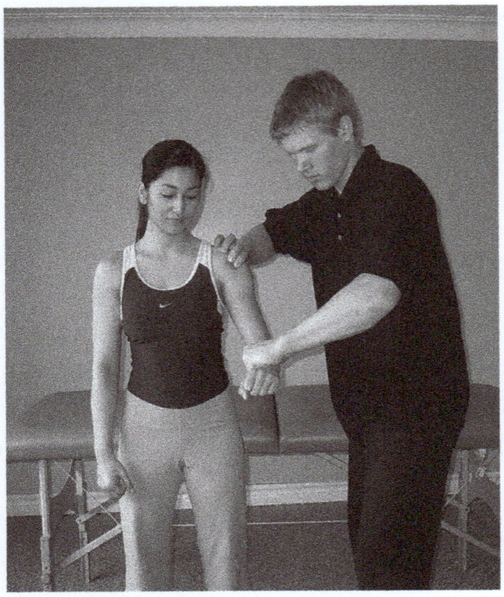

FIGURE 16.92 Yergason's test

Position the patient.

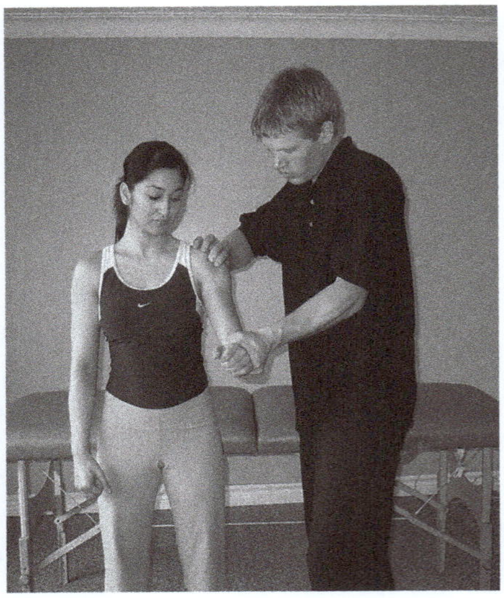

FIGURE 16.93

The therapist applies resistance to prevent any movement by the patient.

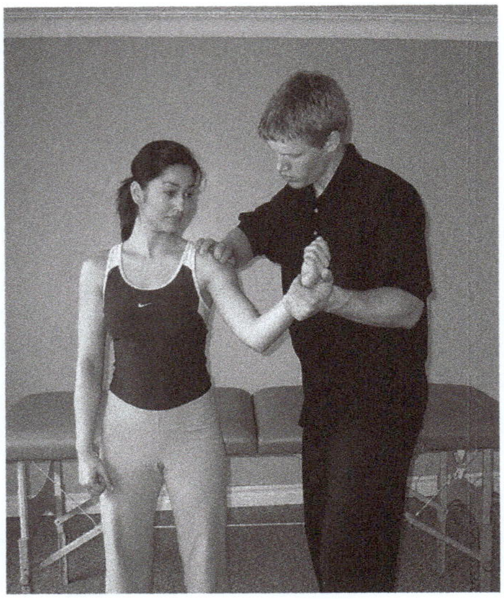

FIGURE 16.94

The patient is allowed to move (under load). Ending position shown.

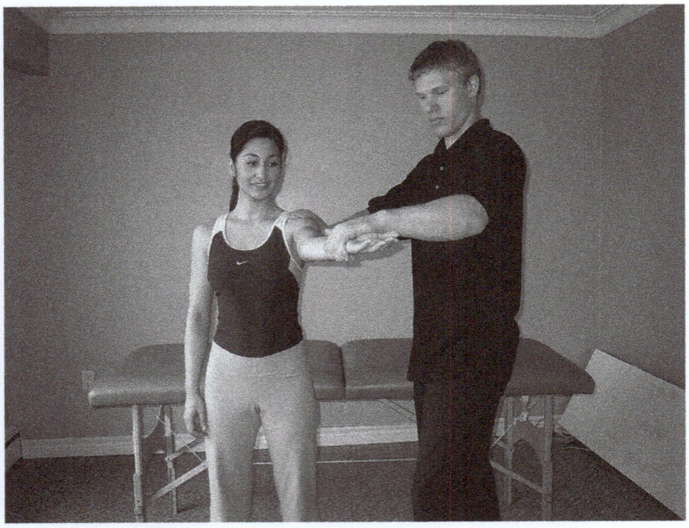

FIGURE 16.95 Classic Speed's test

Have the patient forward flex the shoulder to 90° with the palm up. Apply downward force just above the wrist as the patient resists. Positive test is pain felt in the bicipital groove area.

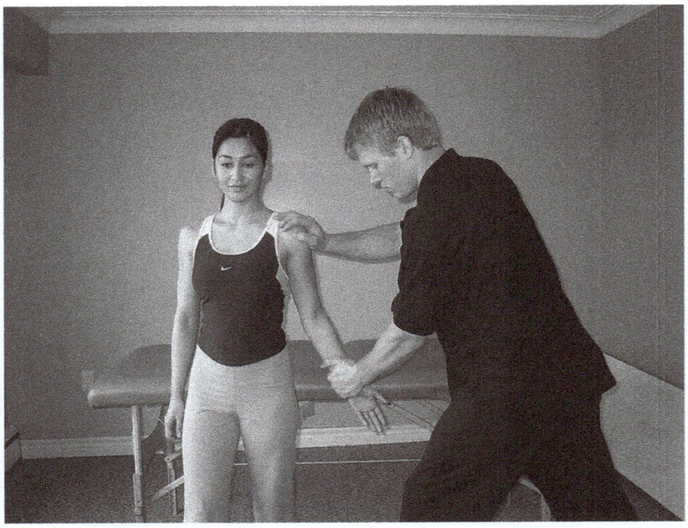

FIGURE 16.96 Alternative Speed's test

1. Performing the test while allowing some arm movement helps clarify the test. With movement the test may be more painful if the patient also has tenosynovitis (where the tendon sheath is also inflamed).

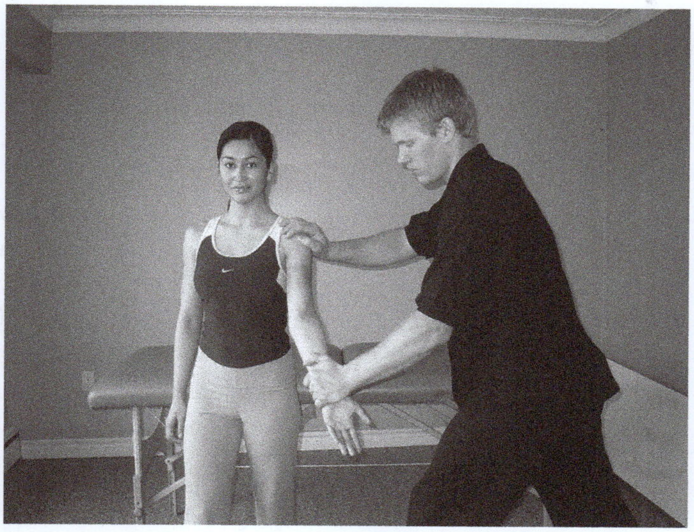

FIGURE 16.97

2. The patient is trying to forward flex the arm while the therapist resists but allows slow movement.

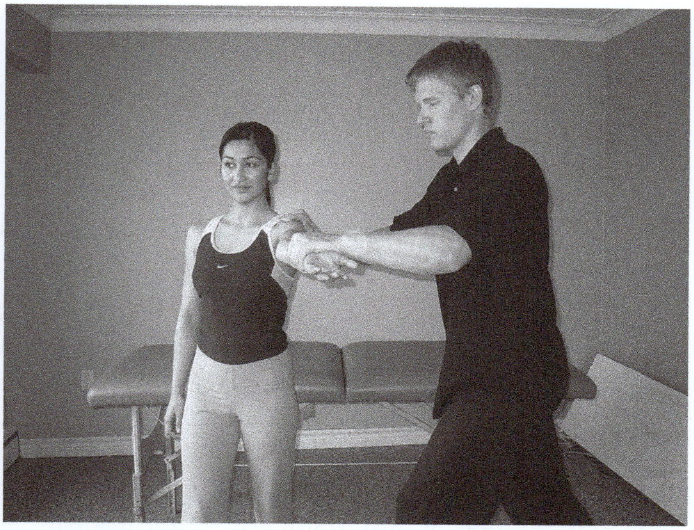

FIGURE 16.98

3. Final position.

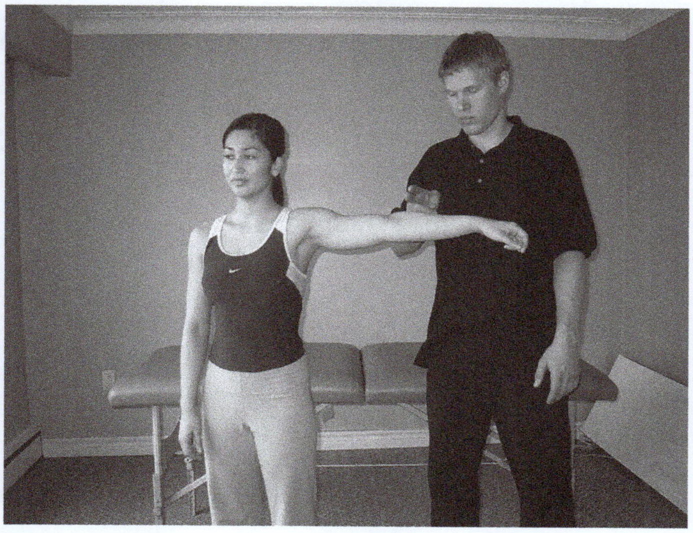

FIGURE 16.99 Drop arm test

Have the patient abduct the arm to 90°. Ask the patient to hold the arm in abduction while you tap or give a slight push downward on the forearm. If a complete rupture is present the patient's arm drops upon the therapist tapping it.

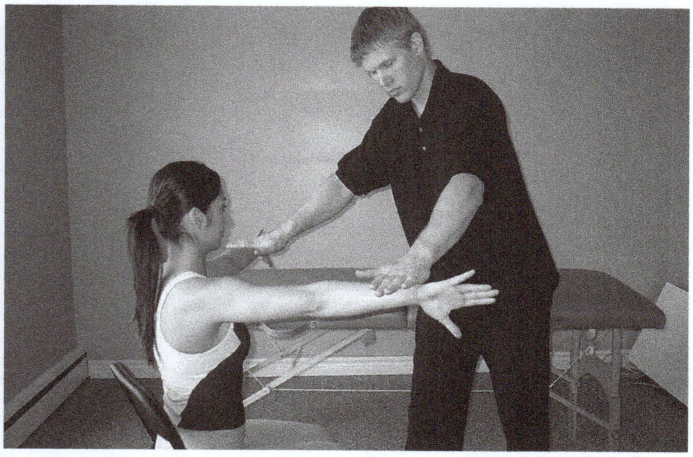

FIGURE 16.100 Empty can test

Have the patient abduct straightened arms to 90° then bring the arms forward at shoulder height about 30°. Finally have the patient point the thumbs toward the ground as if emptying a can. Place your hands just above their wrists and tell the patient to hold this position while you apply pressure downward.

An alternative drop arm test has the patient slowly lowering their arm from the abducted position. If there is a rupture or severe tear the patient's arm will suddenly fall to their side in a jerky or cog-wheel motion. With a rupture or severe tear the patient would even have trouble initiating abduction. If there is a moderate tear the quality of motion will be compromised while lifting or lowering the arm. Once again the motion may appear jerky.

Positive signs for the *empty can test*: if the patient is suffering from supraspinatus tendonitis they will feel pain at either the head of the humerus (insertion point of the muscle) or under the acromial arch (along the course of the tendon). Pain can even refer into the deltoid tubercle area. If tendonitis is severe or a tear is present the patient will not be able to hold this position against resistance. If the patient can hold the position but with some pain the tendonitis is less severe. Weakness without pain can be due either to a reflex protective inhibition as the muscle tries to protect its tendon or there may be neurological involvement. In either case refer out.

Hawkins–Kennedy test (impingement test) (Figure 16.101)

This is to test for tissue being impinged under the acromial arch.

Crank test (apprehension sign) (Figure 16.102)

This is the test for anterior shoulder dislocation, one of many possible tests for the integrity of the glenohumeral joint with respect to its susceptibility to re-dislocate. This test specifically stresses the anterior inferior joint capsule which has an area of natural weakness known as the foramen of Weitbrecht. This is the most common site for shoulder dislocations and should also be done before treating a patient's shoulder if they have a history of dislocation.

Weak serratus anterior test (winging scapula) (Figure 16.103)

For this test designed to check the serratus anterior muscle have the patient push up against the wall. Weakness in the serratus anterior muscle will cause a misalignment of the glenohumeral joint by allowing the whole joint to take on a position of internal

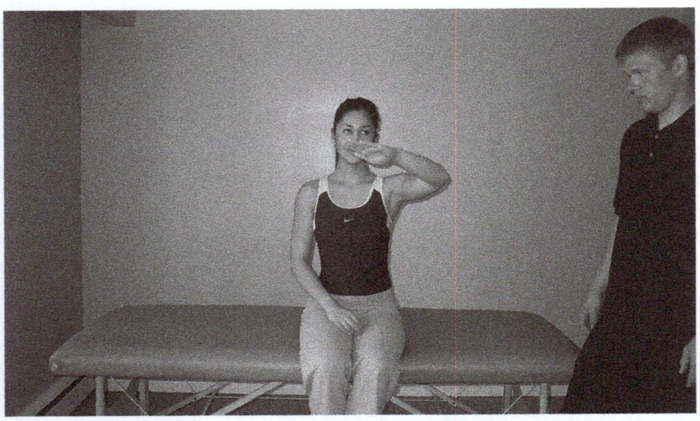

FIGURE 16.101 Hawkins–Kennedy test

The patient abducts the arm to 90° with the elbow flexed also at 90°. Have the patient swing the entire arm into medial rotation (hand swings toward the ground 30–45°). Positive sign is pain felt under the arch. Pain is indicative of bursitis or supraspinatus tendonitis or both. Often if pain is just from bursitis (without supraspinatus involvement) then pain can actually be worse when you stop the test (when you allow the arm to externally rotate back to where you started). However, the tendon is always tender when compressed, less so when compression is released.

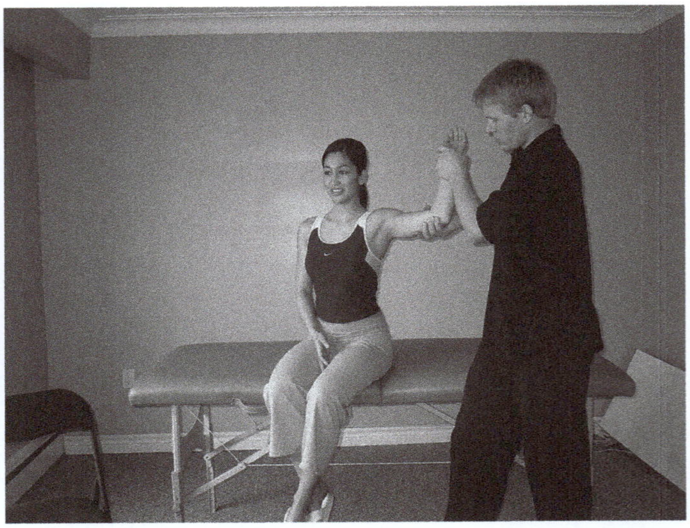

FIGURE 16.102 Crank test

Have the patient abduct the arm to 90° and then flex the elbow to 90°. While standing behind the patient stabilize the scapula with one hand and grasp the forearm with the other hand. Slowly, passively, externally rotate the shoulder. The test is positive if the patient resists movement due to apprehension or if apprehension shows on the patient's face (you may want them facing a mirror so you can see their face).

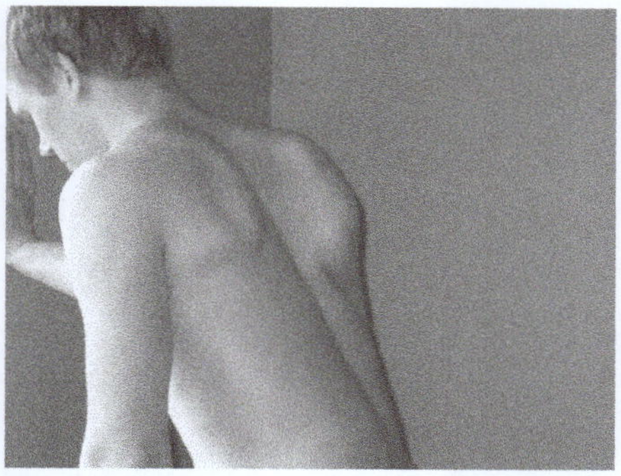

FIGURE 16.103 Weak serratus anterior test (winging scapula)

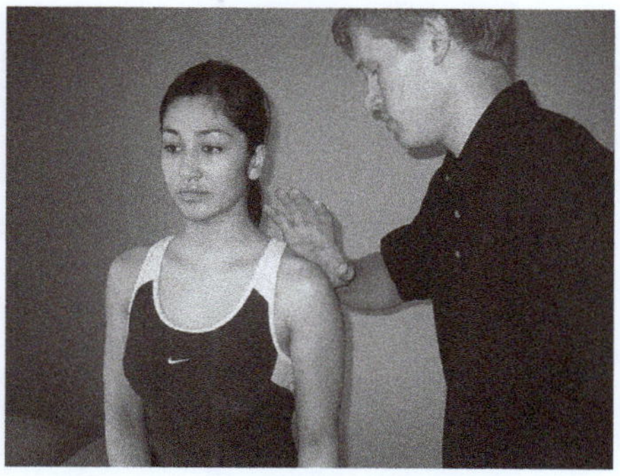

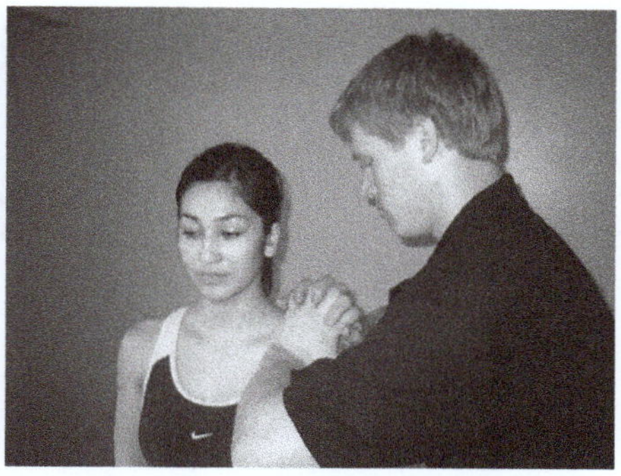

FIGURE 16.104A, B AC joint shear test.

Have the patient seated. Place the base of your hand (pisiform to base of thumb) along the spine of the scapula. Then place the base of the other hand along the middle-to-lateral portion of the clavicle and then interlace the fingers. A squeeze is applied that puts a shear force through the joint. To place more stress on the SC joint move the anterior hand on the clavicle more medially. Positive sign: pain, hypermobility (laxity), or hypomobility (stiffness). Negative sign is a firm springiness.

rotation when performing many movements. This in turn places added strain on the muscles controlling the movement of the scapula and may lead to overworking the muscles of the rotator cuff.

If you notice excessive winging of the scapula bilaterally during this resisted protraction of the scapula the patient may have weak serratus anteriors. If the winging is unilateral there could be two reasons: (1) if there is weakness without pain this is due to an injury to the long thoracic nerve and the patient should be referred out; (2) if there is pain with or without weakness it is reflective of an injury to the muscle.

Acromioclavicular shear tests (Figures 16.104, 16.105)

The alternative shear test is an AF-ROM cross-adduction shoulder motion with over-pressure (O-P) applied at end-range.

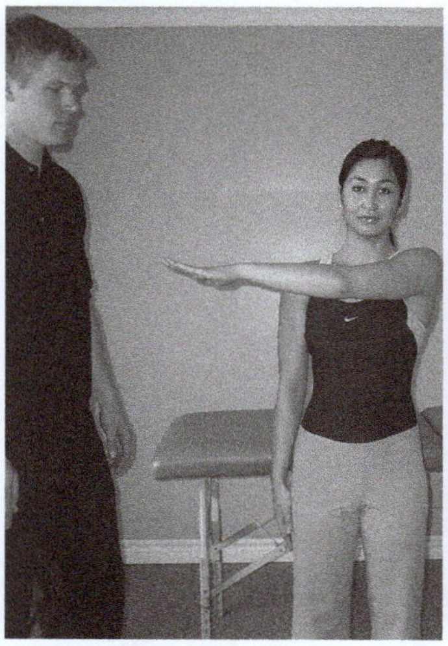

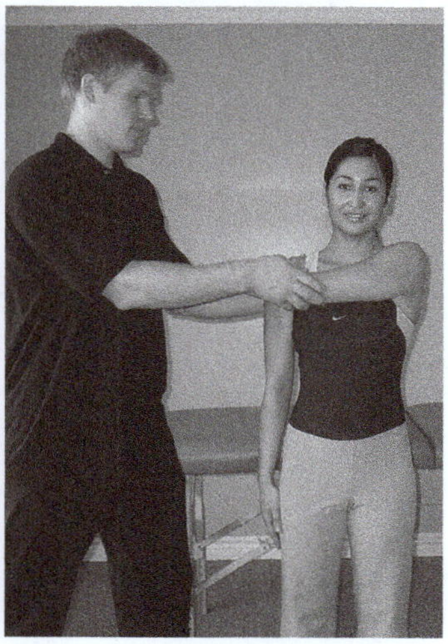

FIGURE 16.105A, B Alternative AC joint shear test

Have the patient cross-adduct the shoulder. With one hand stabilizing the upper back place the other hand above the patient's elbow. Press the arm further into adduction (apply O-P).

Shoulder muscle length testing (Figures 16.106–16.110)

The following are positions in which we can evaluate the length of muscles that may not have already revealed their length during ROM testing done so far.

Latissimus dorsi

Have the patient lie supine on the table with knees extended or bent (whichever is comfortable.)

Note the extent of any lumbar curve. Is the low-back flat against the table or is the low back up off the table? Have the patient lift their arms over their head as far as possible. To show normal length of the latissimus dorsi they should be able to rest their arms above them on the table. If short the arms will remain off the table (Figure 16.107). To reach what appears to be normal length the patient must arch the low back (Figure 16.108).

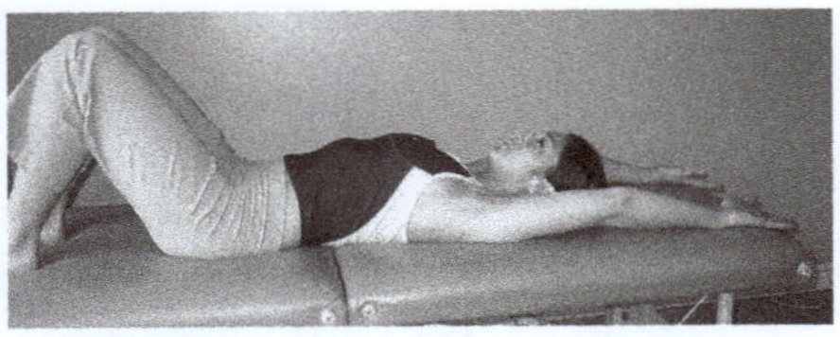

FIGURE 16.106 Latissimus dorsi

1. Within normal length.

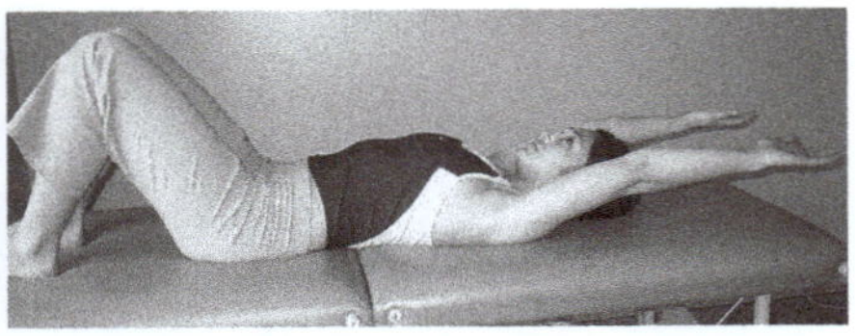

FIGURE 16.107

2. Muscle short. Note arms not fully extended.

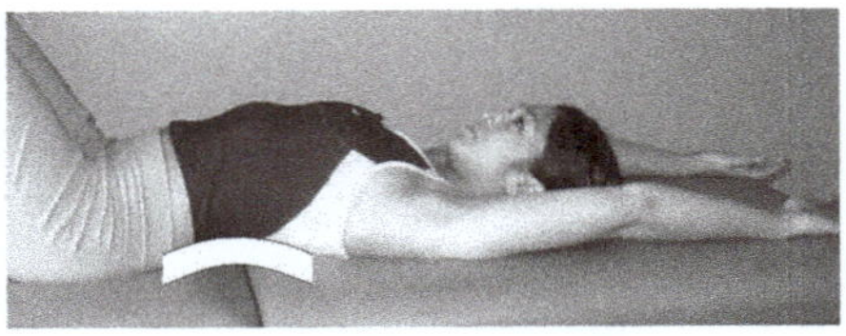

FIGURE 16.108

3. Muscle short. Note arch in lumbar spine.

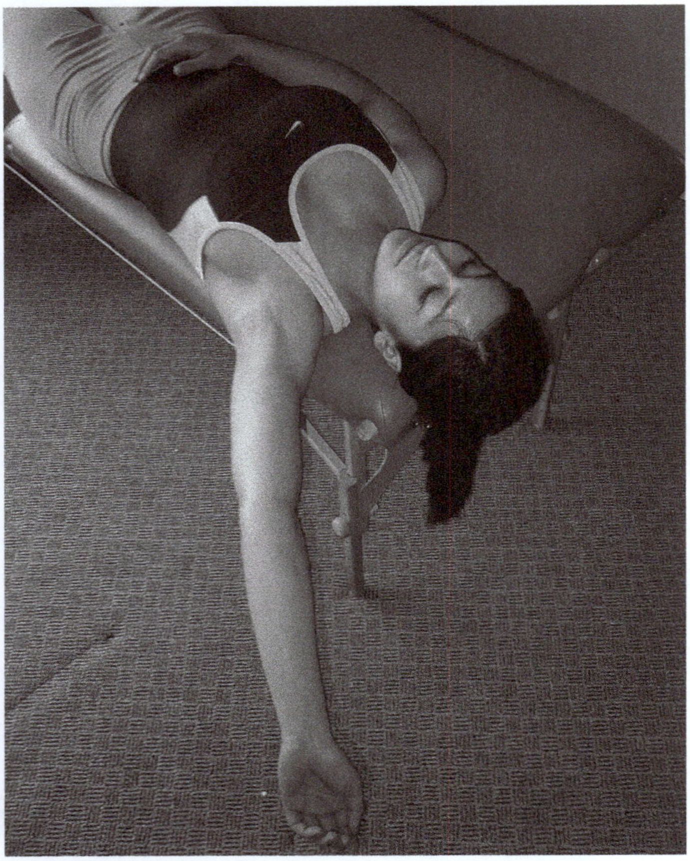

FIGURE 16.109 Pectoralis muscles

If muscle(s) looks short with the arm foreword flexed (from plane of table/ coronal plane) to varying degrees you can gently apply a little O-P toward the ground. The patient can then usually point to where they feel stretch or "burn." This may help clarify the degree to which either muscle is short: pectoralis major often complains at either attachment area on the humerus or down into the sternal area. Pectoralis minor usually complains from the coracoid process area and burn runs down onto ribs 3-4-5 attachment points. Of course, often both can be equally short and equally complaining.

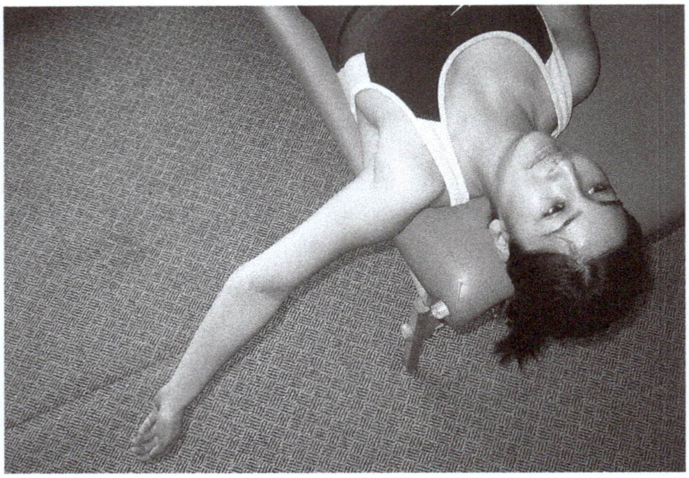

FIGURE 16.110 Pectoralis clavicular portion

With the arm abducted to 80–100° pectoralis major's clavicular attachment/portion can be evaluated. Again, the arm should be able to be at least equal or below the coronal plane established by the table top. Usually a tight and short pectoralis clavicular division does not lift the arm much above the coronal plane. Again, slight over-pressure can be informative. With a shortened clavicular portion a "burn" from stretch or tenderness on light palpation along the inferior border of the medial clavicle will usually be found.

Pectoralis muscle (Figure 16.109, 16.110)

Have the patient supine (it can help if the patient is slightly diagonal so their GH joint is clear of the edge of the table) with the scapula supported by the table, and with the patient generally being supported and secure on the table. Have the patient abduct (or you passively move their arm) to 130–140°. Tell the patient to relax and let the arm sink down so they do not hold it up as it dangles in the air. The arm should be able to be level with the table or even a little extended by 5° toward the ground. This tests both pectoralis majors, sternal, and clavicular attachment/portion.

ELBOW: CHAPTER OVERVIEW

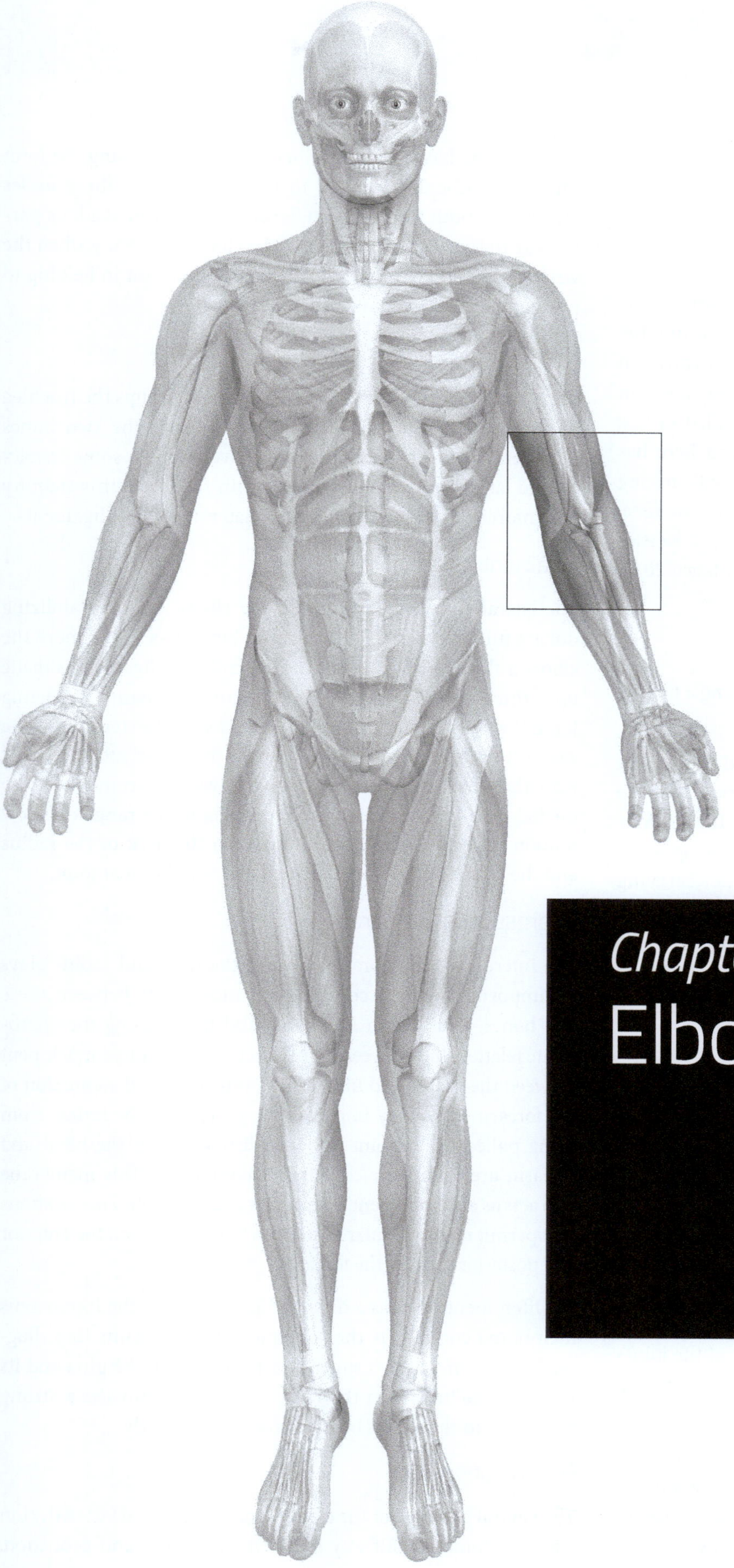

Chapter 17

Elbow

Clinical implications of anatomy and physiology

Understanding the functional relationships (physiology) between structures and tissues (anatomy) helps explain how structures of the elbow can be injured and helps us understand how orthopedic tests work to provide their information. It is suggested that the reader revise the anatomy of the joints and muscles involved in the function of the elbow and that you have an anatomy book on hand to help you understand the information provided in this section. The information that has been summarized here has been chosen because of its direct relevance to orthopedic testing and understanding of mechanical pathologies of the elbow. (See: Agur et al. 2014; Dutton 2012; Hartley 2000a; Hertling & Kessler 2006; Hoppenfeld 1976; Levangie & Norkin 2011; Magee 2014; Schuenke et al. 2014.)

The elbow joint

The elbow is made up of three joints that all share a single fibrous joint capsule, making it a compound synovial joint.

The humeroulnar or trochlear joint is a uniaxial hinge joint that allows only flexion and extension. It is composed of the trochlea of the ulna and capitulum of the humerus. The trochlea is asymmetrical and this results in the forearm moving laterally as the elbow extends. This is referred to as the "carrying angle" of the extended elbow, which ranges, on average, from 10–15° for men and 20–25° for women. This accommodates for the width of the pelvis so that with the elbow fully extended the supinated forearm and hand will be positioned beside but not touching the hip or thigh.

The humeroradial (or radiohumeral) joint is a multiaxial joint that allows flexion and extension while permitting the head of the radius to pivot, or spin on the capitulum in the joint. This occurs in the flexed elbow. In the extended elbow, the radius is no longer in contact with the capitulum.

The superior radioulnar joint, between the radius and ulna, is a uniaxial pivot joint allowing rotation of the radius around the humerus. It provides supination and pronation of the forearm, with the radius moving on the static ulna (and spinning on the capitulum). This is one of the few joints where part of the joint's articular surface is located on a ligament, the annular ligament in this case.

Review the following: brachioradialis, brachialis, biceps brachii, triceps brachii, anconeus, supinator, pronator teres, pronator quadratus; extensor carpi radialis longus/brevis, extensor carpi ulnaris, flexor carpi radialis, flexor carpi ulnaris, palmaris longus.

The elbow has quite a number of muscles crossing the joint that lend muscular support to the elbow joint. The muscles attached to both the common flexor and extensor tendons participate in the general stability of the elbow, especially when the wrist and hand are in use, but also are important in helping to prevent lateral or medial motion of the elbow.

Bony stability

The curved shape of the ulna's trochlear notch cups the trochlea of the humerus, acting like a hook to hold the two bones together. The trochlear ridge and groove provides some restriction to lateral or medial motion within the joint. This stability is reinforced with the lateral and collateral (medial) ligaments.

Ligamentous stability

The lateral collateral ligament of the elbow is most stabilizing during full extension of the forearm, but is less so the more the elbow is flexed. However, the medial collateral ligament is made up of three sections, which allows it overall to remain a stabilizing force throughout the full range of flexion and extension of the elbow. Therefore the lateral collateral is more likely to be injured with the elbow in full extension while various segments of the medial collateral can be injured throughout the range of elbow motion. The quadrate ligament between the neck of the radius and the ulna helps to stabilize the superior radioulnar joint.

Interosseous membrane

The interosseus membrane between the ulna and radius plays an important role in coordinating movements between these two bones, and also in stabilizing and maintaining the appropriate relationship between them. It acts as a soft hinge attachment between the radius and ulna during pronation and supination of the forearm. It is very important in preventing the radius from being pulled out of joint (moving distally) when the hand and forearm are pulling or carrying heavy objects. This membrane also acts as an attachment for muscles and has several perforations that permit neurovascular structures to pass between the anterior and posterior areas of the forearm.

Often mentioned as a distinct ligament from the interosseus membrane complex is the "oblique cord" that runs in a diagonal direction, with its superior attachment on the ulna and its inferior attachment on the radius. This cord provides a strong resistance to the radius being dislocated inferiorly.

Neutral position

The neutral position for the elbow joint is considered 90° of flexion with the forearm half-way between supination and pronation.

This latter position has the thumb of the hand pointing straight up, and is the starting point (0°) from which supination and pronation are measured. However, elbow flexion and extension are measured from the elbow being straight (0°).

End-feel

Extension of the elbow is a bony end-feel: the olecranon process of the ulna comes into contact with the humerus in the olecranon fossa, preventing any further extension of the elbow. The end-feel on flexion of the elbow is tissue approximation. End-feel of supination and pronation is tissue stretch.

Palpation

These landmarks are important for testing purposes, finding joint margins, and locating musculature:

- medial and lateral epicondyles of the elbow, and their supracondylar lines
- olecranon fossa and olecranon process
- ulnar ridge
- sulcus between the medial epicondyle and the olecranon process (ulnar nerve path)
- radial head.

Active range of motion for the elbow joint

Flexion 130–150°

Extension 0–10°

Supination 90°

Pronation 80–90°

The protocol (Box 17.1) begins with the case history.

Box 17.1 Protocol

- Case history (specific questions)
- Observations
- Rule outs
- Active free range of motion (AF-ROM)
- Passive relaxed range of motion (PR-ROM)
- Active resisted range of motion (AR-ROM)
- Special tests

Case history (specific questions)

- Do you have diabetes or any circulatory conditions?
- Do you have any neurological problems in your neck, shoulder, or arm?
- Have you ever injured this arm, or this elbow specifically, before?
- Does one or both of your hands or arms ever feel cold or hot?
- Do you ever feel suddenly weak in the arms, or do you find yourself suddenly dropping things?
- Do you ever feel any tingling that is specific to certain fingers of the hand, or in all of the hand?

Observations

Regional assessment within the context of the whole

As with every area of the body being investigated by orthopedic testing (specific view), remember to always look at that joint or tissue within the context of the surrounding joints and structures (regional view). What is the interplay of impaired tissues or structures with the rest of the tissues in that region? In turn, take into consideration the global view: how is that joint, and region, affecting the whole body? How is the whole affecting or influencing the region and the specific site(s) of impairment(s)? Just as with treatment, the approach to assessment also moves from general-to-specific-to-general. Not all the preconditions for an impairment exist on-site, or in the surrounding region. They can come from the totality of the body, the person and their environment.

REMEMBER: Observation begins the moment a patient enters the clinic. Perform a postural scan from each side and from the front and back. Deformities are visible signs of impairment that result from severe genetic or long-standing conditions. These deformities will have caused clear compensatory changes to the structures in support of those areas. Note obvious deformities and consider their implications. Is the deformity a contributing factor to the patient's chief complaint?

For example, though we are specifically looking to assess the elbow and the patient's chief complaint, we are also looking at the elbow regionally within the context of the arm all the way from the cervical spine, into the shoulder, and down into the fingertips. We also want to have a global view as to how the whole body could predispose the elbow to injury or impairment, and how this impaired elbow may be impacting on the body as a whole.

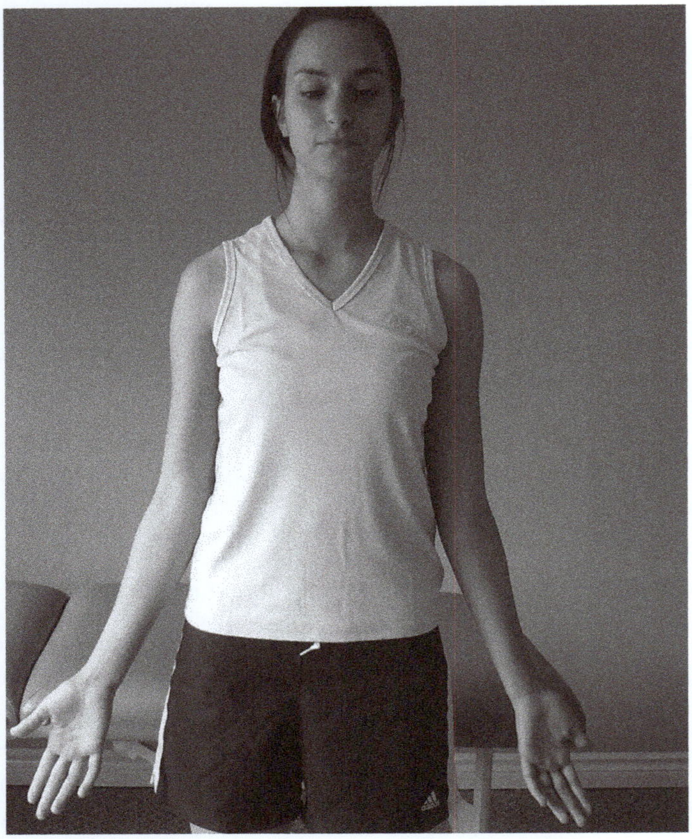

FIGURE 17.1

The carrying angle of the elbow.

The carrying angle of the elbow (Figure 17.1) is the valgus orientation that the forearm has with respect to the upper arm so that the arm clears the hips when walking. The valgus angle, on average, is approximately 10–15° for men and 20–25° for women. Deviations of less than 10° and more than 30° would point to possible bony or joint abnormalities.

Rule outs

General guidelines for ruling out joints above and below the chief complaint

Once you have decided which joint or region of the body you are going to investigate for the source of the patient's chief complaint, you must first rule out the joint above and the joint below. It is imperative to determine whether the joints/areas above and below the primary joint or region could be referring to the impaired joint or tissue. If this rule out testing does not reproduce the patient's chief complaint, then that joint is said to be ruled out and not in need of immediate further testing (Hartley 2000a).

Remember that the patient may experience pain or other symptoms or impairments with the rule out testing, but if they do not provoke or reproduce the chief complaint then they are set aside for now (and may be returned to later). These quick tests stress the principal tissues involved in each of those joints to be ruled out. They primarily focus on the non-contractile elements.

Having applied the over-pressure (O-P), again ask the patient if they feel any pain. If no pain is experienced proceed to the next AF motion and continue as you did above. However, if the patient experiences any pain or impairment then further clarify by asking if it is the same as the pain they have come to see you about, or is if it something different. If you get a positive reproduction of the chief complaint when doing a rule out then that joint now needs to be included in your protocol of testing for the chief complaint; it is considered *ruled in*. Remember, a chief complaint may include more than one joint.

If there is pain with or without other impairments, but it is not part of the patient's chief complaint, then record it. Nonetheless, return to your testing of the area indicated by the patient's complaint. These extra findings can be investigated further at a later date. If neither joint (above or below) rule outs reproduces the patient's chief complaint during either the AF or the PR with O-P portion of testing, then proceed onward to do the regular AF-ROM testing of the joint or structures that are the focus of the day's testing.

The shoulder and wrist joints need to be ruled out before testing the elbow to ensure that their structures are not referring symptoms into the elbow.

Ruling out the shoulder

To rule out the shoulder do two AF movements: forward flexion and abduction, both with O-P. Test the unaffected side first, to establish the normal range and end-feel of the patient, and then the affected side. If there is dysfunction or impairment in the glenohumeral, acromial, sternoclavicular, or scapulothoracic joints these actions with over-pressure will place enough stress on their structures and tissues to elicit a sufficient positive response. This may be pain or reproduction of the patient's chief complaint, which would be enough information to tell us that we need do more thorough testing of these areas.

Ruling out the wrist

This is not really practical as active wrist flexion and extension with over-pressure will activate several muscles that cross the wrist and the elbow via the common flexor tendon or common extensor tendon. (We will use testing that is similar to these rule outs while testing the elbow.)

Range of motion testing (ROM)

Active free range of motion (AF-ROM)

With the patient standing or seated, have them do the actions shown in Figures 17.2–17.6. Whenever possible, do the actions bilaterally at the same time in order to get a better comparison of available ranges. Have the patient begin all actions from the neutral position (Figure 17.2A, B). For testing purposes, neutral position of the elbow is when it is close to, if not touching the body, with forearm flexed to 90°, palm of hand facing medially (thumb is superior), and wrist in mid-position, neither flexed nor extended.

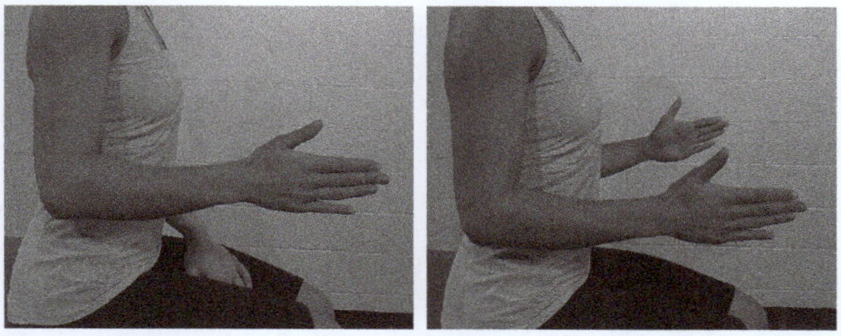

FIGURE 17.2 A,B

Start all actions from neutral.

Demonstrate the actions for the patient (Figures 17.3–17.6)

The therapist should demonstrate the actions and have the patient follow along. Remember that these tests should be placed in an order which will have the patient doing the actions that are known to be the most painful last. Record impairments noticed and ask the patient, after each movement, if any pain or altered sensation is felt and whether you have reproduced the chief complaint.

Passive relaxed range of motion (PR-ROM)

With the patient seated, do the actions in Figures 17.7–17.14 for them as they try to stay relaxed and let you take them through the motions. Remember to begin all movements from a neutral position.

Take hold of the patient's arm and forearm firmly, but gently. Ask them to relax their arm completely and let you do all movements. When you apply over-pressure, make sure that you have stabilized the structures so that movement will only happen at the joint being investigated. Tell the patient to let you know immediately about any pain, or if something does not feel right. When you reach end-range, ask specifically if pain or any symptoms have arisen, and only if none have, proceed to apply over-pressure. If the patient complains of pain do not apply over-pressure and always ask if the pain is the same as the chief complaint.

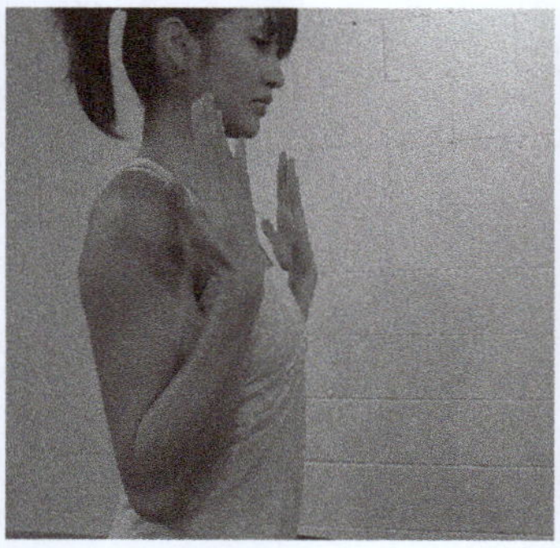

FIGURE 17.3 1. AF flexion 140–150°

The patient brings the hands toward the shoulders. Most functional activities can be done by someone with only 130° of flexion. Many can be done by those who cannot extend the elbow less than 30°.

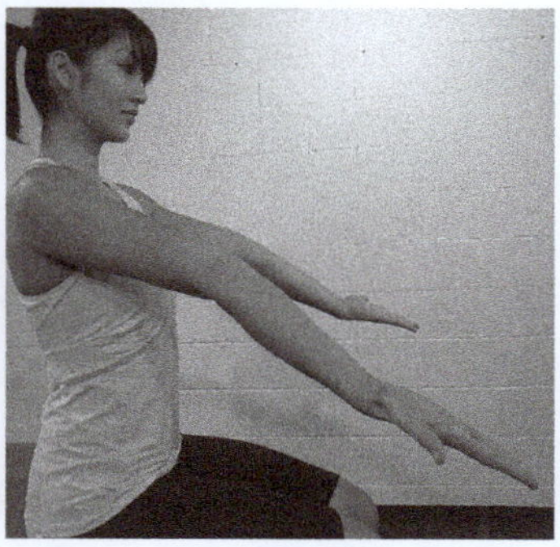

FIGURE 17.4 2. AF extension 0–10°

Have the patient straighten the elbows. Hyperextension is defined as motion greater than 15° of extension.

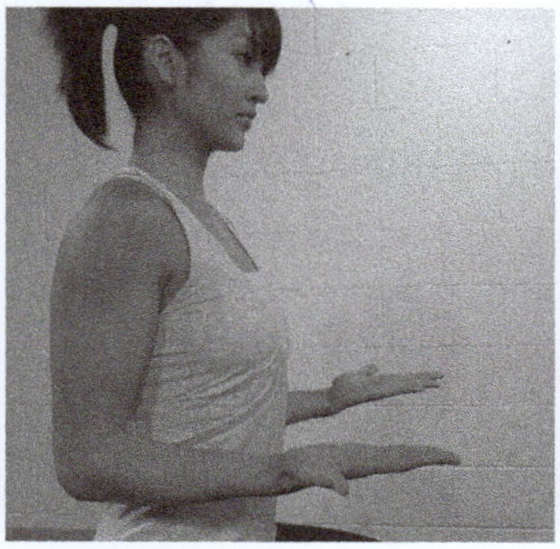

FIGURE 17.5 3. AF supination (forearm) 90°

From the neutral position, the patient turns the palms up. Most functional activities need 50° of supination.

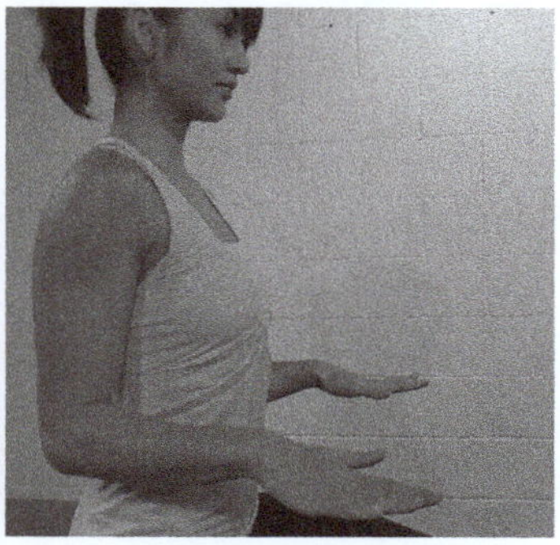

FIGURE 17.6 4. AF pronation (forearm) 80–90°

From the neutral position, the patient turns the palms down. Most functional activities need 50° of pronation.

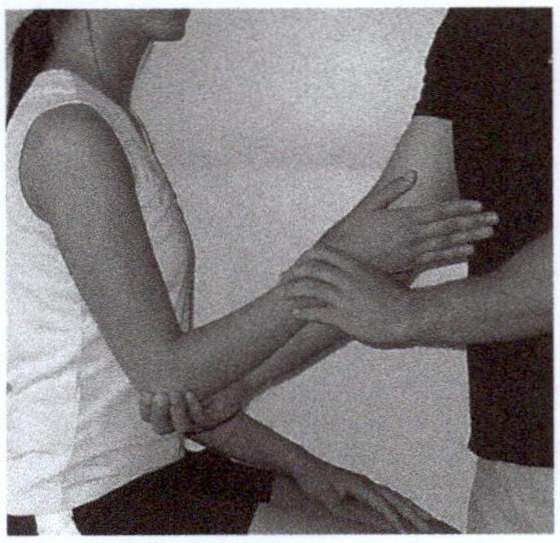
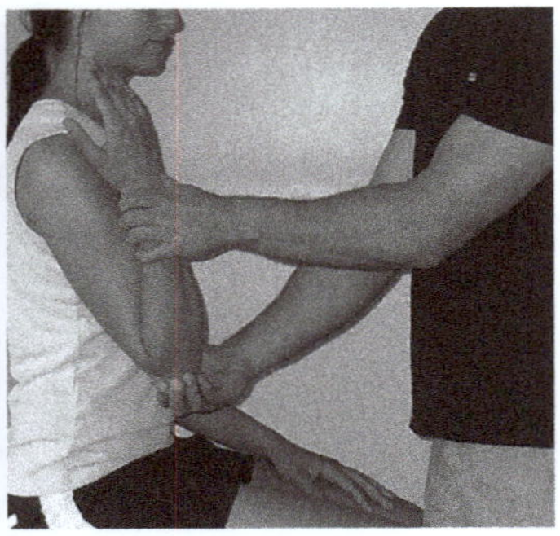

FIGURE 17.7 PR flexion
FIGURE 17.8 PR flexion with O-P

Take the patient's elbow into full flexion and, for O-P, push the forearm into arm. End-feel will be a soft tissue approximation as the forearm meets the biceps brachii.

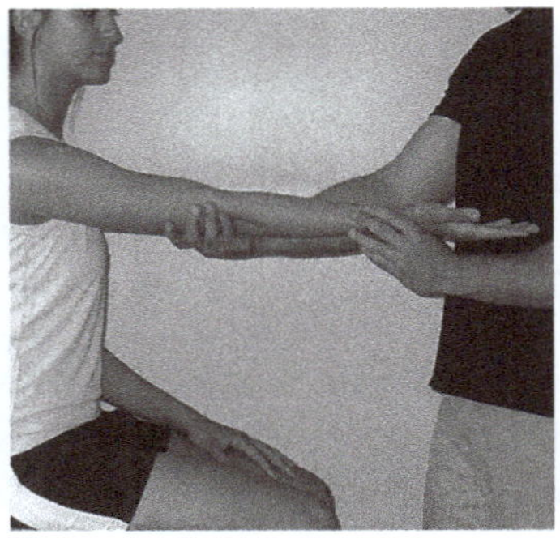
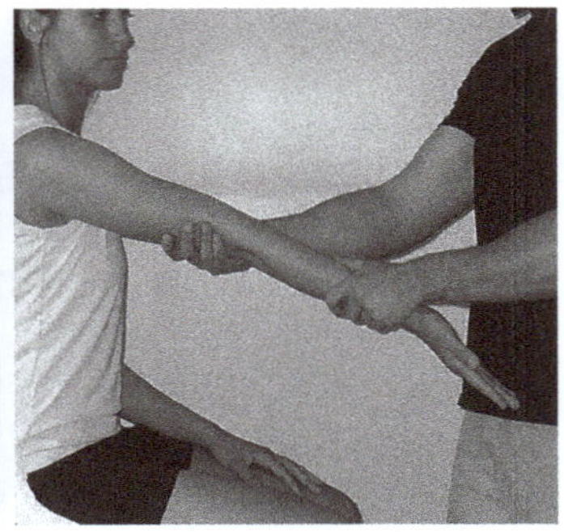

FIGURE 17.9 PR extension
FIGURE 17.10 PR extension with O-P

Extend the patient's elbow. Stabilize the posterior surface of the arm while applying O-P to the forearm to increase extension slightly. End-feel will be bony with a firm, abrupt stop at the humeral-ulnar joint.

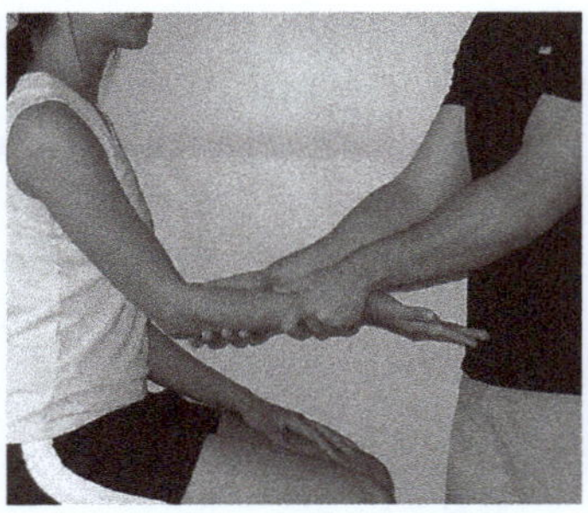

FIGURE 17.11 PR supination of forearm

Relax the patient's elbow out of extension and return the arm to neutral. To supinate the forearm, turn it until the anterior forearm is facing you and the palm is up.

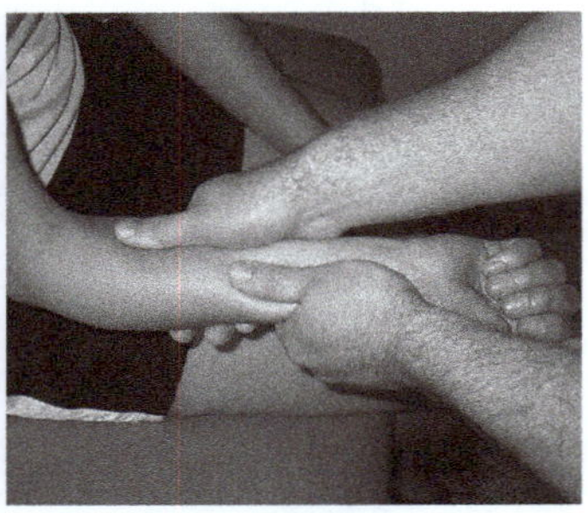

FIGURE 17.12 PR supination with O-P

When applying O-P, you grasp each bone (ulna and radius) separately. Run the thumbs parallel along each. Shown here, the radius, held by the lower hand, is receiving O-P toward further supination, as it is the moving bone in supination and pronation of the forearm and hand. The ulna is being stabilized as the fixed bone. End-feel will be tissue stretch.

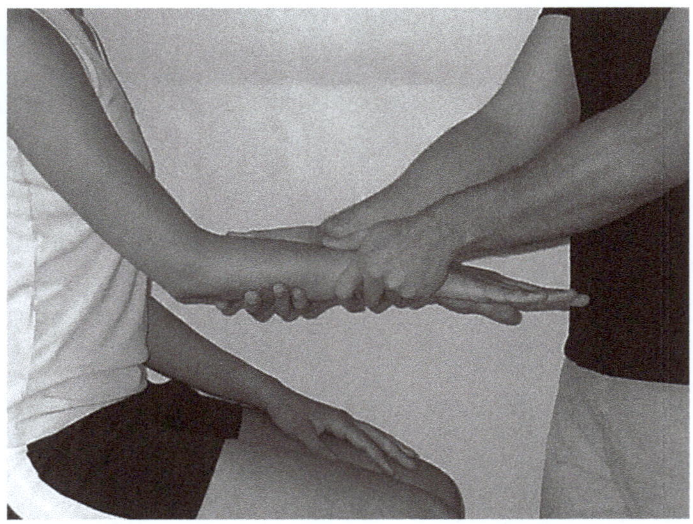

FIGURE 17.13 PR pronation of forearm

Return the forearm and elbow to neutral, and to pronate, continue turning the forearm until the posterior surface of the forearm is up and the palm is facing down.

Joint play inspection of the elbow joint (Figures 17.15–17.21)

Radial and ulnar deviations of the elbow are equal to valgus and varus stress testing.

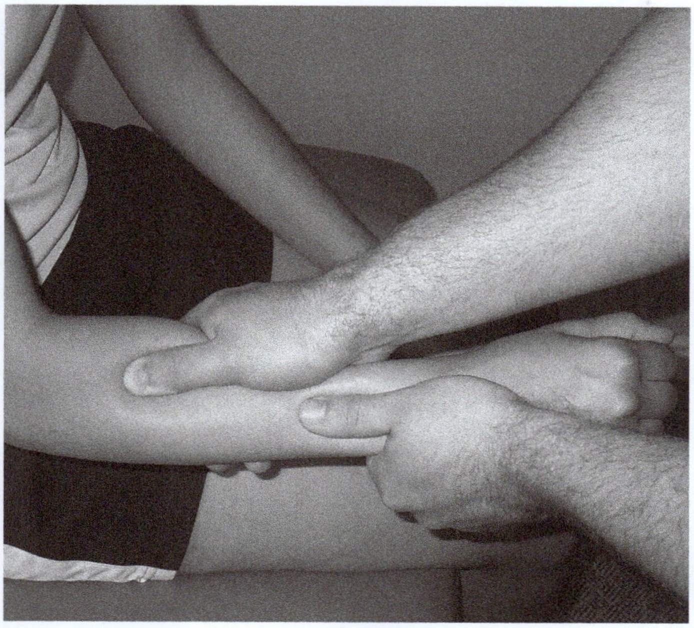

FIGURE 17.14 PR pronation with O-P

As for supination, when applying O-P for pronation, you grasp each bone (ulna and radius) separately. Run the thumbs parallel along each. Here the radius, grasped by the therapist's right hand and thumb, is receiving O-P into further pronation. End-feel will be tissue stretch. With pronation, you need to grasp the ulna and radius at their smallest portions. This is necessary to apply O-P specifically through superior and inferior radioulnar joints. Therefore, careful landmarking and palpation is required to make sure you do not inadvertently grasp both bones with one of your hands. End-feel is normally tissue stretch.

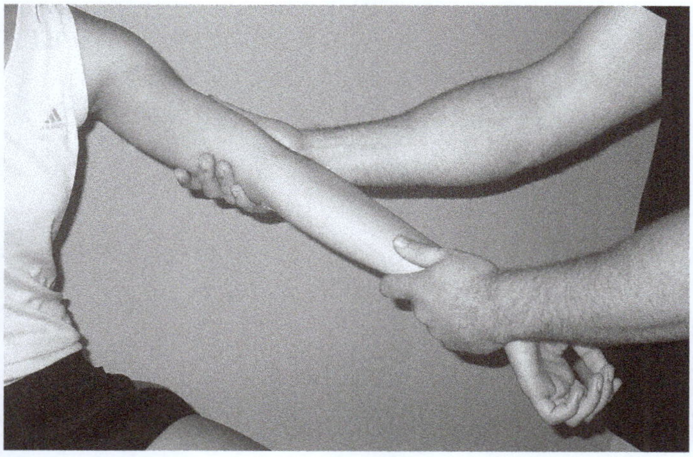

FIGURE 17.15 Radial deviation

To perform radial deviation of the elbow, stabilize the arm above the elbow, take it into extension with the forearm supinated and then move the forearm laterally. Resistance should be firm, with no gapping of the joint on the medial side, and pain-free. If any of these occur, then the medial portion of the elbow is injured/impaired. Pain felt in the posterior portion of the elbow may be due to injury of the olecranon process or fossa. Firmness of a normal elbow in extension comes from the olecranon being wedged into its fossa, and tension in the collateral ligaments.

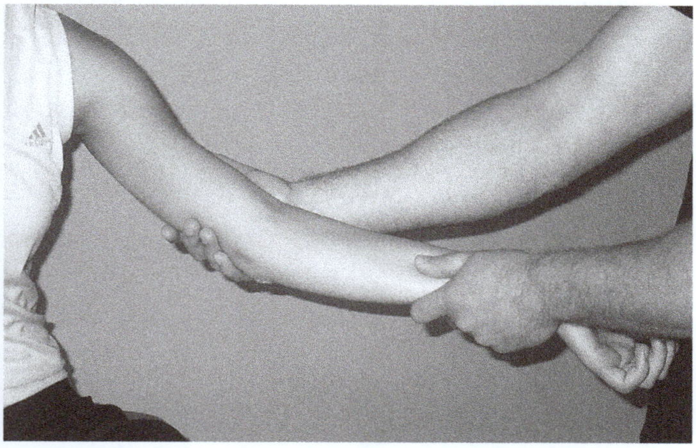

FIGURE 17.16 Radial deviation with unlocked elbow

Unlock the elbow to 10–15° of flexion, apply traction and again radially deviate the supinated forearm. With the joint unlocked, stretch will be placed almost entirely on the soft tissue of the joint (capsule and supportive ligaments), thus testing integrity. It is a valgus stress test. There should be slight laxity palpated initially upon moving bones; however, a strong, leathery feel comes on quickly as slack in the ligaments and capsule is taken up. This position is preferred if you choose to oscillate the joint in a lateral direction (to treat shortened and/or adhering medial ligaments or joint capsule).

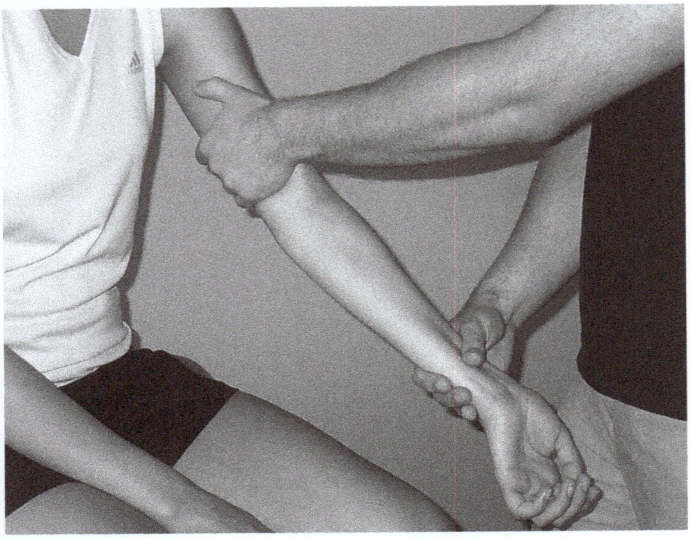

FIGURE 17.17 Ulnar deviation

To perform ulnar deviation take the elbow into extension and while stabilizing the arm above the elbow, draw the tractioned and supinated forearm medially. You should have a firm bony end-feel. Next, take the elbow slightly out of extension (into 10–15° of flexion) and repeat deviation to stress the lateral ligaments and joint capsule, avoiding bony restriction. This is a varus stress of the elbow.

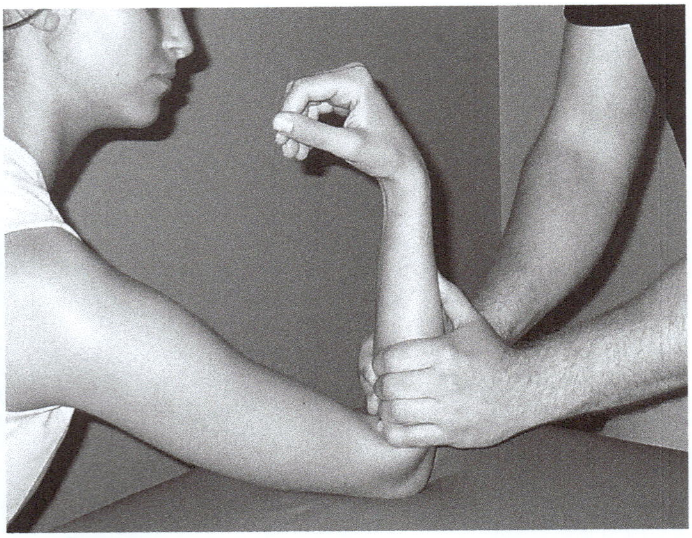

FIGURE 17.18 Distraction of elbow joint

To slightly open or distract the olecranon from the humerus, the elbow should be flexed to rotate the olecranon process out of the olecranon fossa. Use both hands to grasp the forearm, grasping the ulna and radius specifically, and pull the patient's forearm toward you with a scooping action. If you do not feel a slight distraction in the humeral-ulnar joint, this may indicate capsule tightness.

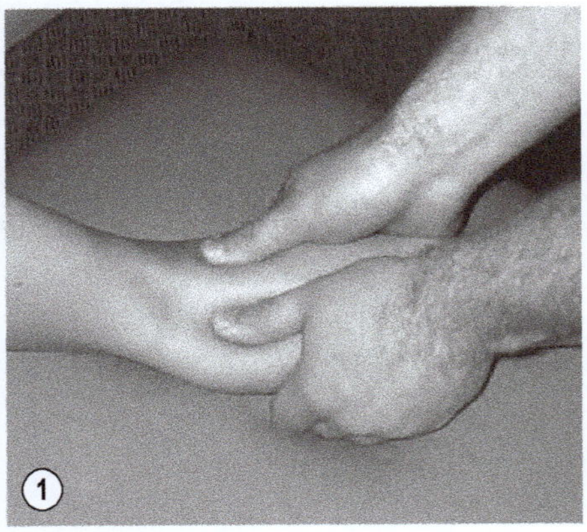

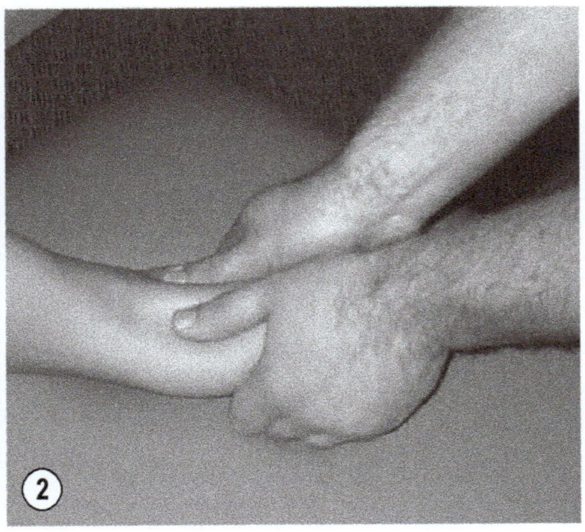

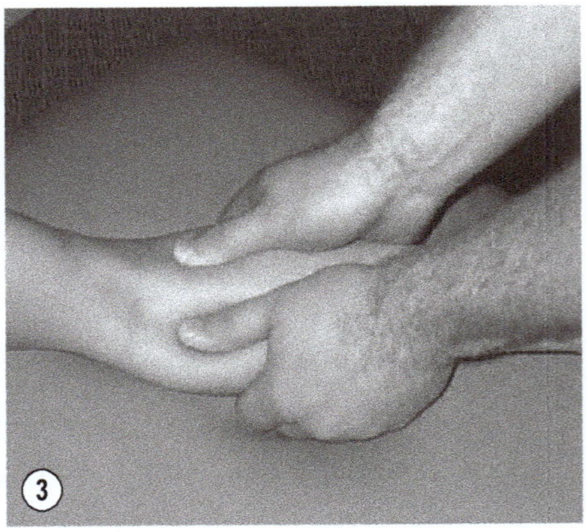

FIGURES 17.19–17.21 Mobilization of radial-ulnar joint

1. To mobilize and test the proximal radial-ulnar joint, have the patient's arm in a resting position at 70° extension with the forearm supinated. You need the forearm supinated so that you are not pushing the radius into the ulna (which would happen if you did this in pronation, where the radius crosses over the ulna). Grasp the proximal end of the forearm, with the ulna and radius each held with one hand. Have the thumbs parallel to each other, with one running along the ulna and other along the radius. Be precise in your landmarking and palpation. Stabilize the ulna, which is the fixed bone. 2. Pull the radius anteriorly and then … 3. push posteriorly, taking up the slack in the soft tissues of the joint. Oscillate back and forth several times. (This can also be used to mobilize the interosseous membrane between the radius and ulna if you repeat as above but then move your hands to the mid-forearm and then just above wrist.)

Active resisted range of motion (AR-ROM) (Figures 17.22–17.27)

See Part I, Chapter 3 for a discussion of active resisted testing and what we learn from such testing, including a grading scale 0 to 5. (See Kendall et al. 2005 for a truly comprehensive exploration and instruction in muscle testing; see also and compare Dutton 2012; Hartley 2000a; Hertling & Kessler 2006; Magee 2014; Petty 2011.)

With the patient seated, do the resisted testing shown in Figures 17.22–17.27, with the elbow in 90° of flexion. Try to keep the patient's elbow close to the body. During testing, watch carefully to see if the patient tries to recruit muscles of the shoulder girdle by internally or externally rotating the glenohumeral joint, or by abducting or slightly flexing and abducting the glenohumeral joint.

Clinical notes on resistance testing can be found in Box 17.2.

NOTE: Because of the large number of muscles that cross both the elbow and the wrist, we should also test the following actions isometrically.

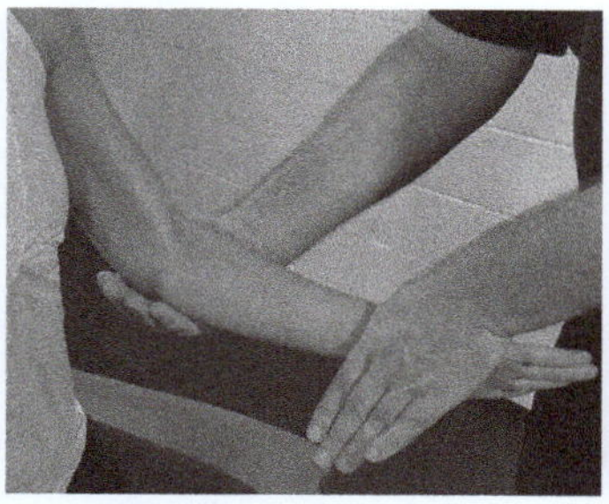

FIGURE 17.22 AR flexion

The patient's elbow is in the neutral position at 90° of flexion, with the arm at the side. Have the patient resist an attempt to extend the elbow. Primarily testing brachioradialis and, secondarily, biceps brachii and brachialis.

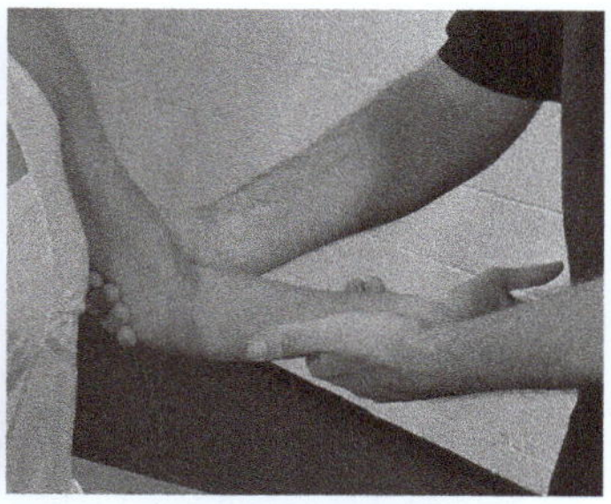

FIGURE 17.23 AR extension

With the patient's elbow in the neutral position, have the patient resist an attempt to flex the elbow. Primarily testing triceps brachii and anconeus.

Box 17.2 Clinical notes

Remember that pain provoked with resistance testing points to injury of the musculotendinous unit. This can show up as pain in the muscle belly, or in the tendinous portion. As with any pain felt by the patient during testing, have them point to exactly where the pain is felt or to circumscribe the area it is felt in if the pain is diffuse. This alone may be enough information for you to be able to distinguish between a strain of the contractile portion of the muscle or injury to the tendinous portion.

The patient should be reminded to immediately tell you when pain is first felt. You should stop the isometric testing to prevent further injury to involved tissues.

Classically, if the patient feels pain during resistance, but is able to generate full strength, then this is recorded as a mild strain. If the patient feels pain and cannot generate full strength, then it is more severe. Note in the records when there is pain, and an approximate value to the percentage of strength the impaired side was able to generate in comparison to the patient's unaffected side.

If the patient shows weakness but experiences no pain this is a **red flag** for a neurological impairment. This should be followed by more extensive scan of myotome, dermatome and, where applicable, deep tendon reflex testing. Regardless, weakness without pain requires you to refer the patient back to the primary physician.

Do not forget that the force being generated during isometric testing is built up over 3–5 seconds, until full strength is reached, or movement is about to occur. The patient needs to reach full exertion, if that is possible, to see if: (1) there is full strength and then pain, indicating a mild tissue strain; (2) if there is loss of strength accompanied by pain, indicating a moderate to severe strain; or (3) if weakness is encountered without any pain, which is a neurological **red flag**. This will require a referral back to their primary physician. If the patient is told use only part of their strength, then both (1) and (2) could be missed.

The therapist can apply the resistance as the patient tries to do the appropriate movement, or if you feel they engage too quickly and strongly, then tell them to hold the starting position while they supply the resistance and you apply the force. (The latter is generally preferred by the author.) If you expect pain or muscle failure to occur, then proceed to increasing the force of your pressure very gradually and very carefully. You want to avoid eccentrically loading any muscle or stretching or tearing any tissue that may be injured.

One further **note:** muscles that cross two joints are more likely to be injured than the one-joint muscles.

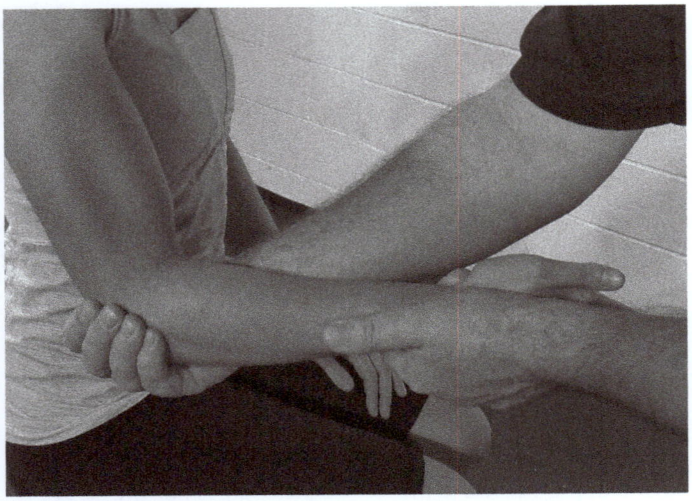

FIGURE 17.24 AR supination of forearm

With the patient's elbow in the neutral position, use one hand to stabilize it against the patient's body. Grasp the forearm with the other hand and run the thumb along the posterior surface of the radius. The patient holds this position and resists your attempt to pronate the forearm. Primarily testing biceps brachii and supinator.

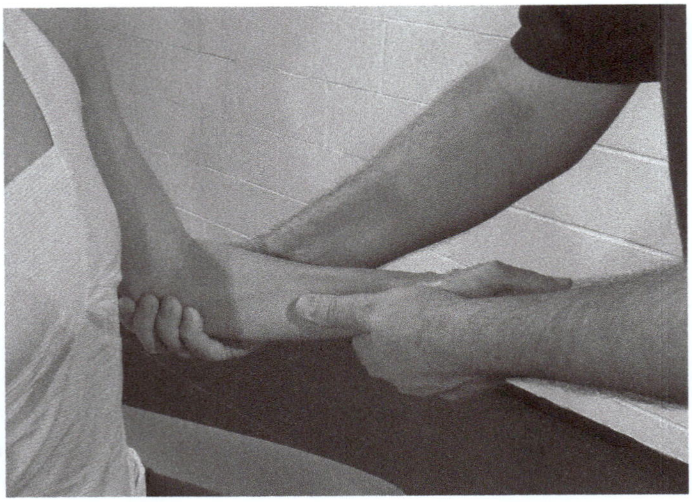

FIGURE 17.25 AR pronation of forearm

With the patient's elbow in the neutral position, use one hand to stabilize it against the patient's body. Grasp the forearm with the other hand and with the thumb running along the anterior surface of the radius. Ask the patient to resist your attempt to supinate the forearm. You are primarily testing pronator teres and pronator quadratus.

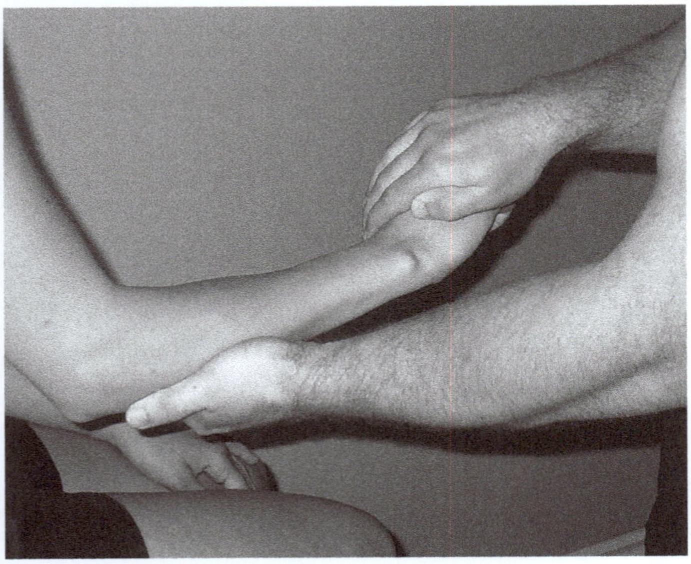

FIGURE 17.26 AR wrist extension

The elbow is flexed to 90°, the wrist is in slight extension, and the forearm is pronated. Stabilize the forearm while the other hand rests on the dorsal surface of the hand. The patient holds the position as you try to flex the wrist. Pain can be in the muscle belly, at the wrist or carpals, and/or the elbow.

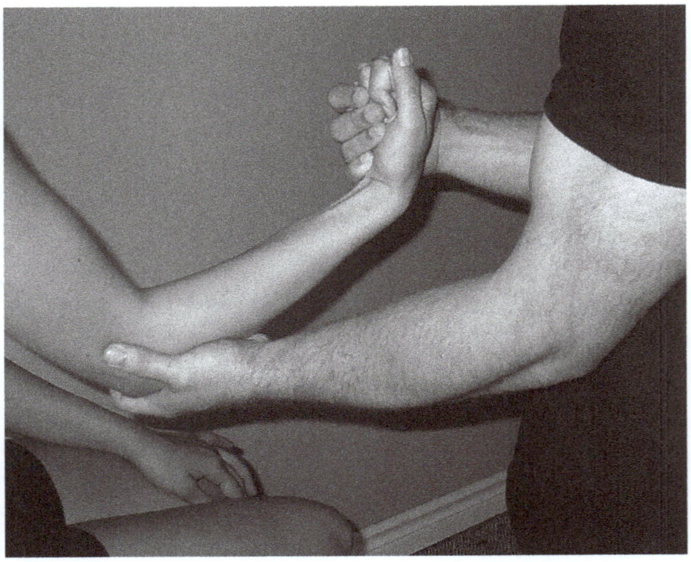

FIGURE 17.27 AR wrist flexion

The patient's elbow is flexed to 90°, the wrist is in slight flexion, and the forearm is supinated. Stabilize the patient's forearm while the other hand rests on the ventral surface of the patient's hand. Have the patient try to flex the wrist while you apply resistance.

Special tests

Differential muscle testing

The therapist uses differential muscle testing on muscles possibly implicated as impaired during AF-ROM or AR-ROM testing, or where the patient's description of pain and/or dysfunction implicates the muscle (Kendall et al. 2005).

Box 17.3 briefly looks at the rationale for testing individual muscles within the tested muscle groups.

Differential testing of brachioradialis, brachialis, and biceps brachii (Figures 17.28–17.30)

We are only performing these tests because we either found pain and/or weakness when performing AR-ROM testing of elbow flexion. To determine which muscles may be impaired

Box 17.3 Where are we in our protocol?

Up to this point we have only tested muscle groups. It is necessary to grade the acuity of impairment of the muscles within that group. It is important to investigate whether there is one muscle of a group that is more impaired than the others. Remember, we are trying to recreate or elicit the patient's chief pain/complaint while taking note of other pain created that may be secondary or compensatory.

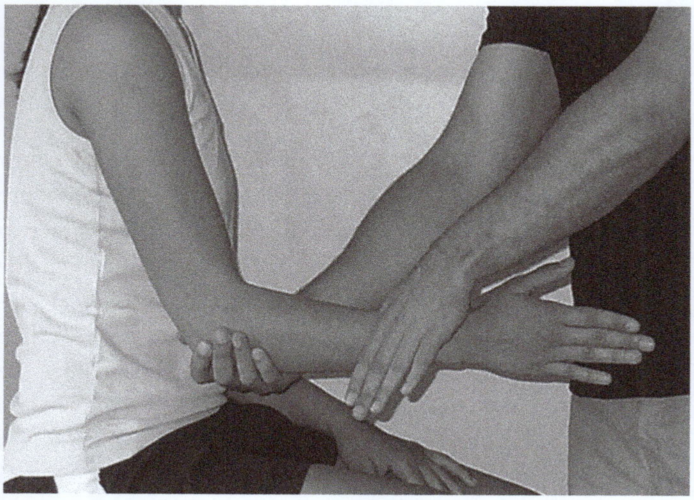

FIGURE 17.28 **1. Stressing the brachioradialis**

With the forearm in neutral (note the position of the hand), having the shoulder slightly flexed and the elbow slightly extended 10–15° isolates brachioradialis more.

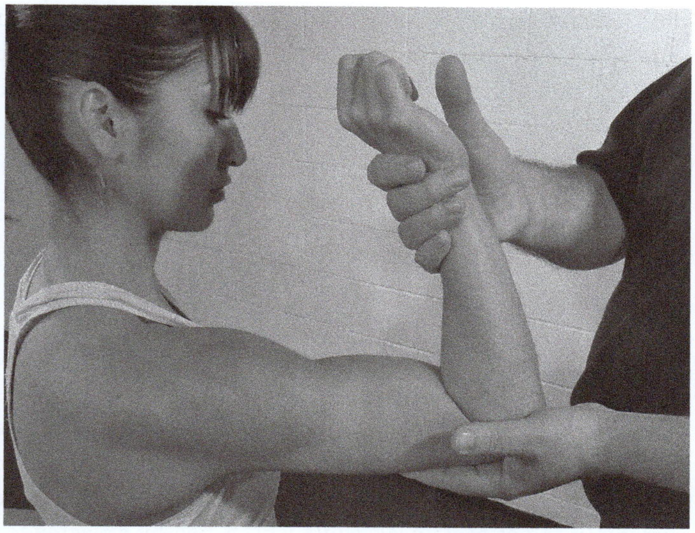

FIGURE 17.29 **2. Brachialis stressed**

With the forearm pronated (note palm is facing down), flex the elbow to 110° and then forward flex shoulder to 80–90° of flexion. Brachialis will now provide most of the resistance. Stabilize the elbow with one hand and try to extend the patient's flexed elbow. Make sure you are not extending the shoulder joint at the same time.

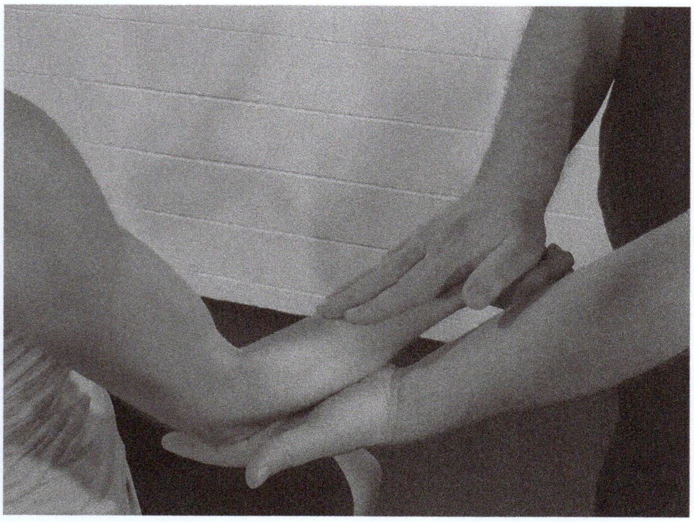

FIGURE 17.30 **3. Biceps brachii**

With forearm supinated (note palm is up), the biceps brachii muscle will assume a more active role than when the elbow/forearm is in neutral. Test flexion of the elbow in this position. If the biceps are highly involved in impaired flexion of the elbow (seen in AR testing), the patient will more clearly complain here.

and to what degree, we need to do several tests in sequence and compare the results as we progress through the tests. We are going to be testing flexion in various positions that will place more stress on some muscles and make them work maximally, while we inhibit and weaken others through lengthening or positioning. We will only be able to decide which specific muscle is impaired and to what degree by seeing which test(s) recreates the pain or weakness of the chief complaint in terms of degree and location.

A positive sign for impaired function is pain felt by the patient along the course of the muscle. The brachioradialis muscle will be generating the most force in this position, since this is the position in which it is most effective and efficient. The biceps brachii and the brachialis will also be working, but the brachialis is not at its peak while lengthened by an extended elbow. Further, the biceps cannot generate its peak force as it is being partially inhibited by not being allowed to supinate the forearm. Record your result regarding pain and strength/weakness.

NOTE: A sign that the brachioradialis is weak and/or impaired is if the arm begins to supinate. This implies that the biceps muscles are being recruited more intently to help replace the weakened brachioradialis. Record if this happens.

The brachioradialis is weakened by the elbow flexion. If there is less pain in this position compared to a positive for test 1 (Figure 17.28), then the brachioradialis may be involved, especially if the pain runs along the muscle in the forearm. The biceps are shortened too much to generate any tension and, as the forearm is pronated, the biceps are further inhibited from working. (If the biceps were the source of pain with AR-ROM testing, the patient would not complain here with this positioning. Or, if acutely injured, they would not have as much pain in the arm as was produced in the neutral position.)

Remember that the brachialis is still the stronger muscle here, in number 3 (Figure 17.30). It is the comparison of the tests that helps generate our decision about which muscle is involved in impairments that were previously noted in AF-ROM. Therefore, if this test produces the most pain of all those done so far, the biceps brachii is implicated as a principal muscle involved in the impaired flexion found in AR-ROM. However, if this position does not generate as much pain/weakness as, or no more pain/weakness than, the previous tests did, the biceps is ruled out as a principal culprit. We then need to think through the results so far in order to deduce which muscle is to be implicated.

Box 17.4 Review of results for tests of elbow flexion done to determine acuity of strain

- If, after doing all these tests, it was the first test that had the most dramatic result (pain and/or weakness), then the brachioradialis is the most injured or impaired of all the muscles involved in elbow flexion.
- If the second test is the one that had the most dramatic results, then the brachialis is the one implicated as the principal cause of the pain that had been seen in AR-ROM testing of flexion of the elbow.
- If the third test is the most dramatic positive result, then the biceps is probably the most injured muscle.

Of course, all, or two of the muscles could be involved but by gauging how each responds in each of the three tests you will be creating the information you will need to differentially assess the degree of each muscle's involvement in the impairment being tested. This will help you decide on a specific treatment plan that can prioritize what is to be treated, in what order, and with what modality or technique, so that the patient is treated effectively and safely. **Note:** As the biceps brachii muscle crosses two joints, it can often be the most injured muscle of the whole group.

Box 17.4 reviews the results for the tests of elbow flexion done thus far.

Differentiating between long head and medial and lateral heads of triceps brachii (Figures 17.31, 17.32)

There are no muscles that we can differentiate with elbow extension. However, the long head of the triceps can be more injured than the medial and lateral heads due to it crossing two joints (the elbow and the shoulder). Note that pain from the long head of the triceps often appears around the lesser glenoid tubercle. When the patient points to this site as the source of pain most therapists will jump to the conclusion that the problem is a rotator cuff tear. To test if the long head is more impaired or is the source of pain, we can do the tests shown in Figures 17.31, 17.32.

Differentiating between the supinator and biceps brachii (Figures 7.33, 7.34)

If the patient had pain upon active resisted (AR) testing of supination, then the following testing can be done to help locate which supinating muscle may be more injured.

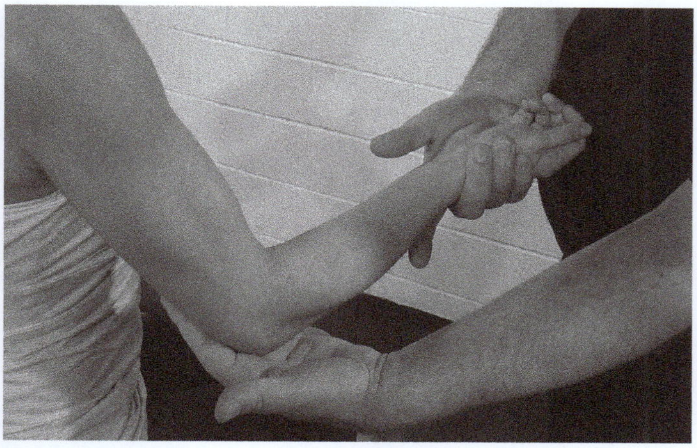

FIGURE 17.31 **Testing all triceps heads**

1. With the elbow in a neutral position, have the patient resist your attempt to flex the elbow. We are primarily testing triceps brachii and anconeus.

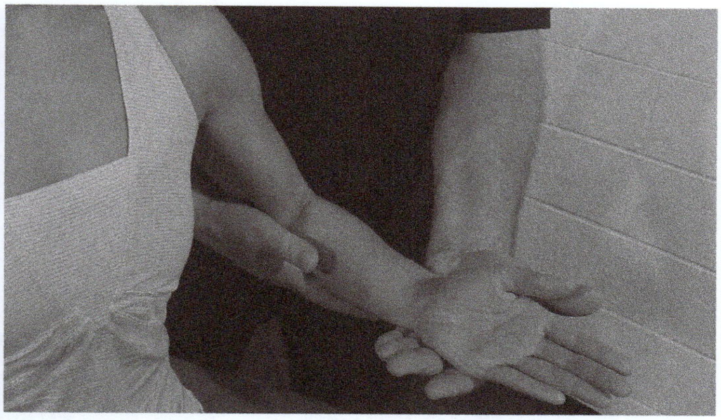

FIGURE 17.32 **Stressing long head of triceps**

2. To place more stress on the long head, place a stabilizing hand on the medial portion of the elbow. This time ask the patient to resist your attempt to simultaneously flex and abduct the elbow. This will add stress to the long head as it not only extends the elbow but assists in the abduction of the arm.

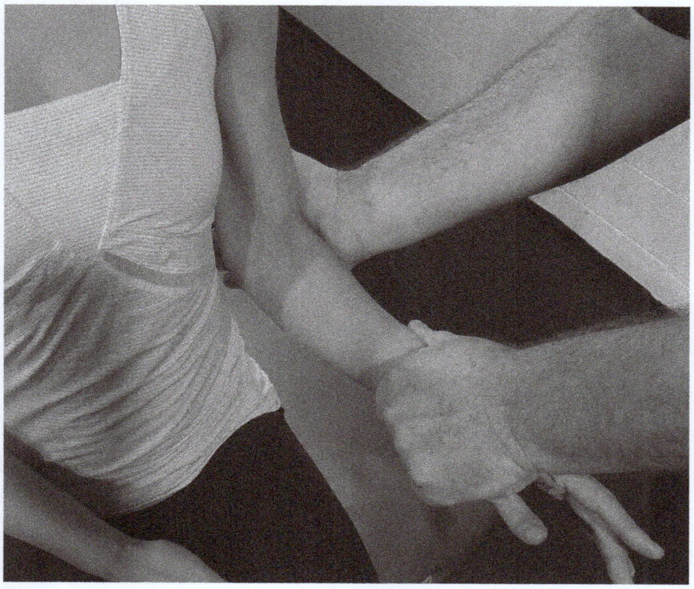

FIGURE 17.33 **1. Testing supinator and biceps brachii**

With the elbow in a neutral position and stabilized against the body with one hand, grasp the forearm just above the wrist with the other hand and have your thumb running along the patient's radius. Ask the patient to hold the position and resist your attempt to pronate the forearm. If the therapist resists the patient's attempt to supinate, the therapist may risk injury to their own wrist.

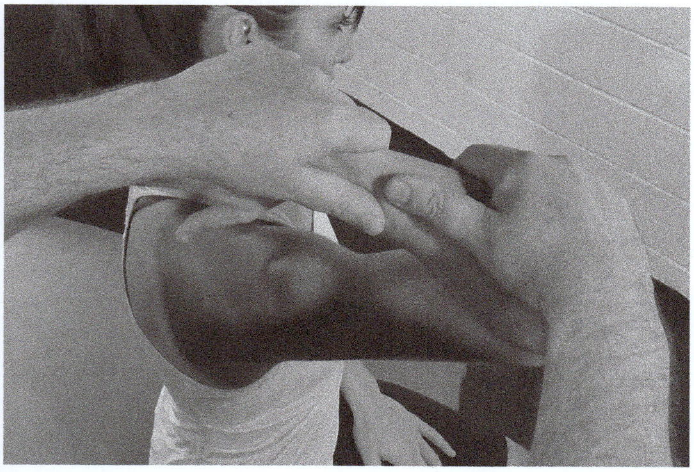

FIGURE 17.34 **2. Stressing supinator more**

To help distinguish which muscle is responsible if pain results from this test, simply repeat the test with the elbow nearly fully flexed and the shoulder flexed 90°, thereby decreasing the role of biceps brachii and leaving the supinator to take on stress. Have the patient's hand positioned so the palm of the hand is facing medially and the thumb points toward the shoulder. Stand beside the patient and stabilize both the radius and the ulnar bones. Ask the patient to try to either turn their hand toward the shoulder as you resist, or to resist your effort to turn the forearm so the palm would be facing away from the shoulder. If resistance is still as painful as in the original test, the supinator is definitely involved. If less painful, then the pain is likely due to the biceps.

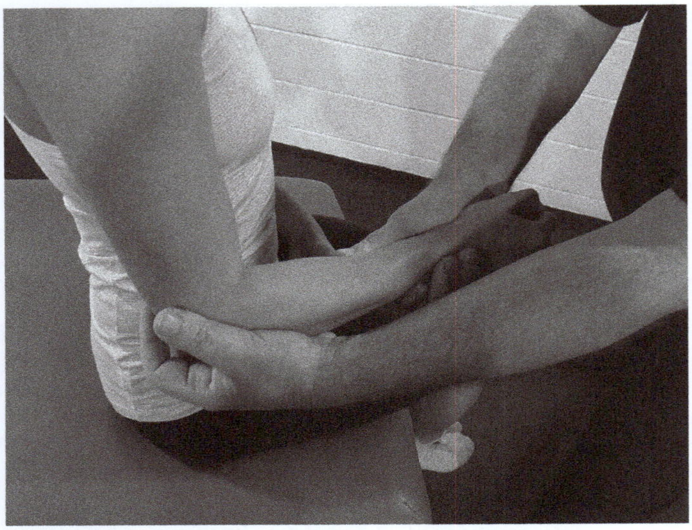

FIGURE 17.35 **1. Testing pronator teres and pronator quadratus**

With the elbow in neutral position and stabilized by the therapist against the body with one hand, grasp above the patient's wrist with your other hand, with the thumb running along the radius. Tell the patient to resist your attempt to supinate their forearm. You are primarily testing pronator teres and pronator quadratus.

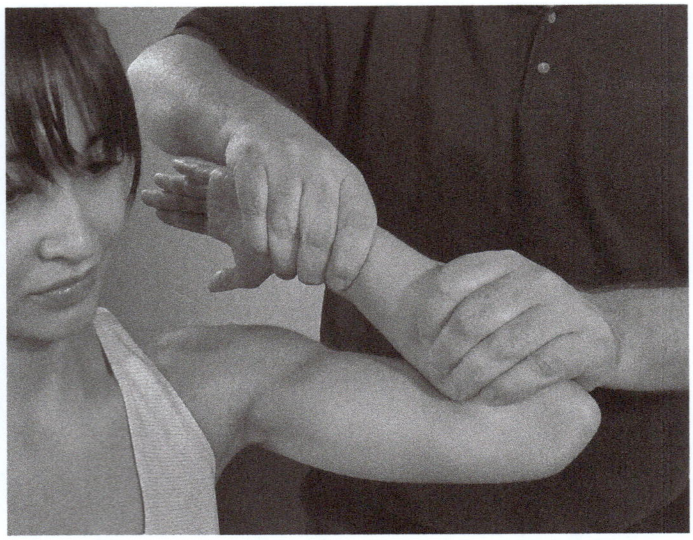

FIGURE 17.36 **2. Stressing pronator quadratus more**

Have the patient fully flex the elbow and have their hand facing their jaw. Stand in front of the patient and stabilize both the radius and ulnar bones. Ask the patient to try to turn their hand toward ceiling as you resist.

Differentiating between pronator teres and pronator quadratus (Figure 17.35, 17.36)

The location of pain will usually aid in distinguishing between these two muscles but, if you wish, you can differentiate between them with testing.

NOTE: Because there are a number of muscles that cross both the elbow and the wrist, we should also test the following actions isometrically. Some of these tests are also tendonitis tests for epicondylitis (medial or lateral) if the pain is felt in the epicondular region of the elbow.

Differentiating between extensor carpi radialis longus and brevis and extensor carpi ulnaris (Figures 17.37–17.39)

The prime movers you are testing are extensor carpi radialis longus and brevis, and extensor carpi ulnaris. Pain can be experienced in the muscle belly in the forearm, at the wrist, or at the elbow attachment sites - or at all three sites. Finding several painful sites usually indicates that the injury is more severe, whether the onset of pain is sudden or gradual.

Differentiating between carpi radialis longus and brevis (Figure 17.40)

Differentiating between flexor carpi radialis and flexor carpi ulnaris and palmaris longus (Figures 17.41–17.43)

Ligamentous stability tests

These test the stability of the collateral ligaments on the medial and lateral sides of the joint. A positive sign can be pain. However, the amount of instability is best determined by palpation during the stress test. Position the patient's arm, and your hands, so the joint margins can be palpated and so that you can feel if the joint space is opening, which implies that the ligaments no longer stabilize the joint. The difference between the joint mobilization tests and these is that the joint margins are specifically palpated.

Valgus stress test for the medial collateral ligaments (Figures 17.44–17.47)

Have the patient high-sitting. The patient's shoulder and elbow should be slightly flexed at 20° each with the arm slightly abducted and the forearm supinated and palm up. We need the

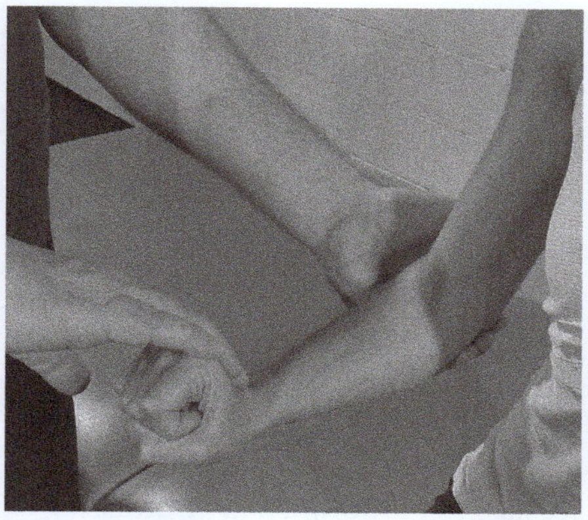

FIGURE 17.37 1. Testing all wrist extensors

Position the patient so the elbow is flexed 90°, the forearm is pronated and the wrist is in slight extension. Stabilize the forearm with one hand while the other rests on the dorsal surface of the patient's hand. Ask the patient to hold the position and not let you move the wrist as you try to flex it. If there is pain, differentiate between extensor carpi radialis longus and brevis and extensor carpi ulnaris by repeating the test with the wrist deviated to either side. Remember to also keep the wrist in slight extension.

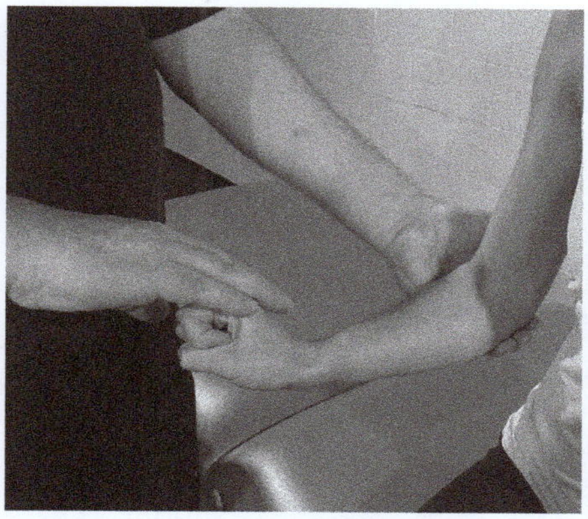

FIGURE 17.38 2. Stressing extensor carpi ulnaris

Have the wrist in ulnar deviation, putting stress more on the extensor carpi ulnaris. Note how the therapist has cupped their fingers over the ulnar border. Ask the patient to hold the position and stop you from trying to bring the wrist into flexion, as you also pull on the ulnar aspect of the hand and try to move it radially. If you only try to flex the wrist in this position, you will still stress ulnaris more than radialis, but trying to also move it radially makes the test even more specific to extensor carpi ulnaris.

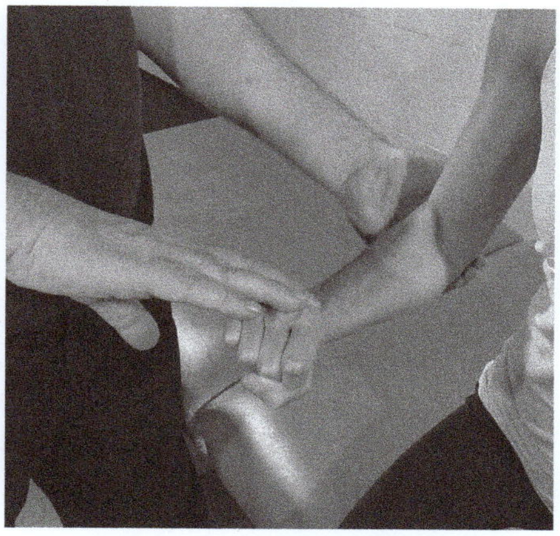

FIGURE 17.39 3. Stressing extensor carpi radialis longus and brevis

With the wrist radially deviated, test the extensor carpi radialis longus and brevis. Note how the therapist's hand covers thumb and radial portion of hand. The therapist tries to apply some ulnar deviation while also trying to flex the patient's wrist. If pain with radial deviation is at the lateral epicondyle, we have a positive test for tennis elbow. If a positive test occurs with radial deviation, you can then also differentiate between the extensor carpi radialis longus and brevis.

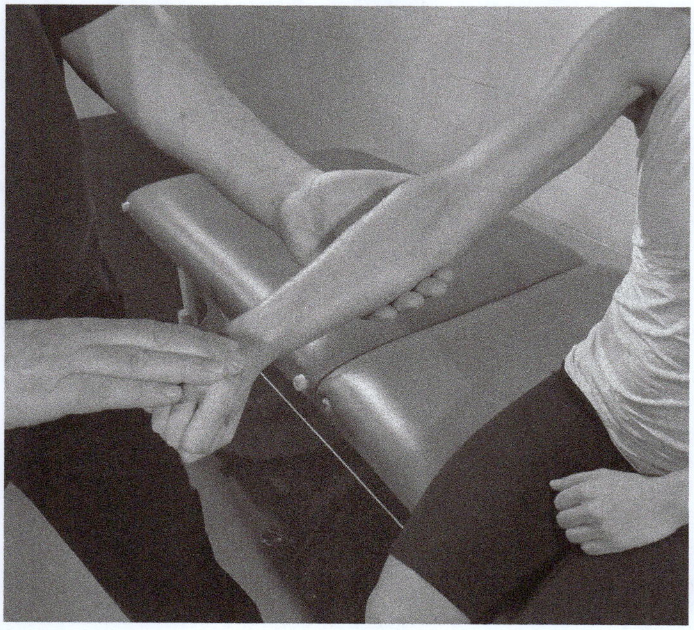

FIGURE 17.40 Extensor carpi radialis brevis

Extend the elbow to almost full extension, radially deviate the wrist and tell the patient to hold as you try to flex the wrist. This position puts the extensor carpi radialis longus at a disadvantage and has the extensor carpi radialis brevis work harder. If pain is now less intense than when testing with the elbow in neutral, then longus is the more injured.

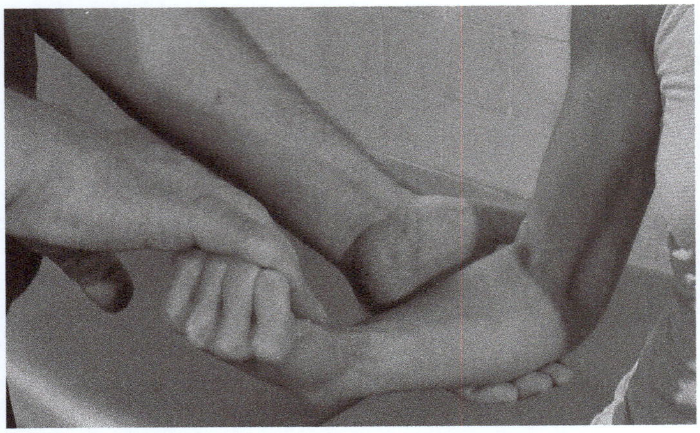

FIGURE 17.41 1. Testing all flexors of wrist

Position the patient so the elbow is flexed 90°, the wrist is in slight flexion (to prevent injury to flexor attachments on the carpal bones) and the forearm is supinated. Stabilize the forearm with one hand while the other rests on the palmar surface of the patient's hand. Have the patient try to flex the wrist while you apply resistance. Prime movers you are testing are flexor carpi radialis, flexor carpi ulnaris, and palmaris longus. To distinguish between the flexor radialis and ulnaris, follow the same principle as with the extensors, except this time have the wrist held in slight flexion with appropriate deviation.

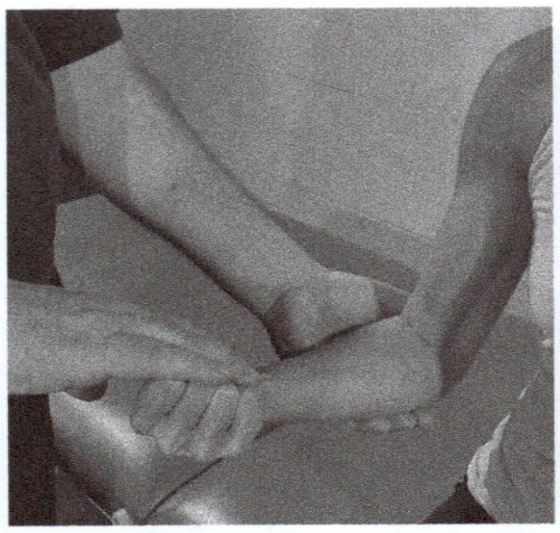

FIGURE 17.42 2. Stressing flexor carpi ulnaris

Put the wrist into ulnar deviation to test flexor carpi ulnaris. If the patient experiences pain at the site of common flexor tendon on the medial epicondyle of the humerus, they may be suffering from medial epicondylitis.

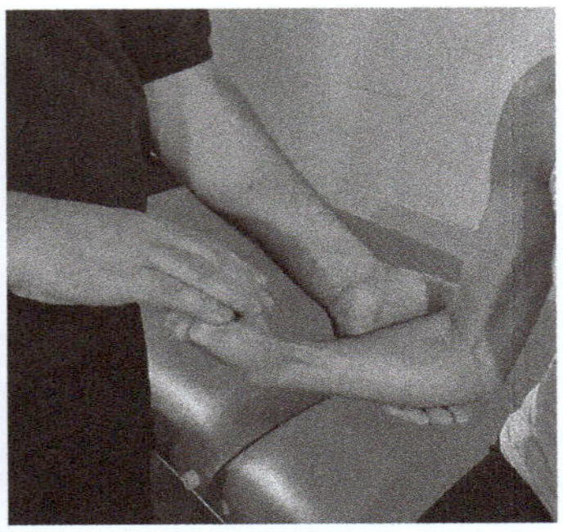

FIGURE 17.43 3. Stressing flexor carpi radialis

Put the wrist into radial deviation to differentiate flexor carpi radialis and perform as above.

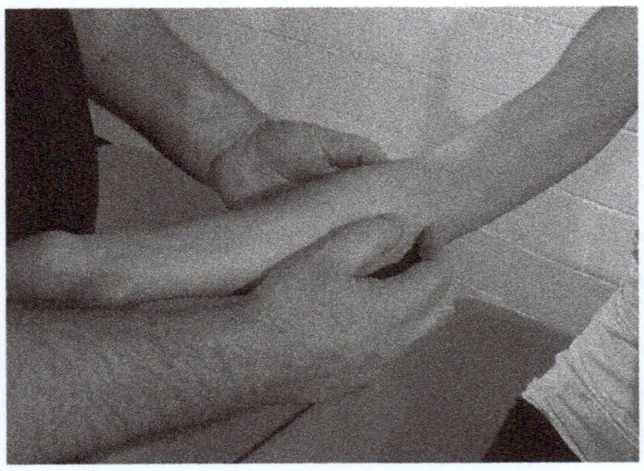

FIGURE 17.44 1. Positioning for valgus stress test

To correctly position your hands to palpate the joint margin, place both hands around the patient's elbow.

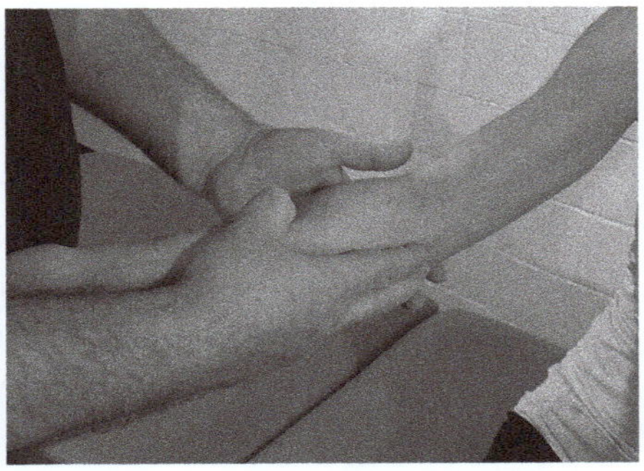

FIGURE 17.45 2. Positioning for palpation and valgus stress test

Slide your hand on the inside of the arm down onto the forearm, but only so far as this leaves the fingertips at the medial joint margin of the elbow. The fingertips will be able to palpate the medial joint capsule and collateral ligament to see if the space opens wider during testing.

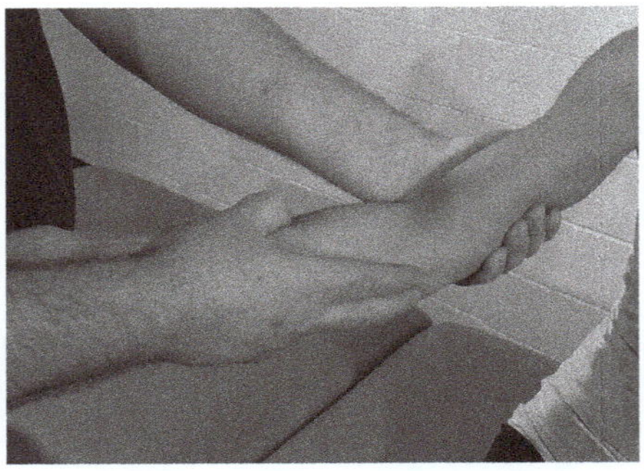

FIGURE 17.46 3. Performing valgus stress test

The outside hand is moved up onto the arm, just above the elbow on the lateral side. The upper hand applies pressure toward the patient's body, while the lower hand pushes the forearm away. By doing this, both hands combine to apply a valgus stress through the joint.

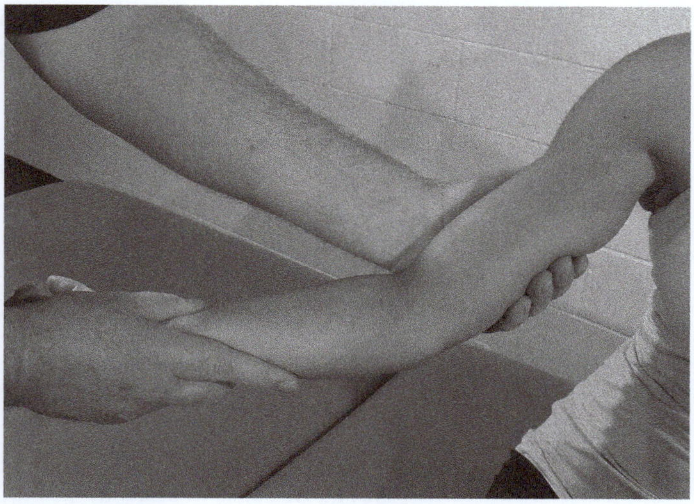

FIGURE 17.47 Alternative positioning for valgus test

Hold the supinated forearm just above the wrist on the medial side; have the elbow in slight flexion and, while stabilizing the arm just above the elbow, draw the tractioned forearm laterally.

elbow slightly flexed so that we do not put a force through the olecranon process when it is in the olecranon fossa, as occurs when the elbow is fully extended.

A positive sign of the valgus stress test is pain at the medial collateral ligament which implies a strain to the medial ligaments or joint capsule. Palpation of the joint opening further implies ligamentous laxity. If the only positive is excessive joint opening, with no pain, this implies laxity in the medial structures of the joint that may have suffered injury (over-stretching) in the past.

NOTE: The joint margin is not palpated here. Therefore, we are not testing the stability of the joint, but only if the medial ligaments and capsule of the elbow are tender. If the ligaments and capsule are stretched but not inflamed, there may be no pain but still excessive opening of the joint. Therefore, with this positioning it is harder to notice laxity in the structures and hence this test is less efficient.

Varus stress test (Figures 17.48–17.50)

This tests the stability of the lateral ligaments and capsule of the elbow joint.

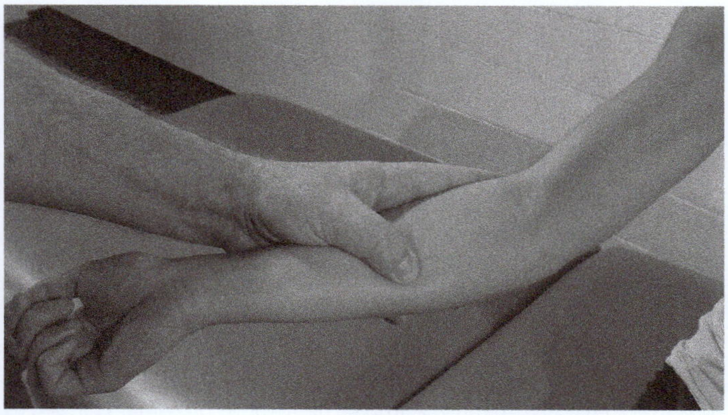

FIGURE 17.48 1. Positioning for varus stress test

With the patient in high-sitting, position the arm as shown with the shoulder and elbow slightly flexed at 20° each, the arm slightly abducted, and the forearm supinated. Reverse your hand position and direction of force from the valgus stress test. To position the hands correctly to palpate the joint margin, place both your hands around their elbow.

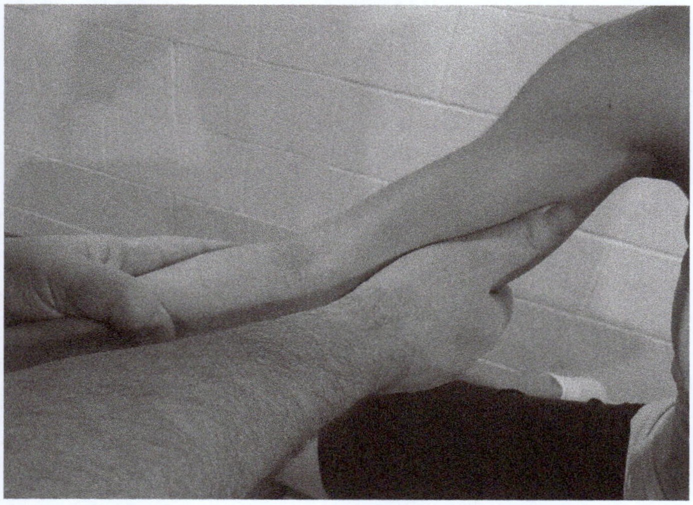

FIGURE 17.49 2. Performing varus stress test

Start by sliding the hand that is on the outside of the patient's arm down onto the forearm, but only so far as this leaves the fingertips at the lateral joint margin of the elbow. These fingertips will be able to palpate the lateral joint capsule and collateral ligament to see if space opens wider during testing. Next, the inside hand is moved up the patient's arm, positioned just above the elbow on the medial side. The upper hand applies pressure away from the patient's body, while the lower hand pushes the forearm toward the patient's body. In this way, both hands combine to apply a varus stress through the joint. A positive sign is pain at the site of the lateral collateral ligament, and palpation of the joint opening.

Alternative positioning for the varus stress test

The varus stress test can also be done as shown in Figure 17.50, but without the palpation of the lateral joint margin we cannot get specific feedback about joint stability, unless it is severe.

Tests for epicondylitis (Figures 17.51–17.56)

Lateral epicondylitis (or epicondylosis) is more commonly known as tennis elbow. This can also be called extensor tendonitis/tendonosis, as it is an impairment of the common extensor tendon attached to the lateral epicondyle of the humerus.

Medial epicondylitis/epicondylosis is also known as golfer's elbow. It is also sometimes referred to as flexor tendonitis/tendonosis since it is an impairment of the common flexor tendon attached to the medial epicondyle of the humerus.

These conditions are further explained in Boxes 17.5 and 17.6.

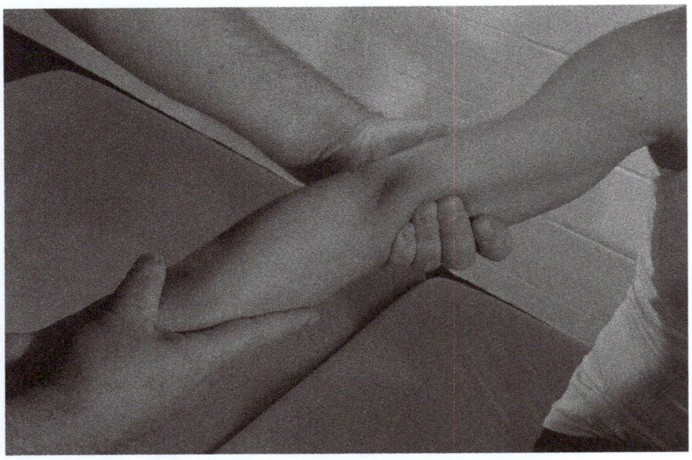

FIGURE 17.50 Alternative varus stress test

Hold the patient's arm just above the elbow with one hand while the other is almost at the wrist. Apply pressure through the distal forearm toward the patient's body while gently pushing away from the body with the hand above the elbow.

Note: Either method for the varus stress test will be less awkward if the patient's forearm and hand are supinated. This helps prevent the upper arm from abducting away from the body.

Box 17.5 Tendonitis versus tendonosis or tendinopathy

Painful and dysfunctional tendons that have previously been diagnosed as tendonitis are now having the term tendonosis being applied, instead. This is due to the findings of histological studies on painful tendons (such as in tennis elbow) showing a lack of neutrophils and other classical inflammatory substances (hence, the move to omitting the "-itis" from the designation). However, saying that inflammation is not part of the tendinopathy may be misleading. While many of the elements of acute inflammation may not be present in chronic cases of tendonosis there is growing evidence from advances in immunohistochemistry and gene expression analysis in the last decades that there are elements of inflammation present in chronic tendinopathies (Rees et al. 2014).

Nonetheless, the term tendonitis is to be reserved for an acute injury that resolves quickly over a week or two; the chronic situation (3–6 months) is being called tendonosis.

Tendonosis is characterized by degeneration of the organized collagen fibers in the tendon into an unorganized condition, accompanied by an excess of ground substance/matrix. Therefore, it has been called angiofibroblastic degeneration. It has been calculated that approximately 20 percent of cases of tendonosis do not resolve on their own. Another complexity to the issue is that without inflammation being present in tendonosis, trying to explain the experience of pain by the patient becomes problematic. The designation of tendonosis may be more accurate, but it actually has made the impairment more puzzling. But, as mentioned above, inflammatory elements may be present and so help explain the presence of pain. Therefore, many of the "older" modalities for tendonitis may still be beneficial to the patient, just as they had been previous to the erroneous blanket statement that no inflammatory chemicals were present in chronic tendonosis.

A diagnosis of either tendonitis or tendonosis technically requires a histological sampling. Manual testing will generate a positive result in either condition. Both can present as painful, usually decrease the range of motion in the joint involved, and may cause weakness in the involved muscles. Therefore, for the time being, both terms (-itis or -osis) may be used in the text, but they are usually meant to imply tendonosis.

Regardless, this issue creates the need for therapists to make an important clinical judgment:

- If there is a clear inflammatory condition (tendonitis) occurring, then treat as such, i.e., less aggressively with ice, drainage, and gentle on-site work when subacute. Over-stretching or loading of the tissue could cause a rupture.
- If it is a chronic condition (tendonosis), and the tendon is disorganized and possibly more fragile (*dis-integrated*, one might say), it may be best to begin with mild or moderate approach to treatment of a suspected tendonosis, and building up slowly as the treatments begin to organize the tissues.

When in doubt, treat as tendonitis for a week or two and, if the condition persists and presents as chronic, then begin treating as tendonosis.

Box 17.6 True epicondylosis

This is experienced by the patient as pain at the epicondyle of the humerus. The more acute the lesion, the more weakness experienced in either the extensors or flexors. Often, during testing, the patient will feel the pain in the proximal forearm, in the extensors or flexors at the musculotendinous junctions of the affected musculature.

There can also be pain at the carpal bones, where the extensors or flexors attach. This speaks to tendonosis being present anywhere along the course of the tendon, which also shows itself as painful; when acute, it produces weakness in the musculature. The differential muscle test presented at the start of this section can sometimes help to identify the principal muscle impaired. You may prefer to use the terms "overuse syndrome" or "repetitive strain" when referring to any of the above mentioned chronic impairments to the tendinous portion of the muscle. Nonetheless, if any of the symptoms mentioned above occur when doing the testing described below, then specifically record if it is lateral/medial epicondylosis, tendonosis, or strain at the musculotendinous junction or tendonosis at the wrist (attachment).

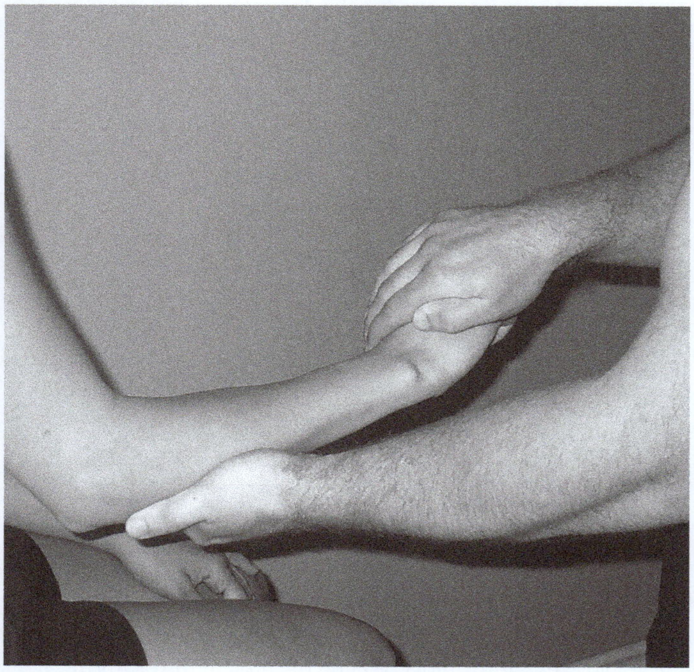

FIGURE 17.51 Lateral epicondylitis/tennis elbow test

Have the patient high-sitting with the shoulder forward flexed 20° and the elbow flexed to 20–30°. Have the patient make a fist and pronate the forearm. Support the elbow by having your thumb, without pressure, over the lateral epicondyle. With your hand over the slightly extended wrist, resist the patient's attempt to further extend. You can add further provocation by applying pressure in a manner that tries to ulnar deviate the wrist as the patient tries to extend it: i.e., resist with greater pressure over the radial side of the hand. A positive sign is a sudden severe pain in the area of the common extensor tendon.

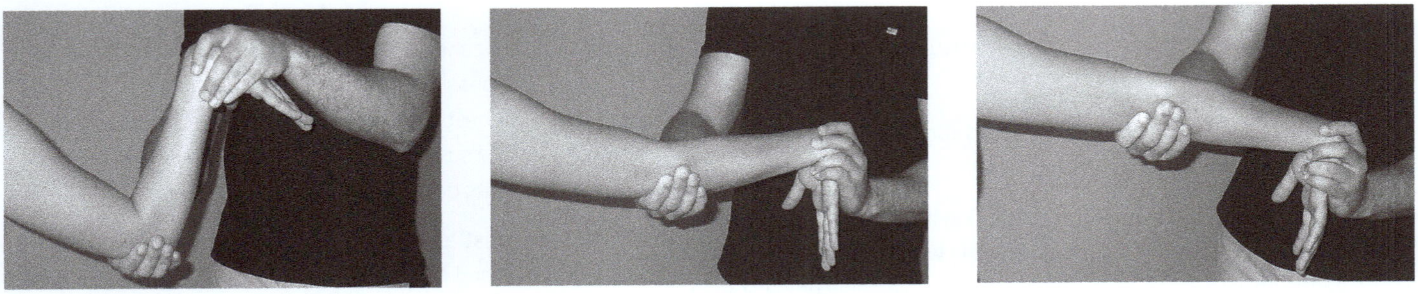

FIGURE 17.52A–C Passive lateral epicondylitis/tennis elbow test

To do a passive test for lateral epicondylitis, have the patient's elbow flexed to 90° with the hand pronated; then passively flex the wrist to the end of range. Now, slowly extend the patient's elbow. This should provoke symptoms at the lateral epicondyle. If further provocation is needed after the elbow is fully extended, then slightly ulnar deviate the wrist. Usually, when this test is positive, the patient will experience pain and will resist the elbow going into extension. Again, tendonitis or tendonosis can also appear during this passive test, as can strain at the musculotendinous junction. However, with this passive test you can also be stretching the radial nerve, which, if injured/inflamed, can exhibit similar symptoms as lateral epicondylitis.

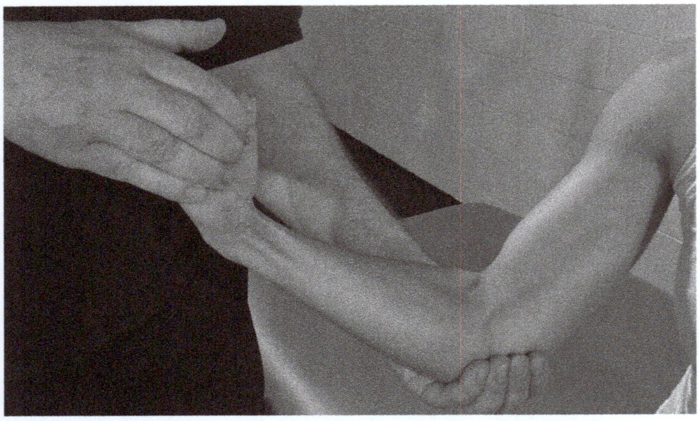

FIGURE 17.53 Medial epicondylitis; golfer's or pitcher's elbow test

Starting with same position as in the previous test, have the patient supinate the forearm. Have the wrist slightly flexed. The fingertips of the hand supporting the elbow should be over the medial epicondyle. Resist the patient's attempt to further flex the wrist. If you resist attempted flexion of the wrist by holding the ulnar border, you will add more provocation. A positive sign is a sudden severe pain in the area of the common flexor tendon (medial epicondyle), which may radiate down into the forearm.

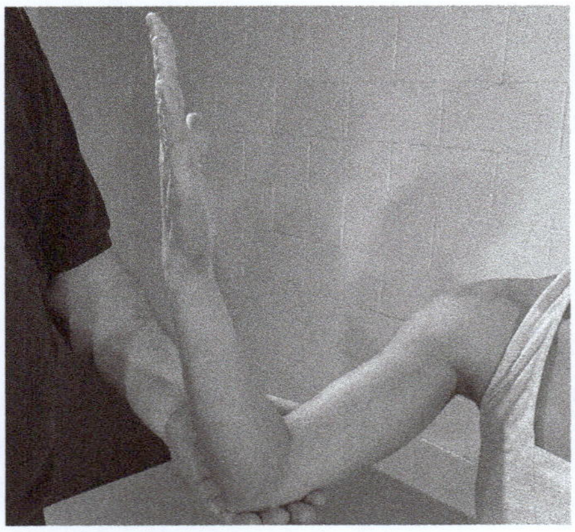

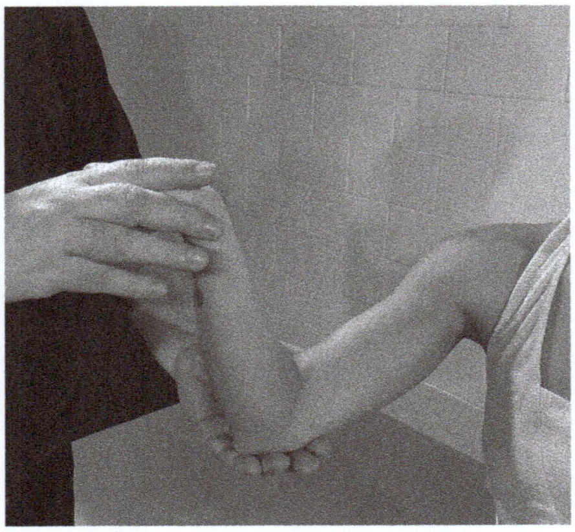

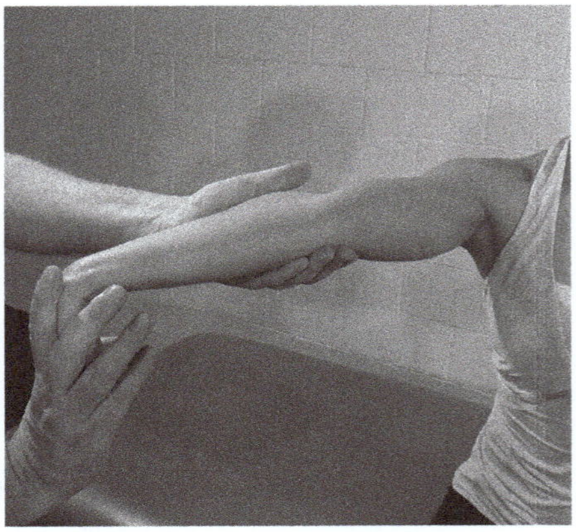

FIGURES 17.54–17.56 Passive medial epicondylitis; golfer's or pitcher's elbow test

To do this test passively, have the patient's elbow flexed, the hand supinated, and then passively extend the wrist to the end of range. Now, slowly extend the patient's elbow. This should provoke symptoms on the medial epicondyle. If further provocation is needed after the elbow is fully extended, then radially deviate the wrist slightly. If pain is felt at the wrist (around the area of the pisiform), then the ulnar nerve may be the source, as it is undergoing stretch. Usually this will "burn" down into the little finger.

Neurological tests for compression syndromes at the elbow (Figures 17.57–17.62)

These neurological tests are designed to confirm nerve entrapment syndromes in the elbow and the forearm. A test is positive if it reproduces the chief complaint, but not positive if you only generate a symptom that the patient has never experienced before. For alternative testing see the upper limb tension tests (ULTT) in Chapter 15.

Ulnar nerve tests

This implies neuritis of the ulnar nerve. Many people who do not suffer from neuritis can feel sensitivity at the point of compression and so this alone should not be taken as a positive sign, i.e., the test needs to reproduce the patient's chief complaint, not just produce a response.

Compression of the median nerve at the ligament of Struthers

The ligament of Struthers is situated on the medial side of the distal end of the humerus. It creates a tunnel across the medial epicondyle of the humerus. The median nerve runs alongside the brachial artery as they pass under the ligament of Struthers on their way to enter the forearm at the cubital fossa. Trauma to this area can directly impact the nerve. Also, an excessive build-up of collagen fibers due to improper healing after a trauma to this ligament can entrap the nerve and cause it to be tractioned as the arm and hand are used in daily activities.

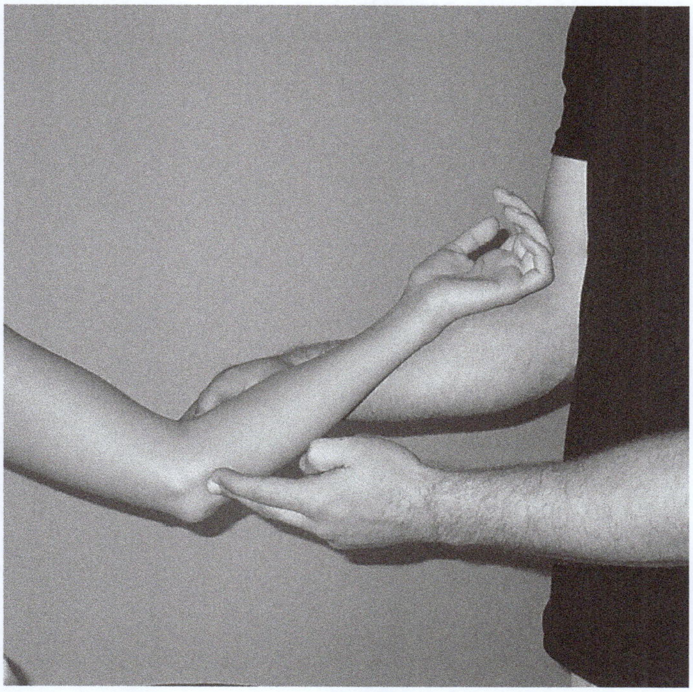

FIGURE 17.57 Tinel's sign at elbow

Tap over the ulnar nerve as it passes between the olecranon process and the medial epicondyle. A positive sign is paresthesia, such as tingling sensation in distribution of the ulnar nerve as it passes down the medial border of the forearm and into the fourth and fifth digits of the hand.

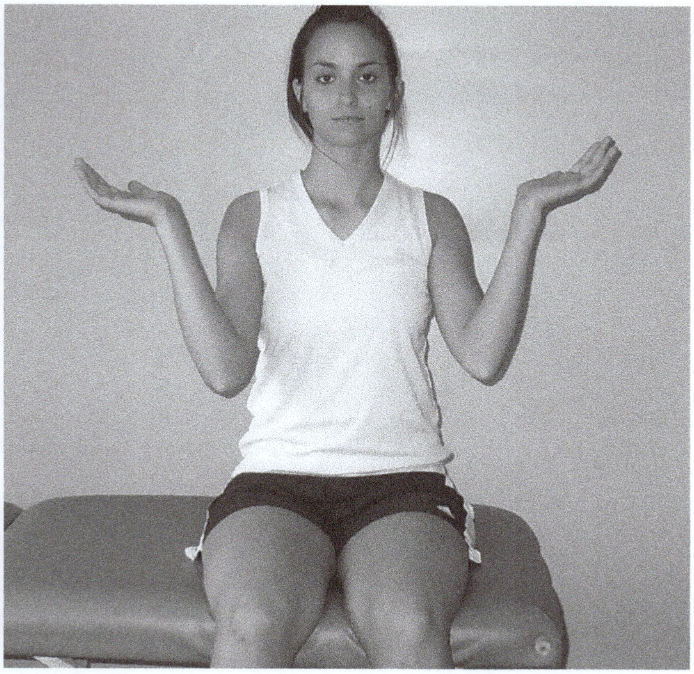

FIGURE 17.58 Ulnar nerve stretch at elbow

This is another way to test the ulnar nerve as it passes between the olecranon process and the medial epicondyle. This test is done by having the patient flex both elbows and extend the wrists. The positive sign is reproduction of the patient's symptoms of paresthesia (e.g., tingling or burning sensation) down the forearm and into the lateral portion of the hand. Symptoms just in the little finger are not conclusive, as compression could be happening closer to the wrist (i.e., tunnel of Guyan between the hook of the hamate and the pisiform).

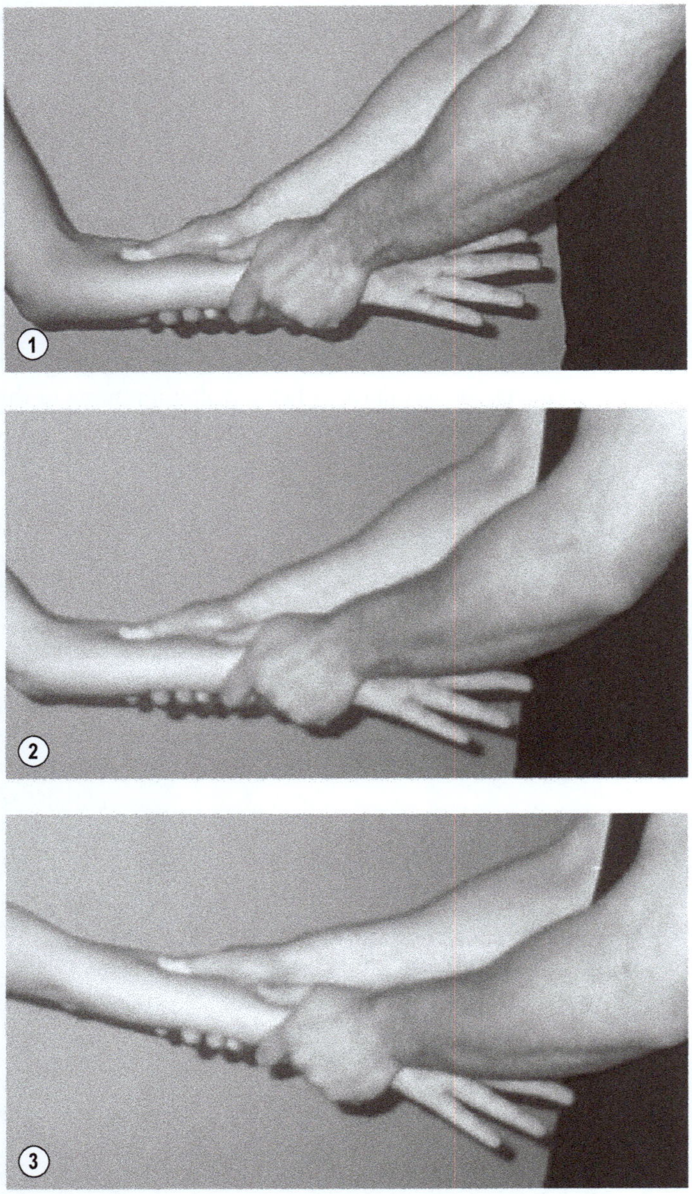

FIGURE 17.59A–C Pronator teres syndrome test or anterior interosseous syndrome test

Have the patient high-sitting with the elbow and forearm in the neutral position. Grasp the patient's forearm with both hands (1) and resist the patient's attempt to pronate the arm. Ask the patient to use only half of their strength, and to continue this while you passively extend elbow (2) over several seconds. The patient keeps trying to pronate the arm (3) while you resist and hold the position for 30 seconds or so. Extension of the elbow increases the chance of the nerve being compressed between the tendons from two heads of the pronator teres as it passes between them. A positive sign is paresthesia traveling down the forearm and into hand along the distribution of the median nerve, especially into the thumb and first two digits and lateral half of the ring finger. Specifically, this is entrapment of the anterior interosseous nerve portion of the median nerve. Often a weakening of pronator teres happens as the test continues, as it compresses its own nerve supply.

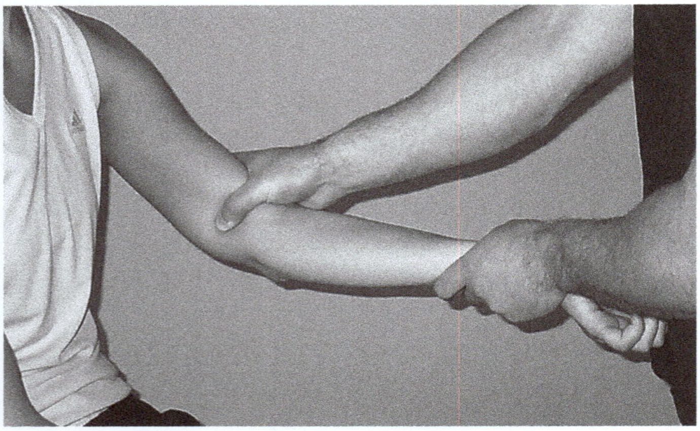

FIGURE 17.60 Test of ligament of Struthers compression

To perform the test, palpate the medial epicondyle area and apply pressure over the ligament. This palpatory test is positive if you re-create the patient's symptoms of median nerve compression.

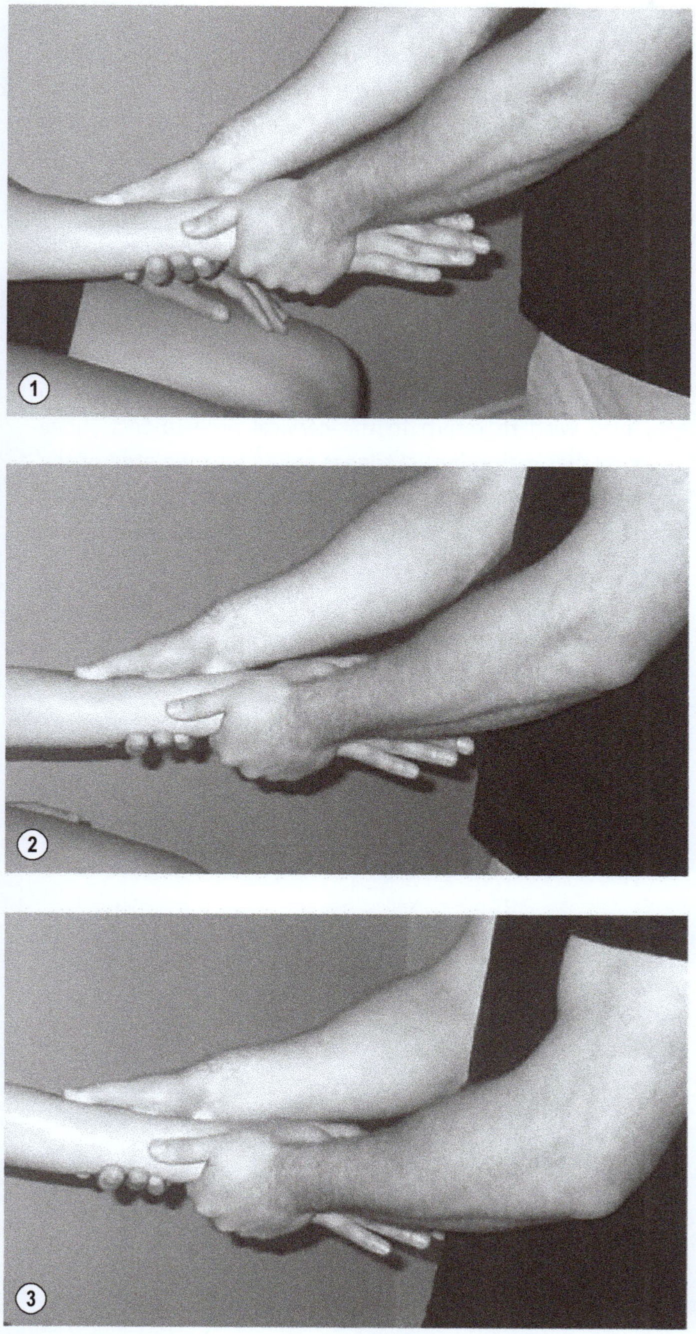

FIGURE 17.61A–C Supinator radial nerve syndrome test

Have the patient high-sitting, with the elbow and forearm in neutral position. 1. Grasp the patient's forearm and resist the patient's attempt to supinate the arm, using only half strength. 2. While the muscle is still being resisted, passively extend the elbow. Ask the patient to continue trying to supinate while you passively extend the elbow over several seconds. 3. The patient continues trying to supinate the arm while you resist and hold the position for 30 seconds or so. This action compresses a portion of the radial nerve (posterior interosseus nerve) as it passes between the heads of deep and superficial muscle portions of the supinator deep into the forearm. Pain or paresthesia spreading from the lateral elbow, distally or proximally, is a positive sign. In the hand, symptoms are usually felt into and around the dorsal radial surface.

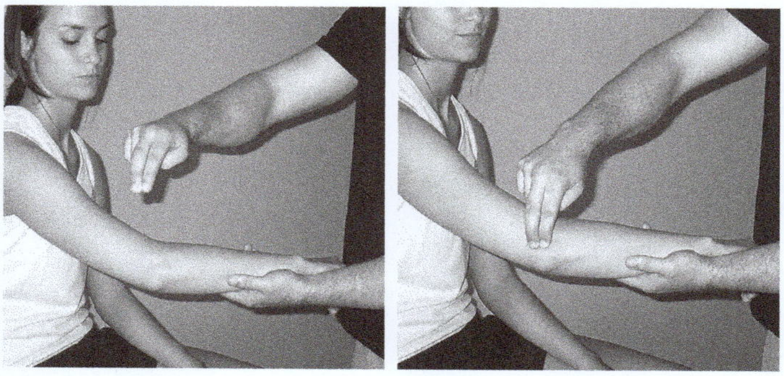

FIGURE 17.62A, B Tinel's sign for radial nerve at the elbow

Tap over the lateral epicondyle area. This is where the radial nerve curls its way around the humerus on its way to the radial tunnel as it passes between the deep and superficial heads of the supinator muscle to course down into the forearm. The positive sign is paresthesia running down the course of the nerve, possibly all the way into the dorsal web space of the hand between the thumb and index finger.

Box 17.7 Source of neurological symptoms not found

If the source of a patient's neurological signs and symptoms has not been found when doing specific neurological tests for compressions syndromes, then a cervical spine assessment should be done (see Chapter 14 for details)

This is done by active free movements – flexion, rotation, and side-bending. If no pain has been felt by the patient as end-range is reached for each range of motion, then each can immediately have over-pressure applied. Finish with extension, which has no over-pressure applied. Then, perform all the appropriate neurological tests: deep tendon reflexes, myotomes, dermatomes, a compression test, Spurling's test bilaterally, and Valsalva's test. Do not forget to do the vertebral artery test if warranted by case history or signs and symptoms that may occur with AF-ROM testing of the cervical spine. Tests of the cervical spine that do not directly test the neurological structures, such as facet joints or specific muscles, could be skipped at this time.

If, however, the neurological tests of the cervical spine do not reveal the source of neurological symptoms, then thoracic outlet syndrome (TOS) testing should be done. Thoracic outlet syndromes should also be ruled out especially if the patient's chief complaint contains any mention of paresthesia in the limb that does not correspond to local compression syndromes at the elbow, peripheral nerve lesions, or cervical lesions, and is not reproduced with cervical testing (see Chapter 15).

If neither of these reveals the cause of the paresthesia, then you may wish to return to the cervical area to test those muscles that may refer via trigger points into the area of the patient's chief complaint. If, after all these tests, you still do not have an answer for the neurological impairments, a referral out may be necessary. Alternately, you may need to take a fresh look by further asking the patient about the onset, symptoms, and other health history questions.

WRIST AND HAND: CHAPTER OVERVIEW

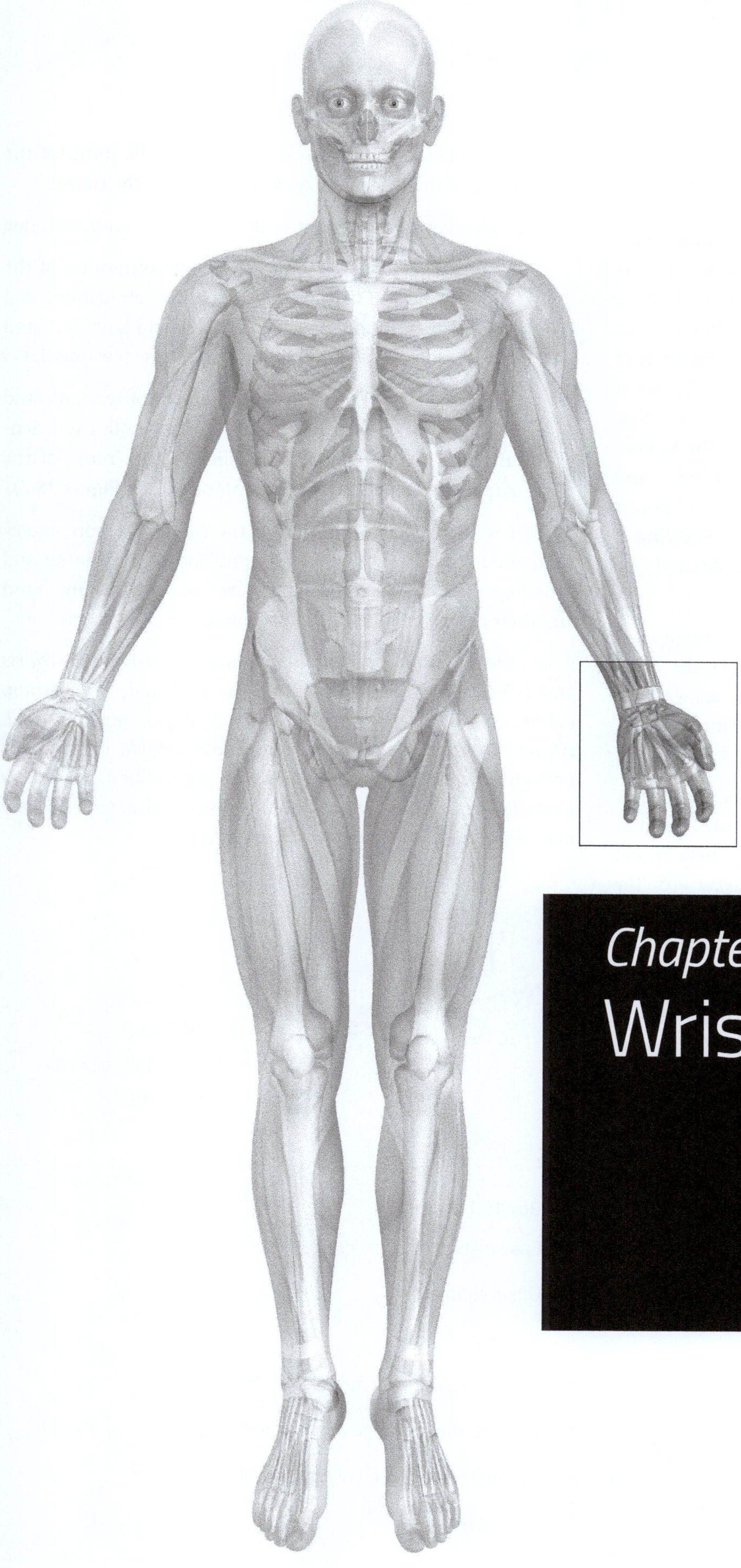

Chapter 18

Wrist and hand

Chapter 18

Clinical implications of anatomy and physiology

This section presents introductory and general information about the wrist and hand together so as to have an overarching understanding of this intricate structure as a functioning whole. This will help inform us in a manner that will be useful in making clinical judgments about how much or what parts of the structure need specific and detailed assessment. The wrist and hand together form one of the most complex structures in the body, especially with respect to understanding the biomechanics of the hand's dexterity. The study of the whole hand can be a text in itself. Here we make only a few brief points (see: Agur et al. 2014; Dutton 2012; Hartley 2000a; Hertling & Kessler 2006; Hoppenfeld 1976; Levangie & Norkin 2011; Magee 2014; Schuenke et al. 2014.)

1. The wrist consists of the radius and the carpal bones; a radiocarpal joint and intracarpal joints. There is also the distal radioulnar joint at the wrist but it does not articulate with any carpal bones hence its function remains supination and pronation of the forearm not wrist articular proper.
2. The carpal joints have more motion than most people imagine (Figure 18.1). For example, the radiocarpal joint and the mid-carpal joints share the task of opening during flexion and extension of the wrist. On average the wrist flexes 90°. The radiocarpal joint provides approximately 60 percent of that flexion with the remainder coming from the mid-carpals.
3. Additional structures that need to be known: metacarpals, phalanges, carpometacarpal joints (CMC), metacarpophalangeal joints (MCPs), proximal interphalangeal joints (PIPs), and the distal interphalangeal joints (DIPs).
4. Review the unique joints and organization of the bones and joints of the thumb:

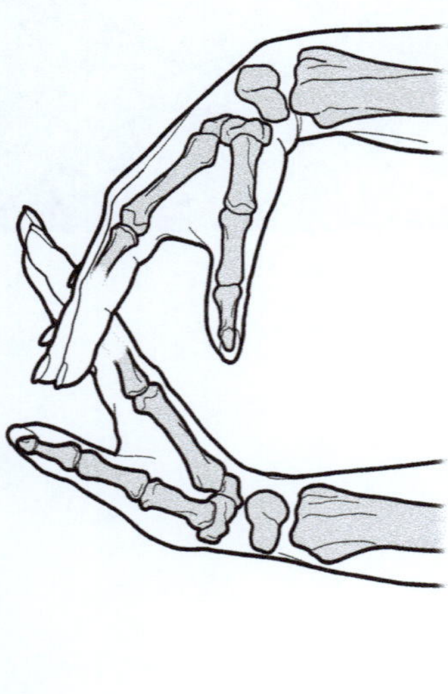

FIGURE 18.1
Flexion and extension of the carpal joints.

- carpometacarpal joint – the unique saddle joint (of the hand) of the trapezium and metacarpal of the thumb
- metacarpophalangeal joint – usually also has a sesamoid bone
- interphalangeal joint: review the ranges of motion of the thumb – flexion, extension, adduction, abduction, and opposition of thumb and finger; be able to landmark and palpate all of the above bones and joints; review muscles
- the carpal tunnel: review the placement of tendons (and their sheaths) blood vessels and nerves; note the orientation of the retinaculum that makes the "roof" of the carpal tunnel and the palpatory landmarks (Figure 18.2).

Review the ranges of motion of the thumb: flexion, extension, adduction, abduction, and opposition of the thumb and little finger. Review the muscles involved in the wrist and hand and their common anatomical placement one to another.

See the Appendices section at the back of this book for charts and tables on muscles (muscle origin, insertion, innervation, action, and synergists) joints (actions, ranges, muscles used, tissues stretched, and compressed; another table on capsular patterns of restriction, open packed/resting positions, and close packed positions) and several charts on neurological testing where any such testing would involve this chapter's region.

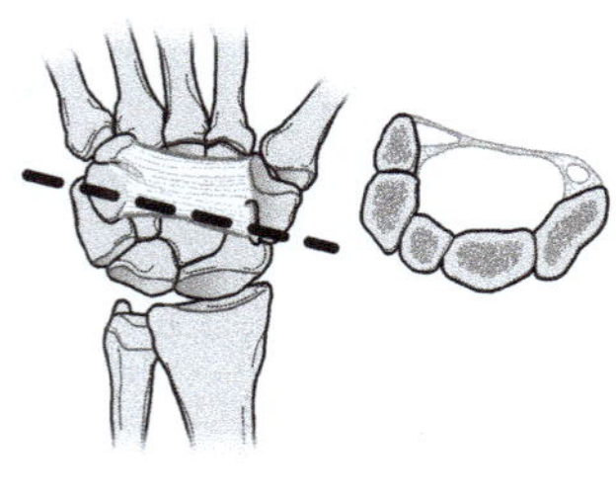

FIGURE 18.2
The orientation of the retinaculum.

Box 18.1 Protocol

Case history (specific questions)

Observations

Rule outs

Active free range of motion (AF-ROM)

Passive relaxed range of motion (PR-ROM)

Active resisted range of motion (AR-ROM)

Special tests

Case history (specific questions)

- Do your hands ever feel cold? Do they ever feel hot or itchy? (If so explore further, e.g., when, for how long, specific activities, etc.)
- Do you find that you suddenly drop things for no apparent reason?
- Do your hands ever tingle or go numb or weak? If so, ask the patient if it is the whole hand (usually related to blood flow) or just part of the hand or certain fingers (implying neurological source). Try to get the patient to be as specific as possible.
- Are there any hand motions or tasks that become difficult to do? Are they repetitive tasks. How long does that take to happen?
- Is this interfering with your tasks of daily living or your work?
- If the patient answers yes to any of the questions above then return to medical history questioning and specifically ask the patient if they have diabetes. Clarify with the patient if they suffer from any systemic pathology.

Observations

Regional assessment within the context of the whole

As with every area of the body being investigated by orthopedic testing (the specific view), remember to always look at that joint or tissue within the context of the surrounding joints and structures (the regional view). What is the interplay of impaired tissues or structures with the rest of the tissues within that region? In turn take into consideration the global view: how is that joint and region affecting the whole body and how is the whole affecting or influencing the region and the specific site(s) of impairment(s)? Just as with treatment, assessment goes from general-to-specific-to-general in its approach. Not all the preconditions for an impairment exist on-site or in the surrounding region. They can come from the totality of the body the person and their environment.

Note the orientation of the hand: at rest the hand is naturally cupped.

When the patient is standing and the hand and arm are at rest the dorsum (back) of the thumb usually points forward anteriorly if the shoulder girdle is properly positioned. However, if the back (dorsum) of the hand is facing forward this is most often due to internal rotation at the shoulder.

This often predisposes the patient to compression syndromes of the neurovascular bundle at the shoulder leading to decreased flow of fluids. This in turn can lead to:

- a blanched appearance to the hand (decreased arterial blood flow); a darkened appearance to the hand (decreased venous return); or an edematous appearance to the hand (decreased lymphatic flow).

A thorough inspection of the hand will provide many clues to what ails the patient. Carefully review the anatomy of the hand. The few points concerning observation of the wrist and hand made below are meant to point out some of the most significant clues about what structures need further investigation, whether through orthopedic testing done by you or by a specialist (such as an orthopedic physician or occupational therapist). For the numerous lesions that can affect the hand you should refer to an appropriate pathology text.

Note the condition of the thenar and the hypothenar eminences. The thenar eminence contains the intrinsic muscles of the hand that provide movement of the thumb while the hypothenar contains those for the little finger. Loss of prominence in either of these denotes atrophy in one or more of those muscles.

Note also the peaks and valleys at the junction between the palm of the hand and the fingers.

These three peaks between the metacarpophalangeal (MCP) joints contain the lumbricals and the neurovascular bundles as they enter into the fingers while the valleys between these peaks contain the flexor tendons of the fingers. Note the size and shape of the joints of the fingers, looking for signs of osteoarthritis or rheumatoid arthritis.

Initially do not hold the patient's hand when inspecting it. Rather show the patient how you would like them to hold the hand as you note both its overall configuration and specific areas of interest.

If you immediately take the hand to inspect it you may miss valuable clues since most people will "un-cup" the hand and flatten it out while they spread their fingers. Therefore, you will not see how the patient naturally holds the hand at rest.

Observe the arches of the palm in the hand's resting position. The two transverse arches of the hand (the proximal arch of the carpal bones and the distal arch through the heads of the metacarpal bones) are sustained by the proper functioning of muscles. Therefore, the loss of the arch in the palm indicates loss of muscular function (Hertling & Kessler 2006; Levangie & Norkin 2011; Magee 2014).

Observing the arches (Figures 18.3, 18.4)

Observe the arches of the palm in the hand's resting position. The two transverse arches of the hand (the proximal arch of the carpal bones and the distal arch through the heads of the metacarpal bones) are sustained by the proper functioning of muscles. Therefore, the loss of the arch in the palm indicates loss of muscular function.

Palpating landmarks (Figures 18.5, 18.6)

Palpate the following two landmarks in and around the wrist while noting any difference in the wrist and palm of the affected hand compared to unaffected limb including edema, temperature, joint, bone malalignment, or nodules etc.

Palpating the motion of the lunate (Figures 18.7–18.9)

Dislocation or subluxation of the lunate is a common reason for loss of extension in the wrist. This usually occurs when the wrist is extended and the person falls onto the hand. The lunate needs to descend when the hand comes out of flexion and into neutral. The lunate moves ventrally (descends) 3/16th of an inch on wrist extension and moves dorsally (ascends) 1/16th of an inch on wrist flexion. Therefore, it can be involved in reduced flexion if it will not elevate.

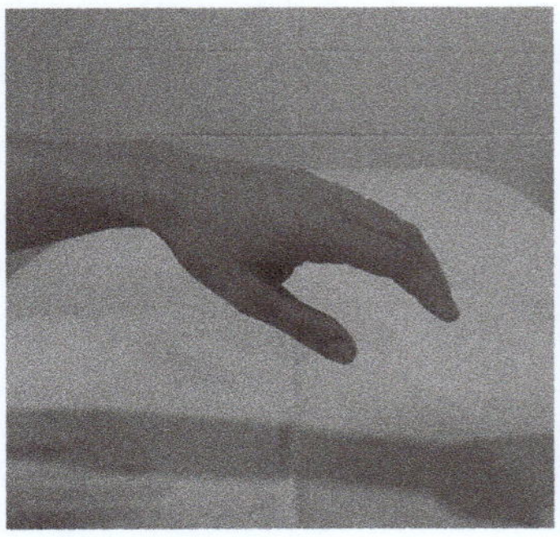

FIGURE 18.3 1. Observing dorsum of hand at rest

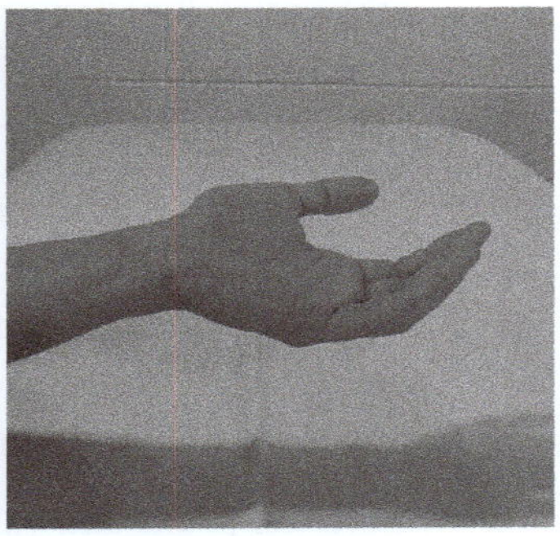

FIGURE 18.4 2. Observing ventral hand at rest

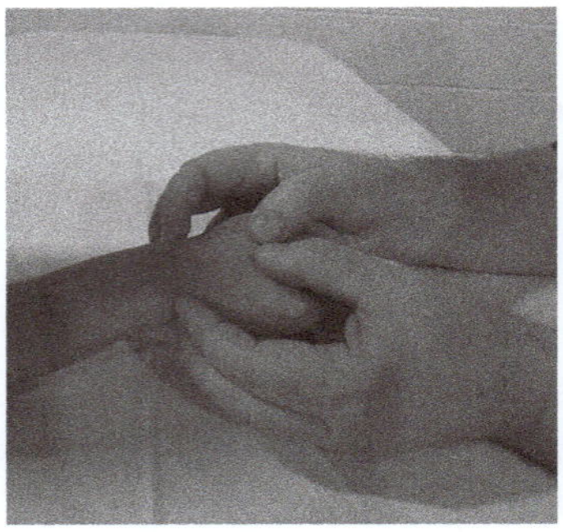

FIGURE 18.5 Medial (ulnar) and lateral (radial) joint margins of radiocarpal joint

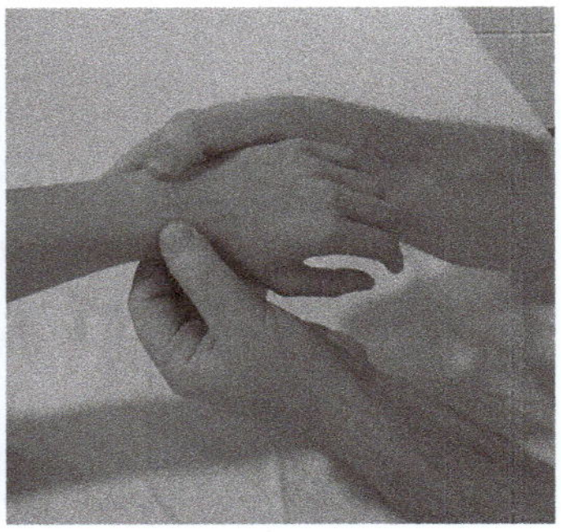

FIGURE 18.6 Radial and ulnar styloid processes

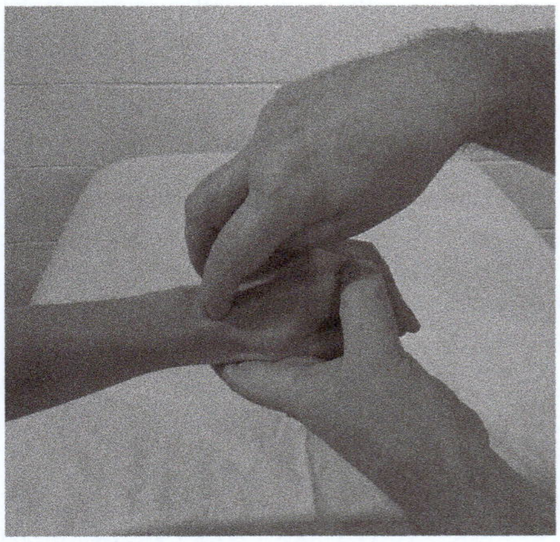

FIGURE 18.7 1. Landmarking position of lunate

Run a finger up the middle metacarpal bone to the hollow just distal to the radius and leave it on that spot.

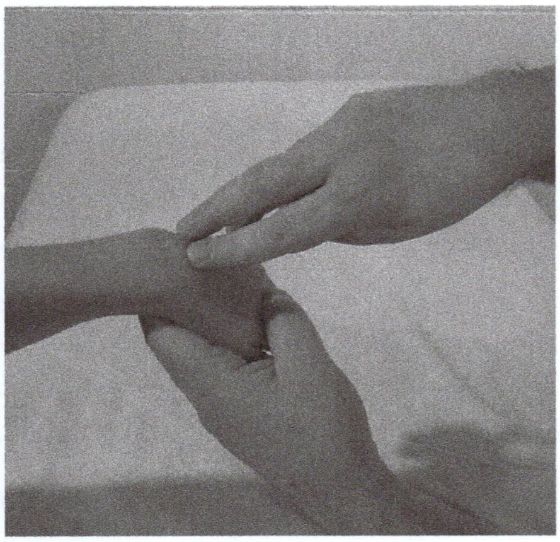

FIGURE 18.8 2. Palpation of lunate

Have the patient flex the wrist and feel the lunate bone take up the space, i.e. elevate.

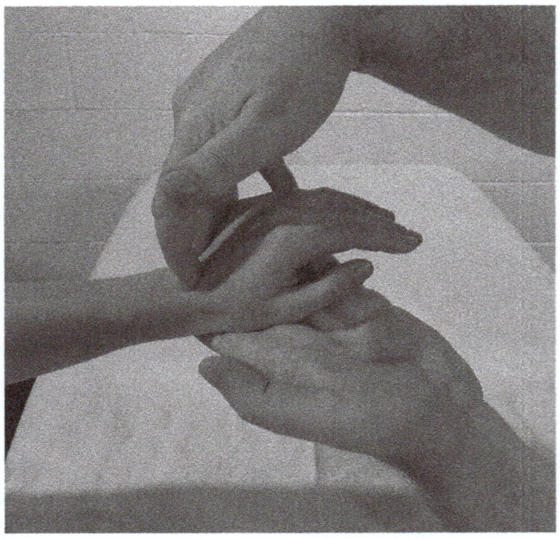

FIGURE 18.9 3. Feeling lunate descend

Bring the wrist back into neutral and feel if the hollow has returned, i.e. lunate has descended. The wrist can also be taken into extension. The lunate may be dislocated if it does not become palpable or will not descend when the patient returns the wrist to neutral (or even into extension).

Palpation of anatomical snuffbox (Figure 18.10)

Inspecting fingers (Figures 18.11–18.14)

When examining the fingers for any abnormal shape or deviations check for edema, tissue texture changes, or nodules.

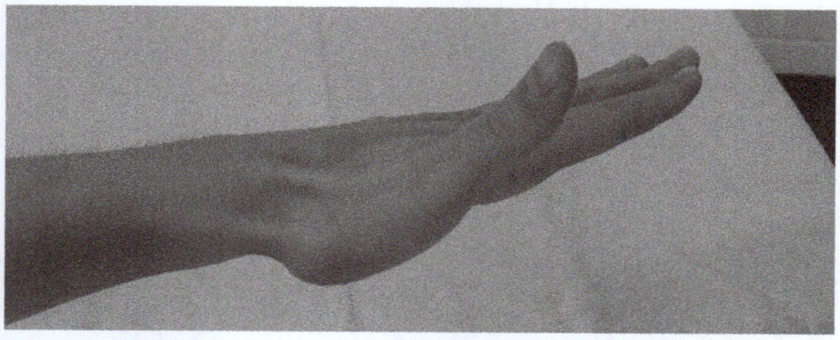

FIGURE 18.10

Have the patient extend the thumb and palpate in the hollow space between the extensor pollicis brevis, abductor pollicis longus, and extensor pollicis longus.

Also, inspect the fingers for any abnormal shape or deviations which could imply structural damage due to trauma or diseases such as osteoarthritis (O-A nodules at joint margins or swollen or tender interphalangeal joints); or rheumatoid arthritis (RA nodules, inflammation, tissue destruction which leads to deformity of the fingers). Use light palpation of fingers (avoid causing discomfort) to feel nodules and other abnormalities in the metacarpophalangeal (MCP) joints; proximal interphalangeal (PIP) joints; and distal interphalangeal (DIP) joints.

Rule outs

The elbow joint should be ruled out by AF-ROM flexion and extension each with O-P (over-pressure) (Figures 18.15–18.18). You should be aware that pronation and supination with O-P, though suggested by many texts, involves too many muscles and joints at the wrist to make it a practical rule out. The two motions can often lead one to believe there is more involvement of the elbow than is actually the case.

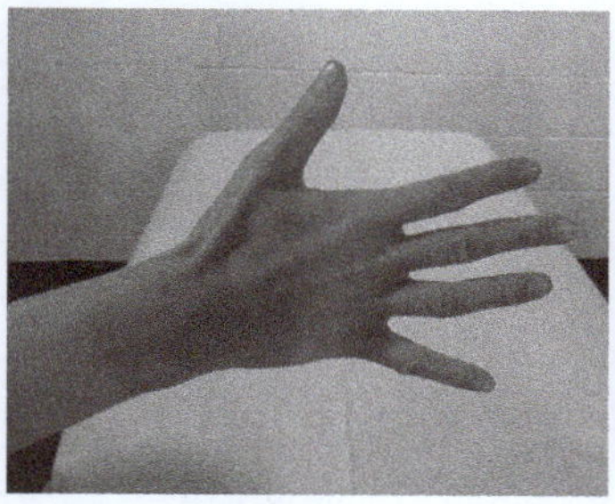

FIGURE 18.11 General observations of fingers

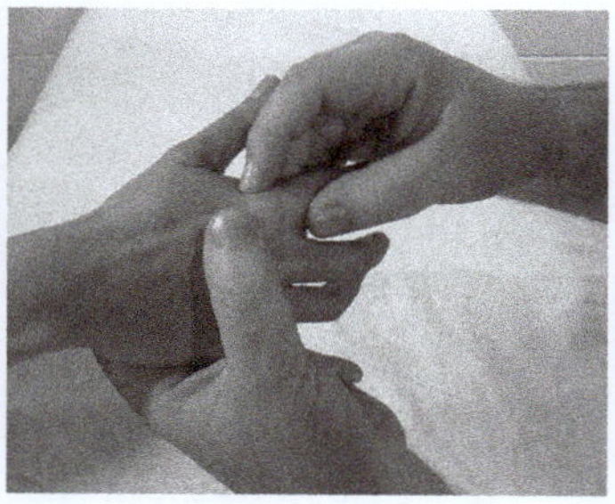

FIGURE 18.12 Palpation of MCP joint

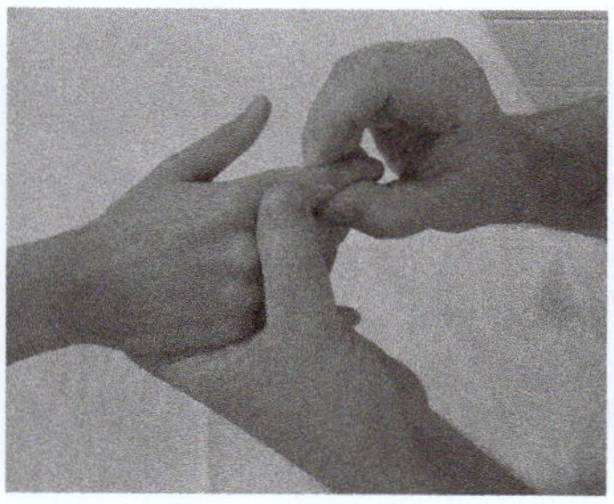

FIGURE 18.13 Palpation of PIP joint

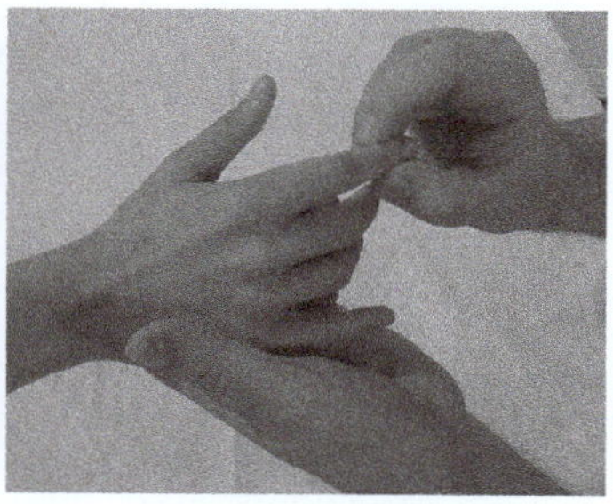

FIGURE 18.14 Palpation of DIP joint

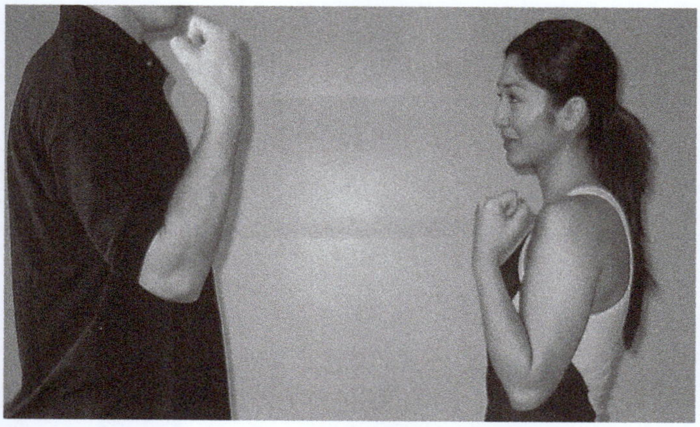

FIGURE 18.15 1. Ruling out elbow flexion

Have the patient first actively flex both elbows.

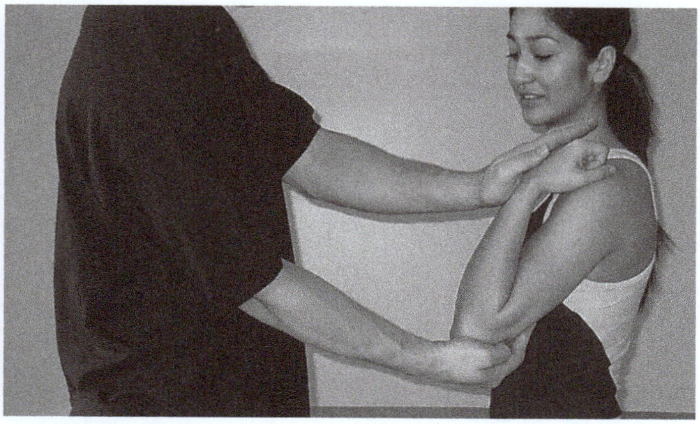

FIGURE 18.16 2. Ruling out elbow flexion with O-P

Grasp the arm and forearm and apply O-P to each elbow (unaffected side first).

REMEMBER: The dominant side will usually differ somewhat from the non-dominant side. Experience gained from testing many patients will enable you to begin to correctly suspect what are compensatory changes as opposed to changes due to handedness.

Ruling out the fingers (Figures 18.19, 18.20)

If the patient's chief complaint is centered upon the wrist (the radiocarpal joints, distal radioulnar joint, or carpal bones) then rule out the fingers by first having the patient make a half-fist causing flexion of the distal and proximal interphalangeal joints only. If there is no pain then have the patient clench this half-fist. Ask the patient if they can do this without pain.

Next have the patient make a full fist flexing the metacarpophalangeal joints. If there is no pain and all the fingers appear to have moved normally have the patient clench their fist tightly for O-P. Note that when the patient makes a tight fist all the MCPs (knuckles) lower and slightly rotate around the middle finger's metacarpal and its MCP becomes prominent. If the patient's chief complaint is not reproduced these joints can be ruled out.

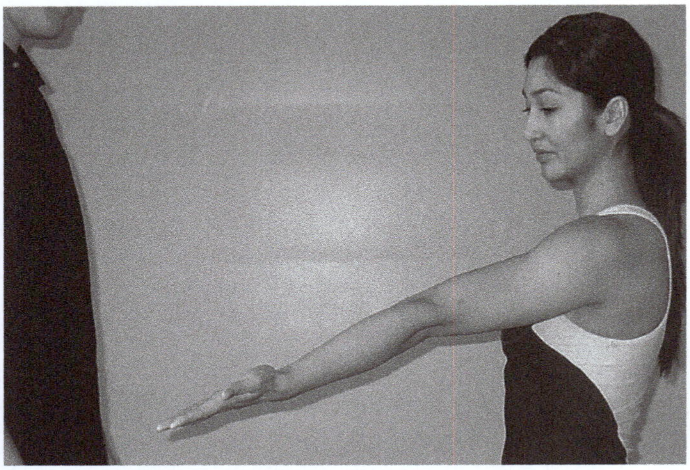

FIGURE 18.17 1. Ruling out elbow extension
Have the patient extend both arms.

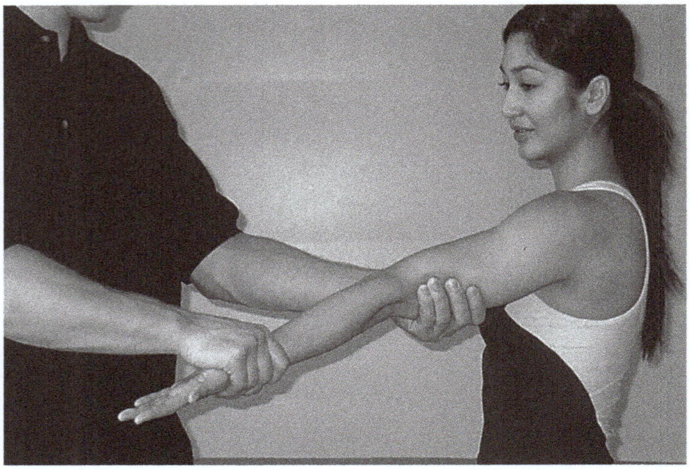

FIGURE 18.18 2. Ruling out elbow extension with O-P
Cup the elbow as shown, have the patient relax, and then apply O-P; first to the unaffected side and then to the affected side.

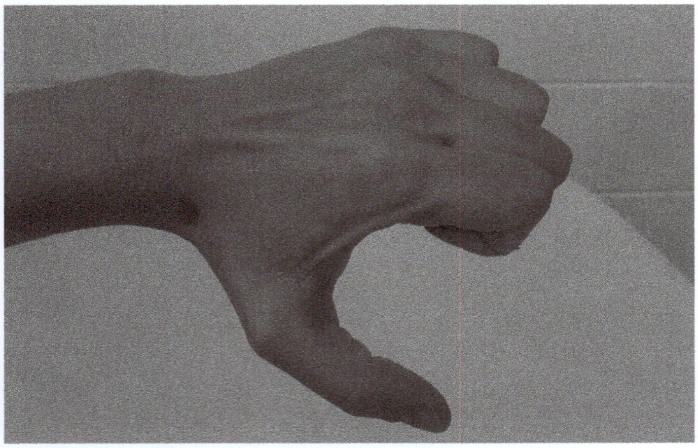

FIGURE 18.19
The patient makes half-fist and applies O-P by clenching.

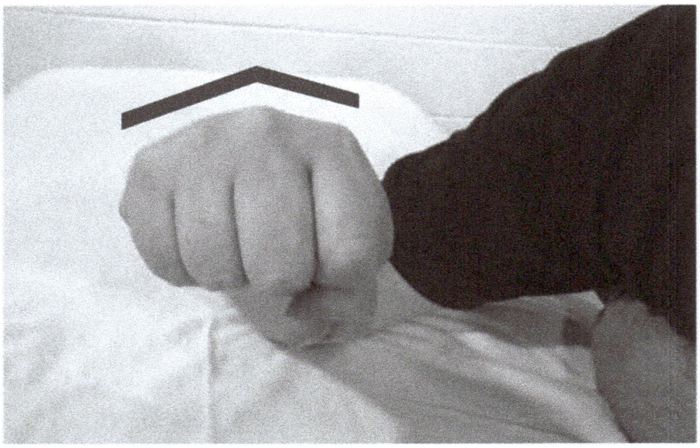

FIGURE 18.20
The patient makes a full fist and applies O-P by clenching.

Neurological issues

If neurological signs and symptoms have come up during case history taking or when doing the rule outs then a cervical spine assessment should be carried out. This is done using AF-ROM (flexion rotation and side-bending) followed by O-P if there was no pain felt. Finish with extension which has no O-P applied. Further, the focus of such testing would be to perform all the neurological tests: deep tendon reflexes, myotomes, dermatomes, a compression test, Spurling's test bilaterally, and Valsalva's test. Remember that you are looking to reproduce the patient's chief complaint by doing this neurological testing. If these tests do not reproduce the neurological symptoms proceed to testing for compression syndromes at the thoracic outlet (TOS testing), and then at the elbow. (See Chapter 14 for these tests.)

Do not forget to do the vertebral artery test if it is warranted by case history or signs and symptoms. There are other tests of the cervical spine that do not directly test neurological structures such as facet joints or specific muscles and these could be skipped at this time. However, if neither the neurological tests nor the thoracic outlet tests etc. reveal the cause of the paresthesia or other neurological impairment then you may wish to return to the cervical area to test those muscles that may refer via trigger points into the area of the patient's chief complaint.

Table 18.1 examines resting positions, close packed and capsular patterns of restriction in the joints of the wrist and hand.

Range of motion testing (ROM)

Active free range of motion (AF-ROM)

With the patient high-sitting, have them perform the actions in Figures 18.21–18.26 bilaterally for ease of comparison (shown here unilaterally for ease of viewing). As determined from their chief complaint and case history, have the patient do any action you would expect to be painful last. When observing motion at the wrist be sure to not to get distracted by the position of the fingers; you should look specifically at the angle made by the forearm and dorsal surface of the hand.

Table 18.1
Wrist and hand: resting positions (position of comfort), close packed and capsular patterns of restriction

Joint	Resting position	Close packed	Capsular pattern of restriction
Distal radioulnar	Slight supination	End of supination	Pain at end-ranges
Radiocarpal	Neutral with slight ulnar deviation	In full extension	Equal limitation in flexion and extension
Intercarpal	Neutral (natural cupping of hand)	In extension (of the wrist)	Not discernable
Mid-carpal	Neutral (natural cupping of hand)	Wrist extension	Equal limitation in flexion and extension
Carpometacarpal: (T) thumb (T) fingers	(t) mid-point of all actions (f) mid-point of flexion and extension	(T) full abduction (F) full flexion	(T) abduction, followed by extension (F) equal in all directions
Metacarpophalangeal	Slight flexion	Full flexion	Flexion, followed by extension
Interphalangeal	Slight flexion	Full flexion	Flexion and extension

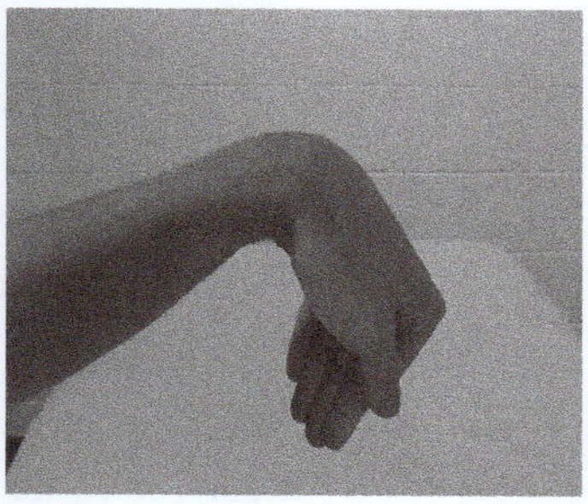

FIGURE 18.21 1. AF flexion of wrist 80–90°

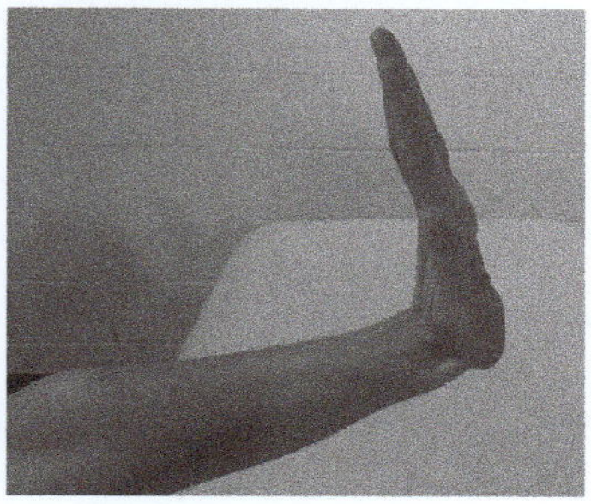

FIGURE 18.22 2. AF extension of wrist 70–90°

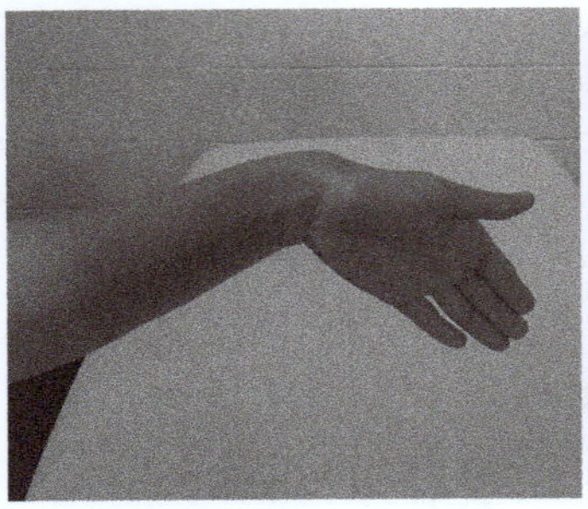

FIGURE 18.23 3. AF ulnar deviation of wrist (adduction) 30–45°

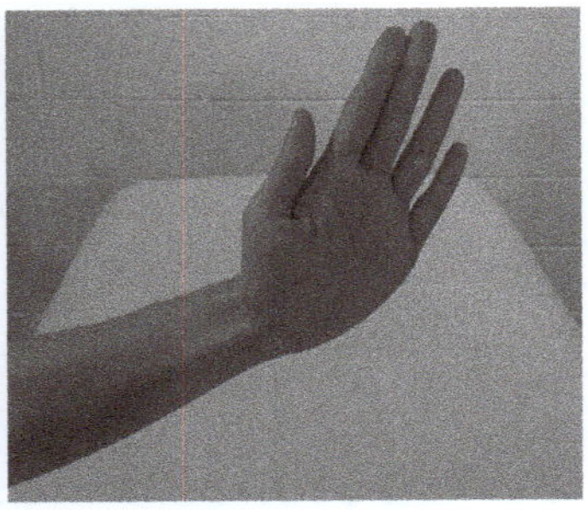

FIGURE 18.24 4. AF radial deviation of wrist (abduction) 15–20°

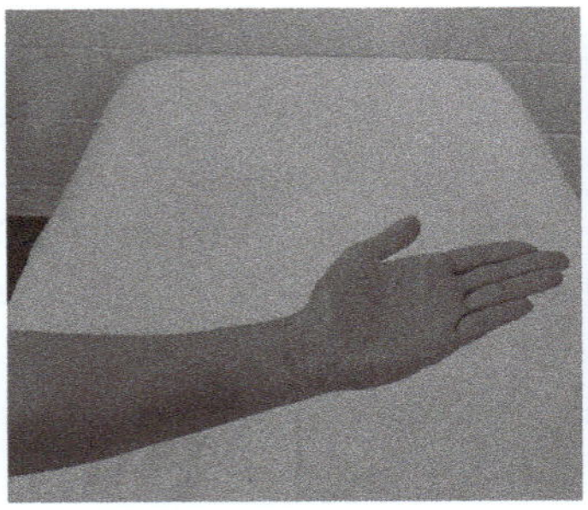

FIGURE 18.25 5. AF supination of forearm 85°

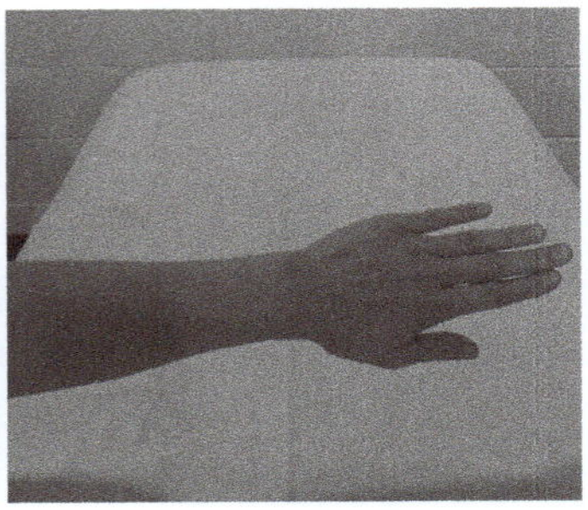

FIGURE 18.26 6. AF pronation of forearm 75–85°

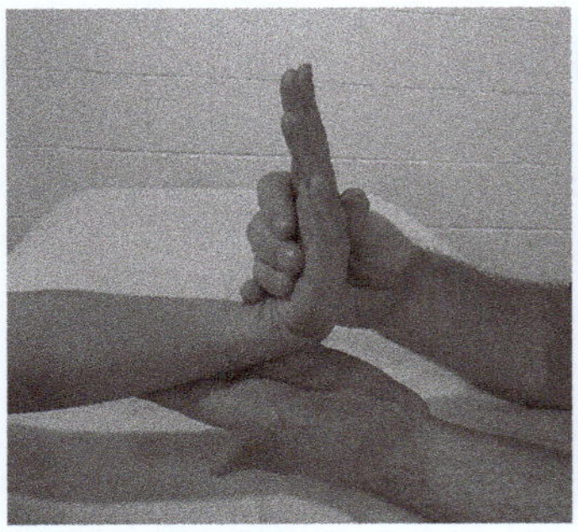

FIGURE 18.27 1. PR wrist flexion

End-feel is tissue stretch. A full 90° of flexion is usually attained.

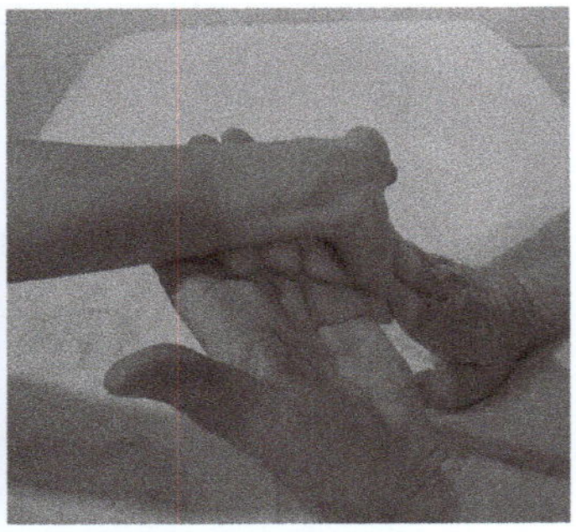

FIGURE 18.28 2. PR wrist extension

End-feel is tissue stretch.

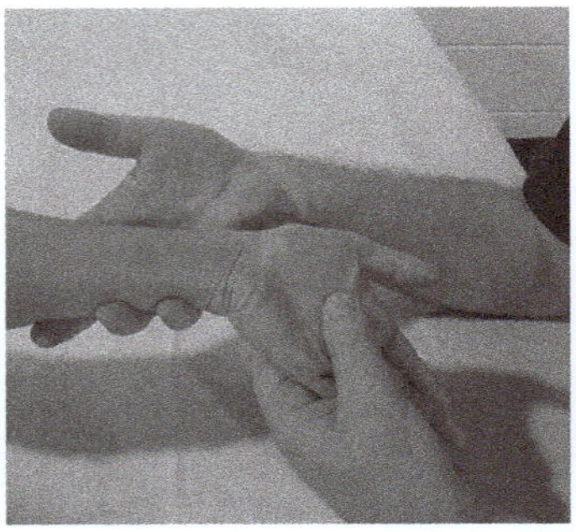

FIGURE 18.29 3. PR ulnar deviation of wrist (adduction)

End-feel is tissue stretch or bony if full end-range is achieved.

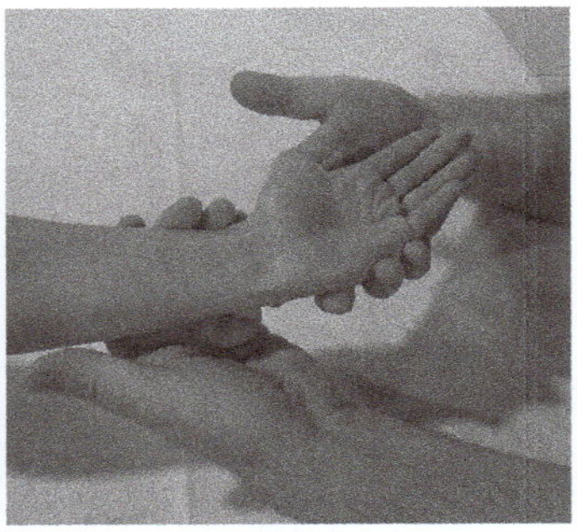

FIGURE 18.30 4. PR radial deviation of wrist (abduction)

End-feel is bony.

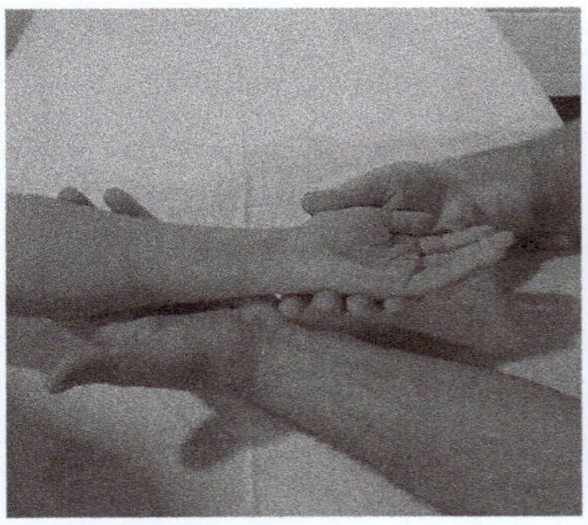

FIGURE 18.31 5. PR supination of wrist

End-feel is tissue stretch.

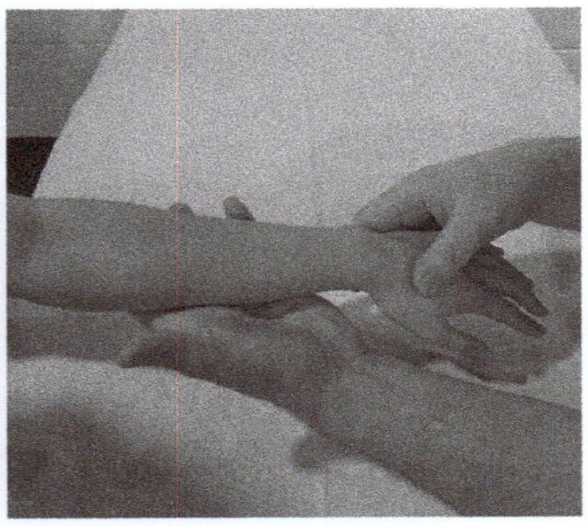

FIGURE 18.32 6. PR pronation of wrist

End-feel is tissue stretch.

NOTE: Most functional activities of daily living require at least 50° of supination and pronation.

Passive relaxed range of motion (PR-ROM) (Figures 18.27–18.32)

With the patient seated and their shoulder and elbow in a position of comfort take the patient's relaxed wrist through its ranges passively.

Joint play inspection the wrist

Note excess motion or a complete lack of motion (or "give"); have the patient tell you immediately about discomfort, pain, or any altered sensation *during and after* each application of mobilization. These tests in general are going to be stressing ligaments and joint capsules. ***REMEMBER:*** Rheumatoid arthritis is a complete contraindication for joint mobilization techniques.

The therapist needs to keep in mind that the restrictions found in joint mobilizations (or assessing joint play) need not necessarily come from intrinsic structures of the joint (joint capsules or ligaments) but may also be restricted by hypertonus in muscle(s) that prevent movement in either general or accessory joint motions under assessment. In the wrist, this can most often be seen in the radiocarpal joint where excessive tone in the flexors and extensors of the wrist and hand interfere with gapping the joint.

(For more details and instruction see Chapter 3. Also see the following for even more information and optional positioning of patient or limb, and variations or additional tests: Edmond 2006; Hertling & Kessler 2006; Kaltenborn 2006; Kisner & Colby 2012; Magee 2014; Starkey & Brown 2015.)

Joint play inspection of the radiocarpal joint (Figure 18.33)

Joint play inspection of the intercarpal joints (Figure 18.34, 18.35)

The intercarpal joints, especially between the two rows of carpals, and the carpal-metacarpal joints have more motion in flexion and extension of the wrist than we usually imagine.

Joint play inspection of the metacarpals (Figure 18.36, 18.37)

Observation experiment

Observe the stability between these two metacarpals in your own hand as you grasp an object, pick up a pen, hold a ball etc.

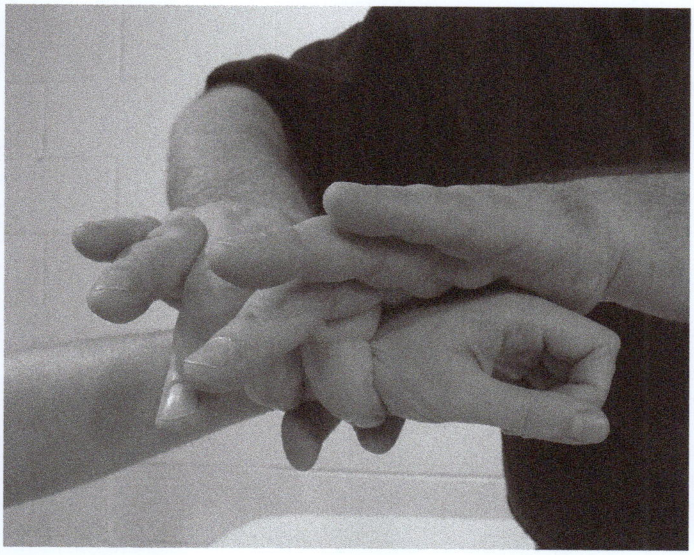

FIGURE 18.33 Positioning to achieve tractioning of wrist

To assess the amount of joint play within the radiocarpal joint encircle the patient's wrist with one hand (using the index finger and thumb) having the index fingers and thumbs pressed snugly up against each other. Apply gentle squeezing with both hands simultaneously and you should feel a space open up between radius and the row of proximal carpals. You have, in fact, tractioned specifically between these bones. Hold this space open gently, and if pain-free for the patient slide the hand/carpals dorsally and then ventrally about 1/8 inch. Check with the patient after each mobilization. Return to neutral but still hold the joint open; slide the hand radially and then ulnarly.

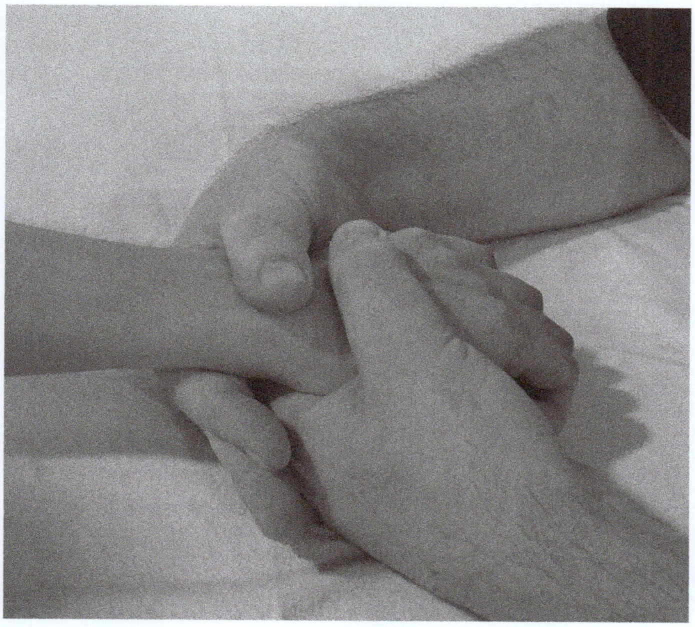

FIGURE 18.34 1. Proximal intercarpal *dorsal* glide

To assess joint play between two rows of carpals place the patient's hand between your hands. The ulnar border of your one hand is along the proximal row of carpals of the dorsal surface of the patient's hand while your other hand's ulnar border runs across the distal carpals on the ventral surface of the patient's hand. Squeeze the hands together focusing on the ulnar border of each hand as you apply pressure. Being "stepped" across carpals you should feel some mobilization between two rows.

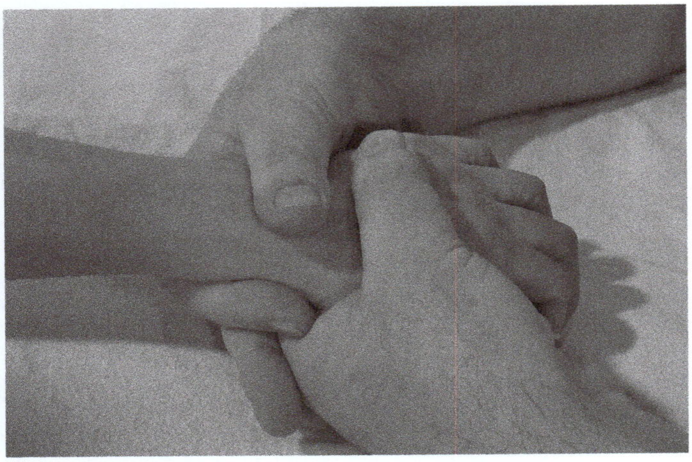

FIGURE 18.35 2. Proximal intercarpal ventral glide

Reverse the positioning of the ulnar borders of your hands (the one that was across the proximal row is now over the distal, and vice versa for other hand) so when you apply pressure you mobilize joints between the two rows in the opposite direction.

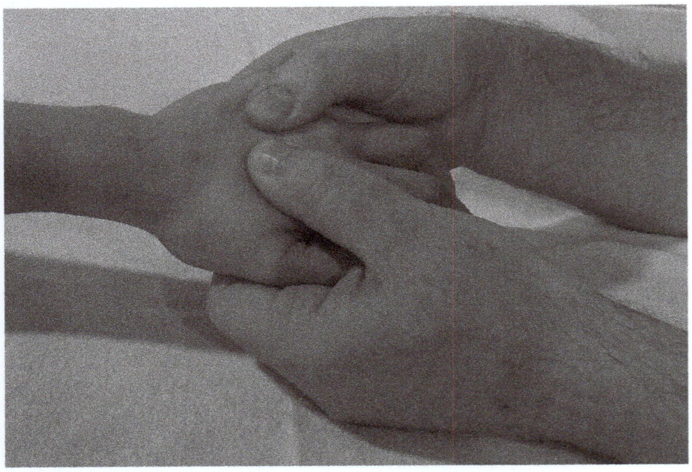

FIGURE 18.36 Palpation of second and third metacarpals

Grasp the index finger's metacarpal with one hand and the middle finger's with the other. Try to wiggle two bones in opposing dorsal-ventral directions. There is little or almost no movement here as these two are considered stable around which two lateral digits and thumb move as hand functions.

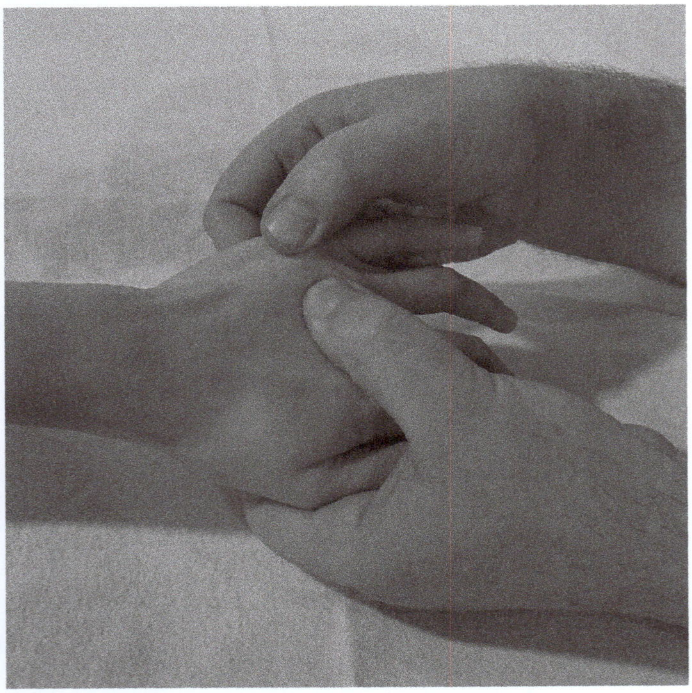

FIGURE 18.37 Palpation of motion between mobile metacarpals

Grasp the third and fourth metacarpals and wiggle them. You should notice significant movement. The same amount of movement or more should occur between the fourth and fifth metacarpals.

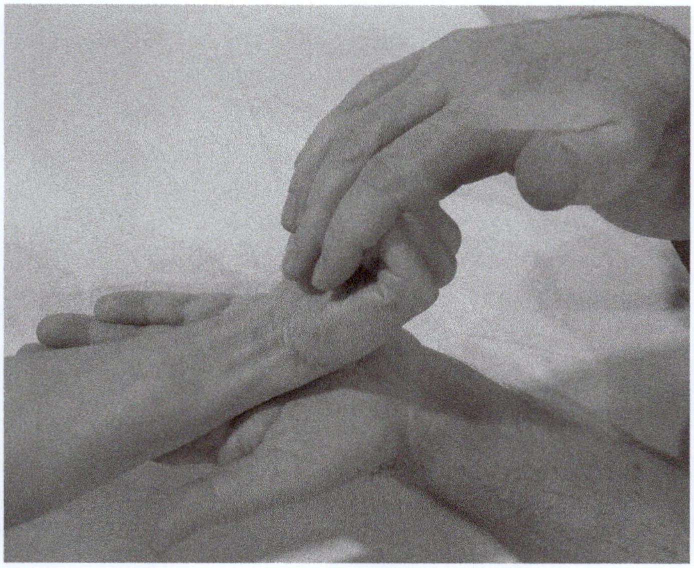

FIGURE 18.38 AR wrist flexion

Position the patient so the elbow is flexed to 90°, the forearm is supinated, and the wrist is in slight flexion (so the flexors can be adequately engaged to reduce the chance of injury). The therapist stabilizes the forearm with one hand while other hand rests on the palmar surface of the patient's hand. Have the patient try to flex their wrist while you provide resistance. Prime movers you are testing are flexor carpi radialis and flexor carpi ulnaris.

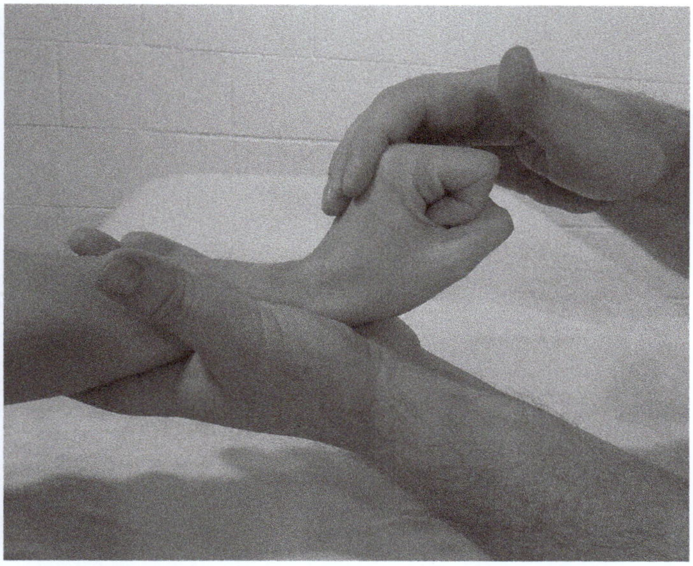

FIGURE 18.39 AR wrist extension

Position the patient so the elbow is flexed 90°, the wrist is in slight extension, and the forearm is pronated. Stabilize the patient's forearm with one hand while the other hand rests on the dorsal surface of the patient's hand. Have the patient try to extend their wrist while you apply resistance. Prime movers you are testing are the extensor carpi radialis longus, brevis, and extensor carpi ulnaris.

We need the hand to be malleable so as to be highly functional but we need this stability to prevent it from being too mobile and unable to grasp or hold things firmly.

Active resisted range of motion (AR-ROM) (Figures 18.38–18.43)

To make sure that you are not excessively compressing the intercarpal, carpal-metacarpal, or the metacarpal-phalangeal joints during isometric testing whenever possible try to have the patient make a half-fist (soft fist) and then position your resisting hand across the phalanges.

Even though the four muscles tested are the same muscles that perform ulnar and radial deviations you still need to test them while performing deviations. Though you may have found a positive result that replicates the patient's chief complaint when testing wrist flexion or extension, nonetheless, test the deviations to see if those actions cause pain and/or weakness as well, and of similar quality. Because the vector of force is different the sensation or weakness may be experienced differently

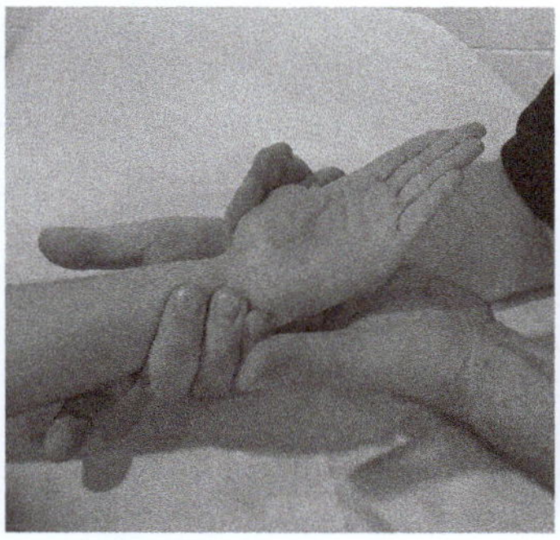

FIGURE 18.40 AR radial deviation

With the forearm supinated and the wrist in neutral resist abduction. Prime movers are the flexor carpi radialis longus, extensor carpi radialis longus and brevis.

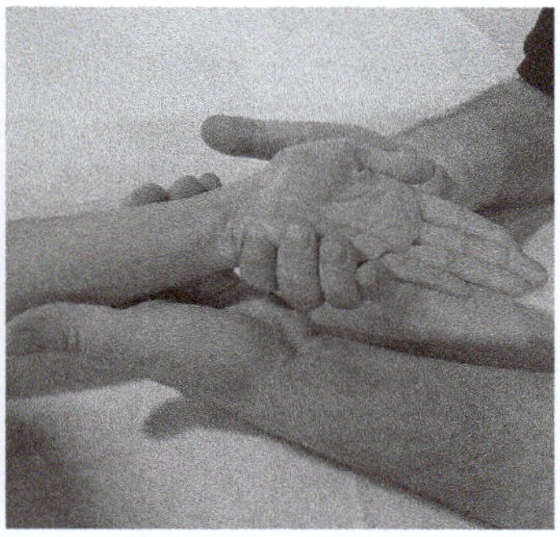

FIGURE 18.41 AR ulnar deviation

In the same position, and stabilizing the elbow against the patient's body, resist wrist adduction. Prime movers are the flexor carpi ulnaris, extensor carpi ulnaris.

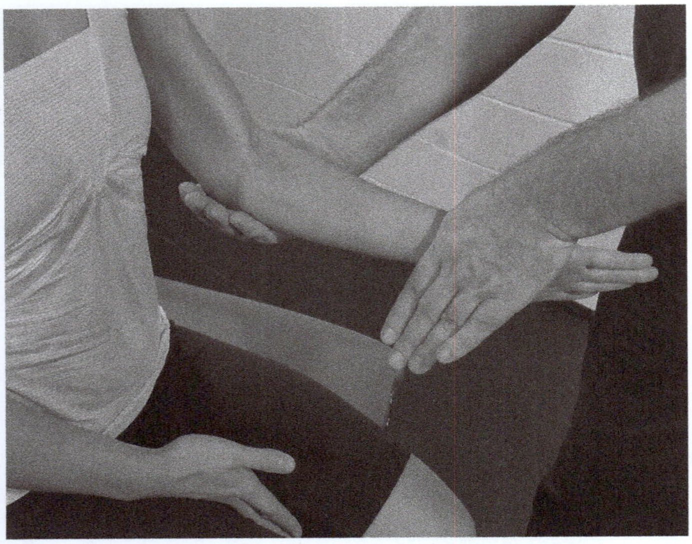

FIGURE 18.42 AR supination

With the elbow in the neutral position use one hand to stabilize it against the patient's body. Grasp the forearm with your other hand and have the thumb running along the posterior surface of the radius. The patient holds this position and resists your attempt to pronate the forearm. If you resist the patient's attempt to supinate you may risk injury to your own wrist. Primarily testing biceps brachii and supinator.

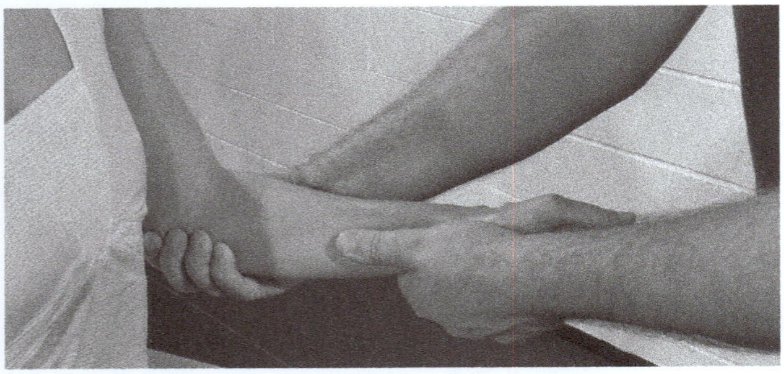

FIGURE 18.43 AR pronation

With the elbow in the neutral position use one hand to stabilize it against the patient's body. Grasp the forearm with your other hand and with the thumb running along the anterior surface of the radius. Ask the patient to resist your attempt to supinate the forearm. You are primarily testing pronator teres and pronator quadratus.

by the patient. Also as the movements employ the same muscles but in different combinations, you may be able to analyze and discover which movements are more impaired. ***REMEMBER:*** Though we may highlight injured and impaired muscle or joints we also need to discover the impairments as defined by the function or motion lost.

Special tests

Differential muscle testing of the wrist

Wrist extensors (Figures 18.44, 18.45)

If the patient had pain on AR-ROM testing of wrist extension (Figure 18.39) then differentiate with the following tests.

1. First test the extensor carpi radialis longus and brevis (Figure 18.44). *If there is pain or weakness* then differentiate between them.
2. Differentiate between longus and brevis (not shown): start with the patient in the same position (Figure 18.44) by keeping the arm parallel to the table and keeping the wrist deviated radially. But now, push their upper arm back so that their shoulder is now slightly extended and the elbow is now

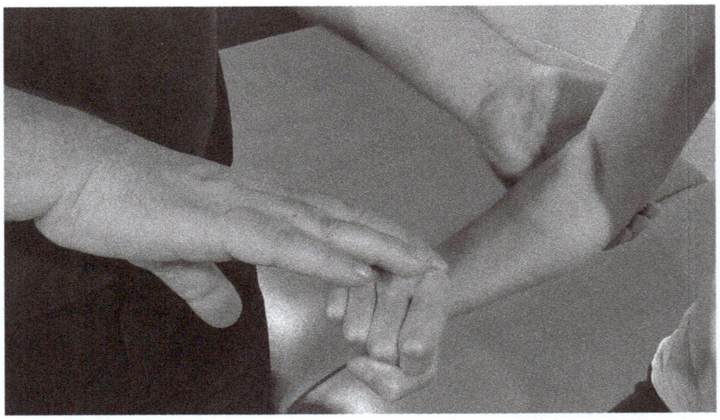

FIGURE 18.44 Extensor carpi radialis longus and brevis

To test the extensor carpi radialis longus/brevis together have the elbow flexed 90°, the shoulder forward flexed 45°, and the forearm pronated. Have the patient radially deviate the slightly extended wrist with the hand in a half-fist. Ask the patient to hold this position while you try to take the wrist into flexion and ulnar deviation. In other words, push down at an oblique angle toward the ulnar side of the wrist.

much more flexed, to 110–120°. This shortens extensor carpi radialis longus enough that brevis must do more work. Ask the patient to hold this position while you try to take the wrist into flexion and ulnar deviation. In other words, push down at an oblique angle toward the ulnar side of the wrist.

Compare results: If the second test is more painful than the first test then the brevis is more acute. If the test is less painful then the longus is more acute. If the pain is the same in both cases we cannot assume that the brevis is the only injured muscle: the test can be considered inconclusive with respect of differentiating since we cannot test the longus by itself. Now, proceed to testing the extensor carpi ulnaris (Figure 18.45).

Wrist flexors (Figure 18.46–18.48)

If the patient had pain on AR-ROM testing of wrist flexion then differentiate with the tests shown in Figures 18.46–18.48.

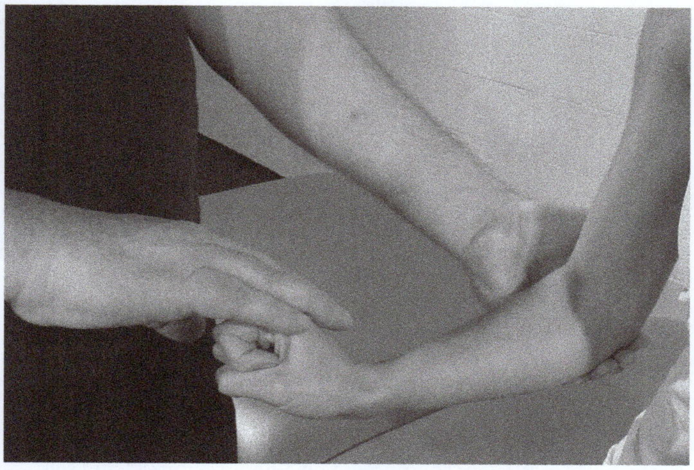

FIGURE 18.45 Extensor carpi ulnaris

To test extensor carpi ulnaris position the shoulder in neutral, the elbow at 90°, the wrist ulnarly deviated and slightly extended. Push the patient's fist into flexion and radial deviation (or obliquely down and toward the radial side of the wrist).

Take all of your results from differential testing of the muscles involved in wrist extension and create a picture of which muscles are impaired (strained), to what degree of severity or which may be ruled out as involved.

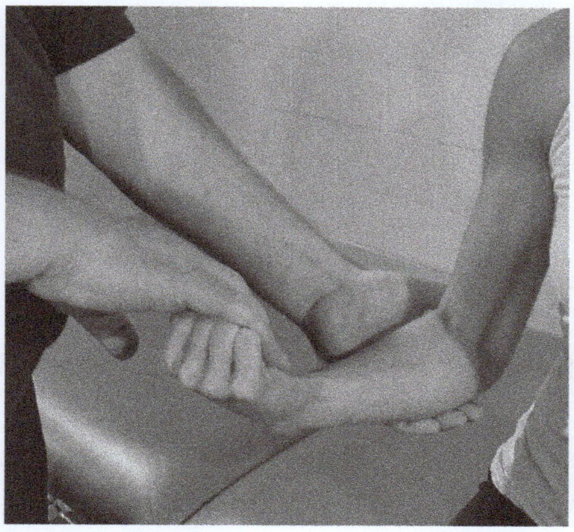

FIGURE 18.46 1. Wrist flexors in general

Position the patient so the elbow is flexed to 90°, the forearm supinated, and the wrist in slight flexion so the flexors can be adequately engaged and the chance of injury is reduced. Stabilize the forearm with one hand while the other hand rests on the distal palmar surface of the patient's hand.

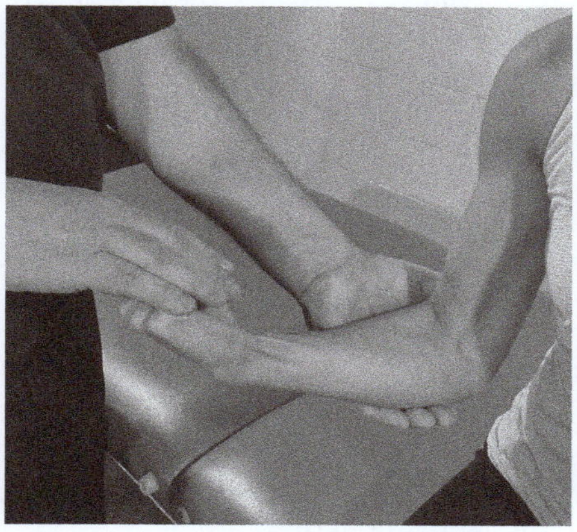

FIGURE 18.47 2. Testing flexor carpi radialis

To test flexor carpi radialis position the patient's wrist so it is radially deviated and apply your force down obliquely into extension and toward the ulnar side of wrist.

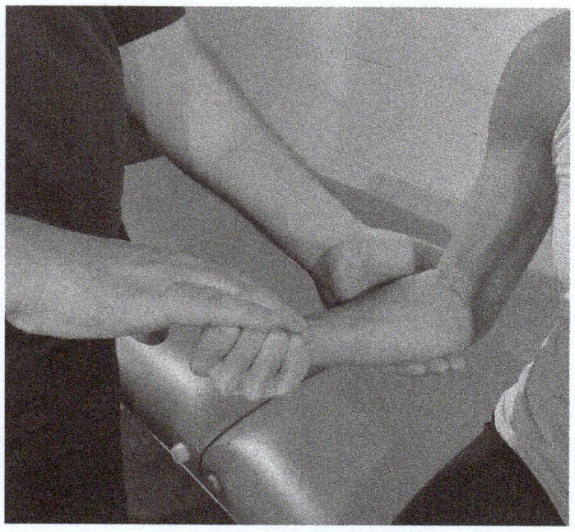

FIGURE 18.48 3. Testing flexor carpi ulnaris

To test flexor carpi ulnaris position the patient's wrist so it is ulnarly deviated and apply your force down obliquely into extension and toward the radial side of wrist.

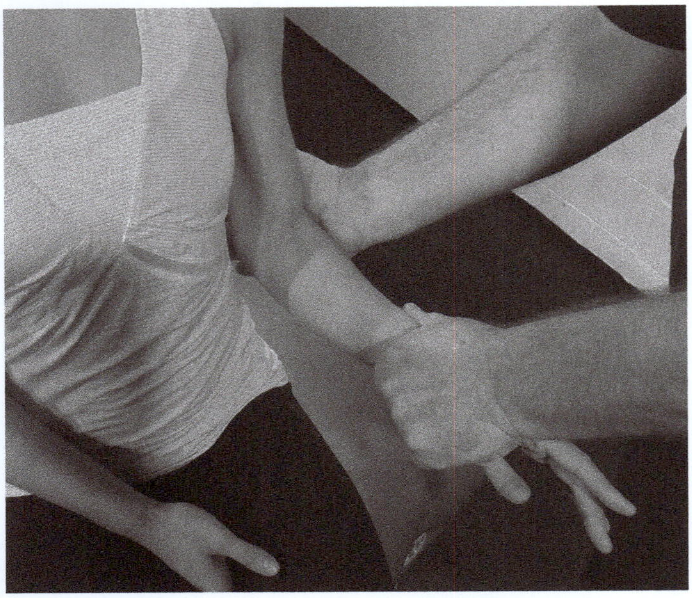

FIGURE 18.49 Testing supination in general

With the elbow in a neutral position and stabilized by the therapist against the body, with one hand grasp the forearm just above the wrist. With your other hand have your thumb running along the patient's radius. Tell the patient to hold the position and resist your attempt to pronate their forearm. If the therapist resists the patient's attempt to supinate they may risk injury to their own wrist. You are primarily testing biceps brachii and supinator.

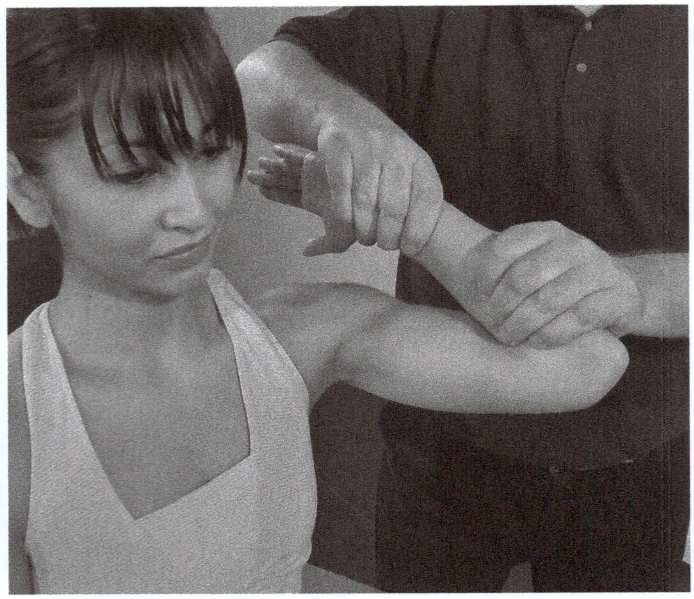

FIGURE 18.50 Specific test for supinator

Have the patient place the affected arm's hand on their shoulder. Then ask the patient to turn their palm so it faces their jaw. Stabilize the elbow and hold the forearm just proximal to the wrist (with your thumb running along the radius) and tell the patient to turn their wrist down towards their shoulder while you resist.

Differentiating between the supinators (Figures 18.49, 18.50)

The following tests are designed to differentiate between the biceps brachii and the supinator.

If this test produces pain distinguish which of the two muscles is responsible for the pain by focusing on the supinator and then making the biceps insufficient by shortening it. We shorten the biceps by having the patient place the affected arm's hand on their shoulder.

You may want the patient to first supinate their forearm without resistance so that you can clearly see how the forearm is going to move. Have the patient reposition for the AR test and place your hands as required. If resistance is still as painful as when testing supination with the elbow in neutral then it is most probably due to the supinator. However, if resisted supination is less painful in the specific test for the supinator then most likely the pain felt during resisted supination in neutral was due to the biceps.

Differentiating between the pronators (Figure 18.51, 18.52)

The following tests differentiate between the pronator teres and the pronator quadratus. The location of pain will aid in distinguishing between these two when testing pronation in general. However, if unexplained weakness without pain occurs (a neurological sign) or the patient received non-specific blows to the arm, then you can do the tests shown in Figures 18.51 and 18.52.

The patient in the second (specific) testing position here (Figure 18.52) is the same as specifically testing the supinator. The only difference is which way you instruct the patient to try and turn their palm.

Tendinopathies: tendonosis, tendonitis, and tenosynovitis

Many wrist impairments such as loss of motion or pain (with or without weakness) that are the result of tendinopathies (including periostitis) at the wrist may have already shown up in AR-ROM testing. Using differential muscle testing (described above) will

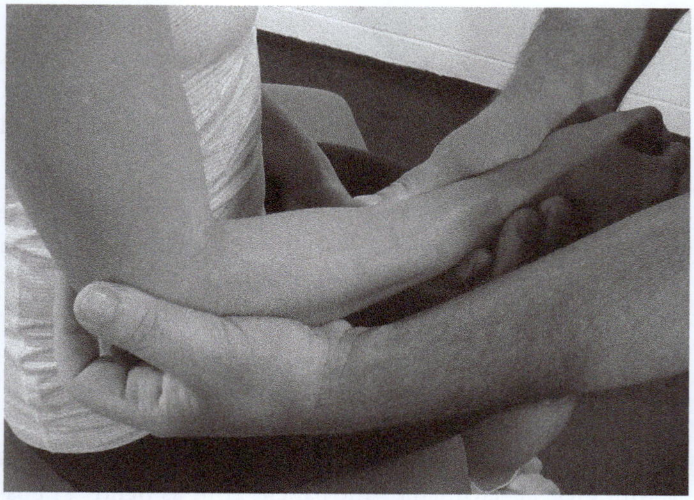

FIGURE 18.51 Testing pronation in general

With the elbow in a neutral position and stabilized by the therapist against the body, with one hand grasp above the patient's wrist with the other hand, with the thumb running along the radius. Tell the patient to resist your attempt to supinate the forearm. Primarily testing pronator teres and pronator quadratus.

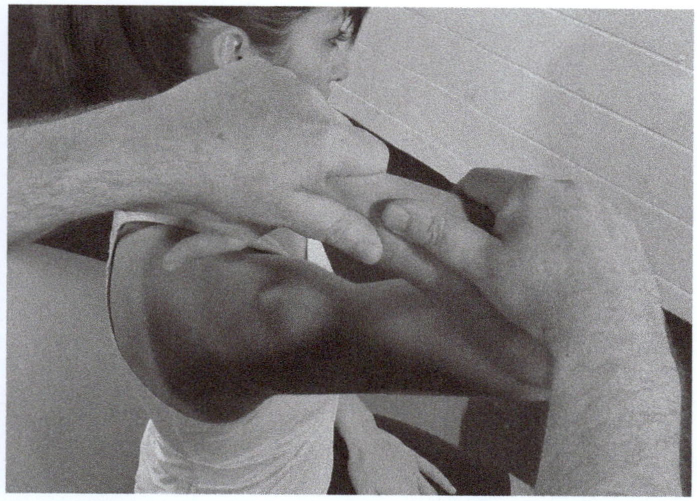

FIGURE 18.52 Specific to pronator quadratus

Have the patient fully flex the elbow and have their hand facing their jaw. Stand in front of the patient and stabilize both radius and ulnar bones. Ask the patient to try to turn the hand toward the ceiling as you resist.

locate the specific muscle/tendon/periosteum involved. Tendon pain in the carpal and metacarpal areas are usually at the insertion sites of forearm muscles. Note that inflamed and/or injured periosteal attachments of muscle are often mistaken for joint injury/disease such as osteoarthritis in the wrist and carpal joints.

An example of this possible confusion between whether it is tendonosis/tendonitis and joint disease is when pain or tenderness appears at the base of the thumb. We need to differentiate between flexor carpi radialis tendinopathy and synovitis of the carpal-metacarpal or the metacarpal-phalangeal joint of the thumb. To repeat comparing our results from differential muscle testing and PR-ROM will often reveal which is which.

One more point regarding tendinopathies: many of the muscles whose tendons are symptomatic at their carpal attachments can also be the same muscles that are involved in elbow (or proximal and mid-forearm) pain from tendonosis/tendonitis. While testing, for example, at the elbow for epicondylitis you get a positive at the lateral epicondyle but you may also get pain at the wrist. Therefore, you should perform those elbow tests that involve such muscles when testing the wrist.

Next, we take a look at some of the common occurrences of tendinopathies (tendonosis, tendonitis, tenosynovitis) specific to the wrist and the special tests developed for them.

De Quervain's syndrome (Finkelstein test)

A stenosing tenosynovitis, De Quervain's syndrome is a specific tendinopathy common in the thumb. Both the extensor pollicis brevis and the abductor pollicis longus tendons share the same sheath as their tendons cross the wrist and travel to the thumb. Repetitive actions such as tapping the space bar with the thumb will cause these two tendons to rub against each other and they can become inflamed; in turn the sheath they share will become inflamed. In an acute phase, it is very painful for the patient to move the thumb at all. There are such impairments as finding it difficult to open doors that have round knobs or to firmly grasp anything like a cup in the affected hand.

The test for this is referred to as the Finkelstein test (Figure 18.53A, B). Like most tests for tendinopathy, stretching the muscle usually recreates the symptoms. Since we have an extensor and an abductor of the thumb involved we take the thumb in the opposite directions.

Positive in acute

In an acute case of tenosynovitis this movement alone will be very painful and the patient may not be able to even complete this initial portion of the test. The pain is felt around the base of the thumb and at the radial border of the wrist in the anatomical snuffbox.

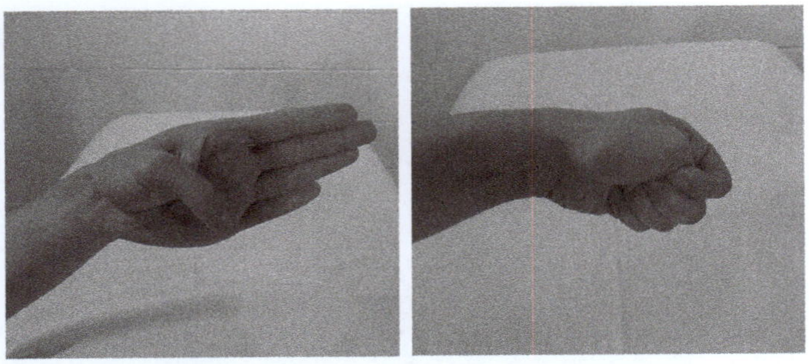

FIGURE 18.53A, B Finkelstein test

The patient flexes the thumb across the palm, which flexes and adducts the thumb. Ask about pain. If it is not painful then have the patient make a fist around their thumb and ulnar deviate the wrist.

Positive in subacute or chronic

If the patient could do the above action, get them to now ulnar deviate the wrist. This is the completed Finkelstein test. This further stretching of the tendons through the sheath would then cause pain in the areas mentioned above. The pain can refer into the whole thumb, radial carpal bones, and up into the radial border of the forearm when the condition is severe.

Flexors digitorum tendinopathy ("mouse hand")

Flexors digitorum tendinopathy is an achy pain throughout the palmar/ventral surface of the fingers which can be due to overuse of the flexors digitorum superficialis and profundus. It arises from either gripping an object (such as a computer mouse) for long periods of time or excessive repetitive flexion of the fingers for long periods of time. The test for this may require extended isometric or concentric muscle testing to get the symptoms to recur.

Intersection syndrome

The extensor pollicis longus tendon travels to the ulnar side of Lister's tubercle on the distal radius. It takes a 45° turn around this tubercle using it like a pulley to course its way to the distal phalange of the thumb. In doing this turn it runs over or intersects with the extensor carpi radialis longus and brevis tendons which lie underneath. Excessive use of thumb extension (e.g., holding the thumb in extension and occasionally hitting the space bar of a computer) can cause the extensor pollicis longus tendon/sheath to friction across the extensor carpi radialis tendons/sheaths.

There is no specific test per se for this syndrome. Use the Finkelstein test above. Usually irritation or inflammation of the extensor carpi radialis longus and brevis tendons is felt less in the anatomical snuffbox area (radial side of wrist) and more over the posterior distal forearm just below the wrist. (A quick look in an anatomy text at the relative positions at the wrist of the extensor pollicis and extensor carpi radialis tendons will make clearer where the symptoms might be.)

After doing the Finkelstein test, do resisted testing of the extensor carpi radialis muscles (resisting wrist extension with radial deviation; see differential testing above). This test will generate a positive result as well, while the extensor and abductor pollicis alone would not.

Flexor digitorum tendinopathies test

The therapist makes a fist with one hand and the patient grasps it with their affected hand. The patient grips as tightly as possible and holds for a minute or two to try to provoke their symptoms. The patient can repeat this two or three times in order to add further provocation. An alternative is to have the patient squeeze a ball repeatedly for several minutes.

Conditions of the hand

NOTE: The following special tests are concerned with the carpals, metacarpals, and phalanges, and should therefore be included later, but we include them here in order to complete the classic organization of the special tests for the wrist and hand.

Fracture of the scaphoid (Figure 18.54)

A fracture of the scaphoid carpal bone could give a false positive for the Finkelstein test. This is the most common carpal bone to be fractured and usually occurs falling onto an outstretched hand. The pain from a fracture of this bone would be exacerbated with radial deviation which would press the bone into the articular surface of the radius.

Extensor expansion test (Bunnel–Littler test) (Figure 18.55A–C)

This tests whether contracturing or other impairment is affecting the elements of the extensor expansion, especially those that would interfere with flexion of the DIPs or PIPs. Understanding what is being tested, how this test works, and what are the positive and negative results requires understanding the extensor expansion. If you are not sure how the test works and what constitutes a positive or negative result then review the anatomy/structure and function of the extensor expansion.

Ligamentous tests of the MCP, PIP, and DIP joints

This testing is done during PR-ROM joint mobilization assessment of the phalangeal joints. (See Appendix B, p. 518.)

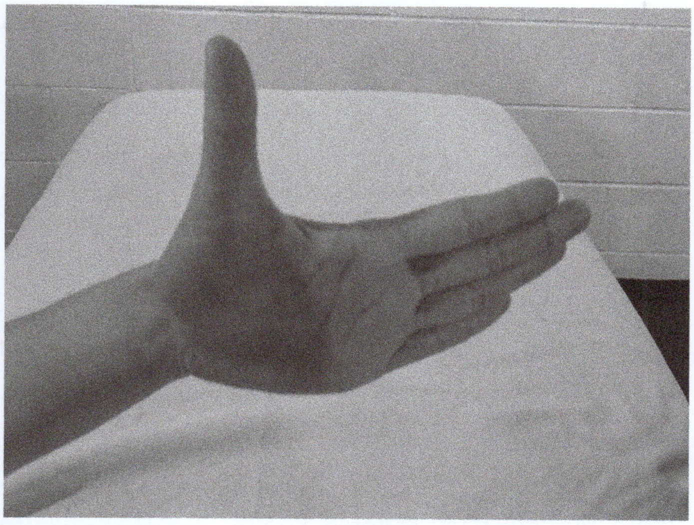

FIGURE 18.54 Testing for fracture of scaphoid

Have the patient extend the distal phalange of the thumb (i.e., close pack joints all the way down the thumb and into the scaphoid) and then tap the thumb lightly at its tip in the direction of the scaphoid. A positive sign is a sudden increase in pain felt at or around the scaphoid carpal bone.

Skier's thumb (Figure 18.56)

This term is sometimes used when the medial collateral ligament of the thumb's MCP joint is strained or torn. An example of how this can happen is when a skier falls and the thumb is hyper-abducted because the thumb of the hand holding the ski pole takes the force of the fall the skier is trying to avoid. There are many other situations where this type of injury can occur. The test should only be used if the injury is in the chronic stage.

Trigger finger (Figures 18.57–18.59)

This describes a situation where a finger "catches" or "locks" when it tries to extend or flex. This is usually due to a nodule or thickening of connective tissue that grows on a flexor tendon as it travels up along the ventral surface of the finger when the nodule is close to either end of a sheath through which it travels past a joint. The cause of the nodule is not usually known.

The common sites are at the MCP and PIP joints. When the patient flexes the finger the nodule gets pulled into the tendon's sheath which transverses the joint. Then when the patient tries to extend the finger the nodule that is now "stuck" in the sheath prevents movement of the tendon and therefore prevents that finger from extending. The finger may suddenly release a few

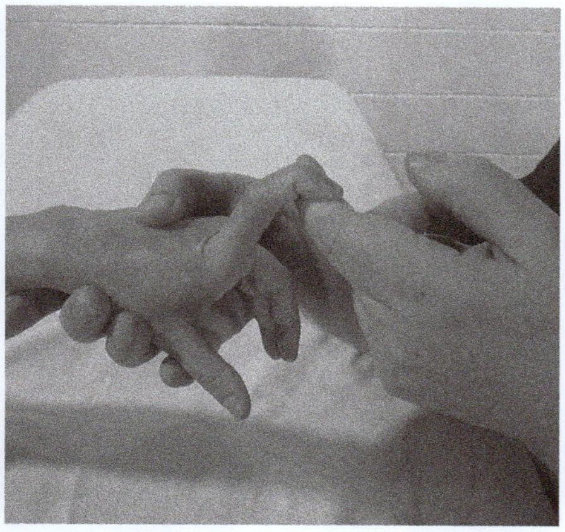

FIGURE 18.55A Extensor expansion test

1. Stabilize the patient's MCP joint of the finger being tested, which is in extension. Ask the patient to then flex the PIP and DIP joints of that finger. The test is negative if the patient can fully flex both joints.

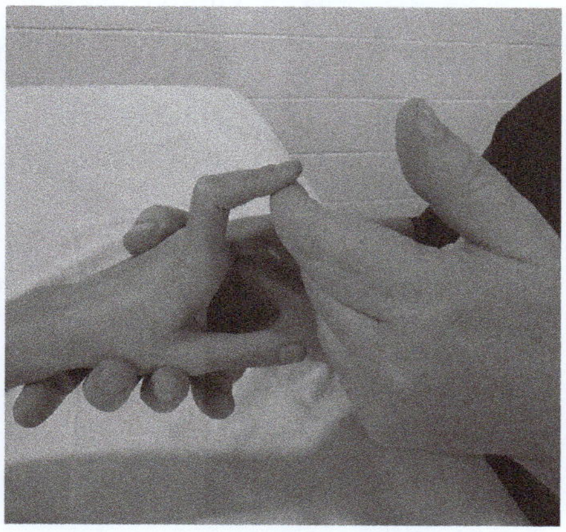

FIGURE 18.55B

2. If one of these joints cannot flex the test may be positive. This may be due to contracturing of the lumbricals and interosseus muscles, which will hold tension on extensor expansion (preventing flexion).

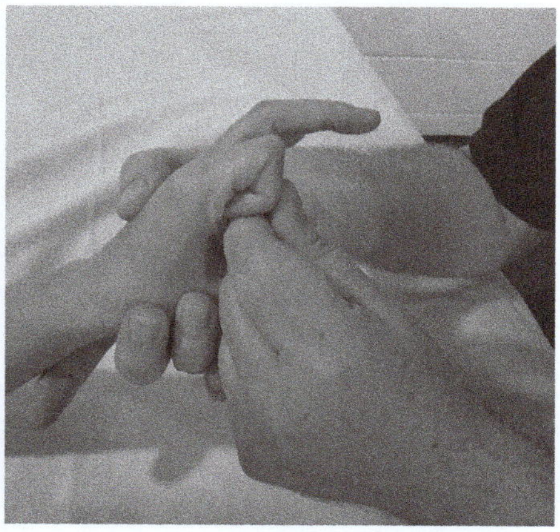

FIGURE 18.55C

3. To ensure it is not some impairment of a joint (e.g., contracture of joint's capsule), stop holding the MCP in extension and see if you can passively flex all joints. If the joints can now all move, this implies a joint capsule contracture. If one or more still cannot flex the extensor expansion is restricted.

seconds later as the tendon slowly makes its way out of the snug sheath or it can get locked and the patient has to use the other hand to straighten out the finger (i.e., force the nodule out of the sheath).

It can have several presentations depending on severity:

- As the patient extends or flexes a finger the finger momentarily cannot complete the movement but it will then suddenly move and finish the action.
- The patient cannot extend a flexed digit, for example, but needs to use the other hand to move the finger into neutral.
- Where the finger becomes fixed and can no longer move.

If the patient has previously received cortisone shots but the condition has returned, the tissue may be frail, and prone to tear or rupture if worked too aggressively. Surgery is usually successful by cutting open the sheath to allow more room.

Assessment for trigger finger: observing the motion of the impaired finger and palpation of a nodule are the means of assessing this condition. The *example here is at the MCP joint.*

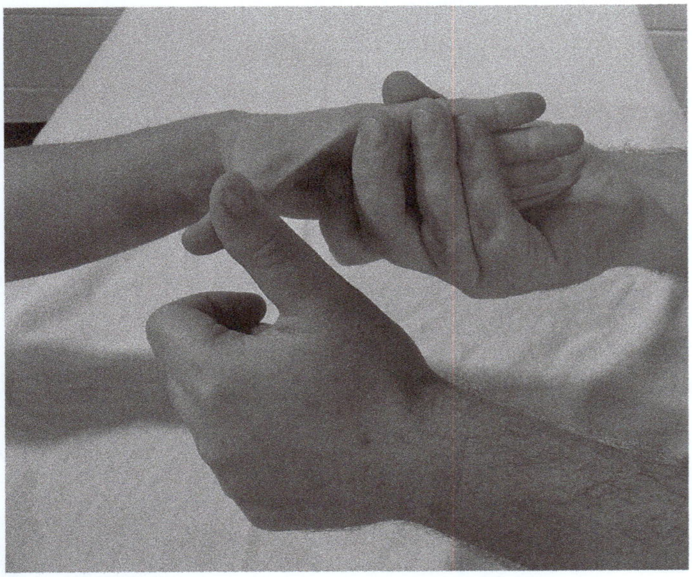

FIGURE 18.56 Skier's thumb test

A stress is put through the MCP ligament of the thumb by abducting the thumb and applying O-P. This is a re-creation of how it was injured. A positive sign is pain.

Nerve compression syndromes at the wrist (Figures 18.60–18.70)

Tests for median nerve impingement

Observations Atrophy of the thenar eminence (which is composed of intrinsic muscles of the hand that are supplied by the median nerve) is an observable sign of median nerve dysfunction. Another observable sign that predisposes the patient to having carpal tunnel syndrome is what is referred to as having a "square wrist." In this instance, a cross-section of the wrist would appear squarer than the usual rectangular look associated with a normal healthier wrist (Pascarelli & Quilter 1994).

It is thought that the so-called square wrist may not only decrease the total area of the carpal tunnel but also cause the tendons and sheaths to stack up on top of each other in a manner that leads to a greater risk of tenosynovitis. It is likely that the swelling of the sheaths is the principal cause of compression on the median nerve as it passes through the carpal tunnel.

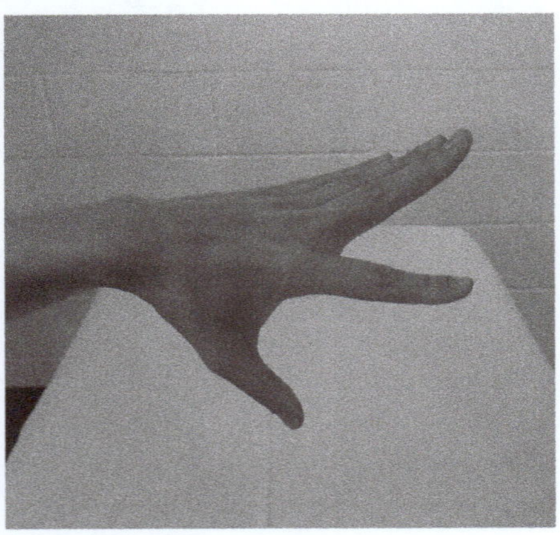

FIGURE 18.57 1. Finger unable to extend

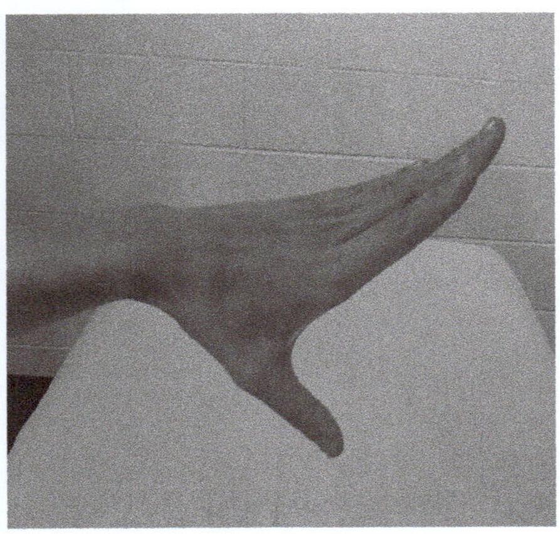

FIGURE 18.58 2. Finger eventually extends

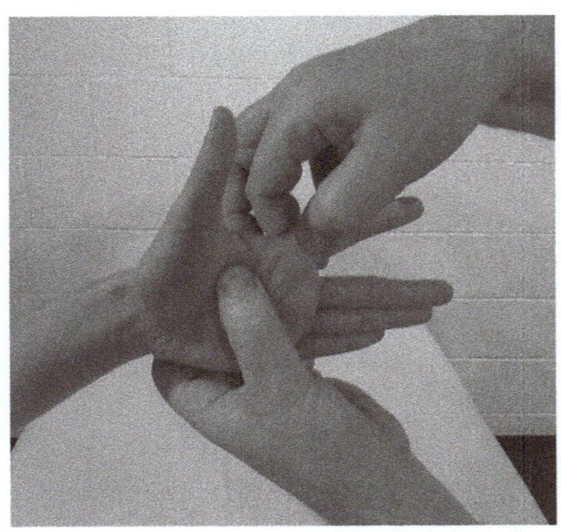

FIGURE 18.59 3. Palpation of nodule

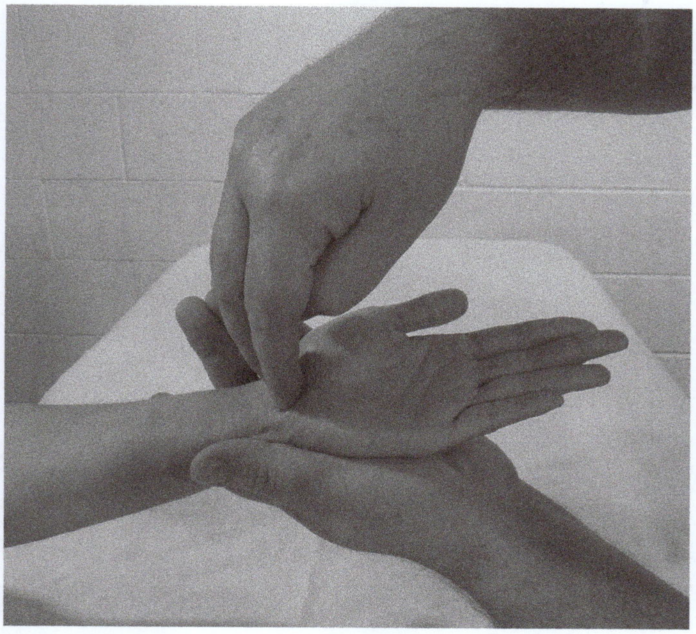

FIGURE 18.60 Tinel's sign at the wrist

This tests for compression or inflammation of the median nerve as it passes through the carpal tunnel. Test to confirm carpal tunnel syndrome. Tap several times over the area of the carpal tunnel (over the volar carpal ligament or retinaculum). A positive sign is tingling or paresthesia into the thumb and first two and half fingers.

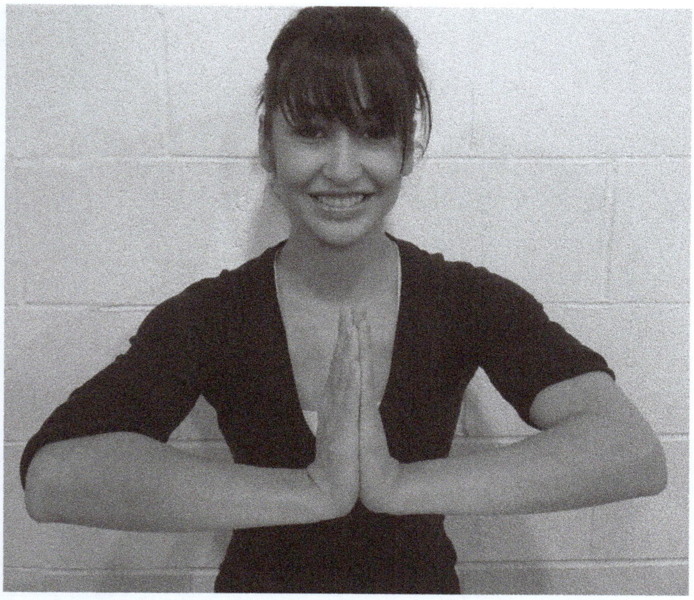

FIGURE 18.61 Phalen's test (Cyriax's variation)

Phalen's test is another test which can used to confirm carpal tunnel syndrome. The patient places the dorsal surfaces of the hands together in front of the chest so the wrists are flexed 90° (not shown). The patient holds the position for one minute. You may then add provocation by having the patient suddenly extend the wrists and bring the palms together, fingers pointing superiorly (Cyriax's suggestion or variation).

Motor test for the median nerve (Figures 18.62, 18.63)

So far, we have only tested the sensory portion of the median nerve and we need to see if motor function associated with the median nerve is compromised. This can be assessed by a "pinch test."

The positive sign for these tests is weakness without pain in the affected hand. It is also positive if you notice that the patient cannot hold or resist using the tips of the finger and thumb but the DIPs of each extend and they can only hold by using the pads of the finger and thumb. (It is actually the thumb that extends and by this change of position the index finger pad also becomes the point of contact.)

Ulnar nerve impingement/compression (Figures 18.64, 18.65)

The ulnar nerve can be compressed under the pisiform or as it passes along the surface of the hamate (under the hook of the hamate). This can be done by a single trauma, as when a fall or blow crushes the nerve bringing on immediate symptoms, or by repetitive trauma, as when the patient has been using the

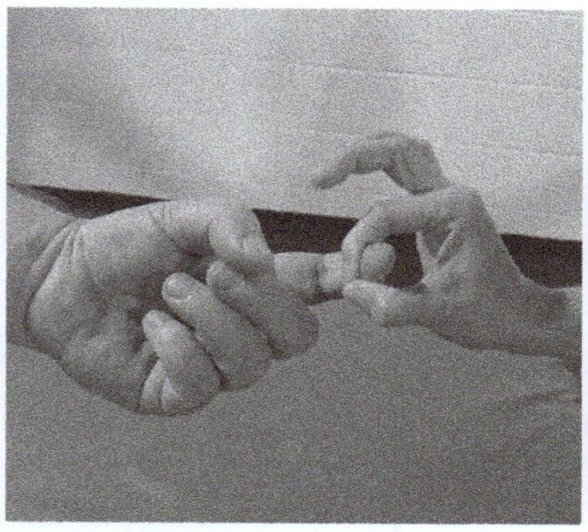

FIGURE 18.62 Pinch test

The patient brings the tips of the thumb and index finger together as if making the "okay" hand gesture. Ask the patient to hold this position while you use your flexed index finger to try and pull through.

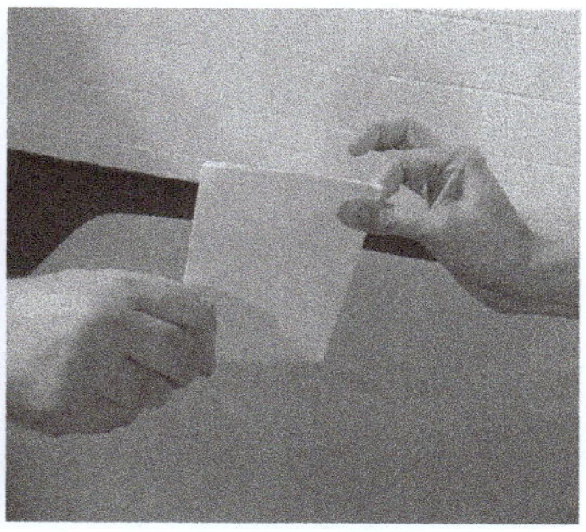

FIGURE 18.63 Alternative pinch test

Have the patient pinch piece of paper between thumb and index finger using only the tips of the thumb and index finger as you try to pull it out of their grasp.

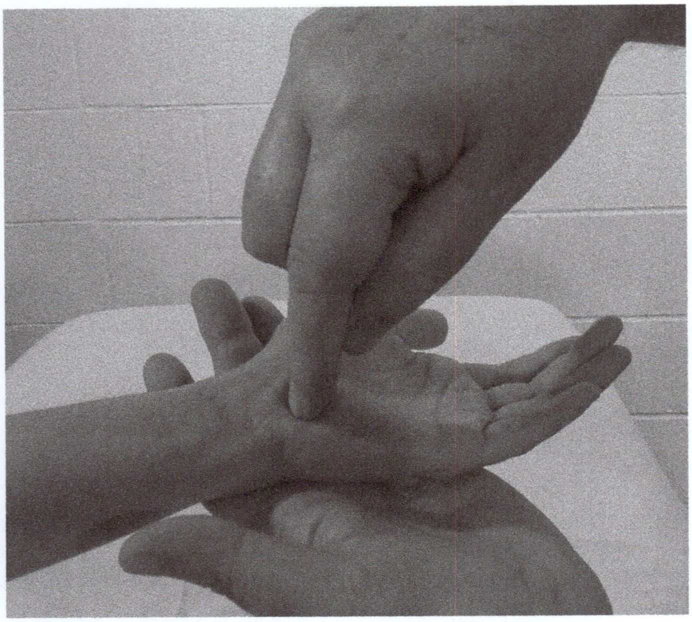

FIGURE 18.64 Tinel's sign for ulnar nerve

The therapist taps over the pisiform/hamate area. An alternative is the therapist compressing the pisiform down into the tissue and holding it there for 30 seconds or so. The positive sign is radiation of pain into the ulnar border of the hand and into the little finger.

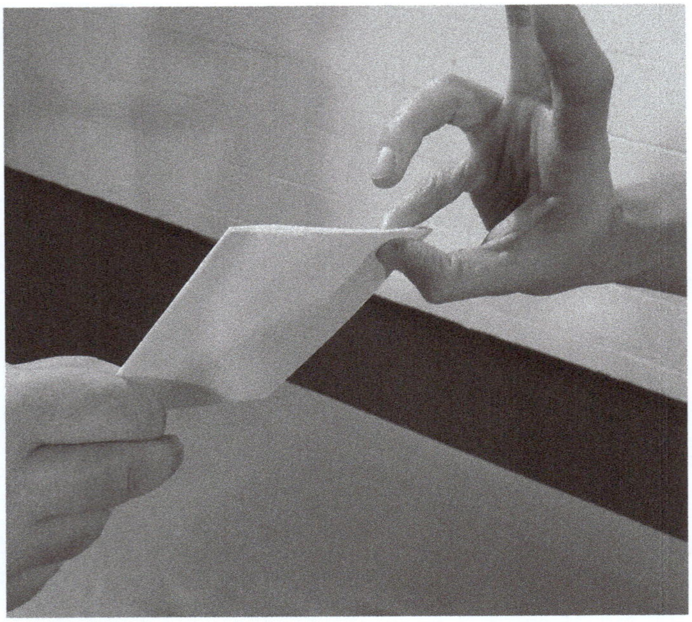

FIGURE 18.65 Frommet's sign/test

This ulnar motor nerve test uses the adductor policis. The patient holds a piece of paper between their thumb and index finger as you try to pull it away. A positive test shows increasing flexion of the distal phalanges of the thumb (as shown).

hypothenar portion of the hand as a tool to shift or move things about (for instance, a carpenter might use it to tap a piece of wood into place before securing it). This can also happen to bike riders who lean on the handlebars with their hypothenar eminences.

NOTE: Local pain without radiation could imply injury to the pisiform or hamate (e.g., a fracture of the pisiform or the hook portion of the hamate carpal bone). In a trauma scenario injury to both the involved carpal bone and the ulnar nerve is possible.

A patient with ulnar nerve palsy (compromised ulnar nerve) may flex the thumb's distal interphalangeal joint to try to maintain a hold on the paper. They will not be able to hold it without this flexing. Hence, they may appear to have full strength by recruiting other musculature but you still have a positive sign showing weakness without pain of the abductor pollicis.

Vascular impairment or compression at the wrist or in the hand (Figures 18.66–18.70)

When there is a vascular problem in the hand the therapist should be able to observe some changes in the affected hand. If the problem is situated in the wrist or hand the following signs are seen in comparison to the unaffected limb:

- Paleness in the hand suggests arterial supply is compromised.
- Darkness implies venous congestion.
- A puffiness of the whole hand may suggest impairment to the lymphatics in the forearm, wrist, and hand.

REMEMBER: Compromised vascular and lymphatic flow can come from many sources in the upper limb including the elbow, upper arm, brachial plexus, and thoracic outlet. While the whole limb could be suffering from decreased flow, the most obvious signs and symptoms of such impairments often appear at the most distal end of the limb (i.e., in the hand).

Be careful not to jump to conclusions about the site of the impairment. You may need to backtrack all the way up the arm and into the neck to find the site of compression (i.e., rule out thoracic outlet syndrome, etc.). Regardless, make sure the patient has spoken to their primary physician about this or refer them back to their physician if they have not or the condition has recently worsened.

Allen's test at the wrist (Figures 18.66–18.70)

This test is for arterial blood flow and especially to test the viability of the anastomosis in the palm of the hand that is fed from both the radial and ulnar arteries at the wrist. This test is to be done only if there appears to be a blood flow issue with the hand. Clues include: paleness in the hand, palpable coolness and/or weakness of any intrinsic musculature of the hand that develops quickly during use.

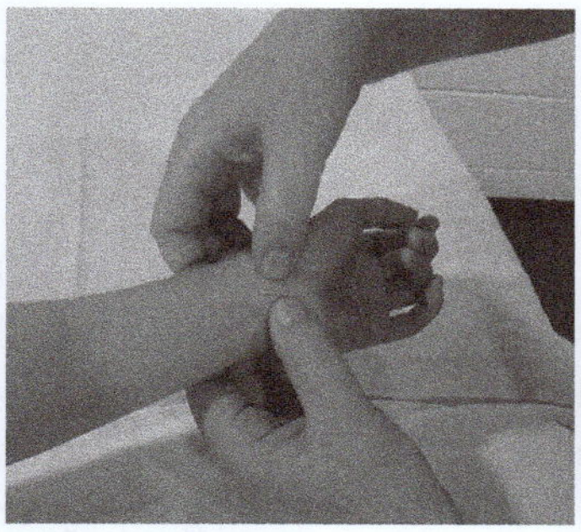

FIGURE 18.66 1. Landmarking arteries

Landmark the radial and ulnar arteries just proximal to the wrist.

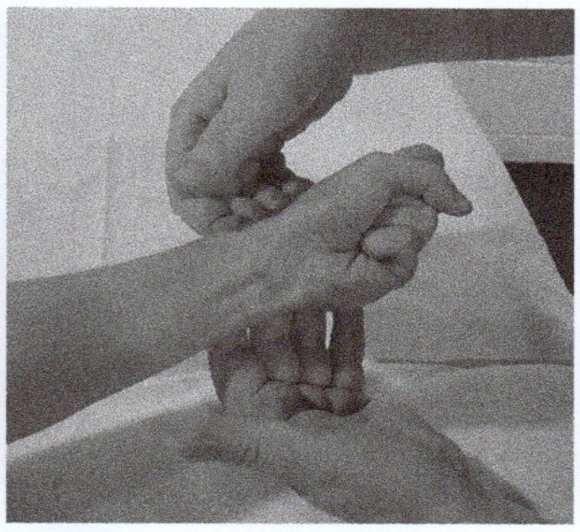

FIGURE 18.67 2. Pumping blood out of hand

The patient opens the hand and makes a fist, repeating this over and over several times as fast as they can.

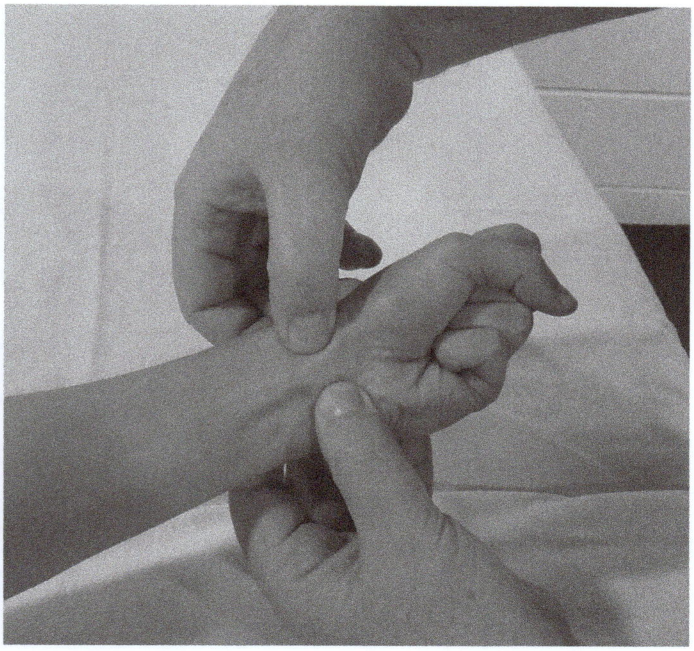

FIGURE 18.68 3. Compression of arteries

Ask the patient to make a tight fist while you quickly compress over the arteries. The patient then opens the hand. The palm of the hand and fingers should look pale.

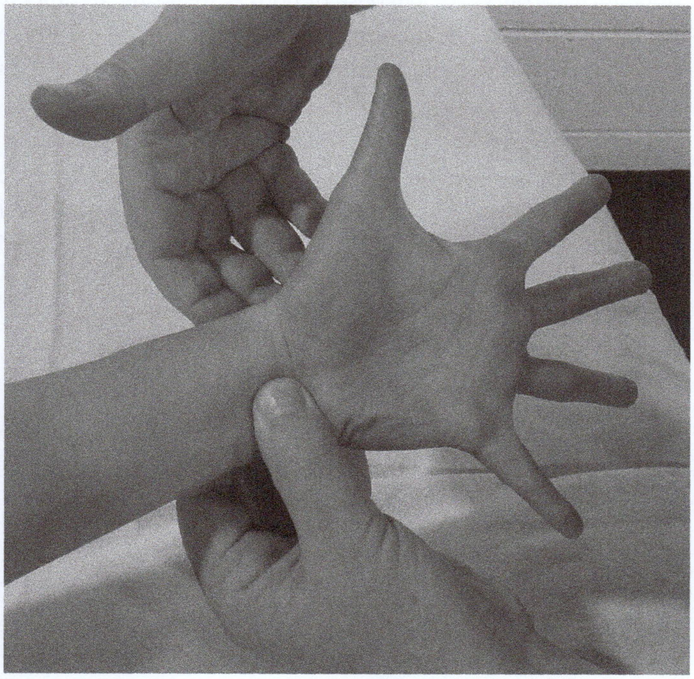

FIGURE 18.69 4. Testing ulnar artery

Release the ulnar artery while sustaining compression on the radial and watch the blood flow back into hand. Normally the blood will enter the hand on ulnar side but should then spread across palm and into the radial side of hand (i.e., anastomosis is functional). Positive sign: the hand flushes on the ulnar side but this does not move to the radial side, or does so very slowly.

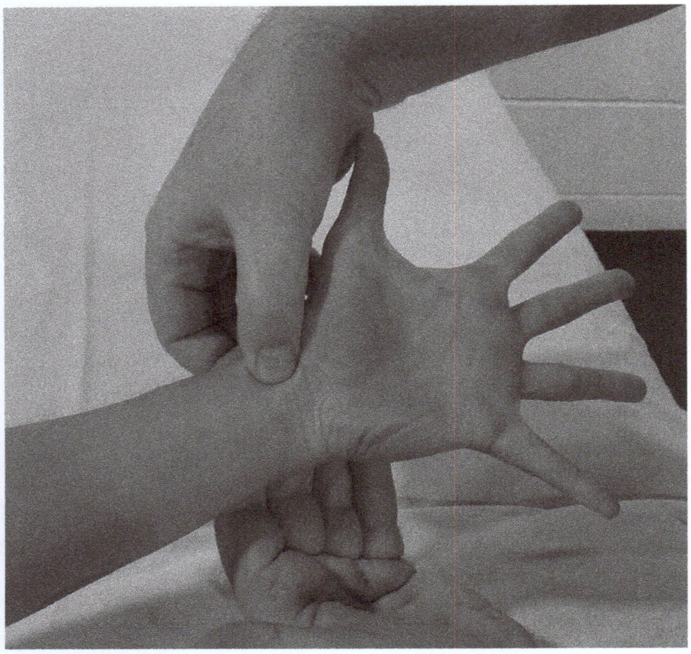

FIGURE 18.70 5. Testing radial artery

Repeat as above with pumping and compression but this time release the radial artery and make your observations. Blood should enter the hand on the radial side but should then spread across the palm and into the ulnar side of hand.

Each finger also has a collateral blood supply. Paleness, etc., may be restricted to just one finger. You can have the patient fully flex the finger several times and then keep it flexed while you pinch the ventral/palmar sides of the finger. Release first on one side then repeat and release the other side. Regardless of whether you find the site of local occlusion or not tell the patient to seek medical attention as soon as possible as tissue health could be quickly compromised.

If the patient has neurological signs and symptoms the cause of which has not been revealed by testing for compression syndromes of the appropriate peripheral nerve(s), then a more complete neurological testing needs to be done. If the neurological impairments appear to belong to peripheral nerves then we need to test for compression syndromes in the elbow and then in the thoracic outlet.

If the presentation of the neurological impairments is radicular (nerve root) in nature then the neurological tests of the cervical spine need to be done: deep tendon reflexes, myotomes, dermatomes; Valsalva's test, compression-decompression test, and Spurling's test bilaterally (see Chapter 14). Remember the vertebral artery test if warranted by case history or signs and symptoms.

Usually tests of the cervical spine that do not directly test neurological structures (such as facet joints or specific muscles) are skipped at this time. If, however, neither the neurological tests nor the thoracic outlet tests reveal the cause of the paresthesia you may wish to return to the cervical area to test those joints and muscles that may refer via trigger points or by other means into the area of the patient's chief complaint.

Chapter appendix A: Brief testing protocol of the hand and fingers

We present here some general or "quick" testing of the hand and fingers. These include AF-ROM, PR-ROM with O-P, and AR-ROM. Note that the thumb is not tested here. It really only requires testing if the patient's complaint specifically includes thumb pain or impairment or if there is difficulty grasping or manipulating objects in general. If this is the case proceed to specific testing of the thumb (see Chapter appendix B below, which also contains more specific testing of the fingers when warranted).

Quick range of motion testing of the hand and fingers: AF-ROM with O-P

Moving from AF-ROM to PR-ROM and applying overpressure (O-P) is done only when the patient reports no pain and no symptoms. This form of quick testing is the same as the testing done for rule outs. The purpose of both is the same: to quickly see if there is involvement or impairment to the fingers. If there is no problem a therapist can quickly move on to other tests rather than getting bogged down unnecessarily (and unproductively) in doing several specific or detailed testing of each finger and running through the special tests. Note, however, that we are going to include AR-ROM testing in our quick test protocol here. If these tests produce no pain or impairment more detailed testing is not needed.

Finger extension (Figures 18.71–18.73)

Finger flexion (Figures 18.74–18.77)

Test for flexion of the DIPs and PIPs of the fingers by having the patient make a half-fist. If the patient has full range then take hold of their hand and apply O-P.

If the testing of the DIPs and PIPs has been pain-free then have the patient make a full but soft fist (flexing the MCP joints as well) and observe if all the fingers function. A soft fist means that the patient is asked not to clench the fist but leave it somewhat loose.

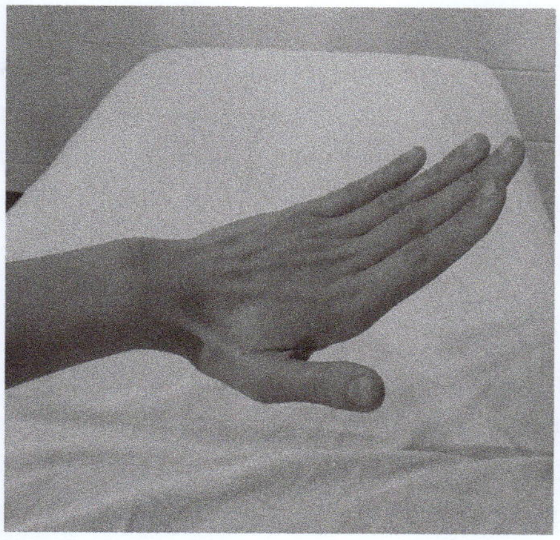

FIGURE 18.71 1. Finger extension 30–45°

For extension of the fingers have the patient place the palms of the hands on the table. Demonstrate and tell the patient to then extend the fingers as far as is possible while leaving the palms on the table.

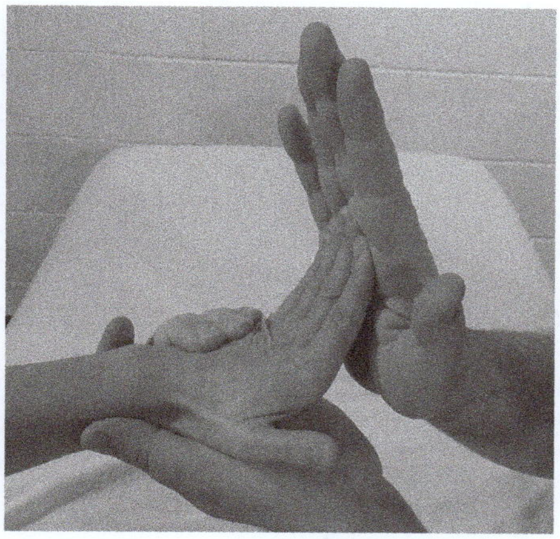

FIGURE 18.72 2. PR-ROM with O-P of extension

If the patient has no pain then while they are holding the fingers in extension slip the fingers of one hand under the patient's. Ask the patient to relax and while stabilizing over the wrist and metacarpals lift the fingers into end-range of extension. Ask the patient once again about pain or reproduction of symptoms associated with their impairment.

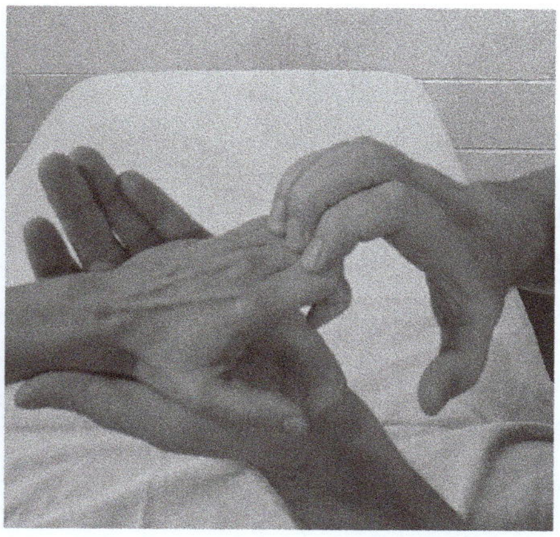

FIGURE 18.73 3. AR-ROM for general finger extension

Stabilizing across the patient's proximal phalanges (half-fist position), resist extension. The main movers are the extensor digitorum, extensor indicis, extensor digiti minimi.

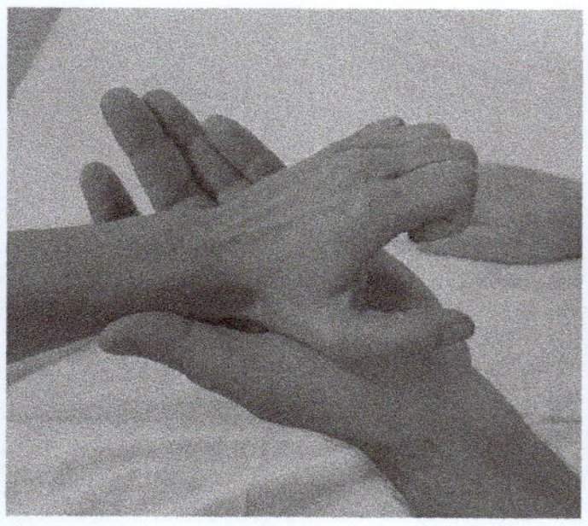

FIGURE 18.74 1. Half-fist for AF-ROM of DIPs and PIPs

Have the patient form a half-fist and observe if all DIPs and PIPs comply.

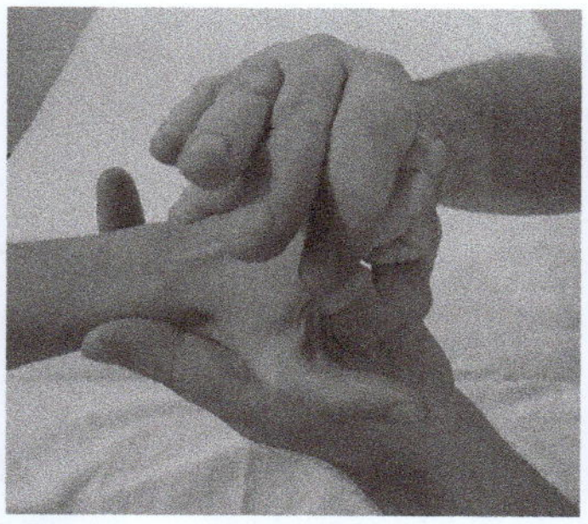

FIGURE 18.75 2. O-P of DIPs and PIPs

The therapist grasps the patient's half-fist and squeezes gently at first then with moderate pressure.

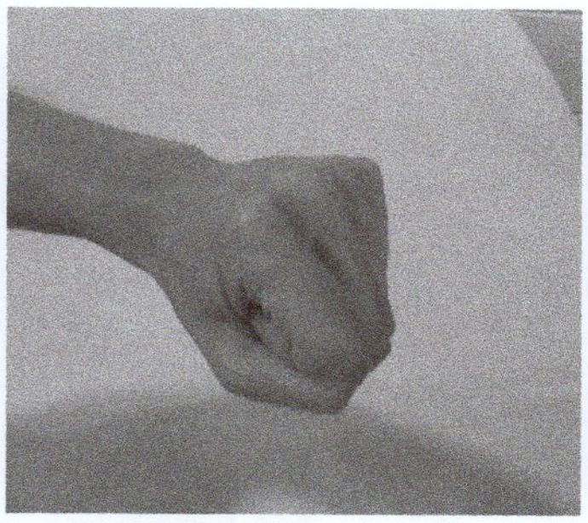

FIGURE 18.76 3. Patient makes soft fist

Observe if all joints participate.

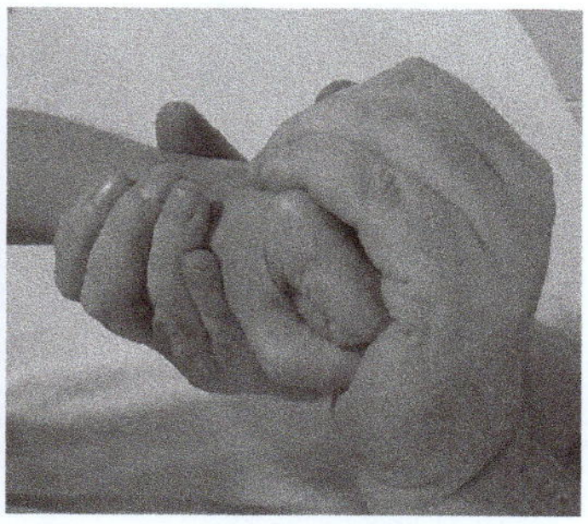

FIGURE 18.77 4. PR-ROM with O-P of MCP joints

Ask the patient to relax their fist. Wrap your hand around theirs and then apply O-P. Ask about pain.

AR-ROM testing (Figure 18.78)

If there is no pain and fingers appear to have moved normally have the patient clench their fist tightly.

Important observation

NOTE: *When the patient makes a tight/hard fist all the MCPs (the knuckles) lower and slightly rotate around the middle finger's metacarpal. The middle finger's MCP becomes more prominent. This implies normal functioning of the metacarpals themselves and the MCP joints specifically. The test also helps to confirm results of the half-fist testing of the phalangeal joints. Even if everything appears normal still ask about reproduction of their chief complaint.*

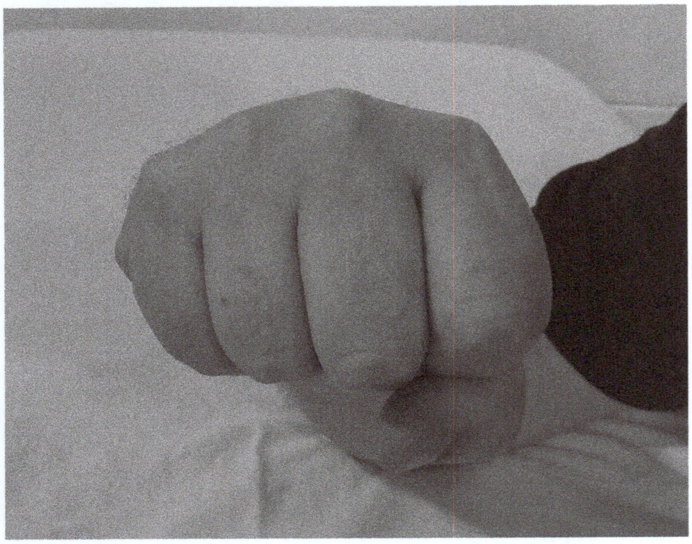

FIGURE 18.78
Observe if all joints function normally and if this causes any pain.

AR-ROM for general finger flexion (Figures 18.79–18.81)

If the patient cannot form a tight/hard fist with the characteristics just mentioned or they mention a sense of weakness then you may wish to perform an AR-ROM test that allows you to palpate the amount of strength that they are able to generate.

Testing adduction and abduction of the fingers (Figures 18.82–18.85)

NOTE: The four tests in Figures 18.82–18.85 could be done quicker if you do not mind breaking a few rules concerning ROM testing. They could be organized as follows:

- AF adduction – the patient adducts the fingers.
- AR abduction – while the patient still has their fingers adducted resist abduction.
- AF abduction – remove resistance and let the patient spread their fingers apart (abduct).
- AR adduction – interlace your fingers between the patient's and ask them to try to bring their fingers together (adduct).

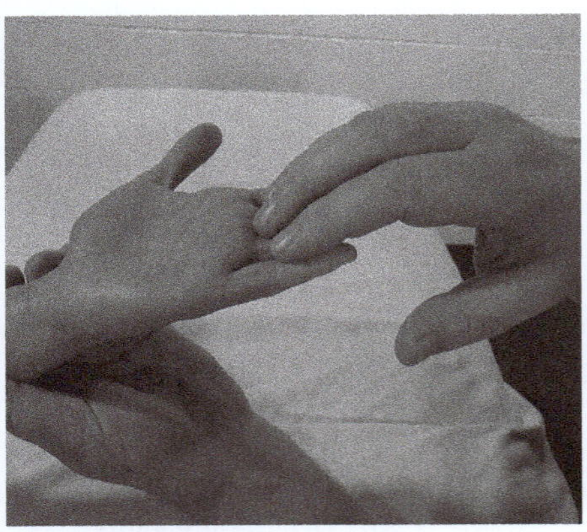

FIGURE 18.79 1. Positioning for test
The therapist places the fingers under the patient's fingers.

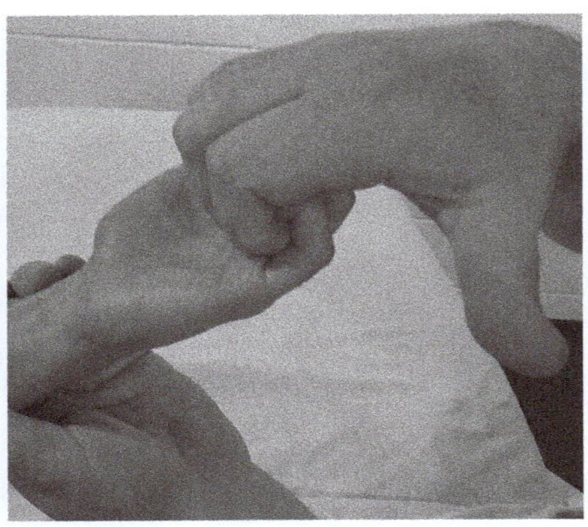

FIGURE 18.80 2. Patient grasps your fingers
The patient slowly makes a soft fist. Roll up your fingers inside the patient's fist.

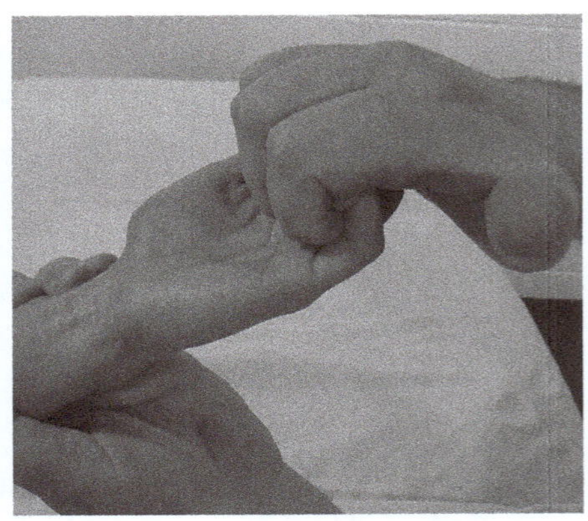

FIGURE 18.81 3. Resistance applied
Have the patient hold the position while you try to straighten out their fingers.

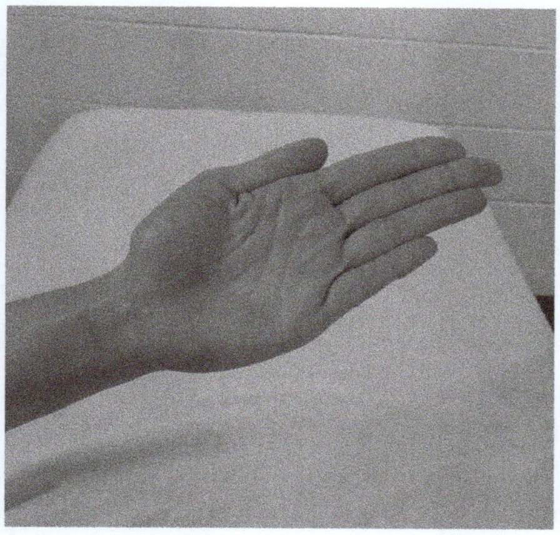

FIGURE 18.82 1. AF-ROM finger adduction to 0°

Have the patient adduct all their fingers.

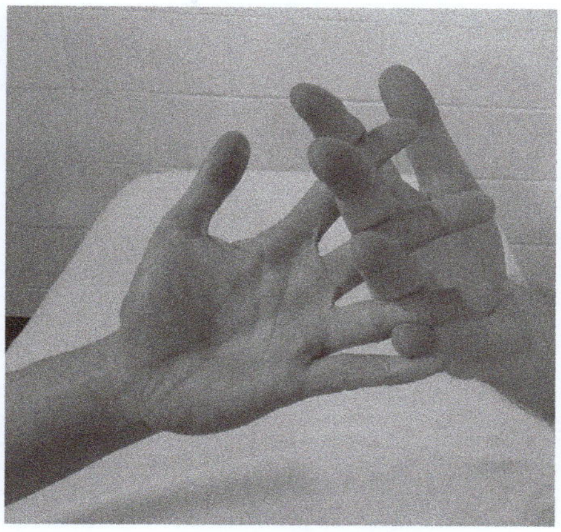

FIGURE 18.83 2. AR-ROM adduction

Ask the patient to spread their fingers apart then place the ends of your fingers between their abducted fingers. Ask the patient to bring (adduct) their fingers together and try to squeeze your fingers.

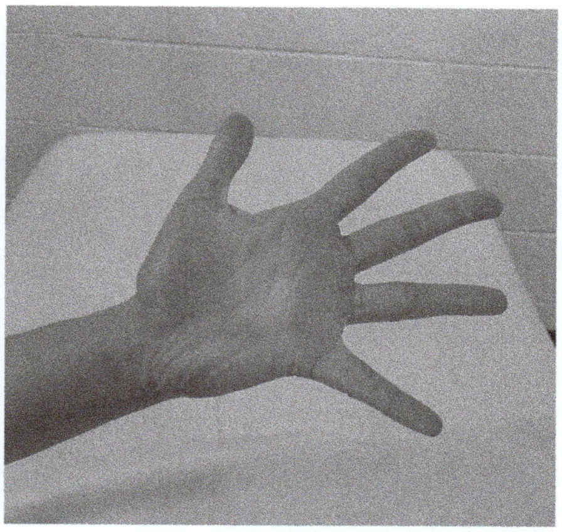

FIGURE 18.84 3. AF-ROM finger abduction 20–25°

Have the patient spread (abduct) their fingers fully.

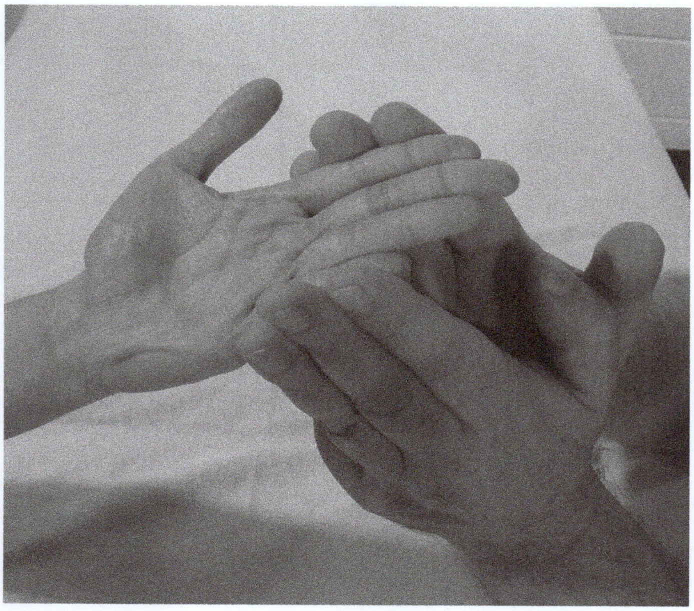

FIGURE 18.85 4. AR-ROM finger abduction

The patient places the hand on the table palm down and bring the fingers together. Resist at the outside of the index finger and little finger as you have the patient try to bring the fingers apart. Tell the patient to avoid cupping the fingers or palm of the hand as they try to abduct fingers to keep their hand and fingers flat.

Chapter appendix B: Testing of the fingers and thumb

AF-ROM of the thumb (Figures 18.86–18.90)

Examination of the fingers

Average joint range for finger flexion

- Distal interphalangeal joints: 80–90°
- Proximal interphalangeal joints: 100–115°
- Metacarpophalangeal joints: 85–90°

Only if there is abnormal movement (or lack of movement) and/or pain at any stage of quick testing do you need to do a more detailed testing of individual fingers and their structures.

AF-ROM testing (Figures 18.91, 18.92)

If pain or impairment occurred for the patient during general extension of the fingers then proceed to test individual extension of each finger separately.

With AF testing of the fingers have the patient supinate their forearm and flex one at a time while they hold the other fingers in neutral. Most people cannot flex their DIPs and PIPs separately. If need be the therapist can hold in neutral those fingers not being tested.

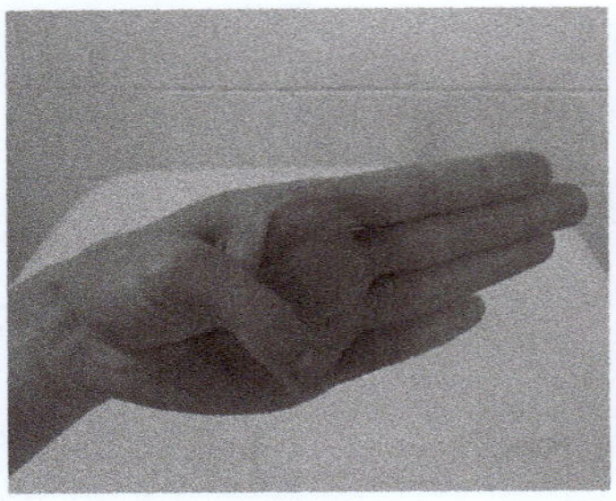

FIGURE 18.86 1. AF-ROM thumb flexion

The carpometacarpal joint is 45–50°; the metacarpophalangeal joint is 50–55°; the interphalangeal joint is 80–90°.

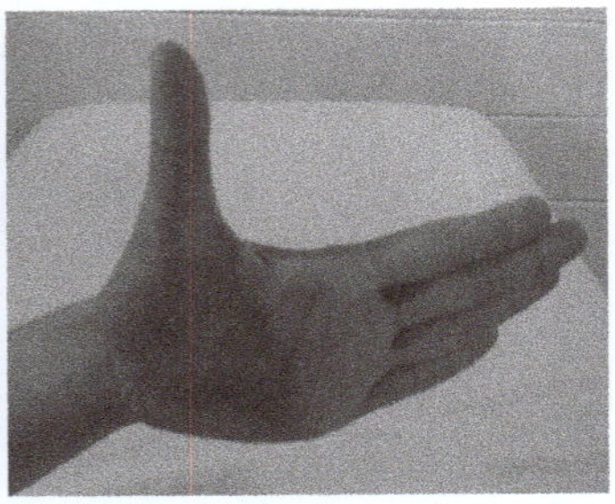

FIGURE 18.87 2. AF-ROM thumb extension

The interphalangeal joint 5–20°. As the hand is held in the anatomical position for its neutral position the motion of the metacarpophalangeal joint is 0°, since it has not really moved.

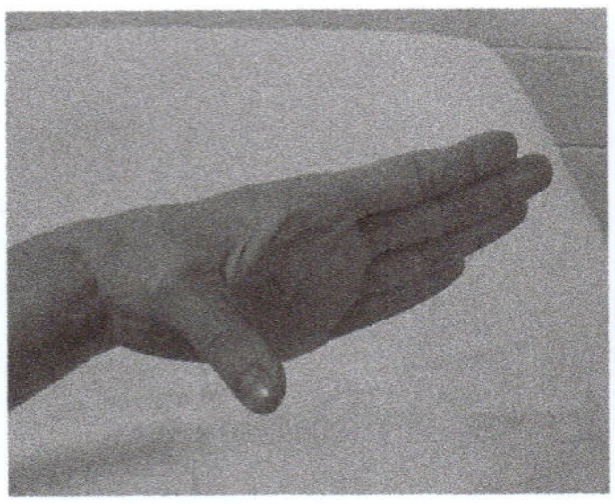

FIGURE 18.88 3. Thumb abduction

On average abduction is 60–70°.

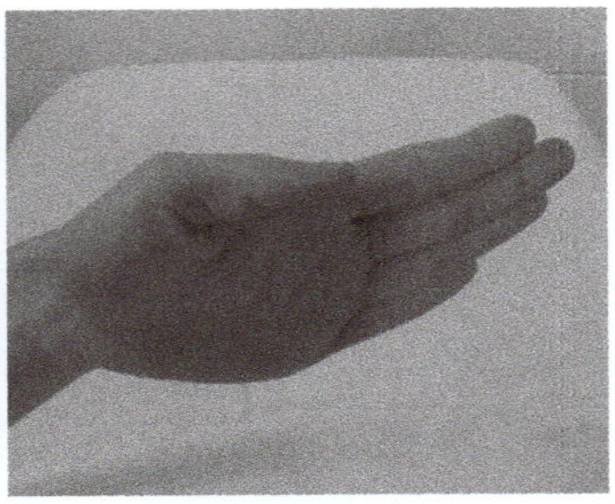

FIGURE 18.89 4. Thumb adduction

Adduction from neutral or resting position is 30°.

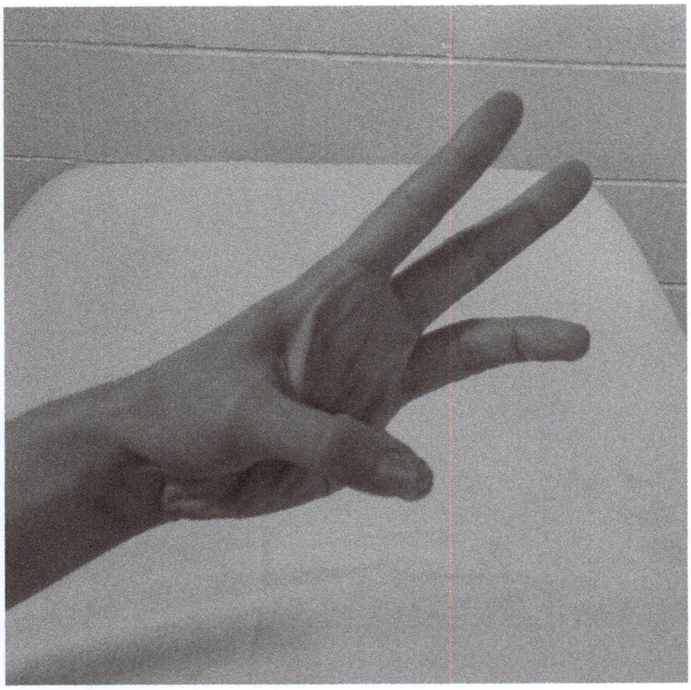

FIGURE 18.90 5. Opposition

An important AF-ROM test is the movement of the thumb and little finger "opposing." Ask the patient to touch the tip of the thumb to the tip of its opposing little finger.

Testing the lumbricals (Figure 18.93)

This test requires the MCP joints to flex while the DIPs and PIPs are extended.

Passive relaxed range of motion (PR-ROM) of the fingers

In this section, the therapist passively repeats all of the actions performed in the previous AF-ROM section. To perform the movements that follow take each finger into extension and flexion and if pain-free apply O-P. The following end-feels are the expected norm for each movement.

Finger extension: the end-feel is firm tissue stretch.

Finger flexion: the end-feel for all the joints may be either tissue approximation or tissue stretch. Finger abduction: the end-feel is tissue stretch.

Thumb movements: the end-feel of all movements is tissue stretch.

Joint play inspection of the fingers and thumb (Figures 18.94–18.96)

Now move your stabilizing hand to the proximal phalange and the mobilizing hand to the middle phalange. Repeat the movements as above. Then move on to the distal phalange – note that the movements here are usually proportionately smaller.

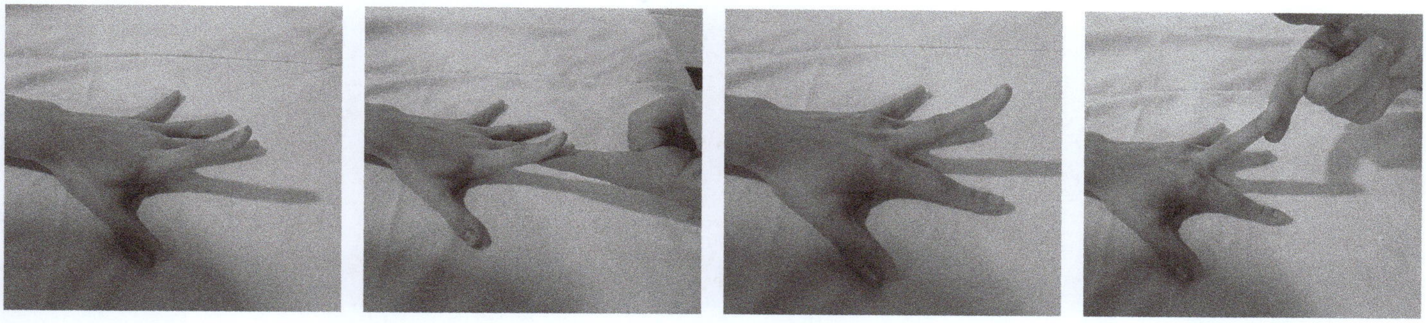

FIGURE 18.91A–D AF-ROM individual finger extension

Have the patient lift the index finger into extension. If pain-free apply O-P. Then have the patient place it back on the table. Repeat through the other three digits. With extension, some patients can only extend the index finger and little finger individually while the third and fourth fingers will lift together. Other patients can lift all fingers individually.

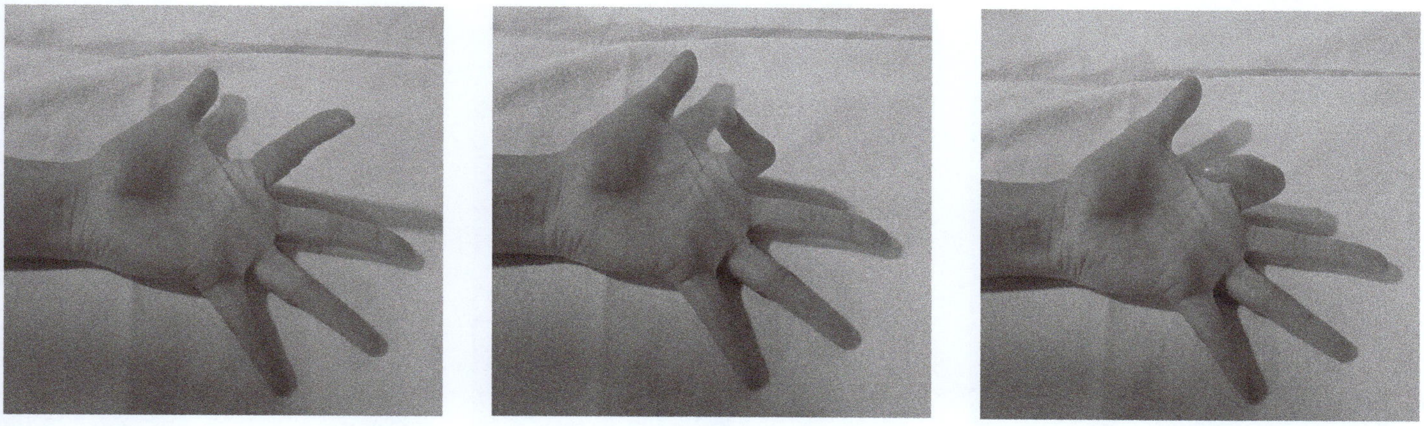

FIGURE 18.92A–C AF-ROM individual finger flexion

Do flexion of the DIPs and PIPs of each affected finger (and its bilateral, unaffected twin). Note loss and whether it is the PIP or DIP that is most affected, or some combination of the two.

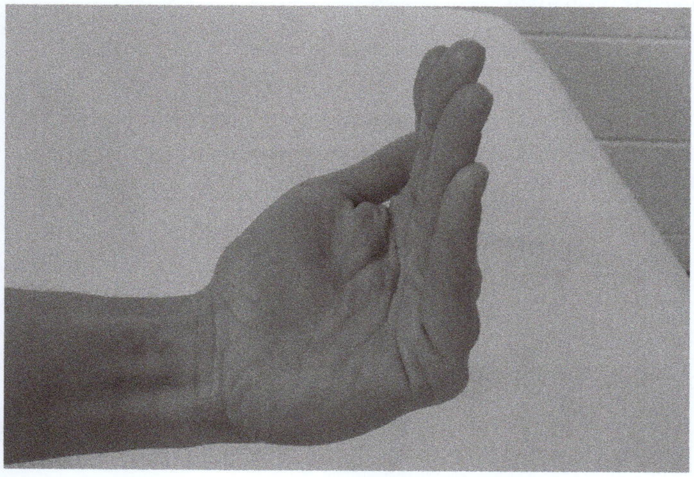

FIGURE 18.93 Testing the lumbricals

Keep the DIPs and PIPs of the fingers as straight as possible and try to have movement come primarily from the MCP alone. If the patient can do this action in each finger with little or no movement of the DIP and PIP joints then we know that extensor expansion for finger is working.

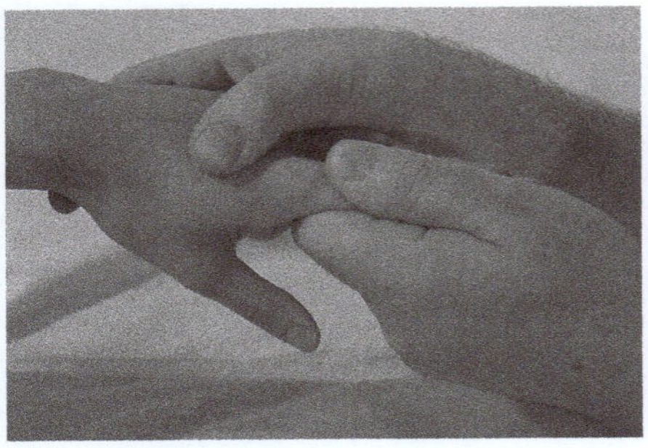

FIGURE 18.94 1. Decompress/ traction the joint

Grasp and stabilize the patient's metacarpal. Grasp the proximal phalange and apply a slight and gentle traction to create space between joints.

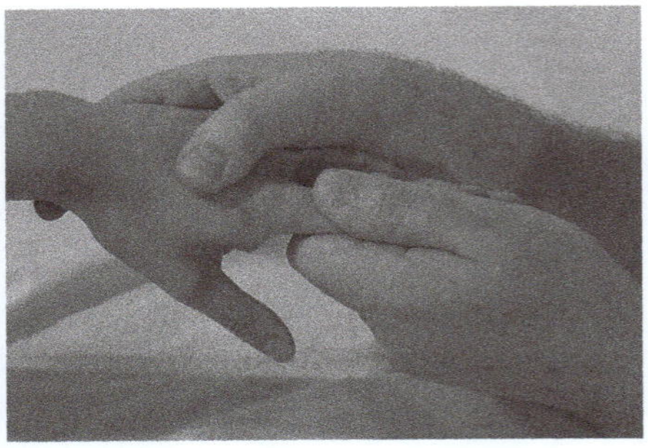

FIGURE 18.95 2. Dorsal-ventral glides

Lift the phalange dorsally, then ventrally to one side and then the other (always pausing for a moment in neutral between these movements).

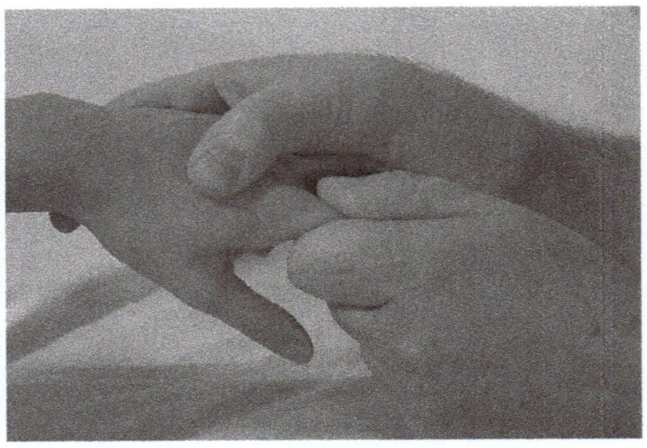

FIGURE 18.96 3. Rotation

Finish off with a gentle clockwise and then a counter-clockwise twist of the phalange. You are expecting minimal pain-free movement.

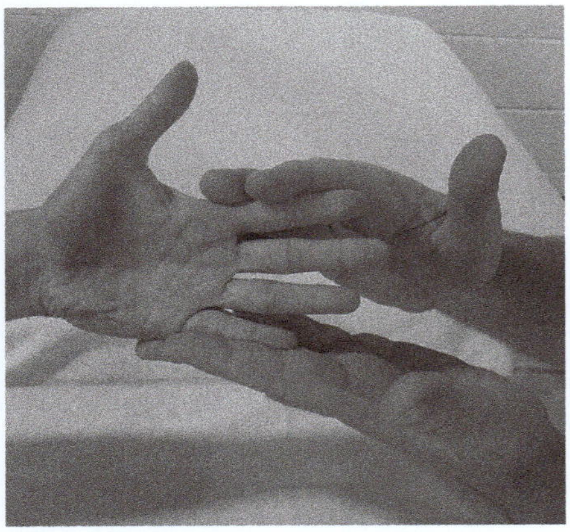

FIGURE 18.97 AR-ROM finger abduction

Grasp the patient's fingers, which are in neutral (i.e., just slightly apart), between your thumb and fingers in order to resist the patient's attempt to abduct the fingers. Prime movers are: dorsal interossei, abductor digiti minimi.

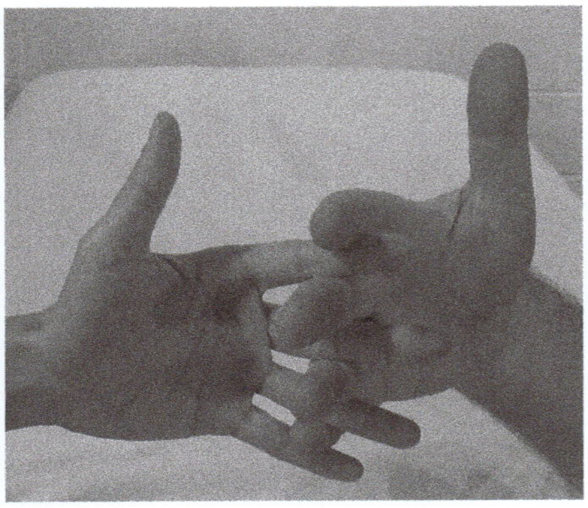

FIGURE 18.98 AR-ROM finger adduction

The therapist interlaces their fingers with the patient's and has the patient attempt to adduct all their fingers. The prime mover is the palmar interossei. If there is pain then do two fingers at a time to locate which of the palmar interossei is the source.

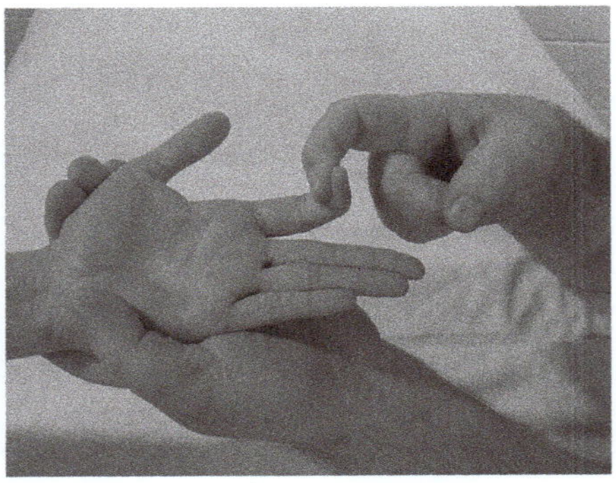

FIGURE 18.99 AR-ROM finger flexors

To test the fingers individually start resisting at the distal phalange of each finger and work across four fingers. Testing the flexor digitorum profundus. Then resist at the middle phalange of each finger and test them working your way across. Now testing the flexor digitorum superficialis.

Active resisted range of motion (AR-ROM) of the fingers (Figures 18.97–18.106)

NOTE: *The extensor expansion apparatus works as an "extensor longus muscle" for all the fingers but especially for the third and fourth digits. Palpatory experiment: resisting extension at the index finger or the little finger recruits those specific muscles and the strain can be felt down into the forearm. Resisting the third and fourth digits at their distal end creates strain felt in the metacarpal area as the lumbricals are doing most of the work.*

AR-ROM testing of the thumb

As anyone one who has injured their thumb knows not being able to use it makes you feel that your hand is of little use to you. The specific testing for the thumb is as in Figures 18.107–18.109.

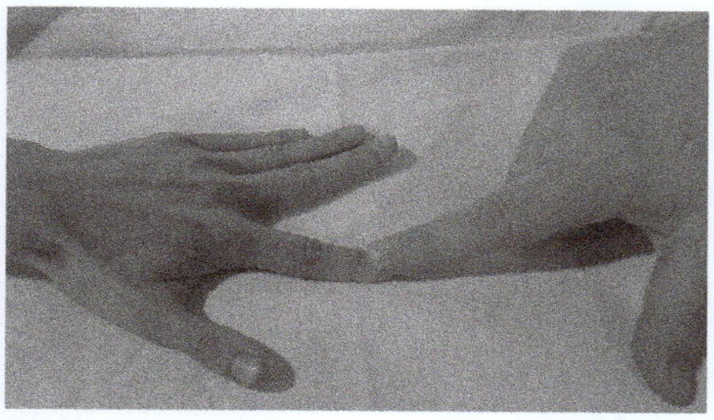

FIGURE 18.100 1. AR-ROM index finger extension

The patient's forearm and hand are resting on the table palm down.
To specifically test extensor indicis place your index finger over the distal phalange of the patient's index finger and have them try to extend just their index finger.

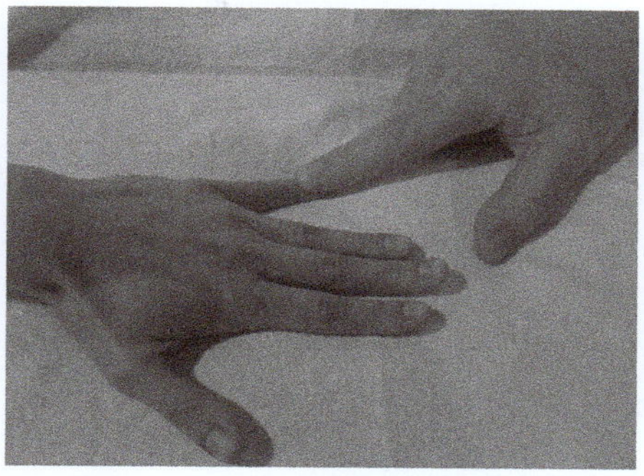

FIGURE 18.101 2. AR-ROM extensor digiti minimi

To specifically test the extensor digiti minimi place your index finger over the distal phalange of patient's little finger and have them try to extend this little finger.

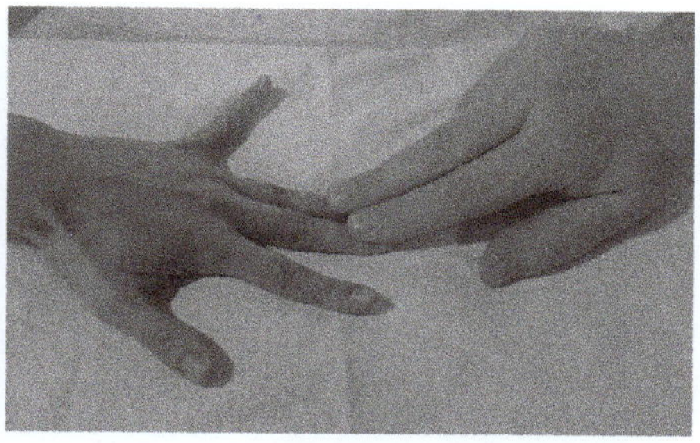

FIGURE 18.102 3. AR-ROM for third and fourth digit extension

Stabilizing across the patient's proximal phalanges (half-fist position), resist extension of the third and fourth digits. The main movers are extensor digitorum.

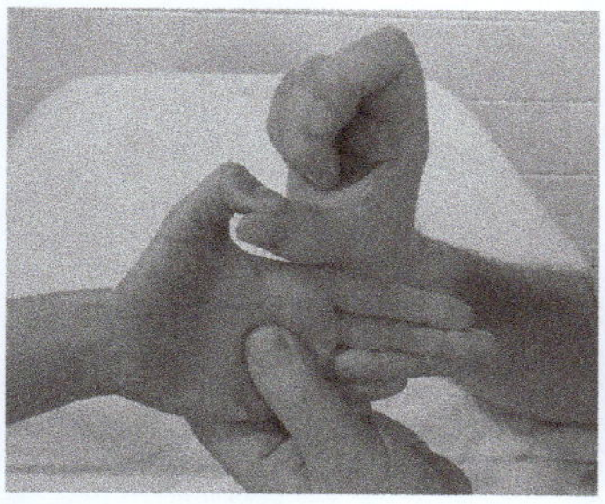

FIGURE 18.103 Flexion at interphalangeal joint

Resist at the most distal phalange. Tests flexor pollicis longus.

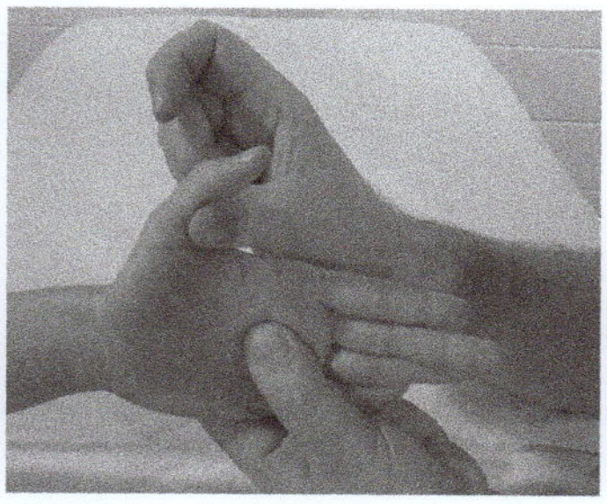

FIGURE 18.104 Flexion at metacarpal-phalangeal joint

Resist at the first phalange. Tests flexor pollicis brevis.

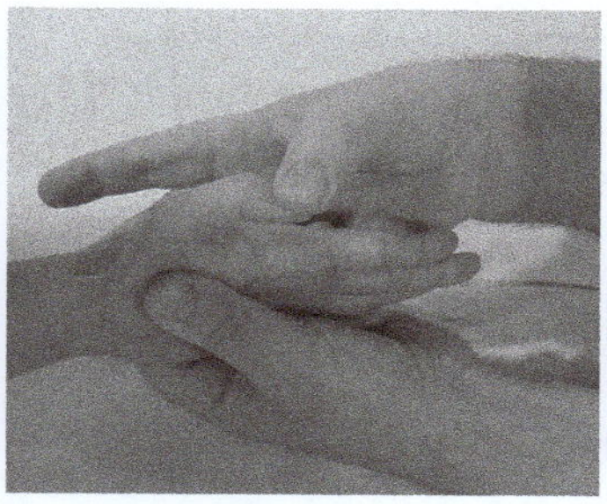

FIGURE 18.105 Extension at interphalangeal joint

Resist at the most distal phalange. Tests extensor pollicis longus.

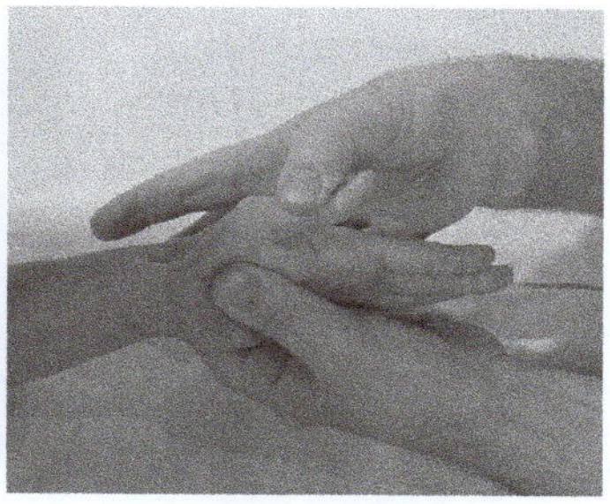

FIGURE 18.106 Extension at metacarpal-phalangeal joint

Resist at the second phalange. Tests extensor pollicis brevis.

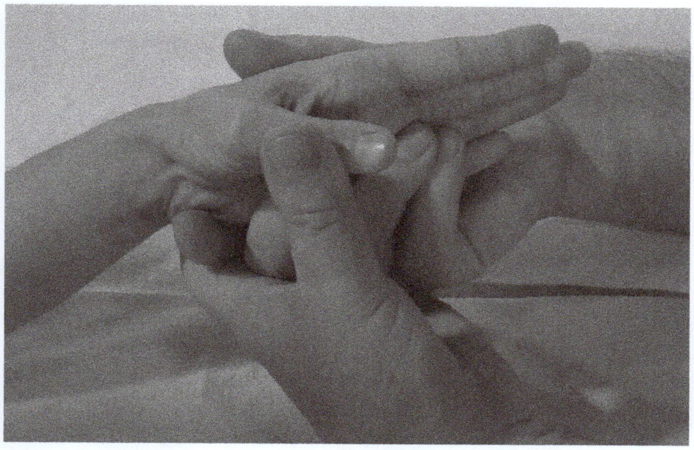

FIGURE 18.107 Abduction of thumb

Resist at the most distal phalange; testing abductor pollicis longus and brevis.

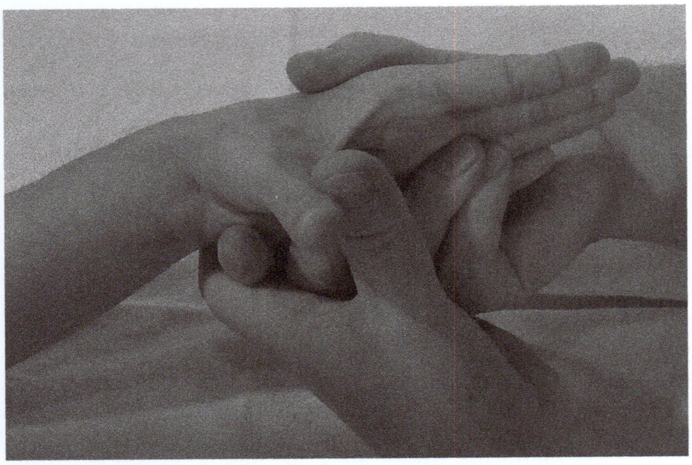

FIGURE 18.108 Adduction of thumb

Resist below the second phalange or place a piece of paper between the index finger and thumb and tell the patient not to let you pull the paper out from between them. Prime mover is adductor pollicis.

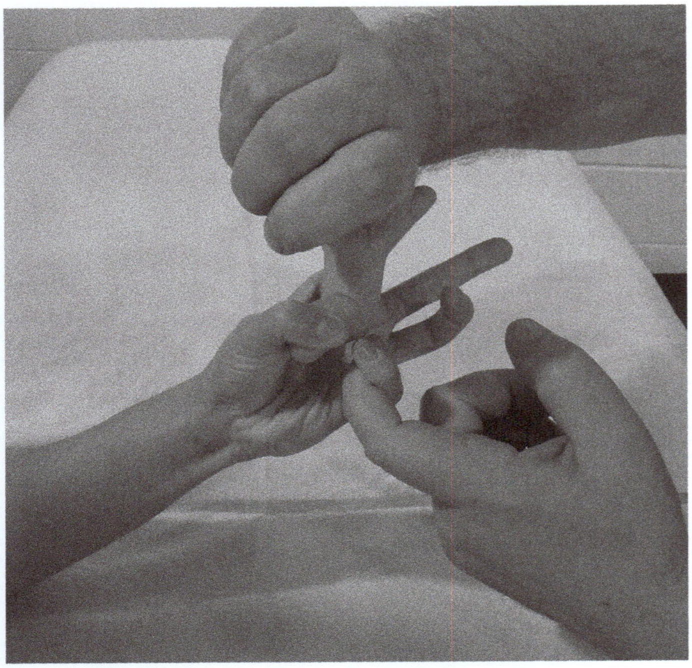

FIGURE 18.109 Opposition of thumb and little finger

Have the patient oppose the thumb and fifth digit. The therapist hooks a finger around their opposed fingertips and tries to pull through their fingers. Or have the patient pinch a piece of paper between the tips of the thumb and index finger. If the patient must extend DIP joints of both thumb and index finger in order to resist and can only pinch paper with the finger pads then this can be a potential neurological sign. The prime movers are opponens pollicis, opponens digiti minimi.

Appendices

The appendices, as well as presenting factual information in tabular format, are also meant to assist the student to consider the nerves, joints, and muscles that could be involved in a musculoskeletal impairment. For example, in the muscle charts there is a list of synergists that may be assisting a specific muscle to perform its function. This list can inform the choice of other muscles to test when a specific muscle is injured. Hence, though it could appear that the patient's biceps brachii is clearly injured, we would need to also look to the brachialis, brachioradialis, supinator, anterior deltoid, pectoralis major, and coracobrachialis.

While much of what is presented is basic information that the student or therapist may find helpful as purely anatomical (structural) or physiological (functional), the reader is also encouraged to consider the relationships between what is listed, and explore others that may not be listed. As discussed in Part I of this manual, assessment by its very nature makes one seek the specific; however, the best use of that information is when the therapist steps back and sees first, a more regional view and then, a global view. Even when seeking detailed knowledge, we must never lose sight of the whole patient.

Bear in mind too that these lists, though correct to the best of the author's knowledge, do not cover every possibility – there may well be some omissions, oversimplifications, controversial/disputed information, or even errors, so approach them as you should approach all information, with your critical faculties alert.

APPENDIX 1 Muscle chart					
			CERVICAL		
MUSCLE	**ORIGIN**	**INSERTION**	**INNERVATION**	**ACTION**	**SYNERGIST**
Upper trapezius	External occipital protuberence Ligamentum nuchae of C7–T12 SPs	Lateral clavicle Acromion	Accessory nerve CN XI (Cranial and C1–4)	Elevation, lateral rotation of scapula Extension and contralateral rotation of head	Levator scapula, lower trapezius, serratus anterior
Levator scapula	C1–4 TVPs	Vertebral border of scapula from superior angle to root of spine	Dorsal scapular nerve (C4, 5)	Elevation, medial rotation of scapula	Upper trapezius, rhomboids, pectoralis minor
Sternocleido-mastoid	Manubrium of sternum, medial clavicle	Mastoid process	Accessory nerve CN XI (Cranial and C1–3)	Bilaterally: flexion of neck Unilaterally: lateral flexion of neck to same side, rotation of head to opposite side	Scalenes, splenius capitis/cervicis, intertransversarii
Anterior scalene **Middle scalene** **Posterior scalene**	TVPs of C3–6 TVPs of C2–7 TVPs of C4–6	First rib Second rib	C3–8	Bilaterally: raise first 2 ribs during forced inspiration or assist neck flexion Unilaterally: assist in lateral flexion of neck to same side	Sternocleidomastoid, intercostals, splenius capitis/cervicis, intertransversarii
Suprahyoids	Mandible, posterior digastric-mastoid process of temporal bone	Hyoid bone	Cranial nerves V, VII, XII, C1, 2	Raises hyoid bone in swallowing or opens the jaw	Platysma
Infrahyoids	Thyroid cartilage, manubrium of sternum, superior border of scapula	Hyoid bone	C1–3	Stabilizes hyoid bone in swallowing by pulling it downward	
Rectus capitis anterior	TVP and anterior body of C1 (atlas)	Inferior basilar part of occipital bone	C1, 2	Flexes head (occipital-atlas)	Superior portion of longus capitis
Longus colli	Anterior tubercles of some cervical and thoracic TVPs and vertebral bodies	Anterior tubercles of some cervical and thoracic TVPs and vertebral bodies	C2–7	Flexes cervical spine	Sternocleidomastoid, scalenes, longus capitis
Splenius capitis **Splenius cervicis**	Ligamentum nuchae, SPs of C7–T3 T3–6	Mastoid process of temporal and occipital bone TVPs of C1–3	Dorsal rami of lower cervical nerves	Bilaterally: extension of neck Unilaterally: lateral flexion and rotation of head to same side	Iliocostalis, longissimus, spinalis, sternocleidomastoid, scalenes, semispinalis, rotators, interspinalis, intertransversarii, multifidus
Longissimus **Spinalis**	Thoracolumbar aponeurosis, lumbar and thoracic TVPs Ligamentum nuchae, cervical and thoracic SPs	Cervical and thoracic TVPs, mastoid process Cervical and thoracic SPs, occipital bone	Dorsal rami of adja-cent spinal nerves	Bilaterally: extension of spine Unilaterally: lateral flexion of spine	Semispinalis, multifidus, rotators, interspinalis, intertransversarii, internal/external oblique, splenius capitis/cervicis

Semispinalis **Multifidus**	Cervical and thoracic TVPs Sacrum, posterior superior iliac spine, TVPs all vertebrae	Cervical and thoracic TVPs, (spans 3–6 vertebrae), occipital bone SPs of all vertebrae, inserting 2–4 vertebrae above origin	Dorsal rami of adjacent spinal nerves	Bilaterally: extension of spine Unilaterally: rotation to opposite side	Iliocostalis, longissimus, spinalis, splenius capitis/cervicis, rotators, interspinalis
Rotatores **Interspinales**	TVPs of all vertebrae SPs of cervical, lumbar and T1–2, T11–12 vertebrae	SPs of all vertebrae, inserting on vertebra directly above origin	Dorsal rami of adjacent spinal nerves	Extension of spine, rotation to opposite side Extension of spine	Iliocostalis, spinalis, longissimus, semispinalis, multifidus, interspinalis Iliocostalis, longissimus, spinalis, semispinalis, multifidus
Intertransversarii	TVPs of cervical, lumbar and T1–12 vertebrae	TVPs directly above origin	Dorsal rami of ventral and dorsal spinal nerves	Lateral flexion of spine	Iliocostalis, longissimus, spinalis, splenius capitis/cervicis, quadratus lumborum
			SHOULDER		
MUSCLE	**ORIGIN**	**INSERTION**	**INNERVATION**	**ACTION**	**SYNERGISTS**
Upper trapezius **Middle trapezius** **Lower trapezius**	External occipital protuberence Ligamentum nuchae of C7–T12 SPs	Lateral clavicle Acromion Spine of scapula Root of spine of scapula	Accessory nerve CN XI (Cranial and C1–4)	Elevation, lateral rotation of scapula Extension and contralateral rotation of head Retraction of scapula Depression, lateral rotation of scapula	Levator scapula, lower trapezius, serratus anterior Rhomboid Pectoralis minor, upper trapezius, serratus anterior
Latissimus dorsi	Thoracolumbar aponeuerosis, lower 6 T/S SPs, sacrum, iliac crest, lower 3–4 ribs Inferior angle of scapula	Bicipital groove of humerus	Thoracodorsal nerve (C6, 7, 8)	Extension, medial rotation, adduction of humerus	Teres major/minor, triceps, subscapularis, pectoralis major/ minor, infraspinatus, coracobrachialis
Teres major	Inferior angle of scapula	Medial lip of bicipital groove of humerus	Lower subscapular nerve (C5, 6, 7)	Extension, medial rotation, adduction of humerus	Latissimus dorsi, posterior deltoid, infraspinatus, teres minor, triceps, pectoralis major, coracobrachialis
Teres minor	Upper axillary border of scapula	Greater tubercle of humerus	Axillary nerve (C5, 6)	Lateral rotation, extension of humerus	Latissimus dorsi, teres major, posterior deltoid, infraspinatus, triceps, pectoralis major
Levator scapula	C1–4 TVPs	Vertebral border of scapula from superior angle to root of spine	Dorsal scapular nerve (C4, 5)	Elevation, medial rotation of scapula	Upper trapezius, rhomboids, pectoralis minor

APPENDIX 1 Muscle chart *continued*

SHOULDER					
MUSCLE	**ORIGIN**	**INSERTION**	**INNERVATION**	**ACTION**	**SYNERGISTS**
Rhomboid major	T2–5 SPs	Medial border of scapula from root of spine to inferior angle	Dorsal scapular nerve (C4, 5)	Retraction, medial rotation of scapula	Middle trapezius, levator scapula, pectoralis minor
Rhomboid minor	C7-T1 SPs	Root of spine of scapula			
Anterior deltoid	Lateral third of clavicle	Deltoid tuberosity	Axillary nerve (C5, 6)	Flexion, horizontal adduction, medial rotation of humerus	Pectoralis major, coracobrachialis, biceps brachii, subscapularis, teres major, latissimus dorsi
Middle deltoid	Lateral acromion			Abduction of humerus to 90°	Supraspinatus
Posterior deltoid	Spine of scapula			Extension, horizontal abduction, lateral rotation of humerus	Infraspinatus, teres major/minor, latissimus dorsi, triceps, pectoralis minor
Coracobrachialis	Coracoid process of scapula	Middle ⅓ of medial surface of humeral shaft	Musculocutaneous nerve (C6, 7)	Flexion, adduction of humerus	Anterior deltoid, pectoralis major, biceps brachii, teres major, latissimus dorsi
Supraspinatus	Supraspinous fossa of scapula	Greater tubercle of humerus	Suprascapular nerve (C5, 6)	Abduction of humerus Stabilization of head of humerus	Middle deltoid
Infraspinatus	Infraspinous fossa of scapula			Lateral rotation, extension of humerus	Teres major/minor, posterior deltoid, latissimus dorsi, triceps, pectoralis minor
Subscapularis	Subscapular fossa of scapula	Lesser tubercle of humerus	Upper and lower subscapular nerve (C5, 6, 7)	Medial rotation of humerus	Anterior deltoid, pectoralis major, teres major, latissimus dorsi
Pectoralis major	Clavicular head: medial ½ of clavicle Sternal head: sternum, cartilages of upper 6 ribs	Lateral lip of bicipital groove of humerus	Clavicular head: lateral pectoral nerve (C5, 6, 7) Sternal head: medial pectoral nerve (C6, 7, 8, T1)	Adduction, horizontal adduction, medial rotation of humerus Clavicular head: flexion of humerus Sternal head: extension of humerus from flexed position	Anterior deltoid, subscapularis, teres major/minor, latissimus dorsi, coracobrachialis, triceps, infraspinatus
Pectoralis minor	Anterior surface of ribs 3–5 near costal cartilage	Coracoid process of scapula	Medial pectoral nerve (C7, 8)	Protraction, depression, medial rotation of scapula	Serratus anterior, lower trapezius, rhomboids, levator scapula
Biceps brachii	Short head: coracoid process Long head: supraglenoid tubercle of scapula	Tuberosity of radius	Musculocutaneous nerve (C5, 6,)	Flexion of elbow, supination of forearm, flexion of humerus	Brachialis, brachioradialis, supinator, anterior deltoid, pectoralis major, coracobrachialis

Triceps brachii	Long head: infraglenoid tubercle of scapula Lateral head: posterior humerus above spiral groove Medial head: posterior humerus below spiral groove	Olecranon process of ulna	Radial nerve (C6–T1)	Extension of elbow Long head: extension of humerus	Anconeus, latissimus dorsi, teres major/minor, posterior deltoid, infraspinatus, pectoralis major
			ELBOW		
MUSCLES	**ORIGIN**	**INSERTION**	**INNERVATION**	**ACTION**	**SYNERGISTS**
Biceps brachii	Short head: coracoid process Long head: supraglenoid tubercle of scapula	Tuberosity of radius	Musculocutaneous nerve (C5, 6)	Flexion of elbow, supination of forearm, flexion of humerus	Brachialis, brachioradialis, supinator, anterior deltoid, pectoralis major, coracobrachialis
Brachialis	Lower ½ of anterior shaft of humerus	Tuberosity and coronoid process of ulna	Musculocutaneous nerve (C5, 6)	Flexion of elbow	Biceps brachii, brachioradialis
Triceps brachii	Long head: infraglenoid tubercle of scapula Lateral head: posterior humerus above spiral groove Medial head: posterior humerus below spiral groove	Olecranon process of ulna	Radial nerve (C6–T1)	Extension of elbow Long head: extension of humerus	Anconeus, latissimus dorsi, teres major/minor, posterior deltoid, infraspinatus, pectoralis major
Anconeus	Lateral epicondyle of humerus	Olecranon process of upper posterior surface of ulna	Radial nerve (C6–T1)	Extension of elbow	Triceps brachii
Brachioradialis	Lateral supracondylar ridge of humerus	Styloid process of radius	Radial nerve (C6–T1)	Flexion of elbow in neutral position	Biceps brachii, brachialis
Supinator	Lateral epicondyle of humerus, annular and radial collateral ligaments, proximal ulna	Between anterior and posterior oblique lines of proximal radius on anterior surface	Radial nerve (C6–T1)	Supination of forearm	Biceps brachii
Pronator teres	Humeral head: medial epicondyle Ulnar head: coronoid process	Middle lateral shaft of radius	Median nerve (C6, 7)	Pronation of forearm, assists elbow flexion	Pronator quadratus
Pronator quadratus	Distal ¼ of anterior ulna	Distal ¼ of anterior radius	Median nerve (C6, 7)	Pronates forearm	Pronator teres
			WRIST		
MUSCLES	**ORIGIN**	**INSERTION**	**INNERVATION**	**ACTION**	**SYNERGISTS**
Extensor carpi radialis longus	Lateral supracondylar ridge, lateral epicondyle of humerus	Base of 2nd metacarpal	Radial nerve (C6, 7, 8)	Extension, radial deviation of wrist	Extensor carpi radialis brevis, extensor carpi ulnaris, flexor carpi radialis

APPENDIX 1 Muscle chart *continued*

WRIST					
MUSCLE	**ORIGIN**	**INSERTION**	**INNERVATION**	**ACTION**	**SYNERGISTS**
Extensor carpi radialis brevis	Lateral epicondyle of humerus	Base of 3rd metacarpal	Radial nerve	Extension of wrist	Extensor carpi radialis longus, extensor carpi ulnaris
Extensor carpi ulnaris	Lateral epicondyle of humerus, posterior proximal ulna	Base of 5th metacarpal	Radial nerve	Extension, ulnar deviation of wrist	Extensor carpi radialis longus/brevis, flexor carpi ulnaris
Supinator	Lateral epicondyle of humerus, annular and radial collateral ligaments, proximal ulna	Between anterior and posterior oblique lines of proximal radius on anterior surface	Radial nerve	Supination of forearm	Biceps brachii
Pronator teres	Humeral head: medial epicondyle Ulnar head: coronoid process	Middle lateral shaft of radius	Median nerve (C7, 8, T1)	Pronation of forearm, assists elbow flexion	Pronator quadratus
Pronator quadratus	Distal ¼ of anterior ulna	Distal ¼ of anterior radius	Median nerve	Pronates forearm	Pronator teres
Flexor carpi ulnaris	Humeral head: medial epicondyle of humerus Ulnar head: proximal posterior ulna and olecranon process	Pisiform, hamate, and base of 5th metacarpal	Ulnar nerve (C7, 8,T1)	Flexion, ulnar deviation of wrist	Flexor carpi ulnaris, palmaris longus, extensor carpi ulnaris
Palmaris longus	Medial epicondyle of humerus	Palmar aponeurosis and flexor retinaculum	Median nerve (C7, 8, T1)	Assists flexion of wrist	Flexor carpi radialis/ ulnaris
Flexor carpi radialis	Medial epicondyle of humerus	Bases of 2nd and 3rd metacarpals	Median nerve	Flexion, radial deviation of wrist	Flexor carpi ulnaris, palmaris longus, extensor carpi radialis longus
HAND/FINGERS					
MUSCLE	**ORIGIN**	**INSERTION**	**INNERVATION**	**ACTION**	**SYNERGISTS**
Extensor digitorum	Lateral epicondyle of humerus	Base of middle phalanges of 4 fingers on dorsal surface	Radial nerve (C6, 7, 8)	Extension of proximal phalanges of 4 fingers of MCP joints	Extensor indicis
Extensor digiti minimi	Lateral epicondyle of humerus	Extensor expansion of little finger	Radial nerve	Extension of proximal phalanx of little finger at MCP joint	
Extensor indicis	Posterior ulna and interosseous membrane	Extensor expansion of index finger	Radial nerve	Extension of proximal phalanx of index finger at MCP joint	Extensor digitorum
Abductor pollicis longus	Posterior radius, ulna and interosseous membrane	Base of 1st metacarpal	Radial nerve	Abduction of 1st meta-carpal of thumb of CM joint	Abductor pollicis brevis

Extensor pollicis brevis	Posterior radius, interosseous membrane	Base of proximal phalanx of thumb	Radial nerve	Extension of proximal phalanx of thumb at MCP joint	
Extensor pollicis longus	Posterior ulna and interosseous membrane	Base of distal phalanx of thumb	Radial nerve	Extension of distal phalanx of thumb at IP joint	
Flexor digitorum superficialis	Humeral head: medial epicondyle of humerus Ulnar head: coronoid process Radial head: anterior oblique line of radius	Sides of shafts of middle phalanges of 4 fingers	Median nerve	Flexion of middle phalanges of 4 fingers at PIP joints	
Flexor digitorum profundus	Middle of anterior ulna and interosseous membrane	Bases of distal phalanges of 4 fingers	Median (C6, 7) and ulnar nerve (C8, T1)	Flexion of distal phalanges of 4 fingers at DIP joints	
Flexor pollicis longus	Middle of anterior radius and interosseous membrane	Distal phalanx of thumb	Median nerve	Flexion of distal phalanx of thumb at IP joint	
Abductor pollicis brevis	Flexor retinaculum, trapezium and scaphoid	Base of proximal phalanx of thumb on radial side	Median nerve	Abduction of 1st metacarpal of thumb at CM joint	Abductor pollicis longus
Adductor pollicis	Transverse head: shaft of 3rd metacarpal Oblique head: base of 2nd and 3rd metacarpals and capitate	Base of proximal phalanx of thumb on medial side	Ulnar nerve	Adduction of 1st metacarpal of thumb at CM joint	
Flexor pollicis brevis	Superficial head: flexor retinaculum and trapezium Deep head: trapezoid and capitate	Base of proximal phalanx of thumb on radial side	Median (C6, 7) and ulnar nerve (C8, T1)	Flexion of proximal phalanx of thumb at MCP joint	
Flexor digiti minimi	Flexor retinaculum and hook of hamate	Base of proximal phalanx of little finger	Ulnar nerve	Flexion of proximal phalanx of little finger at MCP joint	Lumbricals, dorsal/ palmar interossei
Opponens pollicis	Flexor retinaculum and trapezium	Lateral shaft of 1st metacarpal	Median nerve	Opposition of thumb	
Opponens digiti minimi	Flexor retinaculum and hook of hamate	Ulnar border of 5th metacarpal	Ulnar nerve	Opposition of little finger	
Abductor digiti minimi	Pisiform	Base of proximal phalanx of little finger on ulnar side	Ulnar nerve	Abduction of proximal phalanx of little finger at MCP joint	Dorsal interossei
Dorsal interossei (4)	Each interosseous had 2 heads arising from adjacent dorsal surfaces of metacarpals	Base of proximal phalanges to extensor expansion of 2–4 fingers	Ulnar nerve	Abduction of 2nd, abduction and adduction of 3rd and 4th fingers	Abductor digiti minimi, palmar interossei, adductor pollicis

APPENDIX 1 Muscle chart *continued*

HAND/FINGERS					
MUSCLE	**ORIGIN**	**INSERTION**	**INNERVATION**	**ACTION**	**SYNERGISTS**
Palmar interossei (3)	Shaft of 2nd, 4th and 5th metacarpals on palmar surface	Base of proximal phalanges to extensor expansion of 2nd, 4th and 5th fingers	Ulnar nerve	Adduction of 2nd, 4th and 5th fingers	Adductor pollicis
Lumbricals (4)	Flexor digitorum profundis tendon	Extensor expansion of 2nd to 5th fingers at proximal phalanges on radial side	Radial and ulnar nerve	Flexion of fingers at MCP joints, extension of fingers at PIP and DIP joints	Palmar/dorsal interossei
THORACIC SPINE and RIBCAGE					
MUSCLE	**ORIGIN**	**INSERTION**	**INNERVATION**	**ACTION**	**SYNERGISTS**
Latissimus dorsi	Thoracolumbar aponeurosis, lower 6 T/S SPs, sacrum, iliac crest, lower 3–4 ribs Inferior angle of scapula	Bicipital groove of humerus	Thoracodorsal nerve (C6, 7, 8)	Extension, medial rotation, adduction of humerus	Teres major/minor, triceps, subscapularis, pectoralis major/minor, infraspinatus, coracobrachialis
Rhomboid major	T2–T5 SPs	Medial border of scapula from root of spine to inferior angle	Dorsal scapular nerve (C4, 5)	Retraction, medial rotation of scapula	Middle trapezius, levator scapula, pectoralis minor
Intercostals	Between adjacent ribs	Between adjacent ribs	Intercostals nerves	Elevates ribs in inspiration, maintains intercostal spaces	Serratus posterior superior, scalenes
Diaphragm	1st 3 lumbar vertebrae, lower 6 costal cartilages Xiphoid process	Central tendon of diaphragm	Phrenic nerve (C3, 4, 5)	Flattens central tendon and increases vertical diameter of thoracic cavity in inspiration	Intercostals, serratus posterior superior
Serratus posterior superior	Caudal ligamentum nuchae, SPs of C7–T2	Superior borders of ribs 2–5	Intercostal nerves T1–4	Raises ribs to increase thoracic cavity during inspiration	Scalenes, intercostals
Serratus posterior inferior	SPs of T11–L3	Inferior borders of last 4 ribs	Intercostal nerves T9–12	Draws ribs outward and downward, counteracting the inward pull of the diaphragm during expiration	Intercostals
Iliocostalis **Longissimus** **Spinalis**	Thoracolumbar aponeurosis, posterior ribs Thoracolumbar aponeurosis, lumbar and thoracic TVPs Ligamentum nuchae, cervical and thoracic SPs	Posterior ribs, cervical TVPs Cervical and thoracic TVPs, mastoid process Cervical and thoracic SPs, occipital bone	Dorsal rami of spinal nerves	Bilaterally: extension of spine Unilaterally: lateral flexion of spine	Semispinalis, multifidus, rotators, interspinalis, intertransversarii, internal/external oblique, splenius capitis/cervicis

Semispinalis	Cervical and thoracic TVPs	Cervical and thoracic TVPs (spans 3–6 vertebrae), occipital bone	Dorsal rami of spinal nerves	Bilaterally: extension of spine Unilaterally: rotation to opposite side	Iliocostalis, longissimus, spinalis, splenius capitis/cervicis, rotators, interspinalis
Multifidus	Sacrum, posterior superior iliac spine, TVPs all vertebrae	SPs of all vertebrae, inserting 2–4 vertebrae above origin			
Rotatores	TVPs of all vertebrae		Dorsal rami of adjacent spinal nerves	Extension of spine, rotation to opposite side	Iliocostalis, spinalis, longissimus, semispinalis, multifidus, interspinalis
Interspinales	SPs of cervical, lumbar and T1–2, T11–12 vertebrae	SPs of all vertebrae, inserting on vertebra directly above origin		Extension of spine	Iliocostalis, longissimus, spinalis, semispinalis, multifidus
Intertransversarii	TVPs of cervical, lumbar and T1–12 vertebrae	TVPs directly above origin	Dorsal rami of ventral and dorsal spinal nerves	Lateral flexion of spine	Iliocostalis, longissimus, spinalis, splenius capitis/cervicis, quadratus lumborum
		LUMBAR SPINE			
MUSCLES	**ORIGIN**	**INSERTION**	**INNERVATION**	**ACTION**	**SYNERGIST**
Rectus abdominis	Pubic symphysis and crest	Costal cartilates 5–7, xiphoid process	Intercostals nerves T7–T12	Flexion of trunk, supports compression of abdominal contents	External/internal oblique, transverse abdominis
External oblique	Ribs 5–12	Abdominal aponeurosis and linea alba, iliac crest	Intercostals nerves T7–T12 and L1	Bilaterally: flexion of trunk, compression of abdominal contents Unilaterally: lateral flexion, rotation of trunk to opposite side	Rectus abdominis, internal oblique, transverse abdominis
Internal oblique	Inguinal ligament and anterior iliac crest	Costal cartilages of ribs 9–12, abdominal aponeurosis and linea alba	Intercostals nerves T8–T12 and L1	Bilaterally: flexion of spine, compression of abdominal contents Unilaterally: lateral flexion, rotation of trunk to same side	Rectus abdominis, external oblique, transverse abdominis
Transverse abdominis	Inguinal ligament, iliac crest, thoracolumbar aponeurosis, internal surface of costal cartilages 7–12	Abdominal aponeurosis, linea alba, pubis	Intercostals nerves T7–T12 and L1	Compression of abdominal contents	Rectus abdominis, external/internal oblique
Quadratus lumborum	Posterior iliac crest	12th rib, TVPs of L1–4	T12–L4	Lateral flexion of trunk or raises hip	Internal/external obliques, gluteus medius/minimus
Iliocostalis	Thoracolumbar aponeurosis, posterior ribs	Posterior ribs, cervical TVPs	Dorsal rami of spinal nerves	Bilaterally: extension of spine Unilaterally: lateral flexion of spine	Semispinalis, multifidus, rotators, interspinalis, intertransversarii, internal/external oblique, splenius capitis/cervicis
Longissimus	Thoracolumbar aponeurosis, lumbar and thoracic TVPs	Cervical and thoracic TVPs, mastoid process			

APPENDIX 1 Muscle chart *continued*					
			LUMBAR SPINE		
MUSCLES	**ORIGIN**	**INSERTION**	**INNERVATION**	**ACTION**	**SYNERGIST**
Multifidus	Sacrum, posterior superior iliac spine, TVPs all vertebrae	SPs of all vertebrae, inserting 2–4 vertebrae above origin	Dorsal rami of spinal nerves	Bilaterally: extension of spine Unilaterally: rotation to opposite side	Iliocostalis, longissimus, spinalis, splenius capitis/cervicis, rotators, interspinalis
Rotatores **Interspinales**	TVPs of all vertebrae SPs of cervical, lumbar and T1–2, T11–12 vertebrae	SPs of all vertebrae, inserting on vertebra directly above origin	Dorsal rami of adjacent spinal nerves	Extension of spine, rotation to opposite side Extension of spine	Iliocostalis, spinalis, longissimus, semispinalis, multifidus, interspinalis Iliocostalis, longissimus, spinalis, semispinalis, multifidus
Intertransversarii	TVPs of cervical, lumbar and T1–12 vertebrae	TVPs directly above origin	Dorsal rami of ventral and dorsal spinal nerves	Lateral flexion of spine	Iliocostalis, longissimus, spinalis, splenius capitis/cervicis, quadratus lumborum
			SACRUM and PELVIS		
MUSCLES	**ORIGIN**	**INSERTION**	**INNERVATION**	**ACTION**	**SYNERGIST**
Gluteus maximus	Posterior sacrum, ilium, superior gluteal line of ilium	Gluteal tuberosity of femur and iliotibial tract	Inferior gluteal nerve (L5, S1,2)	Extension of femur at hip, lateral rotation of extended hip	Bicep femoris, semitendinosus, semimembranosus, piriformis, iliopsoas, sartorius
Gluteus medius **Gluteus minimus** **Tensor fasciae latae**	Iliac crest, ilium between superior and middle gluteal lines Posterior ilium between middle and inferior gluteal lines Iliac crest	Greater trochanter of femur Anterior surface of greater trochanter of femur Ilitotibial tract	Superior gluteal nerve (L4, 5, S1)	Abduction, medial rotation of femur at hip Prevents collapse of extended knee in ambulation, assists abduction, medial rotation, flexion of femur	Tensor fasciae latae, sartorius, pectineus, adductor longus/brevis, magnus Gluteus medius/minimus, sartorius, pectineus, adductor longus/brevis/magnus, iliopsoas, rectus femoris
Piriformis **Gemellus superior** **Obturator infernus** **Gemellus inferior** **Obturator externus** **Quadratus femoris**	Anterior sacrum, ischium, obturator foramen	Greater trochanter of femur	Branches of sacral plexus (L4, 5, S1,2)	Lateral rotation of femur at hip	Gluteus maximus, iliopsoas, sartorius
Psoas major **Iliacus**	Lumbar vertebrae T12–L5 Iliac fossa inner surface	Lesser trochanter of femur	Lumbar plexus (L1, 2, 3, 4)	Flexion, lateral rotation of femur at hip	Pectineus, tensor fasciae latae, adductor brevis/longus/magnus, rectus femoris, sartorius, piriformis, gluteus maximus

HIP					
MUSCLE	**ORIGIN**	**INSERTION**	**INNERVATION**	**ACTION**	**SYNERGISTS**
Psoas major **Iliacus**	Lumbar vertebrae T12–L5 Iliac fossa inner surface	Lesser trochanter of femur	Lumbar plexus (L1, 2, 3, 4)	Flexion, lateral rotation of femur at hip	Pectineus, tensor fasciae latae, adductor brevis/ longus/magnus, rectus femoris, sartorius, piri-formis, gluteus maximus
Sartorius	Anterior superior iliac spine	Upper medial shaft of tibia	Femoral nerve (L2, 3. 4)	Assist flexion, abduction, lateral rotation of femur at hip and assists flexion, medial rotation of knee	Piriformis, iliopsoas, gluteus medius/minimus, tensor fasciae latae, biceps femoris, semitendinosus, semimembranosus
Rectus femoris	Long head: anterior inferior iliac spine Short head: upper margin of acetabulum	Patella and via patellar ligament to tibial tuberosity	Femoral nerve	Extension of knee, assists flexion of femur at hip	Vastus lateralis/ intermedius/medialis, tensor fasciae latae, iliopsoas, pectineus, adductor longus/brevis/ magnus, sartorius
Vastus medialis **Vastus lateralis** **Vastus intermedius**	Linea aspera on posterior femur Linea aspera on posterior femur and greater trochanter of femur Anterior and lateral femoral shaft	Patella and via patellar ligament to tibial tuberosity	Femoral nerve	Extension of knee	Rectus femoris, tensor fasciae latae
Pectineus	Anterior pubis	Between lesser trochanter and linea aspera of posterior femur	Femoral nerve	Flexion of femur at hip and assists adduction of femur at hip	Iliopsoas, tensor fasciae latae, adductor brevis/ longus/magnus, rectus femoris, sartorius, gracilis
Adductor longus/ brevis	Anterior pubis	Linea aspera on posterior femur	Obturator nerve (L2, 3, 4)	Adduction of femur at hip and assists flexion and medial rotation of femur at hip	Adductor magnus, gracilis, pectineus, gluteus medius/minimus, tensor fasciae latae, pectineus, iliopsoas, rectus femoris, sartorius
Adductor magnus	Pubic ramus, ishcial tuberosity and ramus	Linea aspera of posterior femur, adductor tubercle of medial femur	Obturator nerve (L2, 3, 4) and sciatic nerve (L4, 5, S1)	Adduction of femur at hip, assists medial rotation	Adductor longus/brevis, gracilis, pectineus, gluteus medius/minimus, tensor fasciae latae
Gracilis	Anterior pubis	Medial proximal tibia	Obturator nerve (L2, 3, 4)	Adduction of femur at hip and assists flexion and medial rotation of flexed knee	Adductor brevis/longus/ magnus, pectineus, iliopsoas, tensor fasciae latae, rectus femoris, sartorius
Biceps femoris	Long head: ischial tuberosity Short head: linea aspera	Head of fibula	Sciatic nerve: tibial branch (L5, S1, 2, 3) and peroneal branch (L5, S1, 2)	Long head: extension of hip Both heads: flexion of knee and lateral rotation of flexed knee	Gluteus maximus, semitendinosus, semimembranosus, adductor magnus, sartorius, gracilis, gastrocnemius, plantaris, popliteus

APPENDIX 1 Muscle chart *continued*

HIP					
MUSCLE	**ORIGIN**	**INSERTION**	**INNERVATION**	**ACTION**	**SYNERGISTS**
Semimembranosus **Semitendinosus**	Ischial tuberosity	Posterior medial tibial condyle Anterior proximal tibial shaft	Sciatic nerve – tibial branch (L5, S1, 2, 3)	Extension of hip, flexion of knee, medial rotation of flexed knee	Gluteus maximus, biceps femoris, adductor magnus, sartorius, gracilis, gastrocnemius, plantaris, popliteus

KNEE					
MUSCLE	**ORIGIN**	**INSERTION**	**INNERVATION**	**ACTION**	**SYNERGISTS**
Gastrocnemius	Medial and lateral epicondyle of femur			Plantar flexion of ankle or assists flexion of knee	Soleus, plantaris, peroneus longus/brevis, tibialis posterior, flexor hallucis longus, flexor digitorum longus, biceps femoris, semitendinosus, semimembranosus
Plantaris	Lateral epicondyle of femur	Calcaneus via Achilles tendon	Tibial nerve	Assists plantar flexion of ankle, assists flexion of knee	Gastrocnemius, soleus, biceps femoris, semitendinosus, semimembranosus
Popliteus	Lateral condyle of femur	Posterior proximal tibial shaft	Tibial nerve (L4, 5, S1)	Initiates knee flexion by medial rotation of tibia to unlock the extended knee	Biceps femoris, semitendinosus, semimembranosus
Sartorius	Anterior superior iliac spine	Upper medial shaft of tibia	Femoral nerve (L2, 3, 4)	Assist flexion, abduction, lateral rotation of femur at hip and assists flexion, medial rotation of knee	Piriformis, iliopsoas, gluteus medius/minimus, tensor fasciae latae, biceps femoris, semitendinosus, semimembranosus
Rectus femoris	Long head: anterior inferior iliac spine Short head: upper margin of acetabulum	Patella and via patellar ligament to tibial tuberosity	Femoral nerve (L2, 3, 4)	Extension of knee, assists flexion of femur at hip	Vastus lateralis/intermedius/medialis, tensor fasciae latae, iliopsoas, pectineus, adductor longus/brevis/magnus, sartorius
Vastus medialis **Vastus lateralis** **Vastus intermedius**	Linea aspera on posterior femur Linea aspera on posterior femur and greater trochanter of femur Anterior and lateral femoral shaft	Patella and via patellar ligament to tibial tuberosity	Femoral nerve	Extension of knee	Rectus femoris, tensor fasciae latae
Gracilis	Anterior pubis	Medial proximal tibia	Obturator nerve (L2, 3, 4)	Adduction of femur at hip and assists flexion and medial rotation of flexed knee	Adductor brevis/longus/magnus, pectineus, iliopsoas, tensor fasciae latae, rectus femoris, sartorius
Semimembranosus **Semitendinosus**	Ischial tuberosity	Posterior medial tibial condyle Anterior proximal tibial shaft	Sciatic nerve – tibial division (L5, S1, 2, 3)	Extension of hip, flexion of knee, medial rotation of flexed knee	Gluteus maximus, biceps femoris, adductor magnus, sartorius, gracilis, gastrocnemius, plantaris, popliteus

Biceps femoris	Long head: ischial tuberosity Short head: linea aspera	Head of fibula	Sciatic nerve: tibial branch (L5, S1, 2, 3) and peroneal branch (L5, S1, 2)	Long head: extension of hip Both heads: flexion of knee and lateral rotation of flexed knee	Gluteus maximus, semitendinosus, semimembranosus, adductor magnus, sartorius, gracilis, gastrocnemius, plantaris, popliteus
			ANKLE		
Gastrocnemius	Medial and lateral epicondyle of femur			Plantar flexion of ankle or assists flexion of knee	Soleus, plantaris, peroneus longus/brevis, tibialis posterior, flexor hallucis longus, flexor digitorum longus, biceps femoris, semitendinosus, semimembranosus
Soleus	Soleal line of tibia, posterior head and upper shaft of fibula			Plantar flexion of ankle	Gastrocnemius, plantaris, peroneus longus/brevis, tibialis posterior, flexor hallucis longus, flexor digitorum longus
Plantaris	Lateral epicondyle of femur	Calcaneus via Achilles tendon	Tibial nerve (L5, S1, 2)	Assists plantar flexion of ankle, assists flexion of knee	Gastrocnemius, soleus, biceps femoris, semitendinosus, semimembranosus
Tibialis posterior	Posterior tibia, fibula and interosseous membrane	Navicular, adjacent tarsals and metatarsals on plantar surface	Tibial nerve	Inversion of foot, assists plantar flexion of ankle	Tibialis anterior, gastrocnemius, soleus, plantaris, peroneus longus/brevis, flexor hallucis longus, flexor digitorum longus
Flexor digitorum longus	Posterior tibia	Distal phalanges of 4 lateral toes on plantar surface	Tibial nerve	Flexion of 4 lateral toes at DIP, assists plantar flexion of ankle	Gastrocnemius, soleus, plantaris, peroneus longus/brevis, tibialis posterior, flexor hallucis longus
Flexor hallucis longus	Posterior fibula	Distal phalanx of great toe on plantar surface	Tibial nerve	Flexion of great toe, assists plantar flexion of ankle	
Tibialis anterior	Lateral condyle and lateral shaft of tibia, interosseous membrane	Base of 1st metatarsal, 1st cuneiform	Deep peroneal nerve (L4, 5, S1)	Dorsiflexion of ankle, inversion of foot	Extensor digitorum longus, peroneus tertius, extensor hallucis longus, tibialis posterior
Extensor hallucis longus	Anterior shaft of fibula, interosseous membrane	Base of distal phalanx of great toe	Deep peroneal nerve	Extension of great toe, assists dorsiflexion of ankle	Tibialis anterior, extensor digitorum longus, peroneus tertius
Extensor digitorum longus	Lateral condyle of tibia, proximal ⅔ of anterior shaft of fibula	Middle and distal phalanges of 4 lateral toes	Deep peroneal nerve	Extension of 4 lateral toes, assists dorsiflexion of ankle	Extensor digitorum brevis, tibialis anterior, peroneus tertius, extensor hallucis longus
Peroneus tertius	Anterior distal fibula	Base of 5th metatarsal	Deep peroneal nerve	Eversion of foot, assists dorsiflexion	Peroneus brevis/longus, tibialis anterior, extensor digitorum longus, extensor hallucis longus

APPENDIX 1 Muscle chart *continued*

ANKLE					
MUSCLE	**ORIGIN**	**INSERTION**	**INNERVATION**	**ACTION**	**SYNERGISTS**
Peroneus brevis	Lateral shaft of fibula on lower ⅔	Base of 5th metatarsal	Superficial peroneal nerve (L4, 5, S1)	Eversion of foot, assists plantar flexion of ankle	Peroneus tertius/longus, gastrocnemius, soleus, plantaris, tibialis posterior, flexor hallucis longus, flexor digitorum longus
Peroneus longus	Head and lateral shaft of fibula on upper ⅔	Base of 1st metatarsal and 1st cuneiform on plantar surface	Superficial peroneal nerve	Eversion of foot, assists plantar flexion of ankle	Peroneus tertius/brevis, gastrocnemius, soleus, plantaris, tibialis posterior, flexor hallucis longus, flexor digitorum longus
FOOT/TOES					
MUSCLE	**ORIGIN**	**INSERTION**	**INNERVATION**	**ACTION**	**SYNERGISTS**
Flexor digitorum longus	Posterior tibia	Distal phalanges of 4 lateral toes on plantar surface	Tibial nerve (L5, S1, 2)	Flexion of 4 lateral toes at DIP, assists plantar flexion of ankle	Gastrocnemius, soleus, plantaris, peroneus longus/brevis, tibialis posterior, flexor hallucis longus
Flexor hallucis longus	Posterior fibula	Distal phalanx of great toe on plantar surface	Tibial nerve	Flexion of great toe, assists plantar flexion of ankle	
Tibialis anterior	Lateral condyle and lateral shaft of tibia, interosseous membrane	Base of 1st metatarsal, first cuneiform	Deep peroneal (fibular) nerve (L4,5)	Dorsiflexion of ankle, inversion of foot	Extensor digitorum longus, peroneus tertius, extensor hallucis longus, tibialis posterior
Extensor hallucis longus	Anterior shaft of fibula, interosseous membrane	Base of distal phalanx of great toe	Deep peroneal nerve	Extension of great toe, assists dorsiflexion of ankle	Tibialis anterior, extensor digitorum longus, peroneus tertius
Extensor digitorum brevis	Anterior calcaneus	Extensor expansion of 4 medial toes	Deep peroneal nerve	Assists extension of 4 medial toes at MCP joints	Extensor hallucis longus, extensor digitorum longus
Extensor digitorum longus	Lateral condyle of tibia, proximal ⅔ of anterior shaft of fibula	Middle and distal phalanges of 4 lateral toes	Deep peroneal nerve	Extension of 4 lateral toes, assists dorsiflexion of ankle	Extensor digitorum brevis, tibialis anterior, peroneus tertius, extensor hallucis longus
Peroneus tertius	Anterior distal fibula	Base of 5th metatarsal	Deep peroneal nerve	Eversion of foot, assists dorsiflexion	Peroneus brevis/longus, tibialis anterior, extensor digitorum longus, extensor hallucis longus

Peroneus brevis	Lateral shaft of fibula on lower ⅔	Base of 5th metatarsal	Superficial peroneal (fibular) nerve (L4, 5, S1)	Eversion of foot, assists plantar flexion of ankle	Peroneus tertius/longus, gastrocnemius, soleus, plantaris, tibialis posterior, flexor hallucis longus, flexor digitorum longus
Peroneus longus	Head and lateral shaft of fibula on upper ⅔	Base of 1st metatarsal and 1st cuneiform on plantar surface	Superficial peroneal nerve	Eversion of foot, assists plantar flexion of ankle	Peroneus tertius/brevis, gastrocnemius, soleus, plantaris, tibialis posterior, flexor hallucis longus, flexor digitorum longus
Abductor hallucis	Calcaneus	Base of proximal phalanx of great toe	Medial plantar nerve (L5, S1, 2)	Flexion, abduction of great toe at MCP joint	Flexor hallucis longus, flexor hallucis brevis
Flexor digitorum brevis	Calcaneus	Middle phalanges of 4 lateral toes	Medial plantar nerve	Flexion of PIP joints of 4 lateral toes	
Abductor digiti minimi	Calcaneus	Base of proximal phalanx of little toe	Lateral plantar nerve (L5, S1, 2)	Flexion, abduction of little toe at MCP joint	
Lumbricals	Tendons of flexor digitorum longus	Extensor expansion of 4 lateral toes	Medial and lateral plantar nerve	Flexion of MCP joints, extension of DIP and PIP joints	Quadratus plantae
Quadratus plantae	Calcaneus	Tendons of flexor digitorum longus	Lateral plantar nerve	Assists flexion of DIP joints	Lumbricals
Flexor hallucis brevis	Base of metatarsal of great toe	Base of proximal phalanx of great toe	Medial plantar nerve	Flexion of MCP joint of great toe	Abductor hallucis, flexor hallucis longus
Adductor hallucis	Oblique: base of 2nd, 3rd metatarsals Transverse: 3rd to 5th MCP joint capsules	Base of proximal phalanx of great toe	Lateral plantar nerve	Adduction, flexion of great toe	Flexor hallucis longus, abductor hallucis
Flexor digiti minimi	Cuboid and base of 5th metatarsal	Base of proximal phalanx of 5th toe	Lateral plantar nerve	Flexion of MCP joint of little toe	Lumbricals
Dorsal interossei (4)	Adjacent metatarsals	Extensor expansion of 2nd to 4th toes	Lateral plantar nerve	Abduction of 2nd to 4th toes, assists flexion of MCP and extension of IP joints of 4 lateral toes	Lumbricals
Plantar interossei (3)	Medial side of 3rd to 5th metatarsals	Extensor expansion of 3 lateral toes	Lateral plantar nerve	Adduction of 3 lateral toes, assists flexion of MCP and extension of IP joints of 4 lateral toes	Lumbricals

APPENDIX 1 Muscle chart *continued*

FACE/HEAD					
MUSCLE	**ORIGIN**	**INSERTION**	**INNERVATION**	**ACTION**	**SYNERGISTS**
Nasalis (compressor naris and dilator naris)	Maxilla	Nose	Facial nerve (CN VII)	Dilator: widens nasal opening Compressor: compresses nasal cartilages	
Frontalis	Skin and fascia of eyebrows	Epicranial aponeurosis	Facial nerve	Raises eyebrows and moves scalp	
Occipitalis	Nuchal line of occipital bone				
Platysma	Fascia over pectoralis major and deltoid	Mandible, muscles around mouth	Facial nerve	Depresses mandible, draws lower lip downward	Suprahyoids
Procerus	Nose	Skin between eyebrows	Facial nerve	Wrinkles nose skin	
Corrugator supercilii	Frontal bone	Skin of eyebrow	Facial nerve	Draws eyebrow down in frowning	
Depressor anguli oris **Depressor labii inferioris** **Levator anguli oris** **Levator labii superioris** **Levator labii superioris alaque nasi** **Mentalis** **Risorius** **Zygomaticus major** **Zygomaticus minor**	Bones and fascia around mouth	Lips	Facial nerve	Separates lips	
Levator palpebrae superioris	Roof of orbit	Upper eyelid	Oculomotor nerve (CN III)	Elevates upper eyelid	
Orbicularis oculi	Orbital margin	Eyelid	Facial nerve	Closes eyelid	
Temporalis	Lateral surface of temporal bone	Mandible	Trigeminal nerve (CN V)	Closes and retracts jaw	Masseter, medial pterygoid
Masseter	Zygomatic arch	Mandible	Trigeminal nerve	Closes jaw and assists protraction Unilaterally: lateral jaw motion to same side	Temporalis, medial/ lateral pterygoid
Orbicularis oris	Maxilla, mandible, lips, buccinator	Mucous membranes, muscles inserting into lip	Facial nerve	Lip closure	Buccinator

Buccinator	Maxilla, mandible	Lips	Facial nerve	Maintains cheeks near teeth	Orbicularis oris
Medial pterygoid	Pterygoid plate on medial surface	Mandible	Trigeminal nerve	Closes jaw and assists protraction Unilaterally: lateral jaw motion to opposite side	Temporalis, masseter, lateral pterygoid
Lateral pterygoid	Pterygoid plate on lateral surface	Mandible, temporomandibular joint capsule	Trigeminal nerve	Protracts jaw Unilaterally: lateral jaw motion of opposite side	Temporalis, masseter, medial pterygoid

Note:
SP, spinous process; TVP transverse process; MCP joint, metacarpophalangeal joint; PIP joint, proximal interphalangeal joint; DIP joint, distal interphalangeal joint; IP joint, interphalangeal joint; CM joint, carpometacarpal joint.

APPENDIX 2 Joints: range of motion and tissues involved				
• Tissues stretched and compressed are more capable of sustaining injury when the joint is at or near its end range of motion				
ANKLE JOINT: TALOCRURAL				
ACTION	NORMAL DEGREES OF MOVEMENT	ACTIVATED MUSCLES	TISSUES BEING STRETCHED	TISSUES COMPRESSED
Dorsiflexion Active free **Dorsiflexion Passive**	10–20° 20°	Tibialis anterior Extensor digitorum longus Extensor hallucis longus Peroneus tertius N/A	Gastrocnemius Soleus Tibialis posterior Peroneus longus/brevis Flexor hallucis/digitorum longus Posterior joint capsule Calcaneofibular ligament Posterior talofibular ligament	Anterior joint capsule Anterior joint surface Anterior talofibular ligament
Plantar flexion Active free **Plantar flexion Passive**	40–50° 50°	Gastrocnemius Soleus Tibialis posterior Plantaris Flexor digitorum/hallucis longus Peroneus longus/brevis N/A	Tibialis anterior Extensor digitorum longus Extensor hallucis longus Peroneus tertius Anterior joint capsule Anterior talofibular ligament	Posterior joint capsule Calcaneofibular ligament Posterior talofibular ligament

Notes:
Capsular pattern of restriction: plantar flexion is most notably lost first.
Resting position: 10° plantar flexion, midway between inversion and eversion.
10° dorsiflexion needed for normal locomotion.

KNEE JOINT: TIBIOFEMORAL				
ACTION	NORMAL DEGREES OF MOVEMENT	ACTIVATED MUSCLES	TISSUES STRETCHED	TISSUES COMPRESSED
Flexion Active free **Flexion Passive**	125–135° 125–135°	Semimembranosus Semitendinosus Biceps femoris Sartorius Gracilis Gastrocnemius Plantaris Popliteus N/A	Patellar tendon Anterior cruciate ligament Anterior joint capsule Prepatellar bursa Superficial infrapatellar bursa Vastus lateralis/intermedius/medialis Rectus femoris	Posterior joint capsule Posterior portion of menisci Popliteal lymph nodes Posterior surface of patella
Extension Active free **Extension Passive**	0–10° 5–10°	Vastus lateralis Vastus intermedius Vastus medialis Rectus femoris Tensor fasciae latae N/A	Posterior joint capsule Posterior cruciate ligament Semimembranosus Semitendinosus Biceps femoris Gracilis Gastrocnemius Plantaris Popliteus	Anterior joint capsule Central and anterior portion of menisci Deep infrapatellar bursa

Internal rotation Active free **Internal rotation Passive**	20–30° 25-30°	Semitendinosus Semimembranosus Popliteus Gracilis Sartorius N/A	Biceps femoris Cruciate ligaments	Portions of menisci
External (lateral) Rotation Active free **External rotation Passive**	30–40° 30–40°	Biceps femoris N/A	Collateral ligaments Semitendinosus Semimembranosus Popliteus Gracilis and sartorius Lateral and medial ligaments	Portions of menisci

Notes:
Capsular pattern of restriction: flexion is most notably lost first followed by extension.
Resting position: 25° flexion.

HIP JOINT: ILIOFEMORAL				
ACTION	**NORMAL DEGREES OF MOVEMENT**	**MUSCLES ACTIVATED**	**TISSUES STRETCHED**	**TISSUES BEING COMPRESSED**
Flexion Active free **Flexion Passive**	110–120° 110–130°	Iliopsoas Pectineus Tensor fasciae latae Adductor brevis/longus/ magnus Rectus femoris Sartorius N/A	Posterior joint capsule Sciatic nerve Ischiofemoral ligament Gluteus maximus Biceps femoris Semitendinosus Semimembranosus	Inguinal lymph nodes Iliofemoral ligament Pubofemoral ligament Femoral nerve Anterior joint capsule Ischial bursa
Extension Active free **Extension Passive**	10–25° 25–30°?	Gluteus maximus Biceps femoris Semitendinosus Semimembranosus N/A	Iliofemoral ligament Pubofemoral ligament Anterior joint capsule Femoral nerve Iliopsoas Pectineus Tensor fasciae latae Adductor brevis/longus/ magnus Rectus femoris and sartorius	Ischiofemoral ligament Posterior joint capsule Psoas bursa
Abduction Active free **Abduction Passive**	30–50° 40–50°	Gluteus medius Gluteus minimus Tensor fasciae latae Sartorius N/A	Pubofemoral ligament Adductor brevis/longus/ magnus Medial joint capsule	Lateral joint capsule Psoas bursa Superior portion of hip joint (cartilage and labrum)
Adduction Active free **Adduction Passive**	20–30° 30°	Adductor brevis/longus/ magnus N/A	Gluteus medius Gluteus minimus Tensor fasciae latae Sartorius Lateral joint capsule	Pubofemoral ligament Medial joint capsule Trochanteric bursa Inguinal neurovascular bundle

APPENDIX 2 Joints: range of motion and tissues involved *continued*

HIP JOINT: ILIOFEMORAL

ACTION	NORMAL DEGREES OF MOVEMENT	MUSCLES ACTIVATED	TISSUES STRETCHED	TISSUES BEING COMPRESSED
External rotation **Active free**	40–60°	Pirifomis Gluteus maximus Iliopsoas Sartorius Gemellus superior/inferior Obturator infernus/xternus Quadratus femoris	Gluteus medius Gluteus minimus Tensor fasciae latae Pectineus Adductor brevis/longus/ magnus	Pubofemoral ligament Iliofemoral ligament Ishciofemoral ligament
External rotation **Passive**	50–60°	N/A		
Internal rotation **Active free**	30–40°	Gluteus medius Gluteus minimus Tensor fasciae latae Pectineus Adductor brevis/longus/ magnus	Pubofemoral ligament Iliofemoral ligament Ishciofemoral ligament Pirifomis Gluteus maximus	
Internal rotation **Passive**	30–40°	N/A	Iliopsoas Sartorius Gemellus superior/inferior Obturator infernus/externus Quadratus femoris	

Notes:
Capsular pattern of restriction: flexion, abduction and internal rotation are most notably lost. The order of these restrictions may vary.
Resting position: 30° flexion, 30° abduction and slight lateral rotation.

SHOULDER JOINT: GLENOHUMERAL

ACTION	NORMAL DEGREES OF MOVEMENT	MUSCLES ACTIVATED	TISSUES STRETCHED	TISSUES COMPRESSED
Abduction **Active free** **Abduction** **Passive**	170–180° 180°	Supraspinatus Middle deltoid N/A	Pectoralis major Coracobrachialis Latissismus dorsi Teres major Middle glenohumeral ligament Conoid ligament	Subdeltoid bursa Lateral joint capsule Supraspinatus tendon Coracohumeral ligament
Adduction **Active free**	50–75°	Pectoralis major Coracobrachialis Latissismus dorsi Teres major	Supraspinatus Middle deltoid Coracohumeral ligament	Anterior and superior joint capsule
Adduction **Passive**	60–75°	N/A		
Flexion **Active free**	160–180°	Anterior deltoid Pectoralis major Coracobrachialis Biceps brachii	Latissismus dorsi Teres major/minor Posterior deltoid Infraspinatus Triceps brachii Pectoralis major Posterior coracohumeral ligament	Subacromial bursa Anterior joint capsule Anterior corachumeral ligament
Flexion **Passive**	160–180°	N/A		

Extension Active free **Extension Passive**	50–60° 60°?	Latissismus dorsi Teres major/minor Posterior deltoid Infraspinatus Triceps brachii Pectoralis major N/A	Anterior deltoid Pectoralis major Coracobrachialis Biceps brachii Inferior glenohumeral ligament Anterior coracohumeral ligament Anterior-superior joint capsule	Posterior joint capsule Posterior coracohumeral ligament
Internal rotation Active free **Internal rotation Passive**	60–100° 100°	Anterior deltoid Pectoralis major Subscapularis Teres major Latissimus dorsi N/A	Infraspinatus Teres minor Posterior deltoid	Anterior coracohumeral ligament
External rotation Active free **External rotation Passive**	80–90° 80–90°	Infraspinatus Teres minor Posterior deltoid N/A	Anterior deltoid Pectoralis major Subscapularis Teres major Latissimus dorsi Middle glenohumeral ligament Anterior joint capsule	Posterior coracohumeral ligament
Horizontal adduction Active free **Horizontal adduction Passive**	110–130° 110–130°	Anterior deltoid Pectoralis major N/A	Posterior deltoid Infraspinatus and teres minor	Acromioclavicular joint
Horizontal abduction Active free **Horizontal adduction Passive**	45°	Posterior deltoid N/A	Anterior deltoid Pectoralis major Coracobrachialis (brachial plexus)	

Note:
Capsular pattern of restriction: lateral rotation is most notably lost first, followed by abduction then medial rotation.
Resting position: 55° abduction, 30° horizontal adduction.

ELBOW JOINT: HUMEROULNAR, HUMERORADIAL				
ACTION	**NORMAL DEGREES OF MOVEMENT**	**MUSCLES ACTIVATED**	**TISSUES STRETCHED**	**TISSUES COMPRESSED**
Flexion Active free **Flexion Passive**	140–150° 140–160°	Biceps brachii Brachialis Brachioradialis Pronator teres N/A	Triceps brachii Anconeus Arcuate ligament	Olecranon bursa Anterior joint capsule Ulnar nerve
Extension Active free **Extension Passive**	0–10° 0–10°	Triceps brachii Anconeus N/A	Biceps brachii Brachialis Brachioradialis Pronator teres	Posterior joint capsule

APPENDIX 2 Joints: range of motion and tissues involved *continued*

ELBOW JOINT: HUMEROULNAR, HUMERORADIAL				
ACTION	**NORMAL DEGREES OF MOVEMENT**	**MUSCLES ACTIVATED**	**TISSUES STRETCHED**	**TISSUES BEING COMPRESSED**
Supination Active free **Supination Passive**	90° 90°	Biceps brachii Supinator N/A	Pronator teres Pronator quadratus Superior quadrate ligament Annular ligament	Posterior interosseous nerve
Pronation Active free **Pronation Passive**	80–90° 85–90°	Pronator teres Pronator quadratus N/A	Biceps brachii Supinator Posterior quadrate ligament Annular ligament	Anterior interosseous nerve

Note:
Capsular pattern of restriction: flexion is most notably lost first.
Resting position: 70° flexion, 10° supination.

WRIST JOINT: RADIOCARPAL				
ACTION	**NORMAL DEGREES OF MOVEMENT**	**MUSCLES ACTIVATED**	**TISSUES STRETCHED**	**TISSUES COMPRESSED**
Flexion Active free **Flexion Passive**	75–90° 80–90°	Flexor carpi radialis Flexor carpi ulnaris Palmaris longus N/A	Extensor carpi radialis longus Extensor carpi radialis brevis Extensor carpi ulnaris *And their sheaths over the radiocarpal and intercarpal joints*	Median nerve and carpal tunnel contents Volar portions of radiocarpal and intercarpal joints
Extension Active free **Extension Passive**	70–90° 80–90°	Extensor carpi radialis longus Extensor carpi radialis brevis Extensor carpi ulnaris N/A	Flexor carpi radialis Flexor carpi ulnaris Palmaris longus (and tendon sheaths for all muscles passing through carpal tunnel) Median nerve Ulnar nerve	Dorsal portions of radiocarpal and intercarpal joints
Radial deviation Active free **Radial deviation Passive**	15° 15–20°	Flexor carpi radialis Extensor carpi radialis longus N/A	Extensor carpi ulnaris Flexor carpi ulnaris Ulnar collateral ligament	Radial collateral ligament Scaphoid tubercle Ulnar styloid process
Ulnar deviation Active free **Ulnar deviation Passive**	30–45° 40–45°	Extensor carpi ulnaris Flexor carpi ulnaris N/A	Flexor carpi radialis Extensor carpi radialis longus Radial collateral ligament	Ulnar collateral ligament

Notes:
Capsular pattern of restriction: flexion and extension are equal in limitations.
Resting position: neutral with slight ulnar deviation.

CERVICAL SPINE				
ACTION	**NORMAL DEGREES OF MOVEMENT**	**MUSCLES ACTIVATED**	**TISSUES STRETCHED**	**TISSUES COMPRESSED**
Flexion Active free **Flexion Passive**	50–65° 50–70°	Sternocleidmastoid Scalene anterior/medius/ longus colli N/A	Splenius capitis/cervicis Erector spinae Trapezius; levator scapula Multifidus Interspinalis Nuchal and interspinous ligament, supraspinous ligament Ligamentum flavum Vertebral artery between occiput–C1 Facet joint	Anterior portion of intervertebral disc Hyoid bone and muscles Neurovascular bundle in lower scalene triangle
Extension Active free **Extension Passive**	50–70° 60–70°	Splenius capitis/cervicis Erector spinae Trapezius Levator scapula Multifidus Interspinalis N/A	Sternocleidmastoid Scalene anterior/medius Anterior longitudinal ligament Vertebral artery Vagal and phrenic nerves	Vertebral artery between occiput–C1 Posterior intervertebral disc Intervertebral foramen
Side-bending (lateral flexion) Active free **Side-bending Passive**	20–45° 30–55°	Trapezius Splenius capitis/cervicis Sternocleidomastoid Erector spinae Levator scapula Multifidus Intertransversarii Scalenes N/A	Alar ligament *Same structures as "muscles activated", but opposite side* Contralateral facet joint (and O–C1–2) Contralateral vertebral artery Contralateral uncovertebral joint	Ipsilateral portion of intervertebral disc Ipsilateral facet joint (and O–C1–2) Ipsilateral vertebral Artery between occiput–C1 Ipsilateral uncovertebral joint and intervertebral foramen Vagus and glossopha-rangeal nerves
Rotation Active free **Rotation Passive**	70–85° 80–90°	Trapezius Splenius capitis Sternocleidomastoid Erector spinae Levator scapula Multifidus Intertransversarii Rotatores N/A	*Same structures as "muscles activated", but opposite side* Facet joint contralateral to rotation	Vertebral arteries Ipsilateral facet joint Uncovertebral joints

Note:
Capsular pattern of restriction: lateral flexion and rotation are equally limited, followed by extension.
Resting position: slight extension.

APPENDIX 2 Joints: range of motion and tissues involved *continued*				
LUMBAR SPINE				
ACTION	NORMAL DEGREES OF MOVEMENT	MUSCLES ACTIVATED	TISSUES STRETCHED	TISSUES COMPRESSED
Flexion **Active free** **Flexion** **Passive**	40–60° 40–60°	Psoas major Rectus abdominis External/internal oblique Transverse abdominis N/A	Latissimus dorsi Erector spinae Transversospinalis Interspinales Quadratus lumborum Interspinous ligament Supraspinous ligament Ligamentum flavum Interspinous ligament Facet joints	Anterior portion of intervertebral disc
Extension **Active free** **Extension** **Passive**	20–35° 25–35°	Latissimus dorsi Erector spinae Transversospinalis Interspinales Quadratus lumborum N/A	Psoas major Rectus abdominis External/internal oblique	Posterior portion of intervertebral disc Interspinous and supraspinous ligament Facet joints Intervertebral foramen
Side-bending (lateral flexion) **Active free** **Side-bending** **Passive**	15–20° 15–20°	Latissimus dorsi Erector spinae Transversalis Intertransversarii Quadratus lumborum Psoas major External oblique N/A	*Same structures as "muscles activated", but opposite side* Contralateral facet joint	Ipsilateral lateral portion of intervertebral disc Ipsilateral facet joint Intervertebral foramen
Rotation **Active free** **Rotation** **Passive**	3–18° 5–18°	Transversalis* N/A	*Same structures as "muscles activated", but opposite side* Ipsilateral facet joint	Facet joint contralateral to rotation

Notes:
Capsular pattern of restriction: lateral flexion and rotation are equally limited, followed by extension.
Resting position: midway between flexion and extension.
* Limited rotation occurs at the lumbar spine because of the facet joints.

THORACIC SPINE				
ACTION	**NORMAL DEGREES OF MOVEMENT**	**MUSCLES ACTIVATED**	**TISSUES STRETCHED**	**TISSUES COMPRESSED**
Flexion Active free **Flexion Passive**	20–45° 30–45°	Rectus abdominis External/internal oblique N/A	Spinalis thoracis Erector spinae Multifidus Rotatores Interspinalis Posterior longitudinal ligament Ligamentum flavum Interspinous ligament Facet joints	Diaphragm muscle (by abdominal contents) Anterior longitudinal ligament Anterior portion of intervertebral disc
Extension Active free **Extension Passive**	25–40° 30–40°	Spinalis thoracis Erector spinae Multifidus Rotatores Interspinalis N/A	Rectus abdominis External/internal oblique Anterior longitudinal ligament Sympathetic chain Vagal and phrenic nerves	Posterior longitudinal ligament Posterior portion of intervertebral disc Facet joints Intervertebral foramen
Side-bending (lateral flexion) Active free **Side-bending (lateral flexion) Passive**	20–40° 20–40°	Erector spinae External/internal oblique Multifidus Rotatores Transverse abdominis N/A	*Same structures as "muscles activated", but opposite side* Contralateral intertransverse Ligament	Ipsilateral lateral portion of intervertebral disc Ipsilateral facet joint
Rotation Active free **Rotation Passive**	35–50° 40–55°	Erector spinae External/internal oblique Multifidus Rotatores Transverse abdominis N/A	*Same structures as "muscles activated", but opposite side* Intertransverse ligaments Facet joint (*opposite to those compressed*)	Facet joint (*in higher T-spine ipsilateral to rotation like in the C-spine; in the lower T-spine contralateral to rotation as in the lumbar spine*)

Note:

Capsular pattern of restriction: side flexion and rotation equally limited, followed by extension.

Resting position: midway between flexion and extension.

APPENDIX 3 Joints; capsular pattern, resting position ("open packed") and close packed position

- The capsular pattern of restriction identifies those specific and unique ranges of motion that a joint may lose when the joint capsule is impaired or dysfunctional. This unique pattern of restrictions is seen when testing a joint's range of motion.
- The resting position (sometimes called the open packed position) is the position the joint takes when injured and especially when swelling has occurred. It is a positon of comfort, or the most painless position the patient wants to hold that joint or limb in. Again, seeing this suggests to the therapist that a joint pathology is involved in the patient's impairment.
- The close packed position is when the joint surfaces are most congruent or in contact and in this positon the joint is usually considered to be at its most stable. An example would be extension of the knee. Note: in the case of trauma or excessive force being applied ligaments and other joint structures and tissues will take the full impact of that force and if overpowered, will sustain injury.

JOINT	CAPSULAR PATTERN OF RESTRICTION	RESTING POSITION	CLOSE PACKED POSITION
Glenohumeral	Lateral rotation, abduction, medial rotation	55° abduction, 30° horizontal adduction	Full abduction, lateral rotation
Ulnohumeral	Flexion, extension	70° elbow flexion, 10° supination	Extension with supination
Radiohumeral	Flexion, extension	Full extension and full supination	Elbow flexed to 90°, forearm supinated to 5°
Proximal radioulnar	Equal limitation of supination and pronation	35° supination, 70° elbow flexion	5° supination
Distal radioulnar	Pain at extreme rotation	10° supination	5° supination
Iliofemoral	Flexion, abduction, medial rotation (order may vary)	30° flexion, 30° abduction, slight lateral rotation	Extension, medial rotation and abduction
Tibiofemoral	Flexion, extension	25° flexion	Full extension, lateral rotation of tibia
Tibiofibular	Pain on stress	Plantar flexion	Maximum dorsiflexion
Talocrural	Plantar flexion, dorsiflexion	10° plantar flexion, midway between inversion and eversion	Maximum dorsiflexion
Subtalar	Varus, valgus	Midway between extremes of range of motion	Supination
Midtarsal	Dorsiflexion, plantar flexion, adduction, medial rotation	Midway between extremes of range of motion	Supination
Tarsometatarsal	None	Midway between extremes of range of motion	Supination
Metatarsophalangeal	Big toe: extension, flexion 2nd–5th toe: variable	Midway between extremes of range of motion	Full extension
Interphalangeal (toes)	Flexion, extension	Slight flexion	Full extension

APPENDIX 3 *continued*			
Radiocarpal	Flexion and extension equally limited	Neutral with slight ulnar deviation	Extension
Mid carpal	Equal limitation of flexion and extension	Neutral or slight flexion with ulnar deviation	Extension with ulnar deviation
Intercarpal	None	Neutral or slight flexion	Extension
Thumb	Abduction then extension	Midway between abduction and adduction, plus midway between flexion and extension	Full opposition
Carpometacarpal	Equal limitation in all directions	Midway between flexion and extension	Full flexion
MCP	Flexion then extension	Slight flexion	Full flexion
DIP/PIP (fingers)	Flexion, extension	Slight flexion	Full extension
Cervical spine	Side-flexion/rotation equally limited, followed by extension	Slight extension	Full extension
Facets of thoracic spine	Side-flexion and rotation equally limited, then extension	Midway between flexion and extension	Extension
Lumbar spine	Side-flexion and rotation equally limited, then extension	Midway between flexion and extension	Extension
Sacroiliac	Pain when joints are stressed	Neutral	
Temporomandibular	Limited ability to open mouth	Mouth slightly open, lips together, teeth not in contact	Teeth slightly clenched

APPENDIX 4 Neurological testing of nerve roots: upper extremity				
NERVE ROOT	**DEEP TENDON REFLEX**	**MUSCLES SUPPLIED**	**SENSATION – DERMATOME**	**MOTOR TEST – MYOTOME**
C1 and 2		Deep flexors of the neck and suboccipital muscles	C1 vertex of head C2 cheek bone	Nodding of the head
C3		Lateral muscles of the neck	Under the mandible and down into the neck	Sidebending of the cervical spine
C4		Elevators of the scapula	Under the clavicle	Shoulder shrug
C5	Biceps reflex	Deltoid Biceps	Lateral shoulder and arm down into the lateral elbow	Shoulder abduction
C6	Brachioradialis reflex (Biceps reflex)	Wrist extensors Biceps	Whole thumb, and up into the lateral wrist	Wrist extension
C7	Triceps reflex	Wrist flexors Finger extensors Triceps	Both dorsal and ventral surfaces of the middle finger	Wrist flexion
C8		Finger flexors Hand intrinsics	Ulnar border of little finger and wrist	Finger flexion
T1		Hand intrinsics	Medial forearm up to the elbow	Finger abduction

APPENDIX 5 Neurological testing of nerve roots: lower extremity				
NERVE ROOT	DEEP TENDON REFLEX	MUSCLES SUPPLIED	SENSATION	MOTOR TEST
L2		Iliopsoas	Mid anterior thigh	Hip flexion above 90°
L3		Quadriceps	Anterior thigh above knee cap	Knee extension
L4	Patellar reflex	Anterior tibialis	Medial leg and medial foot	Dorsiflexion and inversion of foot
L5		Extensor hallucis longus	Lateral leg and dorsum of foot	Dorsiflexion of big toe
S1	Achilles reflex	Peroneus longus and brevis	Lateral foot	Plantar flexion and eversion of foot

APPENDIX 6 Testing of major peripheral nerves: upper extremity		
NERVE	**MOTOR TEST**	**SENSORY TEST**
Femoral nerve	Knee extension	Anteromedial thigh and leg
Lateral cutaneous		Lateral thigh
Posterior cutaneous		Posterior thigh
Saphenous branch of femoral nerve		Anteromedial knee and medial leg
Obturator nerve	Hip adduction	Medial thigh
Sciatic nerve	Knee flexion Foot dorsiflexion	Anterior and posterior leg Sole and dorsum of foot
Common peroneal nerve	Foot dorsiflexion with inversion (or eversion)	Anterior leg, dorsum of foot

APPENDIX 7 Testing of major peripheral nerves: lower extremity		
NERVE	MOTOR TEST	SENSORY TEST AREA
Axillary nerve (C5–6)	Deltoid – shoulder abduction	Lateral arm and deltoid area on upper arm – but distinctive is total loss in circular area mid-lateral deltoid – down to the elbow and over to medial forearm
Musculocutaneous nerve (C5–6)	Biceps and brachioradialis – elbow flexion done with elbow in neutral ("thumb up")	Lateral forearm
Median nerve (C6–8)	Thumb-index finger pinch Abduction of thumb	Last phalange and tips of the index, middle and medial side of the 4th digit are distinctive; and the dorsal surface of those fingers and the palm of the hand
Radial nerve (C6–T1)	Wrist extension Thumb extension	Dorsal surface of the lateral hand – thumb and index finger web space is distinctive – and onto the thumb; and also the dorsal surface index , middle finger and lateral portion of the 4th finger, all up to the "DIP" joint but not including the surface of the distal phalanges
Ulnar nerve (C8–T1)	Tip of little finger reaches across to touch the base of the thumb (opposition)	Dorsal and ventral surfaces of the little finger is distinctive; also lateral half of the 4th digit

APPENDIX 8 List of classic orthopedic tests

Below you will find an indexed list of the classic orthopedic tests. These are the most basic "special tests" that all massage therapists should be aware of and know how to do. This knowledge will aid all therapists in communicating with other health care professions.

APPENDIX 8 continued			
Noble's compression test	162	Tinel's sign at the wrist	511
Ober's test	203	Trendelenburg's test	205
Patellar apprehension test	160	Trigger finger	509
Patellofemoral compression testing	161	Valgus stress test elbow	480
Pectoralis minor syndrome test	421	Valgus stress test knee	153
Phalen's tests	511	Valsalva's test: *lumbar*	306
Piriformis test	204	Valsalva's test: *cervical*	385
Pitcher's elbow	486	Varus stress test elbow	483
Posterior displacement test of the hip	258	Varus stress test knee	153
Posterior draw test for the knee	156	Wedge test	121
Scouring test	206	Well leg raise	304
Shoulder impingement test	462	Winging scapula test	462
Skier's thumb	509	Yergason's test	458
Slump test	304		
Speed's test	459, 461		
Spurling's test	385		
Stork test	210, 241		
Straight leg raise test	302		
Supraspinatus tendonitis tests	459		
Swallowing test	386		
Talar tilts (ankle ligament tests)	119		
Thomas test	200		
Thompson's test	121		
Tinel's sign at the ankle	122		
Tinel's sign at the elbow	487, 489		
Tinel's sign at the neck	386		

**Excluded* tests are still described, but are not recommended for use with patients. However, they are still taught to students as their patients may have had them done with other health care practitioners. Reasons for exclusion are given for each in the text.

References

Agur AMR, Moore KL and Dalley AF (2014) Clinically oriented anatomy, 7th edn, Philadelphia: Wolters Kluwer/Lippincott Williams & Wilkins.

Andrade C-K (ed) (2014) Outcome-based massage: Putting evidence into practice. Philadelphia: Lippincott Williams & Wilkins.

Basmajian JV (1985) Manipulation, traction and massage, 3rd edn. Baltimore: Williams & Wilkins.

Bogduk N (2003) The anatomy and pathophysiology of neck pain. Physical Medicine and Rehabilitation Clinics of North America 14 455–472.

Bogduk N (2012) Clinical and radiological anatomy of the lumbar spine and the sacrum, 5th edn. Philadelphia: Churchill Livingstone.

Cailliet R (1996) Soft tissue pain and disability. Philadelphia: FA Davis.

Chila AJ (ed) (2010) Foundations of osteopathic medicine. Philadelphia: Lippincott Williams & Wilkins.

Cleland JA and Koppenhaver S (2011) Netter's orthopaedic clinical examination: An evidence-based approach, 2nd edn. Philadelphia: Saunders Elsevier.

Cook C (2007) Orthopedic manual therapy: An evidence-based approach. Upper Saddle River: Pearson Prentice Hall.

Costi JJ, Stokes Gardner-Morse IA, M Laible JP, Scoffone HM and Iatridis JC (2007) Direct measurement of intervertebral disc maximum shear strain in six degrees of freedom: Motions that place disc tissue at risk of injury. Journal of Biomechanics 40 (11) 2457–2466.

Cyriax J (1982) Textbook of orthopaedic medicine, volume I: Diagnosis of soft tissue lesions, 6th edn. London: Bailliere Tindall.

DeStefano LA (2011) Greenman's principles of manual medicine, 4th edn. Philadelphia: Wolters Kluwer/ Lippincott Williams & Wilkins.

Deyo RA (1998) Low-back pain. Scientific American August 48–53.

Deyo RA (2002) Diagnostic evaluation of low back pain with emphasis on imaging. Annals of Internal Medicine 137 (7) October 586–597.

Deyo RA, Mirza SK, Turner JA and Marting BI (2009) Over-treating chronic low back pain: Time to back off? Journal of the American Board of Family Medicine 22 (1) 62–68.

Dutton D (2012) Manual therapy of the spine: An integrated approach. Pittsburgh: McGraw-Hill.

Edmond S (2006) Joint mobilization/manipulation: Extremity and spinal techniques, 2nd edn. Philadelphia: Elsevier Health Sciences.

Evans RC (2009) Illustrated orthopaedic physical assessment, 3rd edn. St Louis: Mosby.

Forst SL, Wheeler MT, Fortin JD and Vilensky JA (2006) The sacroiliac joint: Anatomy, physiology and clinical significance, a focused review. Pain Physician 9 (1) 61–68.

Grob D, Frauenfelder H and Mannion AF (2007) The association between cervical spine curvature and neck pain. European Spine Journal 16 669–678.

Gross JM, Fetto J and Rosen E (2009) Musculoskeletal examination, 3rd edn. Chichester: Wiley.

Grossman S and Porth CM (2014) Pathophysiology: Concepts of altered health states. Philadelphia: Wolters Kluwer/Lippincott Williams & Wilkins.

Hammer WI (2007) Functional soft tissue examination and treatment by manual methods: New perspectives, 3rd edn. Gaithersburg: Jones & Bartlett.

Hartley A (2000a) Practical joint assessment: Upper quadrant: A sports medicine manual. St Louis: Mosby.

Hartley A (2000b) Practical joint assessment: Lower quadrant: A sports medicine manual. St Louis: Mosby.

Hertling D and Kessler RM (2006) Management of common musculoskeletal disorders: Physical therapy principles and methods, 4th edn. Philadelphia: Lippincott Williams & Wilkins.

Hoppenfeld S (1976) Physical examination of the spine and extremities. Norwalk: Appleton & Lange.

Janda V (1984) Muscles and motor control in cervicogenic disorders, in Grant R (ed) Physical therapy of the cervical and thoracic spine. Edinburgh: Churchill Livingstone, pp 195–215.

Janda V and Jull G (1987) Muscles and motor control in low back pain, in Twomey LT (ed) Physical therapy for the low back: Clinics in physical therapy. New York: Churchill Livingstone, pp 195–215.

Kaltenborn FM (2006) Manual mobilization of the joints, volume 1: The extremities, 7th edn. Norway: Orthopedic Physical Therapy Products.

Kapandji IA (1986a) Physiology of the joints: Annotated diagrams of the mechanics of the human joints, volume 1: Upper limb, 5th edn. New York: Churchill Livingstone.

Kapandji IA (1986b) Physiology of the joints: Annotated diagrams of the mechanic of the human joints, volume 2: Lower limb, 2nd edn. New York: Churchill Livingstone.

Kapandji IA (2008) Physiology of the joints: Annotated diagrams of the mechanic of the human joints, volume 3: The trunk and the vertebral column, 2nd edn. New York: Churchill Livingstone.

Kendall FP, McCreary EK, Provance PG, Rodgers MM and Romani WA (2005) Muscles, testing and function, with posture and pain, 5th edn. Philadelphia: Lippincott Williams & Wilkins.

Kisner C and Colby LA (2012) Therapeutic exercise: Foundations and techniques, 6th edn. Philadelphia: FA Davis.

Levangie PK and Norkin CC (2011) Joint structure and function: A comprehensive analysis, 5th edn. Philadelphia: FA Davis.

Magee DJ (2014) Orthopedic physical assessment, 6th edn. St Louis: Saunders Elsevier.

Maitland J (2001) Spinal manipulation made simple: A manual of soft tissue techniques. Berkeley: North Atlantic Books.

Malanga GA, Andrus S, Nadler SF et al. (2003) Physical examination of the knee: A review of the original test description and scientific validity of common orthopedic tests. Archives of Physical Medicine and Rehabilitation 84 592–603.

Melzack R, Wall PD (1965) Pain mechanisms: A new theory. Science 150 971–979.

Melzack R and Katz J (2013) Pain. WIREs Cogn Sci 4 1–15. doi: 10.1002/wcs.1201.

Mense S and Simons DJ (2001) Muscle pain: Understanding its nature, diagnosis and treatment. Philadelphia: Lippincott Williams & Wilkins.

Mitchell FL, Jr (2001) The muscle energy manual, volume 3: Evaluation and treatment of the pelvis and sacrum. 2nd edn. East Lansing: MET Press.

Mitchell FL, Jr (2004) The muscle energy manual, volume 2: Evaluation and treatment of the thoracic spine, lumbar spine, and rib cage, 2nd edn. East Lansing: MET Press.

Mitchell FL, Jr (2005) The muscle energy manual, volume 1: Concepts and mechanisms, the musculoskeletal screen, cervical region evaluation and treatment, 2nd edn. East Lansing: MET Press.

Myers TW (2014) Anatomy trains: Myofascial meridians for manual and movement therapists, 3rd edn. Philadelphia: Churchill Livingstone.

Oatis CA (2004) Kinesiology: The mechanics and pathomechanics of human movement. Philadelphia: Lippincott Williams & Wilkins.

Okeson JP (1996) Orofacial pain: Guidelines for assessment diagnosis and management. Chicago: Quintessence Publishing.

Palmer ML and Epler ME (1998) Fundamentals of musculoskeletal assessment techniques, 2nd edn. Philadelphia: Lippincott-Raven.

Pascarelli E and Quilter D (1994) Repetitive strain injury: A computer user's guide. New York: John Wiley & Sons.

Petty NJ (2011) Neuromusculoskeletal examination and assessment: A handbook for therapists. Physiotherapy Essentials (Kindle Locations 15130-15131). Elsevier Health Sciences UK. Kindle edition.

References

Pope RE (2003) The common compensatory pattern: Its origin and relationship to the postural model. American Academy of Osteopathy Journal Winter 19–40.

Puledda F, Messina R and Goadsby PJ (2017) An update on migraine: Current understanding and future directions. Journal of Neurology 264 (9) 2031–2039.

Rees JD, Stride M and Scott A (2014) Tendons – time to revisit inflammation. British Journal of Sports Medicine 48 1553–1557.

Schuenke M, Schulte E and Schumacher U (2006) Thieme atlas of anatomy: Neck and internal organs. Stuttgart/New York: Thieme.

Schuenke M, Schulte E and Schumacher U (2007) Thieme atlas of anatomy: Head and neuroanatomy. Stuttgart/New York: Thieme.

Schuenke M, Schulte E and Schumacher U (2014) Thieme atlas of anatomy: General anatomy and musculoskeletal system, 2nd edn. Stuttgart/New York: Thieme.

Schultz RL and Feitis R (1996) The endless web: Fascial anatomy and physical reality. Berkeley: North Atlantic Books.

Snijders CJ, Vleeming A and Stoeckart R (1993) Transfer of lumbosacral load to iliac bones and legs, part 2: Loading of the sacroiliac joints when lifting in a stooped posture. Clinical Biomechanics (Bristol, Avon) 8 (6) 295–301.

Starkey C, Brown SD (2015) Orthopedic and athletic injury examination handbook, 3rd edn. Philadelphia: FA Davis.

Tillmann BN (2007) Atlas of human anatomy. New York: Mud Puddle Books.

Tovin BJ and Greenfield BH (2001) Evaluation and treatment of the shoulder: An integration of the guide to physical therapist practice. Philadelphia: FA Davis.

Travell JG and Simons DG (1992) Myofascial pain and dysfunction: The trigger point manual, the lower extremities, volume 2. Philadelphia: Lippincott Williams & Wilkins.

Travell JG, Simons DJ and Simons LS (1999) Travell & Simons' myofascial pain and dysfunction: The trigger point manual, volume 1: Upper half of body, 2nd edn. Baltimore: Williams & Wilkins.

Upledger JE and Vredevoogd JD (1992) Craniosacral therapy. Seattle: Eastland Press.

van Wingerden JP, Vleeming A, Snijders CJ et al. (1993) A functional-anatomical approach to the spine-pelvis mechanism: Interaction between the biceps femoris and the sacrotuberous ligament. European Spine Journal 2 140.

Vleeming A and Stoeckart R (2007) The role of the pelvic girdle in coupling the spine and the legs: A cinical-anatomical perspective on pelvic stability, in Vleeming A, Mooney V, Stoeckart R (eds) Movement, stability and lumbopelvic pain: Integration and research. Edinburgh: Churchill Livingstone, pp 113–137.

Vleeming A, Snijders CJ and Stoeckart R (1993) Transfer of lumbosacral load to iliac bones and legs, part 1: Biomechanics of self-bracing of the sacro-iliac joints and its significance for treatment and exercise. Clinical Biomechanics 8 (6) 285–294.

Vleeming A, PoolGoudzward A, Hammudoghlu D, Stoeckart R, Snijders CJ and Mens JM (1996) The function of the long dorsal sacroiliac ligament: Its implication for understanding low back pain. Spine 21 (5) 556–562.

Vleeming A, Schuenke MD, Masi AT, Carreiro JE, Danneel L and Willard FH (2012) The sacroiliac joint: An overview of its anatomy, function and potential clinical implications. Journal of Anatomy 221 537–567.

Vleeming A, Schuenke MD, Sturesson B and Willard FH (2013) Authors' response to the letter to the editors by Professor MT Cibulka: A critical interpretation of sacroiliac joint movement studies. Journal of Anatomy 222 391–395.

Ward RC (ed) (2003) Foundations for osteopathic medicine. Philadelphia: Lippincott William & Wilkins.

Waxman SG (2000) Correlelative neuroanatomy, 24th edn. New York: Lange Medical Books/McGraw-Hill.

Weinstein JN, Tosteson TD, Lurie JD, Tosteson ANA, Hanscom B, Skinner JS and Deyo RA (2006) Surgical vs nonoperative treatment for lumbar disk herniation. The Spine Patient Outcomes Research Trial (SPORT): A randomized trial. Journal of the American Medical Association, 296 (20) 2441–2450.

Willard FH, Vleeming A, Schuenke MD, Danneels L and Schleip R (2012) The thoracolumbar fascia: Anatomy, function and clinical considerations. Journal of Anatomy 221: 507–536.

Zink JG, Lawson WB (1979) An osteopathic structural examination and functional interpretation of the soma. Osteopathic Annals 7 12 December.

FURTHER READING

Alix ME Bates DK (1999) A proposed etiology of cervicogenic headache: The neurophysiologic basis and anatomic relationship between the dura mater and the rectus posterior capitis minor muscle. Journal of Manipulative and Physiological Therapeutics 22 (8) 534–539.

Anderson RG, Hayak R and Fogarty MP (1995) Leg length inequality and the side of low back pain: A pilot study. COMSIG review 4 (2).

Andrade Carla-Krystin and Paul Clifford (2014) Outcome-based massage, 3rd edn. Philadelphia: Lippincott Williams & Wilkins.

Bogduk N (2004) Management of chronic low back pain. Medical Journal of Australia 180 (2) 79–83.

Calais-Germain B (1993) Anatomy of movement. Seattle: Eastland Press.

Cameron G (2009) Frozen shoulder and how to survive it: An electronic book by Dr Gordon Cameron. http://wwwcameronmedicalcouk/frozenshoulderbookhtm [6 June 2009].

Cash M (1996) Sport and remedial massage therapy. London: Ebury Press.

Cattley P, Winyard J, Trevaskis J and Eaton S (2002) Validity and reliability of clinical tests for the sacroiliac joint: A review of the literature. Australasian Chiropractic and Osteopathy November 10 (2) 73–80.

Chaitow L (1997) Palpation skills: Assessment and diagnosis through touch. New York: Churchill Livingstone.

Chaitow L (2003) Modern neuromuscular techniques, 2nd edn. New York: Churchill Livingstone.

Clarkson HM (1999) Musculoskeletal assessment: Joint range of motion and manual muscle strength, 2nd edn. Philadelphia: Lippincott Williams & Wilkins.

Comeaux Z (2008) Harmonic healing: A guide to facilitated oscillatory release and other rhythmic myofascial techniques. Berkeley: North Atlantic Books.

Cornwall J and Mercer SR (2004) Anatomy in practice: Lumbar zygapophysial joint palpation. New Zealand Journal of Physiotherapy November 32 (3) 140–142.

Costi JJ, Stokes Gardner-Morse IA, M Laible JP, Scoffone HM and Iatridis JC (2007) Direct measurement of intervertebral disc maximum shear strain in six degrees of freedom: Motions that place disc tissue at risk of injury. Journal of Biomechanics 40 (11) 2457–2466.

Dean NA, Mitchell BS (2002) Anatomic relation between the nuchal ligament (ligamentum nuchae) and the spinal dura mater in the craniocervical region. Clinical Anatomy 15 (3) 182–185.

Dillon DQ (2007) Charting skills for massage therapists: A self-study workbook. wwwMassageTherapistPracticecom [17 April 2016].

Don Tigny RL (2002) Critical analysis of the sequence and extent of the result of the pathological failure of self-bracing of the sacroiliac joint. http://wwwkalindracom/criticalpdf [24 April 4 2008], 18 pages.

Don Tigny RL (2002) Function of the lumbosacroiliac complex as a self- compensating force couple with a variable force-dependent transverse axis: A theoretical analysis. http://wwwkalindracom/dontigny_lumbopdf [24 April 2008], 14 pages.

Foster MA (2004) Somatic patterning: How to improve posture and movement and ease pain. Longmont: EMS Press.

Fritz S (2017) Mosby's fundamentals of therapeutic massage, 6th edn. St Louis: Elsevier.

Galluzzi KE (2005) Management of neuropathic pain. Journal of the American Osteopathic Association Supplement 4, 105 (9) S12–S19.

Gerwin RD (2002) Myofascial and visceral pain syndromes: Visceral-somatic pain representations. Journal of Musculoskeletal Pain 10 (1/2) 165–175.

Goadsby PJ, Holland PR, Martins-Oliveira M, Hoffmann J, Schankin C and Akerman S (2017) Pathophysiology of migraine: A disorder of sensory processing. Physiological Reviews 97 (2) 553–622.

Greenman PE (1996) Principles of manual medicine, 2nd edn. Baltimore: Williams & Wilkins.

Hack GD and Hallgren RC (2004) Chronic headache relief after section of suboccipital muscle dural connections: A case report. Headache 44 84–89.

Hadjipavlou AG, Tzermiadianos MN, Bogduk N and Zindrick MR (2008) The pathophysiology of disc degeneration: A critical review. Journal of Bone and Joint Surgery 90-B (10) 1261–1270.

Hansen HC, McKenzie-Brown AM, Cohen SP, Swicegood JR, Colson JD and Manchikanti L (2007) Sacroiliac joint interventions: A systematic review. Pain Physician 10 (1) 165–184.

Hasset G and Barnsley L (2001) Pain referral from the sternoclavicular joint: A study in normal volunteers. Rheumatology 40 859–862.

Hong C (2000) Specific sequential myofascial trigger point therapy in the treatment of a patient with myofascial pain syndrome associated with reflex sympathetic dystrophy. Australasian Chiropractic and Osteopathy 9 (1) 7–11.

Humphreys BK, Kenin S, Hubbard BB and Crammer GD (2003) Investigation of connective tissue attachments to the cervical spinal dura mater. Clinical Anatomy 16 152–159.

Ingber DE (1993) Cellular tensegrity: Defining new rules of biological design that govern the cytoskeleton. Journal of Cell Science 104 (3) 613–627.

Ingber DE (1997) Tensegrity: The architectural basis of cellular mechanotransduction. Annual Review of Physiology 59 575–599.

Ingber DE (2008) Tensegrity and mechanotransduction. Journal of Bodywork and Movement Therapies 12 198–200.

Jarvik JG, Robertson WD, Wessbecher F, Reger K, Solomon C, Whitten R, Lumley T and Deyo RA (2000) Variation in the quality of lumbar spine MR images in Washington State. Radiology 215 (2) 483–490.

Kahkeshani K and Ward PJ (2012) Connection between the spinal dura mater and suboccipital musculature: Evidence for the myodural bridge and a route for its dissection – a review. Clinical Anatomy 25 (4) 415–422.

Kall LB (2008) Assessment of motion in the cervico-thoracic spine in patients with subacute whiplash-associated disorders. Journal of Rehabilitative Medicine 40 418–425.

Kim SK (2002) Role of injection therapy: Review of indications for trigger point injections regional blocks facet joint injections and intra-articular injections. Current Opinion in Rheumatology 14 52–57.

Kuchera ML (2005) Osteopathic manipulative medicine considerations in patients with chronic pain. Journal of the American Osteopathic Association 105 (9) supplement s29–s36.

Lee D and Walsh M (1996) A workbook of manual therapy techniques for the vertebral column and pelvic girdle, 2nd edn, fully revised. Altona: Friesen Printers.

Maigne J (2004) Towards a model of back pain: The 3 circles of pain. Europa Mediocophysica 40 (1) 21–27.

Palomeque-Del-Cerro L, Arráez-Aybar LA, Rodríguez-Blanco C, Guzmán-García R, Menendez-Aparicio M and Oliva-Pascual-Vaca Á (2017) A systematic review of the soft-tissue connections between neck muscles and dura mater: The myodural bridge. Spine 42 (1) 49–54.

Pastakia K and Kumar S (2011) Acute whiplash associated disorders (WAD). Open Access Emergency Medicine : OAEM 3 29–32.

Radakovich M and Malone T (1982) The superior tibiofibular joint: The forgotten joint. Journal of Orthopaedic and Sports Physical Therapy 3(3) 129–132.

Rattray F and Ludwig L (2000) Clinical massage therapy: Understanding assessing and treating over 70 conditions. Toronto: Talus Press.

Robson HE (1985) Dr James H Cyriax. British Journal of Sports Medicine 19 (3) 164 PMCID: PMC1478256 HE Robson.

Rolf IP (1989) Rolfing: Re-establishing the natural alignment and structural integration of the human body for vitality and well-being. Rochester: Healing Arts Press.

Further reading

Rooks J and Tracey I (2005) From nociception to pain perception: Imaging the spinal and supraspinal pathways. Journal of Anatomy 207 (1) 19–33.

Rubinstein SM, Pool JJM, van Tulder MW et al. (2006) A systematic review of the diagnostic accuracy of provocative tests of the neck for diagnosing cervical radiculopathy. European Spine Journal 16 307–319.

Sahrmann S (2002) Diagnosis and treatment of movement impairment syndromes. St Louis: Mosby.

Scali F, Pontell ME, Enix DE and Marshall E (2013) Histological analysis of the rectus capitis posterior major's myodural bridge. Spine J 13 (5) 558–563.

Schmitt Jr WH and Cuthbert SC (2008) Common errors and clinical guidelines for manual muscle testing: "The arm test" and other inaccurate procedures. Chiropractic and Osteopathy. doi: 10.1186/1746-1340-16-16.

Schuenke MD, Vleeming A, Van Hoof T and Willard FH (2012) A description of the lumbar interfascial triangle and its relation with the lateral raphe: Anatomical constituents of load transfer through the lateral margin of the thoracolumbar fascia. Journal of Anatomy 221: 568–576. doi:101111/j1469-7580201201517x.

Simpson JK and Budge R (2004) Treatment of frozen shoulder using distension arthrography (hydrodilation): A case series. Australasian Chiropractic and Osteopathy 12 (1) 25–35.

Snijders CJ, Vleeming A and Stoeckart R (1993) Transfer of lumbosacral load to iliac bones and legs, part 1: Biomechanics of self-bracing of the sacroiliac joints and its significance for treatment and exercise. Clinical Biomechanics (Bristol Avon) 8 (6) 285–294.

Swartz EE, Floyd RT, Cendoma M (2005) Cervical spine functional anatomy and the biomechanics of injury due to compressive loading. Journal of Athletic Training 40 (3) 155–161.

Tortora GJ, Grabowski SR (2003) Principles of anatomy and physiology, 10th edn. Hoboken: John Wiley & Sons.

Upledger JE and Vredevoogd JD (1992) Craniosacral therapy. Seattle: Eastland Press.

Upledger JE (1993) Craniosacral therapy II: Beyond the dura. Seattle: Eastland Press.

Weinstein JS and Deyo RA (2000) Issues in data collection. Spine 25 (24) 3104–3109.

Werner R (2015) Massage therapist's guide to pathology: critical thinking and practical application. Philadelphia: Wolters Kluwer.

Wilson E et al. (2003) Muscle energy technique in patients with acute low back pain: A pilot clinical trial. Journal of Orthopedic Sports Physical Therapy 33 (9) 502–512.

Wilson JJ and Best TM (2005) Common overuse tendon problems: A review and recommendations for treatment. American Family Physician. wwwaafporg/afp [19 February 2009].

Index

Note: *Page number followed by b, f, and t indicates text in box, figure and table respectively.*

E

F

G

H

L

Q

T

U

V

W

X

Y

Z